Practical Guide to Ultrasound in Obstetrics and Gynecology

A Comprehensive Book

Practical Guide to Ultrasound in Obstetrics and Gynecology

A Comprehensive Book

Sonal Panchal MD
Ultrasound Consultant
Dr Nagori's Institute for Infertility and IVF
Ahmedabad, Gujarat, India

Chaitanya Nagori MD DGO
Director
Dr Nagori's Institute for Infertility and IVF
Ahmedabad, Gujarat, India

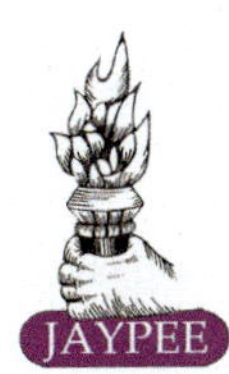

JAYPEE BROTHERS MEDICAL PUBLISHERS
The Health Sciences Publisher
New Delhi | London

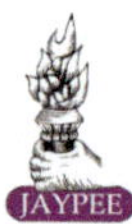

Jaypee Brothers Medical Publishers (P) Ltd

Headquarters
Jaypee Brothers Medical Publishers (P) Ltd
EMCA House
23/23-B, Ansari Road, Daryaganj
New Delhi 110 002, India
Landline: +91-11-23272143, +91-11-23272703
+91-11-23282021, +91-11-23245672
Email: jaypee@jaypeebrothers.com

Corporate Office
Jaypee Brothers Medical Publishers (P) Ltd
4838/24, Ansari Road, Daryaganj
New Delhi 110 002, India
Phone: +91-11-43574357
Fax: +91-11-43574314
Email: jaypee@jaypeebrothers.com

Overseas Office
J.P. Medical Ltd
83 Victoria Street, London
SW1H 0HW (UK)
Phone: +44 20 3170 8910
Fax: +44 (0)20 3008 6180
Email: info@jpmedpub.com

Website: www.jaypeebrothers.com
Website: www.jaypeedigital.com

Practical Guide to Ultrasound in Obstetrics and Gynecology: A Comprehensive Book

First Edition: 2022, Reprint: 2025

ISBN: 978-93-5465-346-9

Printed in India

Dedication

With great honor and respect, I dedicate this book to my mentors:
Professor Asim Kurjak
Dr Chaitanya Nagori
Thank you both for trusting my abilities and always supporting and encouraging me in all my endeavors.

Contributors

Asim Kurjak MD PhD
Professor
Department of Obstetrics and Gynecology
Medical School University of Zagreb
Zagreb, Croatia
Professor Emeritus
University Sarajevo School of Science and Technology
Sarajevo, Bosnia and Herzegovina

Binodini M Chauhan MD (Obst and Gyne) Fellowship in Fetal Medicine
Fetal Medicine Consultant
Department of Fetal Medicine
Government Medical College and New Civil Hospital
Surat, Gujarat, India

Chaitanya Nagori MD DGO
Director
Dr Nagori's Institute for Infertility and IVF
Ahmedabad, Gujarat, India

Darshan Wadekar MS. (Obst and Gyn)
Director
Wadekar Hospital
Surat, Gujarat, India

Kairavi Desai MS (Obst and Gyne) CIMP Fellow in Fetal Medicine
Consultant
Udhna Hospital Private Limited
Assistant Consultant
Government Medical College
Surat, Gujarat, India

Khurshid Alam DNB Radiodiagnosis, Postdoctoral Fellowship in Fetal Medicine (Mediscan, Chennai)
Consultant Fetal Medicine Fetomaternal Foundation and Care IVF
Kolkata, West Bengal, India

KV Sridevi MD (Obst and Gyne) FICOG Fellow in Fetal Medicine, Diploma in Obstetrics Ultrasound (RCOG), UK
Consultant
Department of Fetal Medicine
Pinnacle Women's Imaging Center
Visakhapatnam, Andhra Pradesh, India
President, SFM (Andhra Pradesh Chapter)
Director, Ian Donald USG Training Program (South India)
FOGSI Ultrasound Training Program

Rafat Jamal DNB Pediatrics Postdoctoral Fellowship in Pediatric Neurology
Consultant Pediatrician
Kolkata, West Bengal, India

Sonal Panchal MD
Ultrasound Consultant
Dr Nagori's Institute for Infertility and IVF
Ahmedabad, Gujarat, India

Zalak Mehta MBBS
Consultant Radiologist
New Civil Hospital
Surat, Gujarat, India

Preface

Ultrasound has become a primary tool and modality of choice for assessment and management of the patients with any obstetric or gynecological conditions. From simple B mode ultrasound, advances in technology has led to development of Doppler, 3D and even 4D ultrasound and all these sub-modalities have individually developed like specialty and have been now widely used for the assessment of obstetric, gynecological and infertile patients. Even thinking in terms of their applications, individual application is also developing forth and wide. Obstetric ultrasound has grown up into fetal medicine specialty. Gynecological and infertility ultrasound have also developed as specialty ultrasound. It has become difficult for a practicing obstetrician and gynecologist to master these specialized ultrasound. For that reason, these clinicians have to sacrifice a huge chunk of their practice and limit themselves to a very primary obstetric and gynecological practice only, in spite of the fact that every case will not require a specialist's opinion.

This book is designed therefore to help and assist practicing obstetricians and gynecologists to do ultrasound for their own patients and confidently diagnose normal patients and common abnormalities and to direct only the more complex cases to the respective specialties. It is easy to read and understand and straight forward to apply into practice.

Happy reading and wish you success in practice.

Sonal Panchal
Chaitanya Nagori

Acknowledgments

I sincerely acknowledge the entire team of M/s Jaypee Brothers Medical Publishers (P) Ltd, New Delhi, India, especially Shri Jitendar P Vij (Group Chairman), for believing in me to write this book and Mr Ankit (Managing Director), Mr MS Mani (Group President), Ms Chetna Malhotra (Associate Director—Content Strategy), Ms Pooja Bhandari (Production Head), Ms Kritika Dua (Senior Development Editor) and the entire team, for supporting me during the preparation process of this book.

My sincere thanks to contributors of this book, Dr KV Sridevi (Visakhapatnam), Dr Binodini M Chauhan (Surat), Dr Darshan Wadekar (Surat) and Dr Khurshid Alam (Kolkata), for their kind support and contribution for this book in their field of expertise.

Contents

1

CHAPTER

Basics of Ultrasound and Safety Concerns

Sonal Panchal, Chaitanya Nagori

INTRODUCTION

Ultrasound is the sound with frequencies higher than 20 Hz. These frequencies have least interaction with the body tissues and so can be used for diagnostic procedures. Commonly, the equipment used for diagnostic purposes operate on 1–20 MHz frequencies. Energy applied in ultrasound diagnosis is mechanical energy of the sound wave. It propagates as particle oscillations. As a result of this propagation, sound wave can be presented as regular interchange of regions of compression and rarefaction. So, it requires medium to travel and cannot propagate in space. It propagates as a longitudinal wave. The velocity (acoustic velocity) of the sound wave is determined by elastic properties and density of the medium. Its propagation is slowest in air (344 m/s) and increases in homogeneous liquids and increases with increasing viscosity and in solid elastic medium. The propagation ability of particular tissue is called "acoustic impedance" of a tissue. It is calculated as acoustic velocity in medium multiplied by density of the medium ($Z = p \times v$).

Intensity of the sound wave is the measure of energy that sound wave carries through space. It is the velocity of the energy carries through 1 m^2 area perpendicular to propagation direction. Intensity determines possible consequences of diagnostic ultrasound on body tissues. It measures energy of interaction of sound wave and biological tissue. Intensity and amplitude have inverse relationship. Higher frequency sound has lower amplitude intensity.

In ultrasound scanner, transducer (probe) is the source of and receiver for the sound wave. The active component in the probe is piezoelectric crystal. When exposed to mechanical perturbation of sound wave, crystal this mechanical energy into electrical energy and this is called piezoelectric effect. It has ability to transform the energy of oscillating electric field into mechanical energy of sound waves by a process called "inverse piezoelectric effect".[1] The ability of energy transformation is dependent on the thickness of the crystal. Best energy transformation is achieved when crystal's own frequency is identical to the frequency of the sound wave.

The materials used in ultrasound probe are ferroelectric ceramic, lead zirconate titanate (PZT) or plastic, and polyvinylidene difluoride. The crystal thickness is few 10th of millimeters sandwiched by thin-film silver electrodes on opposite sides of crystals. To produce good quality images, the emitted sound wave bundle should be narrow and directed to a definite direction. This is achieved by a massive attenuator in the background of the crystal wrapped in acoustic insulator **(Fig. 1)**.

Energy of the sound beam decreases as it traverses in the medium due to absorption of the energy by the solid particles that it hits to. This is known as attenuation of the sound wave. When the wave meets an interface between two media, part of the energy will be transmitted and part of it is reflected back. As both the media have different acoustic impedance, the reflected wave retains its velocity but changes direction and transmitted one continues to move forward with minimal

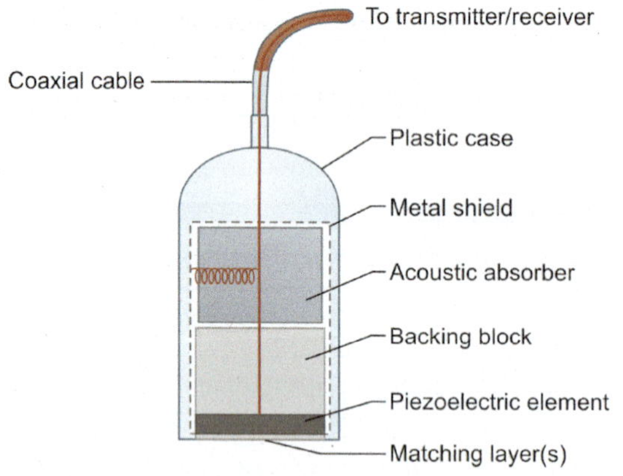

Fig. 1: Basic structure of the ultrasound transducer.

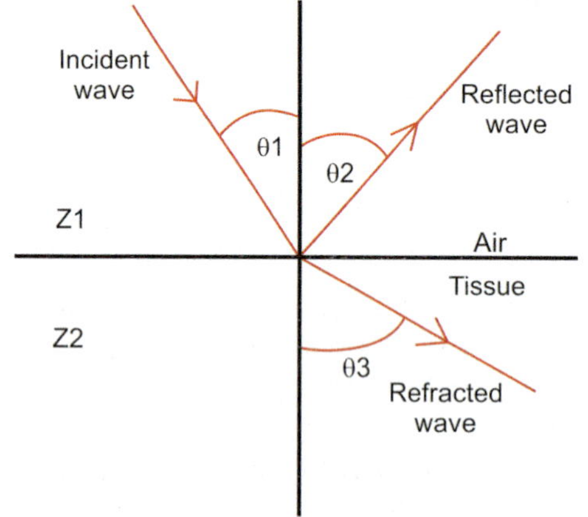

Fig. 2: Reflection and refraction of plane wave on flat boundary. The ratio of acoustic impedances determines the intensities of reflected and of transmitted waves. The angles of reflection and refraction are determined only by the velocity of sound propagation in the media.

change in direction but changes velocity. For the reflected waves, the reflection angle is equal to the incident angle and for transmitted wave, the angle depends on the velocity of propagation in two media **(Fig. 2)**.

Reflection and scattering of the ultrasound wave in heterogeneous biological tissues are the two diagnostic mechanisms. Reflection provides information about size and geometry and scatter about the texture and regular structure of the organ. Distance of the structure from the source is calculated by the time taken for the ultrasound pulse to reach the structure of interest and return back to the probe. Intensity of the returned pulses reflects the ratios of acoustic impedances and is also dependent on the absorption along the path of propagation.

Ultrasound image of the biological tissue is produced by sound waves reflected from the interfaces perpendicular to the direction of propagation. Added information is due to scattering on small inhomogeneities. Scattering and reflection are dependent on the elastic properties of tissues. Elasticity is due to connective tissue and, therefore, it is believed that those tissues with more connective tissue have higher acoustic impedance.

Dimensions and properties of ultrasound pulse are changing with penetration into the body and that primarily determines the quality of image. Quality of the ultrasound image is defined by the resolution, which can be achieved. Resolution is the smallest distance between two details in the tissue that can be separated on the image. It is measured in millimeters. Maximal resolution is limited by wavelength and pulse width. Resolution is in the direction of ultrasound propagation, is axial resolution, and perpendicular to the propagation direction is lateral resolution. Axial and longitudinal resolution is the minimal measurable distance between two reflecting interfaces on the propagating path. Lateral resolution is always less than longitudinal resolution. It is in the range of several wavelengths and depends on the geometry of ultrasound probe, frequency of the wave, and depth of the observed boundary in the body.[2]

SAFETY OF DIAGNOSTIC ULTRASOUND

To use ultrasound safely, it is essential to understand the bioeffects of ultrasound. Ultrasound absorption leads to rise in temperature of the tissues and this is one of the major concerns.[3] Nonthermal effects are inertial cavitation and other mechanical effects.

Safety Limits of Thermal Effects

No hazardous thermal effects are expected when the temperature rise is <1.5°C and local temperature is <38.5°C.[4] If temperature rise is 2°C, the fetus can tolerate it till 50 hours,[5] but temperature of 41°C can cause damage in 5 minutes.[4] In general, B-mode ultrasound does not show any hazardous effect [World Federation for Ultrasound in Medicine and Biology (WFUMB) and International Society of Ultrasound in Obstetrics and Gynecology (ISUOG)].

Thermal effects are quantified by thermal index (TI) and mechanical effects are quantified by mechanical index (MI) and also by output ultrasound power. Thermal effect is a big concern in Doppler ultrasound. In color and power Doppler, the ultrasound intensity is lower than pulsed wave Doppler because of scanning motion of Doppler ultrasound beam in the region of interest. Intensity of Doppler is lower in fetal Doppler scanners as compared to that in adult Doppler devices and is usually in the limit of nonhazardous Food and Drug Administration (FDA) regulation—720 mW/cm^2.

In the Doppler scanners, TI, MI, and transducer temperature are displayed on the monitor screen and to keep watch on maintaining the safety limits of the use of ultrasound and Doppler.[6] Settings should be checked before starting obstetric scans for safety concern. Ideally, the presets should be made to match the safety measures. Considering what should be the TI for safe use of diagnostic ultrasound in obstetrics, basic understanding of calculation of TI is essential. TI is the index to estimate tissue temperature in ultrasound examination and to study ultrasonic thermal effect. One TI indicates 1°C rise in temperature. TIS is used for the rise in temperature in an embryo with no bones. TIB is used for assessment of temperature rise on a fetus with bones. But the ultimate effect depends not on how much is the temperature rise, but how much is the resultant temperature. Therefore, more care should be taken when ultrasound is used in febrile patients. It is safe to use ultrasound or Doppler when TI is <1.

Mechanical Effects of Diagnostic Ultrasound

Mechanical index is used to estimate mechanical bioeffect of ultrasound. It is rarefactional sound pressure expressed in megapascal (MPa) divided by square root of ultrasound frequency. This effect is more in presence of gas bubbles in tissue fluids. MI should also be set to <1.

NORMS FOR SAFE USE OF ULTRASOUND IN 11–14 WEEKS SCAN (WFUMB, ISUOG, AND AMERICAN INSTITUTE OF ULTRASOUND IN MEDICINE)[7,8]

- Pulsed Doppler (spectral, power, and color Doppler) ultrasound should not be used routinely.
- Pulsed Doppler ultrasound may be used for clinical indications such as to refine risks for trisomies.
- When performing Doppler ultrasound, displayed TI should be ≤1.0 and exposure time should be kept as low as possible (usually not longer than 5–10 minutes) and should not exceed 60 minutes.
- When using Doppler ultrasound for research, teaching, and training purposes, the displayed TI should be ≤1.0 and exposure time should be kept as short as possible (not longer than 5–10 minutes) and should not exceed 60 minutes. Informed consent should be obtained.
- In educational settings, discussion of first trimester pulsed or color Doppler should be accompanied by information on safety and bioeffects (e.g., TI, exposure times, how to reduce output power?).
- When scanning maternal uterine arteries in the first trimester, there are unlikely to be any safety implications as long as the

embryo/fetus lies outside the Doppler ultrasound beam.

Safety is the primary concern. Ultrasound, though considered generally safe, must be used with recommended settings. Exposure time should be controlled to minimum possible and should never exceed safe limits.

REFERENCES

1. Dowsett DJ, Johnston RE. The Physics of Diagnostic Imaging. London: Chapman and Hall Medical; 1998. pp. 415-66.
2. Krestel E. Bildgebende Systeme für die medizinische Diagnostik. Berlin: Seimens; 1988.
3. National Council on Radiation Protection and Measurements. (1992). Report No. 113—Exposure Criteria for Medical Diagnostic Ultrasound: I. Criteria Based on Thermal Mechanisms. [online] Available from https://ncrponline.org/shop/reports/report-no-113-exposure-criteria-for-medical-diagnostic-ultrasound-i-criteria-based-on-thermal-mechanisms-1992/. [Last accessed on August, 2021].
4. WFUMB Symposium on Safety and Standardisation in Medical Ultrasound. Issues and Recommendations Regarding Thermal Mechanisms for Biological Effects of Ultrasound. Hornbaek, Denmark, 30 August-1 September 1991. Ultrasound Med Biol. 1992;18: 731-810.
5. AIUM Official Statement Changes: Revised Statements. Clin Saf. 1998;154:6-7.
6. American Institute of Ultrasound in Medicine/ National Electrical Manufacturers Association. (1992). Standard for Real-Time Display of Thermal and Mechanical Acoustic Output Indices on Diagnostic Ultrasound Equipment, Revision 2. [online] Available from https://www.nema.org/standards/view/Standard-for-Real-Time-Display-of-Thermal-and-Mechanical-Acoustic-Output-Indices-on-Diagnostic-Ultrasound-Equipment. [Last accessed on August, 2021].
7. WFUMB/ISUOG. WFUMB/ISUOG statement on the safe use of Doppler ultrasound during 11-14 week scans (or earlier in pregnancy). Ultrasound Med Biol. 2013;39:373.
8. Salvesen K, Lees C, Abramowicz J, Brezinka C, Haar GT, Maršál K, et al. ISUOG statement on the safe use of Doppler in the 11 to 13+6-week fetal ultrasound examination. Ultrasound Obstet Gynecol. 2011;37:628.

2

CHAPTER

Know the Scanner and its Controls to Optimize the Image

Sonal Panchal, Chaitanya Nagori

INTRODUCTION

Ultrasound is the prime diagnostic tool for all obstetric and gynecological patients. It is a very cost-effective, easily repeatable, and a patient friendly modality. But, it is operator dependent also. To get the best results, therefore, it is essential to master the technique to produce best quality images. It is essential therefore to understand the functions of the scanner and how to adjust these to produce best possible images.

High quality images on ultrasound means high resolution image with a high frame rate. Resolution is assessed by number of pixels in a unit area. More the pixels, better is the resolution. Since the two-dimensional (2D) scan that is done is a live real-time scan, it can be truly real time, if there are more 2D still frames coming one after the other in a unit time. Number of frames being changed in a unit time is frame rate. Higher the frame rate, better is the quality of the scan. But, very interestingly when more pixels are used to create an image, the processing time increases and, therefore, the frame rate decreases. Therefore, there always need to be a compromising balance between the two.

EQUIPMENT SETTINGS

Usually, there are presets on all the equipments for different scans. The advantage of using correct preset is that one does not have to manipulate multiple knobs with every scan. The probes now available are multifrequency probes and the frequency setting changes with the depth of scanning selected. Lower frequency sound beam has longer wavelength and gives better penetration but lower resolution and higher frequency sound beam has shorter wavelength and gives lesser penetration but higher resolution. So, to evaluate superficial structures, high frequency probe is selected and for evaluation of deeper structures, low frequency probes are selected.

OPTIMIZING THE IMAGE

The basis of correct diagnosis on B-mode, Doppler study, and three-dimensional (3D) ultrasound is a good quality B-mode image. Good image quality on B-mode or 2D ultrasound means better resolution and higher frame rate. The understanding of the settings and optimization of the image equally applies to any route of the scan and whichever probe one uses.

BASIC UNDERSTANDING OF KNOBS AND THEIR SETTINGS

- *Scanning angle*: The scanning angle decides the width of scanning area. The scanning angle is kept open, to its full limits when the scan is started, so that a pilot view of anatomy can be studied. The maximum scanning angle for different probes vary from 120 to 180°. Once the general anatomy is understood and one needs to concentrate on a particular organ, then the scanning angle is narrowed to accommodate a particular structure and marginal surroundings. This improves the frame rate and, in turn, resolution of the image **(Figs. 1A and B)**.

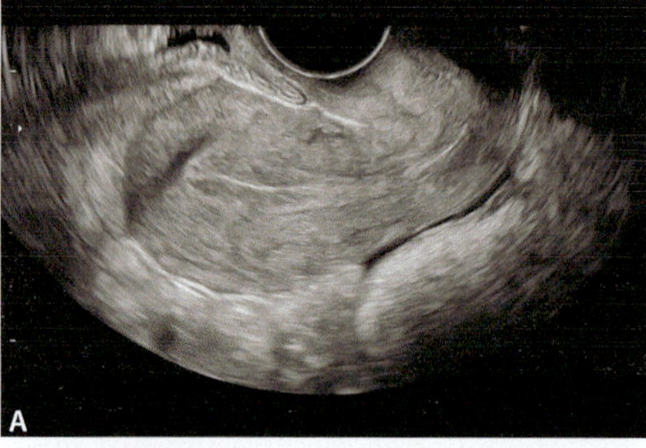

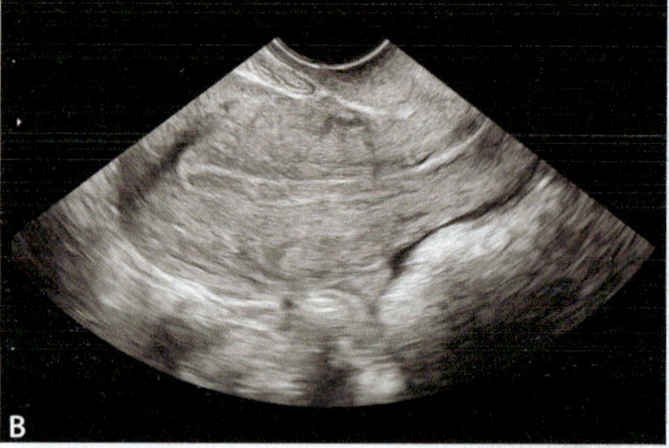

Figs. 1A and B: 2D ultrasound image of the uterus in sagittal section with wide scanning angle (A) and with narrow scanning angle (B).

- *Scanning depth*: Same as for scanning angle, the scanning depth also is set several times during each scan depending on the organ or lesion of interest. At the start of the scan, the scanning depth is high, but after the overview of the general anatomy, when one concentrates on a particular organ or lesion, the scanning depth is also decreased like angle, so that the region of interest fills two-thirds of the image. This also increases the frame rate and improves resolution **(Figs. 2A and B)**.
- *Zoom*: After the overview scanning, decreasing the scanning angle and depth, image should be zoomed large enough to fill up two-thirds to three-fourths of the screen. One may zoom the whole image (panzoom) or may use a zoom box to define which part of the image needs to be zoomed (HD zoom). This improves resolution of the image **(Figs. 3A and B)**. But, it is important here to mention that panzoom just increases the distance between the pixels and does not improve the image quality, though it may improve the visibility of smaller details due to magnification. So, panzoom is not to be used while doing live scans. When used

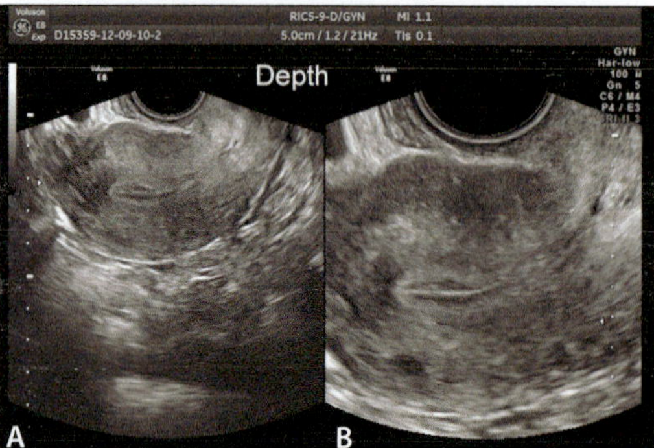

Figs. 2A and B: 2D ultrasound image of the sagittal section of the uterus on transvaginal scan with more scanning depth (A) and less scanning depth (B).

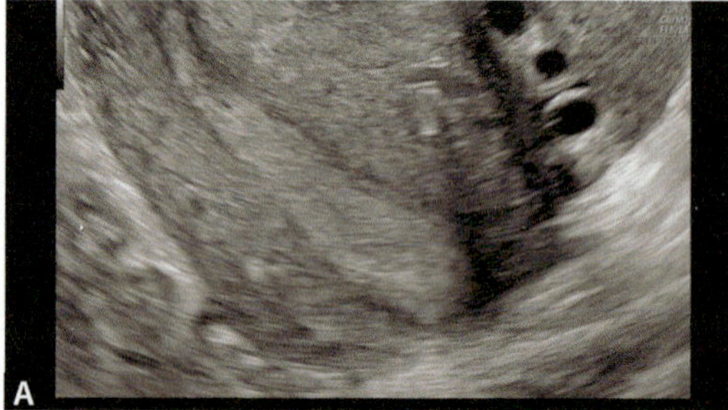

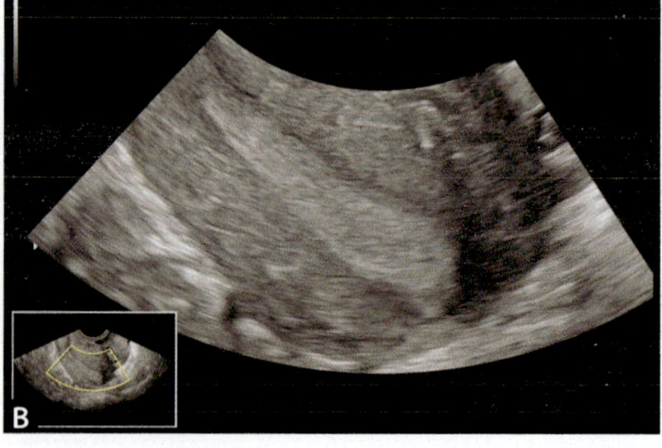

Figs. 3A and B: 2D ultrasound image of the uterus using pan zoom (A), and using HD zoom (B).

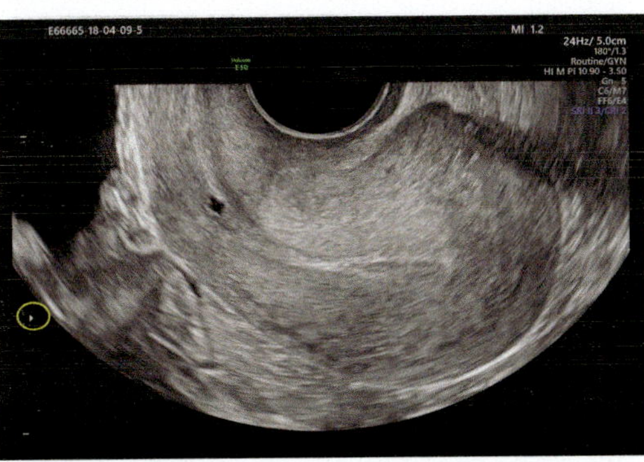

Fig. 4: 2D ultrasound image of the sagittal section of the uterus showing single focal zone marked by yellow circle on left side of the image.

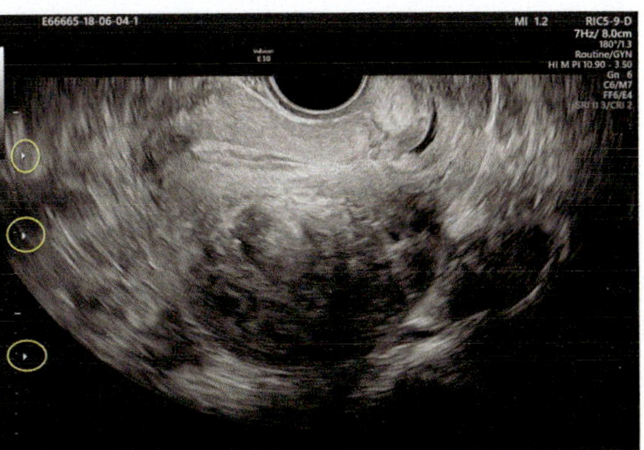

Fig. 5: 2D ultrasound image of the sagittal section of the uterus showing three focal zones marked by yellow circles on left side of the image.

on a frozen image, it does not damage the image quality which is already fixed. For live scan, therefore, it is best to use HD zoom and panzoom is spared for frozen or stored images.

- *Setting the focal zone*: The arrowhead on right side of the image indicates the focal zone **(Fig. 4)**. Focal zone is the level at which the ultrasound beam converges to become narrowest and, therefore, the image is the sharpest. So, focal zone is always set at the level of area of interest. There is also an option of having more than one focal zone when there are multiple levels at which the image needs to be sharp. But, increasing the number of focal zones decreases the frame rate because the same ultrasound beam needs to be processed several times. Therefore, usually single focal zone is selected, except when large lesions are scanned or anatomical relationship of pelvic organs is required **(Fig. 5)**.
- *Gains*: It is known that structures far from the probe appear hypoechoic (darker) than what they are. This is because as the ultrasound beam traverses through the tissues, it loses its intensity. This is because at every solid particle that the sound beam hits to, some energy is absorbed lost. This may cause an error of diagnosis due to decreased visibility. When the image is too dark or unclear, the examiner may be tempted to change the gains of the image, but changing gains inadvertently may lead to erroneous diagnosis. With increased gains, even the anechoic structures may appear echogenic. Therefore, the gains are set in such a way that the urinary bladder appears anechoic, but its walls do not lose thickness **(Figs. 6A and B)**.

  To compensate for the loss of intensity of the sound beam traversing to and returning from the deeper structures, "time gain compensation (TGC)" is used. This enables to adjust the gains of the returning sound beam depthwise **(Figs. 7A and B)**.
- *Contrast/Dynamic range*: Contrast or dynamic range indicates the number of gray shades displayed in the image. Higher the contrast, less number of gray shades is seen and with lower contrast, more numbers of gray shades are seen. This means that when contrast is high, soft-tissue details will be obliterated and when contrast is low, there are so many shades of gray that it is virtually difficult to differentiate one from the other.

  Harmonics, speckle reduction imaging (SRI), and compound resolution imaging (CRI) are more advanced tools used to further enhance the image quality.
- *Harmonics*: This is selective regulation of chosen frequency of sound waves from the

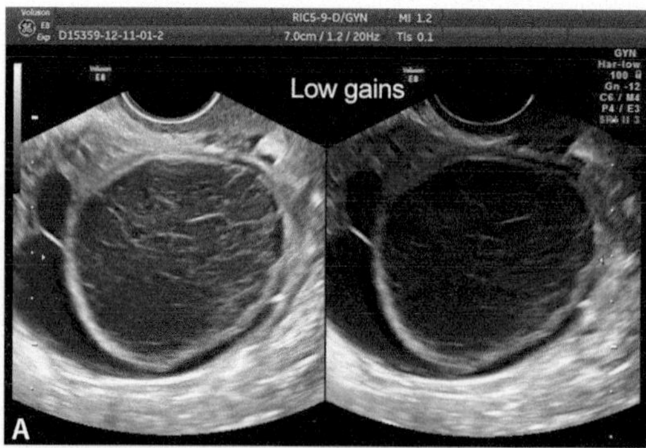

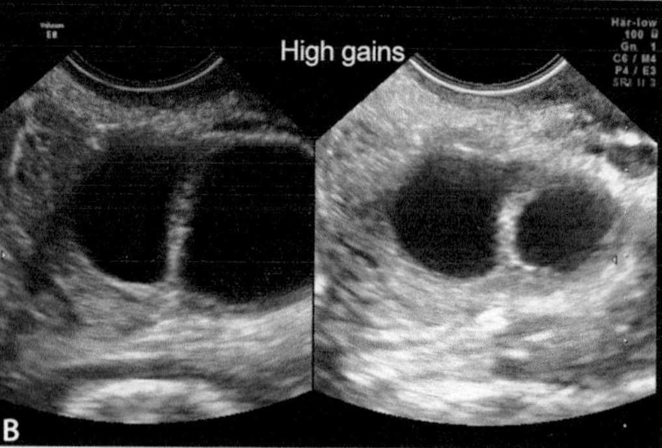

Figs. 6A and B: (A) B mode ultrasound image of the corpus luteum with optimum gain settings (on left) and low gain settings (image on right); (B) B mode ultrasound image of the follicles with optimum gain settings (on left) and high gain settings (image on right).

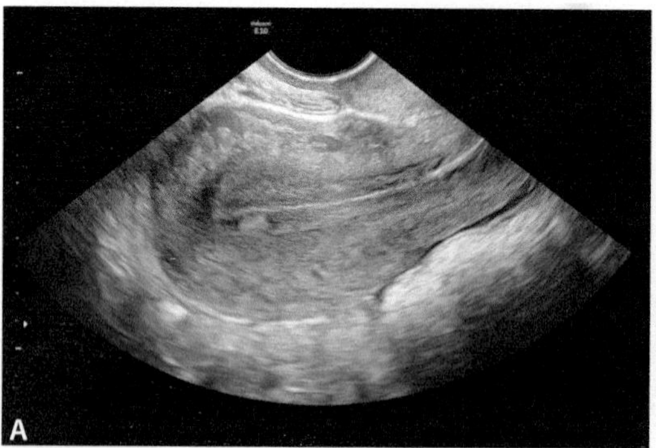

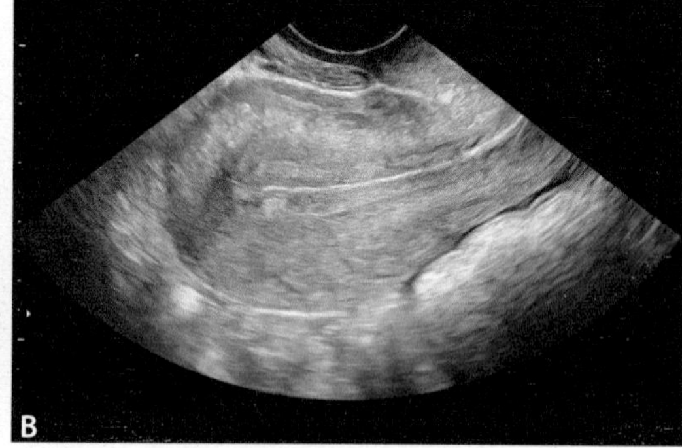

Figs. 7A and B: B mode ultrasound image of the uterus with routine TGC settings (A) and with increased gain settings at the level of endometrium (B).

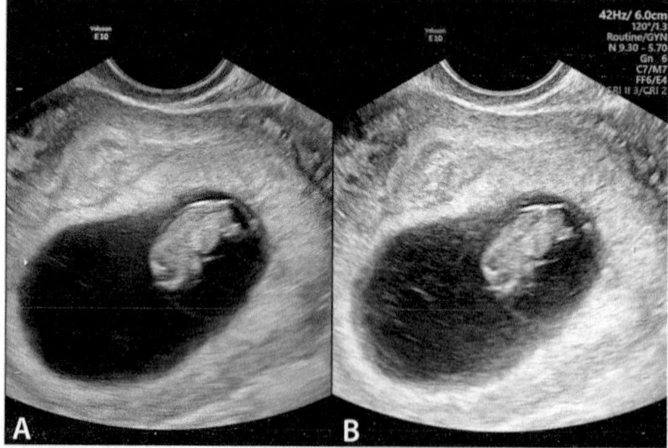

Figs. 8A and B: B mode image of the fetus in gestational sac, with harmonics (A) and without harmonics (B).

returning signals. This reduces artifacts and enhances image quality **(Figs. 8A and B)**.

While conventional ultrasound uses the same frequency bandwidth for both the transmitted and received signals, tissue harmonic imaging (THI) uses a low frequency for the transmitted signal and a high frequency for the received signal. When echoes return after being reflected, they do so not only at the basic frequency but also at multiples of the basic frequency. This leads to less attenuation, less scatter, and less side lobe artifact and more clearer images.

- *Speckle reduction imaging*: *Speckles* are inherent artifacts to ultrasound imaging and are created by refracted sound waves from any solid particle that the sound beam hits. SRI—cuts off this undesired refracted sound beam information and improves edge definition **(Figs. 9A and B)**.

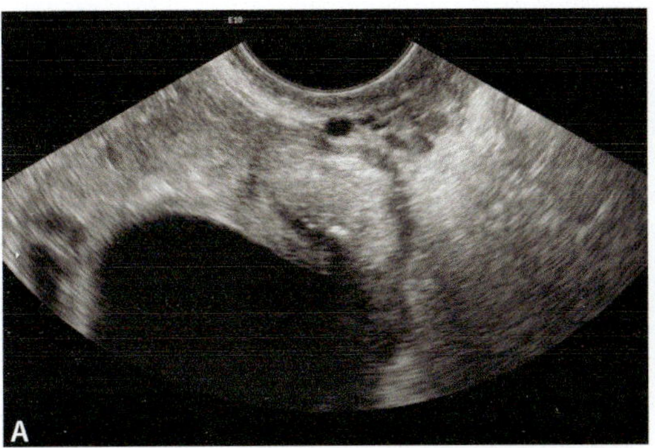

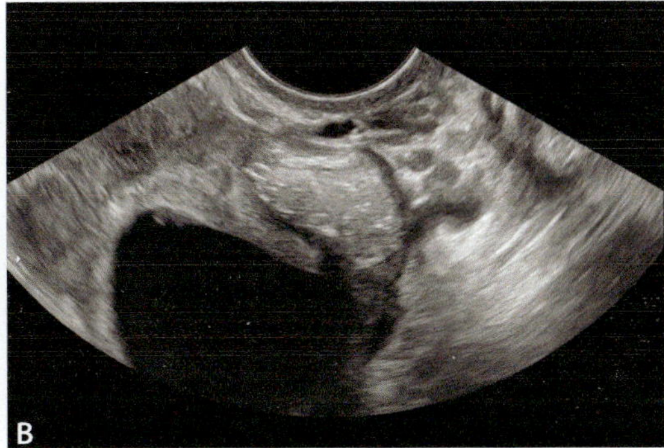

Figs. 9A and B: B mode ultrasound image of the female pelvis concentrate on the hypoechoic vertically oriented tissue layers (muscularis of bowel). Figure A without SRI shows less sharpness of this layer and Figure B with SRI shows clear definition of this layer.

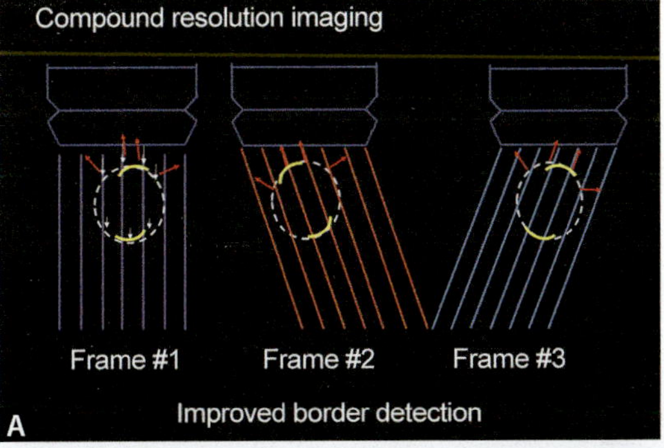

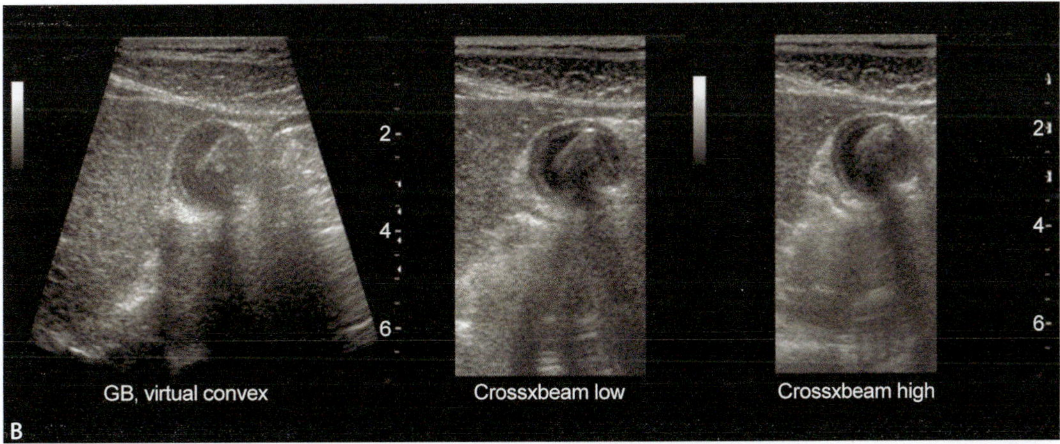

Figs. 10A and B: B mode images of cystic structure showing fairly defined margins of a cystic lesion in image on left. The two images on right of these show much better clarity of the image where CRI is used.

- *Compound resolution imaging*: CRI is a result of multiple coplanar images from different angles combined into a single image in real time. Though the borders for each steering angle are the same, the noise and speckle position change for each frame and average out noise and smoothen borders **(Figs. 10A and B)**. It is especially of use for definition of margins of cystic structures. It is also of use to visualization of the tissue details across hyperechoic structures such as bones.

SUMMARY

Production of good quality B-mode imaging is the basis of good Doppler and 3D ultrasound imaging. Only well-optimized B-mode image can give correct diagnosis. This can be achieved by adjusting scanning angle, scanning depth, focal zone, zoom, and several times scanning a single patient. Gains and contrast settings are not to be changed as far as possible. Harmonics, SRI, and CRI improve the image quality, should be used with B-mode imaging, and should be adjusted in presets.

3

CHAPTER

Doppler Basics for a Gynecologist

Sonal Panchal, Chaitanya Nagori

WHAT IS DOPPLER?

Doppler is an effect produced on the frequency of a sound wave when it hits a moving object. This can be most simply explained by the difference in the sound quality perceived by an individual who is standing on the road and hears the voice of the siren of the moving ambulance. The intensity of the sound increases as the sound source moves toward the individual and decreases as it moves away from the individual. When the receiver and the sound source move toward each other, the frequency of the heard sound wave is higher than sent by the sound source and if the two move away from each other, the frequency of the heard sound is lower than that produced by the sound source. The difference in the emitted and the received frequency is known as Doppler shift. This effect was first described by Christian Johann Doppler in 1842. But, it was only in 1959 that Satumora demonstrated the use of this technology for demonstration of blood flow.

Translating the Doppler effect in the body for blood flow assessment: The sender and receiver are both static (the ultrasound transducer) and the target [red blood cells (RBCs)] move. The first frequency shift occurs when the sound beam hits the moving RBC and the frequency shift again occurs when it returns.

The shift depends on the angle at which the sound beam hits the moving object.

$$\text{Doppler frequency } (f_d) = \frac{2.f_1.V.\text{Cos}\theta}{c}$$

f_d = Doppler shift
f_1 = transmitted beam
c = speed of sound in tissue
V = velocity of blood flow
θ = angle of incidence between the ultrasound beam and the direction of flow.

Considering this equation, it is important to notice that the frequency of the received beam is dependent on the frequency of incident beam, velocity of the moving object, and the angle of incidence. But, more importantly, it is not dependent on the absolute value of the angle of incidence, it is on the "cos" value of this angle. Therefore, for correct calculation of the frequency or any one of the unknown variable out of these above-mentioned four, the cos value of the angle (cos θ) should be within acceptable limits (one or closest to one) **(Table 1)**.

The precise Doppler frequency is calculated taking into account an angle correction factor of 1/cos θ **(Table 2)**.

The Doppler effect can be displayed as color Doppler, power Doppler, and spectral Doppler.

COLOR DOPPLER

Doppler is most commonly used term for color Doppler. It displays the blood flow in

TABLE 1: The angle of incidence of the sound beam, their cos values, and the percentage deviation that lead to the velocity value.[1]

Angle	*Cos value*	*% deviation*
0°	1	0
30°	0.866	13
45°	0.707	29
60°	0.5	50
90°	0	100

two colors and these are conventionally red and blue. The color indicates the direction of the flow. Flow toward the probe is red and away from the probe is blue **(Fig. 1)**. But, these can be interchanged by using the invert switch **(Fig. 2)**. When the flow is perpendicular to the sound beam not towards or away from the probe, no color will be displayed in spite of presence of the flow. When the flow is perpendicular to the sound beam, the Doppler angle is 90° and the cos θ value is 0, so the flow cannot be displayed. The arterial flow is pulsatile and the venous flow is nonpulsatile. The brightness of the color depends on the velocity of the flow. The higher flow velocities display bright colors and the lower flow velocities display dull colors **(Fig. 3)**, though color Doppler does not give exact velocity values. So, it is a directional semiquantitative Doppler.

TABLE 2: Table showing the angle of incidence of the sound beam, correction factors used for calculation of velocity, and the correction error.[1]

Angle	*Correction factor 1/cos θ*	*Correction error*
30°	1.15	±3%
45°	1.41	±6%
60°	2.00	±9%
70°	2.92	±14%
75°	3.86	±21%
80°	5.76	±30%

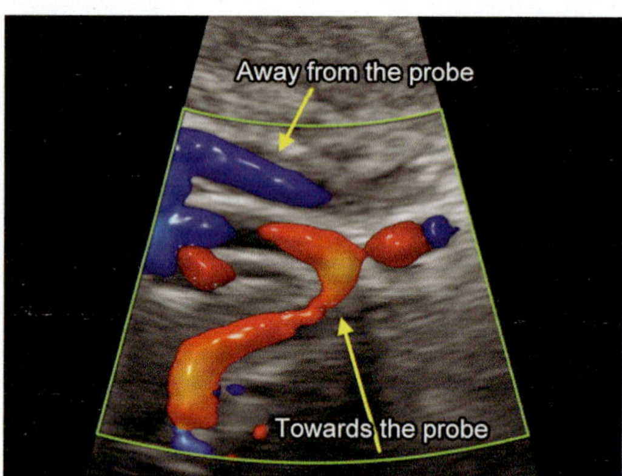

Fig. 1: Color Doppler image showing flow toward the probe is red and away from the probe is blue.

POWER DOPPLER

Though a Doppler, power Doppler is not an angle-dependent technology. It is known that movement of any object produces energy and this is used to depict the blood flow signals in power Doppler. This means that wherever there is a movement of blood or of body tissues, color signals will be generated. It is not an angle-dependent technology and so the advantage is that it displays color signals even in vessels are perpendicular to the sound beam. But, the disadvantage is that it is a single color display and does not show the flow direction. It indigenously potentiates the

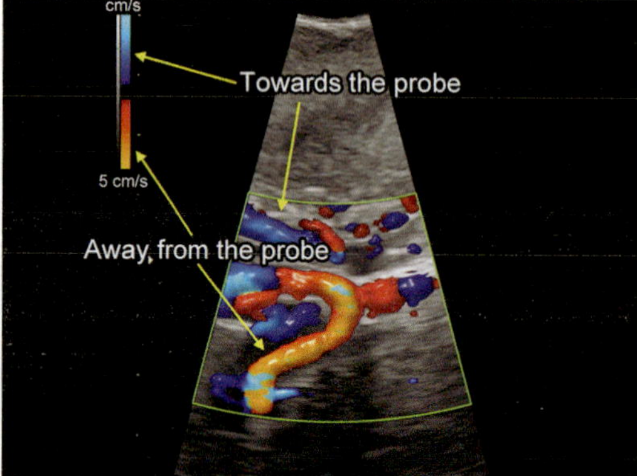

Fig. 2: Color Doppler image showing reversal of the flow color against direction. The inversion can be seen on the color bar also as shown by the arrow.

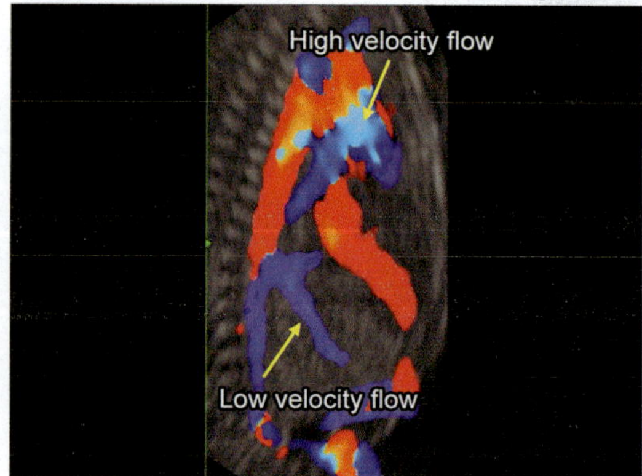

Fig. 3: Color Doppler image showing brighter color for high velocity flow and dull color for low velocity flow.

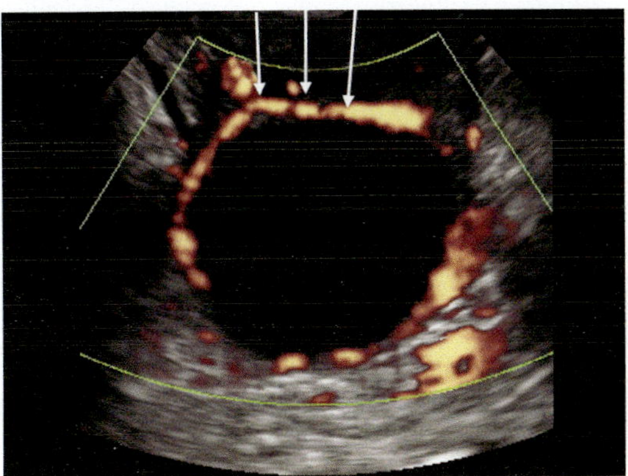

Fig. 4: Power Doppler image showing color in the vessels perpendicular to the sound beam—sound beam is shown by white arrows.

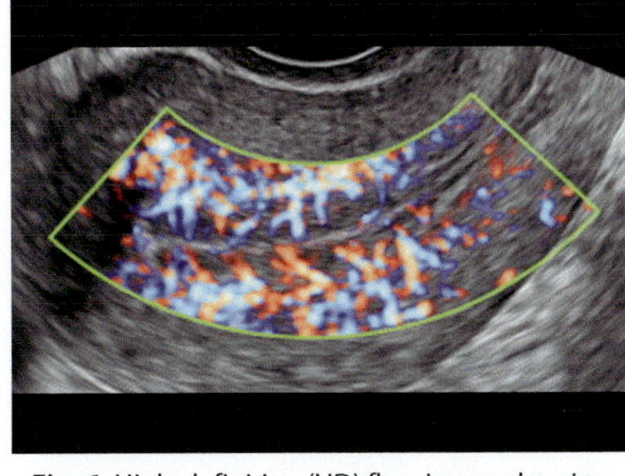

Fig. 6: High-definition (HD) flow image showing color of the flow according to its direction.

signals and, therefore, is a useful technology for documentation of low velocity blood flow. The main application of the power Doppler, therefore, is to pick up flow in low velocity blood vessels and the blood flows in the vessels perpendicular to the sound beam **(Fig. 4)**.

Like color Doppler, the brightness of color display of the power Doppler signals also varies depending on the velocity of the moving object. High velocity movements show a bright color and the low velocity movements display dull color **(Fig. 5)**.

High-definition (HD) flow is a new addition to the basic power Doppler technology. It is a directional power Doppler. Apart from high flow sensitivity, HD flow also has a color coding for the flow toward or away from the probe as in color Doppler **(Fig. 6)**. Like color and power Doppler, the brightness of the color correlates with the velocity of the moving object.

SPECTRAL DOPPLER

Spectral Doppler is the spectral display of the flow/movement of a moving object. Trace above the baseline in the spectrum is the flow toward the probe and the trace below the baseline is the flow away from the probe **(Fig. 7)** on the spectrum. Like in color Doppler, the invert switch can reverse the flow display. On the spectral Doppler, the arterial flow appears

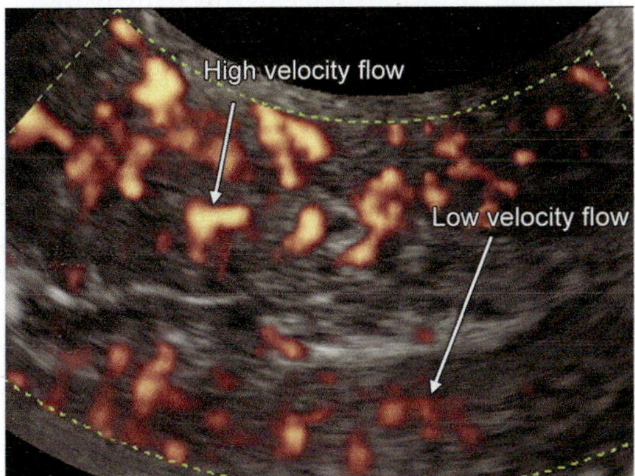

Fig. 5: Power Doppler image shows high velocity movements that show a bright color and the low velocity movements display dull color.

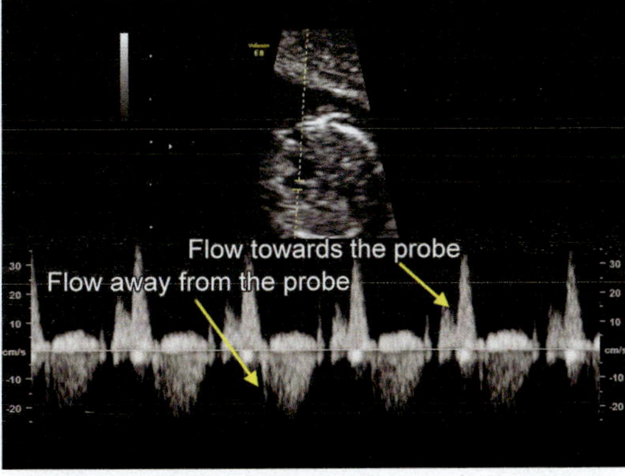

Fig. 7: Spectral Doppler image showing trace above the baseline in the spectrum is the flow toward the probe and the trace below the baseline is the flow away from the probe.

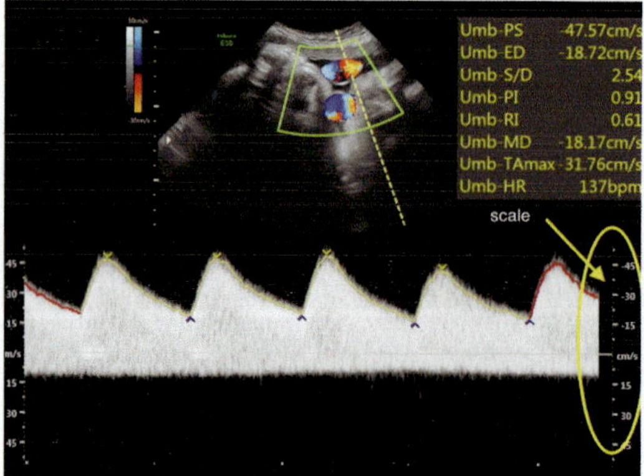

Fig. 8: Spectral Doppler showing scale on the side of the spectrum for calculation of the flow velocities.

spiky and the venous flow appears flat. There is a scale on the side of the spectrum and it is by this scale that the exact velocities of the blood flow can be calculated **(Fig. 8)**.

The spectrum can be displayed for pulsed wave Doppler and the continuous wave Doppler. In pulsed wave Doppler, the transducer is dedicatedly used for emitting the sound wave and then dedicatedly to receive the sound wave alternatively. As the sound waves are emitted in pulses, it is called a pulsed wave Doppler. The limitation of the pulsed wave Doppler is that the maximum frequencies recorded correctly are smaller than half that of the pulse repetition frequency (PRF). This limit of any PRF is called Nyquist limit/frequency. The PRF, therefore, should at least be double the frequency to be measured. Therefore, to record different velocities, the PRFs have to be accordingly selected. Pulsed Doppler, therefore, has a limitation to maximum velocities that it can record. This can be overcome by continuous wave Doppler. This uses dedicated elements for emitting and receiving sound waves and, therefore, has no higher limit for velocities recorded. This is used chiefly for adult echocardiography as the velocity of blood in the heart is very high. Since continuous wave Doppler is not used for the Doppler studies in gynecology and obstetrics, we shall not include it in further discussion here.

To obtain the correct information about flow velocities with Doppler, certain settings and adjustments on the scanner are required. Though most of these are set on the dedicated presets, it is important to understand how we can manipulate certain switches/knobs to achieve best flow information.

These are the Doppler box size, color gains, PRF, wall motion filter (WMF) and balance on color and power Doppler and sample volume, and angle correction for the pulsed wave Doppler.

COLOR/POWER DOPPLER SETTINGS

Box Size

When one switches on the color Doppler, a box appears on the screen on the B-mode image. This box defines in which area of the B-mode image, the blood flow information will be displayed. It is important to consider here that when the Doppler is switched on, the machine has to process the B-mode information as well as the flow information and, therefore, the frame rate significantly decreases. What is this frame rate?

The ultrasound scan that we are doing gives us continuous live, real-time information of the area scanned. This is called real time because it matches with the live movements of the human body. This is done by compilation of multiple B-mode images. Only if the B-mode images are processed fast enough to match the real-time changes, this scan can be seen like a continuous scan as in a video. This number of B-mode images produced in a unit time is called a frame rate. This clearly means that the higher the frame rate, better would the scan quality be considered. This frame rate can be increased, if the machine has to process less. Though it is known that starting the color Doppler decreases the frame rate, the frame rate with color Doppler can be optimized. The color box size is planned just large enough to cover the area of interest. I would add here that before switching on the color Doppler, the B-mode image also should be optimized

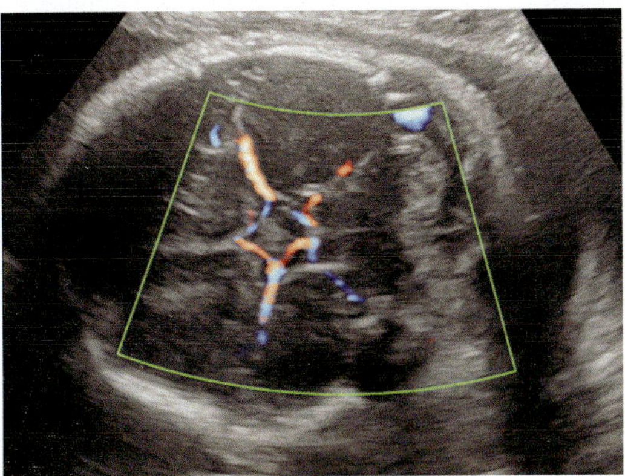

Fig. 9: Color Doppler image showing the box in green outline in which the flow is assessed.

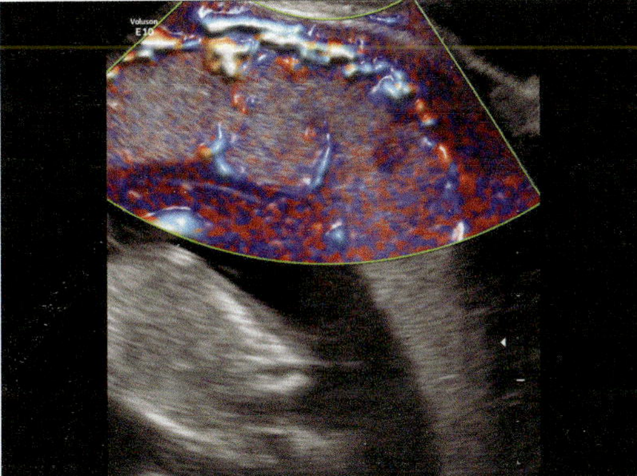

Fig. 10: High-definition (HD) flow image shows high gains and the color is seen spilling out of the vessels.

for its angle and depth to concentrate only on the area of interest. The color box can be moved all across the B-mode image and the size can be altered based on the requirement **(Fig. 9)**. Apart from this, using the color box just adequate for the study, it also decreases the color artifacts.

Gains

When the Doppler is switched on, it should show the blood vessels filled up with color and no color spilling out of the vessels. This is done by gain adjustment. When the gains are too high, the color will be seen spilling out of the vessels **(Fig. 10)**, whereas when the gains are low, the color will not completely fill up the vessels **(Fig. 11)**. There is a black empty space seen between the color column

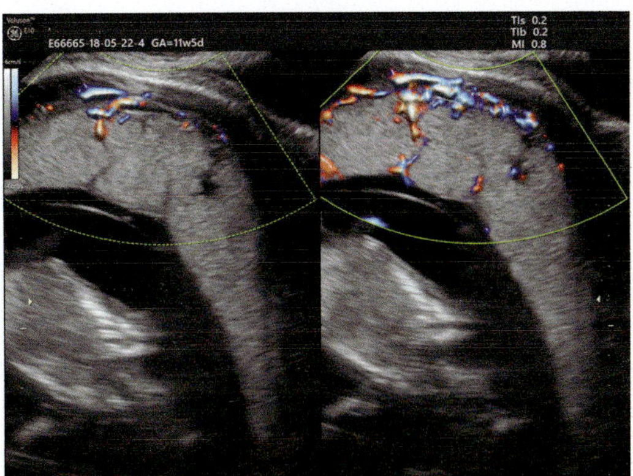

Fig. 11: High-definition (HD) flow image: the image in the left shows hardly any vessels as the gains are low, whereas that on the right shows adequate filling of the vessels.

and the vessel wall or low velocity vessels may not be filled at all. This is because when the gains are low, the low velocity signals will not be picked up by Doppler. It is important to mention at this stage that in a vessel, the central stream has the highest velocity flow, whereas close to the walls, the velocity is lower due to friction with the walls. The correct gain, therefore, is when the entire lumen of the vessel is filled with color and there is no spill outside.

How to set?

To increase the gains to maximum, there will be a lot of spill of color almost entire box is filled with mixed colors. Start decreasing the gains till the color is contained in the vessel further decreases the gains and there will be black (anechoic) areas between the color column and the vessel wall **(Fig. 12)**. You have over-reduced the gains. Increase till the vessel again fills up fully and this is your correct setting. Gain settings for color and power Doppler once set and placed in the presets are not to be changed.

Pulse Repetition Frequency

It has already been discussed that the PRF decides what is maximum receiving frequency of the sound wave (indirectly velocity) that is recordable at a particular setting (Nyquist

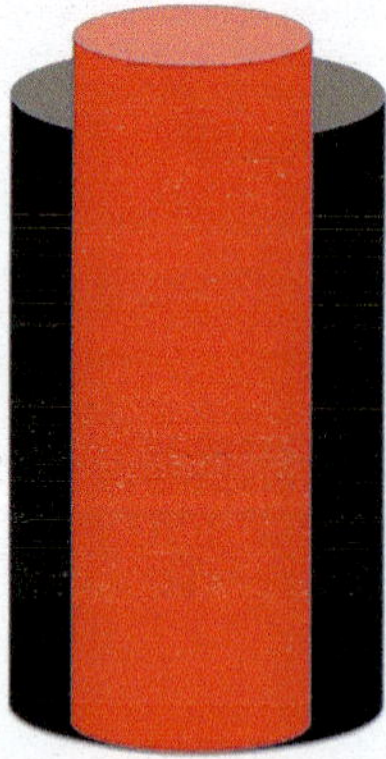

Fig. 12: Diagrammatic demonstration of the color flow in presence of low gains—black area between the vessel wall and the color column due to nonvisibility of the low velocity flow information close to the walls due to low gains or high wall filter.

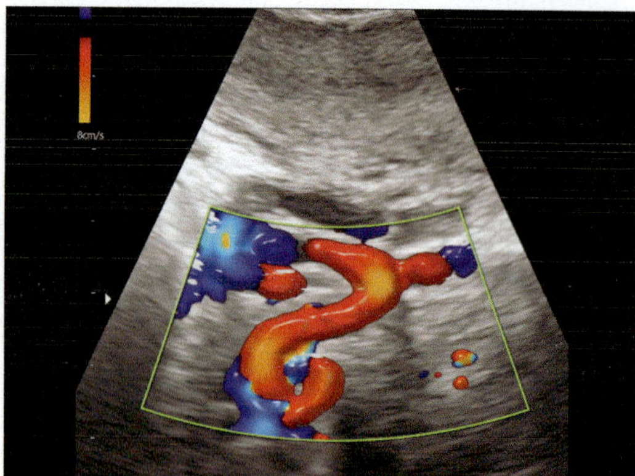

Fig. 14: Low pulse repetition frequency (PRF) when used for high velocity flow shows mixing of colors.

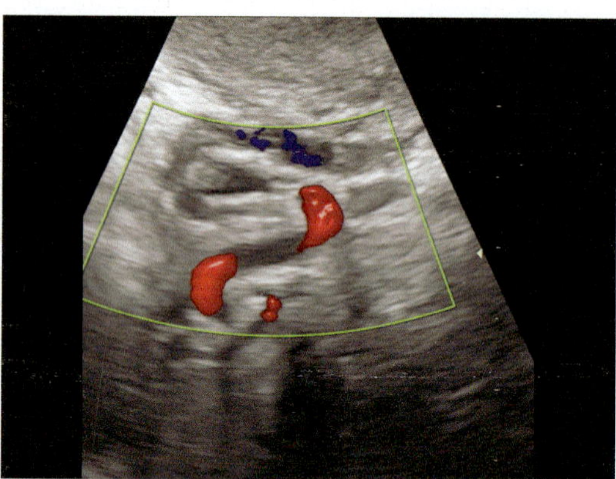

Fig. 13: High pulse repetition frequency (PRF) for low velocity flow showing empty vessel lumen without the flow.

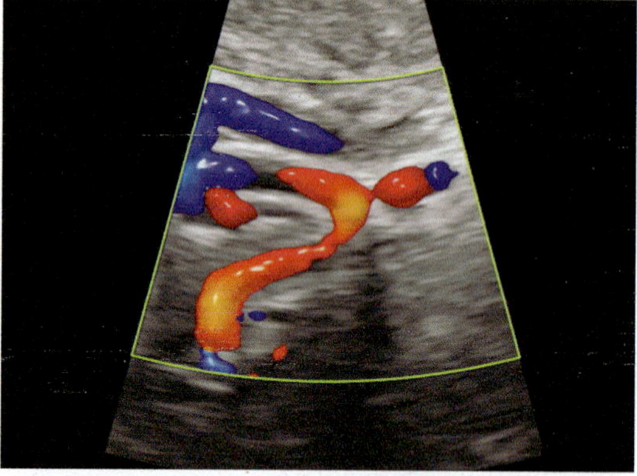

Fig. 15: Optimum pulse repetition frequency (PRF) setting gives unicolor filling of the vessel.

frequency).[2] Therefore, it is important to select an optimum PRF for the velocity of the blood vessels flow studied. High PRF, if used for low velocity flow, will not be possible to pick up the color where there are flows **(Fig. 13)**. Instead, if low PRF is used for high velocity flow, there will be aliasing—mixing of red and blue colors—appears like turbulence **(Fig. 14)**. The PRF setting would be optimum when the color homogeneously fills the entire vessel with single color—red or blue **(Fig. 15)**.

Wall Motion Filter (WMF)

It is known that Doppler produces color signals wherever there is a movement and the brightness of the color depends on the velocity of the moving object. This means that the color signals are produced by the RBCs in the blood, but are also produced by the wall movement of the artery and also by the pulsations transmitted to the surrounding tissues. The color signals of the blood flow are the brightest, those of wall motion are dull, and those due to transmitted pulsations from the surrounding tissues are the dullest for the reasons explained earlier in this chapter. But, these dull signals produced by low velocity movements corrupt the flow information and can be eliminated only if a low velocity filter is used. This filter is named as WMF.

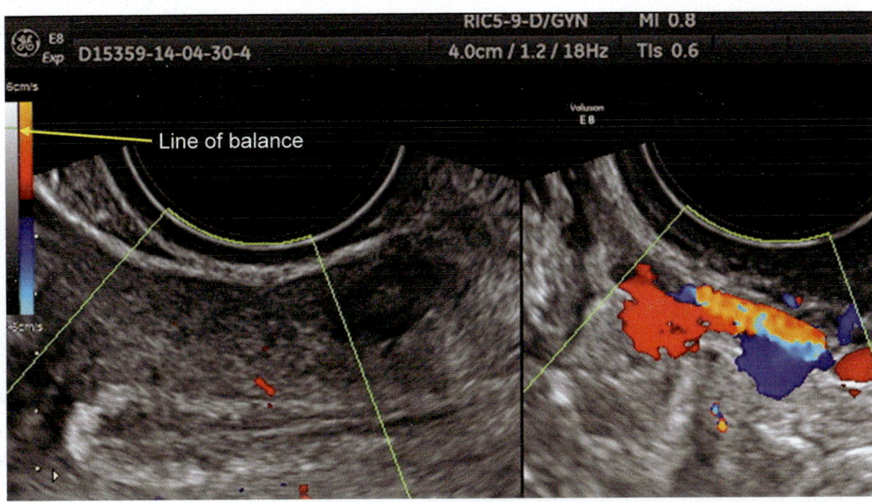

Fig. 16: Color Doppler image showing gray bar and the color bar on the left upper corner of the image with gray bar showing green "line of balance".

WMF can be adjusted at various levels depending on the level of sound signals that need to be eliminated to produce clear flow velocity signals. For larger vessels with high velocity flow, the arterial flow movement is more and higher WMF is required, whereas for small vessels with low velocity signals, the arterial wall movements are less and so low wall filters are required. Using higher wall filter for a low velocity blood flow vessel, it will eliminate the slow flow information. This will lead to a typical color flow signal with a color column seen in the center of the vessel and there is a black line seen on both the sides between the vessel wall and the color column similar to that produced by low gains **(Fig. 12)**.

Balance

As the name suggests, this is a balancing tool between the two modalities—(1) the B-mode and (2) the color Doppler. As discussed earlier, when Doppler is switched on the scanner, computer processing is doubled and so scanner is to be advised as to which of the two modalities should be given predominance. This can be decided by the balance. When color/power Doppler is switched on a gray bar, and a color bar appears on the left side of the screen. On the gray bar is a green line **(Fig. 16)**.

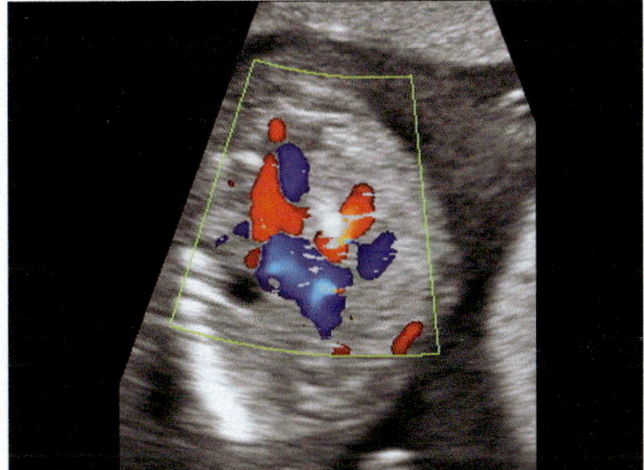

Fig. 17: Color Doppler image showing white patches in the color due to low balance.

This line indicates the balance adjustment. When the brightness of the gray scale on the image matches the brightness below the green line on the gray bar, the color predominates and the color filling is normal, but when the brightness on the gray scale image matches the brightness above the green line on the gray bar, the B-mode predominates and, therefore, in these areas, if the color is present to show the flow, the color will be patched up with white (this looks like snow on the color) **(Fig. 17)**. Increasing color gains is surely not an answer to this problem.

Very importantly, when this happens, the correct thing to do is to change the balance to

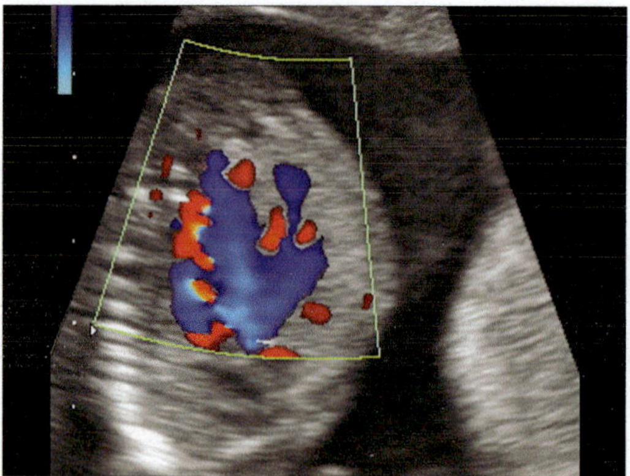

Fig. 18: Decreasing the gains of B-mode in the same case as in Figure 17, the color pickup becomes bold and smooth.

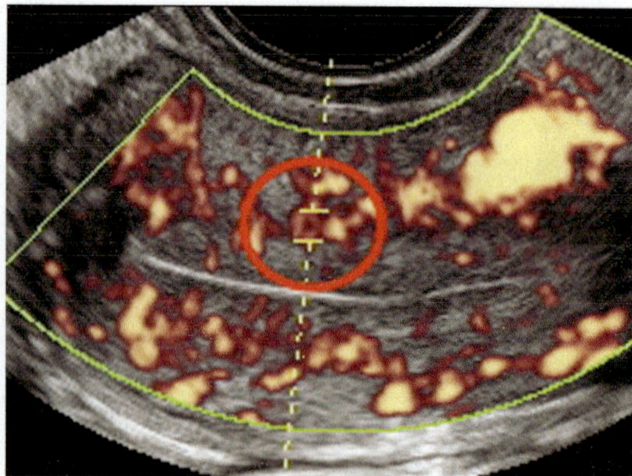

Fig. 19: Two parallel short horizontal lines (= sign) is seen on the dotted line on activation of the spectral Doppler.

higher that allows the color pick up even with bright gray scale. But, the balance setting on many scanners is on the submenu of color Doppler. This makes it clumsy, because when the operator is assessing flow in a relatively small vessel on the scan, to open the submenu and change the balance is difficult. Therefore, a practical solution to this is to reduce the B-mode gains that will match the brightness of the image to a gray shade below the green line on the gray bar and allows good color pickup **(Fig. 18)**.

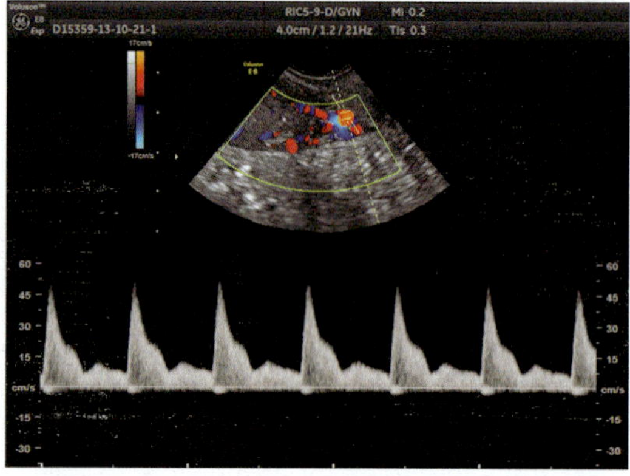

Fig. 20: A sample volume smaller than the diameter will not evaluate the flow in the entire stream and will give erroneously higher velocity.

SETTINGS FOR PULSED WAVE DOPPLER

Sample Volume

Sample volume is the selected length of the vessel to assess the flow. When pulsed wave Doppler is switched on, a dashed line appears on the screen. This line is perpendicular to the sound beam that can be swapped across the entire image. Two parallel short horizontal lines (= sign) appear on this line **(Fig. 19)**. This "= sign" can be moved up and down on the dotted line anywhere. This sign is to be placed on the vessel in which the flow is to be measured. The distance between the two lines decide what length of the vessel will be evaluated for the flow assessment. If the vessel is not absolutely parallel to the sound beam (overlapping on the dashed line), the distance between the two lines (sample volume) should be equal to the diameter of the vessel. A sample volume smaller than the diameter will lead to error in the velocity assessment because it will not evaluate the flow in the entire stream, but may measure it only in the central part of the stream **(Fig. 20)**. When that happens, correct velocity readings are not possible because it is known as flow velocities in the central stream and at the sides are not the same. If the sample volume is larger than the diameter of the vessel, the vessel wall movement or flow information from neighboring vessels may corrupt the flow information details **(Fig. 21)**.

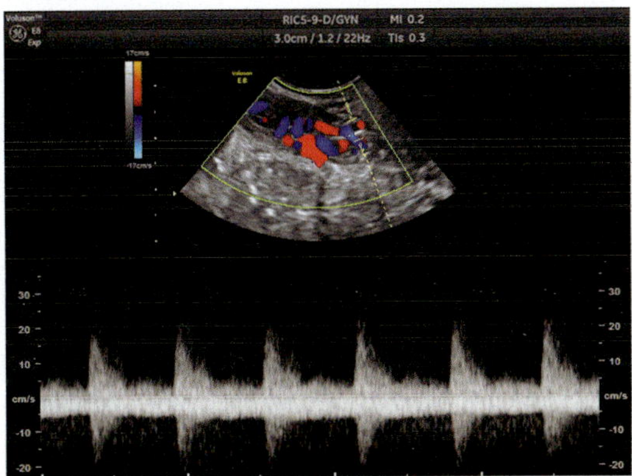

Fig. 21: Sample volume, larger than the diameter of the vessel, shows flow information from neighboring vessels.

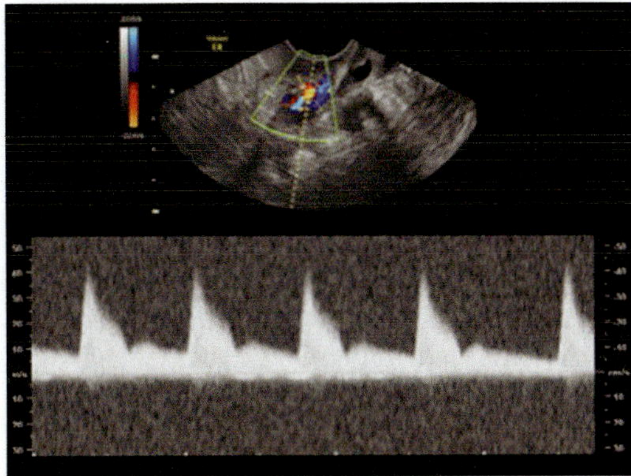

Fig. 23: High gains on spectral Doppler show noise on the spectrum.

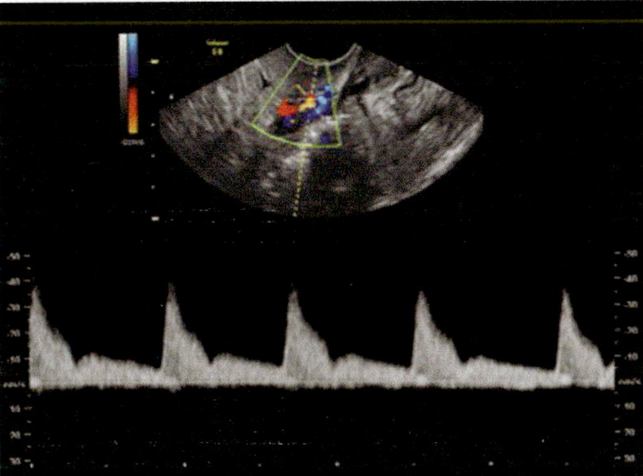

Fig. 22: Bold spectrum on the spectral Doppler showing the flow information.

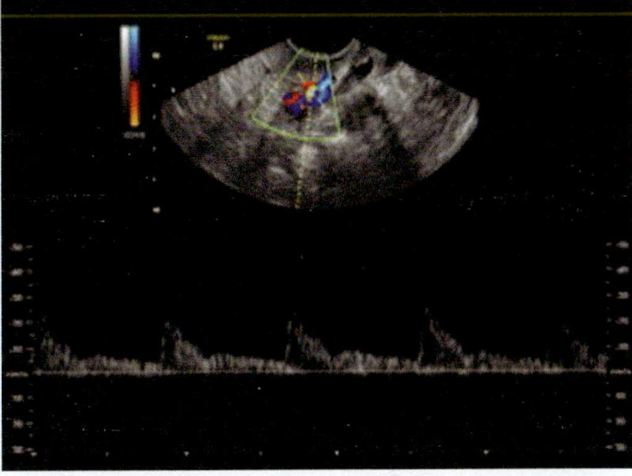

Fig. 24: Low gains on the spectral Doppler show scattered spectrum.

Gains

Gain settings on the pulsed wave Doppler should be such that it produces a clear well-defined bold spectrum of blood flow **(Fig. 22)**. If the gains are too high, the flow information will be corrupted by lot of noises **(Fig. 23)**. If the gains are too low, the entire spectrum will appear scarce and scattered **(Fig. 24)**.

Pulse Repetition Frequency

As it has been discussed earlier, the Nyquist frequency of a sound wave decides what maximum flow velocities can be recorded by a sound wave of certain frequency. Therefore, the PRF is adjusted according to flow velocity to be assessed. If high PRF is used for low velocity flow, it will not be possible to differentiate between the systolic and diastolic flows, as the systolic flow recordings will be subdued **(Fig. 25)**. If low PRF is selected for high velocity blood flow, there will be overlapping of systolic and diastolic signals and is known as aliasing **(Fig. 26)**. The correct PRF setting would, therefore, be when the spectrum will fill up two-thirds of the spectral area (above the baseline) **(Fig. 27)**. Though when there is minimal adjustment required to achieve this, moving the baseline up or down would also serve the purpose.

Wall Motion Filter

Like in color and power Doppler, the function of WMF in pulsed Doppler also is to eliminate signals from low velocity movements, chiefly

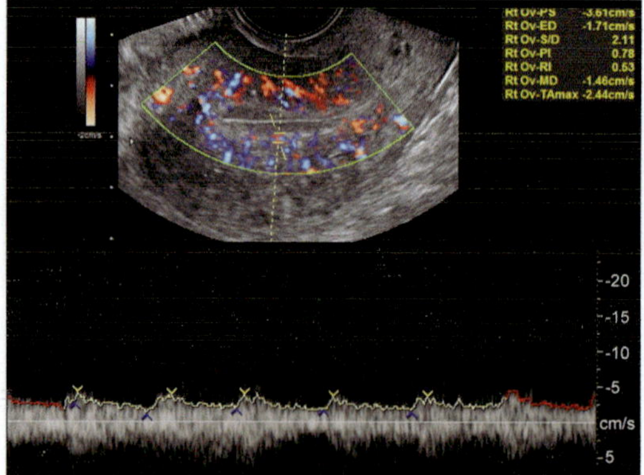

Fig. 25: Spectral Doppler image of a low velocity flow documented by high pulse repetition frequency (PRF) showing minimal difference in the systolic peak and diastolic flow.

not to corrupt the image with wall motions and also with venous flow adjoining the artery. Again, same as for color and power Doppler, the settings are low for low velocity vessels and high for high velocity vessels. But, the wall filter setting in a pulsed Doppler spectrum is known to be correct only, if the spectrum touches the baseline (**Fig. 28**). When there is a black line or a gap between the baseline and the spectrum (**Fig. 29**), this trace is not to be accepted as this clearly indicates high wall filter for the case. In that case, if we say it eliminates low velocity information, it means that it interferes with the diastolic flow information and may lead to false diagnosis of absent end-diastolic flow

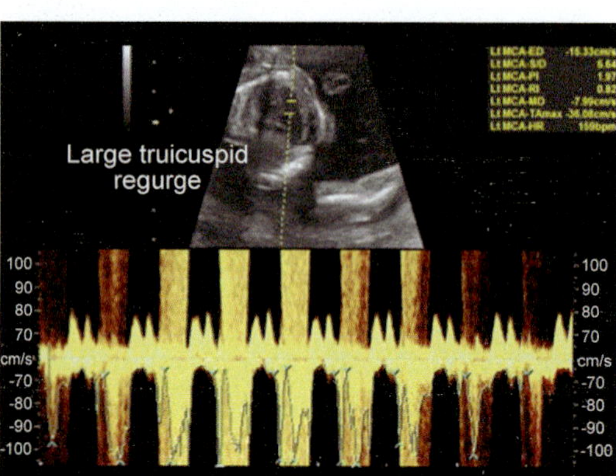

Fig. 26: If low pulse repetition frequency (PRF) is selected for high velocity blood flow, there will be overlapping of systolic and diastolic signals.

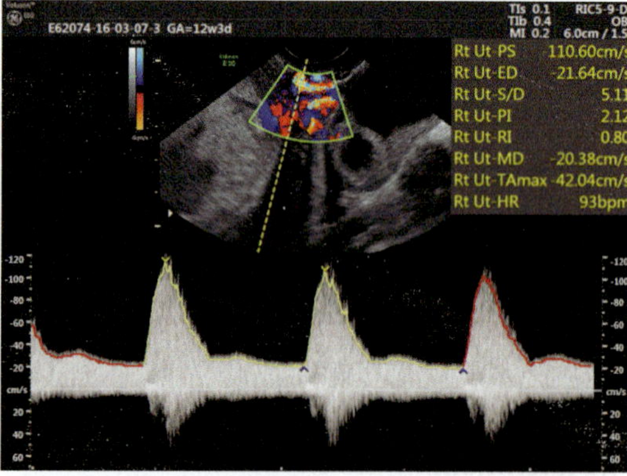

Fig. 28: Spectral Doppler image showing the spectrum touching the baseline and that is optimum setting of wall filter.

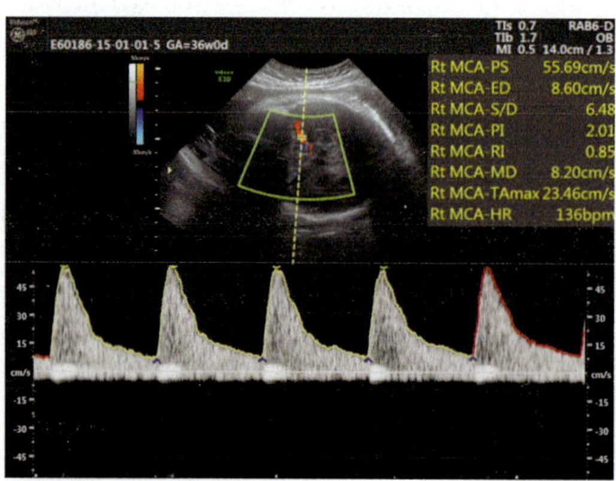

Fig. 27: Spectral Doppler showing the spectrum above the baseline using two-thirds of the area dedicated to spectrum.

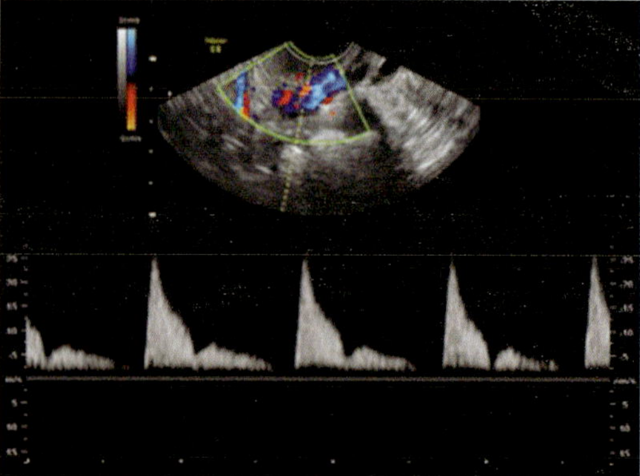

Fig. 29: Spectral Doppler image showing the spectrum not touching the baseline and that is high setting of wall filter.

and naturally, therefore, wrong interpretations. In spectral Doppler, being a quantitative Doppler, the wall filter settings on this modality are in numbers—30, 60, 90 Hz, etc. Wall filters, as a rule for gynecological and infertility assessment, are set at the lowest 30 Hz and for fetal echocardiography, this is set high may be 90–120 Hz depending on the fetal gestational age.

As it is discussed earlier, considering the equation for derivation of the blood flow velocity from frequency of incident sound beam, frequency of received sound beam, and cos θ of the angle of incidence, if the angle of incidence is 90°, then the cos θ being 0, the velocity value will be 0 and also that with increasing angle from >60°, the percentage of error in calculation is highly significant and so the Doppler angle is always set between 0 and 60°, preferably <30°. When the pulsed wave Doppler is switched on, the dashed line and the "= sign" appear. The Doppler angle can be considered or set at 0 when the vessel is parallel to the dashed line. This is often times possible because the dashed line can be swapped across the entire B-mode image and the probe manipulation may also help in the alignment of the two. But, if it is still not possible, after achieving the smallest angle between the vessel and the dashed line, angle correction is used. This deviates out a short line from the dashed line and is tried to align this short line to the vessel **(Fig. 30)**. In trying to do this, the angle between the dashed line and the short line is the Doppler angle. It is displayed on the screen or the touch pad of the scanner **(Fig. 31)**. This angle is to set as <30° preferably and maximum of 60° may be allowed. With angle of up to 30° the value deviation is up to 30% but goes to more than 50% with angle of more than 60°.

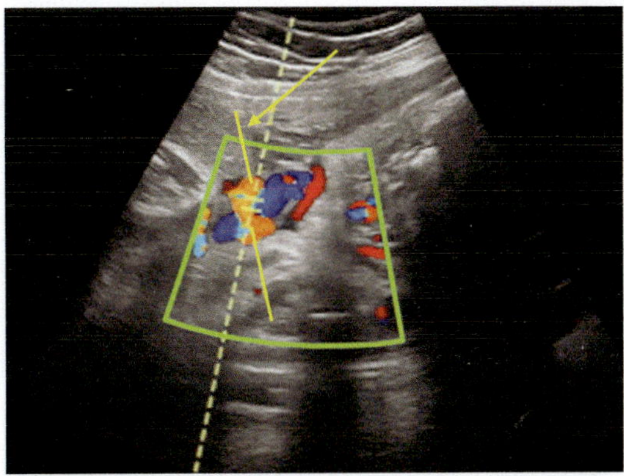

Fig. 30: Activation of the spectral Doppler shows a dotted line, the sample volume seen as an "= sign," and the short yellow line is the line that can be aligned to the long axis of the vessel.

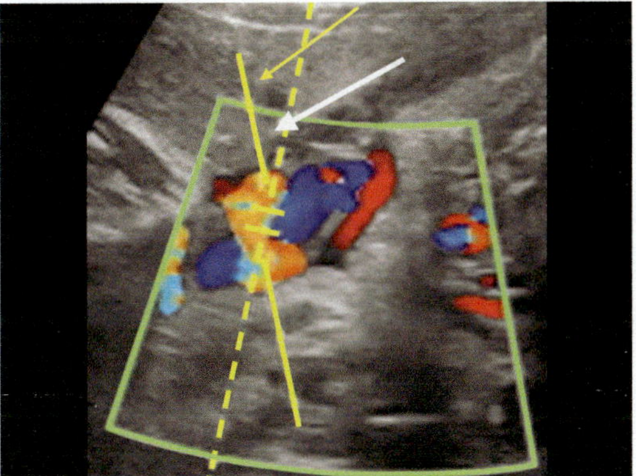

Fig. 31: The angle between short line and the dotted line is shown by the white blocked arrow.

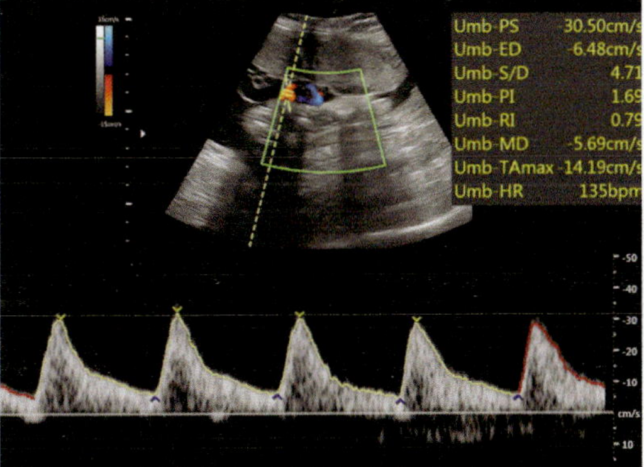

Fig. 32: Spectral trace showing four to five cardiac cycles on a single trace.

SETTING THE SPEED OF THE TRACE

An ideal spectral trace is when there are four to five cardiac cycles **(Fig. 32)** recorded on any one spectrum image. This can be done by scaling the time axis, or in simpler words, setting the speed of the trace. For most scans,

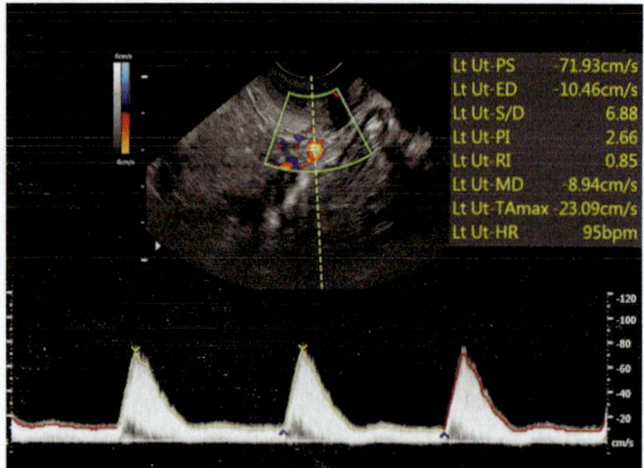

Fig. 33: Spectral Doppler traced on higher speed showing trace of multiple cardiac cycles.

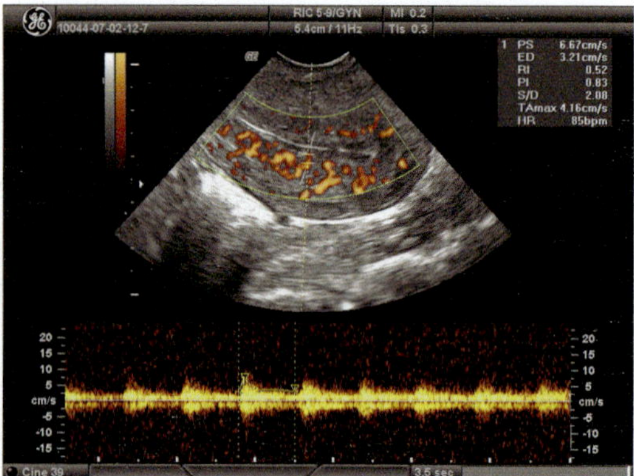

Fig. 34: Spectral Doppler traced on lower speed showing trace of less than five cardiac cycles.

this is possible when the speed is set as 4 or 5. Higher speed gives trace of too few cardiac cycles **(Fig. 33)** and lesser speed gives too many cardiac cycles traced **(Fig. 34)**.

ARTIFACTS

In spite of all these settings used to optimize the Doppler images, certain artifacts still cannot be completely eliminated. These are aliasing, mirror image artifact, and artifacts due to electrical interferences.

Aliasing

When the Doppler frequency exceeds the Nyquist frequency, it results in aliasing. This is overlapping effect of systolic and diastolic velocities across the baseline on both the sides of the spectrum. This effect is similar

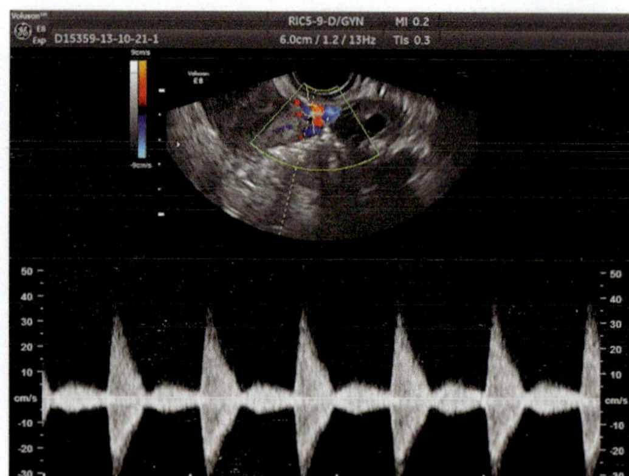

Fig. 35: Mirror image artifact showing similar flow trace on both the sides of baseline.

to what we have often observed especially in movies. The car wheels suddenly appear to start rotating in the opposite direction when the car speeds up. This can be explained diagrammatically here.

If the frequency of the oscillations is 5 Hz, but the PRF is 2 Hz/s, therefore, this signal will see this movement only twice in a second and not only miss the intermittent information, but also will interpret that the flow is in both directions. Adjusting the optimum PRF sorts out this problem.

Mirror Image Artifact

Mirror image artifact is when a similar spectrum is seen on both the sides of the baseline. This is especially possible when the sample volume is large and is tracing the flow in two vessels or two loops of the same vessel positioned side-by-side **(Fig. 35)**. Second possibility is that a large sample volume is placed on the curve of the loop; when in the proximal half of the loop, the blood flow is observed away from the probe by the transducer and in the distal half of the sample volume, the flow is perceived toward the probe. Decreasing the sample volume and planning to place it on one vessel only sort out this problem.

Electrical Interferences

These may appear as random signals on color, power, or spectral Doppler **(Fig. 36)**, especially

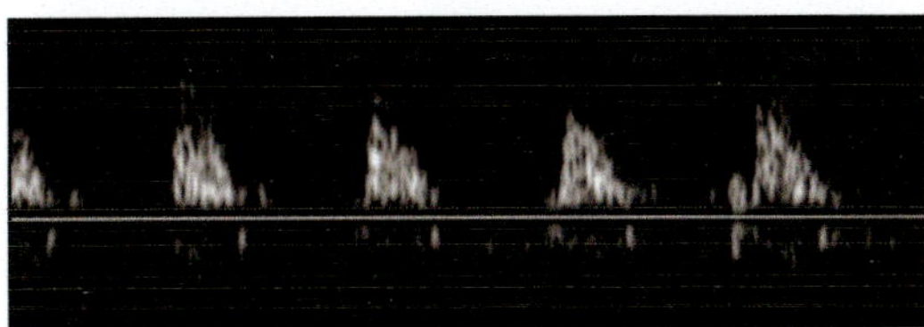

Fig. 36: Scattered shadows seen on the spectral Doppler possibly due to electrical interference.

when the scanner is sharing the same electrical line as some high voltage gadget and the only way to get rid of this is to plan the electrical supply to the scanner wisely.

SAFETY OF DOPPLER

There is a big scare against using Doppler in the people who are aware of the ill effects of Doppler and a false sense of safety in those who are not aware of these side effects. The two major effects of sound wave when it passes through the human body are:

1. *Thermal effect*: Production of heat that may damage the cells.
2. *Mechanical effect*: Due to pressure changes on the molecule.

Thermal Effects

As the sound waves pass through the body tissues, there is absorption of energy and transformation of ultrasound energy into heat. The energy absorption is minimal in fluid and maximum in bones. It is also dependent on the frequency of the ultrasound waves. The absorption is higher with higher frequency sound waves and lower with low frequency sound waves. A temperature rise up to 1°C is considered absolutely safe, whereas if it is >2.5°C, it can lead to significant tissue damage. This thermal effect is measured and displayed as thermal index on the screen. It is generally found that the temperature rise of 2°C is thermal index 2. We know that the temperature rise of 1°C is safe, so thermal index should be limited at maximum 1. Though it is important here to understand that with higher thermal indices also, the damage can occur only after exposure of a certain period of time. Unfortunately, this time is difficult to define confidently. Moreover, since the energy absorbing capacity of different tissues is different, thermal index for soft tissues (TIs) and bones (TIb) is different.[3]

Mechanical Effect

When the sound wave passes through the body tissues, it leads to oscillations of the body molecules resulting in cavitating (low pressure) phase and a compressing (high pressure) phase. In the negative pressure phase or the cavitation phase, large microbubbles are formed. Once the oscillations reach a certain level, fluid medium incorporating gas microbubbles is set in motion called microstreaming. This generates very strong pressure and leads to bursting of cell membranes. This effect is pronounced if the high frequency, high intensity ultrasound is aimed on a small focus.[1]

The second possible mechanism leading to tissue damage explained is as follows: existing microbubbles or cells undergoing cavitation inflate under the influence of negative pressure and implode abruptly. This takes microseconds but causes sudden rise in temperature/pressure and results in tissue destruction. This is transient cavitation and occurs only when energy levels are beyond certain thresholds. This threshold may be quantitatively documented as **mechanical index** (MI). MI is defined as "maximum estimated in situ rarefaction pressure or maximum negative pressure (in MPa) divided by the square root of the frequency (in MHz)." MI up to 0.3 can be considered safe and >0.7 can lead to cavitation.[4]

CONCLUSION

Doppler is a very useful modality for assessment of circulation in the human body. Correct settings on the scanner only can give optimum results and, therefore, it is very important to understand the basic principles and settings of the ultrasound scanner before starting to use Doppler for interpretation of vascular flow and information of oxygenation in human fetus. Ultrasound and Doppler are generally safe modalities. Their safety can be related to frequency used and the length of exposure. Therefore, Doppler should not be used for long time on a single focus and, therefore, as low as reasonably achievable (ALARA)[5] principle is now applied for all ultrasound scan.

REFERENCES

1. Frey H. Physical and technical fundamentals of ultrasound and Doppler ultrasound. In: Sohn C, Voigt HJ, Vetter K (Eds). Doppler Ultrasound in Obstetrics and Gynecology. Germany: Thieme Medical Publishers; 2004.
2. Burns PN. Principles of Doppler and color flow. Radiol Med (Torino). 1993;85:3-16.
3. Duck FA, Wladimiroff JW, Nes SHE. Ultrasound in Obstetrics and Gynecology. New York: Elsevier; 2009. pp. 21-30.
4. British Medical Ultrasound Society (BMUS). (2020). Safety of ultrasound. [online] Available from: www.bmus.org/public-info/pi-safety01.asp. [Last accessed on August, 2021].
5. Auxier JA, Dickson HW. Guest editorial: concern over recent use of the ALARA philosophy. Health Phys. 1983;44:595-600.

4

CHAPTER

Ultrasound in First Trimester Pregnancy

Sonal Panchal, Chaitanya Nagori

INTRODUCTION

First trimester of pregnancy is the most eventful time of human life. Study of the first trimester of pregnancy by ultrasound (US) is sonoembryology. Embryology has always been a study of specimens. It was very difficult to understand the development of human embryo until the advent of volume US. Volume US with transvaginal probe has brought a revolution in the study of embryology.

Transvaginal sonography (TVS) is so far the method of choice for earliest visual documentation of pregnancy and volume US has added value to that by various rendering modes and the multiplanar mode to understand the anatomy better.

Using transvaginal US, study of pregnancy can be started even before the sac appears. It is known that the blastocyst implants in the endometrium, 5 days after the fertilization of the ovum in the fallopian tube, i.e., approximately 18th–20th day of the 28 days cycle. With implantation, the progesterone secretion is enhanced from corpus luteum and this is reflected as increased blood flow to the corpus luteum. The receptive organ to this progesterone and proteolytic and other factors is the endometrium. It thickens due to the decidual reaction. New blood vessels develop to provide nutritional support to the embryo. On US, these changes are represented as:

- Two-dimensional (2D) US:
  - *Asymmetrical endometrial thickening*: One of the endometrial lips is thickened as compared to other because of implanting embryo **(Fig. 1B)**.
  - Corpus luteum **(Fig. 1A)**
- Color Doppler:
  - High-velocity, low-resistance trophoblastic flow [peak systolic velocity (PSV) > 6] in the thickened endometrial lip. This is typically described as a color comet sign by Honemeyer et al. **(Fig. 2B)**.[1]
  - Corpus luteum vascularity with low RI < 0.5 **(Fig. 2A)**

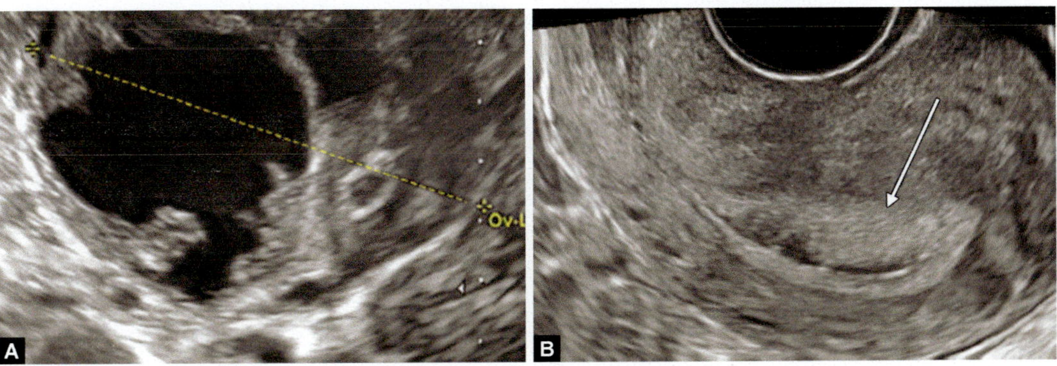

Figs. 1A and B: Corpus luteum and secretory endometrium with asymmetrical thickening on B mode (arrow).

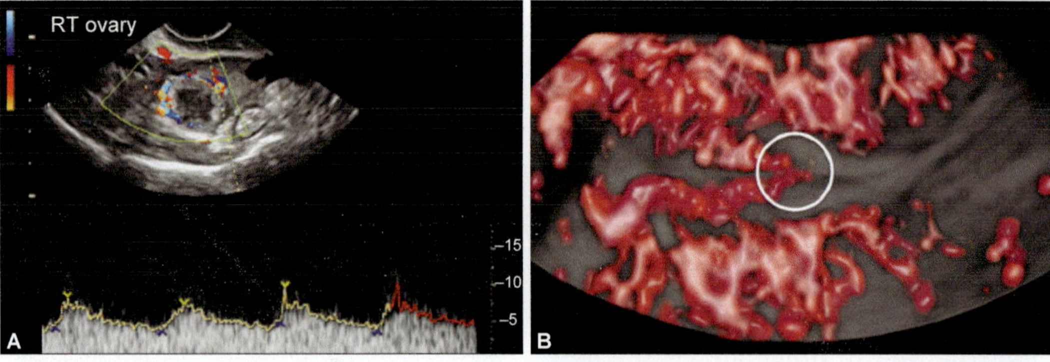

Figs. 2A and B: Corpus luteal and endometrial color comet sign on power Doppler (circle). (RT: right)

- *Three-dimensional (3D) US*:
  - Asymmetrical endometrial thickening is more evident on 3D US, with thickened part showing increased echogenicity due to decidual reaction and increased vascularity **(Fig. 3)**.

Endometrial thickness of <6 mm and non-hyperechogenic endometrium with scanty vascularity in mid-luteal phase are negative predictors of conception.

Embryo is a very fast growing structure and therefore its anatomy changes every day or may be even faster. It is very difficult to keep a day-to-day track of these changes. Therefore, changes in the embryo are described week-to-week. Scans are done during early pregnancy for:

- Confirmation of pregnancy
- Location of pregnancy
- Early detection of multiple gestation
- Assessment of progress of pregnancy
- Evaluation of early abnormal pregnancy.

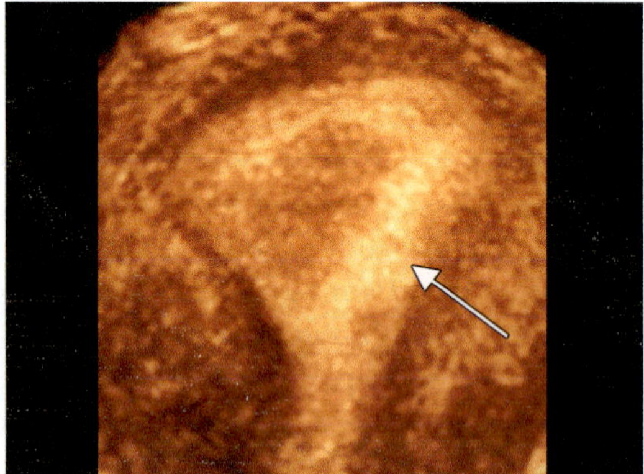

Fig. 3: Three-dimensional ultrasound—possibly conception cycle, mid-luteal phase (arrow).

CONFIRMATION OF PREGNANCY

Since the use of transvaginal US has become popular, documentation of pregnancy has become earlier. Presence of gestational sac can be confirmed in the endometrial cavity as early as 4 weeks and 3–4 days and is diagnostic of intrauterine pregnancy. Gestational sac is a round anechoic structure with thick hyperechoic margins. This echogenic margin is because of decidual reaction and is known as double decidual ring sign. The true gestational sac must be differentiated from pseudo-sac that may often be seen in patients with ectopic pregnancies and the differentiating points between true gestational sac and pseudogestational sac are shown in **Table 1**.

TABLE 1: Difference between true sac and pseudo-sac.

Features	***True sac (Fig. 4)***	***Pseudo-sac (Fig. 5)***
Situation	Eccentric in endocavity	Central in endocavity
Margins	Double decidual ring	No hyperechoic ring
With uterine peristalsis	No change in shape	Changes shape
On Doppler	Peripheral vascular ring	No peripheral vascularity

β-human chorionic gonadotropin (β-hCG) is the earliest and the first marker for confirmation of pregnancy and gestational sac must be detected in the endometrial cavity on transvaginal scan when β-hCG levels are > 1,000 IU/mL.

In absence of which the possibilities are—(1) ectopic pregnancy, (2) early multiple pregnancy, and (3) early missed abortion. At appearance, gestational sac is 2–3 mm in diameter. It grows at a rate of 1 mm/day and at 7 weeks, it occupies one-third of endometrial cavity. As it is implanted in one of the endometrial leaves, the endometrial cavity still persists till the sac grows large enough to abut the endometrial cavity. This residual cavity may be seen till 7 weeks and fluid seen surrounding the sac till this time should be first considered as a residual cavity, rather than perisac bleeding **(Fig. 6)**. Its continuity with the endometrial central line toward fundus or with cervical canal toward cervix confirms that it is residual endometrial cavity.

A gestational sac that is not circular, does not have thick echogenic margins, appears late, is too large or too small for dates, has internal echogenicities, and does not show peripheral vascularity is considered abnormal **(Figs. 7A to C)**.

A gestational sac that grows <0.7 mm a day is also considered to have a bad prognosis.

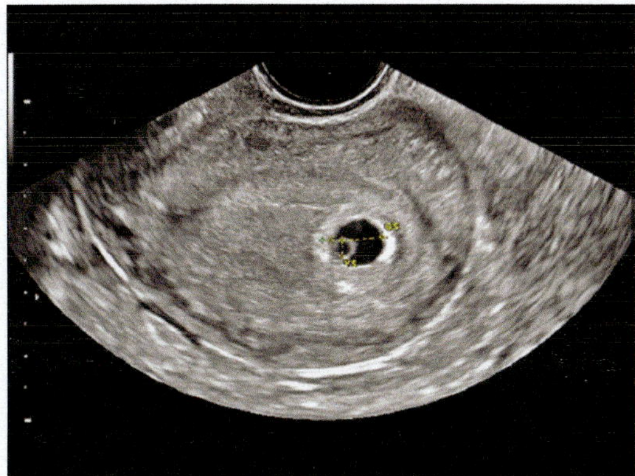

Fig. 4: True gestational sac (GS).

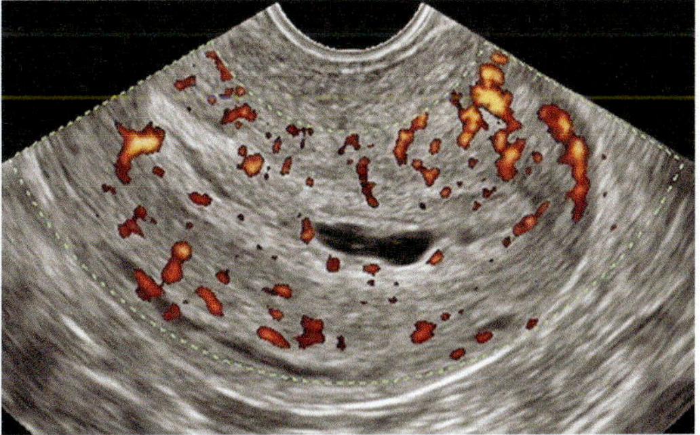

Fig. 5: Pseudo-sac.

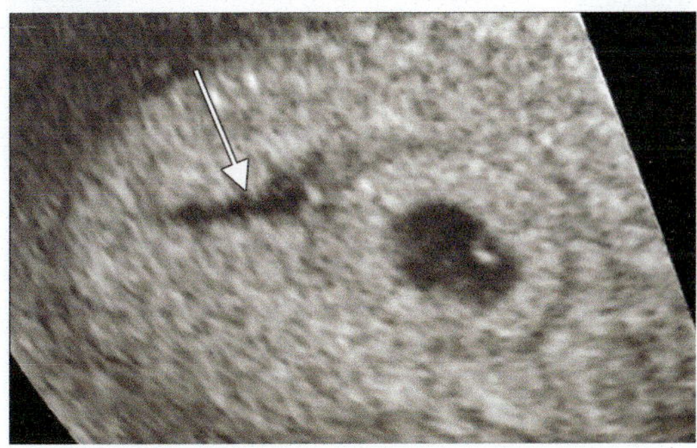

Fig. 6: Residual endometrial cavity (arrow).

LOCATION OF GESTATIONAL SAC

Usually, the gestational sac is implanted in the fundal area **(Fig. 8)**. Gestational sac that is implanted at any other location than this is considered abnormal or ectopic. Gestational sac that is implanted low **(Fig. 9)** in the endometrial cavity though may not be called ectopic but has increased chance of abortion.

Other locations of gestational sac in uterine cavity that are not considered normal are angular and interstitial pregnancy. Pregnancy in the lateral angle of the endometrial cavity is called angular pregnancy and the one in the interstitial part of the fallopian tube is interstitial pregnancy. Gestational sac in angle of the endometrial cavity usually grows inside the endometrial cavity **(Fig. 10A)**. Pregnancy in this location is usually observed closely. The risk is only possibility of adherent placenta. Interstitial part of the tube is covered by myometrium and gestational sac in this location cannot distend beyond 6–7 weeks. Differentiation between the two is also important **(Fig. 10B)**.

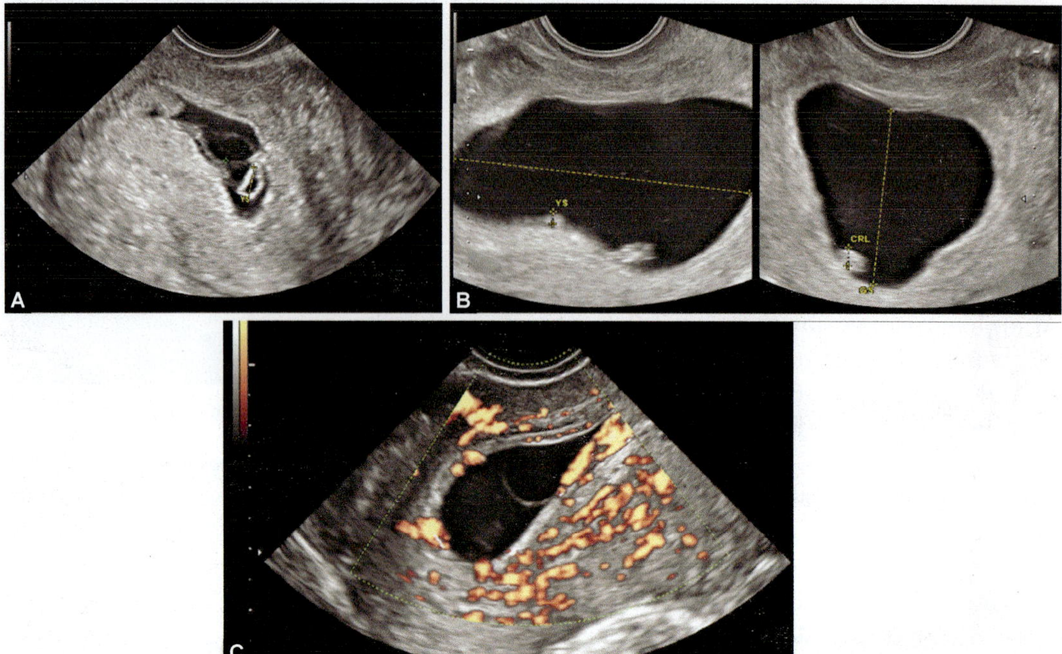

Figs. 7A to C: (A) Irregular sac with internal echogenicities; (B) Large gestational sac (GS); (C) Gestational sac with yolk sac (YS) and minimal vascularity. (CRL: crown-rump length)

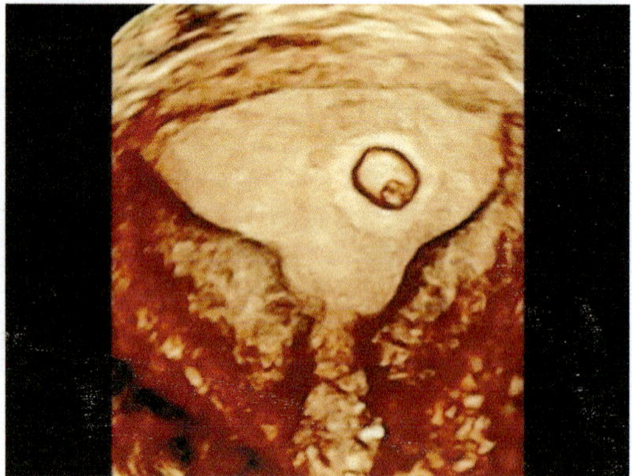

Fig. 8: Normally implanted gestational sac.

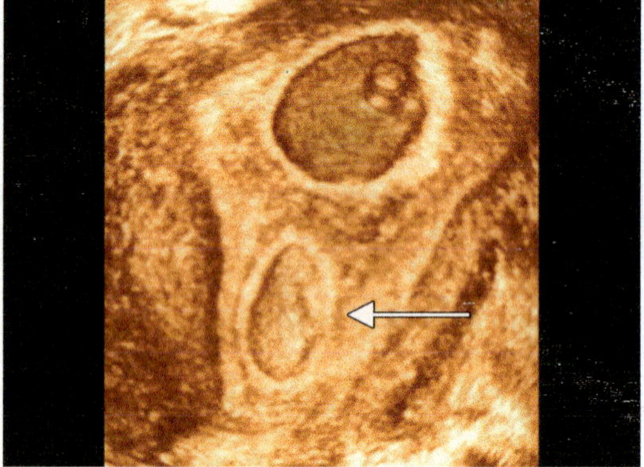

Fig. 9: Three-dimensional ultrasound image of the uterus with twin gestational sacs, one is normal in fundus and the other is low implanted (arrow).

In interstitial pregnancy, myometrial interface is seen between the endometrium and gestational sac on transverse section of uterus that is cut at the level of the gestational sac. Whereas in angular pregnancy, transverse section of the uterus at the level of gestational sac shows endometrial shadow covering the gestational sac medially but no endometrium is seen lateral to gestational sac **(Figs. 10C and D)**. Cornual pregnancy was the term earlier used for angular pregnancy. But now, that term is reserved for the pregnancies in abnormal uterine cornu.

Gestational sac may also implant in the cervix and is known as cervical pregnancy and is typically seen as ballooning of the cervix and hourglass shape of the uterus **(Fig. 11A)**.

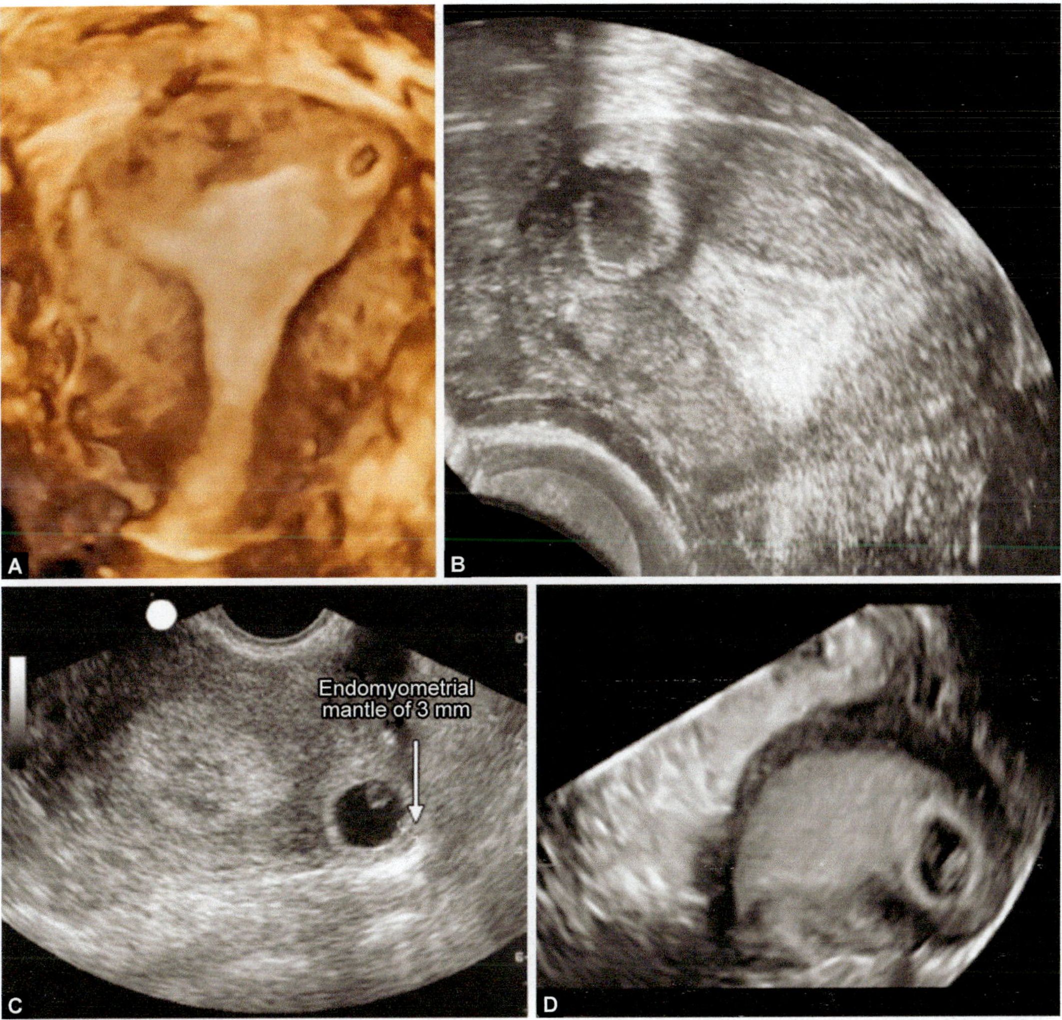

Figs. 10A to D: (A and B) Cornual pregnancy on two-dimensional (2D) and three-dimensional (3D) ultrasound; (C and D) Interstitial pregnancy on 2D and 3D ultrasound interstitial pregnancy.

Cervical pregnancy can be differentiated from gestational sac in process of abortion by its eccentric location and the surrounding vascularity **(Fig. 11B)**.

Rarely, one may also see a gestational sac in the scar. It is called scar pregnancy and the incidence is increasing because of increased rate of cesarean sections. Scar pregnancy may be implanted in the scar or over the scar **(Fig. 11C)**. Gestational sac, which implants in the scar, is more dangerous, as it can tear off the scar. But the gestational sac that is implanted over the scar can grow in the endometrial cavity, though there is a risk of adherent placenta **(Fig. 11D)**. In this case the gestational sac is still in the endometrial cavity, but the chorionic tissue extends into the scar.

Abnormal location of pregnancy that is extrauterine is in the tube, ovary, or free in the peritoneal cavity. Tubal ectopics are the most common of all ectopic situations.

Patients with ectopic pregnancy typically present with a history of missed period with either fainting attacks, dizziness, or acute lower abdominal pain with raised β-hCG levels. The US diagnostic signs are discussed

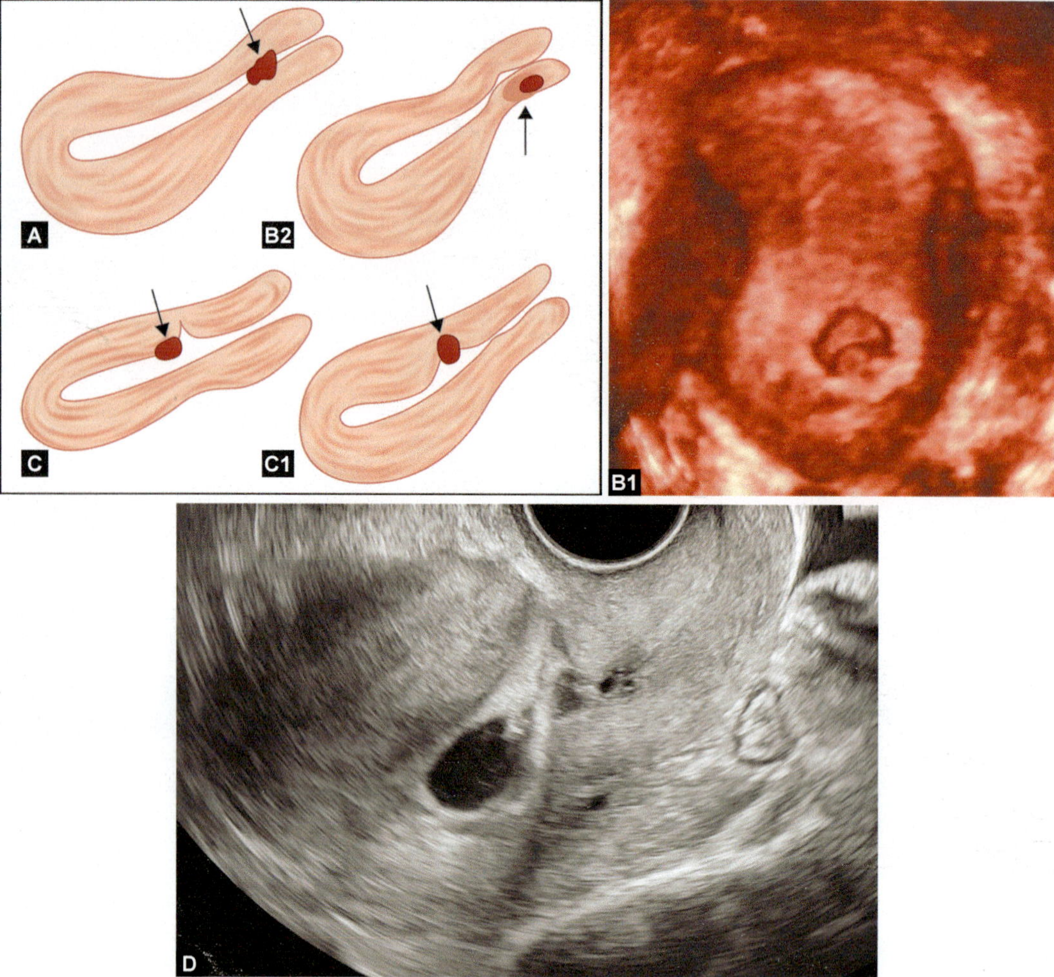

Figs. 11A to D: (A) Diagrammatic presentation of gestational sac in the cervical canal in case of abortion in process in the left side image, diagrammatic presentation of gestational sac in the cervical wall indicating cervical pregnancy in the right image; (B) Three-dimensional (3D) ultrasound image of cervical pregnancy; (C) Diagrammatic presentation of scar pregnancy, over the scar in image on left and in the scar in image on right; (D) B mode ultrasound image of pregnancy in the scar.

here. Typically the beta hCG level is lower than expected for the duration of amenorrhea. It also rises at a slower pace than normal, that means the values do not double in 48 hours.

Tubal Ectopic Pregnancy

- No intrauterine gestational sac with symmetrical endometrial cavity **(Fig. 12A)**.
- Adnexal mass with peripheral low resistance vascularity with or without gestational sac, which is tender on probe pressure **(Fig. 12B)**. In earlier stages of ectopic pregnancy, the adnexal mass only appears as an isoechoic mass, in extraovarian location with peripheral vascularity. A central hyperechoic shadow then becomes visible, followed by central anechoic area (gestational sac). It is important to diagnose ectopic pregnancy early. This can minimize the risk to the patient. It is also true that this ectopic pregnancy can be followed up closely

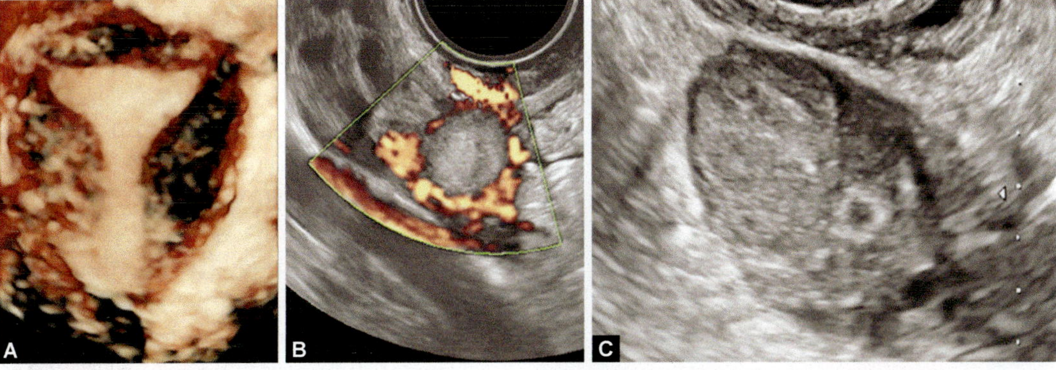

Figs. 12A to C: (A and B) Tubal ectopic pregnancy; (C) Ovarian ectopic pregnancy.

without any intervention. If the mass size increases, gestational sac appears with cardiac activity, or patient becomes unstable, intervention is justified.

- Ipsilateral active corpus luteum
- *Free fluid in pelvis*: This sign is seen only when the pregnancy completely invades the tubal wall and bleeding starts from the tube.

Ovarian Ectopic Pregnancy (Fig. 12C)

- No intrauterine gestational sac with symmetrical endometrial cavity
- Anechoic circular gestational sac in ovary with typical hyperechoic decidual reaction such as rim, with peripheral vascularity
- This can be differentiated from a corpus luteum only by its hyperechoic rim which is not seen in corpus luteum.

Abdominal/Peritoneal Ectopic Pregnancy (Fig. 13)

- No intrauterine gestational sac with symmetrical endometrial cavity
- Gestational sac is seen lying free outside uterus, tubes, or ovaries and does not show any myometrium around.
- It is usually surrounded by fluid.
- Is it very difficult to locate, as it can be placed anywhere in the peritoneal cavity.

It must be remembered that ectopic pregnancy may coexist with intrauterine pregnancy and is then known as heterotopic pregnancy.

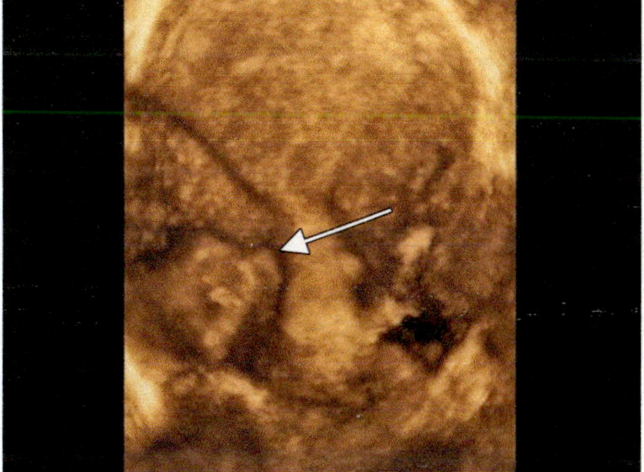

Fig. 13: Abdominal ectopic pregnancy (arrow).

EARLY DETECTION OF MULTIPLE GESTATIONS

Multiple gestations have much higher complication rate than singleton pregnancy. The complication rate and management are different for monochorionic and dichorionic and monoamniotic and diamniotic pregnancies. It is therefore essential to confirm the chorionicity and amnionicity of any multiple gestations. This can be best done at 8 weeks of pregnancy. This is the time when gestational sacs are small and therefore individual sac margins can be confidently identified **(Fig. 14)**. Without mentioning the chorionicity and amnionicity, no report of multiple gestations is to be considered complete.

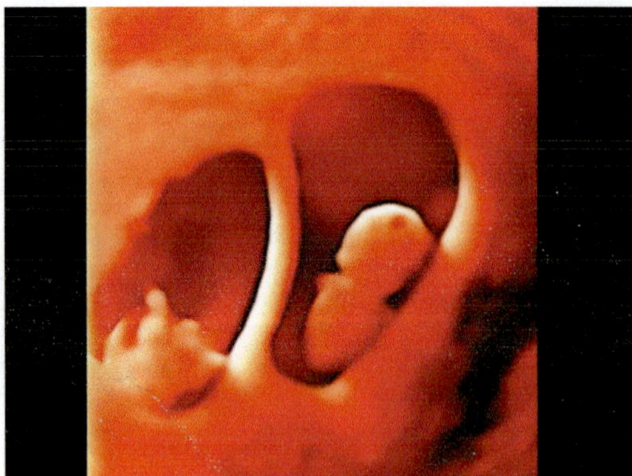

Fig. 14: Multiple gestations (dichorionic diamniotic twins).

GROWTH AND PROGRESS OF PREGNANCY

Growth of pregnancy is assessed by increase in the size of gestational sac or fetal pole and development of new structures in the fetus. Gestational sac, yolk sac, amniotic sac, and fetal pole, all have a definite time of appearance and pace of growth. These growth rates are very precise in first trimester and do not have genetic or individual variation. The technique for these measurements therefore should be standardized.

Gestational Sac (Fig. 15)

- Gestational sac appears at 4 weeks 5/6 days.
- It should grow at a rate of 1 mm per day.
- It is measured from "inner to inner" edge.
- Always take a mean of 3 largest orthogonal diameters. After locating the gestational sac, the probe is rotated to find the longest diameter. The second measurement is the longest diameter perpendicular to the longest diameter. The probe is rotated 90° and the side-to-side longest diameter parallel to X-axis is transverse diameter is measured. Mean of these three is the mean gestational sac diameter or one may also calculate the volume of the gestational sac from these three diameters. Nomograms are available for both mean sac diameter and of gestational sac volume.

Volume is now considered more reliable **(Fig. 16)**.

Abnormal gestational sac:

- Irregular gestational sac—gestational sac may appear irregular due to:
  - Myoma
  - Uterine contraction

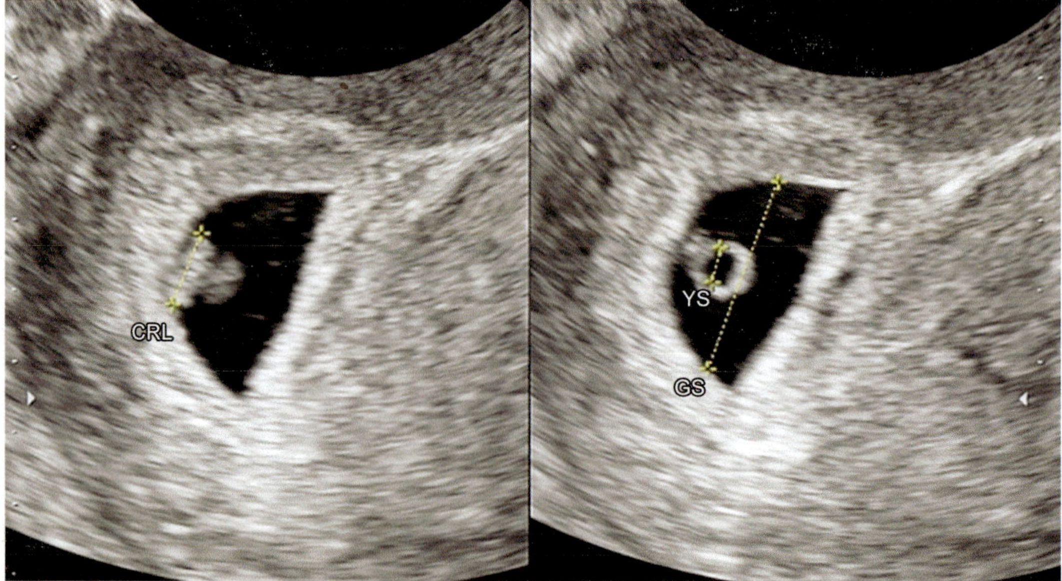

Fig. 15: Measuring gestational sac (GS), yolk sac (YS), and crown-rump length (CRL).

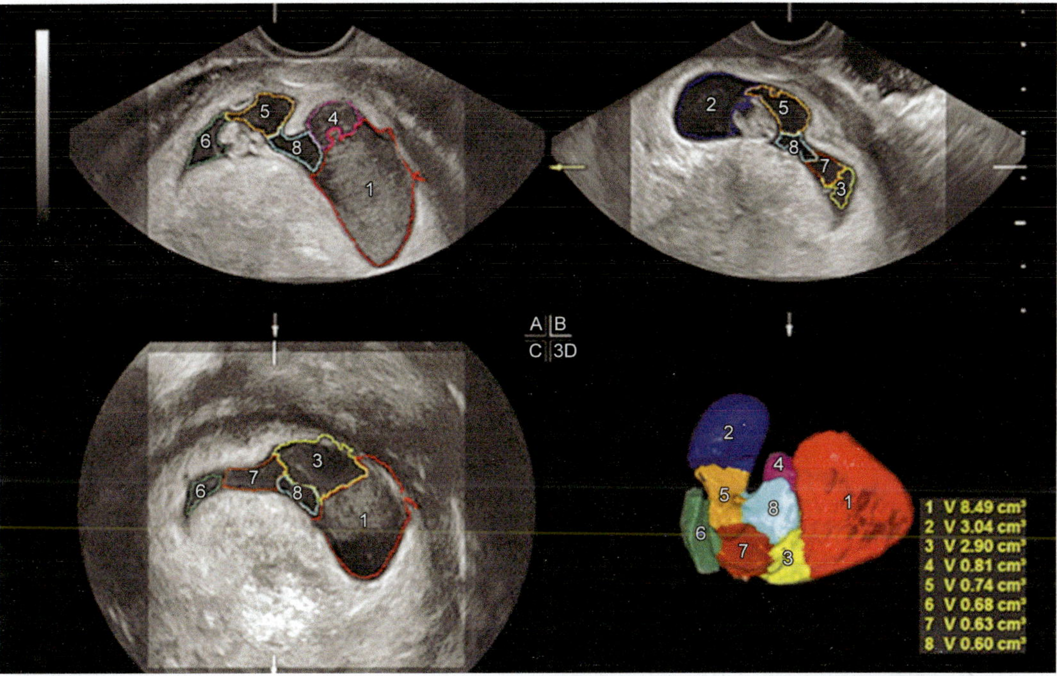

Fig. 16: Gestational sac volume measured by three-dimensional ultrasound.

  - Perisac bleeding
  - Overdistended bladder
- Decidual wall thickness <3 mm
- Large/small sac (in relation to the duration of amenorrhea)
- Sac >10 mm in size with no yolk sac
- Sac >16 mm with no fetal pole.[2]
- Abnormal sac and early embryo failure should be considered when gestational sac fails to increase at a rate of 0.7 mm/day.
- Abnormal gestational sac size is associated with trisomy and triploidy.[3]

But, it has been suggested that one should declare a failed pregnancy when:

- An empty gestational sac >25 mm or if a sac is smaller than that but is not increasing at a rate of at least 4 mm in a week.
- Missing yolk sac with gestational sac >20 mm or even when the yolk sac is not seen in a smaller sac when the sac is not growing at least 4 mm in a week.
- Crown-rump length (CRL) of 7 mm with no cardiac activity[4]

Though perisac blood flows are not different in normal or abnormal pregnancy.

Perisac bleeding: According to the location, it is classified as subchorionic, marginal, and supracervical. It may or may not be associated with vaginal bleeding. With absence of vaginal bleeding, it is an incidental finding. When bleeding is present, it is termed a threatened abortion.

- Sonography can identify perigestational hemorrhage in 5–22% as a cause of vaginal bleeding in women with threatened abortion.
- Inhibin A, activin A, human chorionic gonadotropin (hCG), pregnancy-associated plasma protein-A (PAPP-A), and follistatin concentrations were all significantly lower in women who subsequently miscarried when compared with live births.
- At 6–7 weeks gestation, plasma inhibin A (~fourfold, $p < 0.01$), hCG (~fourfold, $p < 0.01$), and estradiol (~twofold, $p < 0.001$) levels were significantly lower in women

who went on to have another miscarriage than those with a live birth.[5]

Prognosis of pregnancy in patients with perisac bleeding depends on:

- Size of perisac bleed
- Location of perisac bleed (hematoma on the chorion frondosum side has more risk of abortion than the one on the chorion leave side).
- Location of hematoma is more predictive of pregnancy outcome than the size of the hematoma. Hematomas that are at the cephalic end of the implanted sac have a higher risk to end into abortion than those at the caudal end
- Subchorionic hematomas lead to compression of spiral arteries and therefore increased resistance in the spiral arteries.
- These hematomas have a tendency to get absorbed and then the circulation normalizes.
- Improvement of blood flow indices is therefore predictive of normal pregnancy outcome.[6]
- It is important to differentiate perisac hematomas from an endometrial that is still not obliterated.

Yolk Sac

Yolk sac has nutritive, metabolic, endocrine, immunological, and hematopoietic functions. It must be seen after 7–8 days of visualization of the gestational sac. Yolk sac appears toward the end of the 4th week or when gestational sac is 10 mm in diameter. Fetal pole must be seen when gestational sac is 15 mm in diameter. It is a confirmatory sign of true gestational sac:

- Measured inner wall to inner wall
- Increases 0.1 mm/day till 10 weeks—maximum normal diameter is 5–6 mm

Its yolk sac is an indicator of poor pregnancy outcome, if it is **(Figs. 17A to D)**:

- Too small yolk sac <2 mm
- Too large yolk sac >6 mm
- Thick walled yolk sac
- Irregular yolk sac
- Solid yolk sac.

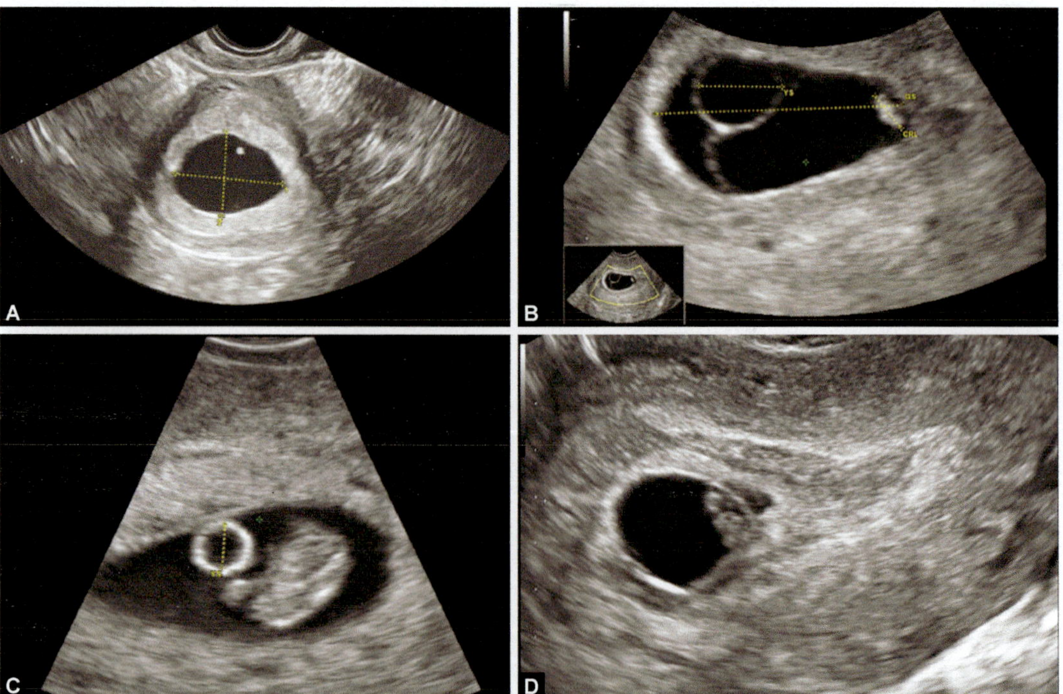

Figs. 17A to D: (A) Tiny yolk sac; (B) Large yolk sac; (C) Thick-walled yolk sac; (D) Solid yolk sac.

Fetal Pole

Fetal pole is the structure to follow the appearance of yolk sac. Detection of the fetal pole is actually by visualization of the cardiac activity. By transvaginal US, fetal cardiac activity can be detected at 5.6 weeks approximately, when the fetal pole appears like a linear structure by the side of the yolk sac approximately 1–2 mm in length. Its length is measured from end to end. Fetal pole grows at a rate of 1 mm/day. Size-to-date discrepancy of up to 5 days can be considered to be within normal limits in first trimester. Difference in crown-rump length (CRL) of >7 mm of normal indicates three times higher risk of aneuploidy.

Cardiac activity must always be seen at all times after 6 weeks of pregnancy. Appearance of a fetal pole without cardiac activity is a sign of abnormal pregnancy prognosis.

Cardiac Activity (Rate at Different Gestational Age)

- 5th week—slow-like peristalsis—60-80/min
- End of 5th week—100/min
- End of 6th week—105-130/min
- 9 weeks—160-170/min, then120-160/min
- Heart rate of >200/min is termed as tachycardia and <100/min is termed as bradycardia in the first trimester.

Persistently abnormal heart rate or irregular rhythm and late appearance of cardiac activity also indicate pregnancy with bad prognosis.

Structures then to appear by completion of each following week after 5 weeks are as follows:

Six weeks ***(Fig. 18)***:

- Fetal pole is seen and cephalic and caudal poles of the fetal pole are identified.
- Omphalomesenteric duct is seen.

Seven weeks:

- Cephalic pole shows the first brain vesicle—rhombencephalon
- Amnion is seen around the fetal pole

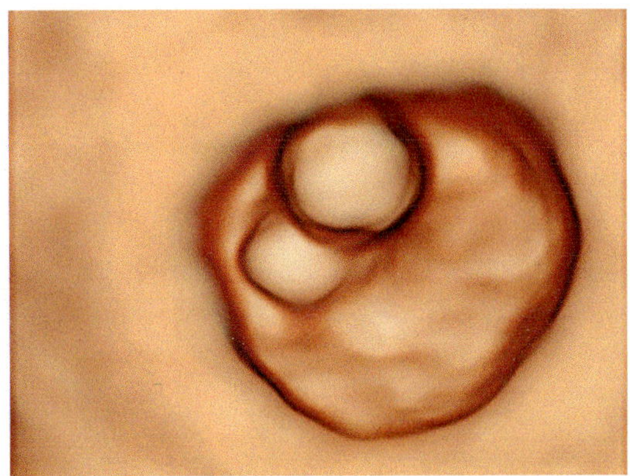

Fig. 18: Six weeks pregnancy.

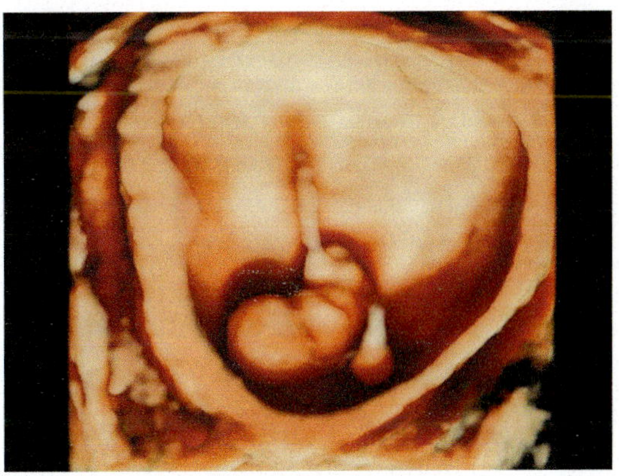

Fig. 19: Eight weeks pregnancy.

- Chorionic tissue around the gestational sac starts differentiating into chorion frondosum and chorion leave.

Amniotic membrane:

- It is seen when CRL is 5–7 mm.
- When it starts appearing with tiny fetal pole, it appears to be the same size as the yolk sac and is mistaken by some as double yolk sac. But, presence of fetal pole in this cyst like structure confirms it is amniotic sac.
- It grows at a rate of 1 mm/day.
- It fuses with chorion at about 14 weeks.
- If it does not fuse, it may suggest a higher risk of chromosomal abnormality.

Normal US at 8 weeks of pregnancy is a positive prognostic sign for a normal pregnancy outcome.

Eight weeks ***(Fig. 19)***: Fetal trunk straightens, rhombencephalon becomes evident, limb

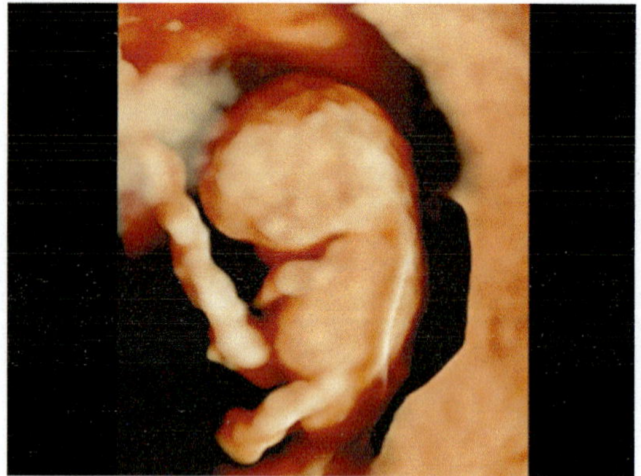

Fig. 20: Ten weeks pregnancy.

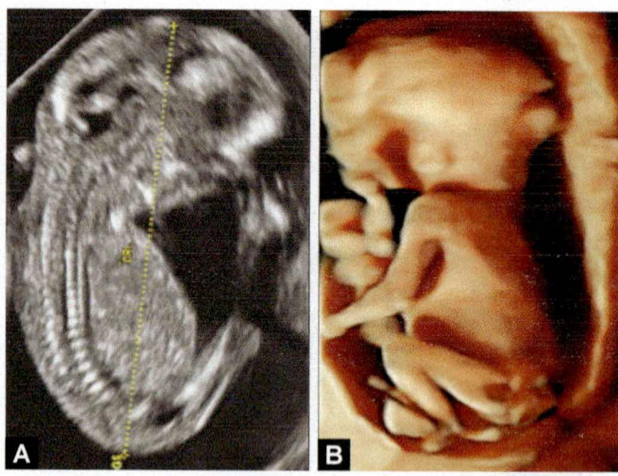

Figs. 21A and B: Twelve weeks pregnancy.

buds appear, and physiological umbilical hernia develops by the end of this week.

Nine weeks: Fetal neck, upper end of spine, and coccyx lower end of spine are clearly seen. Limb buds develop further and elbows and knees are formed. Facial details start appearing. Falx and choroid plexus start showing. Pulsations appear in the umbilical vessels.

*Ten weeks **(Fig. 20)**:* Brain further develops and now three brain vesicles—prosencephalon, mesencephalon, and rhombencephalon are seen. The limb buds start showing fingers and toes. With that, the knees bend and the two feet approach each other in midline. There is further development of the circulatory system and ossification of the spine starts.

Eleven weeks: Spinal column is well seen. Facial details are well developed; abdominal organs, liver, and stomach are seen. Umbilical hernia starts getting smaller and disappears almost completely at 11 weeks and 5 days.

*Twelve weeks **(Figs. 21A and B)**:* Kidneys and urinary bladder are developed. Ears, nose, orbits, lens, lips, and jaws can be seen. Heart is well seen.

Thirteen weeks: Facial features and individual vertebrae in the spine are seen. Diaphragm can be appreciated; heart clearly shows four chambers and umbilical hernia is no more seen.

Beyond 12 weeks, fetus is fully formed and therefore that is the time for nuchal scan. This shall be discussed in **Chapter 19** of this book. But, there are abnormalities that can be suspected or even at times diagnosed earlier in the first trimester.

These include:

- *Acrania **(Fig. 22)***: Acrania is lack of skull bone development. This leads to abnormal head shape as the developing brain tissue is directly exposed to amniotic fluid. This can be diagnosed as early as 9–10 weeks of gestation.
- *Holoprosencephaly **(Fig. 23)***: This is absence of development of falx. It has been discussed earlier that falx can be

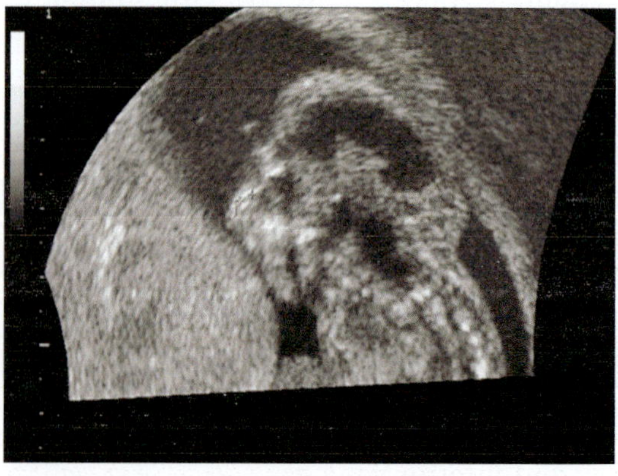

Fig. 22: Acrania.

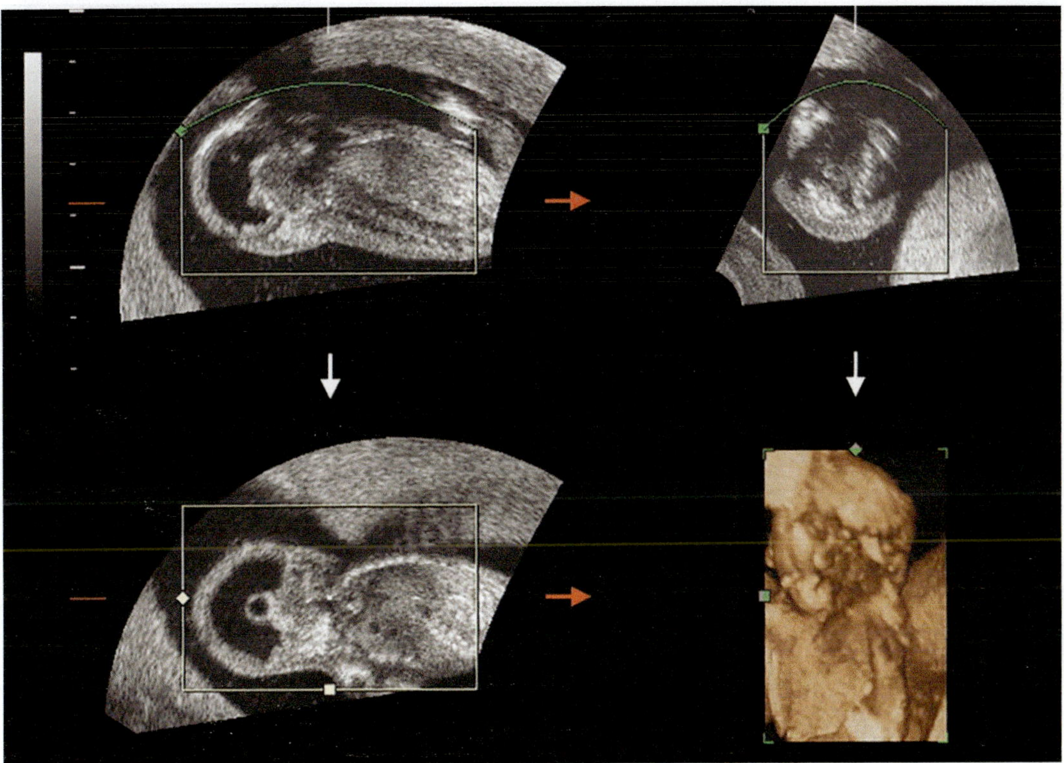

Fig. 23: Holoprosencephaly.

seen at all times after completion of 9th week. If it is not seen beyond 10th week, holoprosencephaly must be suspected.

- *Anencephaly*: A major neural canal defect with complete absence of brain development leads to absence of any tissue above the forehead, due to which the face appears like a frog and the condition is not compatible with life.
- *Major limb abnormalities:* All limb buds appear at 8 weeks and by the end of 10 weeks, all the segments of all four limbs are formed. Complete or partial absence of any of the limbs can be detected at all times after 10 weeks.
- *Situs inversus*: Situs inversus is complete reverse position of all fetal organs: a mirror image, where heart, aorta, and stomach are on right side and liver, gallbladder, and inferior vena cava (IVC) are on left side. As heart and stomach are developed and are evident at 10 weeks, their position can be checked and situs inversus can be diagnosed in first trimester. All situs abnormalities can be diagnosed.
- *Dextrocardia*: Solitary dextrocardia is heart in the right hemithorax. This can be diagnosed in first trimester of pregnancy.
- *Major cardiac abnormalities* ***(Figs. 24A and B)***: By 11 weeks, four-chambered heart is formed and can be seen clearly on transvaginal scan. Major cardiac abnormalities, such as single ventricle, and truncus arteriosus, can be diagnosed on first trimester scans.
- *Major spinal defects*: Ossification centers of the spine are formed at the end of 10 weeks. Major spinal defects, multiple vertebral abnormalities, hemivertebrae, etc. can be diagnosed on first-trimester scans.
- *Chorioangioma* ***(Fig. 25)***: Chorioangioma is an overgrowth, tumor of the chorionic

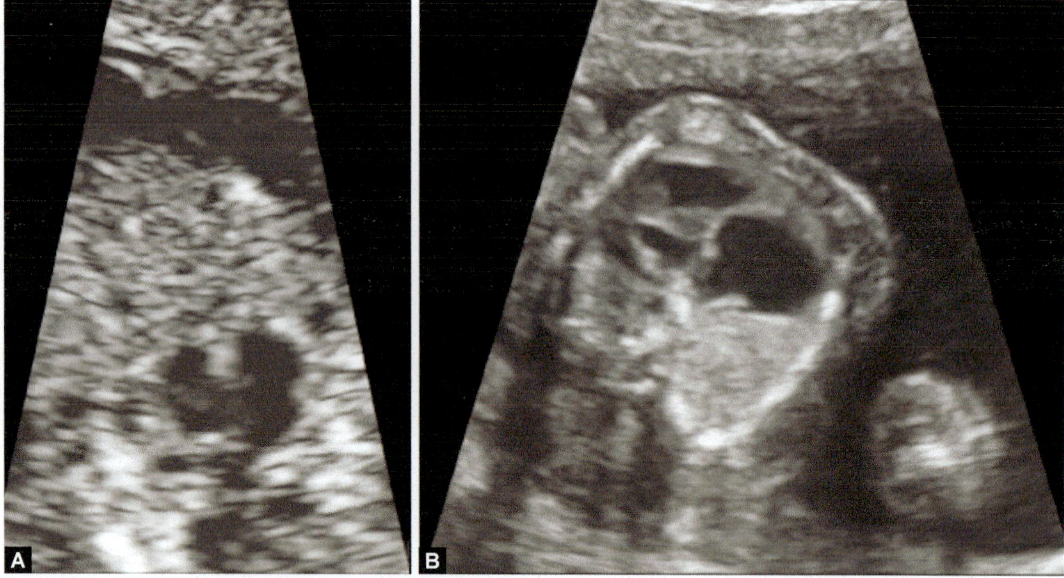

Figs. 24A and B: (A) Major septal defect; (B) Ebstein's anomaly.

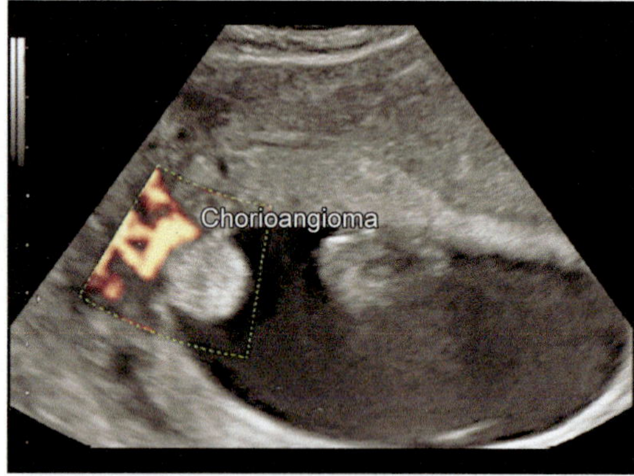

Fig. 25: Chorioangioma.

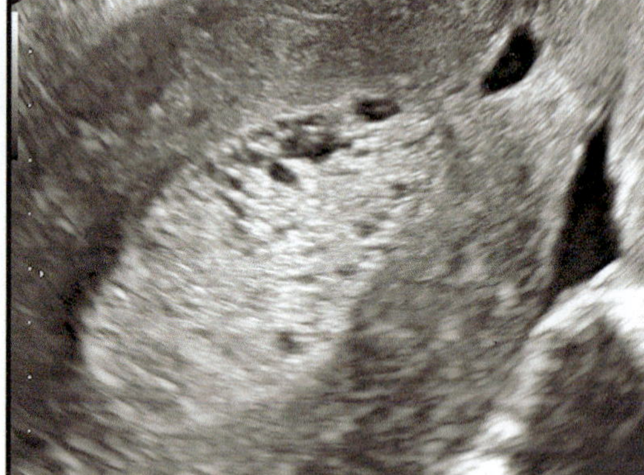

Fig. 26: Vesicular mole.

tissue. Chorioangiomas can be seen very early in pregnancy, 7–8 weeks of pregnancy. Small chorioangiomas do not affect the pregnancy, but larger ones may lead to overload circulatory failures in fetus.

- *Vesicular mole* **(*Fig. 26*)**: This is another chorionic lesion. High β-hCG levels with absent gestational sac with thick echogenic endometrium that has small anechoic areas are diagnostic of vesicular mole. In early phases, vascularity may not be picked up on Doppler studies due to low velocity flow. Only when it becomes invasive, it disrupts the endometriomyometrial junction and then is usually large enough to show abundant low-resistance vascularity.

Umbilical cord cyst is another not so uncommon lesion that can be picked up in first trimester, but is not clinically significant **(Fig. 27)**. Amniotic bands also can be picked up by the end of the first trimester.

Detailed and careful systematic scanning technique can therefore help in early diagnosis

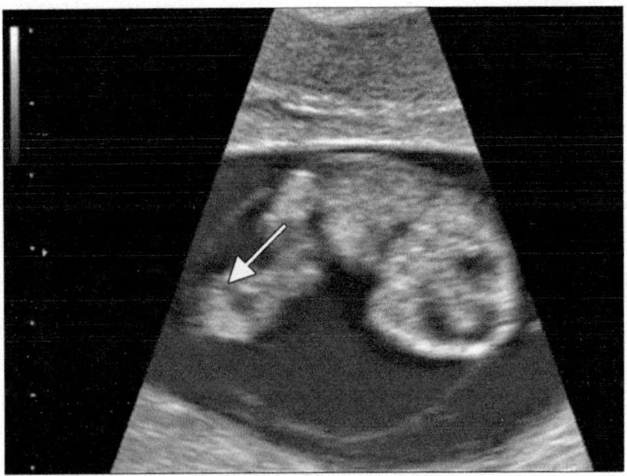

Fig. 27: Umbilical cord cyst (arrow).

of several fetal abnormalities. Volume US is very informative for first-trimester scanning.

REFERENCES

1. Honemeyer U, Kurjak A, Monni G. Normal and abnormal early pregnancy. In: Kurjak A, Chervenak FA (Eds). Donald School Textbook of Ultrasound in Obstetrics and Gynecology, 2nd edition. New Delhi: Jaypee Brothers Medical Publishers (P) Ltd.; 2008. pp. 106-29.
2. Levi CS, Lyons EA, Lindsay DJ. Early diagnosis of nonviable pregnancy with endovaginal US. Radiology. 1988;167:383-5.
3. Nyberg DA, Mack LA, Laing FC, Patten RM. Distinguishing normal from abnormal gestational sac growth in early pregnancy. J Ultrasound Med. 1987;6:23-7.
4. Jeve Y, Rana R, Bhide A, Thangaratinam S. Accuracy of first-trimester ultrasound in the diagnosis of early embryonic demise: a systematic review. Ultrasound Obstet Gynecol. 2011;38(5):489-96.
5. Muttukrishna S, Lygnos M, Groome N, Jauniaux E, Johns J. Maternal serum hormone concentrations for prediction of adverse outcome in threatened miscarriage. Reproductive Biomedicine Online. 2007;15(4):413-21.
6. Kurjak A, Schulman H, Zudenigo D, Kupesic S, Kos M, Goldenberg M. Subchorionic hematomas in early pregnancy: clinical outcome and blood flow patterns. J Matern Fetal Med. 1996;5(1):41-4.

5

CHAPTER

11–14 Weeks Scan

Sonal Panchal, Chaitanya Nagori

INTRODUCTION

As seen in sonoembryology, at 12–13 weeks, the fetus is a fully developed human being and naturally; therefore, if only one scan is to be done in the first trimester to detect abnormalities, it should be done after 10 weeks, preferably 11–12 weeks. The purpose of this scan is to look for structural abnormalities, but more importantly for chromosomal abnormalities and the most feared of the chromosomal abnormalities is trisomy 21 (T21) or Down's syndrome. Though trisomy 13 (T13) and trisomy 18 (T18) are not uncommon, fetuses with these abnormalities either die intrauterine or soon after birth. T21 babies wherein have a nearly normal lifespan, and because of the marked mental retardation that they have as a result of their aneuploidy, they are not capable of independent existence and so they suffer a lot and also are burden on the society. For this reason when we discuss about fetal screening for chromosomal abnormalities, it is chiefly about Down's syndrome, though we shall also discuss the markers for the other two aneuploidies.

It is important here to understand that screening means segregating the high-risk patients from the low-risk patients. Screening does not diagnose an aneuploidy; it only tells as to how much is the risk of a particular fetus being chromosomally abnormal. There are different tests offered for screening. The most primary is the age of the patient.

It has been studied that the risk of chromosomal abnormalities increases as the maternal age advances and is very high when maternal age is more than 35 years. These women are considered high-risk mothers. But, that does not mean that only the fetuses of the mothers of 35 years of age or more are at risk, because as seen on the graph **(Fig. 1)**, only 30% of the babies having Down's syndrome have been born to the mothers of more than 35 years of age. This clearly means that 70% of the Down's babies are born in the low-risk group mothers.

The risk of chromosomal abnormalities is higher in those fetuses whose siblings have chromosomal abnormalities, or mother has a family history of chromosomal abnormalities, or if the fetus has any structural abnormalities, etc. Apart from the history, other screening tests include hematological investigations such as dual marker, triple marker, and quadruple marker. Though triple marker is not commonly used now, a dual marker test consisting of free β-human chorionic gonadotropin (β-hCG) and pregnancy-associated plasma protein-A (PAPP-A) can be done from 10 to 14 weeks. Free β-hCG and PAPP-A increase and decrease with the gestational age, respectively. In order

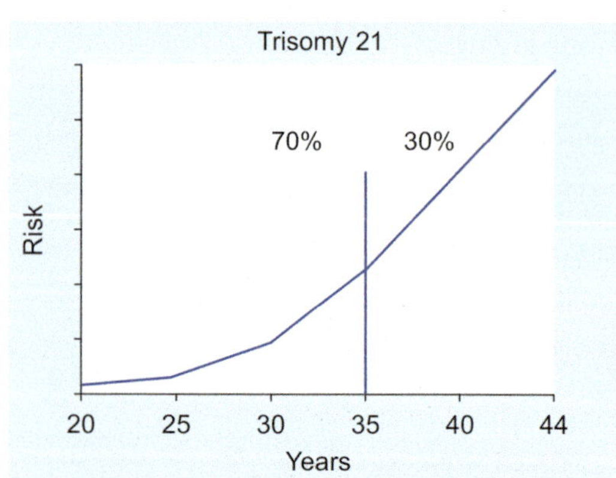

Fig. 1: From Fetal Medicine Foundation, 11–13^{+6} weeks scan.

to standardize and eliminate the variation associated with gestational age, they are converted to multiples of median (MoM). In euploid pregnancies, the average free β-hCG is 1.0 MoM and PAPP-A is 1.0 MoM. In T21 at 12 weeks, the maternal serum concentration of free β-hCG is about twice as high (2 MoMs) and PAPP-A is reduced to about half (0.5 MoM) compared to chromosomally normal pregnancies. In T18 and T13, both the serum markers are reduced. The individual risk is derived by the laboratories using software and this risk is compared to the cut-off risk for final interpretation, follow-up, and management. But, the testing and risk assessment should be done by the laboratories that are conscious for their quality of work.

Quadruple marker includes α-fetoprotein, unconjugated estriol (uE3), free β-hCG, and inhibin A, and is done between 15 and 19 weeks. The detection rate (DR) for quadruple tests is 65–75% respectively, for a false-positive rate (FPR) of 5%.

Ultrasound (US) is also used as an important modality for screening these fetuses. If by screening a particular fetus proves to be at high risk then diagnostic test is done. These include chorion villous biopsy, amniocentesis, etc.

Down's or any other chromosomal abnormalities can be most confidently diagnosed by invasive testing such as amniocentesis and chorion villous biopsy followed by chromosomal study. But, these invasive tests have 1% risk of abortion. Moreover, being invasive can be offered only to the high-risk mothers, which means detecting only 30% of Down's babies, and if this method was preferred, 70% of the Down's babies will be missed on antenatal screening if only age is considered as a factor to screen high-risk patients.[1]

ULTRASOUND AS A SCREENING MODALITY

In early 90s, some subtle anatomical variations were detected in the fetuses with chromosomal abnormalities. Though these subtle variations could be detected in about 2% of normal fetuses, their frequency was very high in fetuses with aneuploidies. These subtle anatomical variations are called markers for aneuploidies. It is important to remember here that markers are subtle variations in the usual features and these are not abnormalities.

Based on this knowledge of markers, a detailed scan was designed that could be best done between 11 and 13^{+6} weeks for detection of aneuploid fetuses and was called a *genetic scan*.

By definition, a genetic sonogram is defined as a US scan that can modify the *a priori* risk of fetal aneuploidy, typically based on a panel of US markers. The background risk, which depends upon the maternal age and gestational age, is referred to as the "a priori risk". To this, the risk (0.75%) of previous chromosomally abnormal fetus is added, if the patient has such a history. Screening is started after that. Depending on the positive or negative likelihood ratio (LR) of present or absent abnormal marker,[2,3] the risk calculation for a particular aneuploidy is done. This scan is done for detection of:

- *Major structural anomalies in aneuploidies:*
  - Compatible with life
  - Incompatible for independent existence
- *Chromosomal markers:*
  - Most indicative or major markers
  - Soft markers.

Structural abnormalities that must be looked for and are detectable on early 11–13^{+6} weeks scan can be listed as follows:

- *Neural tube abnormalities:*
  - Holoprosencephaly
  - Anencephaly and/or acrania
  - Iniencephaly
  - Spina bifida
- *Facial abnormalities:*
  - Cleft palate
  - Ocular abnormalities
  - Micrognathia
  - Short/low-placed ears

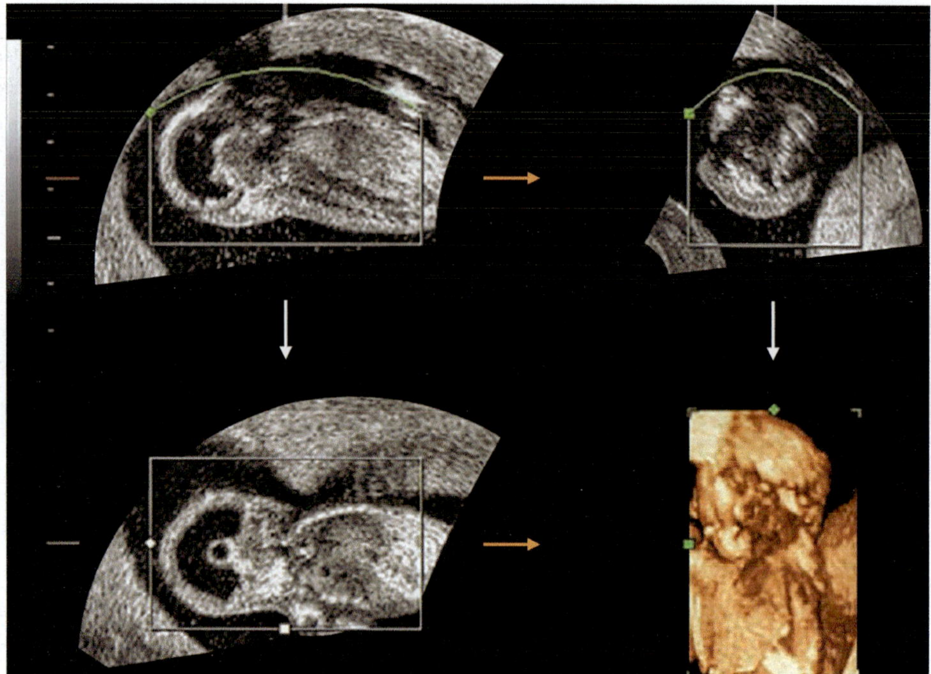

Fig. 2: Holoprosencephaly.

- Cardiovascular abnormalities
- *Abdominal abnormalities:*
  - Diaphragmatic hernia
  - Duodenal atresia
  - Omphalocele
  - Mega cystitis
- Limb reduction abnormalities
- Hydrothorax—ascites.

NEURAL TUBE ANOMALIES

Holoprosencephaly (Fig. 2)

This abnormality is complete or partial deficiency of falx leading to alobar, semilobar, or lobar type of holoprosencephaly. Lobar is the mildest form with defect of the falx only in mid-hemispheric region and often not diagnosed till late pregnancy and also has least neurological implications. Whereas alobar is the most extensive defect leading to severe neurological deficits and can be diagnosed as early as 12–14 weeks of gestational age. This shows single spherical cerebral structure, with single common ventricle, posterior large cyst of third ventricle known as dorsal sac, absent olfactory bulbs, and tracts and single optic nerve. Septum pellucidum is always absent with midline fusion of cingulated gyrus and frontal horns of lateral ventricles. These have flat roof and freely communicate with third ventricle.

About 40–60% of the holoprosencephalic fetuses have chromosomal abnormalities, of which 50% are T13. Of those which are euploids, 90% have facial abnormalities. The commonly seen abnormalities include cyclopia, hypotelorism, proboscis, and median cleft lip.[4,5] About 70% have other structural abnormalities.[6] Alobar and semilobar holoprosencephaly are more likely to be associated with aneuploidies, rather than the lobar ones.

Acrania/Exencephaly and Anencephaly (Figs. 3A and B)

Acrania is total nonossification of skull vault bones and exencephaly is partial (above the orbits) nonossification of skull vault bones. Acrania may evolve from exencephaly.

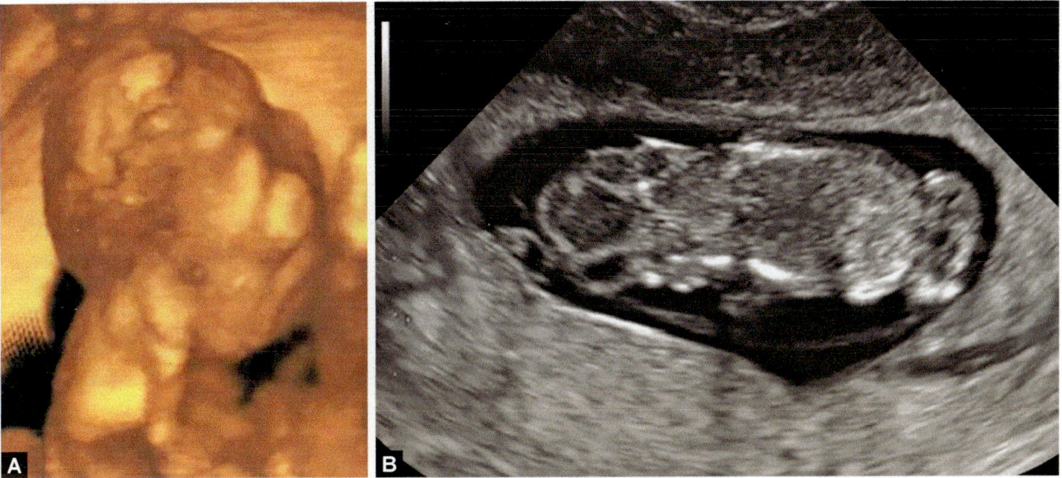

Figs. 3A and B: Exencephaly and acrania.

Ossification of the skull bones starts and accelerates at 9 weeks of gestation. Acrania can, therefore, be diagnosed after 10–11 weeks. In acrania, brain matter lies free in the amniotic cavity and shows abnormal shape of the head due to disintegration of brain matter. Typical shape of the head is described as Mickey Mouse head when majority of the brain matter is disintegrated.

Smaller defects in skull vault with herniation of the meninges or brain matter is described as cephaloceles **(Fig. 4)**.

Anencephaly is a neural tube defect. Total disintegration of brain matter and appearance is described as frog face as the orbits become the most protruding structures. There is no forehead or calvarium **(Fig. 5)**.

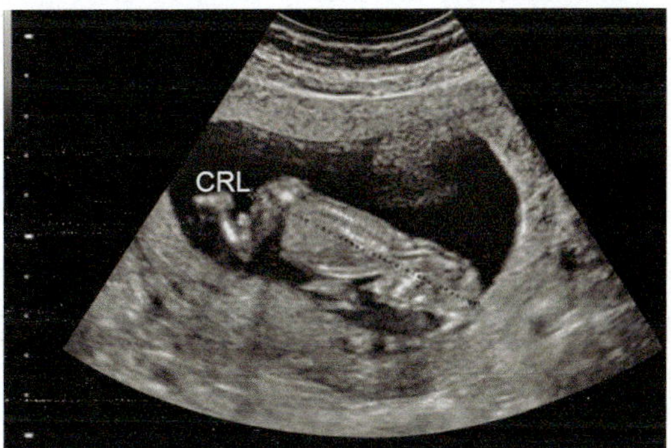

Fig. 5: Acrania.
(CRL: crown rump length)

Iniencephaly (Fig. 6)

This is a lethal anomaly with defect in occiput involving foramen magnum, a complete spina bifida, retroflexion of entire spine—stargazing

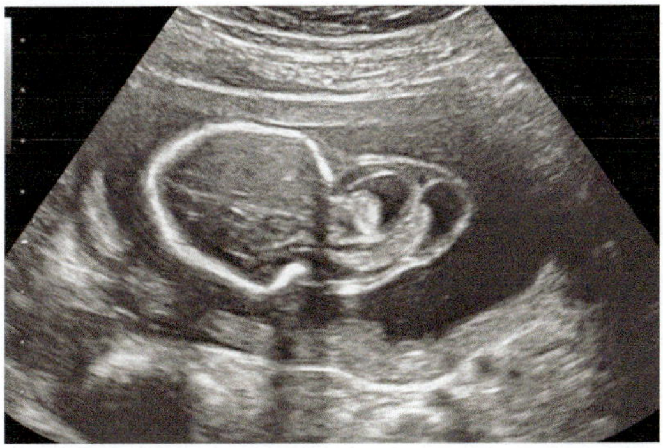

Fig. 4: Encephalocele.

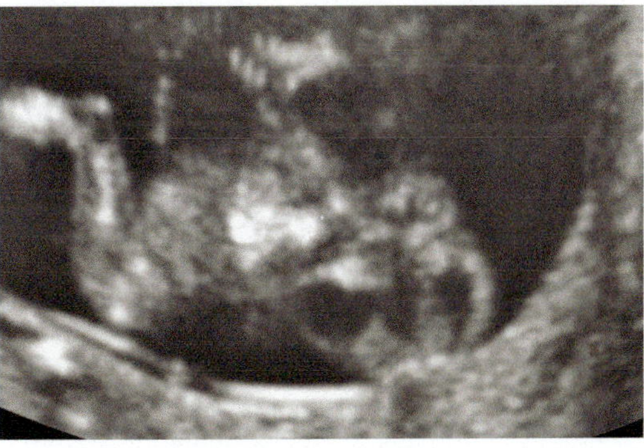

Fig. 6: Iniencephaly.

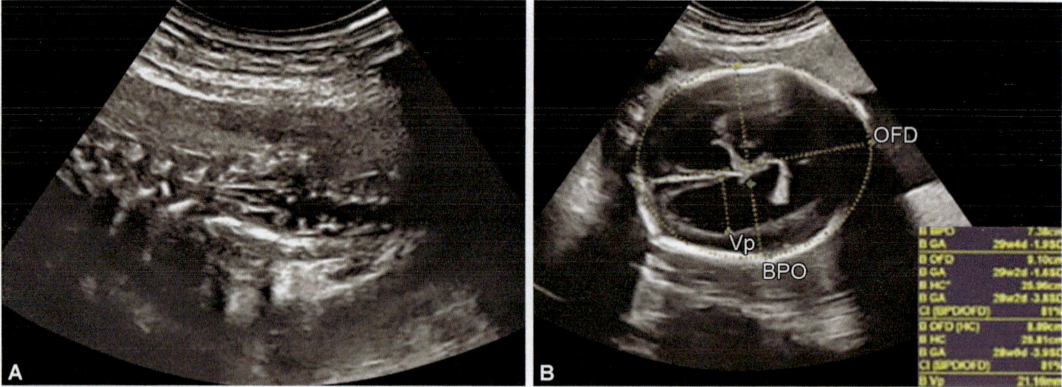

Figs. 7A and B: Spina bifida with hydrocephalus.

fetus, and open spinal canal defects of variable degrees. Associated abnormalities such as hydrocephaly, microcephaly, ventricular atresia, and holoprosencephaly are also known. It may also be associated with diaphragmatic hernia, urinary tract abnormalities, cleft lip and palate, omphalocele, and thoracic cage abnormalities with polyhydramnios; though these associated abnormalities may be more evident only in second trimester.

Spina Bifida and Hydrocephalus (Figs. 7A and B)

The most common abnormality of spine, detectable in first trimester, is open spinal canal defects or spine bifida. About 14% fetuses with spina bifida have aneuploidy, most commonly trisomies 18, 13, triploidy, and translocation.[7] Hydrocephalus is a common association and consequence. About 22% of the fetuses with chromosomal anomalies may present only with spina bifida and hydrocephalus in first trimester.

The earliest sign for open spinal canal defects is measuring intracranial translucency (IT). This requires the same section as that for nuchal translucency (NT) and, therefore, we shall discuss it later in this chapter.

FACIAL ANOMALIES

The midline facial anomalies especially with holoprosencephaly are commonly associated with trisomies 18 and 13 and so, whenever found, detailed study for chromosomal abnormalities is mandatory. Facial abnormalities are best diagnosed by volume US, rendered imaging as coronal view of the face is required, which is more easily obtainable on three-dimensional (3D) US.

Cleft Lip and Palate

Lip becomes continuous at 8 weeks and, therefore, a cleft can be diagnosed at 11–14 weeks scan. On nuchal scan, on the coronal plane of the face, prenasal triangle is seen, on a plane just anterior to the coronal section of orbits. This triangle is formed of two tiny nasal bones (NBs) at the apex, sides formed by frontal process of maxillary bone, and base formed by maxillary plate. Incomplete base on this plane indicates cleft palate. The imaging plane for this is considered correct when the two echogenic dots of ossification centers of mandibular bone are placed within the width of the base of this triangle **(Fig. 8A)**.

The chances of aneuploidy with cleft palate are:

- 20–30%, if unilateral cleft palate (more common on left side and in females)
- 30–50%, if bilateral cleft palate
- 50–80%, if median cleft palate.

Isolated cleft lip without a cleft palate is not commonly associated with aneuploidies.[8] Three-dimensional ultrasound is an impressive

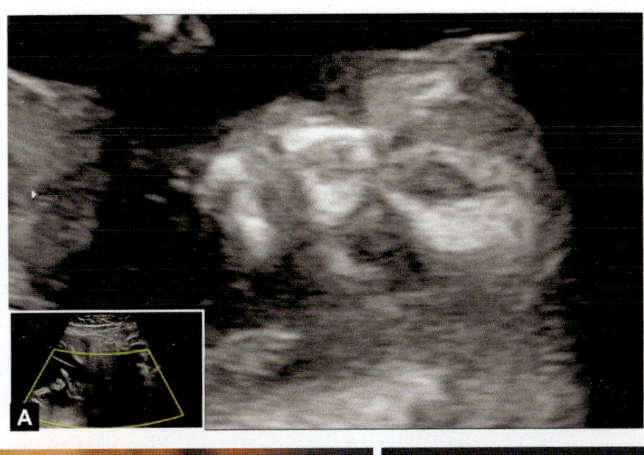

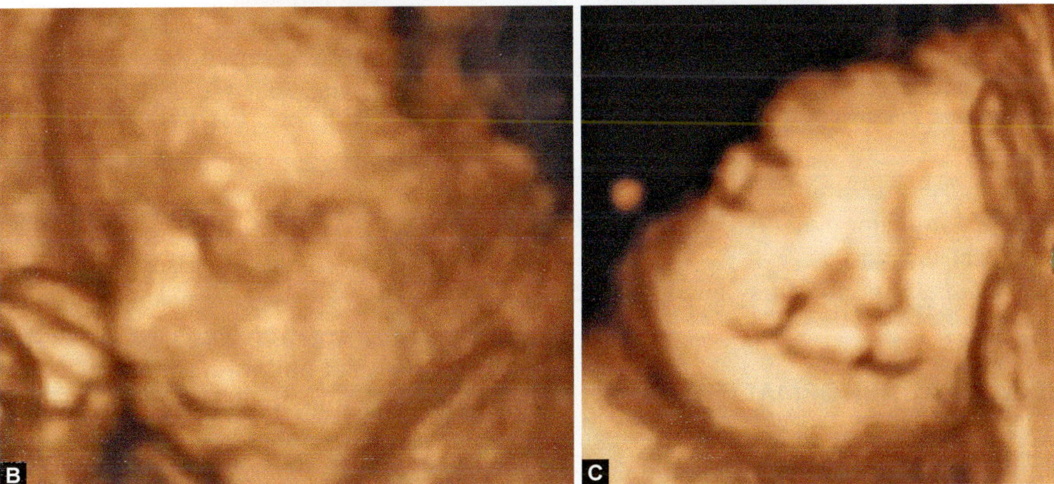

Figs. 8A to C: (A) B mode ultrasound image of the coronal section of the face showing retronasal triangle; (B and C) Cleft lip and cleft palate on three-dimensional ultrasound.

modality to demonstrate this abnormality **(Figs. 8B and C)**.

OCULAR ABNORMALITIES

Cyclopia (single orbit in the center), hypotelorism (closely placed orbits), or hypertelorism (widely placed orbits) is associated with trisomies 13, 18, 21 and nonchromosomal syndromes. These are best demonstrated on coronal or transverse plane of the face.

Micrognathia (receding small chin) may be an indicator of T18 or triploidy **(Fig. 9)**. This is best seen on the midsagittal plane, which is same as the plane for NT. It indicates a small mandible and the chin and the lower lip appear small and displaced posteriorly.

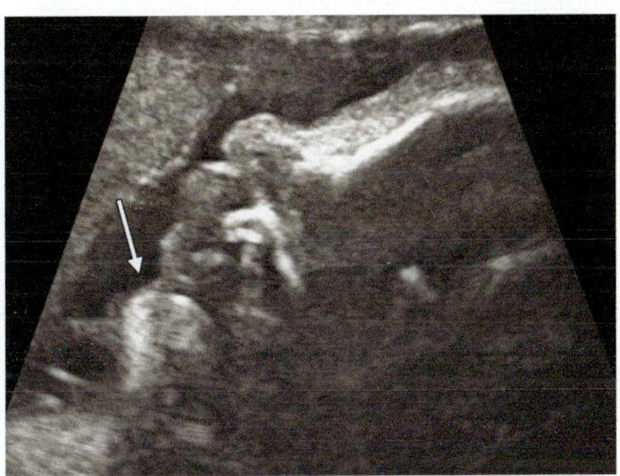

Fig. 9: Micrognathia.

Short low-placed ears **(Fig. 10)** are typically associated with trisomies 21, 18, and 13 and have similar value as increased NT in detection of fetal aneuploidies. But, these are not easy

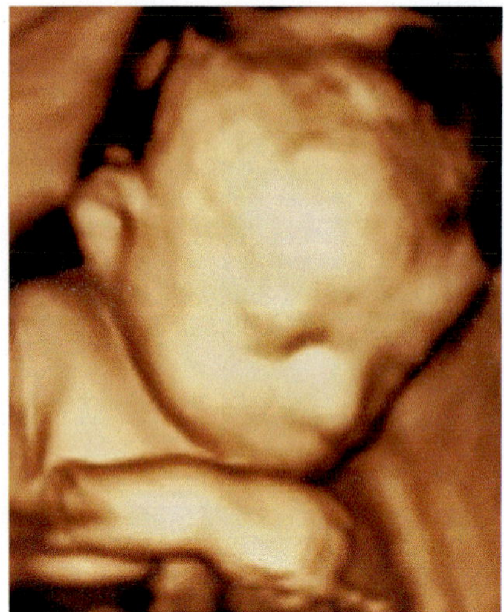

Fig. 10: Low-placed ear.

to diagnose on B-mode US and so are not included in major markers. Though volume US can be diagnostic.

Prominent occiput may be seen in T18 fetuses.

CARDIAC ABNORMALITIES

About 22–32% of fetuses with cardiac anomalies have chromosomal anomalies.[9] Only 0.1% of euploid neonates have cardiac abnormalities but 13% of the aneuploid neonates have cardiac abnormalities.

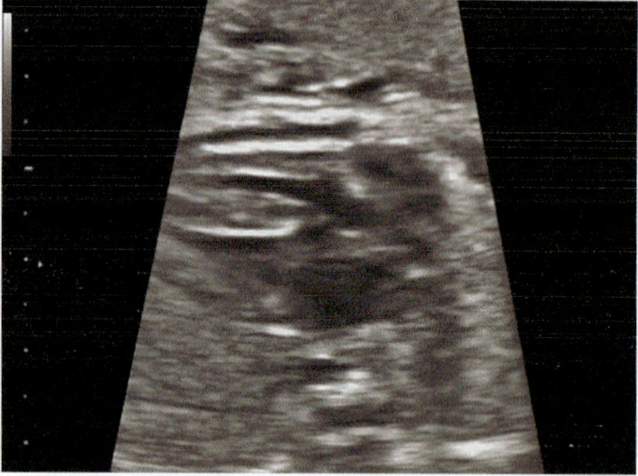

Fig. 12: Fallot's tetralogy.

Atrioventricular septal defects (AVSDs) **(Fig. 11A)**, ventricular septal defect (VSD), Ebstein's anomaly **(Fig. 11B)**, Fallot's tetralogy **(Fig. 12)**, and hypoplastic left heart are often associated with aneuploidies.[10] Ectopia cordis, only when associated with pentalogy of Cantrell, is associated with trisomies.

(Pentalogy of Cantrell has a panorama of abnormalities, which consist of median supraumbilical abdominal defect, defect in lower sternum, defect of diaphragmatic pericardium, defect of anterior diaphragm, and intracardiac abnormality.)

Isomerism, transposition of great arteries, pulmonary atresia, and stenosis are never associated with aneuploidies.

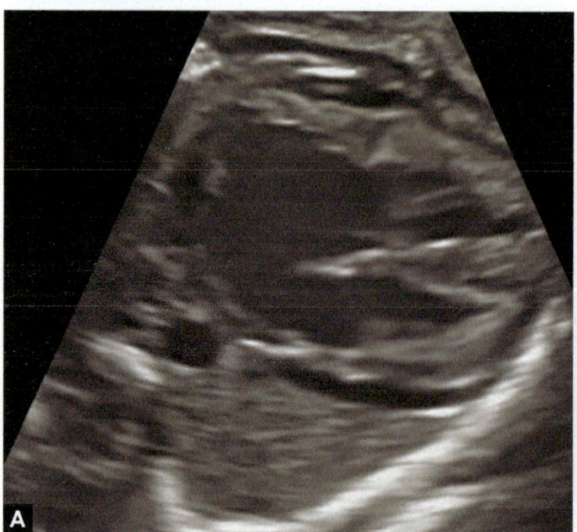

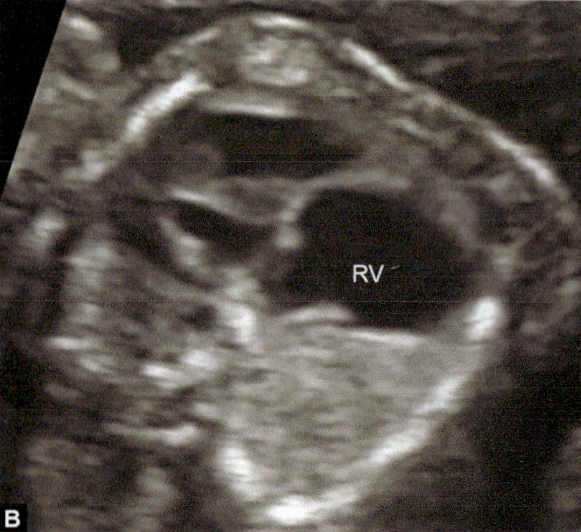

Figs. 11A and B: (A) Complete atrioventricular septal defect; (B) Ebstein's anomaly. (RV: right ventricle)

The incidence of cardiac abnormalities in fetuses with chromosomal abnormalities is:

- 90% in T13
- 40–50% in T21
- 15–20% in Turner's syndrome.

Detailed echocardiography is out of the scope of this chapter. But, it is still essential to emphasize at this point that with advancing technology of US, it is now possible to study fetal heart transvaginally in late first trimester in detail.

ABDOMINAL ABNORMALITIES

Diaphragmatic Hernia (Fig. 13A)

About 10–20% of fetuses with diaphragmatic hernias have chromosomal anomalies, the most common being T18, but are more significant when associated with other abnormalities, especially increased NT. Diaphragmatic hernia is diagnosed on US by assessing the transverse section of the thorax at the level of four-chamber heart. Heart is displaced to right side and stomach shadow or bowel shadows are seen at the same level as the four-chamber heart. Stomach shadow may not be seen in the abdomen. Though liver herniation in the thorax is rare, if present, it displaces the heart to extreme left side. In cases of diaphragmatic hernia, prognosis depends on the resultant pulmonary hypoplasia.

Duodenal Atresia (Fig. 13B)

One-third of the fetuses with duodenal atresia have T21.[11] Typical sign described to diagnose duodenal atresia is "double-bubble sign", where one bubble is the distended stomach and the other one is the distended duodenal cap. But, duodenal atresia is very difficult to diagnose before 20–24 weeks. Karyotyping is a must when duodenal atresia is diagnosed.

Omphalocele (Fig. 14)

It is physiologically present from 8th to 12th weeks of gestation but is considered abnormal, if it persists after 12th week of gestation. It increases the risk of T18. Even before 12th week, an omphalocele may be considered abnormal, if:

- Has a neck of more than 7 mm
- It is larger than or of the size of the abdomen
- There is herniation of the liver.

An omphalocele may contain bowel or liver, but those containing liver are usually not associated with aneuploidies.[12] The bowel containing omphalocele is commonly associated with syndromes and 50% of bowel

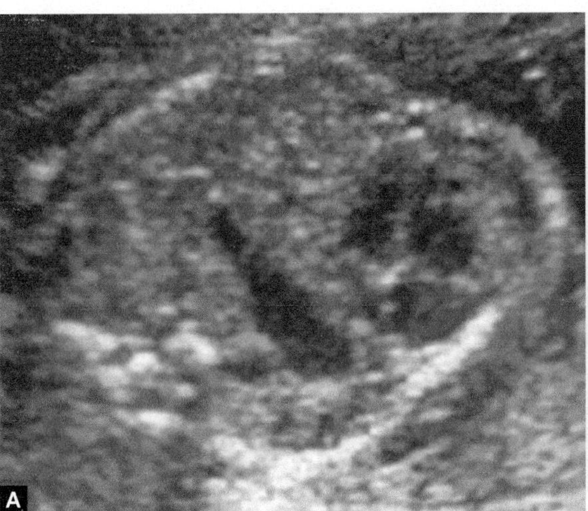

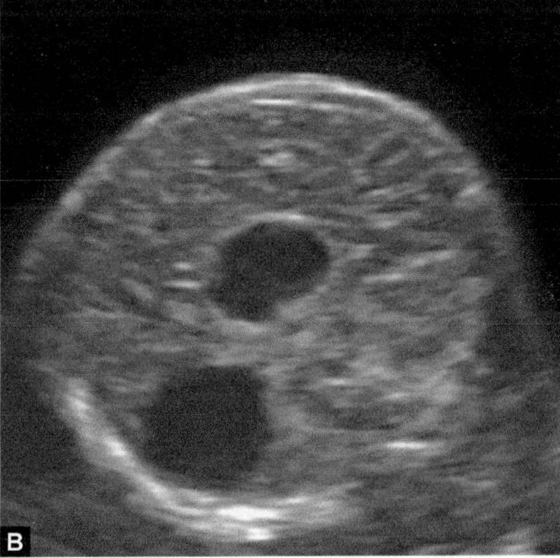

Figs. 13A and B: (A) Diaphragmatic hernia; (B) Double bubble sign—duodenal atresia.

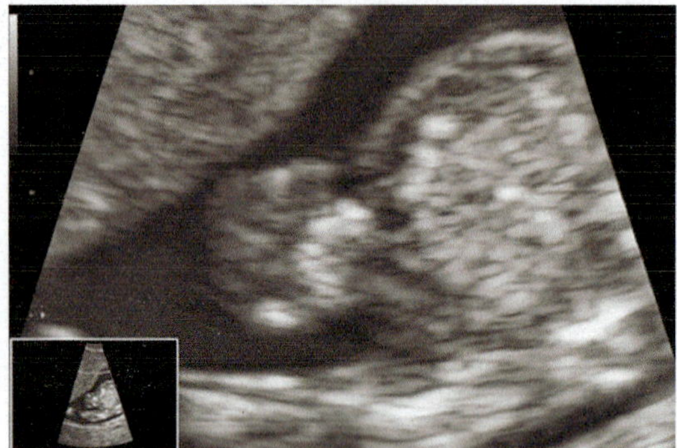

Fig. 14: Omphalocele—three-dimensional and two-dimensional ultrasound.

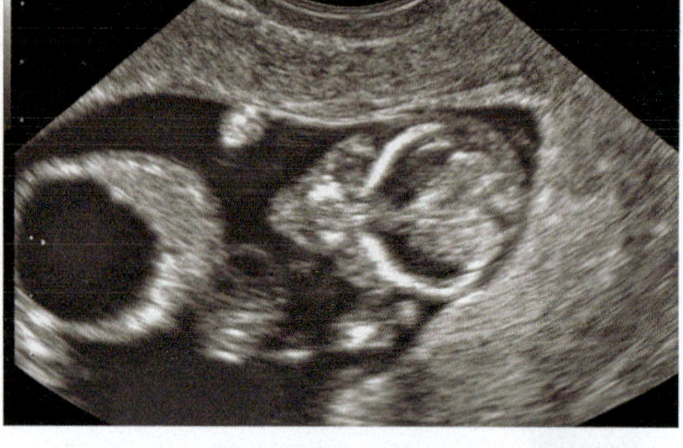

Fig. 16: Megacystis.

containing omphaloceles are associated with cardiac anomalies also.

When it contains bowel, it appears more echogenic than abdomen, which contains liver, and when it contains liver, abdomen is more echogenic, which contains bowel.

About 40–60% of the fetuses with omphalocele have chromosomal anomalies and are 10 times more common in fetuses with increased NT. Others are likely to have nonchromosomal syndromes such as Turner's syndrome or uniparental disomies.

Gastroschisis (Fig. 15)

This is another anterior abdominal wall defect. This defect is usually to the right of the umbilicus with evisceration of abdominal organs. Gastroschisis can be diagnosed as early as 12 weeks of gestation. This condition is not often associated with chromosomal abnormalities, but is associated with other structural abnormalities such as exstrophy of bladder, intrauterine growth restriction (IUGR), and malrotation of gut.

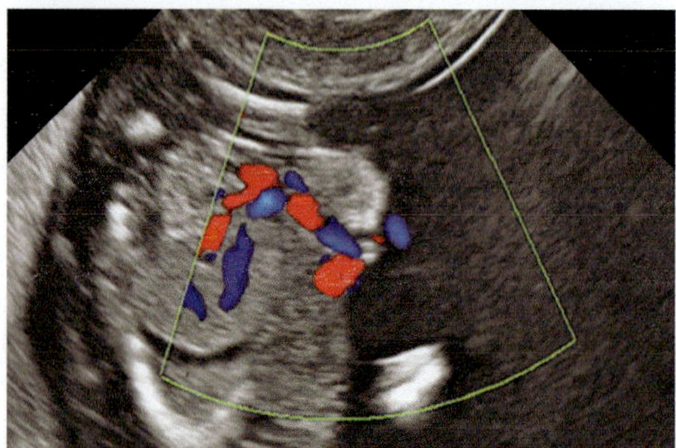

Fig. 15: Gastroschisis—cord insertion is seen by the side of the anterior abdominal wall defect.

Genitourinary Anomalies

The most common ones associated with chromosomal abnormalities are bladder outlet obstruction and megacystis **(Fig. 16)** and are most commonly associated with trisomies 18 and 13.[13] More proximal genitourinary tract malformations are less associated with chromosomal abnormalities, and the risk is still lower with unilateral affections. Moreover, these are less likely to be diagnosed in the first trimester.

Fetal kidneys are consistently seen after 11 weeks of gestation normally. Their absence may indicate agenesis, which may be confirmed by absence of renal vessels also (unilateral or bilateral) on Doppler examination. Kidneys are hyperechoic oval structures at 12 weeks. Dysplastic kidneys though may appear large with cystic lesions. Renal pyelectasis has been discussed with chromosomal markers.

SKELETAL ABNORMALITIES

Limb reduction deformities and radial aplasia indicate a risk of T18. Isolated clubfoot is not commonly associated with chromosomal abnormality, especially in an otherwise low-

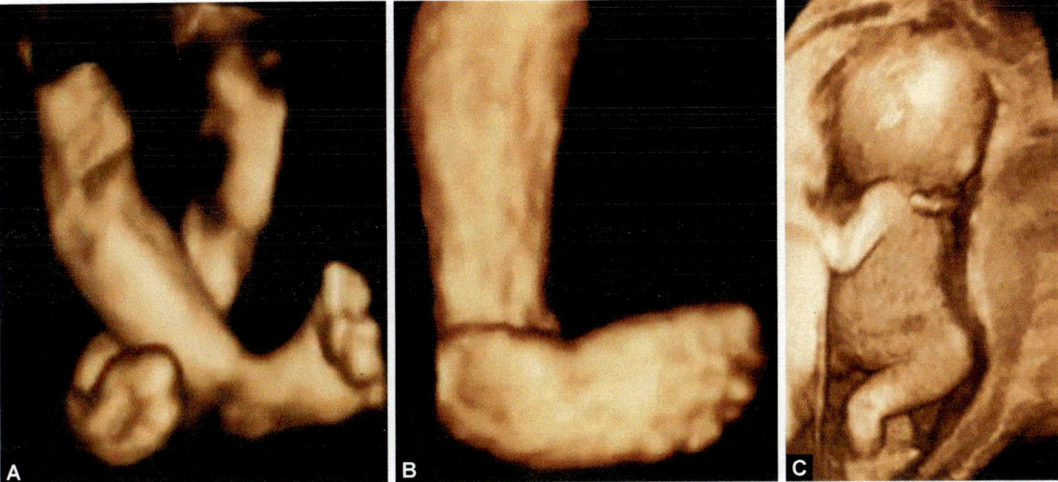

Figs. 17A to C: (A and B) Clubfeet; (C) Achondroplasia.

risk patient. But, there is a consensus that whenever a clubfoot **(Figs. 17A to C)** is seen, a fetal karyotyping must be done because there is a possibility of presence of many other subtle abnormalities, which are very likely to be missed on first trimester scan, if a very careful detailed search is not done.

Hand makes an important landmark for chromosomal abnormalities. Clinodactyly is seen in T21, clenched hands in T18, polydactyly in T13, and syndactyly in triploidy.

Generalized skeletal dysplasias such as achondroplasia **(Fig. 17C)** and achondrogenesis can be diagnosed on late first trimester scan by disproportionately short long bones. It is easy to note that this disproportion in the first trimester as the whole fetus can be seen in a single frame. Osteogenesis imperfecta is diagnosed by nonossified bones. This may be seen as less echogenic bones of skull and limbs.

Sirenomelia (fusion of lower limbs), if present, can be diagnosed as early as 10–11 weeks and is commonly associated with other abdominal structural abnormalities and single large umbilical artery.

MISCELLANEOUS ABNORMALITIES

Ascites and hydrothorax suggest possibility of aneuploidy or infection, especially when present without hydrops.

As such, any abnormalities in the fetus should lead the sonographer toward the search for the chromosomal anomalies, except the acquired disorders, which are a result of tissue or vascular disruption, e.g., tumors, hydranencephaly, amniotic band syndrome, limb body wall complex, jejunal atresia due to vascular insufficiency, and gastroschisis and complex anomalies such as cardiosplenic syndrome. The identification of a major anomaly obviates the need for further screening tests and calls for diagnostic invasive test because:

- If the abnormalities are lethal or associated with severe handicap, invasive testing and fetal karyotyping may determine the possible cause and predict the risk of recurrence in future pregnancy.
- If pregnancy is to be continued in case of a potentially correctable defect, it is essential to exclude chromosomal defect.

CHROMOSOMAL MARKERS

Markers, as already been discussed, are not structural abnormalities but are subtle variations in the normal anatomy that indicate the presence of chromosomal abnormalities. If sonographic markers for fetal anomalies are taken into consideration with other sonographic findings, 50–70% of T21, 80% of

T18, and 90% of T13, fetuses will show positive genetic sonogram.

These markers are divided into major and soft markers depending on their sensitivity for the diagnosis of aneuploidies.

Major or most indicative markers are:

- Nuchal translucency—cystic hygroma
- Ductus venosus flow
- Nasal bone length.

Nuchal Translucency

Nuchal translucency refers to the sonographic appearance of subcutaneous accumulation of fluid behind the fetal neck in the first trimester. Normally, NT is 1.5–2.5 cm between 10 and 12 weeks and 2–3 mm between 12 and 14 weeks. NT increases by 17% every week. It must be remembered that there is no cut-off value for NT. It has definite values for definite gestational age, so ideally the calculated values must be placed on the nomograms for correct risk assessments. Though any value above 3 mm surely requires counseling, these nomograms are based on the NT values in relation to crown-rump length (CRL). Therefore, correct assessment of CRL is essential. CRL is measured in midsagittal plane of the fetus, when the fetal trunk and neck are neither extended nor flexed. In the correct plane, the proximal long bones (femur and humerus) are never seen. Both crown and the rump must be clearly seen and the straight distance from crown to rump is measured **(Fig. 18)**. The prevalence of defects increases from 0.8 to 65.8 per thousand, as the NT increases from below 95th percentile to above 99th percentile **(Fig. 19)**.

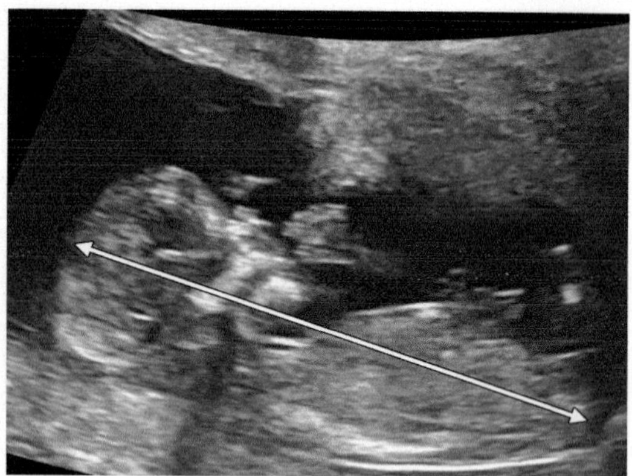

Fig. 18: Measurement of crown-rump length.

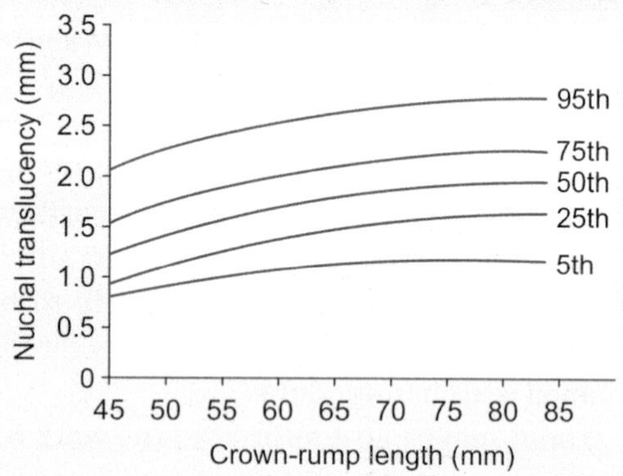

Fig. 19: Chart of 95th, 75th, 50th, 25th, and 5th centile values of nuchal translucency varying with crown-rump length (CRL).

Measuring Nuchal Translucency (The Fetal Medicine Foundation) (Fig. 20A)[14]

Nuchal translucency can be measured accurately by transabdominal route in 95% of cases; while in others, transvaginal ultrasonography would be required.

- When CRL is between 45 and 84 mm, preferably 45–84 cm
- In true sagittal section, in which:
  - Echogenic tip of the nose
  - Nasal bone
  - Rectangular shape of palate anteriorly
  - No bone is seen between NB and palate (zygoma)
  - Fluid in third ventricle between thalami
  - Diencephalon is seen
  - Aqueduct of Sylvius in-between cerebral peduncles
  - Mandible is seen as a point.
- With maximum magnification—75% of the screen should be covered by head and upper chest (caliper 0.1 mm).
- Neutral position—neither extension, nor flexion of the head, because NT increases by 0.6 mm on extension and reduces up to 0.4 mm on flexion of the fetal neck. Cord

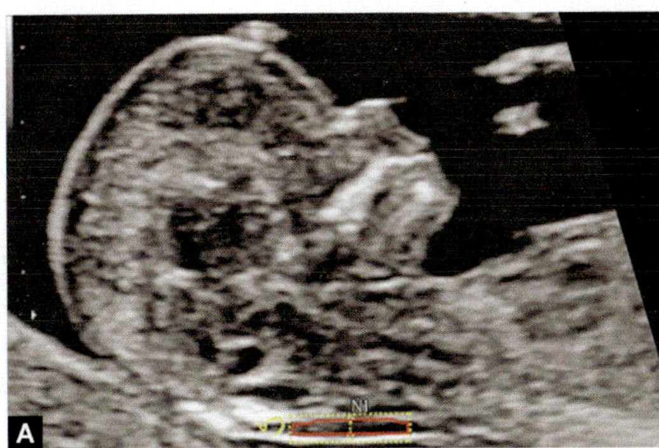

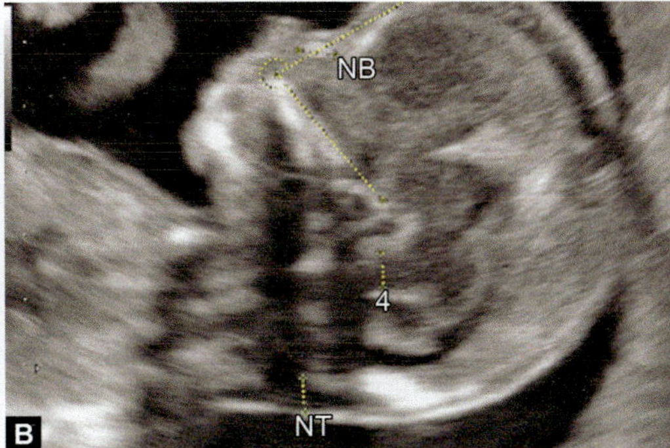

Figs. 20A and B: Measuring nuchal translucency (NT).
(NB: nasal bone)

round neck leads to false increase in NT up to 0.8 mm measurements above and below the cord depending on how tight is the loop tied.

- Maximum width of the translucency between the skin and soft tissues posterior to the cervical spine
- The calipers should be placed on the interface between the tissue (white line) and nuchal fluid that describes the NT—the horizontal line of the crossbar of the caliper should merge with the white line of the margin and not seen in the nuchal fluid.
- It is important to take more than one measurement and record the maximum one **(Fig. 20B)**.
- Care must be taken to distinguish between fetal skin and amnion.

When NT is measured in this way, the interobserver and intraobserver errors are only of <0.5%. Accurate measurement of NT requires adequate training, expertise, and adherence to the standard protocols laid by the Fetal Medicine Foundation (FMF), UK. The individual measuring NT should be ideally certified by FMF and his/her performance should be regularly audited.

About 75–80% of the fetuses with trisomy 21 and 5–10% of euploid fetuses may show increased NT. But, even in euploid fetuses with increased NT, prevalence of major defects was 7.3%. NT may be increased due to several causes apart from aneuploidies.

Causes of Increased Nuchal Translucency

- *Chromosomal anomalies*: Altered extracellular matrix composition is seen in chromosomal abnormalities as the component proteins of extracellular matrix are encoded on chromosomes 21, 18, and 13. The diagnosis can be guided by a few associated features and dual marker tests.
- *Trisomy 18:* Early intrauterine growth restriction (IUGR), relative bradycardia, and omphalocele (both free β-hCG and PAPP-A are low)
- *Trisomy 13:* IUGR, relative tachycardia, omphalocele, and holoprosencephaly
- *Turner's syndrome:* Early IUGR and tachycardia
- *Triploidy:* Asymmetrical IUGR, bradycardia, holoprosencephaly, omphalocele, posterior fossa cyst, and molar changes in placenta.

It has also been found in other genetic syndromes such as achondrogenesis type II due to altered collagen metabolism in achondroplasia and thanatophoric dysplasia due to abnormal fibroblast growth factor receptors and in Zellweger's syndrome due to disturbed metabolism of peroxisome biogenesis factor.

- *Cardiac abnormalities and overload in T-T transfusion*: The prevalence of the cardiac defects was increased from <3% at NT of <3 mm at 14 weeks, to 15% if it was >5.4 mm.[15]

- *Venous congestion* due to fetal constriction due to amniotic rupture or superior mediastinal compression due to diaphragmatic hernia or narrow chest due to skeletal dysplasias.
- *Delayed development of lymphatic drainage*: Neuromuscular defects such as fetal akinesia sequence leading to impaired lymphatic drainage.
- *Congenital infection* causing fetal anemia and cardiac dysfunction.
- *Anemia and hypoproteinemia*: Increased NT may resolve at and after 16 weeks. Moreover, the subcutaneous fat deposition starts after 16 weeks and then the significance of NT decreases. What we measure after 16 weeks is Nuchal fold thickness and not NT. It is very important to remember here that spontaneous resolution of increased NT does not exclude chromosomal defects. A normal karyotype in the fetuses with increased NT also does not exclude structural abnormalities, especially cardiac abnormalities and abnormalities of abdomen.

Significance

- Nuchal translucency only picks up Down's syndrome in 85% of high-risk patients and in 75% of low-risk patients.
- Maternal age + NT + NB + serum parameters 97% sensitivity with 5% false negative (FMF, London 2004)

The Fetal Medicine Foundation Multicenter Project Report

Assessment of risk by combination of maternal age and NT followed by invasive diagnostic testing for 5% of pregnancies with screen positive result and selective termination of affected fetuses would reduce the live birth incidence of T21 by 75%.[16]

Nuchal translucency scan with dual marker test for risk assessment can be done according to following two schedules depending on the convenience of the doctor and the patient:

1. Both the NT measurement and the biochemical markers can be analyzed at the same time at 12 weeks. This option is employed in United Kingdom at OSCAR (One-Stop Clinic for Assessment of Risk) clinics, where the results of the combined screen are available in 30 minutes. The DR is 85–90% for a FPR of 5%.
2. Serum biochemical analytes are measured at 10 weeks and NT is done at 12 weeks in two separate visits. It has been estimated that this approach would improve the DR to 93–94%. But, the disadvantage will be an increase in the noncompliance rate that is associated with this method. In twin babies with twin-to-twin transfusion, NT is frequently increased.

In recipient fetus, it is a manifestation of heart failure due to hypervolemic congestion. As the gestation advances, there would be diuresis, which will correct the hypervolemia, decrease the heart strain, and resolve the NT.

Limitations

- If normal NT is considered as the sign for a normal embryo, chances are there to miss a significant percentage of abnormal babies, so detailed structural scan is always a must.
- Increased NT, as a single sign, may be rarely seen in a normal baby also.

Nuchal Fold Thickness (Fig. 21)

Nuchal fold thickness is measured as the total soft tissue thickness behind the cervical spine. It is measured in axial plane on transcerebellar section. It is to be measured only between 15 and 20 weeks when the skin thickness is constant. It is normally ≤5 mm, though if plotted on graphs as MoM, it has specific LRs at a particular thickness and particular gestational age. It is found to be increased in 0.1% of normal but 80% of Down's fetuses, and is also seen in fetuses with Noonan's syndrome and cardiac abnormalities. Like NT, this also

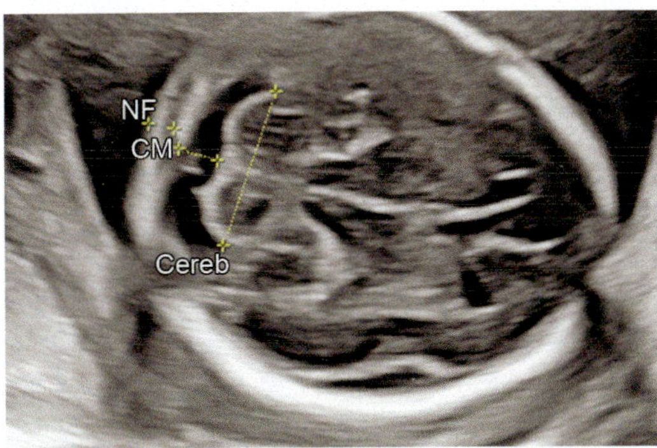

Fig. 21: Nuchal thickness.
(Cereb: cerebellum; CM: cerebral matastases; NF: nuchal fold)

may be a transient sign or may be present after resolution of cystic hygroma, but that does not decrease the risk of aneuploidy and must be considered as important as NT for the suspicion of aneuploidy or cardiac defect.

Cystic Hygroma (Figs. 22A and B)

It is grossly increased nuchal edema, which extends beyond neck to involve the back and the head also. Cystic hygroma may or may not be septated. Nonseptated nuchal edema increases the risk of cardiac defects or trisomies, whereas septated cystic hygroma is almost invariably associated with Turner's syndrome.

Cystic hygroma is the one isolated abnormality, where invasive testing is a must because 47–73% of fetuses with cystic hygroma have cytogenetic anomalies and one-third fetuses have nonimmune hydrops. But isolated cystic hygromas in atypical location are not notably associated with chromosomal abnormality.

In 37% of fetuses, cystic hygroma will resolve in second trimester. If it progresses to lymphangiectasis or persists in second trimester, chances of Turner's syndrome are more and it may be fatal.

Milder cases of cystic hygroma have better prognosis. Surgical correction after birth is possible. But even after surgery for correction of cystic hygroma, bony abnormalities of mandible, occipital bone, and vertebrae and facial palsy may persist. Counseling for cystic hygroma therefore should be done very carefully.

Ductus Venosus Flow

Ductus venosus is a vessel that connects the umbilical vein to the right atrium of the fetal heart. It has no anatomical continuity with the umbilical vein but connects portal sinus to the umbilical sinus. It is only 2 mm in diameter at its inlet into the umbilical sinus but carries 56% of the total fetal oxygenated blood. Ductus venosus flow velocity is approximately three times higher than the flow velocity in the umbilical vein or inferior vena cava. This vessel can be visualized in midsagittal longitudinal

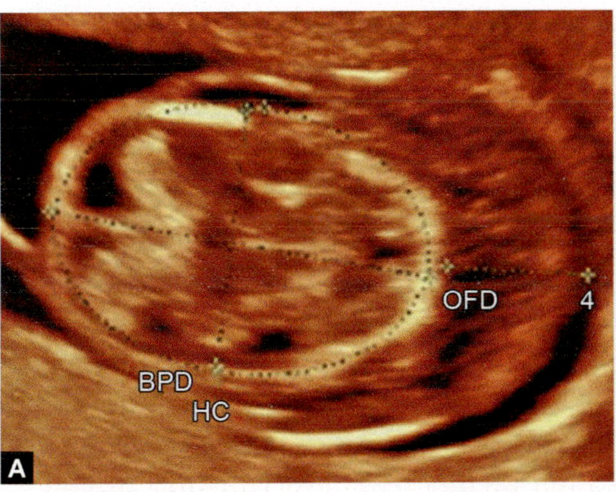

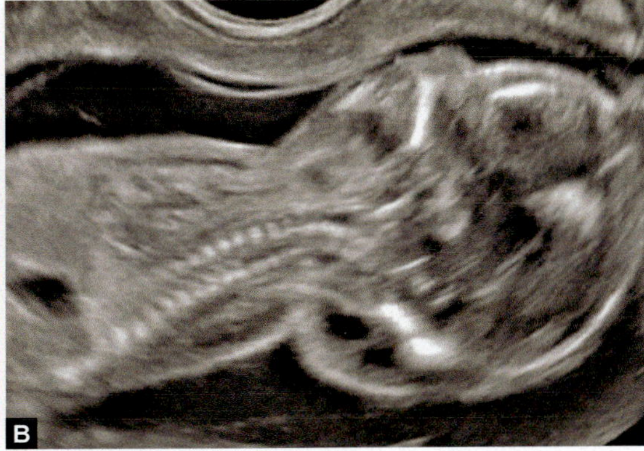

Figs. 22A and B: Cystic hygroma.
(BPD: biparietal diameter; HC: head circumference; OFD: occipitofrontal diameter)

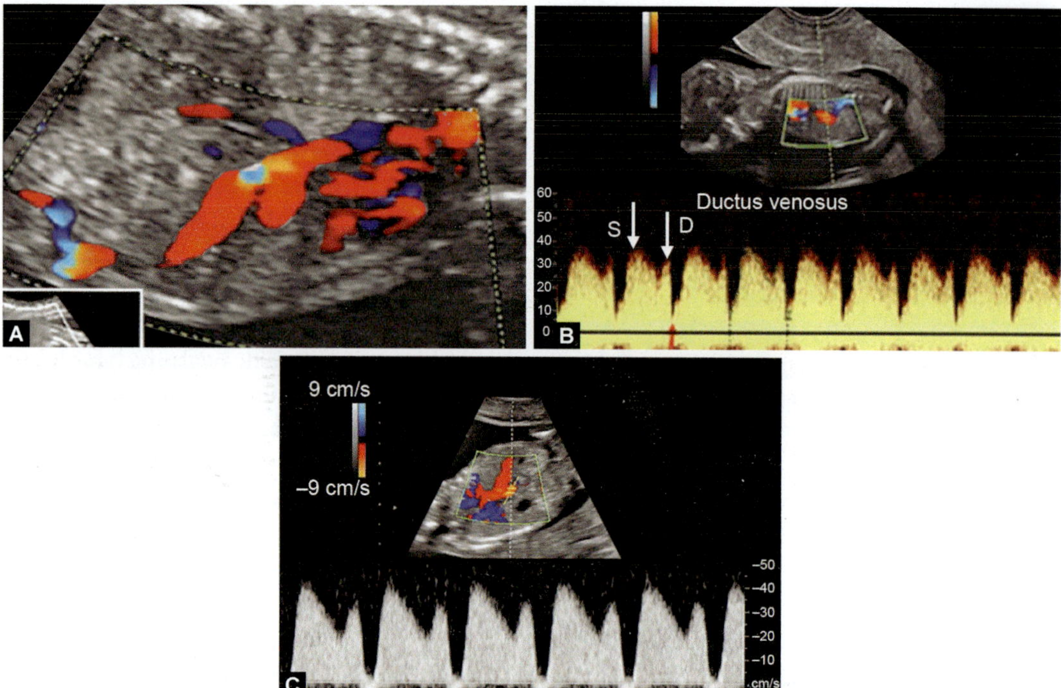

Figs. 23A to C: (A and B) Ductus venosus flow; (C) Abnormal ductus venosus flow.

section or oblique transverse section through upper abdomen as a most bright spot on color Doppler. It shows a continuous forward triphasic flow **(Figs. 23A and B)** normally, where the first peak indicates the ventricular systole, the second peak corresponds to ventricular diastole, and the deepest point after the second peak corresponds to the atrial systole and is known as the A wave. Reversed diastolic flow, which means an absent flow or flow reversal at A wave, indicates chromosomal or cardiac anomalies **(Fig. 23C)**. Though early in first trimester, an immature sphincter of ductus venosus would give a reversal of A wave due to backflow of blood into the ductus with atrial systole. Absent/inverted A wave has been seen in about 70–90% with chromosomal anomalies.[17] About 40% fetuses having an abnormal ductus venosus waveform show increased NT. Evaluating it inversely, fetuses with increased NT showed abnormal ductus flow in 90% of chromosomally abnormal fetuses or with cardiac defects. With the addition of new sonographic markers to the combined test, the detection rate (DR) would be 93–96% for a false positive rate (FPR) of 2.5%.[18]

An abnormal ductus flow in T21 can be explained by increased levels of atrial and brain natriuretic peptide messenger ribonucleic acid in fetal heart suggesting heart strain. This abnormal waveform may be in the form of reversal of the A wave or increased pulsatility index.

But, this alteration in the waveform must be very carefully evaluated, as it is very common to make a mistake of examining the hepatic vein instead of ductus venosus, which would show a reversal of A wave normally. Ductus venosus is best picked up in midsagittal plane as the brightest color spot below the diaphragm on color Doppler. Doppler sample should be small (0.5–1.0 mm) to avoid contamination from the adjacent veins. The insonation angle should be less than 30°. The filter should be set at a low frequency (50–70 Hz) to allow visualization of the whole waveform. The sweep speed should be high (2–3 cm/s) so that the waveforms are assessed better.

Nasal Bone (Figs. 24A and B)

As it is often observed that Down's syndrome babies have a flat nasal bridge and a flat nose. This observation was applied into the fetal evaluation for diagnosis of Down's syndrome. It was observed that 40% of Down's syndrome fetuses have absent nasal bone (NB) but no euploid fetuses showed this finding.[19] LR of absent NB for Down's syndrome is as high as 83.

So that it makes NB a very important marker, independent of NT for diagnosis of aneuploidies. The NB is nonossified in 60% of fetuses with T21. In the normal population, the frequency of nonossified NB is related to the ethnicity of the mother. It is 2.2% in Caucasians, 5% in Asians, and 9% in the Afro-Caribbeans. This needs to be taken into account while evaluating the individual patient risk.

Earlier, NB length was considered important but since the huge variation according to ethnicity has been recognized, it is now believed that it is presence or absence (ossification or nonossification of the NB that is important rather than the length of the NB). Its presence is confirmed in the same plane as for NT. Looking at the profile of the face, the top line represents the skin, and the underlying line, which is thicker and more echogenic than the overlying skin, represents the NB. These two parallel lines of echogenicity have the shape of an "equal sign". A third line in front of the bone and at a higher level than the skin represents the tip of the nose. But the recent school of thoughts now is that the NB can be short in certain ethnic groups and it is only the presence of the NB that is important at Nuchal scan. Of course further in second and third trimester then, the values of NB length are to be plotted on the nomogram. It must be remembered that the more recent studies have shown that 0.5% of normal patients have absent NB and if a detailed US and a marker test do not show any indication of T21, follow-up scans should be done and any structural abnormalities must be looked for.

It must be remembered that incidence of absent NB decreased with fetal CRL, increased with NT thickness, and was substantially high in Afro-Caribbeans than in Caucasians.[20]

Though the sensitivity for Down's syndrome as individual marker is as follows:

- Nuchal translucency—80.4%
- Nasal bone—58.7%
- Ductus venosus flow—93.5%.

All three together have sensitivity for Down's syndrome of 94% with LR for negative test only 0.08%.

Apart from these, there are some new markers for aneuploidies that are gaining

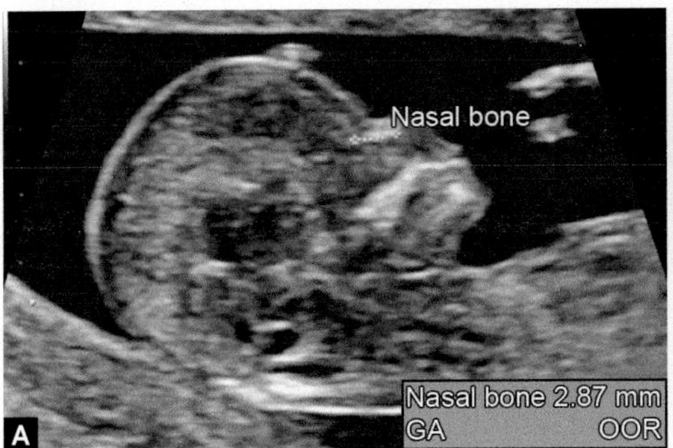

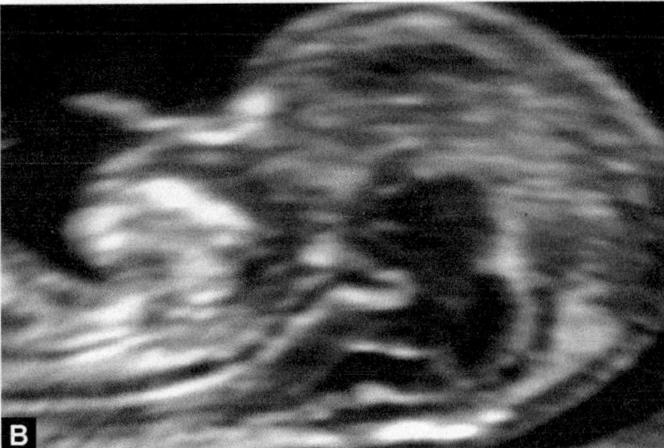

Figs. 24A and B: Nasal bone.

a lot of importance and significance lately. These are:

- Facial angle or frontomaxillary facial (FMF) angle
- Tricuspid regurgitation
- Intracranial translucency: Though not a marker for chromosomal abnormalities, it is also an important measurement to exclude open spinal defects that may be a part of chromosomal abnormality.

Frontomaxillary Facial Angle (Fig. 25)

In midsagittal plane of the face, a line is drawn on the superior surface of the maxilla that is rectangular in shape and a second line is drawn from the anterior point of maxilla to the nasion. But, it needs to be a true midsagittal plane. Rotation of even 5–15° will lead to error of 2–3°. In normal fetuses, this angle is 66.6–89.5°, mean 78.1°, but it decreases with increase in CRL. It is 84° at CRL 45 mm and 76.5° at CRL 84 mm.

Incorporating FMF angle in first trimester combined screening *increased the estimated DR of T21 from 90 to 94% at FPR 5%* and from 85 to 92% at FPR of 3%.[21]

Tricuspid Regurgitation (Fig. 26)

Four-chamber heart view is the section required for assessing the tricuspid valve flow. With the new advances in US technology, now this view can be achieved at the nuchal scan. The sample volume of pulse Doppler is placed across the tricuspid valve with a sample volume of 2–3 mm and the spectrum of flow is documented. The insonation angle to the direction of flow should be <30° from the direction of the interventricular septum. The sweep speed should be high (2–3 cm/s) so that the waveforms are widely spread for better assessment. Tricuspid flow is a positive flow during ventricular diastole and is absent during ventricular systole. Reverse flow during ventricular systole that involves more than half of the systolic phase and has a velocity of 60 cm/s or more is defined as tricuspid regurgitation. This is a marker for chromosomal and/or cardiac abnormality in the fetus **(Figs. 27A to D)**.

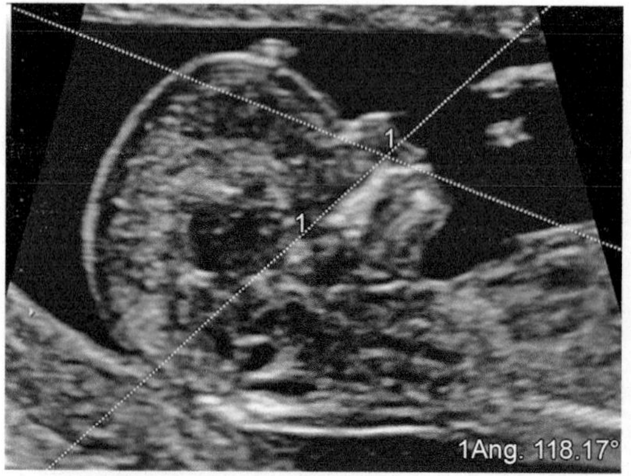

Fig. 25: Frontomaxillary facial angle.

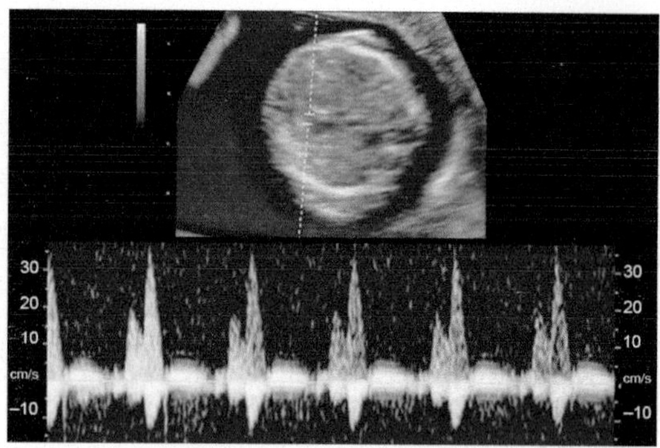

Fig. 26: Normal tricuspid flow.

Incidence of tricuspid regurge is as follows:[22]

- *Euploid*: 0.9%
- *T21*: 55.7%
- *T18*: 33.3%
- *T13*: 30.0%
- *Turner's*: 37.5%.

Intracranial Translucency (Fig. 28)

Midsagittal plane is absolutely essential. This is the space between the posterior margin of the brainstem and anterior margin of choroid plexus of fourth ventricle. It is measured in the same plane as that for NT and parallel to NT. It is a curved translucency, widest in the middle of the fourth ventricle. It is normally 2–3 mm, anything <2 mm, open spinal canal defect is suspected.

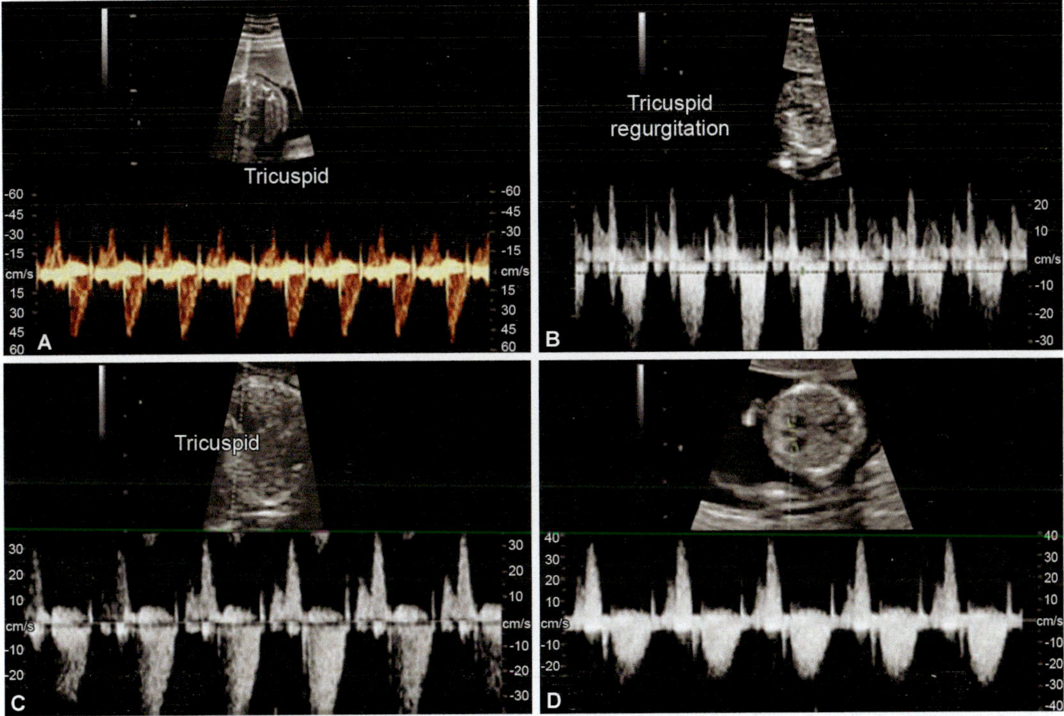

Figs. 27A to D: (A to C) Tricuspid regurgitation, but (D) is not true tricuspid regurgitation.

Narrowed or absent intracranial translucency indicates a possibility of spina bifida. This is because of downward and posterior displacement of the cerebellum.

Apart from this, there are other signs also that are seen on nuchal scan that may indicate spina bifida:

*On midsagittal plane (**Fig. 28**):* Displacement of the brainstem posteriorly and inferiorly, and decreased brainstem to occipital bone distance leading to increased BS-BSOB (brainstem to brainstem-occipital bone) ratio. This also leads to compression of the cisterna magna and on midsagittal plane therefore instead of four lines as seen on the nuchal section, as shown in **Figure 28**, only three lines are seen. This also leads to reduced frontomaxillary facial angle due to downward displacement of the cranial contents and flattening of frontal bones. Brainstem width may also be decreased. These distances are measured by drawing a line on the superior margin of the maxilla, extending posteriorly to the occipital bone. If the diencephalon is outlined, as is known, it has two convexities—upper anterior and lower posterior. The line drawn on the superior margin of maxilla normally crosses through the posterior lower convexity and anterior margin of anterior convexity divides the line into two equal halves. In cases of spina bifida, as the brainstem is pushed posteriorly and inferiorly, this line crosses the upper

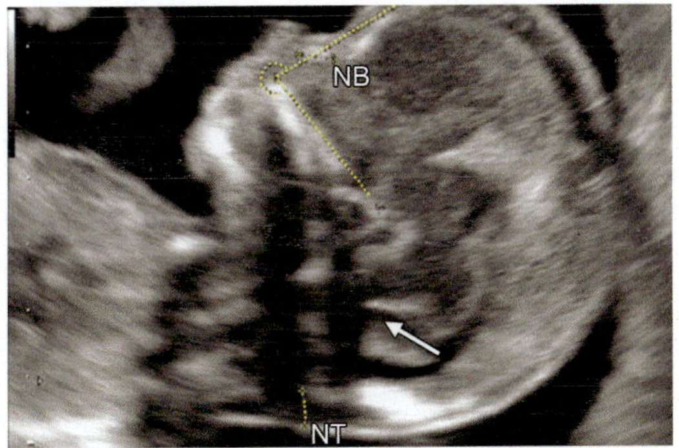

Fig. 28: Intracranial translucency (arrow). (NT: nuchal translucency; NB: nasal bone)

convexity and distance of anterior margin of brainstem to the occipital bone is decreased. Since intracranial translucency is absent or decreased severely, it merges with posterior margin of the brainstem and therefore only three instead of four lines are seen on this plane **(Fig. 28)**.

On axial plane: Due to posterior displacement of the brainstem, the cerebral peduncles are pushed posteriorly and extend almost to the occipital bone in severe cases leading to obliteration of the aqueduct shadow **(Fig. 28)**. As the cerebral peduncles are pulled posteriorly, their lateral margins also become parallel to each other instead of converging posteriorly. Choroid plexuses fill up the entire ventricle and collapse of the frontal bones leads to lemon-shaped skull.

Apart from these markers, some other markers, which though have a lower sensitivity for aneuploidies than the major markers, are seen much more often in the aneuploidies rather than normal fetuses. It should be noted that in the absence of major congenital anomalies and normal karyotype of the fetus, they do not carry any significance and do not affect the fetal prognosis, as they are not pathological except for ventriculomegaly.

These markers are picked up in second trimester except echogenic cardiac focus, megacystis, echogenic bowel, clinodactyly/syndactyly/polydactyly, and aberrant right subclavian artery (ARSA).

Women, who found to be at low risk through first trimester combined test or second trimester quadruple test, should not be referred for further assessment. Such low-risk women would require further assessment only if the following markers are identified:

- Nuchal fold >6 mm
- Ventriculomegaly (atrium >10 mm)
- Echogenic bowel
- Renal pelvic dilatation >7 mm
- Small measurements <5th centile.

These are soft markers and can be listed as follows:

- Ventriculomegaly
- Choroid plexus cyst (CPC)
- Strawberry-shaped head
- Echogenic cardiac focus
- Renal pyelectasis
- Megacystis
- Hyperechoic bowel
- Clinodactyly/syndactyly/polydactyly
- Short long bones
- Aberrant right subclavian artery
- Umbilical cord abnormalities
- Extrafetal abnormalities

*Ventriculomegaly **(Fig. 29)**:* The ventricular size remains relatively constant throughout gestation at 6.1 ± 1.3 mm, though it is slightly larger in males and smaller in females.[23] As a rule, ventricular width <8 mm is considered as normal. 8–10 mm is borderline and 10–12 mm is mild ventriculomegaly. The ventricular size larger than that is called a hydrocephalus and not a ventriculomegaly. Visually, when the choroid plexus of the dependent ventricle is seen hanging away from the medial ventricular wall (separation of >3 mm), it is considered as ventriculomegaly. Ventriculomegaly as an isolated sign is not a very significant marker and demands only a close follow-up, but may be one of the markers of trisomies 18, 13, and 21 and triploidy. The odds ratio of mild ventriculomegaly for chromosomal abnormality is 4.4%.[24]

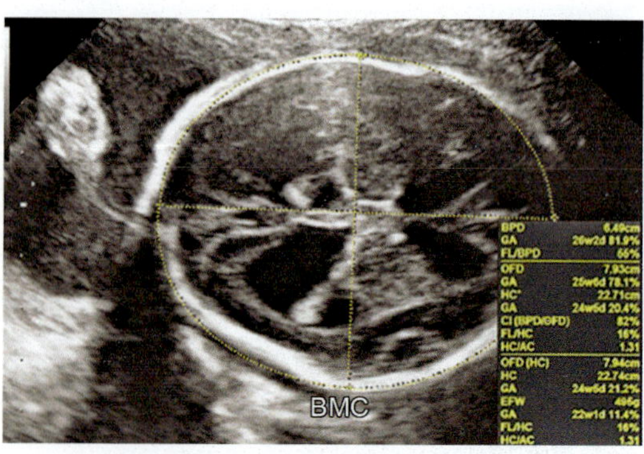

Fig. 29: Ventriculomegaly and measurement.

Strawberry-shaped skull **(Fig. 30)** is anteroposteriorly flattened head which on transthalamic section looks like a strawberry in shape. It is seen in T18, but associated findings must be looked for. Its combination with choroid plexus cyst (CPC) increases the risk of T18.

Choroid plexus cyst ***(Fig. 31)***: CPC is seen in 0.3–3.6% of the population between 16 and 24 weeks. These are transient in 80–94% and disappear at 24 weeks in euploid or aneuploid fetuses. CPCs have no adverse fetal outcome, if the karyotype is normal.

Though CPCs are seen in 1% of normal fetuses but are seen in 50% of T18 fetuses **(Table 1)**. Single CPCs that are <3 mm in size and that are transient are less likely to be associated with aneuploidies. Multiple or bilateral CPCs and especially which persist for a longer time or disappear late have higher risk for aneuploidies, but any associated abnormality with CPC increases the LR by as much as 20 times.[25] The LR of CPC is 13.8 for T18 and for T21.[26]

TABLE 1: Approximate risk of trisomy 18 in fetuses with choroid plexus cyst.[25]

Gestation weeks	*Baseline*	*Isolated cyst*	*Other abnormalities*
20–24	1:4,500	1:2,950	1:225
25–29	1:3,600	1:2,300	1:175
30–34	1:2,000	1:1,300	1:100
35–39	1:750	1:470	1:35
40–44	1:400	1:100	1:10

A quadruple marker must be done for fetuses with isolated CPC, to select the ones which need amniocentesis. If karyotyping is not done, there is no point in doing a follow-up scan for CPCs, as they are almost always transient. A follow-up scan only helps to detect other abnormalities, which may be missed.

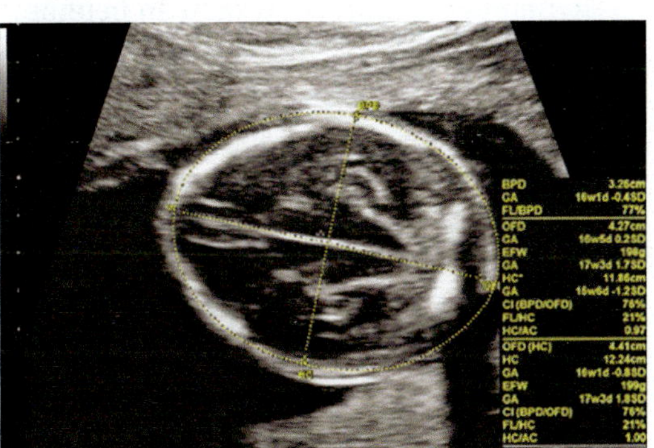

Fig. 30: Strawberry-shaped skull.

Echogenic cardiac focus ***(Fig. 32)***: An echogenic dense spot of 1–6 mm is sometimes seen in the cardiac ventricles, which move in the heart like a golf ball with each ventricular contraction, as it is attached to the papillary muscle or chordae tendineae. A single such focus may be seen in the left ventricle in 3–10% of the population and is more often seen in fetuses of Asian mothers than in fetuses with Down's syndrome. The sensitivity and the specificity of this marker are low. It has an LR for Down's syndrome of 1.8–4.2%.[27] But when such foci

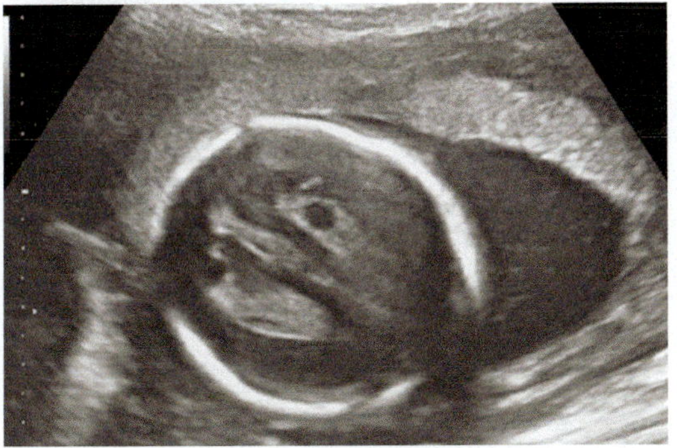

Fig. 31: Choroid plexus cyst.

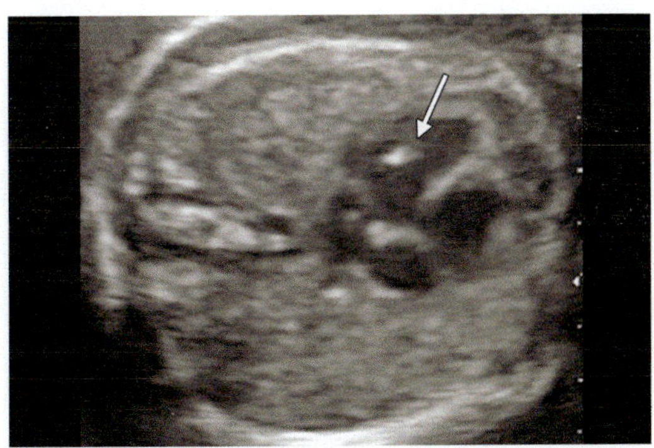

Fig. 32: Echogenic focus in left ventricle.

are multiple or are in the right ventricle or bilateral, the risk increases to double. Less than 20% of aneuploid fetuses have echogenic cardiac focus. It is seen in 16% of fetuses with T21, 39% of fetuses with T13, and in 2% of normal fetuses.[28]

Its significance as a marker for aneuploidies is very low especially when isolated.

Renal pyelectasis **(*Fig. 33*)***:* Renal pelvis diameter is 3–4 mm at 14–15 weeks in antero-posterior (AP) plane when fetal abdomen is seen in transverse section. It must be a true transverse section when renal pelvis is seen but stomach or bladder is not seen. The measurement is taken from inner margin to inner margin of renal pelvis. When this diameter increases to >4 mm, it is called pyelectasis and it increases the risk for T21 by 1.6-folds.[29] Though 2–3% of normal fetuses have pyelectasis, it is seen in 17–25% of Down's syndrome fetuses. Though often a transient sign, renal pelvic diameter of:

- >4 mm between 16 and 20 weeks,
- >5 mm between 20 and 30 weeks, and
- >7 mm between 30 and 40 weeks is considered abnormal.

Megacystis: Normally in all fetuses beyond 67 mm CRL, the bladder is visible. Normal emptying time cycle is 30–155 minutes CRL. Megacystis is defined when the bladder vertically measures >8 mm or bladder diameter/CRL >13%. About 20% of the fetuses with megacystis have aneuploidies. It resolves in second trimester, but that does not exclude the risk of aneuploidy. Risk is significant when due to megacystis, which is due to obstructive uropathy, and associated with other abnormalities.

Hyperechoic bowel **(*Fig. 34*)***:* The bowel is normally a little hyperechoic to the liver due to multiple tissue interfaces, but when it is as dense as bone, it is termed hyperechoic bowel and is a marker for aneuploidies. Hyperechoic bowel increases the risk for T21 by 6–7-folds.[30] It is found in 12% of fetuses with T21.

It is seen in late trimester in presence of fetal growth restriction or intrauterine death in second trimester.

According to the density and the uniformity, it can be graded as:[31]

- *Grade I*: Homogeneously mildly hyperechoic
- *Grade II*: Focal hyperechogenicities
- *Grade III*: As echogenic as bone, hyperechoic bowel may be seen in fetuses with:
  - Aneuploidies
  - Meconium ileus—due to cystic fibrosis
  - Bowel atresia
  - Congenital infections such as cytomegalovirus (CMV)

Phalangeal abnormalities:

- *Clinodactyly*: T21 [ratio of middle phalanx of fifth digit to middle phalanx of fourth digit in Down's is 0.59 (median), normal 0.85]

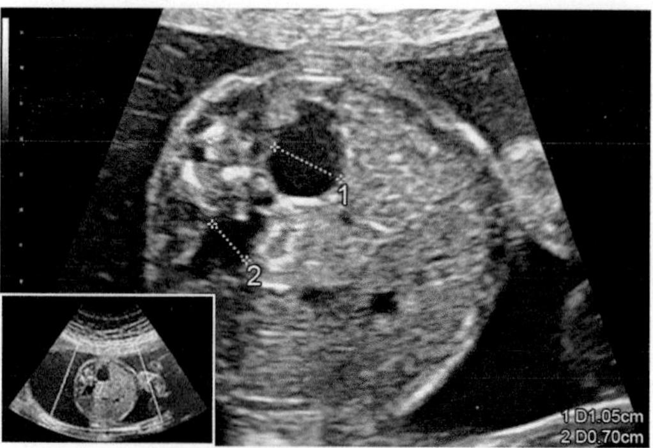

Fig. 33: Renal pyelectasis.

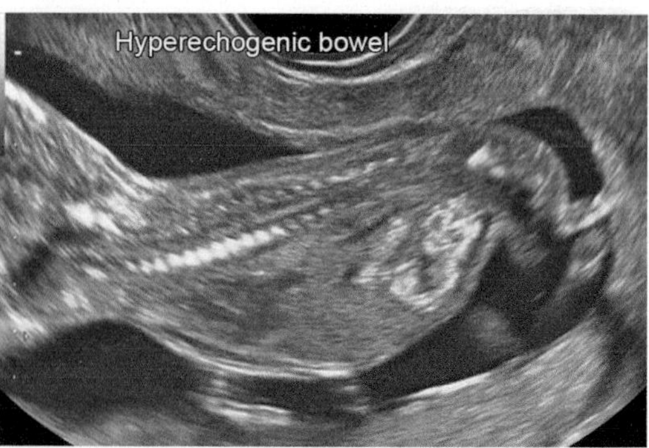

Fig. 34: Hyperechoic bowel.

- *Polydactyly*: T13
- *Syndactyly*: Triploidy.

Short long bones: When femoral length shows a difference of 2 weeks or more than the other biometric parameters, it has a significant risk of aneuploidies, especially T21 and T18. But, short humerus is considered to be more sensitive for T21 than short femur.

Umbilical cord abnormalities: Umbilical cord diameter, though is not normally measured routinely, has its own nomographic values. When it is above 95th percentile, it is considered as abnormal and may increase the risk of aneuploidy.[32] Single umbilical artery **(Fig. 35)**, though once considered a very significant marker, is often seen in normal fetuses also. Single umbilical artery should definitely lead to a detailed search for chromosomal or cardiac abnormalities, but has a significant value only when associated with other abnormalities.

Reversed end-diastolic flow in umbilical artery at 10–14 weeks is thought to be associated with chromosomal anomalies.

Extrafetal markers: Placental thickening or cystic areas (placental lakes) are associated with aneuploidies. Cystic areas in the placenta suggest a possibility of trisomies 18 and 13, especially when associated with oligohydramnios or IUGR.

The risk for aneuploidies increases when:

- Multiple markers are present.

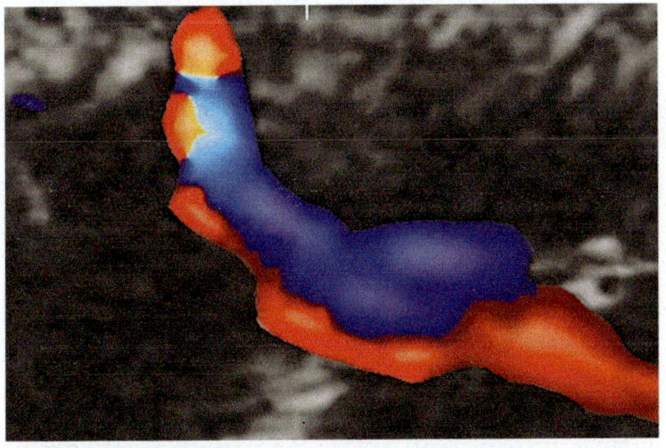

Fig. 35: Single umbilical artery.

- Markers are seen at the higher age of gestation.
- Fetus shows delayed development—the risk of aneuploidy increases by 9.04 odds ratio, if the CRL was 14 mm or more decreased than the expected. Early onset FGR is usually associated with T18 or T13. About 96% of the fetuses with FGR have multisystem abnormalities, characteristic of type of aneuploidy. Though usually symmetric IUGR is seen in most chromosomal abnormalities, triploidy shows asymmetric FGR. FGR with polyhydramnios/oligohydramnios has higher risk for aneuploidies.
- Gestational sac is large for dates.
- Cardiac anomaly or duodenal atresia is present.

But when we say that the risk is increased, it does not suffice. It is important to exactly calculate the risk in order to allow the patient to take a balanced and informed decision regarding the continuation or termination of pregnancy.

Calculating the Risk

- Background risk × LRs of the risk factors or markers.
- *Likelihood ratio of positive scan*: Sensitivity/FPR, LR for a normal scan:false negative rate/specificity. Positive LR of a marker is derived by dividing the percentage of confirmed Down's syndrome having the marker by the percentage of normal fetus with the same marker. Negative LR results from dividing the number of T21 fetuses that do not exhibit the marker by the number of normal fetuses that do not exhibit the marker.
- *Background risk*: Maternal age + gestational age + previous pregnancy with aneuploidy.

Background Risk Factors

- Maternal age >35
- Paternal age >39—three times increased risk

- *Previous chromosomal anomaly*: Previous aneuploid child increases an additional risk of 0.75% to the risk otherwise calculated as background risk
- Biochemical screening—positive
- *Increasing gestational age*: About 30% of T21 fetuses die between 12 weeks of gestation and full-term and 20% between 16 weeks and full-term. That means with increasing age of gestation, the number of aneuploid fetuses decreases due to nature's law of existence of the strongest. So, if the markers for chromosomal abnormality are detected at the higher gestational age, it means that the likelihood of this fetus being abnormal increases
- The actual sensitivity of a genetic sonogram depends on various factors, including the markers sought, gestational age, reasons for referral, and quality of US. The increasing DR of cardiac abnormalities has increased the DR of aneuploidies by sonography from 60 to 90%.

TABLE 2: Likelihood ratios of different markers for trisomy 21.

Marker	*Isolated*	*In combination*
Increased NT	15	60–95
Short humerus	05	15–23
Short femur	04	06–10
Echogenic cardiac focus	04	06–08
Hyperechoic bowel	03	15–33
Choroid plexus cyst	1.5	Same
Mild hydronephrosis	1.5	05–09
Normal scan	0.2	—

(NT: nuchal translucency)

TABLE 3: Number of markers and likelihood ratio for trisomy 21.

Number of markers	*Likelihood ratio*
1	0.2
2	1.9
3	6.2
4	80

Chart of Likelihood Ratios

Likelihood ratio = Cases%/Controls%

Likelihood ratio is calculated for a particular finding by dividing the percentage of abnormal fetuses/percentage normal fetuses with that particular finding/measurement. Each marker has independent LR and increases the risk of aneuploidy accordingly **(Table 2)**.

Moreover, more the markers, more is the risk **(Table 3)**. A single marker increases the risk two-fold, two markers increase the risk nearly ten-fold, and three or more markers increase the risk to more than 100-folds. Though the actual risk depends on the type and number of markers that are present.

A normal US has a LR for aneuploidy of only 0.2-0.4 and decreases the risk by 60–80%.[30] About 45% of risk of chromosomal anomalies is decreased, if US is normal, though the biochemical markers are positive.[30]

The pooled estimates of DR, FPR, and positive and negative LR for T21 for each marker are summarized in **Table 4**.

Ventriculomegaly, nuchal fold thickness, and aberrant right subclavian artery (ARSA) each one of them increases the risk by three to four times. All the other markers in isolation do not have significant effect on the risk, while the presence of two or more markers will produce significant modification of the risk.

Another method of risk assessment based on US is age-adjusted US risk assessment. Here, a priori risk of the maternal age is multiplied by the LRs of the individual sonographic marker. This in low-risk group gives a sensitivity of 61.5% with an FPR of only 4%.

NONINVASIVE PRENATAL TESTS

Since the discovery of cell-free fetal deoxy-ribonucleic acid (cffDNA) in the maternal

TABLE 4: Screening performance of second-trimester soft markers.

Marker	*DR%*	*FPR%*	*LR+*	*LR–*	*LR isolated marker*
Intracardiac echogenic focus	24.4	3.9	5.83	0.80	0.95
Ventriculomegaly	7.5	0.2	27.52	0.94	3.81
Increased nuchal fold	26.0	1.0	23.30	0.80	3.79
Echogenic bowel	16.7	1.1	11.44	0.90	1.65
Mild hydronephrosis	13.9	1.7	7.63	0.92	1.08
Short humerus	30.3	4.6	4.81	0.74	0.78
Short femur	27.7	6.4	3.72	0.80	0.61
ARSA	30.7	1.5	21.48	0.71	3.94
Absent or hypoplastic nasalbone	59.8	2.8	23.27	0.46	6.58

(ARSA: aberrant right subclavian artery; DR: detection rate; FPR: false positive rate; LR: likelihood ratio: LR+: positive likelihood ratio; LR–: negative likelihood ratio)

(*Source*: Adapted from Agathokleous M, Chaveeva P, Poon LCY, Kosinski P, Nicolaides KH. Meta-analysis of second-trimester markers for trisomy 21. Ultrasound Obstet Gynecol. 2103;42:247-61.)

plasma, there has been major progress in the field of prenatal diagnosis. cffDNA is employed in noninvasive prenatal testing (NIPT). NIPT has been endorsed by the American College of Obstetricians and Gynecologists and the Society for Maternal-Fetal Medicine as screening option for aneuploidy in 2011.

The majority of cell-free DNA is maternal in origin, with the fetal origin constituting about 3–13% after 10 weeks of gestation. The fetal DNA is derived from the placental trophoblasts. Testing can be performed at any period of gestation after 10 weeks. Results are generally available within 7–10 days of maternal sampling. NIPT has a sensitivity of 99.3% and a specificity of 99.8% for the detection of T21.

The reported FPR is 1% and is due to vanishing twin, confined placental mosaicism, and maternal malignancy.

Prerequisites

- Baseline US is mandatory to determine the viability, number of fetus, and gestational age.
- The couple should be counseled about the benefits and limitations of NIPT. A negative test does not assure a chromosomally normal fetus in a very small percentage of patients.

Limitations

- NIPT is expensive and is not applicable for screening general obstetric population. It is not universally available.
- Only T21, T18, and T13 can be detected. Information about sex chromosomal aneuploidies and other trisomies (T16 and T22) would be available only if requested for.
- It cannot determine if the trisomy is due to translocation. This information would be important for predicting the risk of recurrence.
- NIPT cannot routinely be offered for the detection of microdeletions. Hence, for the above reasons, NIPT cannot replace conventional karyotype.
- Laboratories require a minimum of 4% fetal fraction for a reportable result, irrespective of the methodology used. Maternal obesity is associated with lesser fetal fraction, leading to 1–8% screen failure.

Recommendations

- *NIPT can be offered* ***(Table 5)***:
  - As a follow-up test for pregnant women with a high or intermediate risk from a conventional screening test before proceeding for invasive tests. But a normal NIPT result does carry a

TABLE 5: Sensitivity and specificity of noninvasive prenatal testing (NIPT).

Condition	Sensitivity	Specificity
Trisomy 18	97.4%	99.8%
Trisomy 13	91.6%	99.9%
Sex chromosome aneuploidy	91%	99.6%

residual risk of 2% of a chromosomal abnormality in such a situation.
  - To any pregnant woman, provided she understands the benefits and drawbacks of this screening strategy in the context of alternative screening tests. But the use of NIPT to the general obstetric population may produce higher screen false-positives because the positive predictive value is lower in this population due to the lower prevalence of aneuploidy in the general obstetric population.
- *NIPT cannot be offered in the following situations*:
  - In the event of identification of a structural anomaly by US which needs a diagnostic test
  - Multiple pregnancy as it provides only a single composite result for the entire gestation
  - Couple is unaffordable
  - Nonavailability of NIPT
- Women with a positive test should undergo invasive diagnostic test since NIPT does not replace the accuracy of invasive tests. Knowing the type of trisomy from the karyotype becomes essential for purposes of prediction of recurrence. Management decisions should not be based solely on NIPT results.
- Women, whose NIPT results are not reported or indeterminate, should be offered comprehensive US evaluation, genetic counseling, and invasive diagnostic test for confirmation.
- In addition to NIPT, parallel or simultaneous testing with multiple screening methodologies for aneuploidy is not necessary and should not be performed. But comprehensive anomaly scan should be offered, as NIPT does not diagnose structural malformations.

Over and above this, every screening procedure for aneuploidy should commence with a counseling session. The aim of pretest counseling is to facilitate the couple to make informed choices concerning the pregnancy outcome. It is the prime responsibility of the clinician and his/her team to explain to the couple about the condition to be screened (Down's syndrome) and the disabilities and morbidities which the child would face. Information about the screening options relevant to their gestational age and the screening process should be provided. Patient should be explained the difference between screening and diagnosis and should also be explained the consequences in case the fetus turns out to be at high risk, or aneuploid at the end of invasive testing.

The scanner's aim should be to minimize the false-positive results in low- risk group and maximize the sensitivity in the high-risk group. With this aim, a scoring index system has been devised by Benacerraf et al. She decided a score of 2 for structural abnormalities and nuchal thickening and 1 point for other markers. All those having a score of more than 2 were offered amniocentesis. Some prefer to modify this system by adding 1 point for maternal age of 35 or more and 2 points for the age of 40 and more.

Though being so significantly helpful for the diagnosis of aneuploidies, sonography is not useful for diagnosis of single gene disorders such as thalassemia or muscular dystrophy, which show no structural variations or abnormalities.

A detailed, well-performed anomaly scan can reduce the rate of invasive testing and less number of abnormal births.[33]

TABLE 6: Performance of different screening protocols for Down's syndrome.

Screening test	*Detection rate*	*False +ve rate*
First-trimester tests:		
MA + NT	75–80%	5%
MA + first trimester serum markers	60–70%	5%
Combined test (MA + NT + serum markers)	85–90%	5%
Contingent first trimester test (combined test + NB/TR/DV flow)	93–96%	2.5%
Second-trimester tests:		
Triple test	60–70%	5%
Quadruple test	65–75%	5%
Genetic sonogram	56%	NA
Quadruple test + genetic sonogram	80%	NA
Combined first- and second-trimester tests:		
Integrated test	90–94%	5%
Stepwise sequential test	90–94%	5%
Contingent sequential test	90–94%	5%
Combined test + genetic sonogram	88%	NA
Noninvasive prenatal test (NIPT)	99%	NA

(DV: ductus venosus; MA: maternal age; NA: not available; NB: nasal bone; NT: nuchal translucency; TR: tricuspid regurgitation)

Source: Benn P, Borrell A, Chiu RW, Cuckle H, Dugofff L, Faas B, et al. Position statement from the Chromosome Abnormality Screening Committee on behalf of the Board of the International Society for Prenatal Diagnosis. Prenat Diagn. 2015;35:725-34.

Nicolaides KH. Screening for fetal aneuploidies at 11–13 weeks. Prenat Diagn. 2011;31:7-15.

The combined first- and second-trimester screening strategies that have been developed in our country are as follows **(Table 6)**:

- *Integrated screening*: It incorporates the results of the combined test and quadruple test into a single risk. The integrated test has the highest DR and least FPR, thereby reducing unwanted amniocentesis in normal pregnancies. The disadvantage associated with integrated screening strategy lies in ethical issue of not conveying the first trimester result and denying them the option of chorionic villus sampling (CVS).
- *Sequential screening*: First trimester combined test is the primary screening modality. The results of the combined test are stratified into low (risk <1:1,000), intermediate (risk ≥1:1,000 and ≤1:51), and high (risk >1:50) risk groups. The results are informed only to women at high risk, thus allowing them to choose the option of CVS. There are two testing strategies in this category:
  1. *Stepwise sequential screening*: Both the low- and intermediate-risk group would be offered the quadruple test in the second trimester.
  2. *Contingent sequential screening*: No further testing would be required for low-risk group. For those in the intermediate-risk group, quadruple test will be offered. This approach is the most effective for population screening, as it obviates the need for second trimester screening in low-risk group, who constitute about 85%.

Following the quadruple test, the final risk is calculated after incorporating both the first and second trimester results. When the risk is below the established cut-off, no further screening would be required. When the risk is above the established cut-off, amniocentesis should be offered.

One must also confirm patient's wish in case the abnormality detected turns out to be incompatible with life, will she be ready for termination. The information should be in simple language, balanced, and nondirective. The couple should be given every opportunity to discuss with the clinician before they make a final decision. This counseling is as important as post-test counseling where the results and their meanings are explained to the patient, the directive is suggested but the final proceedings should be a joint decision of the couple and the doctor.

During this scan, uterine artery flow assessment is also done and this along with mean arterial pressure of the mother and other biochemicals are used to screen the patients with high risk of preeclampsia. Recently, the genome-wide association study (GWAS) has suggested a dysregulation at the FMS-like tyrosine kinase-1 (FLT1) locus in the fetal genome, likely in the placenta, as a fundamental molecular defect in PE, reinforcing the role of genetic predisposition in the phenotypic manifestation of PE.[34] The estimates of mean arterial pressure (MAP), placental growth factor (PLGF), PAPP-A, and mean uterine artery pulsatility index (UtAPI) are converted to log10 transformed multiple of medians (MoM). In the first trimester, spectral Doppler analysis of the ascending branch of the UtA at the level of internal os is preferred over its apparent crossover over of the iliac vessels, as it is more readily obtainable and reproducible at the former site.[35] The UtAPI values at the internal cervical os are higher than the iliac crossover site.[36] The UtA alone has a DR of 40–50% (FPR of 5–10%) for early PE (requiring delivery <34 weeks), while the addition of maternal medical history enhances the DR to 70–80% (FPR of 10%). The UtAPI values for the transvaginal route are higher than the transabdominal route and hence the appropriate nomogram mentioning the route and site of insonation should be used.[37] UtAPI of 2.35, which represents the 95th centile for 11–13.6 weeks, can be used a rough estimate of UtA flow adequacy. The combined multimarker screening for pre-eclampsia encompassing documentation of maternal medical history, measurement of mean arterial pressure, estimation of the maternal serum levels of placental growth factor, pregnancy-associated plasma protein-A, and recording the UtAPI, performed in the first trimester between 11 and 13.6 weeks has proven to be an effective screening strategy. The above model has shown to detect 77% of preterm preeclampsia (<37 weeks), 96% of early preterm pre-eclampsia (<34 weeks), 38% of term preeclampsia, and 54% of all pre-eclampsia, at a false-positive rate of 10%. Uterine artery Doppler is a key to preeclampsia screening. Currently, a risk of >1:100 for preeclampsia developing before 37 weeks (preterm preeclampsia) is regarded as screen positive. Aspirin at a dose of 150 mg at bedtime given to screen positive subjects is associated with a significant reduction of preterm preeclampsia and early preeclampsia. Aspirin acts by diminishing stores of constitutive cyclooxygenase enzyme in the non-nucleated platelets without disturbing systemic prostaglandin production. Selective use of aspirin in screen positive women is associated with a very low incidence of adverse maternal, fetal, and neonatal side effects. Hence, screening for preeclampsia in first trimester, which is now endorsed by the Federation of International Obstetrical and Gynecological Societies, should be offered universally to all women at 11–13.6 weeks of gestation, followed by the administration of aspirin and serial maternal-fetal surveillance in the screen positive woman.[38]

According to International Federation of Gynecology and Obstetrics (FIGO) guidelines: All pregnant women should be screened for preterm PE in the first trimester by a combined test, which incorporates maternal risk factors and biomarkers as a one-step procedure. The best combined test includes maternal risk factors, measurements of MAP, serum PLGF, and the UtAPI.

When it is not possible to measure PLGF and/or UtAPI, a baseline screening should comprise maternal risk factors and measurement of MAP. A woman is considered high risk when the risk is 1:100 in the full combined test. In low-resource setting, a contingent approach for screening can be used wherein, first step comprises of maternal factors and MAP for all pregnancies followed by measurement of PLGF and UtAPI in only the high-risk women. Screen-positive women should receive prophylaxis with low-dose aspirin at a dose of 150 mg commenced at 11–13.6 weeks to be taken at night until 36 weeks/till delivery/PE is diagnosed. Low-dose aspirin should not be advised for all pregnancies.

In women with low calcium intake (<800 mg/day), either calcium replacement (1 g elemental calcium/day) or calcium supplementation (1.5–2 g elemental calcium/day) may reduce the burden of both early and late-onset PE.

REFERENCES

1. Evans MI, Galen RS, Drugan A. Biochemical screening. In: Evans MI, Johnson MP, Yaron Y (Eds). Prenatal Diagnosis: Genetics, Reproductive Risks, Testing and Management. New York: McGraw-Hill; 2006. pp. 277-88.
2. Snijders RJ, Sundberg K, Holzgreve W, Henry G, Nicolaides KH. Maternal age- and gestation-specific risk for trisomy 21. Ultrasound Obstet Gynecol. 1999;13:167-70.
3. Snijders RJ, Nicolaides KH. Sequential screening. Ultrasound Markers for Fetal Chromosomal Defects. Carnforth, UK: Parthenon Publishing; 1996. pp. 109-13.
4. Blaas HG, Eriksson AG, Salvesen KA, Isaksen CV, Christensen B, Mollerlokken G, et al. Brains and faces in holoprosencephaly: pre- and postnatal description of 30 cases. Ultrasound Obset Gynecol. 2002;19:24-38.
5. Blass HG, Eik-Nes SH, Vainio T, Isakesen CV. Alobar holoprosencephaly at 9 weeks gestational age visualized by two- and three-dimensional ultrasound. Ultrasound Obset Gynecol. 2000;15:62-5.
6. Bullen PJ, Rankin JM, Robson SC. Investigation of the epidemiology and prenatal diagnosis of holoprosencephaly in the North of England. Am J Obstet Gynecol. 2001;184:1256-62.
7. Babcook CJ, Goldstein RB, Filly RA. Prenatally detected fetal myelomeningocoele: Is karyotype analysis warranted? Radiology. 1995;1949:491-4.
8. Nyberg DA, Sickler GK, Hegge FN, Kramer DJ, Kropp RJ. Fetal cleft lip with and without cleft palate: US classification and correlation with outcome. Radiology. 1995;195:677-84.
9. Benacerraf BR, Pober BR, Sanders SP. Accuracy of fetal echocardiography. Radiology. 1987;165:847-9.
10. Chaoui R, Körner H, Bommer C, Göldner B, Bierlich A, Bollmann R. Prenatal diagnosis of heart defects and associated chromosomal aberrations. Ultraschall Med. 1999;20:177-84.
11. Fonalsrud EW, DeLorimier AA, Hays DM. Congenital atresia and stenosis of the duodenum. A review complied from the members of surgical section of the American Academy of Pediatrics. Pediatrics. 1969;43:79-83.
12. Nyberg DA, Fitzsimmons J, Mack LA, Hughes M, Pretorius DH, Hickok D, et al. Chromosomal anomalies in fetuses with omphalocele. Significance of omphalocele contents. J Ultrasound Med. 1989;8:299-308.
13. Nicholaides KH, Snijders RJ, Gosden CM, Berry C, Campbell S. Ultrasonographically detectable markers of fetal chromosomal abnormalities. Lancet. 1992;340:704-7.
14. Nicolaides KH. The 11–13+6 weeks scan. London: Fetal Medicine Foundation; 2004.
15. Zosmer N, Souter VL, Chan CS, Huggon IC, Nicolaides KH. Early diagnosis of major defects in chromosomally normal fetuses with increased Nuchal translucency. Br J Obstet Gyneacol. 1999;106:829-33.
16. Snijders RJ, Noble P, Sebire N, Souka A, Nicolaides KH. UK multicentre project on assessment of risk of trisomy 21 by maternal age and fetal Nuchal-translucency thickness at 10–14 weeks of gestation. Fetal Medicine Foundation First Trimester Screening Group. Lancet. 1998;352:343-6.
17. Zoppi MA, Putzolu M, Ibba RM, Floris M, Monni G. First-trimester ductus venosus velocimetry in relation to Nuchal translucency thickness and fetal karyotype. Fetal Diagn Ther. 2002;17:52-7.

18. Nicolaides KH. Nuchal translucency and other first-trimester sonographic markers of chromosomal abnormalities. Am J Obstet Gynecol. 2004;191:45-7.
19. Bromley B, Lieberman E, Shipp TD, Benacerraf BR. Fetal nose bone length: a marker for Down's syndrome in second trimester. J Ultrasound Med. 2002;21:1387-94.
20. Cicero S, Longo D, Rembouskos G, Sacchini C, Nicolaides KH. Absent nasal bone at 11–14 weeks of gestation and chromosomal defects. Ultrasound Obstet Gynecol. 2003;22:31-5.
21. Borenstein M, Persico N, Kagan KO. Frontomaxillary facial angle in screening for trisomy 21 at 11+0 to 13+6 weeks. Ultrasound Obstet Gynecol. 2008;32:5-11.
22. Kagan KO, Valencia C, Livanos P, Wright D, Nicolaides KH. Tricuspid regurgitation in screening for trisomies 21, 18 and 13 and Turner's syndrome at 11+0 to 13+6 weeks of gestation. Ultrasound Obstet Gynecol. 2009;33:18-22.
23. Patel MD, Goldstein RB, Tung S, Filly RA. Fetal cerebral ventricular atrium: difference in size according to sex. Radiology. 1995;194:713-5.
24. Sohl BD, Scioscia AL, Budorick NE, Moore TR. Utility of minor ultrasonographic markers in prediction of abnormal fetal karyotype at prenatal diagnostic center. Am J Obstet Gynecol. 1999;181:898-903.
25. Snijders RJ, Shawa L, Nicolaides KH. Fetal choroids plexus cysts and trisomy 18: assessment of risk based on ultrasound findings and maternal age. Prenat Diagn. 1994;14:1119-27.
26. Yoder PR, Sabbagha RE, Gross SJ, Zelop CM. The second-trimester fetus with isolated choroids plexus cysts: a meta-analysis of risk of trisomies 18 and 21. Obstet Gynecol. 1999;93:869-72.
27. Achiron R, Lipitz S, Gabbay U, Yagel S. Prenatal ultrasonographic diagnosis of fetal heart echogenic foci: no correlation with Down's syndrome. Obstet Gynecol. 1997;89:945-8.
28. Roberts DJ, Genest D. Cardiac histologic pathology characteristic of trisomies 13 and 21. Hum Path. 1992;23:1130-40.
29. Snijders RJ, Sebire NJ, Faria M, Patel F, Nicolaides KH. Fetal mild hydronephrosis and chromosomal defects: relation to maternal age and gestation. Fetal Diagn Ther. 1995;10:349-55.
30. Nyberg DA, Souter VL, El-Bastawissi A, Young S, Luthhardt F, Luthy DA. Isolated sonographic markers for detection of fetal Down's syndrome in second trimester of pregnancy. J Ultrasound Med. 2001;20:1053-63.
31. Nyberg DA, Resta RG, Mahony BS, Dubinsky T, Luthy DA, Hickok DE, et al. Fetal hyperechogenic bowel and Down's syndrome. Ultrasound Obstet Gynecol. 1993;3:330-3.
32. Ghezzi F, Raio L, Di Naro E, Franchi M, Buttarelli M, Schneider H. First-trimester umbilical cord diameter: a novel marker of fetal aneuploidy. Ultrasound Obstet Gynecol. 2002;19:235-3.
33. Nicholaides KH, Bindra R, Heath V, Cicero S. One-stop clinic for assessment of risk of chromosomal defects at 12 weeks of gestation. J Matern Fetal Neonatal Med. 2002;12:9-18.
34. McGinnis R, Steinthorsdottir V, Williams NO, GOPEC Consortium, Thorleifsson G, Shooter S, et al. Variants in the fetal genome near FLT1 are associated with risk of preeclampsia. Nat Genet. 2017;49:1255-60.
35. Akolekar R, Syngelaki A, Poon L, Wright D, Nicolaides KH. Competing risks model in early screening for preeclampsia by biophysical and biochemical markers. Fetal Diagn Ther. 2013;33:8-5.
36. Lefebvre J, Demers S, Bujold E, Nicolaides KH, Girard M, Brassard N, et al. Comparison of two different sites of measurement for transabdominal uterine artery Doppler velocimetry at 11–13 weeks. Ultrasound Obstet Gynecol. 2012;40:288-92.
37. Plasencia W, Barber MA, Alvarez EE, Segura J, Valle L, Garcia-Hernandez JA. Comparative study of transabdominal and transvaginal uterine artery Doppler pulsatility indices at 11–13 + 6 weeks. Hypertension Pregnancy. 2011;30:414-20.
38. Vikraman SK, Elayedatt RA. Pre-eclampsia screening in the first trimester - preemptive action to prevent the peril. J Matern Fetal Neonatal Med. 2020;1-9. Online ahead of print.

6

CHAPTER

Screening for Aneuploidy

Darshan Wadekar, Zalak Mehta

INTRODUCTION

Screening is a process of surveying a population with specific markers in order to identify those individuals with a higher risk for a particular disorder. For high-risk individuals, a diagnostic test is applied to diagnose the disorder. A successful screening program should be complemented with an accurate diagnostic test to identify those who are truly affected and also with a clear strategy of how to treat the affected individuals.

Every fetus has a chance of having a chromosomal or genetic condition. 20% of all the pregnancies are affected by a chromosomal or genetic condition. But, most of them are not viable and hence they do not lead to a live birth. Only some of them (most common Trisomy 21, 13, and 18) can at times lead to live birth. These aneuploidies are caused by errors during the meiotic cellular division. Down's syndrome (Trisomy 21), most common aneuploidy, leads to mental restriction and functional disability. In Trisomy 13 and 18, fetuses have developmental defects in cardiac and central nervous system defects.[1]

Screening for fetal aneuploidy in pregnancy began in the 1960–1970s with maternal age as the only available marker. As maternal age increases, the chance of delivering a child with Down syndrome (DS) or other major autosomal trisomies such as trisomy 18 (T18; Edwards syndrome) or 13 (T13; Patau syndrome) increases. However, screening with maternal age alone (cut-off >35 years) could detect about 30% of trisomies. But, majority of the babies with DS are born by women <35 years of age.

The first breakthrough in screening for fetal chromosomal abnormalities ocurred in 1988 with the introduction of a multiple marker screening test, based on a "risk" calculation for each pregnant woman using her age and the concentrations of three biochemical markers—human chorionic gonadotropin (hCG), αFP (alpha-fetoprotein), and unconjugated estriol (uE3), commonly known as triple marker test from blood samples in the 2nd trimester of pregnancy.

In 1992, fetal nuchal translucency (NT), by far the single best individual marker, was introduced with the improvement of ultrasound machine and knowledge about first trimester in pregnancy by Professor Kipros Nicolaides. In 1997, a new multiple marker screening test commonly knowns as combined test, using NT, free β-hCG, and pregnancy-associated plasma protein-A (PAPP-A) was started.

Since 2010, cell-free fetal DNA (cffDNA) in maternal plasma, in combination with the next generation sequencing techniques, made a big breakthrough step in screening for Down syndrome and other aneuploidies.

Diagnosis of major fetal chromosomal aneuploidies is done by karyotype of fetal cells, obtained through amniocentesis after the 15th week of pregnancy, or chorionic villus sampling (CVS) between the 12th and 14th weeks.

There are various parameters, which act as markers of aneuploidy in a pregnancy, which includes maternal markers, ultrasound markers, and biochemical markers. The details of each are described below.

MARKERS OF ANEUPLOIDY (TABLE 1)

Maternal Risk Factors

- *Maternal age*: The maternal age is directly proportional to the risk of aneuploidy. The real reason for such relationship could lie in the fact that in advanced maternal age group women, the residual follicles rupture lead to the increased risk in aneuploidy. Although the risk of trisomy 13, 18, and 21 rises with maternal age, the risk of Turner syndrome is independent of the maternal age.
- *Gestational age*: The in utero (fetal) death rate of aneuploidic fetuses is 30% in case of trisomy 21 and 80% in case of trisomy 13 and trisomy 18. Hence, the risk of aneuploidy decreases with the increasing gestational age **(Fig. 1)**.
- *Maternal comorbidities and body mass index*: The risk of aneuploidy increases with maternal comorbidities such as diabetes, hypertension, and increased maternal weight.
- *Previous history of aneuploidy fetus*: Risk of aneuploidy increases in a female having previous history of aneuploid fetus.

TABLE 1: Markers of aneuploidy.

Maternal risk factors	• Maternal age • Maternal comorbidities • Maternal height and weight • Previous history of aneuploidy fetus
Maternal serum markers	*Screening in the first trimester:* • Serum-free β-hCG and PAPP-A • Serum PLGF • Serum αFP *Screening in the second trimester:* Total or free β-hCG, αFP, uE3, and inhibin A
Ultrasound markers	• Nuchal translucency • Nasal bone • Fetal heart rate • Tricuspid flow • Ductus venosus • Other sonographic soft markers of aneuploidy

(αFP: α-fetoprotein; β-hCG: β-human chorionic gonadotropin; PAPP-A: pregnancy-associated plasma protein-A; PLGF: placental growth factor; uE3: estriol)

Ultrasound Markers

In today's scenario, ultrasound is the most important investigation during pregnancy. It not only gives maximum information about the fetus, placenta, and pregnancy as a whole, it is also majorly harmless to the fetus. Hence, we perform three major ultrasounds during pregnancy:

- First-trimester scan (genetic/nuchal translucency scan)

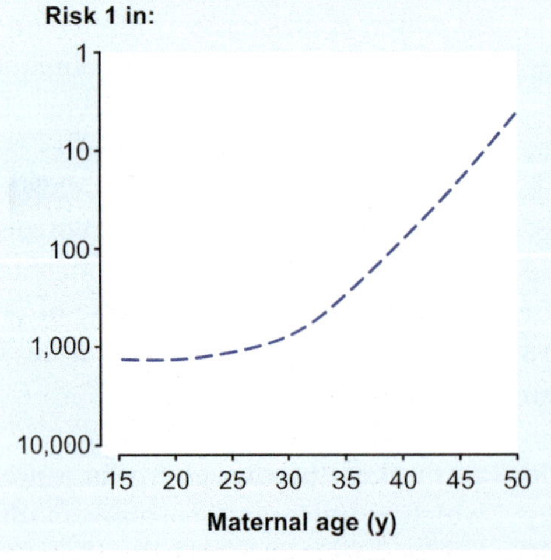

Age (y)	Gestational age		
	12 w	20 w	40 w
20	1100	1300	1500
25	1000	1100	1400
30	650	750	900
31	550	650	800
32	450	550	650
33	400	450	550
34	300	400	450
35	250	300	350
36	200	250	300
37	150	185	220
38	120	140	160
39	90	110	130
40	70	80	100

Fig. 1: Maternal age versus the risk of aneuploidy.

- Second-trimester scan (anomaly scan)
- Third-trimester scan (growth scan)

They help us to identify structural abnormalities (which will affect the fetus in the life ahead) and nonstructural abnormalities/soft markers (which will not affect the fetus structurally), both of which are markers of aneuploidy.

Soft markers are frequently seen in normal fetuses, often transient and insignificant in regard to outcome; however, their presence points us to look for other anomalies or genetic disorders.

Following are the soft markers of aneuploidy.

Nuchal Translucency

Nuchal translucency is a fluid-filled subcutaneous space at the back of the neck of the fetus **(Fig. 2B)**. It may or may not be septated. However, the size rather than its appearance is of importance.

In the 1990s, it was realized that the excess skin of individuals with Down's syndrome can be visualized by ultrasonography as increased nuchal translucency in the 3rd month of intrauterine life.

Fetal Medicine Foundation (FMF) criteria for nuchal translucency measurement (as points) **(Table 2)**:

The NT is to be measured between 11 and 13 + 6 weeks, i.e., crown-rump length (CRL) of 45–84 mm **(Fig. 2A)**.

TABLE 2: Fetal Medicine Foundation (FMF) criteria for measurement of nuchal translucency.

Timing gestational age	11–13+6 weeks
Crown-rump length	45–84 mm
Magnification	Face thorax occupies the entire screen
Midsagittal view	A midsagittal view of fetus is taken: • Tip of nose and nasal bone should be visible • Diencephalon should be visible • Palate is also visible • However maxilla should not be present
Fetal neck position	Neutral
Caliper placement	Inner border of horizontal line of the caliper should be placed on the line that defines NT
Gain	Optimize gain

- CRL of 45–84 mm
- *Midsagittal view*: A midsagittal view of fetus is taken **(Fig. 2C)**:
  - Tip of nose and nasal bone should be visible.
  - Diencephalon should be visible.
  - Palate is also visible.
  - However, maxilla should not be present.
- *Zoom*: Appropriate zooming so that only head and upper thorax are visible.

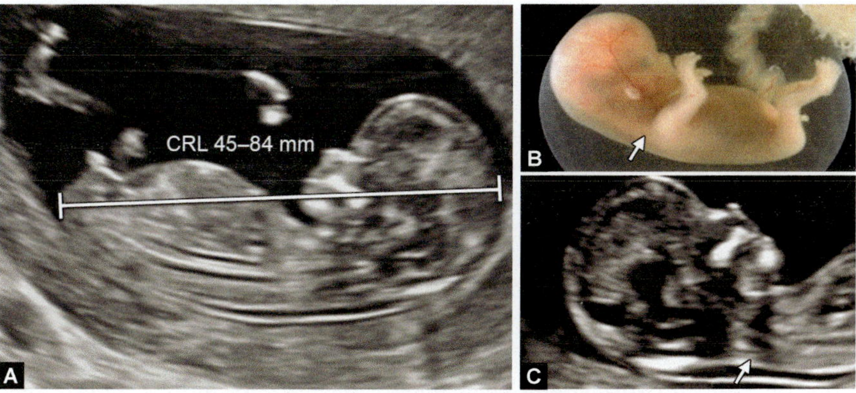

Figs. 2A to C: (A) Measuring correct CRL; (B) Image of the embryo showing nuchal translucency; (C) Nuchal translucency shown on ultrasound image.

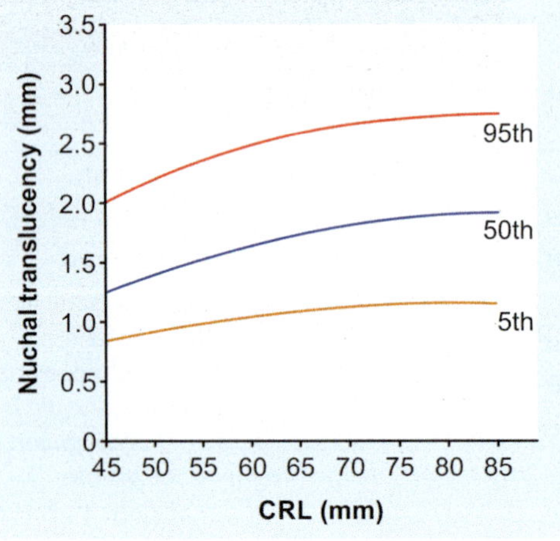

CRL	Median	95th percentile	99th percentile
45 mm	1.2	2.1	3.5
84 mm	1.9	2.7	3.5

Fig. 3: Nuchal translucency versus crown–rump length (CRL).

- *Neutral position*: Fetus should neither be extended (falsely increases NT) nor flexed (falsely decreased NT). The idea is to have a small pocket of liquor between the neck and chin for a neutral position.
- *Caliper placement*: The caliper placement is such that inner borders of calipers are put on echogenic line.
- *Maximum measurement*: The NT is measured in the widest part usually behind the mandible or maxilla.
- *In case of cord around neck*: If there is an amniotic cord around the neck, then NT is measured above and below the cord and the average is taken.

The NT increases as the CRL increases **(Fig. 3)**.

In 75–80% of trisomy 21 fetus, the NT is above the 95 percentile for the given CRL. As gestational age advances, most of the times, increased nuchal translucency may decrease. However, in few cases, they may advance to nuchal thickness or cystic hygroma.

Causes of increased NT: The most common causes of increased nuchal translucency are trisomy 21, trisomy 18, trisomy 13, Turner syndrome, and cardiac abnormalities **(Fig. 4)**.

There are multiple other single gene disorders or syndromes in which nuchal translucency can increase. Hence, in these

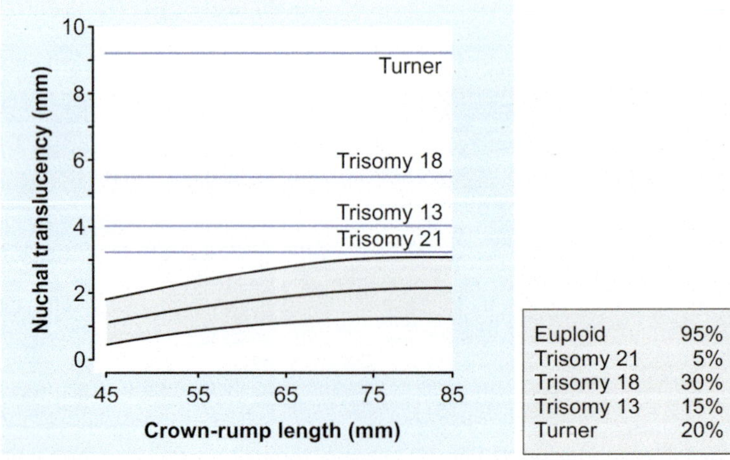

Fig. 4: Nuchal translucency nomogram against CRL, showing normal and abnormal values.

days along with karyotype, microarray is also recommended.

In cases of isolated increased nuchal translucency and normal karyotype, more than 90% of the fetuses are normal. When additional association with any other markers or congenital anomaly is present, the outcome may not be normal.

Although increased NT thickness is associated with abnormalities and fetal death, the majority of babies survives and develops normally.

After the diagnosis of increased NT, the aim must be to distinguish as accurately and quickly as possible between those that are likely to have problems from those where the baby is likely to be normal.

Tips to measure nuchal translucency:

- *First master profile in anomaly scan:* Fetus in first trimester moves much faster than in second. Hence, your probe movement needs to be swift.
- If you get correct crown rump length image, it is the same image zoomed for NT.
- Try keeping nasal bone horizontal and you will get clear nuchal translucency.
- Keep the probe pressure least so that the fetus can move.
- Best time to get NT is after the fetal jump.

Nasal Bone (Fig. 5)

It was in 1866, that absent or hypoplastic nasal bone was noted as a common characteristic of Down's syndrome. There is defective ossification in Down's syndrome fetuses. However, the nasal bone ossification is maternal race dependent. More than 50% of euploid Asians have unossified nasal bone. In the midsagittal section (nuchal translucency image), nasal bone should be visualized. The three echogenic lines represent tip of nose, skin, and nasal bone.

Nasal bone is unossified or hypoplastic in 60–70% of trisomy 21 fetuses, 50% of trisomy 18 fetuses, and 30% of trisomy 13 fetuses.

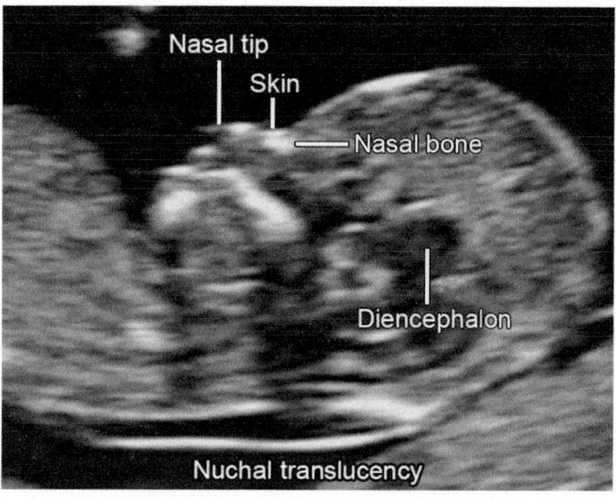

Fig. 5: Midsagittal plane of head and neck.

The length of nasal bone is more important in second trimester. Less than 2.5 mm at 15–21 weeks of gestation is considered hypoplastic.

Tips to measure nasal bone:

- Nasal bone should be kept horizontal to the probe
- Maxilla to be avoided
- Turning the probe 90° from premaxillary triangle image
- Good CRL or NT image should show nasal bone.

Ductus Venosus

Ductus venosus is a small vessel connecting the umbilical vein with the inferior vena cava (IVC).

Its main function is to provide the oxygenated blood to brain.

It shunts oxygenated blood to brain from umbilical vein (IVC to right atrium to left atrium via foramen ovale. From here, blood flows through right ventricle and aorta to fetal organs.)

After birth, when fetal lungs begin to function, there is closure of ductus venosus within few minutes after birth. However, it may be delayed in preterm neonates.

Criteria:

- *Fetus quiescent*: The fetus should not be moving.
- *Midsagittal plane*: Ductus venosus Doppler is performed in midsagittal plane (same as NT an CRL)

- *Zoom*: Only the thorax and abdomen should cover the whole of screen.
- *Doppler gate*: 0.5–1 mm, larger gate will cause contamination of waves with hepatic vein.
- Angle of insonation—should be <30.
- *Filter*—should be set at low (50–70 Hz), so as to view the whole waveform.
- *Sweep speed*—should be high for better assessment of the a-wave.

The high-velocity S wave is due to ventricular systole and D wave is due to diastole. The forward A wave is due to atrial contraction.

A positive or absent A wave is normal **(Figs. 6A to C)** while reversal of A wave is abnormal **(Figs. 7A and B)**. It is associated with cardiac abnormalities, chromosomal abnormalities, and fetal death.

Tips for measuring ductus venosus:

- Apart from fetal quiescence, ask mother to hold breath.
- On best CRL image place the color box, and apply pulse wave Doppler on the brightest color just below the fetal heart.

Fetal Heart Rate

Fetal heart rate is measured in transverse section of heart.

The normal heart rate is 110 beats/min at 5 weeks and increases to 170 beats/min at 10 weeks and then gradually decreases to 140 beats/min at 14 weeks.

There is an association of fetal heart rate and trisomy 21, 18, and 13.

In trisomy 21 and 13, fetal heart rate increases, whereas in trisomy 18, fetal heart rate decreases **(Table 3 and Fig. 8)**.

This is very important in trisomy 18 and 13 because this is the only feature to differentiate them, as both have increased NT and decreased serum β-hCG and PAPP-A levels in maternal serum.

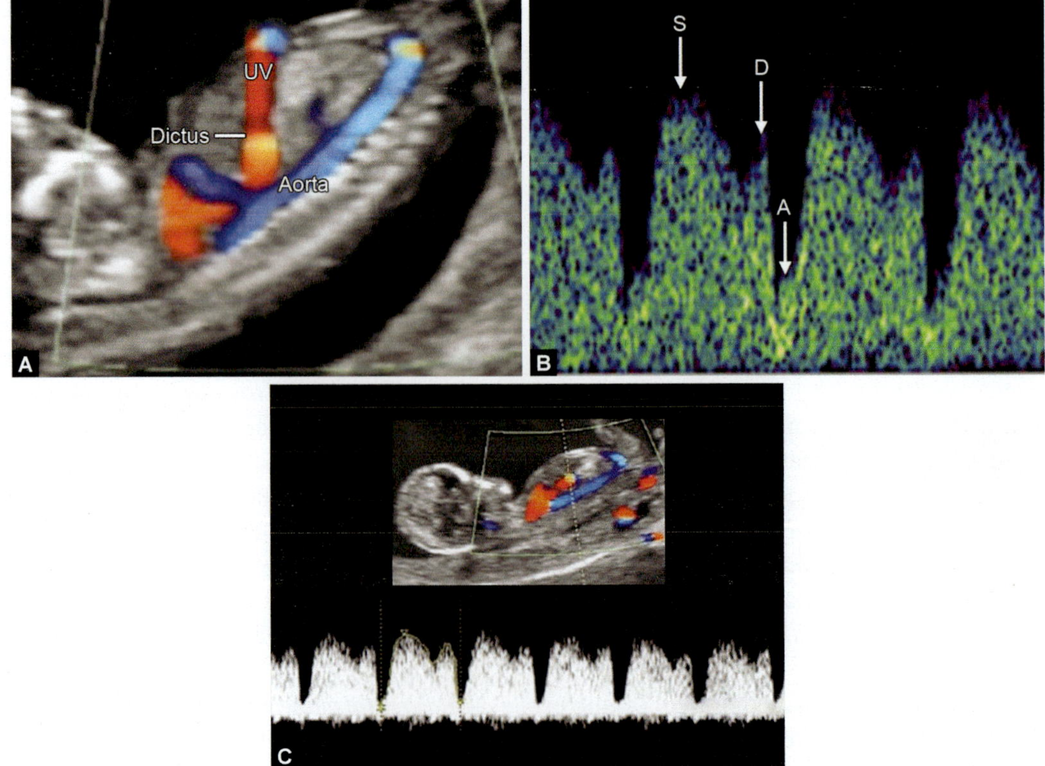

Figs. 6A to C: Normal ductus venosus flow on spectral Doppler.

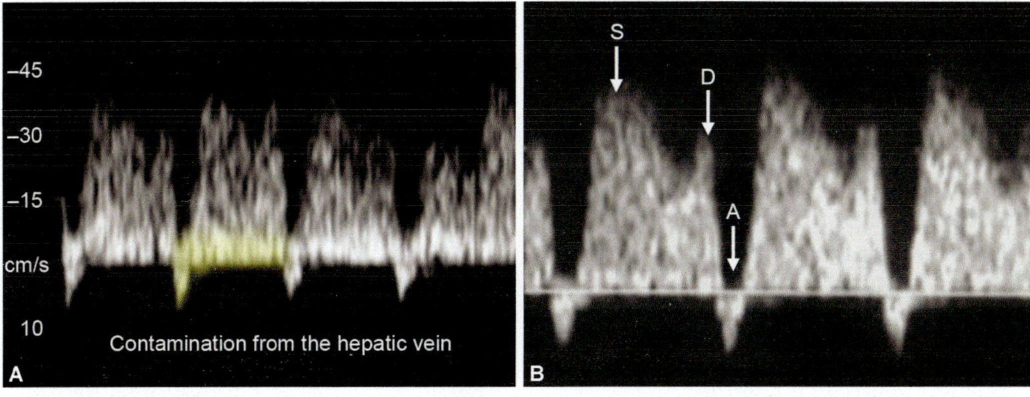

Figs. 7A and B: (A) Ductus venosus flow on spectral Doppler with contamination from the hepatic vein; (B) Abnormal ductus venosus flow on spectral Doppler with reverse A wave.

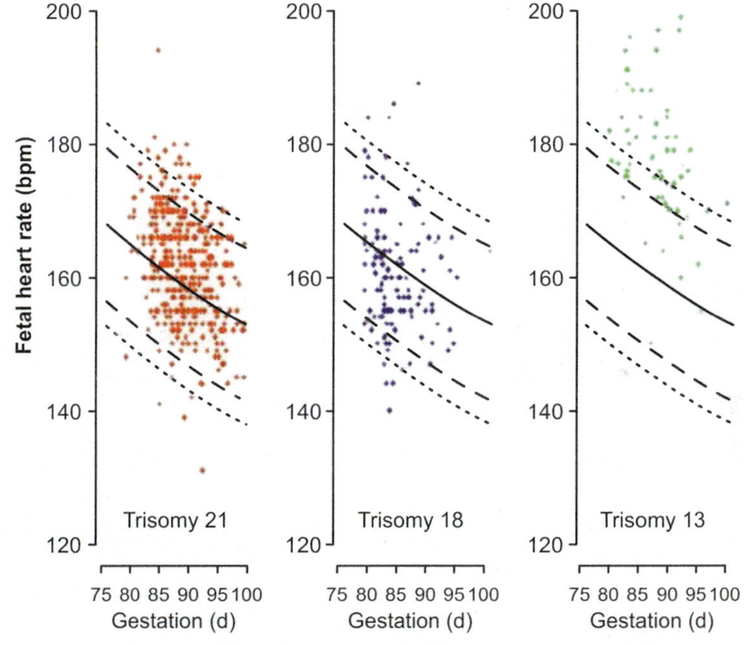

Fig. 8: Distribution of fetal heart rate in different trisomies at different CRL.

TABLE 3: Fetal heart rate variation in trisomy 18, 21, and 13.		
Trisomy 21	FHR increased and is above the 95th centile	In 15% of cases
Trisomy 18	FHR is mildly decreased and is below the 5th centile	In 15% of cases
Trisomy 13	FHR increased and is above the 95th centile	In 85% of cases

(FHR: fetal heart rate)

Fetal Tricuspid Flow

Tricuspid valve is located in the right of fetal heart between the atria and ventricle. It is more apical than mitral normally.

FMF criteria:

- The gestation should be 11^{+0} to 13^{+6} weeks and the CRL should be 45–84 mm.
- The fetus should not be moving.
- The magnification of the image should be such that the fetal thorax occupies the whole screen.

- An apical four-chamber view of the fetal heart should be obtained.
- Color flow mapping should not be used, because it is unreliable for the diagnosis of tricuspid regurgitation in the first trimester.
- The pulsed Doppler sample should be large (2–3 mm) and positioned across the tricuspid valve.
- The insonation angle to the direction of flow should be <30° from the direction of the interventricular septum.
- The tricuspid valve could be insufficient in one or more of its three cusps, and therefore the sample volume should be placed across the valve at least three times, in an attempt to interrogate the complete valve.
- The sweep speed should be high (2–3 cm/s) so that the waveforms are widely spread for better assessment.

Tricuspid regurgitation (TR) is diagnosed when there is reversal of flow with the velocity more than 60 cm/s. However, sometimes, the aortic and pulmonary arterial blood flow may intervene; however, their maximum velocity is not more than 50 cm/s.

Tricuspid regurgitation is seen in fetus with trisomy 21, 18, and 13 and fetal cardiac defects **(Figs. 9A to C)**.

There are other markers like facial angle, which are not much used for screening now.[2]

Second Trimester Soft Markers

The most common soft markers for fetal anomalies (SMFAs) in second trimester are nuchal thickening, hyperechoic bowel, shortened extremities, renal pyelectasis, echogenic intracardiac foci, choroid plexus cyst, strawberry-shaped skull, small, low-set ears, clubfoot, single umbilical artery,

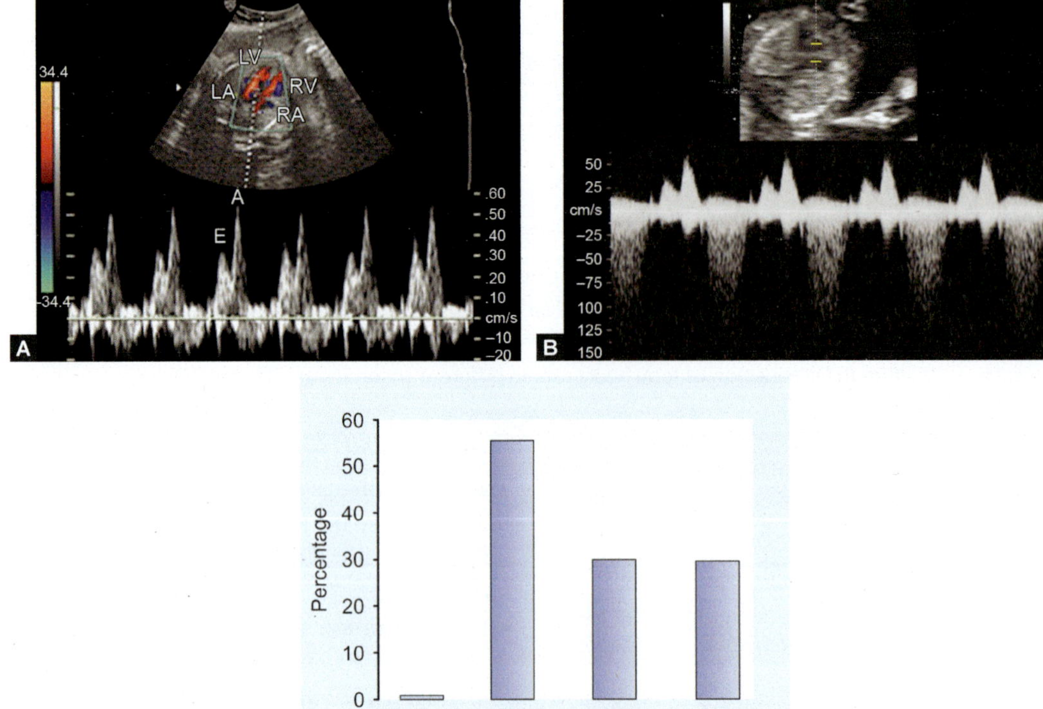

Figs. 9A to C: (A) Normal tricuspid flow with contamination from aorta on spectral Doppler; (B) Tricuspid regurge on spectral Doppler; (C) Incidence of tricustod regurge in normal and aneuploid fetuses.

TABLE 4: Pooled estimates of detection rate (DR), false positive rate (FPR) and positive and negative likelihood ratios (LR+ and LR-) of sonographic markers for trisomy 21 and estimated likelihood ratio (LR) of individual isolated markers.

Marker	*DR (95% CI) (%)*	*FPR (95% CI) (%)*	*LR+ (95% CI)*	*LR– (95% CI)*	*LR isolated marker**
Intracardiac echogenic focus	24.4 (20.9–28.2)	3.9 (3.4–4.5)	5.83 (5.02–6.77)	0.80 (0.75–0.86)	0.95
Ventriculomegaly	7.5 (4.2–12.9)	0.2 (0.1–0.4)	27.52 (13.61–55.68)	0.94 (0.91–0.98)	3.81
Increased nuchal fold	26.0 (20.3–32.9)	1.0 (0.5–1.9)	23.30 (14.35–37.83)	0.80 (0.74–0.85)	3.79
Echogenic bowel	16.7 (13.4–20.7)	1.1 (0.8–1.5)	11.44 (9.05–14.47)	0.90 (0.86–0.94)	1.65
Mild hydronephrosis	13.9 (11.2–17.2)	1.7 (1.4–2.0)	7.63 (6.11–9.51)	0.92 (0.89–0.96)	1.08
Short humerus	30.3 (17.1–47.9)	4.6 (2.8–7.4)	4.81 (3.49–6.62)	0.74 (0.63–0.88)	0.78
Short femur	27.7 (19.3–38.1)	6.4 (4.7–8.8)	3.72 (2.79–4.97)	0.80 (0.73–0.88)	0.61
ARSA	30.7 (17.8–47.4)	1.5 (1.0–2.1)	21.48 (11.48–40.19)	0.71 (0.57–0.88)	3.94
Absent or hypoplastic NB	59.8 (48.9–69.9)	2.8 (1.9–4.0)	23.27 (14.23–38.06)	0.46 (0.36–0.58)	6.58

*Derived by multiplying the positive LR for the given marker by the negative LR of each of all other markers, except for short humerus

(ARSA: aberrant right subclavian artery; NB: nasal bone)

clenched hands, omphalocele, and polydactyly **(Table 4)**.

In a meta-analysis of second trimester ultrasound markers for trisomy 21, Professor Nicolaides suggested that the combined negative LR of all markers, including short femur but not short humerus, was 0.13, implying that if a systematic ultrasound examination is carried out and all markers are excluded, there is a 7.7-fold reduction in risk.[3]

The most common and most important markers for aneuploidy include absent/unossified nasal bone, aberrant right subclavian artery, and increased nuchal fold thickness.

Soft Markers and their Implication (Table 5)

Absent/Unossified or Hypoplastic Nasal Bone

Absent of hypoplastic nasal bone is defined as one that is not visible in first trimester or with a length of <2.5 mm in the midsagittal section of the fetal profile in second trimester. The absence of a fetal nasal bone warrants a detailed evaluation of fetal anatomy. If there are no other anomalies and normal karyotype, it is reasonable to reassure that the likelihood of a good neonatal outcome is high. However, case reports have described an absent fetal nasal bone in B-cell immunodeficiency, cri-du-chat (5p–) syndrome, and partial trisomy 20q. Considering these cases, microarray studies could be performed in addition to a fetal karyotype when an absent fetal nasal bone occurs with additional sonographic anomalies.[16]

Aberrant Right Subclavian Artery

In aberrant right subclavian artery (ARSA), the usual pattern of development is slightly changed, preventing the typical formation of the three blood vessels. This leads to there being four branches rather than the normal three arising from the left aortic arch, one being the ARSA. It is present in 0.4% of the

TABLE 5: Proposal of a simple clinical summary for management of specific soft markers in pregnancies.

Marker	*Incidence (%)*	*Conditions*	*Considerations and follow-up*
Ventriculomegaly	3.0–15	• Aneuploidy • Genetic syndrome • Primary brain abnormalities • Congenital infection (CMV and toxoplasma) • Cerebrovascular accidents • Intracranial hemorrhage	• TORCH screening • Follow up scans to look for progression • Consider brain magnetic resonance imaging, if moderate-to-severe ventriculomegaly for detection of additional brain abnormalities
Choroid plexus cyst	2–4	Aneuploidy	Detail evaluation for other markers of aneuploidy
Absent or hypoplastic nasal bone	0.5–2.8	• Aneuploidy (especially trisomy 21) • B-cell immunodeficiency • Cri-du-chat syndrome • Partial trisomy 20q	• Detailed evaluation of fetal anatomy • Consider microarray studies (if with additional sonographic anomalies)
Thickened nuchal fold	0.4–0.6	• Down syndrome • Congenital heart disease	Evaluation of fetal heart, consider fetal echocardiography
Intracardiac echogenic focus	3–4	Down syndrome	• Detail evaluation for other markers of aneuploidy • More attention in multiple and right ventricle involved
Echogenic bowel	0.2–1.8	• Aneuploidy • Intrauterine growth restriction • Intrauterine fetal demise • Cystic fibrosis • Congenital infection (especially CMV) • Gastrointestinal anomaly	• Evaluation for cystic fibrosis • TORCH screening • 32-week ultrasound to assess for bowel dilatation or obstruction
Shortened humerus and femur length	0.4–3.9	• Aneuploidy • Structural abnormalities • Skeletal dysplasia • Preeclampsia • Preterm delivery • Oligohydramnios • Intrauterine growth restriction • Intrauterine fetal demise	• 32-week ultrasound to assess growth and to rule out certain skeletal dysplasia • Frequent blood pressure measurement • Study umbilical and uterine artery Doppler flow • Surveillance in timing of delivery
Pyelectasis	0.1–2.4	• UPJ obstruction • Vesicoureteral reflux • Posterior urethral valves • Ureteral obstruction • Other renal anomalies	• 32-week ultrasound to assess kidneys • Follow-up scans to look for progression • Postnatal follow-up, if >7 mm
Single umbilical artery	0.5–5	• Controversial aneuploidy • SGA • Preterm birth • Increased cesarean section rate	• Undergo targeted anatomical survey (level II ultrasound) • Controversial ultrasound to assess growth

(CMV: cytomegalovirus; TORCH: toxoplasmosis, rubella, cytomegalovirus, and herpes simplex; UPJ: ureteropelvic junction; SGA: small for gestational age) fetuses. Recent studies indicate it is not associated with increased risk of aneuploidy.

Increased Nuchal Fold Thickness

Thickened nuchal fold (NF) **(Fig. 10)** is defines as—thickening of the skin and the subcutaneous tissues on the posterior aspect of the fetal neck measuring 6 mm or greater before 20+6 weeks' gestation. Its prevalence is 1–6 per 1,000.[5] It is measured in axial section at the level of the transcerebellar diameter just behind the posterior fossa. It is associated with chromosomal and genetic disorders. It can also be a pointer to cardiac disorders.

Ventriculomegaly (Fig. 11)

Fetal ventriculomegaly (VM) is defined as a dilatation of the lateral ventricle atrium to a width of 10 mm or more. A measurement of 10–12 mm is commonly referred to as mild VM, while measurements of 12–15 and >15 mm are defined as moderate and severe VM. Its prevalence varies between 0.3 and 1.5 per 1,000 births.[11] VM has been associated with normal variant, aneuploidy, genetic syndromes, primary brain abnormalities, congenital infection such as cytomegalovirus (CMV) and toxoplasma, cerebrovascular accidents, and intracranial hemorrhage.[11-13]

Isolated mild and moderate VM regresses or becomes stable in diameters contrast to severe VM. In the systematic review and meta-analysis of Scala et al.,[11] the fetuses with isolated unilateral VM had 0% chromosomal abnormalities, 8% congenital infection, and in about 5% of fetuses, there is progression of VM during the course of the pregnancy. The prevalence of neurodevelopmental delay in cases of apparently isolated unilateral mild or moderate VM was 6%, and in severe VM, it was 7%. High rates of cerebral palsy, seizures, and impaired motor capabilities were observed in severe VM.[11-13] The prevalence of neurodevelopmental delay in bilateral mild and moderate VM varies between 8 and 12%.[14] Magnetic resonance imaging can be used for further elucidation of cases with ventricular enlargement.[13]

The overall prognosis of VM strongly depends on both the extent of enlargement and/or the presence of other abnormal findings or structural malformations. Also, asymmetric pattern of VM is a potential risk factor for anomalies of neuropsychological development.[13]

Screening for congenital infection should be part of prenatal workup, especially if VM with increased periventricular echogenicity, calcification, periventricular pseudocysts, and intraventricular synechia.[20] Diagnosis of toxoplasma and CMV infection is based on positive specific immunoglobulin M results with confirmatory immunoglobulin G avidity test. In case of a positive result for

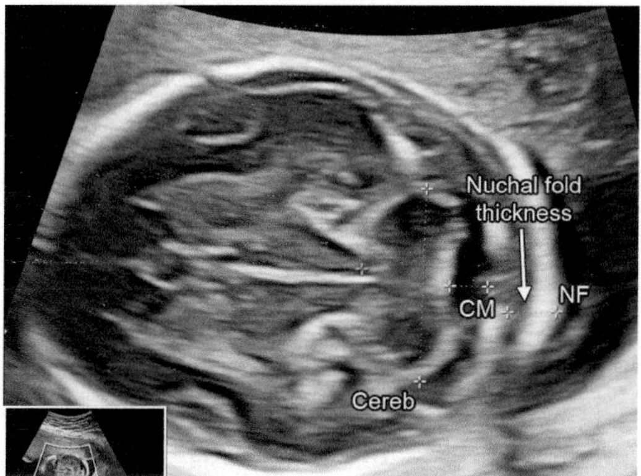

Fig. 10: B mode image showing nuchal fold thickness measurement.

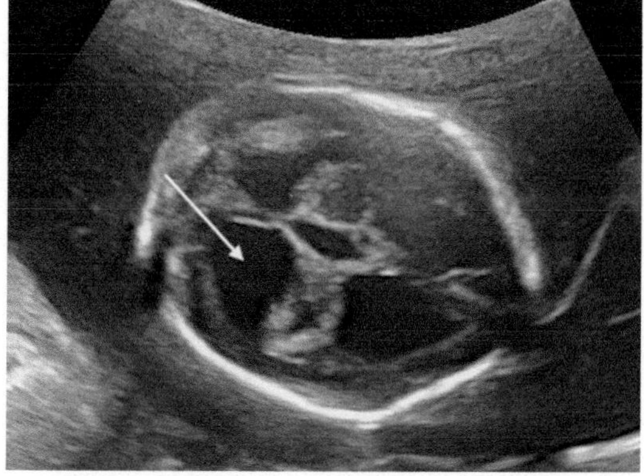

Fig. 11: B mode image of axial section of fetal head showing ventriculomegaly.

toxoplasma infection in maternal serum, amniocentesis is performed to determine the presence of the pathogen in the amniotic fluid by amplification of DNA, using polymerase chain reaction.[21]

Repeated ultrasound scans to follow VM size or extension of VM are recommended because it is correlated with the prognosis.[11-14]

Echogenic Bowel (Fig. 12)

Echogenic bowel is defined as fetal bowel of similar or greater echogenicity than the surrounding bone or fetal liver. The prevalence is ranging from 0.2 to 1.8%. Echogenic bowel resolves spontaneously in 19.7% of cases and the association with Down syndrome reports likelihood ratio of 5.5–6.7.[8]

Echogenic bowel has been described as normal variant, but may be associated with congenital viral infections (particularly CMV), aneuploidy, intra-amniotic bleeding, severe uteroplacental insufficiency, meconium peritonitis, cystic fibrosis, anemia, and fetal growth restriction (FGR).[3,6,13] Therefore, a comprehensive examination and evaluation for CMV infection is suggested, in addition to correlation with aneuploidy testing results.

Serial growth assessment is advocated, as it is associated with FGR and sometimes sudden intrauterine fetal demise [relative risk (RR) 1.6 for FGR and 8.6 for intrauterine fetal demise].

Fetal Pyelectasis

Fetal pyelectasis is defined as an anteroposterior measurement in a transverse scanning plane of 4 mm or larger in second trimester and/or 7 mm **(Fig. 13)** or larger in third trimester, whereas pelvic anteroposterior diameter of 10 mm or larger is criterion for hydronephrosis.[23] The prevalence of pyelectasis varies from 0.1 to 2.4% in low-risk populations.[4]

While most commonly fetal pyelectasis is a transient physiologic state, it can be a marker for aneuploidy and be a precursor of potential urinary tract pathology. The majority of cases of pyelectasis detected in the second trimester will resolve either before delivery or within the first year of postnatal life.[8-10]

Isolated mild pyelectasis in low-risk population is not the evidence of increased risk of aneuploidy and, therefore, it cannot be considered as an indication for the determination of the karyotype.[10]

A prenatal progression of dilatation of pyelectasis was directly related to a worse outcome. Therefore, a follow-up ultrasound at 32 weeks of gestation to rule out persistent pyelectasis should be performed. At this time, approximately half of cases will be normal,

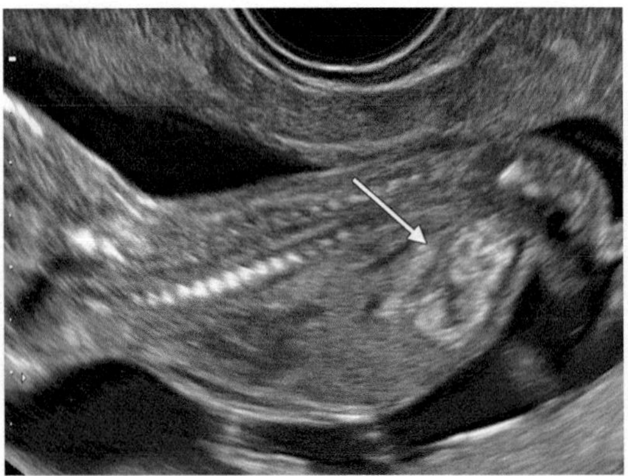

Fig. 12: B mode image of fetus in long axis showing hyperechoic bowel.

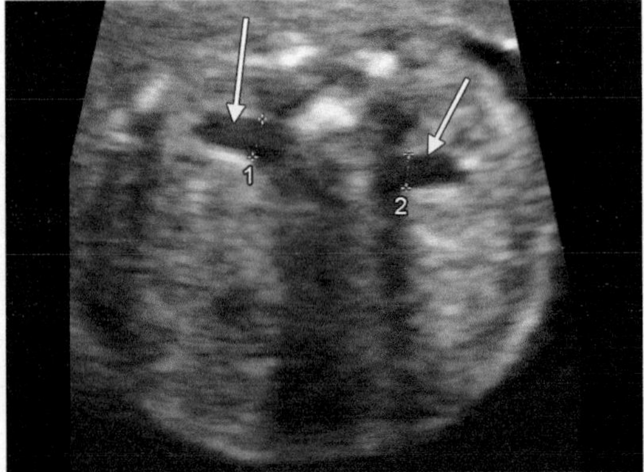

Fig. 13: B mode image of axial section of fetal abdomen showing renal pelvis and their measurement done on both the sides.

30% will continue to have mild pyelectasis, and 15% will have more significant hydronephrosis. If the renal pelvis measures >7 mm at 30 week examination, postnatal follow-up is suggested.[9,10]

Intracardiac Echogenic Foci (Fig. 14)

Intracardiac echogenic focus (IEF) is defined as an echogenic small spot inside the heart having brightness equivalent to that of the bone. It is most commonly located in the left ventricle of heart. They are found in about 3–4% of normal fetuses and in about 25% of those with trisomy 21.[6,22]

Isolated IEFs are associated with an increased risk of Down syndrome, with likelihood ratios generally ranging from 1.5 to 5.0.[17] In about 90% of cases, they resolve by the third trimester of pregnancy.[6] Isolated IEF in low-risk first-trimester combined screening (FTS) or negative noninvasive prenatal testing (NIPT) cases is considered as a normal variant. Hence, it is not an indication for direct testing.

Short Femur and Short Humerus

Shortened humerus and femur are defined as bone length below the 5th percentile for gestational age.[30] Shortened humerus length (HL) and femur length (FL) were observed in 0.4–3.9% of normal fetus.[26] Fetal short long bones have been associated with aneuploidy, skeletal dysplasia, fetal structural anomalies, pre-eclampsia, stillbirth, and FGR. Trisomy 21, 18, 13, or an unbalanced autosomal structural abnormality is associated with relative short FL (risk: 1:123; 95% CI: 79–192).[18,19]

Choroid Plexus Cyst

Choroid plexus cyst (CPC) is a small sonographically discrete fluid-filled space **(Fig. 15)** ≥5 mm within the choroid plexus and CPC is seen as black echo-free areas. CPC is found in approximately 0.3–3.6% of fetuses.

In women with isolated CPC and negative FTS and NIPT, the finding of CPC may be described as not clinically significant or as a normal variant.[7] CPC is not considered a structural nor functional brain abnormality. Isolated CPCs in fetuses with normal karyotypes do not affect child mental and motor development after birth.[15]

Thus, we can divide the soft markers into soft markers for aneuploidy (unossified nasal bone, increased nuchal fold thickness, ventriculomegaly, and short long bones) and likely normal variants (echogenic bowel, mild hydronephrosis, intracardiac echogenic foci, ARSA, and single umbilical artery).

Apart from the above soft markers, in case of any structural abnormalities, further testing is needed. Some of them are described in **Table 6**.

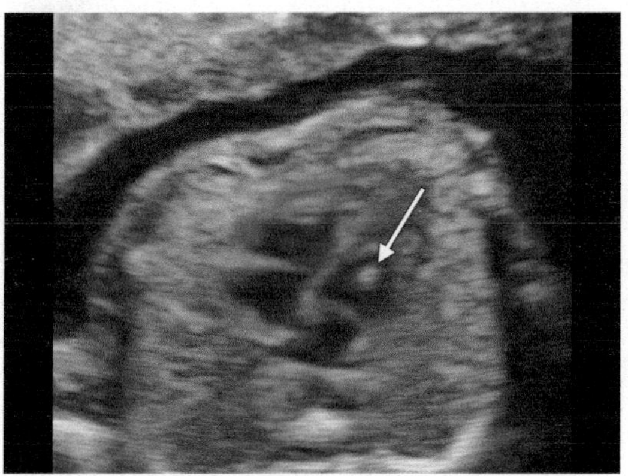

Fig. 14: 4 chamber heart view showing echogenic focus in left ventricle.

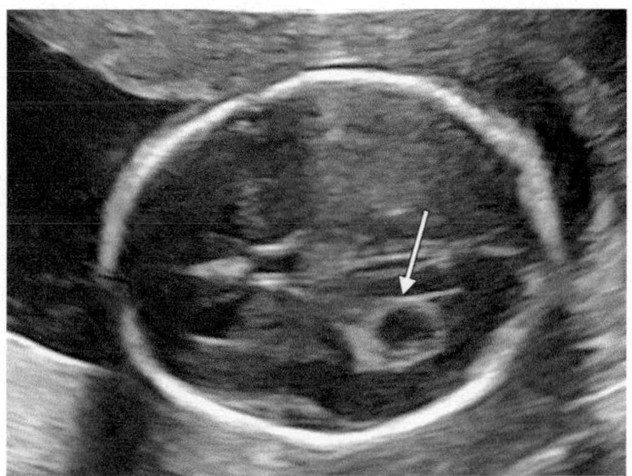

Fig. 15: B mode image of axial section of the fetal head showing choroid plexus cyst.

TABLE 6: Other soft markers that need further testing.[29]	
Diaphragmatic hernia	• There is herniation of intra-abdominal organs and bowel loops into the thorax • The cause of fetal demise is fetal pulmonary hypoplasia
Strawberry-shaped head	Brachycephaly is a common pathologic feature of trisomy 18
Polydactyly	Associated with trisomy 13
Clinodactyly	• Associated with trisomy 21 • Curved little finger and small middle phalanx of little finger
Clenched hand	Clenched hand is associated with trisomy 18
Radial aplasia	
Clubfoot	Associated with trisomy 18
Omphalocele	• Herniation of midgut by anterior abdominal wall • Omphaloceles with bowel only carry much greater risk for aneuploidy than do omphaloceles that contain liver
Duodenal atresia	• Associated with trisomy 21 • Double-bubble sign and polyhydramnios appear mostly after 20–24 weeks
Single umbilical artery/umbilical cord abnormalities	• SUA is characterized by absence of one of umbilical arteries and it occurs in 0.2–1% of pregnancies • When isolated, it is not associated with aneuploidy in low-risk FTS or negative NIPT population. Its association with fetal growth restriction is still under doubt[24]
Umbilical cord cysts/pseudocysts	
Placental abnormalities	• Appropriate gestational age (in weeks) = placental thickness ± 10 mm • Thickened placenta and cystic changes in placenta with oligohydramnios and early onset IUGR—chromosomal abnormality should be suspected
Polyhydramnios	• Idiopathic polyhydramnios is most commonly associated with a large for gestational age fetus, with or without maternal diabetes • Amniotic fluid index more than 25 mm
Oligohydramnios	Amniotic fluid index <8 mm
Spina bifida	• Failure of closure of neural tube resulting into neural tube defects • Spina bifida occulta and aperta are the two types representing close and open type of neural tube defects, respectively • Maternal use of folate can decrease the risk of developing neural tube defects • Risk factors for spina bifida are—maternal diabetes mellitus and previous fetus with neural tube defect
Holoprosencephaly	Absent or partial segmentation of fetal brain parenchyma with facial defects and cyclopia
Anencephaly	Absent cranial vault and cerebral hemisphere
Megacystis	• Length >7 mm at 11–14 weeks FMF (fetal medicine foundation) • Associated with trisomy 18 and 13
Agenesis of the corpus callosum	
Cleft lip and cleft palate	An upper lip or lower lip defect may be seen and is best appreciated on angled coronal scanning
Cystic hygroma	• *Cystic hygroma*, also known as *cystic* or *nuchal lymphangioma*, is a congenital lymphatic malformation that most commonly occurs in the posterior cervical triangle in infants • They are now called as macrocystic lymphatic malformation • Features of fetal anasarca or hydrops may be present • Associated with cardiac defects, chromosomal abnormalities, and fetal demise

(FTS: first-trimester combined screening; IUGR: intrauterine growth restriction; NIPT: noninvasive prenatal testing; SUA: single umbilical artery)

BIOCHEMICAL MARKERS

First Trimester

- *Serum-free beta-hCG*: Human chorionic gonadotropin is a glycoprotein produced by the placenta, composed of two subunits—α and β. Maternal serum contains intact as well as free α- and free β-hCG. In case of anomalies of placenta leading to disturbance in fluid homeostasis are associated high levels of free β-hCG in maternal serum.
- *Pregnancy-associated plasma protein-A (PAPP-A)*: PAPP-A is produced by placental trophoblasts. Lower values of PAPP-A is observed in trisomy 21. Hence, it is of value for screening for aneuploidy. It has also been observed that low values of PAPP-A is correlated with pre-eclampsia and fetal growth restriction.
- *Alpha-fetoprotein (α-FP)*: The α-FP is produced by fetal liver, but its biological functions and the reason why the α-FP level is lower in Down syndrome pregnancies remain unclear. Placentas of affected pregnancies show a high level of α-FP suggesting a defect in the secretion of α-FP into the maternal circulation.[30]
- *Placental growth factor (PLGF)*: PLGF is a human protein encoded by the *PGF* gene, which is implicated in the angiogenesis and trophoblastic invasion of the maternal spiral arteries during placentation in early pregnancy.[1]

Maternal serum levels of PLGF at 11–13 weeks' gestation are decreased in pregnancies with impaired placentation resulting in increased risks for pre-eclampsia and delivery of small for gestational age (SGA) and growth restricted (intrauterine growth restriction) neonates.[2,25,26]

Second Trimester

Alpha fetoprotein and free β-hCG are also utilized in second trimester screening. Other markers include unconjugated estriol and inhibin A.

Unconjugated Estriol

The placenta uses 16α-hydroxydehydroepiandrosterone sulfate (DHEAS) as the precursor of μE3. In Down syndrome pregnancies, both μE3 and DHEAS present lower levels in different tissues, including placenta.[31] During the second trimester, the concentration of μE3 rises quickly and this marker can identify pregnancies with a small or underdeveloped fetus at the time of screening.[27]

Inhibin A

Inhibin is a glycoprotein synthesized by gonads and placenta. The functional protein is dimeric with two subunits—α and β. Inhibin-A (INH-A) is increased in pregnancies with trisomy 21. INH-A allows a good distinction between affected and unaffected pregnancies, alone or in combination with hCG.[32]

SCREENING POLICY FOR ANEUPLOIDY

Screening policy for any disorder depends primarily on the disease prevalence, the morbidity and mortality due to the disease, screening test ability to detect the disease, the false positive, and false negative.

In case of Down's syndrome, the need arouse when all appeared normal on sonography and yet children were seen with morbidity and unable to live a normal life. The screening began with maternal age, triple marker test, and then quadruple marker test, improvising to dual marker test, and nuchal translucency.

The two important aspects we need to understand while using a screening protocol are the detection rate and false-negative rate. Utilizing various permutations, we aim to improve the detection rate while minimizing the false-positive and false-negative rates. Also, it is important to note that the financial considerations and availability of the screening test also play an important role.

TABLE 7: Screening policies for fetal aneuploidies.

Policy	*Detection rate*	*cfDNA*	*False-positive rate*	*Cost per sample (approximate)*	*Cut-off*
Maternal age	58%	NA	18%	No	
Triple marker test[28]	56% 70% 77%	NA	1% 3% 5%	2,500–3,000	
Quadruple marker test	66% 79% 84%	NA	1% 3% 5%	2,500–3,000	1:250
Nuchal translucency	71%	NA	3.5%	1,200–1,500	
Combined first trimester screening (dual marker with NT)	90%	NA	5%	2,500–3,000	1:250
Dual marker with NT, NB, DV, and TR	93.8%	NA	3.4%	2,500–3,000	1:250
Extended FTS (free B-hCG, PAPP-A, aFP, PLGF + NT, NB, and DV)	93.8% 96%	NA	1.2% 2.5%	4,000	1:100 1:250
NT scan with NIPS	99%	100%	0.1% (4% failure rate)	12,000	
Combined FTS followed by NIPS for intermediate risk	94.6% (intermediate risk 1:1,000) 96.3% (intermediate risk 1:2,000) 96.9% (intermediate risk 1:3,000)	cfDNA rate: 12.1% 19.2% 24.5%	0.1%	Most— 2,500–3,000 Few—12,000	1:100 invasive testing (0.37–0.39%)
eFTS followed by NIPS for intermediate risk	96.9% (intermediate risk 1:1,000) 97.6% (intermediate risk 1:2,000) 98% (intermediate risk 1:3,000)	cfDNA rate: 6.4% 9.8% 12.8%	0.1%	Most—4,000 Few—12,000	1:100 Invasive testing (0.34%)

(β-hCG: β-human chorionic gonadotropin; cfDNA: cell-free DNA; PAPP-A: pregnancy associated plasma protein A; aFP: alpha-fetoprotein; PLGF: placental growth factor; NT: nuchal translucency; NB: nasal bone; DV: Du+ctus venosus; NIPS: noninvasive prenatal screening)

The incidence of Down's syndrome is 1:800. The screening policies are described in **Table 7**.

What the **Table 7** guides us to is—combined first trimester screening is a great policy for a detection rate of 90% for a reasonable cost. Importance is for the nuchal translucency to be correctly measured and dual marker test to be measured with 48 hours.

The triple and quadruple marker test is costlier and also has a lower detection rate. Hence, it should not be encouraged.

Noninvasive prenatal screening (NIPS) is very promising in detection rate but has a failure rate of 3%. The lowering of cost will make it for all population.

In spite of NIPS, nuchal translucency and dual marker have additional advantages; hence, their presence is inevitable in screening.

Twin Pregnancies

Chromosomal Abnormalities

As in single pregnancy, in twin pregnancy also, we will measure maternal age related a prior risk.

- *In monozygotic twins*, the risk for a chromosomal abnormality affecting both fetuses is the same. The risk for trisomy 21 is calculated for each fetus and then the average risk between the two fetuses is considered to be the risk for the pregnancy as a whole.
- *In DC twins*, the patient-specific risks for trisomy 21 are different for the two fetuses because of differences in NT.
- In triplets and quadruplets, *maternal serum markers cannot be used hence only ultrasound-based risk is calculated.*

Final Consensus:

- Aneuploidy screening is definitely indicated for all pregnancies.
- Triple marker test is an outdated one.
- First-trimester screening is the best form of screening for aneuploidy.
- When in doubt, direct testing is warranted.
- NIPS has no role, if any abnormal ultrasound marker is present.
- Microarray is preferred choice over karyotype.

Best form of aneuploidy screening policy in descending order:

- eFTS + NIPS
- eFTS followed by NIPS/direct testing for intermediate screening
- FTS followed by genetic sonogram for intermediate screening
- Quadruple marker test (if patient comes directly in 2nd trimester)
- Genetic sonogram
- Triple marker test (only if quadruple marker test is not available)

In case of high-risk or when in doubt, direct testing is advisable. Microarray is preferred test in case of abnormal ultrasound marker to rule out single gene disorders. Karyotype is still the standard genetic test performed.

REFERENCES

1. Rizos D. Prenatal screening for chromosomal abnormalities: Where do we stand today in Mediterranean countries? EJIFCC. 2018;29(4):274-9.
2. Nicolaides KH. The 11-13+6 weeks scan. London: Fetal Medicine Foundation; 2004.
3. Agathokleous M, Chaveeva P, Poon LCY, Kosinski P, Nicolaides KH. Meta-analysis of second trimester markers for trisomy 21. Ultrasound Obstet Gynecol. 2013;41:247-61.
4. Ahman A, Axelsson O, Maras G, Rubertsson C, Sarkadi A, Lindgren P. Ultrasonographic fetal soft markers in a low-risk population: prevalence, association with trisomies and invasive tests. Acta Obstet Gynecol Scand. 2014;93:367-73.
5. Hurt L, Wright M, Brook F, Thomas S, Dunstan F, Fone D, et al. The Welsh study of mothers and babies: protocol for a population-based cohort study to investigate the clinical significance of defined ultrasound findings of uncertain significance. BMC Pregnancy Childbirth. 2014;14:164.
6. Cicero S, Sacchini C, Rembouskos G, Nicolaides KH. Sonographic markers of fetal aneuploidy—a review. Placenta. 2003;24(Suppl B):S88-98.
7. Norton ME, Biggio JR, Kuller JA, Blackwell SC; Society for Maternal- Fetal Medicine (SMFM). The role of ultrasound in women who undergo cell-free DNA screening. Am J Obstet Gynecol. 2017;216:B2-7.
8. Norton ME. Follow-up of sonographically detected soft markers for fetal aneuploidy. Semin Perinatol. 2013;37:365-9.
9. Mallik M, Watson AR. Antenatally detected urinary tract abnormalities: more detection but less action. Pediatr Nephrol. 2008;23:897-904.
10. Signorelli M, Cerri V, Taddei F, Groli C, Bianchi UA. Prenatal diagnosis and management of mild fetal pyelectasis: implications for neonatal outcome and follow-up. Eur J Obstet Gynecol Reprod Biol. 2005;118:154-9.
11. Scala C, Familiari A, Pinas A, Papageorghiou AT, Bhide A, Thilaganathan B, et al. Perinatal and long-term outcomes in fetuses diagnosed with isolated unilateral ventriculomegaly: systematic review and meta-analysis. Ultrasound Obstet Gynecol. 2017;49:450-9.
12. Bar-Yosef O, Barzilay E, Dorembus S, Achiron R, Katorza E. Neurodevelopmental outcome of isolated ventriculomegaly: a prospective cohort study. Prenat Diagn. 2017;37:764-8.
13. Weichert J, Hartge D, Krapp M, Germer U, Gembruch U, Axt-Fliedner R. Prevalence, characteristics and perinatal outcome of fetal ventriculomegaly in 29,000 pregnancies followed at a single institution. Fetal Diagn Ther. 2010;27:142-8.
14. Pagani G, Thilaganathan B, Prefumo F. Neurodevelopmental outcome in isolated mild fetal ventriculomegaly: systematic review and

meta-analysis. Ultrasound Obstet Gynecol. 2014;44:254-60.

15. DiPietro JA, Cristofalo EA, Voegtline KM, Crino J. Isolated prenatal choroid plexus cysts do not affect child development. Prenat Diagn. 2011;31:745-9.
16. Dukhovny S, Wilkins-Haug L, Shipp TD, Benson CB, Kaimal AJ, Reiss R. Absent fetal nasal bone: what does it mean for the euploid fetus? J Ultrasound Med. 2013;32:2131-4.
17. Nyberg DA, Souter VL, El-Bastawissi A, Young S, Luthhardt F, Luthy DA. Isolated sonographic markers for detection of fetal Down syndrome in the second trimester of pregnancy. J Ultrasound Med. 2001;20:1053-63.
18. Kaijomaa M, Ulander VM, Ryynanen M, Stefanovic V. Risk of adverse outcomes in euploid pregnancies with isolated short fetal femur and humerus on second-trimester sonography. J Ultrasound Med. 2016;35: 2675-80.
19. Mathiesen JM, Aksglaede L, Skibsted L, Petersen OB, Tabor A; Danish Fetal Medicine Study Group. Outcome of fetuses with short femur length detected at second-trimester anomaly scan: a national survey. Ultrasound Obstet Gynecol. 2014;44:160-5.
20. Malinger G, Lev D, Lerman-Sagie T. Imaging of fetal cytomegalovirus infection. Fetal Diagn Ther. 2011;29:117-26.
21. Pasquini L, Seravalli V, Sisti G, Battaglini C, Nepi F, Pelagalli R, et al. Prevalence of a positive TORCH and parvovirus B19 screening in pregnancies complicated by polyhydramnios. Prenat Diagn. 2016;36:290-3.
22. Wax JR, Donnelly J, Carpenter M, Chard R, Pinette MG, Blackstone J, et al. Childhood cardiac function after prenatal diagnosis of intracardiac echogenic foci. J Ultrasound Med. 2003;22:783-7.
23. Odibo AO, Marchiano D, Quinones JN, Riesch D, Egan JF, Macones GA. Mild pyelectasis: evaluating the relationship between gestational age and renal pelvic anterior-posterior diameter. Prenat Diagn. 2003;23:824-7.
24. Kim MS, Kang S, Cho HY. Clinical significance of sonographic soft markers: A review. J Genet Med. 2018;15(1):1-7.
25. Nyberg DA, Mahony BS, Luthy D, Kapur R. Single umbilical artery. Prenatal detection of concurrent anomalies. J Ultrasound Med. 1991;10(5):247-53.
26. Coultas L, Chawengsaksophak K, Rossant J. Endothelial cells and VEGF in vascular development. Nature. 2005;438(7070):937-45.
27. Schlembach D, Wallner W, Sengenberger R, Stiegler E, Mörtl M, Beckmann MW, et al. Angiogenic growth factor levels in maternal and fetal blood: correlation with Doppler ultrasound parameters in pregnancies complicated by pre-eclampsia and intrauterine growth restriction. Ultrasound Obstet Gynecol. 2007;29(04):407-13.
28. Reynolds T. The Triple test as a screening technique for down syndrome: reliability and relevance. Int J Womens Health. 2010;2:83-8.
29. Wald NJ, Rodeck C, Hackshaw AK, Walters J, Chitty L, Mackinson AM. First and Second Trimester Antenatal Screening for Down's Syndrome: the results of the Serum, Urine And Ultrasound Screening Study (SURUSS). J Med Screen. 2003;10:56-104.
30. Nicolaides KH, Wright D, Poon LC, Syngelaki A, Gil MM. First-trimester contingent screening for trisomy 21 by biomarkers and maternal blood cell-free DNA testing. Ultrasound Obstet Gynecol. 2013;92:41-50.
31. DNewby, Aitken DA, Howatson AG, Connor JM. Placental Synthesis of Oestriol in Down's Syndrome Pregnancies. Placenta. 2000;21(2-3):263-7.
32. Wald NJ, Cuckle HS, Densem JW, et al. Maternal serum screening for Down's syndrome in early pregnancy. BMJ, 1988;297:883-7.

7

CHAPTER

Second Trimester Scan

Sonal Panchal

INTRODUCTION

By 18–19 weeks, most of the fetal organs become functional and so is considered to be a good time to assess the fetus in detail to exclude any anomalies. Moreover, the bones are also not too dense at this stage to obstruct the view of the soft tissues of the fetus. By this time, the process of placentation is also complete and so this scan is usually also combined with Doppler of uterine and umbilical arteries. It carries the importance almost equal to 11–13+6 weeks scan. This scan is usually done between 18 and 20 weeks and maximum up to 22 weeks. The optimum time period of doing this scan may vary a little in different parts of the world depending on the local rules for permission of legal abortions.

Though usually this scan is not done before 18 weeks, it may be planned at 16–18 weeks especially for fetuses at a higher risk of abnormalities. This group may include those with abnormal ultrasound findings or abnormal biochemical markers in the first trimester, fetuses of mothers with previous abnormal babies, old age mothers, mothers with metabolic derangements, etc.

How to proceed?

As mentioned earlier, this scan is done to assess the complete fetal anatomy and a systematic approach is required. Before starting the scan, it is essential to confirm the date of last menstrual period and document it. Document also age, body mass index (BMI), and the vitals such as blood pressure and heart rate. Confirm that patient does not have a history of any infection in the first trimester, bleeding during first trimester, or any history of abortions during previous pregnancy. Along with, it is also essential to know in detail about any other genetic, metabolic, or endocrinal diseases that may be present in maternal or paternal family of the fetus or in siblings. A dating scan is expected to be done in the first trimester but if no scan is done earlier, dating must be done with this scan using biparietal diameter, head circumference, abdominal circumference and femur length as primary biometric parameters.

PRIMARY ESSENTIALS OF SCANNING

Scan may be done in lying down position or in a recumbent position in reclining examination chair/bed. Confirm that patient is in comfortable position and it is possible to assess the maternal abdomen adequately and comfortably for the sonographer. Patient must be adequately covered and her privacy should be maintained. The scan must be started by primary survey of the entire maternal abdomen to find out the number of fetuses and the position of the fetus/fetuses (lie, spine position, and presentation). Placental location is confirmed and mentioned. Any abnormalities in the uterus such as fibroids must be mentioned with its location in relation to placenta and its size and echogenicity must be documented.

As the fetal assessment is started, it is ideal to move from crown to feet or feet to crown in any fetus, so that no part of the body would remain unassessed. But, it is known that fetus is moving and sometimes may be very active to allow to assess the intended part of its body. Therefore, when doing fetal assessment, one has to be opportunistic and start with imaging the part of the fetal body that is readily seen. In this case, it might be possible to skip or forget to image and assess certain parts of the fetal body; therefore, it is best to make a checklist of the sections and measurements of the fetal body required and confirm that all the items on the checklist are assessed before the scan is declared complete.

A list of mandatory sections suggested by the Fetal Medicine Foundation (FMF), UK and most authentic workers in the field for this scan is as follows:

- *Head and face*:
  - Axial sections:
    - Transventricular plane
    - Transthalamic plane—optional
    - Transcerebellar plane
    - Transorbital plane
    - Maxillary plane
  - *Coronal plane*:
    - Lips
    - Lenses
  - *Midsagittal plane*:
    - Nasal bone and frontomaxillary facial angle
- *Trunk*:
  - *Axial sections*:
    - *Thorax*:
      - Four-chamber view of the heart
      - Right ventricular outflow tract (RVOT)
      - Left ventricular outflow tract (LVOT)
      - Three-vessel view
    - *Abdomen*:
      - Stomach section for abdominal circumference
      - Kidneys
      - Umbilical cord insertion
      - Transverse sacrum
  - *Sagittal plane*:
    - Spine
    - Bladder
    - Aortic arch—optional
    - Ductus arch—optional
  - *Coronal plane*:
    - Spine
  - *Limbs*:
    - All four limbs and all three segments
    - Sagittal leg and foot
    - Forearm with hand

It is very essential that all these sections are imaged in a standardized manner to be reliable and comparable with least interobserver and intraobserver variations. It is also important for optimal anatomical analysis and also for the measurements (biometry) that are to be used for assessment of fetal growth or prediction of any abnormalities of the fetus. To minimize the errors in anatomical details and measurements, it is also essential that the image is optimized and area of interest must be in the center of the screen and sufficient zoom should be used, so that the image covers at least two-thirds of the screen.

So, let us discuss the details of each of these sections and the fetal anatomy that these demonstrate.

Head: Axial Sections

Transventricular Plane

This plane cuts through the ventricles as shown in **Figure 1** as line a. The optimum section must show posterior horns of lateral ventricles, choroid plexus, lateral sulcus, falx, cavum septum pellucidum, and anterior horns

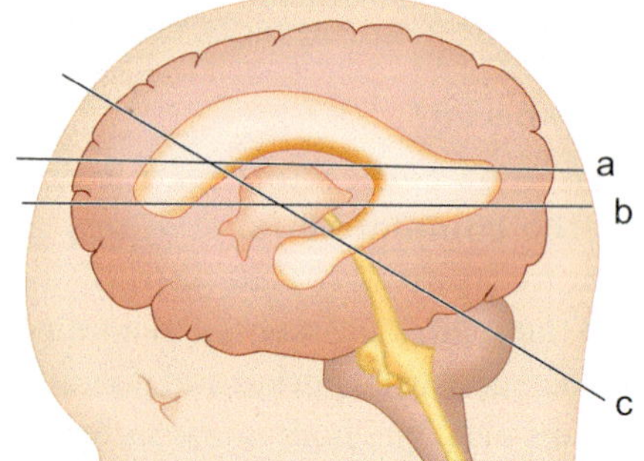

Fig. 1: Diagram showing the three basic axial sections of the head. (a) transventricular section, (b) transthalamic section, and (c) transcerebellar section.

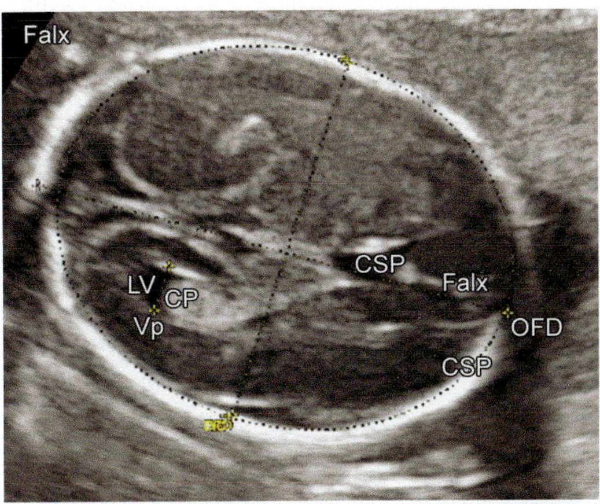

Fig. 2: Transventricular section of the fetal head showing falx, cavum septum pellucidum (CSP), and choroid plexuses (CPs) in posterior horns of lateral ventricles (LVs).
(OFD: occipitofrontal diameter)

of lateral ventricles **(Fig. 2)**. The oval shape of the skull vault is seen in this section and the calvarial thickness should be symmetrical all around and not >3 mm in second trimester. Thicker calvarial thickness and especially asymmetrical may suggest an oblique section.

Thalami must not be seen in this section, as this section cuts higher up in the head. This is an ideal plane for assessment of the ventricles and choroid plexus. The abnormalities that can be picked up on this section are ventriculomegaly, hydrocephalus, choroid plexus cysts, holoprosencephaly, corpus callosal defects, skull vault defects leading to meningocele, encephalocele, exencephaly or acrania, and anencephaly, abnormal skull shape such as strawberry-shaped skull, and brachy- or dolichocephaly **(Figs. 3A to H)**.

Transthalamic Plane (Line b in Fig. 4)

This plane cuts through the thalamus. The optimum section must show the thalami, cavum septum pellucidum, anterior horns of lateral ventricle, falx cerebri, and lateral sulcus. It also shows hippocampal gyrus, posterolateral to the thalami **(Fig. 5)**. The complete oval skull vault should be seen with symmetrical skull thickness all around and it should not be >3 mm. This plane must not show cerebellum or orbits. This plane shows abnormalities of cavum septum pellucidum and corpus callosum and midline shift, if present, is evident on this plane. Absence of lateral sulcus is an earliest indicator of lissencephaly. Coronal sutures can be identified in this plane and, therefore, abnormalities such as craniostenosis can be diagnosed.

Cavum septum pellucidum: Cavum septum pellucidum is a cavity in the midline inferior to the corpus callosum. It is visible at 16 weeks and obliterates near term. This means that it must always be visualized between 18 and 37 weeks, which means when biparietal diameter (BPD) is between 44 and 88 mm.

Both of these above-mentioned planes can be used for the quantitative assessment of the head. This consists of BPD, occipitofrontal diameter (OFD), and head circumference (HC) **(Fig. 6)**. Though conventionally these were measured in transthalamic plane, the FMF suggests to measure these in transventricular plane. Transventricular plane is also used to assess the ventricular diameter.

There is also a suggestion that transthalamic plane may be omitted from the routine protocol of second trimester targeted scan. But, another consideration is that in the late trimester as the brain matter develops, there is compression on the ventricles and ventricular size decreases. This might at times make identification of ventricles difficult and, therefore, transventricular plane may be difficult to obtain. In this case, if head parameters were measured in transventricular plane during second trimester scan, its comparison for growth assessment might become difficult or less accurate in third trimester.

Biparietal diameter: This measurement is taken perpendicular to falx cerebri at the broadest part of the oval skull vault; this is usually at the midpoint between the frontal and the occipital end of the oval skull vault as seen in this axial section. The measurement

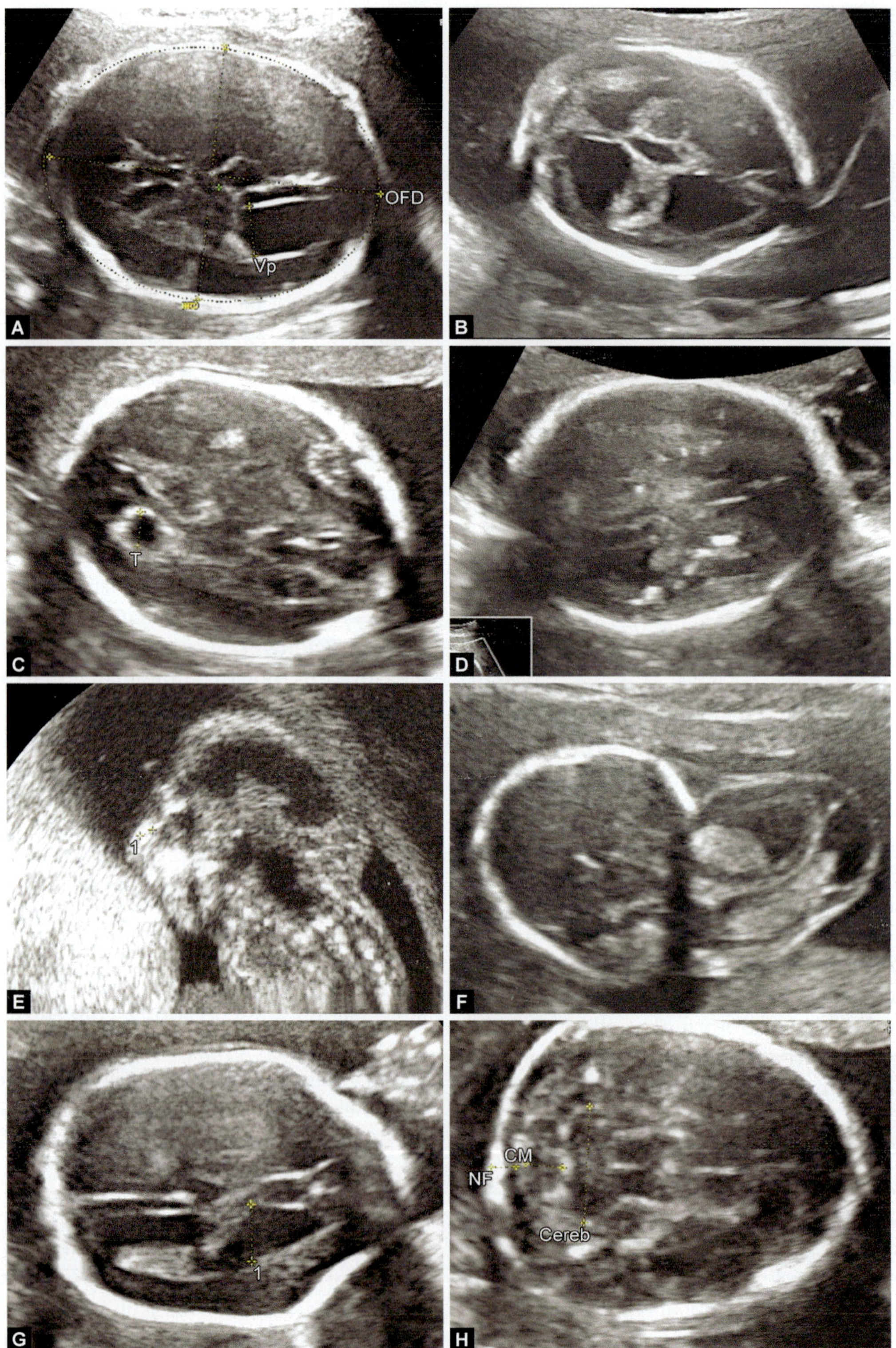

Figs. 3A to H: (A) Ventriculomegaly; (B) Hydrocephalus; (C) Choroid plexus cyst; (D) Ventricular calcifications; (E) Anencephaly; (F) Exencephaly; (G) Lemon skull; (H) Brachycephaly.
(OFD: occipitofrontal diameter; CM: cisterna magna; NF: nuchal fold)

is taken from outer margin of the proximal parietal bone to the inner margin of the distal parietal bone.

Biparietal diameter increases by:

- 3 mm/week till 30 weeks
- 1.5 mm/week at 30–38 weeks
- 1 mm/week after 38 weeks
- Nil at 42 weeks

Fetal growth restriction (FGR) is documented if growth rate is decreased to <5th percentile. There is a high chance of error when the measurements are between 5th and 10th percentile.

Sensitivity of BPD is considered as only 45% at 34–36 weeks for prediction of gestational age, though its sensitivity for growth assessment is much higher in earlier pregnancy. As the pregnancy advances, the genetic factors play a role in controlling the growth pattern and so with advancing pregnancy, the accuracy of growth assessment with all biometric parameters decreases. This measurement is not much affected by placental insufficiency or nutritional deprivation and so is more reliable than abdominal circumference, though it is variable with change in skull shape such as brachycephaly or dolichocephaly. In such cases, it is considered reliable only when cerebral index (CI) is 70–85 (CI: BPD/OFD × 100). As long as the CI is within normal limits, the head shape is considered normal. But, when CI is <70 or >85, these are indicators of pathologically abnormal head shape.

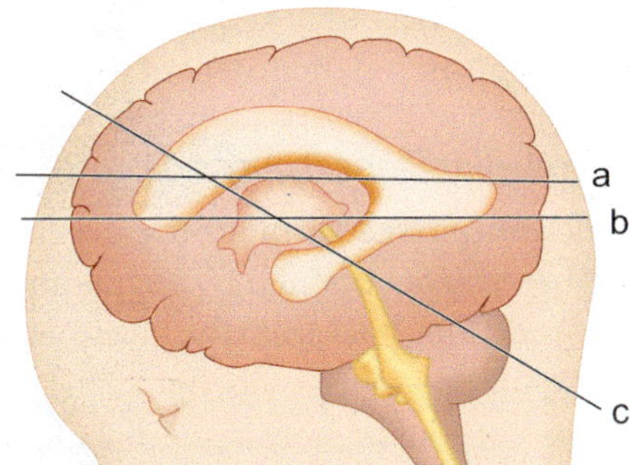

Fig. 4: Diagram showing the three basic axial sections of the head. (a) transventricular section, (b) transthalamic section, and (c) transcerebellar section.

Head circumference: It is measured on the outer edges of calvarium and not the scalp on the same plane as BPD. It is the better predictor of gestational age as compared to other commonly used predictors.

This parameter is not affected by change in head shape as long as CI is within limits (70–85). Its sensitivity is 52% and specificity is 80% for prediction of age in the third trimester.

It is altered in trisomy 18 where the head is strawberry shaped or in craniosynostosis.

Ventricular atrium: It is the measurement of the diameter of the lateral ventricles. It

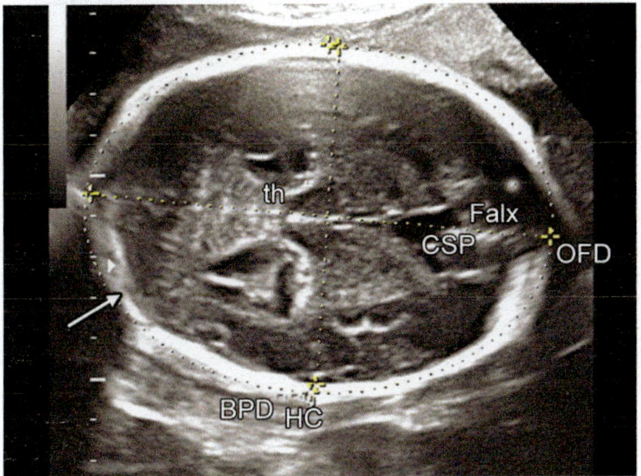

Fig. 5: Transthalamic section showing falx, cavum septum pellucidum (CSP), thalami (th), and occipitoparietal suture (arrow).
(BPD: biparietal diameter; HC: head circumference; OFD: occipitofrontal diameter)

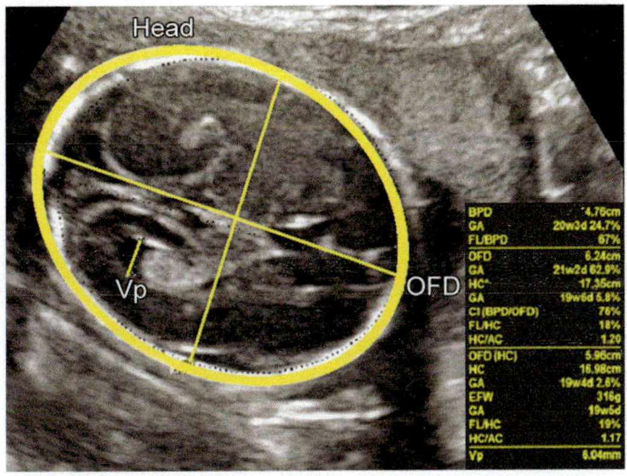

Fig. 6: Transventricular section of the head showing the assessment of biparietal diameter (BPD), occipitofrontal diameter (OFD), head circumference (HC), and ventricular width.

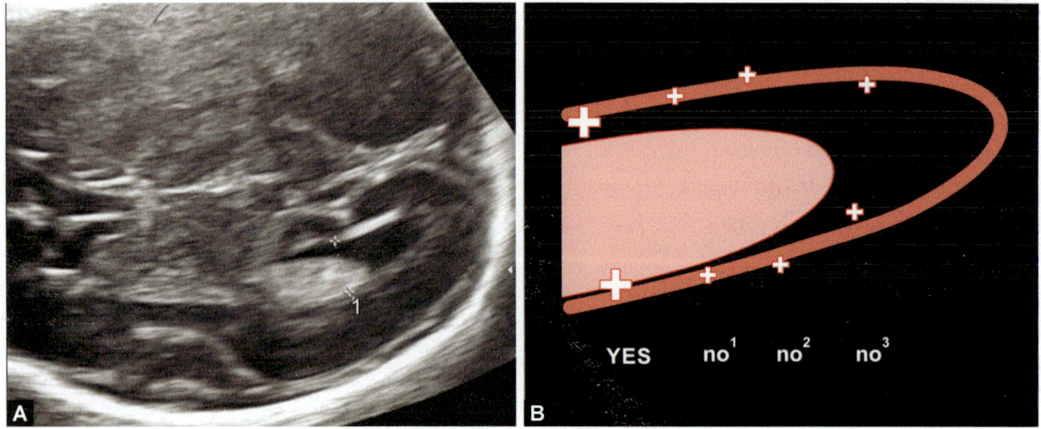

Figs. 7A and B: Ultrasound image and diagram showing assessment of ventricular width.

is measured at the level of parieto-occipital sulcus perpendicular to the medial ventricular wall and not perpendicular to the midline. Calipers are so placed that the horizontal line of caliper cross touches the inner margins of ventricular walls **(Figs. 7A and B)**.

The lateral ventricle to hemisphere ratio decreases from 70% at 18–20 weeks to 30% at 28–29 weeks and remains steady thereafter. In second and third trimesters, it measures 6–8 mm, 8–10 mm is borderline ventriculomegaly, and >10 mm is ventriculomegaly. Ventricular diameter of up to 10 mm is treated expectantly, if it is a solitary finding. Larger ventricular diameters may be considered as a soft marker for chromosomal abnormality. Ventricular diameter of 10–12 mm is ventriculomegaly and >15 mm with increased pressure is called hydrocephalus and may be associated with thinning of skull vault and widening of sutures. It is also a marker of abnormal cerebral development. This may require in utero or immediate postnatal treatment of the fetus.

Transcerebellar Plane (Line c on Fig. 8)

This section passes through the cerebellar hemispheres. It is obtained by angulating the probe toward fetal back from the transthalamic plane. Optimum transcerebellar section will show the cerebellar hemispheres, cisterna magna, falx cerebri, cavum septum pellucidum, and also cuts through the thalamus **(Fig. 9)**. Lateral sulcus also extends to this level. As for the previous two sections, the skull vault should

a
b
c

Fig. 8: Diagram showing the three basic axial sections of the head. (a) transventricular section, (b) transthalamic section, and (c) transcerebellar section.

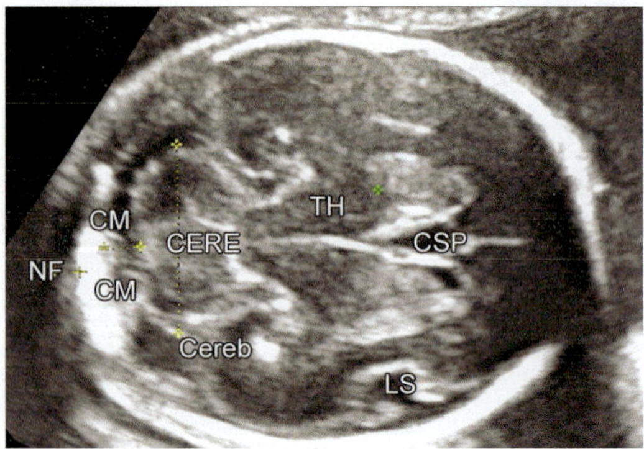

Fig. 9: Transcerebellar section of fetal head showing falx, cavum septum pellucidum (CSP), thalamus (TH), cerebellum (CERE), cisterna magna (CM), and nuchal fold (NF) (space between two yellow lines).

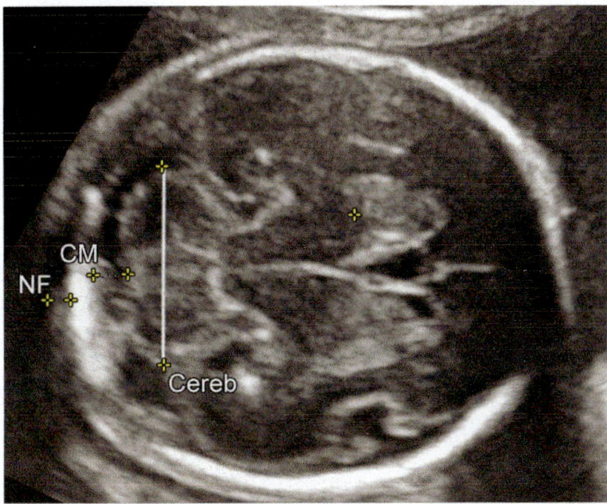

Fig. 10: Transcerebellar section of the head (magnified view) showing measurements of cerebellum (Cereb), cisterna magna (CM), and nuchal fold (NF) thickness.

be seen as a complete oval outline and should be symmetrical. Orbits should not be seen on this section. Cerebellar hypoplasia, mega cisterna magna, Dandy-Walker syndrome, and variant Blake's pouch cyst are the lesions diagnosed on this section. It also gives clue to open spinal canal defect.

Cerebellum: It is measured from outer to outer margin of the cerebellum on transcerebellar section. Transverse cerebellar diameter increases by 1 mm every week from 14 to 21 weeks. Diameter corresponds to the weeks of gestation in second trimester and is not affected by IUGR. Therefore, in cases of severe intrauterine growth restriction (IUGR), it can be used as a parameter for estimation of correct gestational age **(Fig. 10)**.

Cisterna magna: It is measured from posterior margin of cerebellar vermis to the anterior margin of overlying occipital bone **(Fig. 10)**. Cisterna magna is traversed by thin septa and this is a normal appearance. These represent remnants of the walls of Blake's pouch. These are markers of development of roof of rhombencephalon.

It measures 2–10 mm, but is slightly more in dolichocephaly. It is enlarged in cerebellar pathologies, especially in vermian pathologies such as vermian hypoplasia, Dandy-Walker malformations, or variants, but in neural canal defects when cerebellum is pulled caudally and cisterna magna is obliterated. This is known as "banana sign" of cerebellum. This is also associated with collapsed frontal bones and makes the skull shape like a lemon and is called "lemon sign" **(Figs. 11A and B)**.

Major open spinal canal defects can be suspected as early as the 11–13+6 weeks scan. Cisterna magna is seen as intracranial translucency in the midsagittal section of 11–14 weeks fetus **(Fig. 12)**.

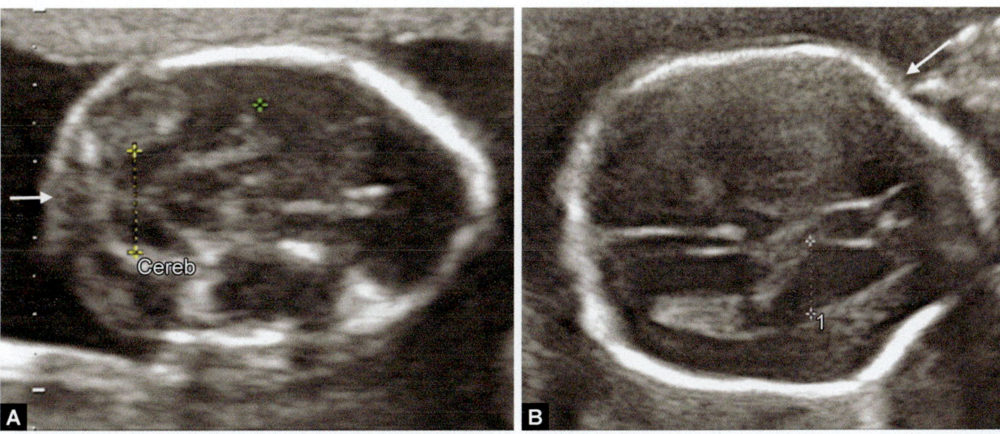

Figs. 11A and B: (A) Obliteration of the posterior concavity of the cerebellum due to open spinal canal defect making cerebellum look like a banana; (B) Collapsing of the frontal bones due to open spinal canal defect make the calvarial shape look like a lemon skull.

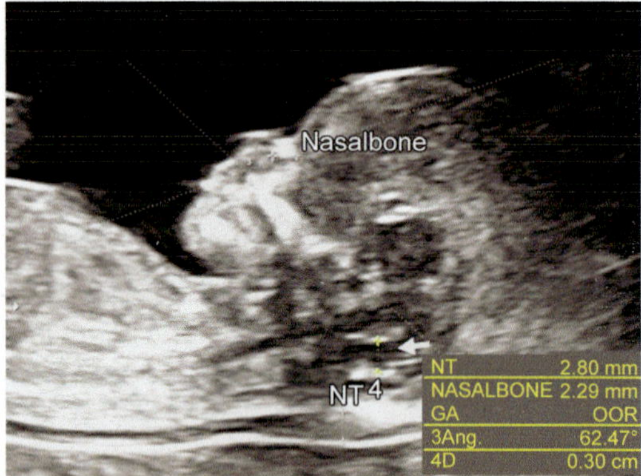

Fig. 12: Midsagittal section of 11–14 weeks fetus showing intracranial translucency.

Transorbital Plane

This plane cuts through the middle of the orbits. It is obtained by slight angulation of the probe toward fetal anterior aspect. It shows both bony orbits in transverse section with nasal bones in between. It might cut through the upper part of the thalamus, but should not show the cerebellum. Bony orbits on this plane show lens—one in each orbit and may also show the artery posterior to it as a single thin line **(Fig. 13A)**.

The quantitative assessment on this plane includes the binocular diameter, interocular diameter, and ocular diameter **(Fig. 13B)**.

Binocular diameter is measured as the largest distance between from lateral inner wall of one orbit to the lateral inner wall of another orbit. Interocular diameter is measured as broadest diameter from medial inner bony wall of one orbit to medial inner bony wall of another orbit. Ocular diameter is measured as broadest diameter of orbit from medial inner bony wall to lateral inner bony wall. Interocular diameter and ocular diameter are almost always equal. This plane is used to diagnose abnormalities of the orbits such as hypotelorism, hypertelorism, single orbit, and anophthalmia.

Increased interocular diameter is hypertelorism and decreased interocular diameter is hypotelorism. It is best to take the measurements when the fetus is facing the probe, though lenses are best seen when the fetal face is not toward the probe but on one of the sides.

Plane of Maxilla

This plane is just slightly caudal to the transorbital plane. This plane shows the tooth line of maxilla. This plane is best achieved in a fetal position where the fetus faces the probe. It is used to exclude maxillary abnormalities such as cleft palate. The soft tissues seen anterior to the maxilla is the upper lip and it is one of the views suggested for diagnosis of cleft lip and palate **(Fig. 14)**.

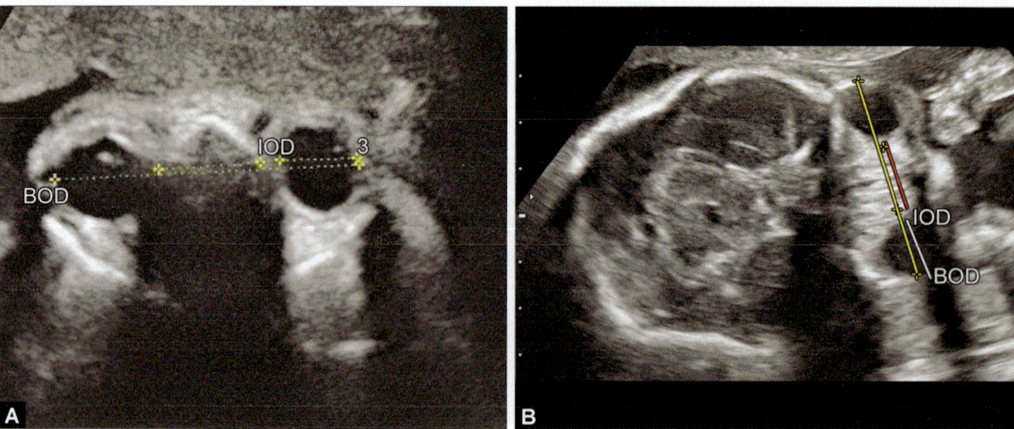

Figs. 13A and B: (A) Transorbital section showing both orbits with lenses; (B) Transorbital section showing the binocular (yellow), interocular (red), and ocular diameters (white).
(BOD: binocular diameter; IOD: interocular diameter)

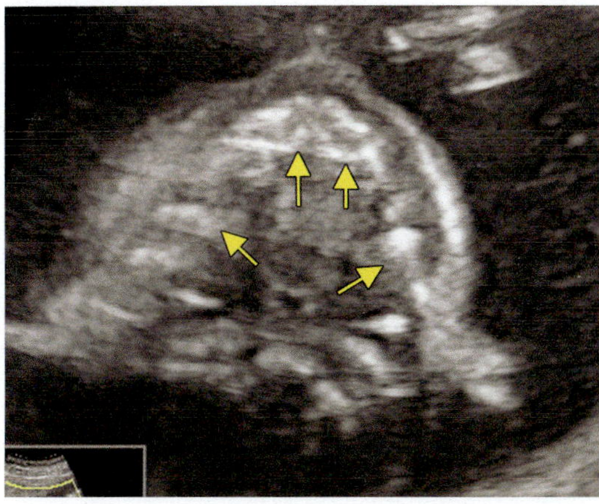

Fig. 14: Maxilla in transverse section (white arrows).

Head: Coronal Section

Lips (Figs. 15A and B)

From the previous plane, 90° rotation of the probe shows coronal or sagittal plane. If sagittal plane is seen on this rotation, lift up the probe to place it on one of the sides of the abdomen to see the coronal plane. Move the probe then toward anterior aspect of the fetus and this will show the tip of the nose/nostrils, upper lip, and the lower lip. This plane is used for diagnosis of cleft lip. Fetuses with cleft lip may also show asymmetry of the nostrils, which may be seen on this section as well.

Midsagittal Plane

This plane is same as the midsagittal plane taken for nuchal translucency on nuchal scan. A true plane will show the tip of the nose, nasal bone and overlying skin maxilla in sagittal section as a bold line and not as a triangle, and mandible is seen as a dot, and no zygoma between nasal bone and maxilla. Because of the ossification of the frontal bone, brain anatomy is not much seen on this section at this stage of pregnancy. This plane is obtained in a fetal position when the fetus is preferably facing the probe. Nasal bone length and frontomaxillary facial angle are the two measurements taken on this plane **(Fig. 16)**. Nasal bone length is measured end to end. Frontomaxillary facial angle is measured by drawing one line on the superior surface of the maxilla and the other line is a line joining anterior superior end of maxilla to the nasion.

Nasion is the point where the nasal bone is attached to the frontal bone. Frontomaxillary facial angle is 66.6–89.5° in normal fetus with a mean of 78.5°. In trisomy 21 fetuses, because of the flat face or a flat nasal bridge, this angle is increased to 75.4–104° with a mean of 88.7°. Even a rotation of the fetal face of 2–3° can lead to a measurement error of 5–15°. Therefore, a correct fetal position is very essential. Prenasal thickness (thickness of the skin anterior to the nasion) is also assessed now as one of the markers for trisomy 21.

It is this section which will also demonstrate micrognathia **(Fig. 17)**. This can also be quantitatively assessed. Cephalometric analysis

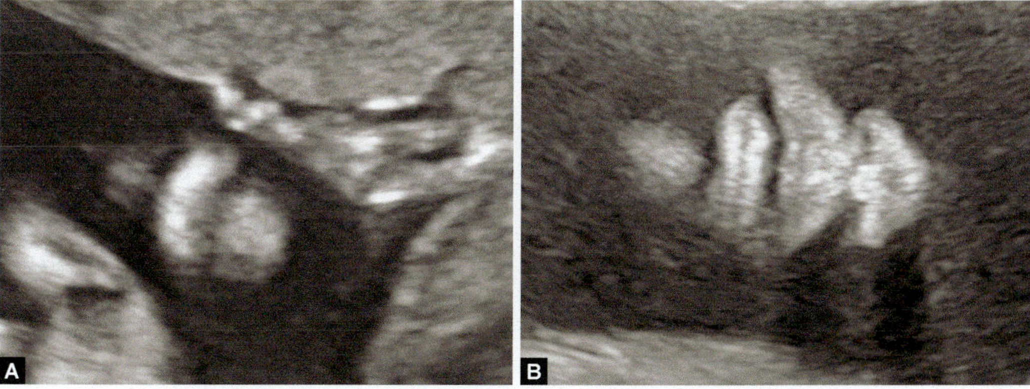

Figs. 15A and B: Nostrils, upper lip, lower lip, and chin are seen in coronal section.

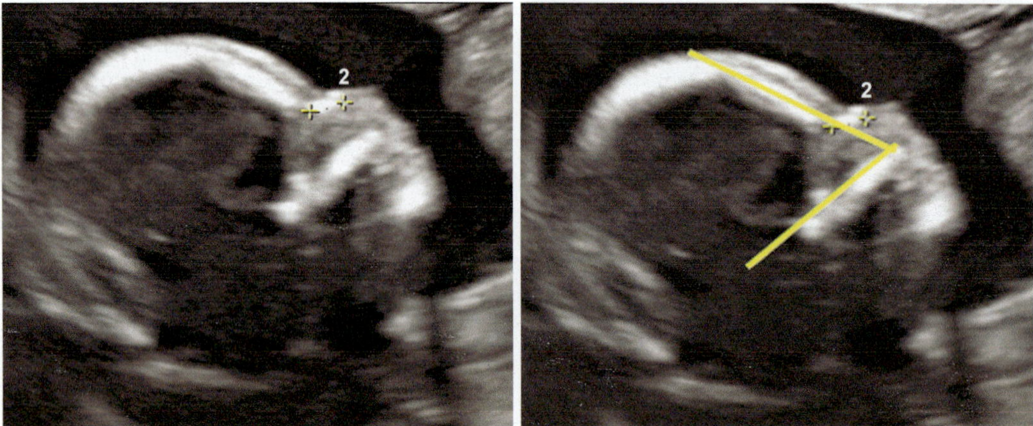

Fig. 16: Midsagittal section of the head showing nasal bone assessment in figure on the left side and frontomaxillary facial angle assessment in figure on the right side.

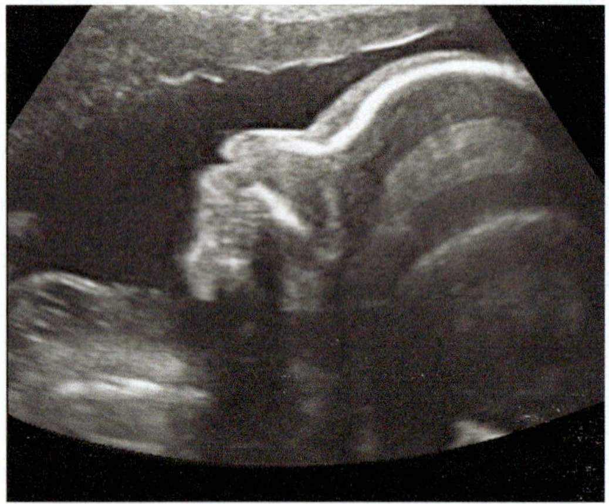

Fig. 17: Midsagittal section of the head showing a small receding chin—micrognathia.

by prenatal sonography can be performed to study the anteroposterior jaw relationship. We think that this procedure could be useful to improve prenatal diagnosis of retrognathism in high-risk pregnancies.[1] Inferior facial angle (IFA) and the frontal nasomental angle have been used on stored grayscale images to objectively establish the diagnosis. The mean values for IFA and frontal nasomental angle were 44.8° and 123.3°, respectively.[2]

Inferior Facial Angle

This angle is measured in the midsagittal view of the fetal profile and is formed by the crossing of a line orthogonal to the vertical part of the forehead drawn at the level of synostosis of nasal bones and a line through the tip of the mentum and the more protrusive lip, usually the upper lip.

Frontal Nasomental Angle

This is the angle between the line drawn from the tip of the nose and frontal bone, intersecting the line from the nasal tip to the mentum.[3]

Trunk

Axial Sections: Thorax

- Four-chamber view of the heart **(Fig. 18)**
- Left ventricular outflow tract **(Fig. 19)**
- Right ventricular outflow tract **(Fig. 20)**
- Three-vessel view **(Fig. 21)**

The above-mentioned four planes will be discussed in detail in Chapter 12 of this book.

Axial Sections: Abdomen

- Section through stomach
- Section through renal pelves
- Section through umbilical cord attachment
- Section through sacrum (transverse sacrum section)

Section through the stomach for abdominal circumference: As mentioned, this section passes through the stomach and entry of

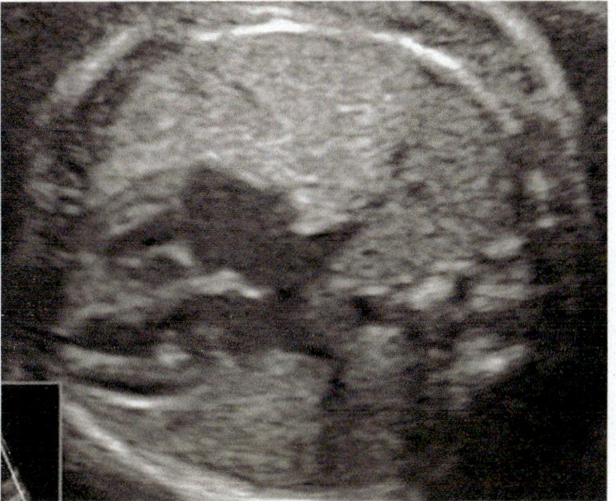

Fig. 18: Four-chamber view of the heart.

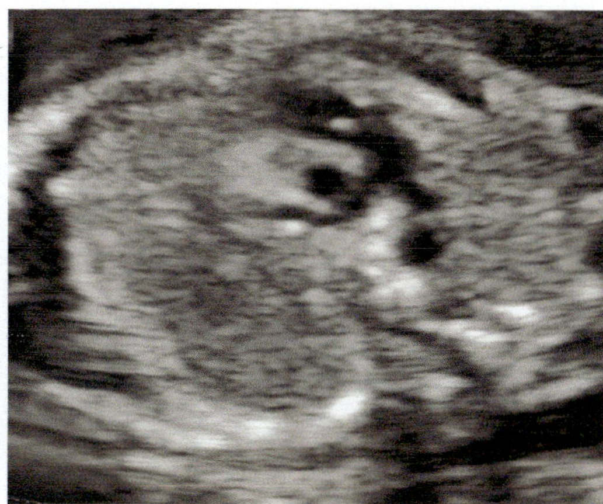

Fig. 20: Three-vessel view.

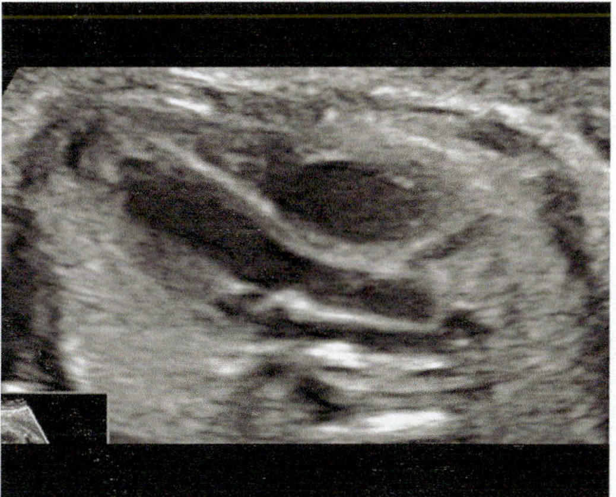

Fig. 19: Left ventricular outflow tract.

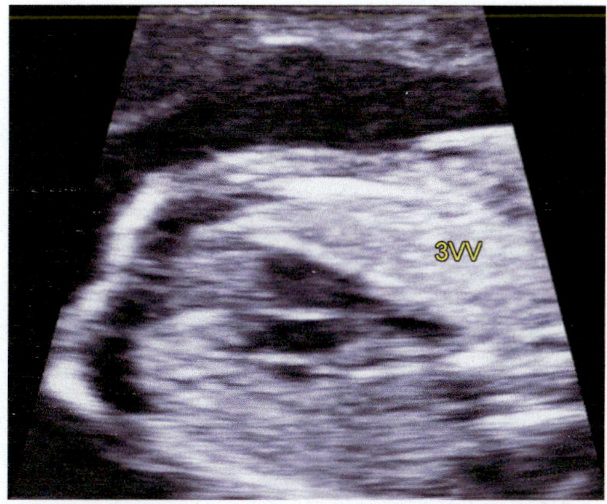

Fig. 21: Right ventricular outflow tract.

umbilical vein to ductus venosus (DV) seen as a J with curve of the J concave toward fetal right **(Fig. 22)**. The ribs cover the contour symmetrically on both sides. This ensures that it is a true transverse section and the section is achieved during fetal apnea. Kidneys must not be seen on this plane.

Abdominal circumference is measured on the outer margin of this section. Most accurate is the smallest measurement. It shows linear rise till 36 weeks of 11–12 mm/week and fall thereafter. It is the first measurement to show alteration in IUGR. This is the single most sensitive measure of fetal growth and it is better to measure it accurately than to add other parameters.

Umbilical cord insertion plane: This plane is a true transverse plane again and is caudal to the abdominal circumference plane. It is at the level where the umbilical cord enters the fetal abdomen.

This plane may be imaged on B mode or with Doppler **(Fig. 23)**. Doppler has an advantage of showing the entry of cord vessels into fetal abdomen more clearly. This plane helps to exclude abnormalities such as omphalocele and gastroschisis **(Fig. 24)**.

Alternatively, some workers would prefer to demonstrate the cord vessels with the urinary bladder to confirm the presence of two umbilical arteries.

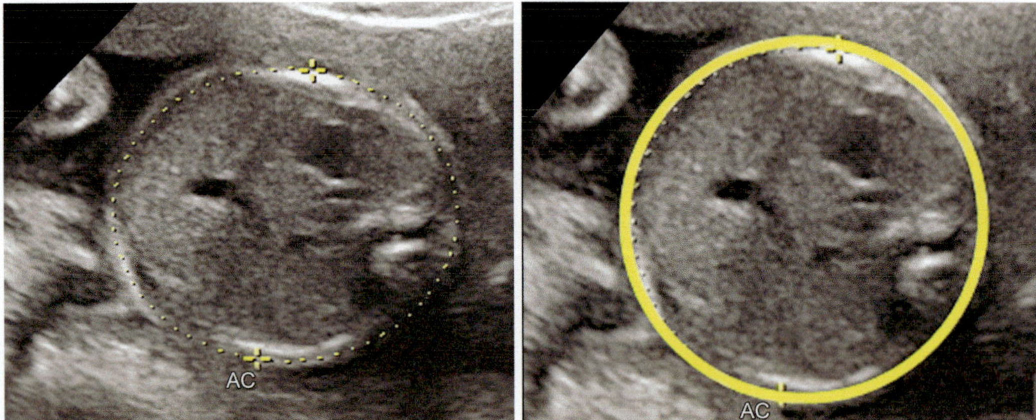

Fig. 22: Axial section of the abdomen showing stomach and mid-third of the vein mentioned in the text above. Figure on the right side shows the same plane with the measurement of abdominal circumference (AC).

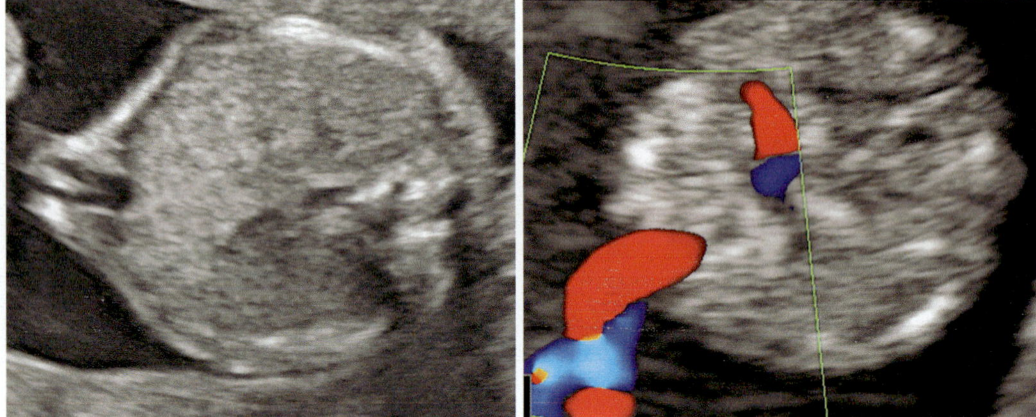

Fig. 23: Axial section of the abdomen showing insertion of the umbilical cord. Figure on the left shows B mode and figure on the right shows color Doppler demonstration of the same.

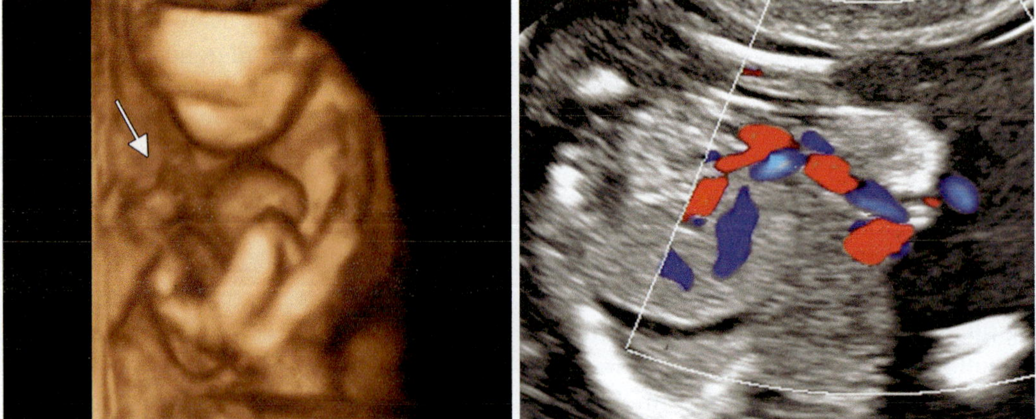

Fig. 24: Figure on the left side shows omphalocele with the umbilical cord arising from the dome of the herniation and figure on the right side shows gastroschisis where the cord is seen arising from the side of the herniation in color Doppler.

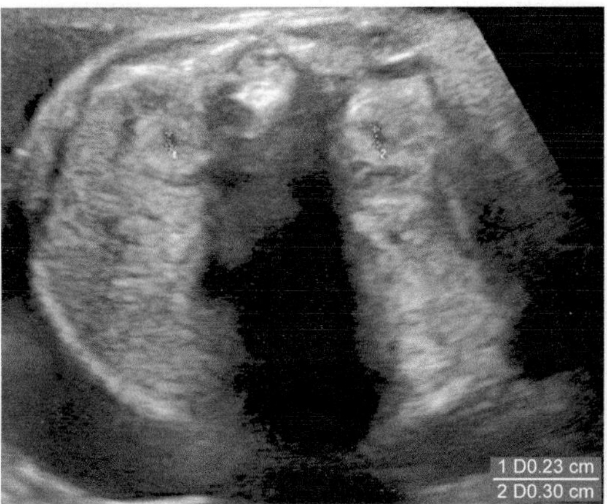

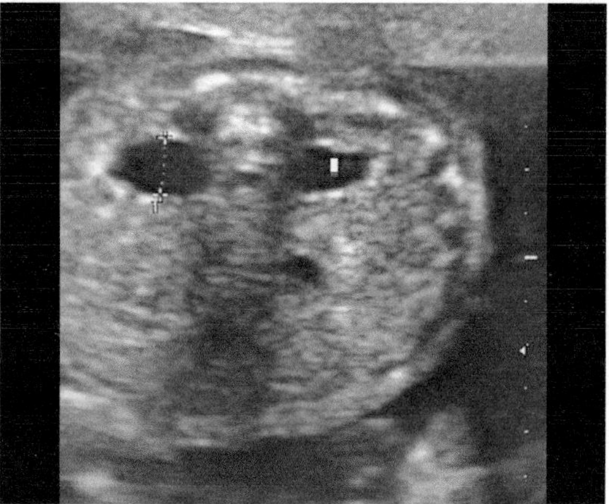

Fig. 25: Both figures show transverse section of the abdomen at the level of renal pelves. Figure on the right shows assessment of renal pelvic diameter.

Renal pelvis plane: This plane is caudal to the plane of cord insertion and it cuts the abdomen through both renal pelves. This plane should not include the stomach shadow and should be symmetrical and circular. This plane is used to measure the diameter of the renal pelvis. It is best to obtain this section with the fetus in a position spine anterior or spine posterior. The renal pelvis diameter is measured anteroposteriorly from inner margin to inner margin **(Fig. 25)**.

Normal measurements:
- 16–20 weeks, 4 mm
- 20–30 weeks, 5 mm
- 30–40 weeks, 7 mm

Dilated renal pelvis may be indicative of chromosomal abnormality. There may also be an obstructive lesion in the ureter or bladder leading to dilatation of renal pelvis and may be unilateral or bilateral.

*Transverse sacral plane **(Fig. 26)**:* This is the lowest transverse section through the fetal trunk. Two iliac bones are seen with three ossification centers of the sacrum seen in the center. This helps to confirm absence of spina bifida or open sacral defects at the level of the sacrum.

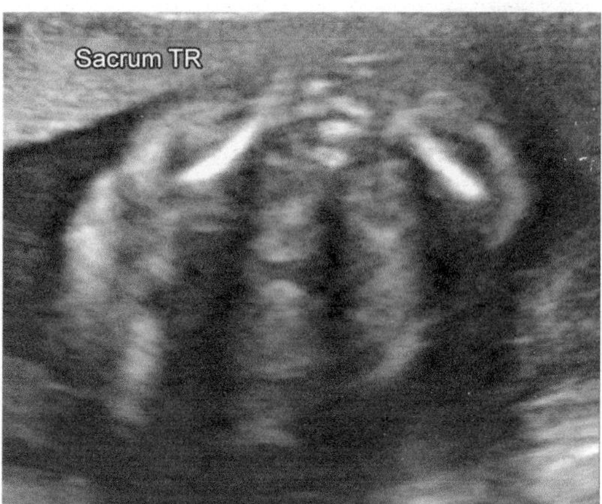

Fig. 26: Axial section of the pelvis or transverse section of sacrum.

Trunk: Abdomen

*Midsagittal section **(Fig. 27)**:* This section is taken to assess the spine in sagittal section. It is seen as two parallel lines of echogenic dots (ossification centers). It is essential to establish the continuity of the overlying skin. It is also important to observe the whole spine, establish the continuity, and also to confirm tapering of ossification centers of the sacrum. Though chiefly aimed to assess the spine, this plane also shows the bladder.

Trunk: Abdomen

Coronal plane: A posterior coronal plane section is essential to observe the whole spine in coronal section **(Fig. 28)**. At the level of vertebral bodies, it is seen as a single line of ossification centers and at the transverse

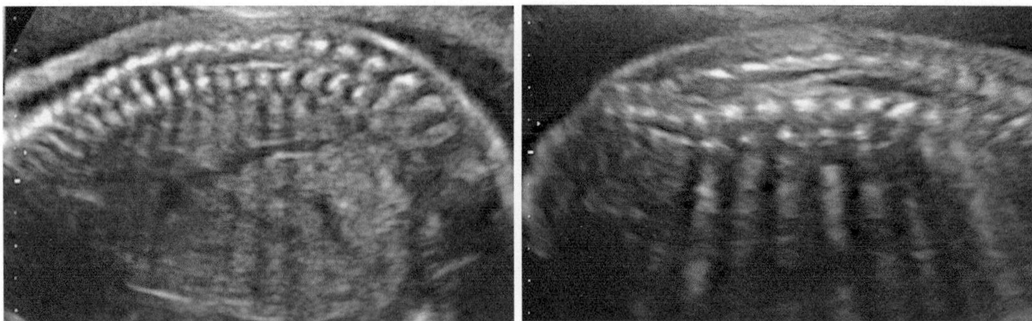

Fig. 27: Sagittal section of the trunk showing spine in sagittal plane. Left image shows the cervicothoracic and upper lumbar spine and the right image shows lumbosacral spine. White arrow shows the sacral tapering.

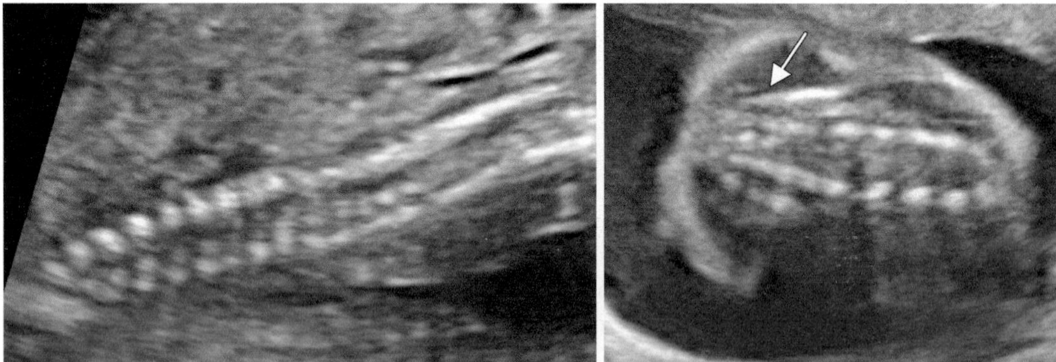

Fig. 28: Coronal section of the spine showing transverse processes of vertebral bodies. Image on left shows thoracolumbar spine and image on right shows lumbosacral spine with sacral tapering (white arrow).

process level, it appears like two parallel lines. Widening of the distance between two lines may be indicative of spina bifida or open spinal canal. Both lines if do not make pairs of ossification centers, it may be indicative of hemivertebrae. On this plane also, it is essential to establish the tapering of ossification in the sacral spine. The vertebral body plane that is a slightly anterior to this plane may also show kidneys in coronal plane.

Seeing kidneys in this plane is especially important for diagnosis of renal parenchymal disorders and renal dysplasias **(Fig. 29)**.

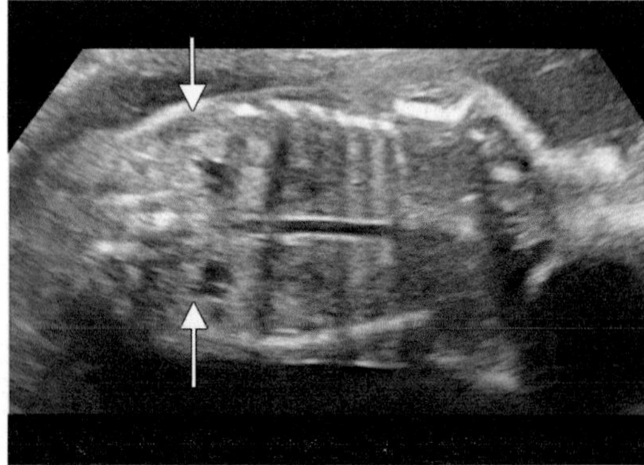

Fig. 29: Coronal section of the abdomen showing renal pelves on both the sides (white arrows).

Limbs: It is essential to document the presence of all four limbs and all three segments of all the limbs. It is best to demonstrate both forearms and hands in a single image and both legs and feet in a single image to establish both limbs have been assessed.

In leg and forearm, presence of two long bones must be documented. Relation of foot to leg and forearm to hand must be established **(Fig. 30)**. Long bones must be measured end-to-end **(Fig. 30)** excluding the epiphysis. Though counting fingers and toes may be

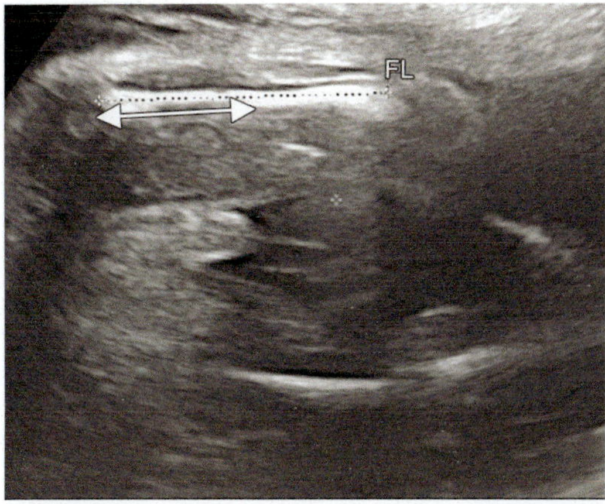

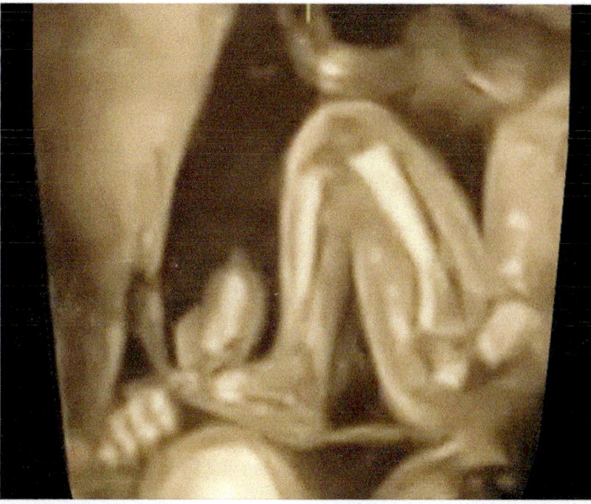

Fig. 30: Image on the left side shows the femur and its longitudinal measurement and image on the right side shows the full lower limb. The special attention is toward the normal relationship of leg to foot.

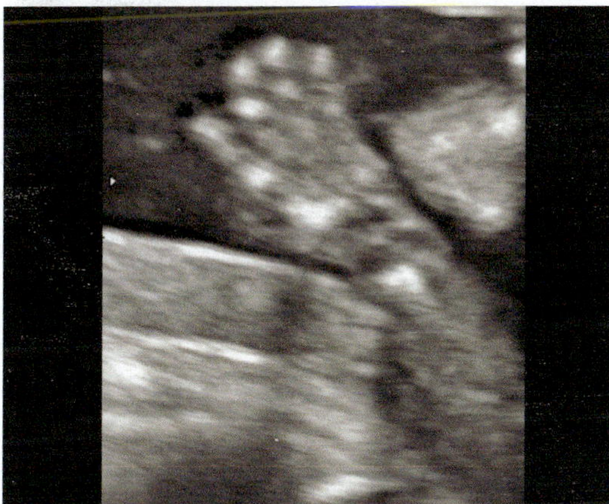

Fig. 31: Image shows open hand with fingers and thumb seen individually.

done, it is not mandatory for the detailed second trimester scan. If an open hand can be demonstrated with the thumb outside, is an image which would be of significance **(Fig. 31)**.

When measuring the femur length, long axis of femur should be aligned with the transducer and only osseous part of diaphysis and metaphysis is measured. Femur grows 3 mm/week from 14 to 27 weeks and 1 mm/week in third trimester.

It shows moderate curvature from 18 weeks onward giving a typical "golf club"-like appearance. But, as compared to femur length (FL) only, FL/abdominal circumference (AC) has been considered to be more reliable. This is so because independent of gestational age, the ratio remains constant after 22 weeks. Its sensitivity is 63% and positive predictive value is 30% for FGR.

We prefer to measure femur, humerus, and tibia in all fetuses.

Apart from assessment of the fetus, it is preferable to assess the placenta and the umbilical cord insertion in the placenta. Though the placenta and umbilical cord will be discussed more in detail in Chapter 8 of this book, the points essential to document are placental location, its texture (presence of lakes/calcification), and uteroplacental interface. Though thickness of the placenta is not always measured, if evidently looks thin or thick, it must be measured and documented. Number of vessels in umbilical cord is always documented. If cord appears evidently thick or thin, hypocoiled, or hypercoiled, it must be quantitatively assessed and documented. Location of cord insertion on placenta also needs a mention.

Amniotic fluid index is assessed as vertical fluid pouch in all four quadrants. The probe must be always kept vertical during assessment of the amniotic fluid index and the deepest pouch clear of umbilical cord loops or fetal limbs is selected **(Fig. 32)**. Many

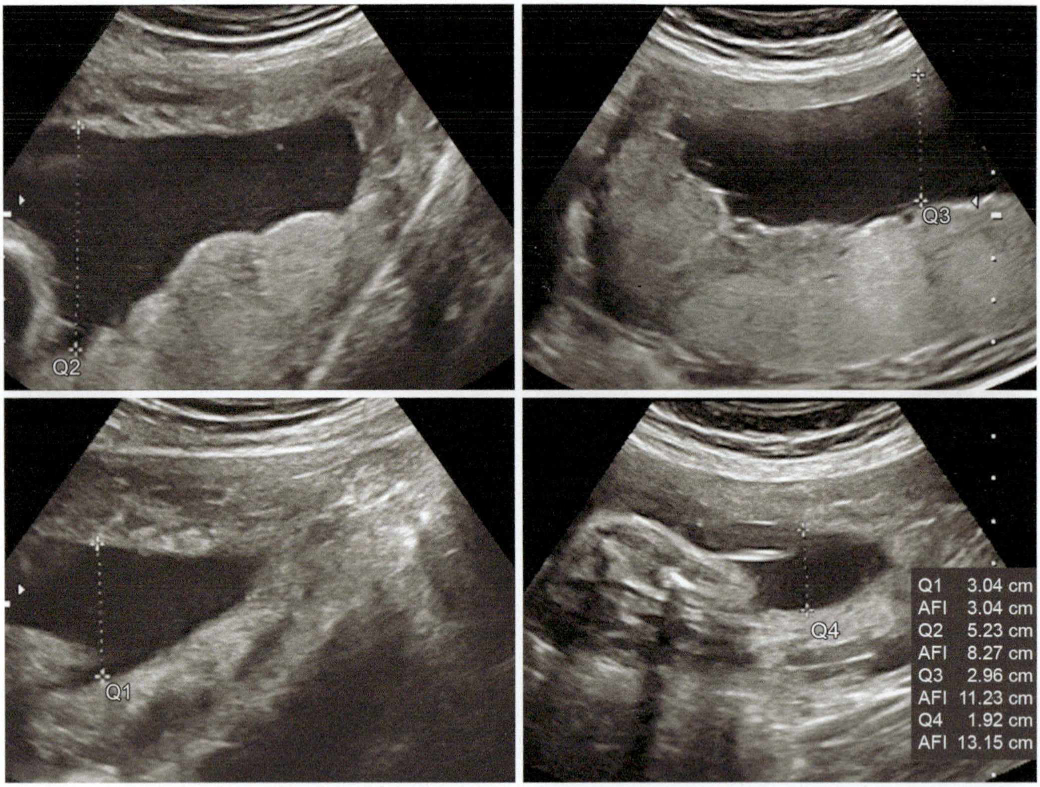

Fig. 32: Image shows assessment of the amniotic fluid index in four quadrants.

workers would prefer to assess the depth of only one largest pocket of amniotic fluid and a single pocket of 5–8 cm may be considered adequate.

Apart from this, the second trimester scan must include assessment of the uterine artery and umbilical artery Doppler. Umbilical artery flow can be assessed in any free loop of umbilical cord but in very mobile fetus, the cord insertion at the placenta may be selected as a site of preference for Doppler assessment of the umbilical artery. Though is thought that the resistance is a little different at the fetal end and the placental end, this difference is not of much clinical significance.

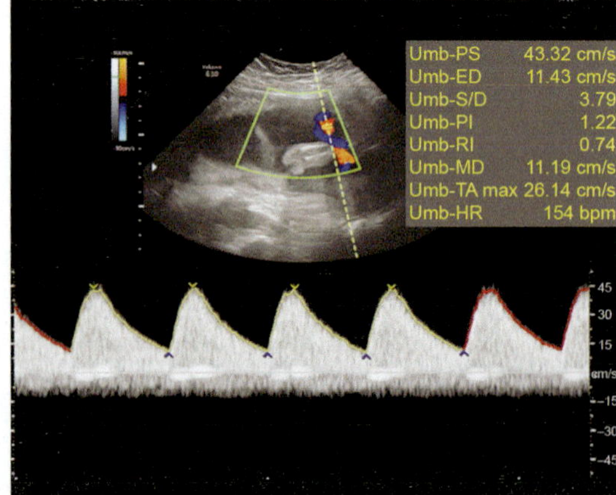

Fig. 33: Spectral Doppler of umbilical artery showing its normal waveform.

Umbilical artery flow is usually a moderate resistance flow **(Fig. 33)** and normally the resistance keeps on decreasing as age advances.

The uterine artery is localized by moving the probe from the symphysis pubis laterally without angulating it. Where the iliac vessels are seen in long axis, a slight medial angulation of the probe shows uterine artery crossing iliac vessels perpendicular to the iliac vessels. Uterine arteries usually have high resistance flow in the early pregnancy, but show fairly low

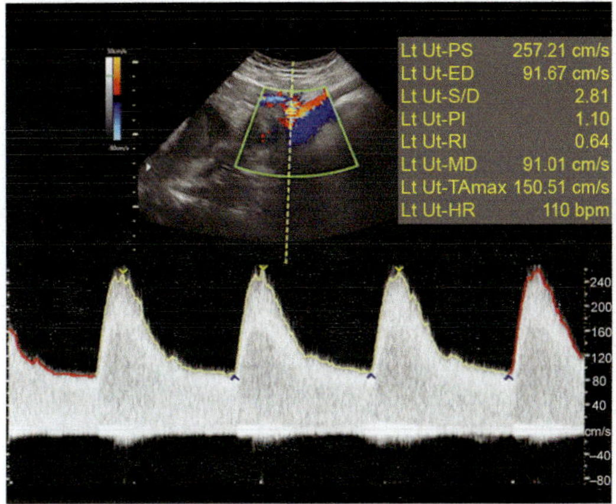

Fig. 34: Spectral Doppler of uterine artery normal waveform in second and third trimesters.

resistance vessels in later pregnancy **(Fig. 34)**, especially on the side of the placenta, if the placenta is not central. It means that uterine artery is of significance for assessing the risk of pregnancy-induced hypertension (PIH) and FGR.

A systematic scan, thus, done in the second trimester is capable to excluding almost all major abnormalities of the fetus. But, it must be remembered that certain anomalies are progressive and may only become evident late in the second trimester or in the third trimester. So, even if second trimester scan is normal, a quick survey of the entire fetus during follow-up scans should be a protocol.

REFERENCES

1. Captier G, Faure JM, Bäumler M, Canovas F, Demattei C. Prenatal assessment of the antero-posterior jaw relationship in human fetuses: from anatomical to ultrasound cephalometric analysis. Cleft Palate Craniofac J. 2011;48:465-72.
2. Rotten D, Levaillant JM, Martinez H, le Pointe HD, Vicaut E. The fetal mandible: a 2D and 3D sonographic approach to the diagnosis of retrognathia and micrognathia. Ultrasound Obstet Gynecol. 2002;19:122-30.
3. Antonakopoulos A, Bhide A. Focus on prenatal detection of micrognathia. J Fet Med. 2019;6:107-12.

8 CHAPTER

Placental Evaluation and Trophoblastic Tumors

Sonal Panchal, Chaitanya Nagori

ABNORMALITIES OF PLACENTA AND UMBILICAL CORD

Placenta is the chief circulatory unit that supports the growing fetus through its low-resistance blood flow.

Formation and Development of the Placenta

With implantation of the embryo in one of the endometrial lips, there are several changes occurring in the endometrium that chiefly include proteolytic and immunosuppression mechanisms for acceptance of the foreign body—the embryo. Progesterone secretion from the corpus luteum and human chorionic gonadotropin (hCG) produced by the implanting embryo together lead to the formation and development of the chorionic tissue, which is the first step toward placentation. In the earlier stages, the chorionic tissue is all around the gestational sac but as the embryo grows, there is a self-selection of the most vascular area expected. It is in this area of the endometrium that the chorionic tissue tries to invade deeper and therefore it appears more thick. The chorionic tissue in the rest of the area surrounding the gestational sac starts regressing. The regressing part of the chorionic tissue then is known as chorion leave, whereas the part which becomes thicker and penetrates deeper and is functionally active in allowing the uterine blood flow to reach the embryo is known as chorion frundosum **(Fig. 1)**. It is the chorion frundosum that will develop ultimately into placenta.

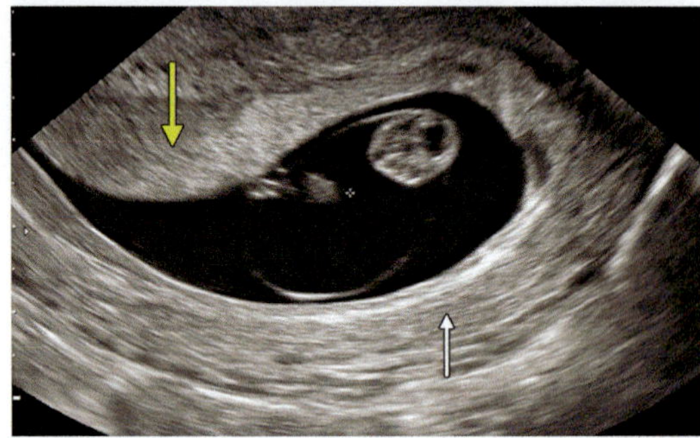

Fig. 1: B-mode image of the gestational sac showing thickened chorion frundosum (yellow arrow) and thin chorion leave (white arrow).

After 3–4 weeks of implantation, intermediate trophoblast invades maternal spiral arteries. This leads to disruption of extracellular matrix and replacement of maternal endothelium by cells of trophoblastic origin. This leads to development of low resistance vascular bed with large capacitance.[1] There is conversion of highly muscular spiral vessels into nonmuscular placental vessels **(Fig. 2)**. Conversion of the vasculature occurs in two phases. First phase starts at around 8 weeks and the second one at around 18 weeks.

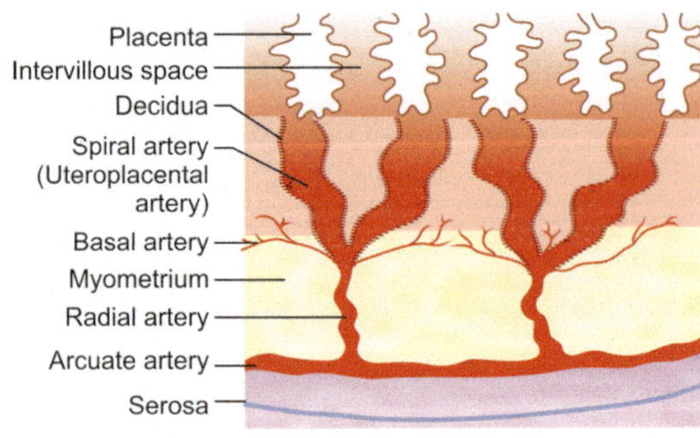

Fig. 2: Diagrammatic representation of vascular changes of normal placentation.

The fall in resistance is fast till 12 weeks, with the initial phase of conversion in the type of vasculature and then slows down till 22 weeks. Beyond 22 weeks till term, further changes in the placental vasculature in terms of lowering resistance are minimal.

Failure of this conversion of high resistance to low resistance vascular system leads to secretion of vasoactive substances from placenta and induces maternal hypertension **(Fig. 3)**. Though a complete failure of this conversion will lead to first trimester abortions most commonly due to inability to support the vascular and nutritional needs of the growing fetus, partial failure of conversion will lead to pregnancy-induced hypertension (PIH) and intrauterine growth restriction (IUGR) in late 2nd and 3rd trimester, depending on the severity.

It is a consequence of multiple factors:

- Primary defect in invasive trophoblasts
- Endocrine, immunological, and inflammatory phenomena, which regulate the interplay between maternal and fetal factors

The pathophysiology that works in development of IUGR is as follows:

- Inadequate trophoblastic invasion, which leads to nondilatation of the uterine vessels; as a result, the placental perfusion is reduced, leading to inadequate villous circulation in turn leading to low oxygen levels in umbilical cord blood and therefore vascular changes in the fetus as a result of stimulation of chemoreceptors. This means the cause is diagnosed by high resistance in the uterine arteries and the results are shown as vascular changes in umbilical cord and fetal vessels.

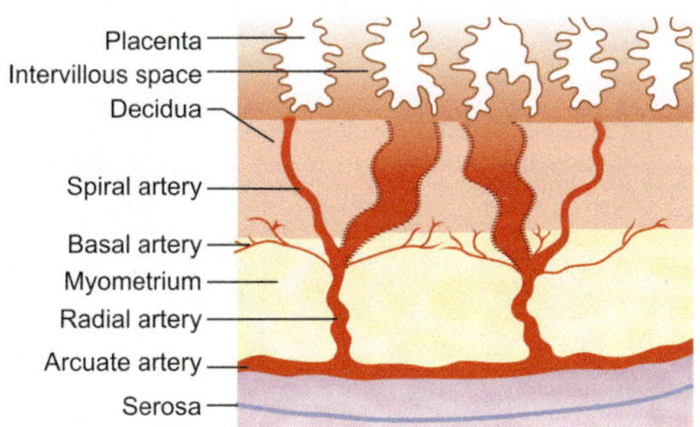

Fig. 3: Diagrammatic representation of vascular changes of abnormal placentation.

Though this chapter is dedicated to abnormalities of placenta and the umbilical cord and not on PIH and IUGR, no mention about the vascular abnormalities may leave the discussion incomplete.

During pregnancy, there is a persistent fall in the resistance of uterine and umbilical arteries, whereas, there is a slow but steady rise in the resistance of middle cerebral artery (MCA), which is considered a representative of fetal circulation. A reverse trend in any of these vessels is indicative of placental insufficiency and may lead to PIH or IUGR **(Figs. 4 and 5)**.

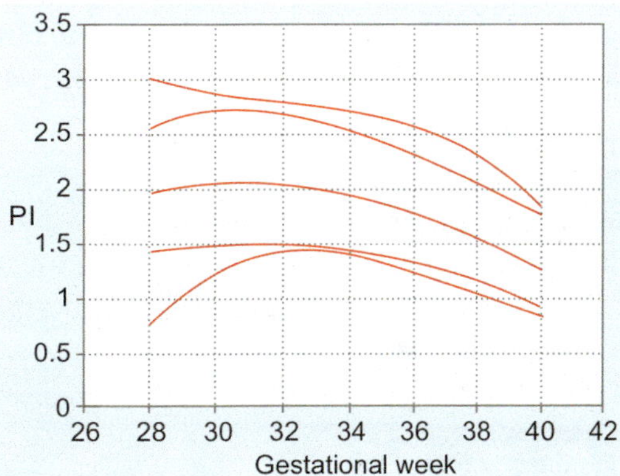

Fig. 4: Nomogram of values of middle cerebral artery (MCA) PI (pulsatility index) with changing gestational age.

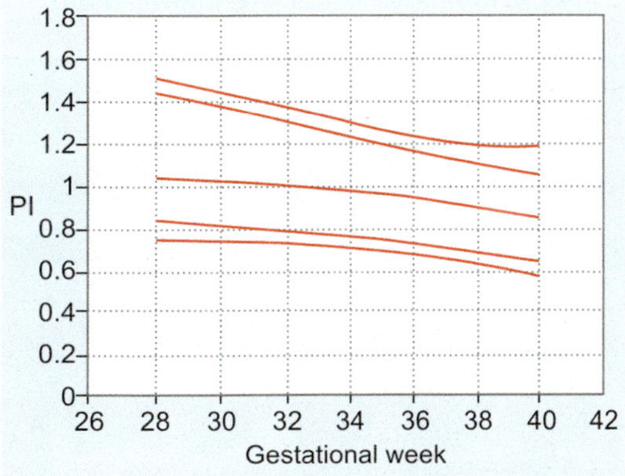

Fig. 5: Nomogram of values of umbilical artery PI (pulsatility index) with changing gestational age.

Placenta has about 50% reserve and so these changes will become evident only when there is compromise of more than 50% of placental circulation. In the initial phases, it is only dilatation of the middle cerebral arteries and reduced resistance that compensates for increased resistance of the umbilical arteries. When umbilical artery resistance increases significantly and the diastolic flow is significantly reduced, the resistance index ratio of MCA to umbilical artery (CPR) becomes one or less than one. This can be taken as a cut off for prediction of bad pregnancy prognosis. An absent or reverse diastolic flow in the umbilical artery is taken as a strongly suggestive sign of fetal morbidity and a high risk of fetal mortality **(Figs. 6 to 9)**. MCA resistance persistently falls to compensate for this reduced oxygenated blood supply through the umbilical cord, but fails at a certain point. When this happens, there is lactic acidosis, cerebral edema, and paradoxical reversal of MCA resistance to normal. This phase is considered to be an irreversible stage of fetal cerebral damage. There is also a circulatory paralysis and fetal or neonatal death is almost always suspected.

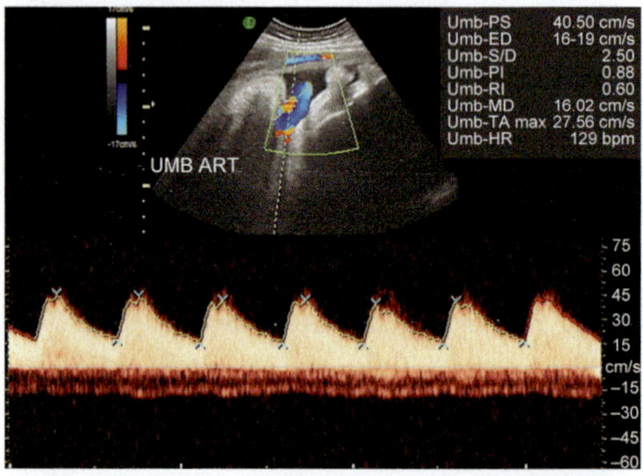

Fig. 6: Normal umbilical artery flow pattern.

After that, short discussion on placental vascular abnormalities now considers other abnormalities of the placenta and umbilical cord.

Abnormalities of placenta may be divided under following heads:

- Size
- Texture
- Shape
- Location
- Penetration
- Cord attachment

Abnormalities of Placental Size

The size of the placenta can be assessed as its extent or thickness. Normal placental thickness in mm is equal to gestational age in weeks ± 10 mm at the thickest part of the placenta, which is at the point of cord insertion usually[2] **(Fig. 10)**.

There are no criteria defined on the normal or abnormal extent of the placenta, but generally narrow placenta is thick and broad placenta is thin. Ideally, both parameters must be combined.

3D ultrasound can be used to calculate placental volume.

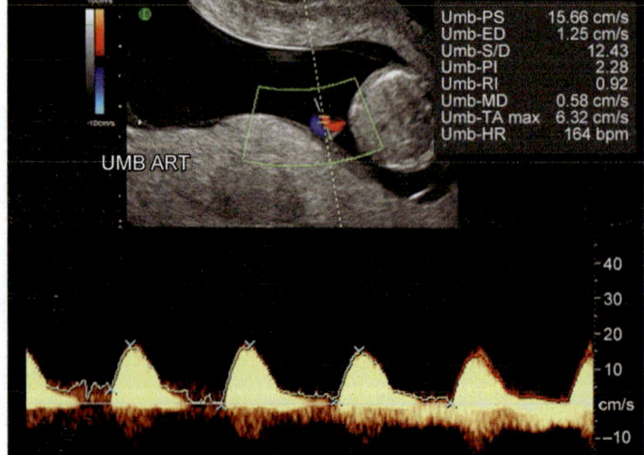

Fig. 7: Absent diastolic flow in umbilical artery.

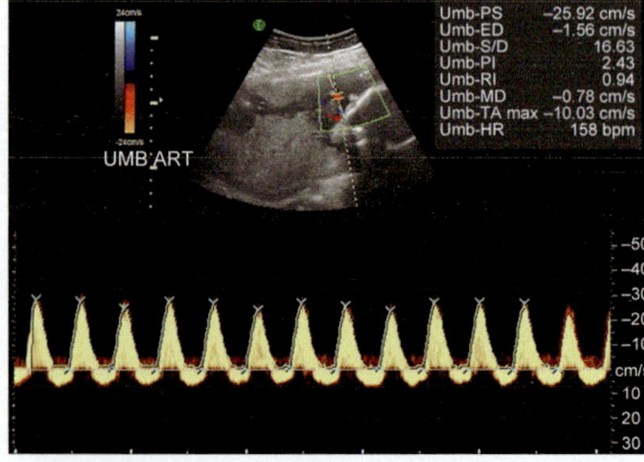

Fig. 8: Reversed diastolic flow in umbilical artery.

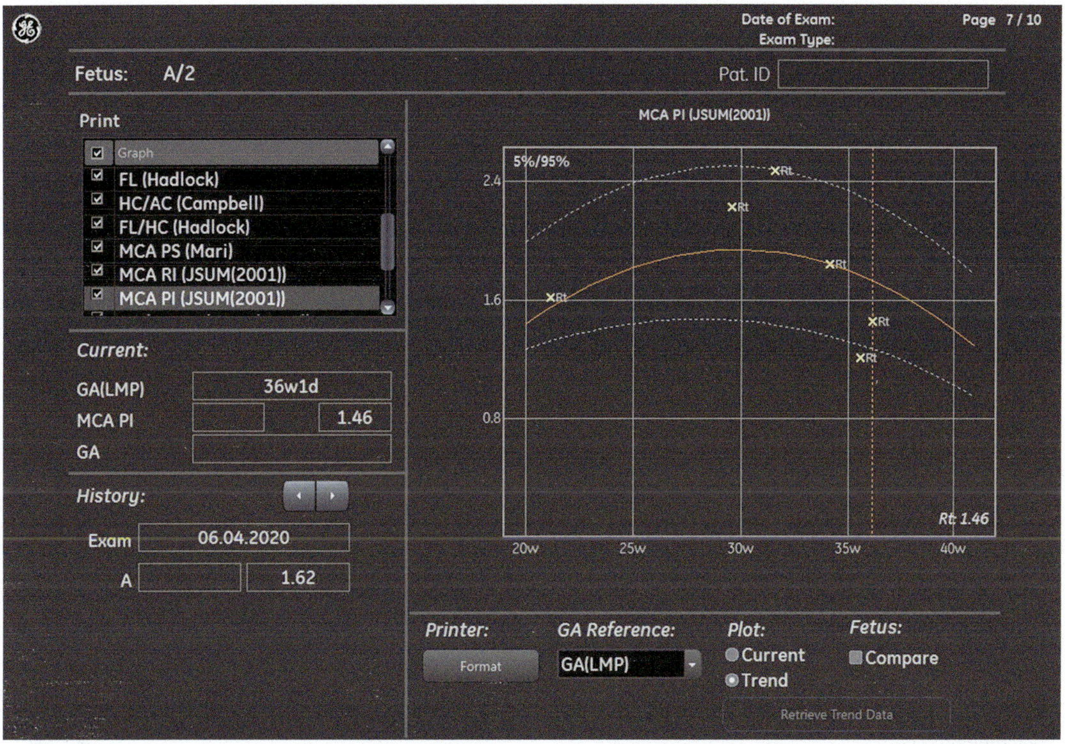

Fig. 9: Plotting of middle cerebral artery (MCA) PI (pulsatility index) on the nomogram shows paradoxical reversal (rise) of the MCA resistance.

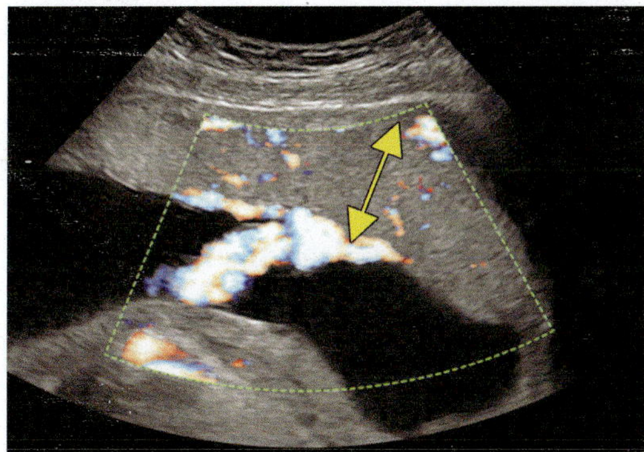

Fig. 10: Normal placenta with cord insertion. Measurement of placental thickness is shown by double-sided arrow.

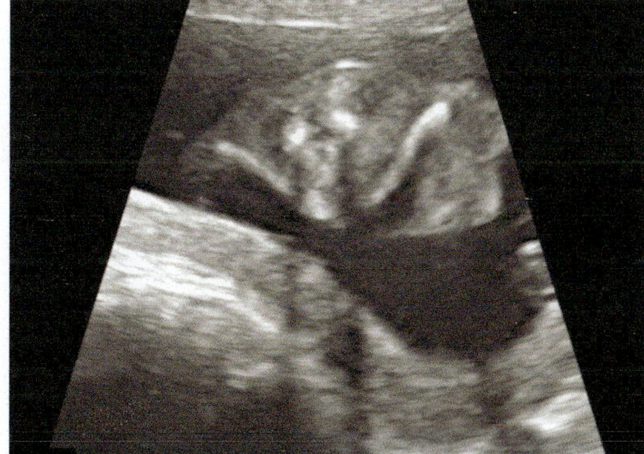

Fig. 11: B-mode ultrasound image shows thin placenta.

Small placenta is seen in:

- Intrauterine infections—chronic
- First trimester or preconceptional diabetes mellitus or glucose intolerance
- Chromosomal abnormalities
- IUGR of any cause
- *Severe polyhydramnios*: In these patients, placenta is not actually thin but because of abundant fluid, it gives an erroneous feel of thin placenta **(Fig. 11)**.

Large placenta is seen with ***(Fig. 12)***:

- Fetal hydrops
- Acute gestational infections
- Maternal anemia
- *Placental mesenchymal dysplasia*: These patients have a high incidence of growth

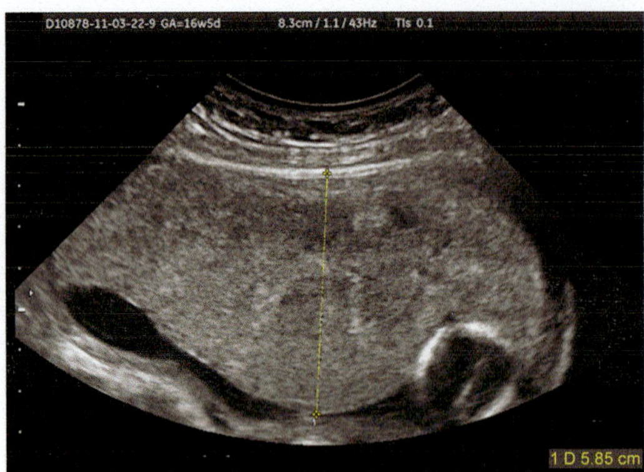

Fig. 12: B-mode ultrasound image of thick-large placenta.

restriction and fetal demise. The placenta shows anechoic areas due to cystic changes in stem villi.

- Aneuploidies
- Triploidy
- Placental hemorrhage
- Molar pregnancy
- Beckwith-Wiedemann syndrome—macrosomia, macroglossia, visceromegaly, and increased susceptibility to childhood tumors.

Texture Abnormalities of the Placenta

Normal placenta has a homogenous texture. Abnormal texture may be in the form of:

- Calcifications
- Lakes.

Placental calcification and grading: Calcifications in the placenta were thought to be related with the circulatory status of the placenta. It is known that toward the end of the 3rd trimester as a preparatory process for delivery of the fetus and the placenta, the placental vasculature starts regressing by calcification of the vascular walls. This means more calcification in the placenta means more mature placenta and this can be graded as **(Figs. 13A to C)**:

- *Grade 0*: Homogenous placenta
- *Grade 1*: Indentations in chorionic plate
- *Grade 2*: Basal stippling of placenta
- *Grade 3*: Calcification is more commonly seen in smokers and in patients on aspirin or heparin prophylaxis.

Stating placental grading is not required in current scenario, as calcification is no longer regarded as consistently associated with growth restriction, fetal distress in labor, PIH, diabetes, or lung maturity.[3]

Placental lakes ***(Fig. 14)****:* Placental lakes are anechoic areas in the placenta. These are almost universally seen after 25 weeks and are of no clinical significance. Lakes are formed by fibrin deposits that are a result of pooling of blood in perivillous spaces. These are more common in peripheral parts of placenta.

But, anechoic areas in the placenta may be also due to:

- Subchorionic hematoma
- Intervillous thrombosis
- Septal cysts
- Infarcts from retroplacental hematoma.

Subchorionic fibrin deposits: These are triangular or rectangular hypoechoic spaces with convex borders. These are of no clinical significance.[4]

Intervillous thrombosis: This is due to fetal hemorrhage in intervillous spaces. These are of significance in fetuses with Rh incompatibility.[5]

Septal cysts: Septal cysts are cystic areas in-between cotyledons and again are of no clinical significance. Though if >45 mm across, these may be associated with growth restriction.

Placental infarcts: Infarcts in the placenta may result from retroplacental hematomas or thrombotic occlusion of fetal arteries.

Small ones are of no clinical significance, but the larger ones may cause severe growth restriction and sometimes also fetal demise[6] **(Fig. 15)**. These are echogenic when fresh but become anechoic later. During the transition process, these may be at times difficult to

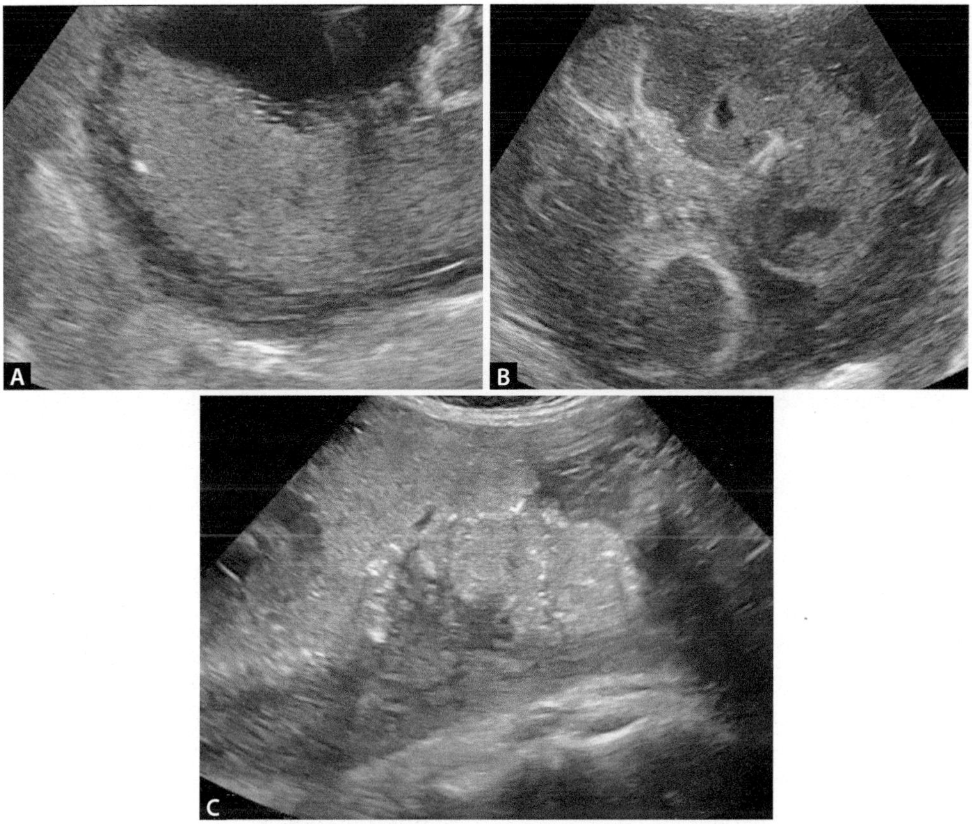

Figs. 13A to C: Placenta grade 0, 1, and 2.

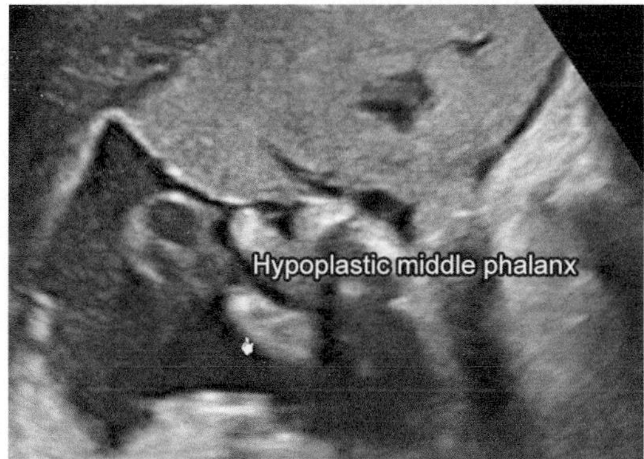

Fig. 14: Anechoic areas in the placenta—known as placental lakes.

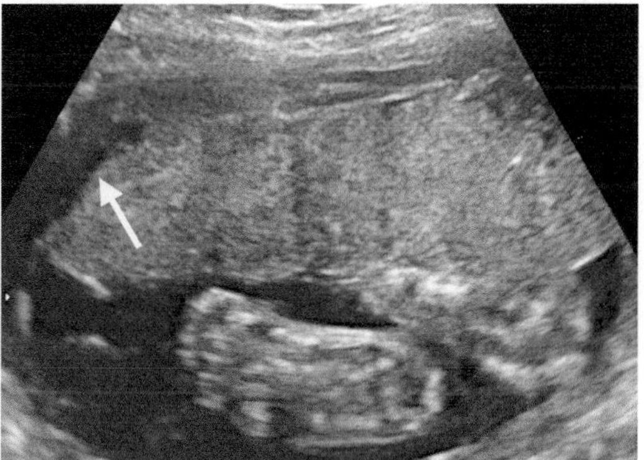

Fig. 15: Anechoic area seen between the placenta and the myometrium—retroplacental hematoma.

identify on scan. Some of these may also calcify and become densely hyperechoic.[6]

Placental Shape

Normal shape of the placenta is biconvex, with one surface attached to the uterine wall and another convex surface is its free surface **(Fig. 16)**. It is thickest in the center, where the umbilical cord is normally attached and thins out toward periphery.

Abnormalities of the placental shape may be:

- Placenta membranacea
- Circumvallate placenta

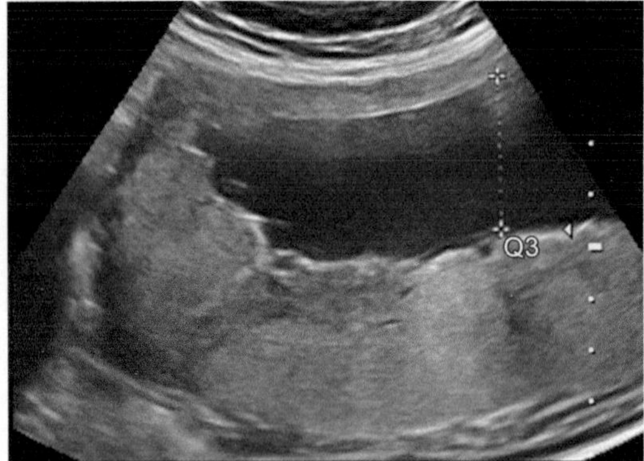

Fig. 16: Normal placenta.

- Horseshoe placenta
- Annular or ring shaped placenta

Placenta membranacea: This is a rare entity. The entire chorion is covered by villi and large part of this placenta is dysfunctional.[7] About one-third of these placentas are abnormally adherent. It often covers the internal os. Because of these two reasons, these placentas are commonly associated with recurrent antepartum hemorrhage, growth restriction, and postpartum hemorrhage.[8]

Circumvallate placenta: In this type of placenta, the chorion plate is smaller than basal plate and therefore membranes insert close to the center instead of at periphery **(Fig. 17)**. It may be complete or partial.

Partial variety is clinically insignificant. The complete variety may lead to placental abruption, growth restriction, perinatal mortality, and fetal growth restriction.[9]

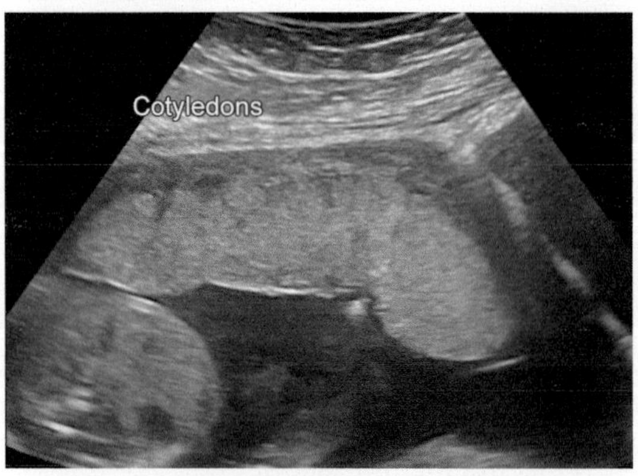

Fig. 17: Circumvallate placenta.

It has thickened rolled ridge of membranes with uplifted placental shelf.[2] It often shows lucent areas in the extrachorial part of placenta due to infarcts and hematomas.

Placental Location

Normally, the placenta is located in the fundus or upper part of the body of the uterus. In this region of the uterus, it may be located anteriorly, posteriorly, or on the sides. Positions other than this are considered abnormal. When located in the lower segment of the uterus, these placentas have higher risk of hemorrhagic complications. These placentas are known as placenta previa.

Depending on how low the lower edge of the placenta extends, these placentas may be graded as **(Figs. 18 and 19)**:

- *Grade 0*—lower segmental—distance from internal os < 10 mm.
- *Grade 1*—marginal, when the lower margin of the placenta is at the margin of the internal os.
- *Grade 2*—incomplete, when the lower margin of the placenta, partially covers the internal os.
- *Grade 3*—complete, when the internal os is fully covered by the placenta.

Risk of postpartum hemorrhage (PPH) is higher when the distance between the internal os and lower edge of placenta is <4 cm.[10]

Risk of placenta previa is more with:

- Previous CS
- Previous surgeries on uterus
- Previous vigorous curettage
- Multiparity
- Advanced maternal age
- But, approximately 90% of low-lying placentas at 20 weeks have a tendency to migrate up to normal position at term. Therefore, diagnosis of placenta previa and its grade must not be made before the end of 2nd trimester.[11] Placentas with thin lower edge are less likely to migrate as compared to those with thick edge.[12]

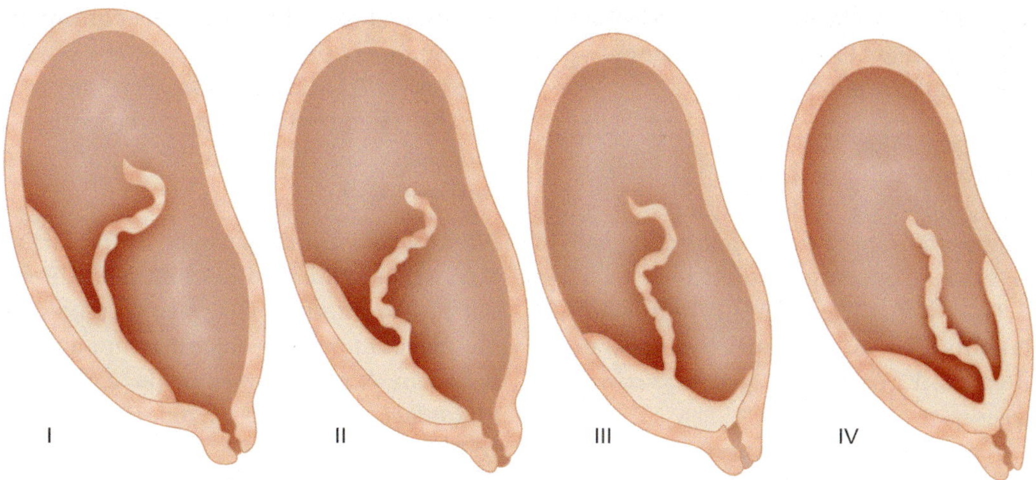

Fig. 18: Diagrammatic representation of grades of placenta previa.

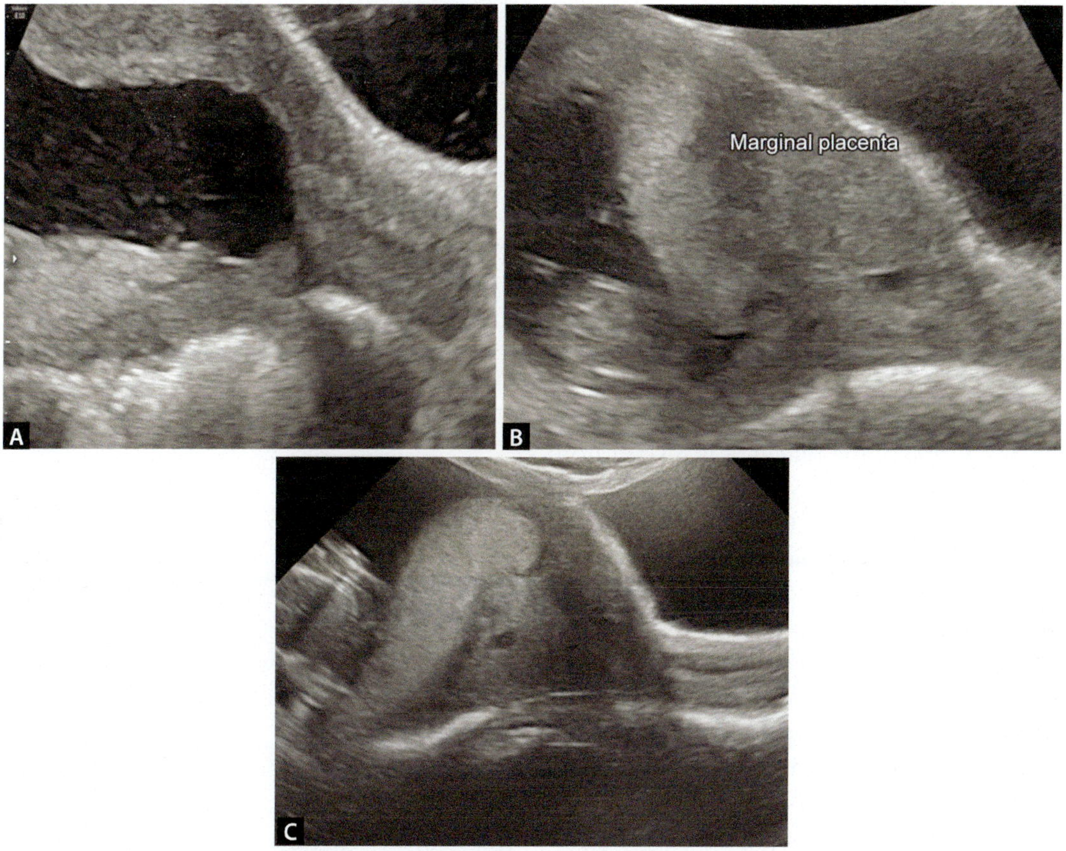

Figs. 19A to C: (A) Low-lying placenta; (B) Marginal placenta previa; (C) Complete placenta previa.

Placental migration is a consequence of:

- Formation of lower uterine segment
- Placental trophotropism.

Placental trophotropism: This term is used to describe preferential proliferation of trophoblastic villi in regions of better endometrial supply and atrophy of the villi in the region of poor blood supply.[13]

This theory can explain regression of placenta previa, succenturiate placental lobes, and abnormal cord insertions in placenta.

When placenta migrates, the raw/just opened up surface of the uterus may bleed leading to antepartum hemorrhage. But, bleeding with placental migration is not life threatening and will not lead to the need of premature delivery usually. Antepartum bleeding can be more correlated with the cervical length and presence of echo-free space in lower edge of placenta, overlying the internal os.[14,15]

Management strategy for pregnancies with low-lying placenta:

- Distance >20 mm—vaginal delivery is possible
- Distance between 10–20 mm—most times vaginal delivery is possible

Succenturiate placental lobe ***(Fig. 20)****:* This means a lobe of the placenta is distant from main placenta. This may be a lobe with vessels not commencing out of this lobe. But, at times, fetal vessels may commence from these lobes to merge with main placenta to form the cord.[16] These vessels are more likely to rupture at labor or at the time of rupture of membranes and can lead to fetal demise. This is especially likely because these vessels may be close to or pass over the internal os and get damaged and also because these may not be protected by Wharton's jelly. Retained placenta and PPH are common complications with succenturiate lobe of placenta.[16]

Vasa previa ***(Fig. 21)****:* When the cord vessels are the presenting structures, it is known as vasa previa. It is different from placenta previa.

This is commonly associated with succenturiate lobe, velamentous, or marginal cord insertion.

Placental invasion: Normally, the placenta is attached to the myometrium of the uterus, but a clear interface is always seen between the placenta and the myometrium and this is known as retroplacental space **(Fig. 22)**. Retroplacental space is a hypoechoic space of 10–20 mm in thickness.

Retroplacental space is irregular or interrupted in conditions such as retroplacental

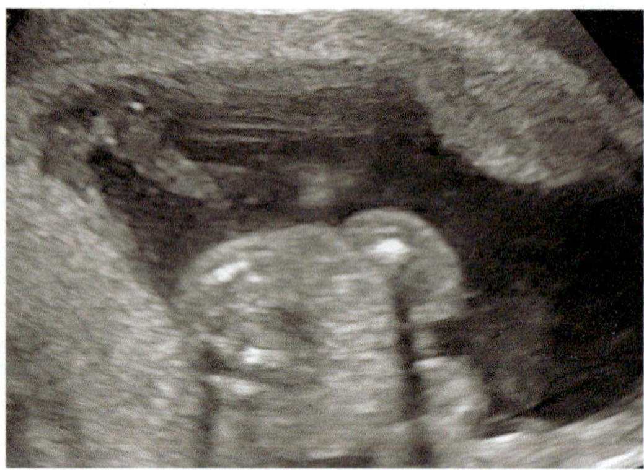

Fig. 20: Succenturiate lobe of placenta seen on the anterior wall with the main placenta on posterior wall.

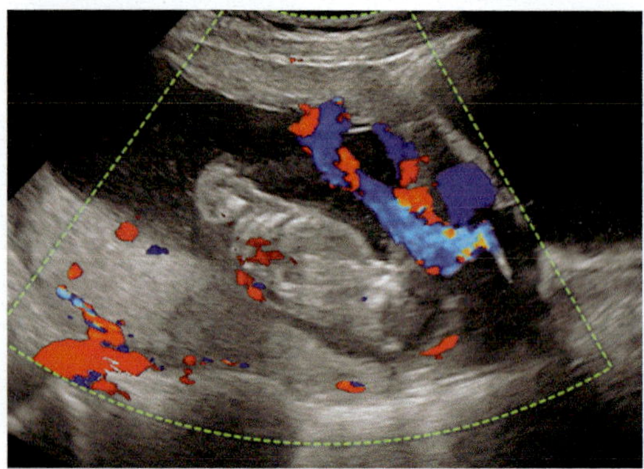

Fig. 21: Vasa previa.

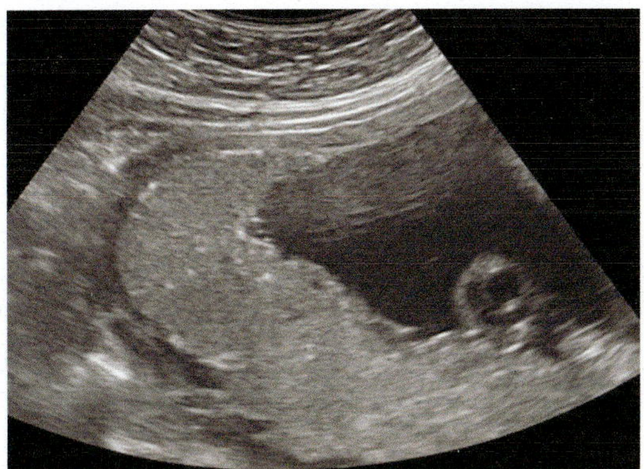

Fig. 22: Normal placenta with intact retroplacental space (hypoechoic area between placenta and myometrium).

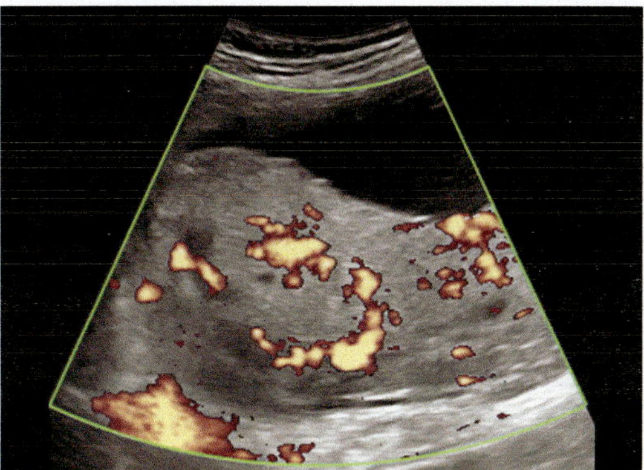

Fig. 24: Placenta increta.

hematoma, placental abruption, and placental adherence. The retroplacental space becomes irregular in placental hematomas and abruption but is obliterated in abnormal placental invasion and abrasion. Whenever this space is not consistent, assessment of the underlying myometrium is mandatory to exclude myomas, adenomyosis, or calcifications. Myomas need to be differentiated from uterine contractions, which disappear in 20–60 minutes.

Placental invasion abnormalities ***(Fig. 23)****:*

- Placenta accreta
- Placenta increta **(Fig. 24)**
- Placenta percreta.

Placenta accreta: It is abnormal adherence of the placenta to myometrium. The placenta is adherent to but not invading the myometrium.

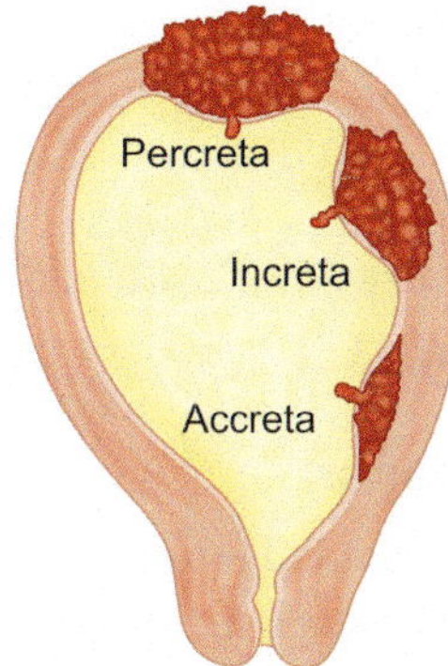

Fig. 23: Diagrammatic representation of types of placental invasion.

It is consequential to a defect in the fibrinoid (Nitabuch's) layer of decidua underlying the placenta.[17] Placenta previa is more commonly seen in patients with placenta accreta.

Diagnosis of placenta accreta on US:

- Normal retroplacental hypoechoic space is 10–20 mm thick, this reduces to <2 mm.
- Interface between placenta and myometrium is lost.
- Multiple anechoic lacunae are seen in the placenta.
- Blood vessels running perpendicular to the myometrial vessels in a normal placenta are also seen running across in to the myometrium.[18]

Placenta percreta: When the placental tissue invades into the myometrium, it is called placenta percreta. On ultrasound, the retroplacental space is obliterated and on Doppler; placental vessels that are perpendicular to myometrial fibers and myometrial surface are seen penetrating into half or more thickness of the myometrium.

Placenta increta: When the placental tissue invades the entire thickness of the myometrium through to serosa and beyond, it is called placenta increta. Ultrasound diagnosis is by obliteration of the retroplacental space and extension of placental vessels across the myometrium, through to the serosa and may be even to the surrounding tissues.

Placenta percreta and increta are the more worse forms of an adherent placenta. These placental abnormalities may often cause uterine inversion and severe bleeding. These may almost always demand a hysterectomy at delivery of the baby.

Accuracy of ultrasound for antenatal detection of invasive placenta is fairly high and diagnosed antenatally, which can plan delivery better and also save the mother from fatal complications.

The diagnostic accuracies of adherent placenta on B-mode and color Doppler studies are as follows:

B-mode:

- Sensitivity—90.72%
- Specificity—96.94%
- Positive LR—11.01
- Negative LR—0.16

Color Doppler:

- Sensitivity—90.74%
- Specificity—87.68%
- Positive LR—7.77
- Negative LR—0.17

Hematomas around placenta:

- Retroplacental hematoma
- Subamniotic hematoma
- Subchorionic hematoma
- Concealed hematoma.

Retroplacental hematomas: Hematoma seen between basal plate of placenta and uterine wall is called a retroplacental hematoma. The fresh ones are isoechoic to placenta and difficult to identify. But, the old ones are hypoechoic and cause evident widening of the retroplacental space on ultrasound. These may lead to villous infarction.

*Subamniotic hematoma **(Fig. 25)**:* Hematoma between amnion and chorion is called a subamniotic hematoma. The most common location is at the placental cord insertion. It often occurs as a result of pulling of cord during delivery and therefore not an antenatal ultrasound diagnosis.

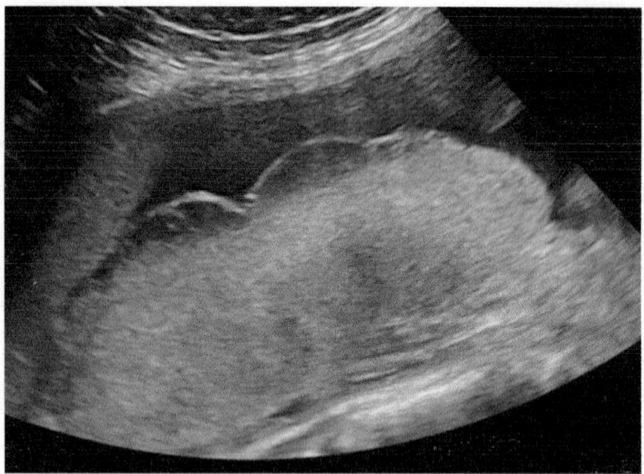

Fig. 25: Subamniotic hematoma.

Only rarely, it may be diagnosed antenatally and when large, it is termed as Breus mole. This is commonly associated with growth restriction and fetal demise. On US, it appears as an avascular hypoechoic lesion between chorion and amnion.[19]

Subchorionic hematoma: Hematoma between fetal aspect of placenta and overlying chorionic membrane is termed as a subchorionic hematoma. It is more often seen in patients with cocaine abuse, smoking habits, hypertension, preeclampsia, anticardiolipin antibodies, and may also occur due to blunt trauma. Its clinical presentation and significance are related to size of hematoma and gestational age. It is associated with uterine irritation due to blood and may lead to preterm labor.[20]

Patients with subchorionic hematoma have a higher risk of abortion, fetal growth restriction (FGR), preterm labor, placental abruption or fetal distress, when associated with vaginal bleeding or uterine contractions.[20]

It can be treated with tocolytics and progesterone.

Placental Tumors

These can be divided into:

1. Nontrophoblastic tumors
2. Placental site trophoblastic tumor (PSTT) and epithelioid trophoblastic tumor (ETT)

Nontrophoblastic Tumors

Gestational trophoblastic disease: In patients with complete mole, the possibility of development of choriocarcinoma or invasive mole increases and this can be diagnosed by persistently high beta-hCG levels after evacuation of the mole. 20% of all complete mole patients may have this risk. Though gestational trophoblastic neoplasia (GTN) may also arise after normal pregnancy, miscarriage, or ectopic pregnancy. This group of tumors includes more common choriocarcinoma and invasive mole and less common placental site trophoblastic tumor (PSTT) and epithelioid trophoblastic tumor (ETT). These may be malignant or potentially malignant. The malignant ones have a tendency to metastasize into vagina or lung. Patients present with high beta-hCG levels, vaginal bleeding, hyperthyroidism, and pelvic pain. The history and clinical presentation are so typical that biopsy is usually not required for confirmation of diagnosis.

- Complete or partial moles
- Invasive mole

Invasive mole: When hydropic villi invade into the myometrium, it is invasive mole. On ultrasound, it appears as ill-defined solid mass in the myometrium with multiple fluid-filled anechoic areas **(Fig. 26)**. These lesions show high score of vascularity with low-resistance flow (RI: 0.4–0.45). Dilated vessels may also be seen in the surrounding myometrium. The neoangiogenesis of the mass lesion shows arteriovenous shunts and therefore turbulent flows. Ovaries show multiloculated cystic lesions with thin septae (theca lutein cysts).

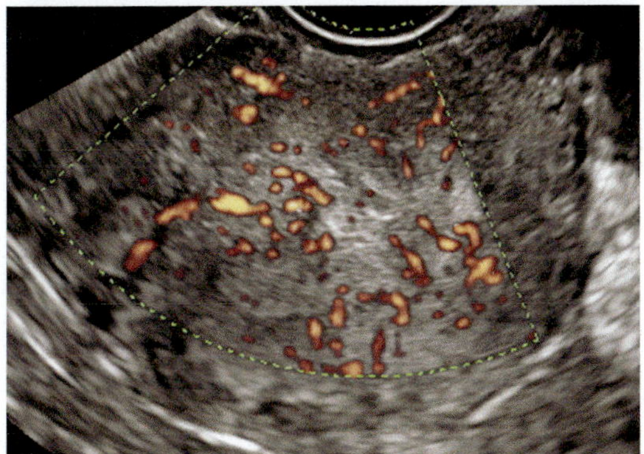

Fig. 26: Ill-defined solid mass in the myometrium with multiple fluid-filled anechoic areas as seen on transvaginal ultrasound with power Doppler showing blood vessels with irregular caliber.

The positive response to treatment may be indicated by decreasing size and vascularity of the lesion.

- *Choriocarcinoma*: This tumor usually follows a molar or a nonmolar pregnancy, invades into the myometrium, consists of cytotrophoblast and syncytiotrophoblast, and has a high malignant potential.

  On ultrasound: These tumors present as ill-defined solid mass lesions with heterogeneous echogenicity consisting of solid components and anechoic areas **(Fig. 27A)** that consist of vascular channels and cystic areas secondary to hemorrhage and necrosis. These tumors are highly vascular and, on Doppler, show moderate-to-high vascularity (score 3–4), with vessels of irregular caliber, arteriovenous shunts, and vascular lakes **(Fig. 27B)**. The uterine artery also shows low resistance flow. In more wide spread tumor, there may be enlargement of the uterus also, with entire myometrium showing heterogeneous echogenicity. The tumor, if extends into the parametrium, may show similar echogenicity and Doppler findings till the extension of the tumor. Theca lutein cysts are also seen in ovaries as multiloculated cystic lesions with thin septae.

Placental Site Trophoblastic Tumor (PSTT) and Epithelioid Trophoblastic Tumor (ETT)

These tumors arise from intermediate cells of extravillous trophoblast of nonmolar pregnancy and secrete low levels of hCG but high levels of human placental lactogen (HPL).

These tumors have indistinct margins and show multiple cystic spaces **(Figs. 28A to C)**. The vascularity is low and the amount

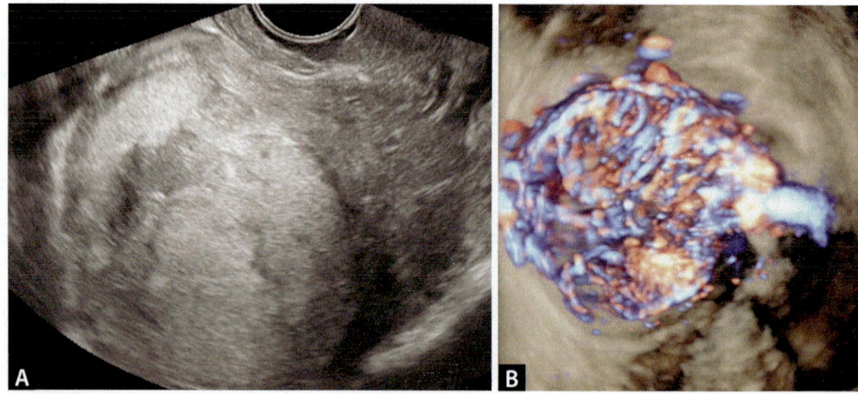

Figs. 27A and B: (A) Ill-defined solid mass lesions with heterogeneous echogenicity consisting of solid components and anechoic areas seen on transvaginal B-mode scan; (B) Doppler shows moderate-to-high vascularity (score 3–4), with vessels of irregular caliber, arteriovenous shunts, and vascular lakes.

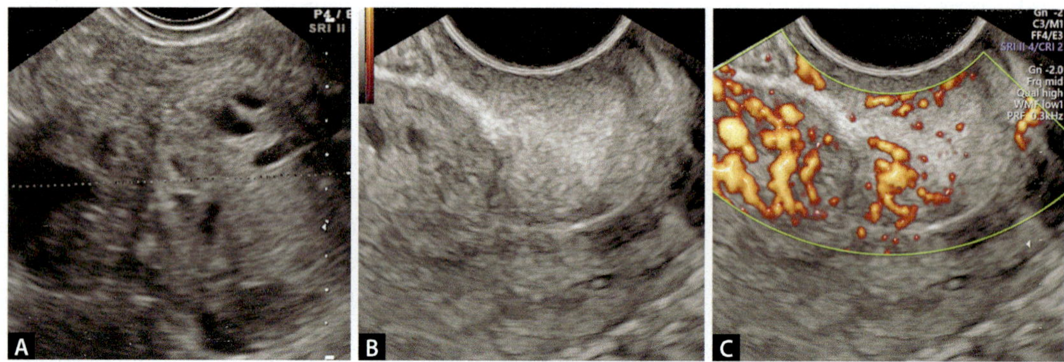

Figs. 28A to C: Tumor with ill-defined margins and multiple small cystic spaces of variable sizes.

of vascularity represents its sensitivity to chemotherapy.

Nontrophoblastic placental tumors:

- Chorioangiomas
- *Placental teratomas* are cystic and solid lesions, variably vascular and on surface of placenta. These may represent an unsuccessful twin pregnancy.[21]
- Metastasis from melanoma, lymphoma, leukemia and breast lesions, though very rare may be seen in the placenta.[22]

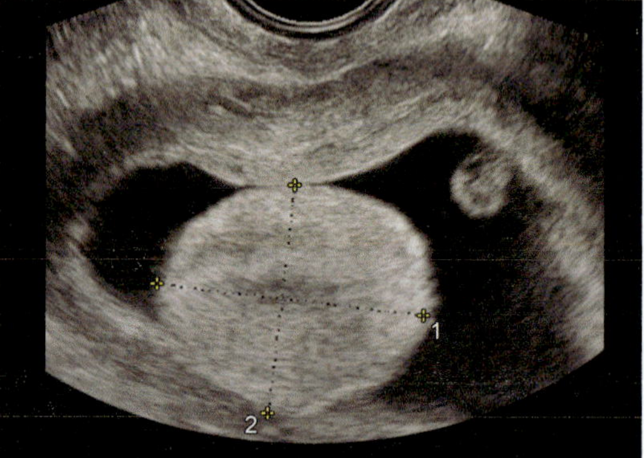

Fig. 29: Chorioangioma.

Chorioangiomas ***(Fig. 29)****:* These are the most common of nontrophoblastic placental tumors. These are benign tumors. They usually arise from close to the cord attachment on the placenta. These are well-defined tumors but variably vascular. The smaller ones are nonsignificant, but the larger ones, especially those larger than >50 mm across, may lead to nonimmune hydrops, fetal cardiomegaly, polyhydramnios, or growth restriction.[23]

Umbilical Cord

Umbilical cord is the vascular and nutritional link between the mother's uterus and the fetus. It chiefly constitutes of two umbilical arteries and an umbilical vein and Wharton's jelly and all these covered in a single layer of amniotic epithelium. It has a helical structure with arteries and vein arranged as a spiral **(Figs. 30A and B)**. At term, it is about 50–60 cm long and has a helical course with 10–11 coils in all.

Structure of the umbilical cord can be influenced by:

- Gestational age
- Amniotic fluid amount
- Composition of amniotic fluid
- Fetoplacental hemodynamics
- Maternal complications

Like all other fetal parts, umbilical cord also follows a sort of a growth pattern and has a definitive consistent pattern that it follows. Its diameter progressively increases till 32 weeks and then plateaus. Its thickness is because of the caliber of arteries and the vein and also because of the amount of Wharton's jelly **(Table 1)**. The umbilical cord vessels also have an increasing caliber with the growing pregnancy **(Fig. 31)**.

TABLE 1: Diameter of umbilical cord vessels at 16 weeks and at term.

	16 weeks	*At term*
Umbilical artery	1.2 ± 0.4 mm	4.2 ± 0.4 mm
Umbilical vein	2.0 ± 0.6 mm	8.2 ± 0.8 mm

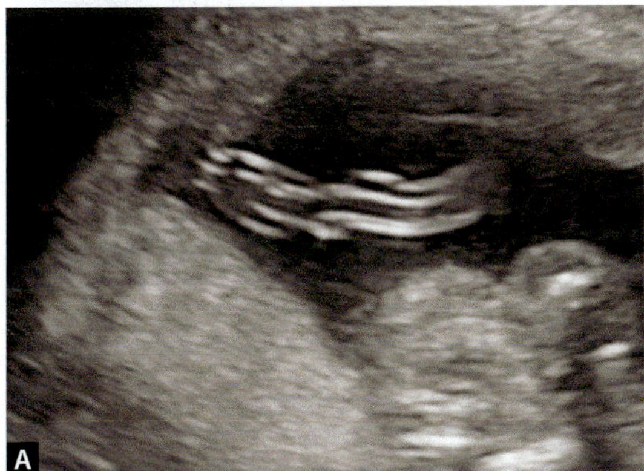

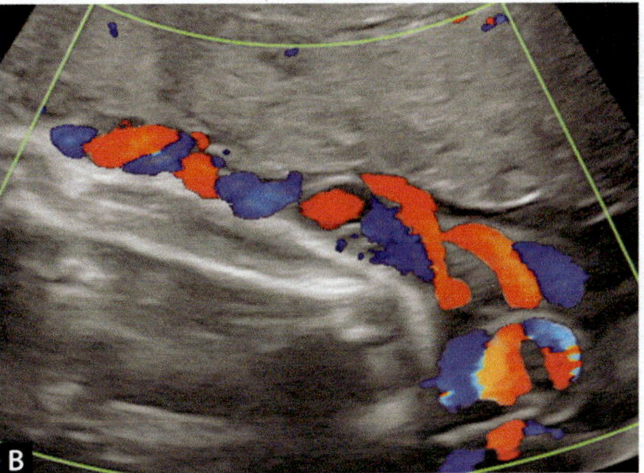

Figs. 30A and B: Normal umbilical cord on B-mode and color Doppler.

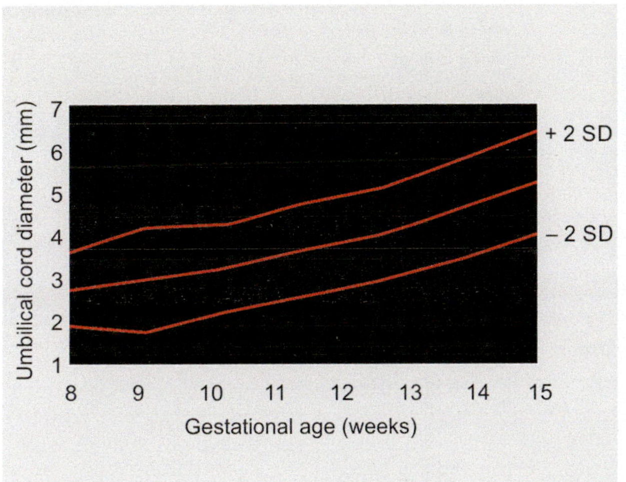

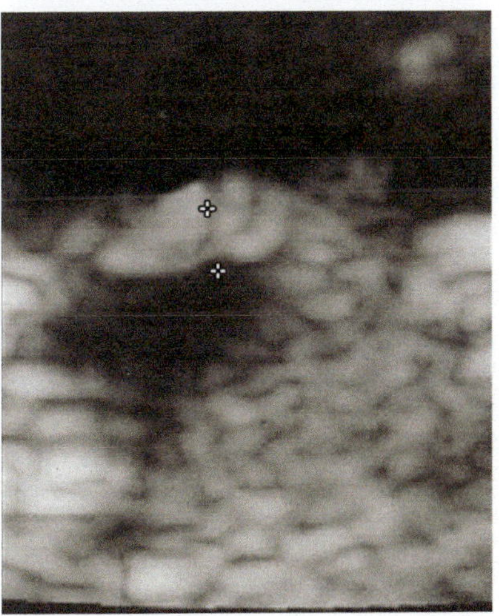

Fig. 31: Graph showing increasing umbilical cord diameter with increasing gestational age.

Wharton's jelly: Wharton's jelly consists of a collagen fibrillar network formed by canalicular structures and cavernous and perivascular spaces.[24] It is also supposed to have contractility comparable to smooth muscle cells and so participates in regulation of blood flow in the cord vessels.

It may have a role in bidirectional transfer of fluid and metabolites between amniotic fluid and cord vessels and also has metabolic functions. It protects the umbilical vessels from external pressure changes and minor injuries.

Abnormalities of the umbilical cord may be:
- Abnormal cord thickness
- Abnormal number of umbilical arteries
- Discordant umbilical arteries
- Abnormal length of the cord
- Abnormal coiling pattern of the cord.

Abnormal Cord Thickness

Cord may be thin because of thin vessels and less amount of Wharton's jelly **(Fig. 32)**. It is known that thin umbilical cord vessels mean less blood flow to the fetus **(Tables 2 and 3)**.

Lean umbilical cord after 20 weeks of gestation had *4.4-fold higher risk of having a small for gestational age (SGA) infant* than the one with normal cord (95% confidence interval, 2.16–8.85).[26] Cord thickness of *<10th centile for gestational age is an early marker of SGA infant and occurrence of intrapartum complications.*[27]

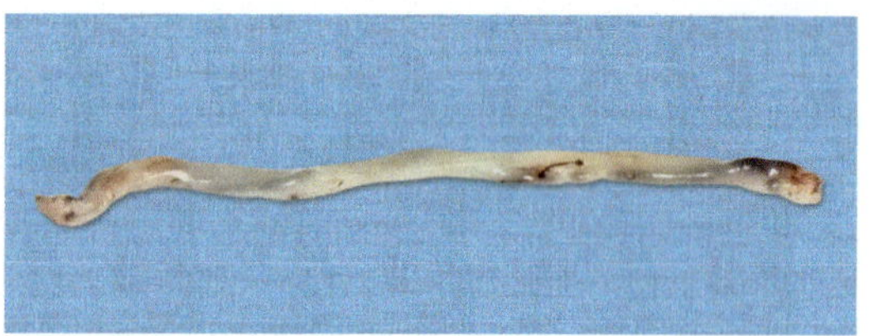

Fig. 32: Thin umbilical cord.

It is shown in this study by Bruch et al. that fetuses with thin cord and IUGR have significantly less amount of Wharton's jelly and also smaller vessels as compared to normal fetuses **(Table 4)**.[28]

Amount of Wharton's jelly may be reduced due to reduction in extracellular fluid or matrix in patients with hypertensive disorders and gestational diabetes.

Thick cord may be due to:
- Cord tumor
- Urachal cysts
- Mucoid degeneration of cord
- Omphalomesenteric cyst

TABLE 2: Cord morphology in normal and thin cord.[25]

Characteristics	***Normal cord***	***Lean cord***	***p***
Cord length (cm)	57.6 ± 10.3	57.2 ± 11.5	NS
Coiling index	0.29 ± 0.09	0.18 ± 0.08	<0.001
Cord area (mm^2)	200.6 ± 34.6	87.6 ± 5.1	<0.001
Art area (mm^2)	14.3 ± 5.4	13.3 ± 5.3	NS
Vein area (mm^2)	50.5 ± 20.2	35.2 ± 11.5	<0.01
Jelly area (mm^2)	122.1 ± 33.4	25.7 ± 10.3	<0.001

TABLE 3: Flow parameters in normal and thin cord.[25]

Characteristics	***Normal cord***	***Lean cord***	***p***
Artery PI	0.83 ± 0.14	0.85 ± 0.09	NS
Absolute vein blood flow	423.5 ± 93.2	293.6 ± 81.8	<0.001
Vein flow for fetal weight	126 ± 23.4	93.7 ± 17.8	<0.001
Vein flow velocity	9.0 ± 3.6	6.6 ± 2.7	<0.05

TABLE 4: Cord parameters in intrauterine growth restriction.

Cord parameters	*Normal*	*IUGR normal Doppler*	*IUGR abnormal Doppler*
Wharton's jelly	49.4 ± 2.2	40.4 ± 3.7	33.4 ± 2.6
Vessel areas	7.8 ± 0.3	6.6 ± 0.3	4.8 ± 0.3
Art wall thickness	654 ± 20	645 ± 23	525 ± 24
Vein wall thickness	465 ± 18	465 ± 18	390 ± 14

- It has also been used as one of the parameters to predict fetal macrosomia.[29]
- Increased amount of Wharton's jelly is seen in patients with gestational diabetes mellitus (due to increased accumulation of fluid and plasma proteins and is seen after 24 weeks of gestation).[30]

Abnormal Number of Umbilical Arteries

This is almost always a single umbilical artery. More than two umbilical arteries are not known. Single umbilical artery can be picked up on long section of the umbilical cord also, but is always better demonstrated on the transverse section of the cord. The normal cord that has two umbilical arteries and one umbilical vein shows a typical Mickey Mouse face appearance on transverse section **(Fig. 33)**. This is not seen in case of a single umbilical artery **(Fig. 34)**.

Incidence of single umbilical artery is:

- 0.5–2.9% in euploid fetuses
- 1.5–7% in aborted fetuses
- 9–11% in aneuploid fetuses

There have been several studies on consequences of single umbilical artery and various studies have shown higher risk of chromosomal abnormalities and higher risk of IUGR. As for the risk of chromosomal abnormality, the current concept is that as an isolated finding, this is of not much importance but when associated with other soft markers, this may increase the risk of chromosomal abnormalities.

Fetuses with single umbilical artery have a higher risk of:

- *IUGR—controversial*: As for the risk of IUGR, the current concept does not agree that the single umbilical artery increases the risk of IUGR. Though fetuses with single umbilical artery have been shown to have a higher risk of intrapartum accidents and stillbirths.
- Risk of congenital anomalies is calculated to be approximately 7 times higher. But, unfortunately only 37% of these anomalies can be identified on prenatal scans.[31]

Fig. 33: Normal cord in transverse section.

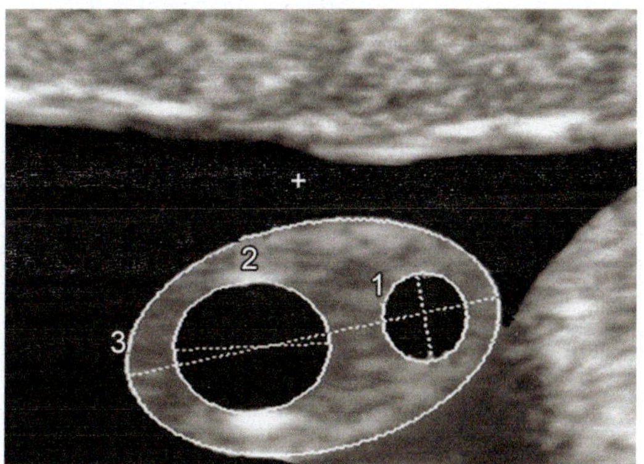

Fig. 34: Cord with single umbilical artery in transverse section.

- Intrauterine death, the risk is more in third trimester.
- There is also an increased risk of intrapartum death.

Intrauterine death and intrapartum death may be attributed to two reasons. First is the absence of Hyrtl anastomosis, therefore, no safety valve mechanism to fight sudden severe pressure changes. Second is that these cords have less Wharton's jelly, which further decreases in third trimester.

Single umbilical artery actually is thought to be an extreme form of discordant umbilical arteries.[31]

Discordant Umbilical Arteries (Fig. 35)

These arteries have difference in diameter of umbilical arteries of at least 1 mm in three different parts of cord. These arteries also show difference in impedance to blood flow.[32] But, discordant umbilical arteries have not shown effect on the development of the fetus.

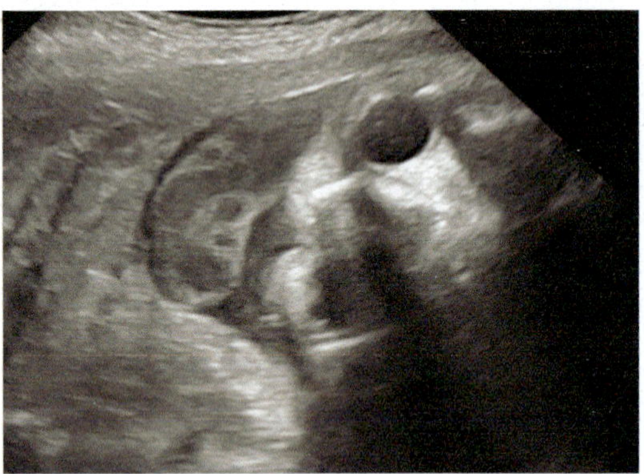

Fig. 35: Discordant umbilical arteries.

Discordant umbilical arteries are common with:

- Placenta bipartite (placenta divided into two parts)
- Placenta succenturiate (succenturiate lobe of placenta)
- Absent Hyrtl anastomosis
- Marginal cord insertion in placenta
- Velamentous cord insertion

Hyrtl anastomosis: Hyrtl anastomosis is the only vessel that connects the two umbilical arteries or their branches on placental surface, close to the site of cord insertion, and equalizes the blood pressure between the territories of two arteries **(Figs. 36A and B)**. As it equalizes the pressure in the two umbilical arteries, it actually works as a pressure release valve and protects the fetus and the cord from damages due to pressure changes. It is present in 95% of normal placentas. Absent Hyrtl anastomosis is more frequently seen apart from fetuses with single umbilical artery, in patients with discordant umbilical arteries and in fetuses with velamentous cord insertion.

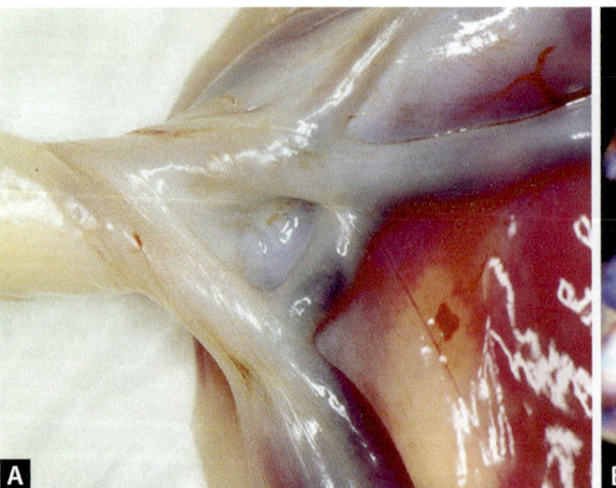

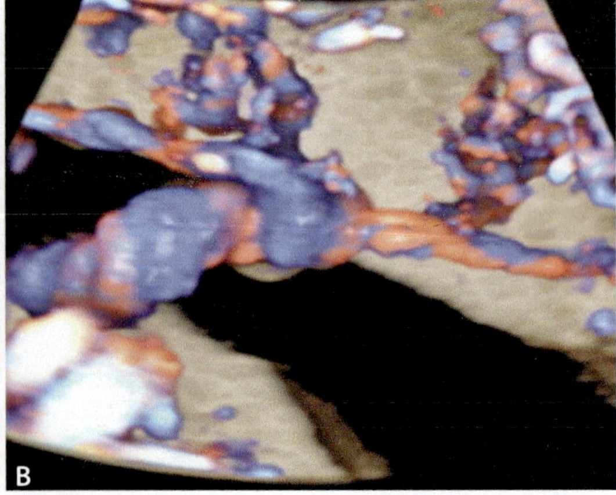

Figs. 36A and B: Normal Hyrtl anastomosis: (A) On dissection; (B) On ultrasound.

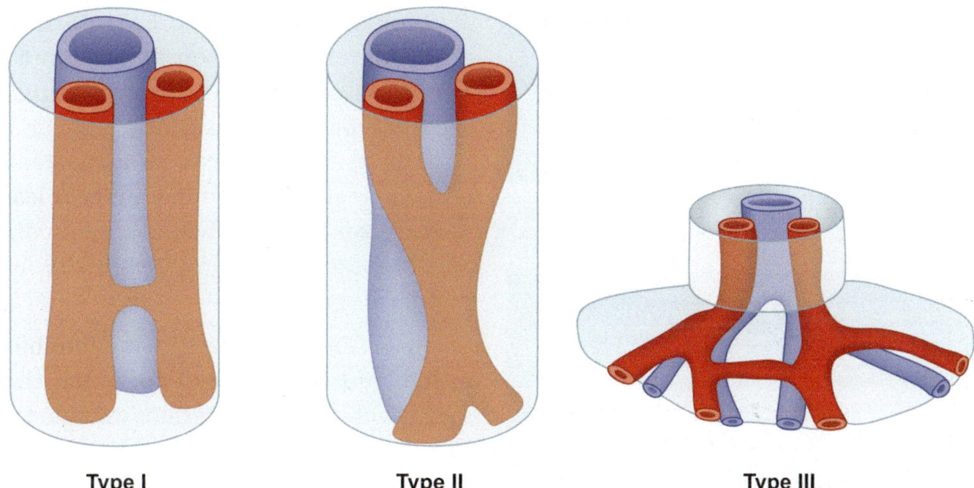

Fig. 37: Diagrammatic demonstration of three types of Hyrtl anastomosis.

Hypothesis on the function of Hyrtl anastomosis:

- It equalizes the pressure between the two umbilical arteries.
- It allows uniform distribution of blood in the different regions of the placenta.
- It acts as a safety valve for the placenta in case of compression or occlusion of one of the umbilical arteries or during uterine contractions.

Hyrtl anastomosis can be of three different types **(Fig. 37)**.

Velamentous cord insertion: Velamentous insertion of the cord is insertion of the cord in the membranes distant from placenta with vessels running in the membranes without being protected by Wharton's jelly **(Fig. 38)**.

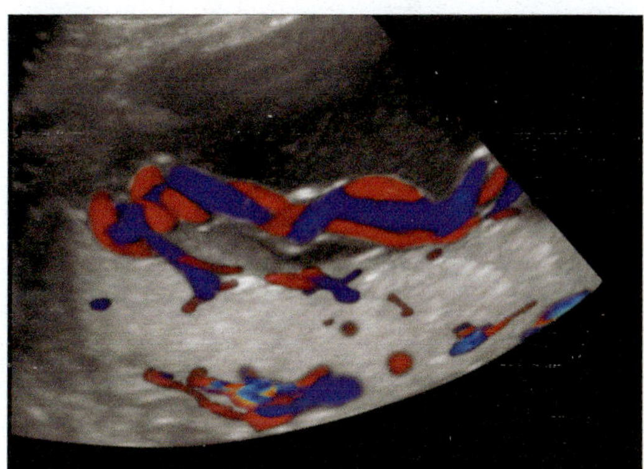

Fig. 38: Velamentous insertion of cord.

Helical pattern of the umbilical cord:

- Umbilical cord starts coiling at 8 weeks. The number of coils at the end of 1st trimester is the same as at term. More cords are left twisted, though the significance of side is not yet understood.
- Single coil is distance between the right outer surface of consecutive arterial coils.
- Umbilical coil index (UCI) is reciprocal of this value and represents the number of coils in the cord. Umbilical coiling index is calculated as: Number of coils/Cord length in cm **(Fig. 39)**.

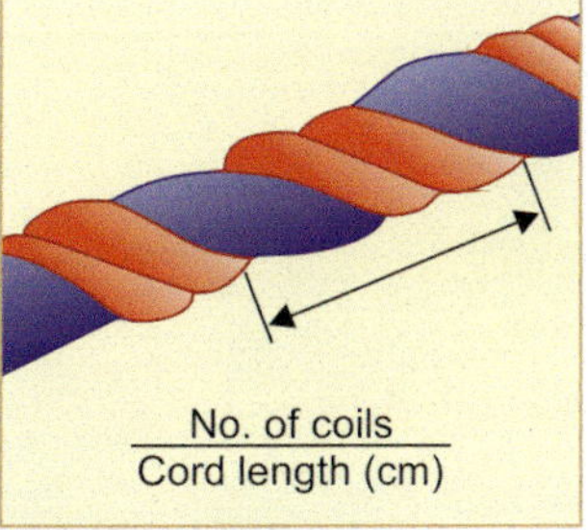

Fig. 39: Calculating umbilical cord coiling index.

Abnormal Coiling Pattern (Fig. 40)

- *Uncoiled*: No coils—straight umbilical arteries

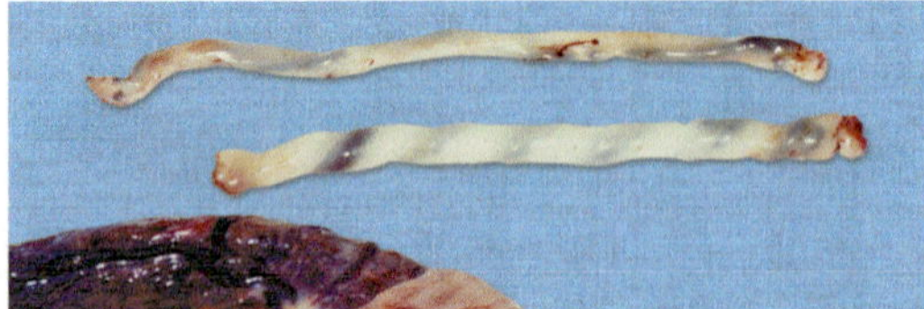

Fig. 40: Less coiled and highly coiled cord at birth.

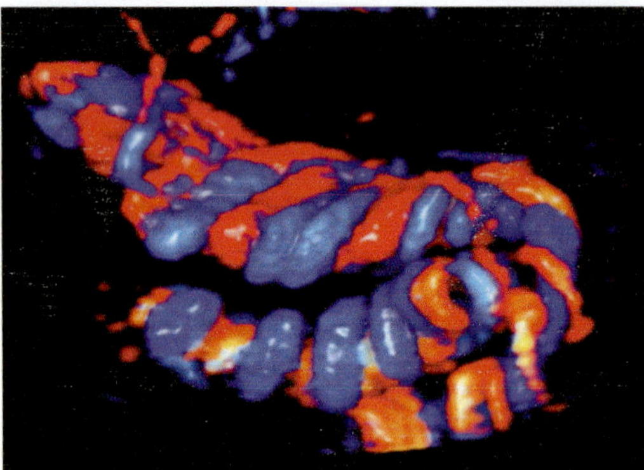

Fig. 41: Hypercoiled cord.

- Uncoiled or hypocoiled cords are more seen in fetuses with IUGR, maternal hypertensive disorders, and aneuploidies
- *Hypocoiled*: UCI <10th centile
- *Hypercoiled*: UCI >90th centile **(Fig. 41)**
- *Atypical coiling*:
  - Uncoordinated or aperiodic coiling
  - Supercoiling or spring-like cord.

Though no definite correlations to pathologies have been established yet, abnormal coiling patterns are thought to influence perinatal outcome.

Supercoiled cords can be associated with pathologic intra-abdominal process leading to increase in resistance at umbilical ring and venous congestion in extra-abdominal umbilical vein.

Cord cyst ***(Figs. 42A and B)****:* Cysts may be seen in the cord. These are of not much clinical significance, though was once thought to be a soft marker for T21.

Cord round the neck: This is commonly seen. Single loop is not of much importance as usually is not a complete circle. When there are two or more loops **(Fig. 43)**, it can strangulate the fetus. But, at times, even a single loop can cause strangulation when there is a knot **(Figs. 44A and B)**.

Knot in the cord may lead to severe fetal hypoxia and intrapartum death. This is usually difficult to identify on B-mode image. Though 3D power Doppler can be diagnostic. But, it is important to remember that it must be suspected to identify. Very important sign that would suggest a possibility is intermittent fetal bradycardia.

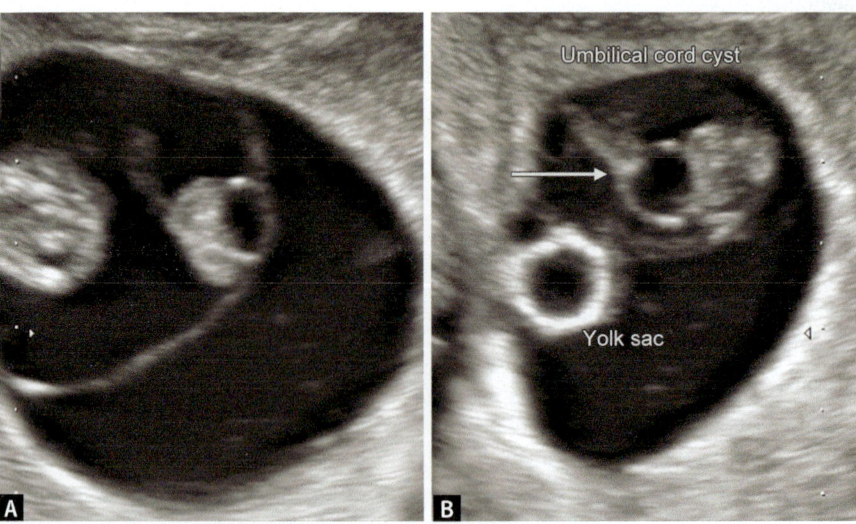

Figs. 42A and B: Umbilical cord cyst (arrow).

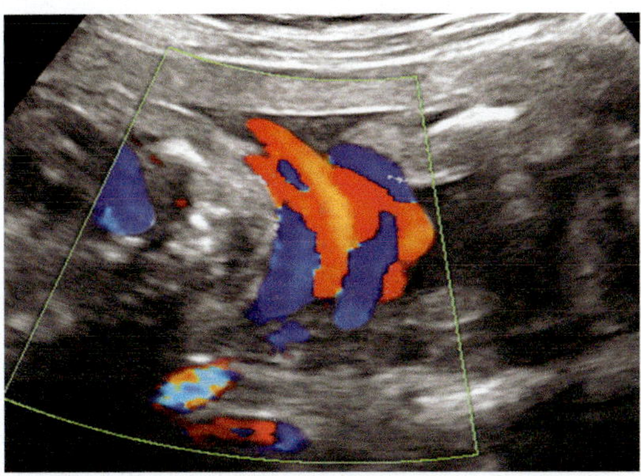

Fig. 43: Two loops of cord round the neck.

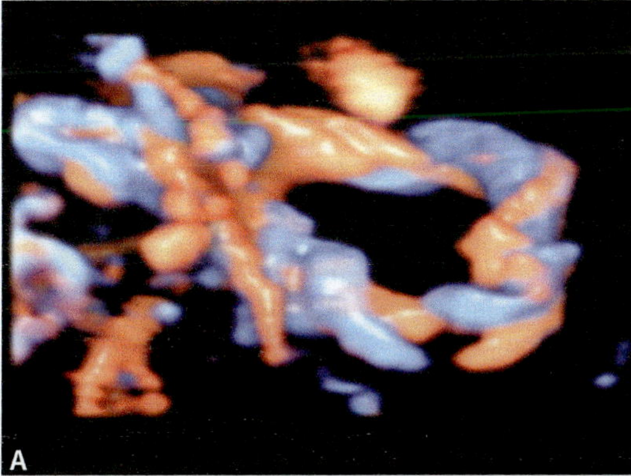

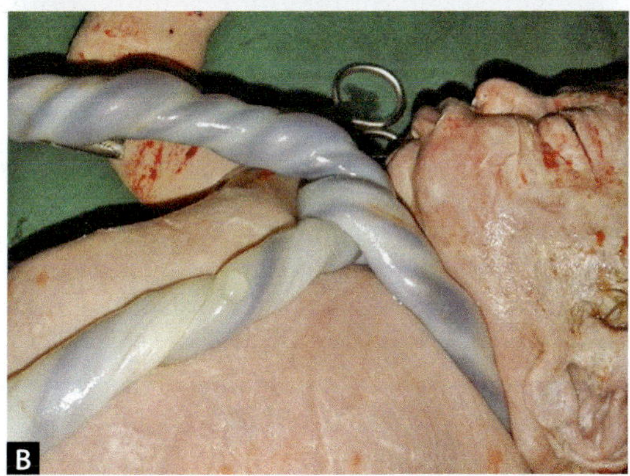

Figs. 44A and B: Single loop of cord round the neck with knot (A) on color Doppler and (B) in the neonate.

To conclude, placenta and the cord, though most times neglected on the scan, can be important indicators of fetal status and must become a part of routine anomaly scans.

REFERENCES

1. Kliman HJ. The placenta revealed. Am J Pathol. 1993;143(2):332-6.
2. Harris RD, Alexander RD. Ultrasound in Obstetrics and Gynecology, 4th edition. Philadelphia: WB Saunders Co.; 2000. pp. 597-625.
3. McKenna D, Tharmaratnam S, Mahsud S, Dornan J. Ultrasonic evidence of placental calcification at 36 weeks' gestation: maternal and fetal outcomes. Acta Obstet Gynecol Scand. 2005;84(1):7-10.
4. McGahan JP, Goldberg BB. Diagnostic Ultrasound: A logical approach, 1st edition. Philadelphia: Lippincott-Raven Publishers, 1998. pp 181-200.
5. Salafia CM, Minior VK, Pezzullo JC, Popek EJ, Rosenkrantz TS, Vintzileos AM. Intrauterine growth restriction in infants of less than thirty-two weeks' gestation: associated placental pathologic features. Am J Obstet Gynecol. 1995;173(4):1049-57.
6. Jauniaux E, Campbell S. Antenatal diagnosis of placental infarcts by ultrasonography. J Clin Ultrasound. 1991;19:58-61.
7. Greenberg JA, Sorem KA, Shifren JL, Riley LE. Placenta membranacea with placenta increta: a case report and literature review. Obstet Gynecol. 1991;78(3 pt 2):512-4.
8. Wilkins BS, Batcup G, Vinall PS. Partial placenta membranacea. Br J Obstet Gynecol. 1991;98(7):675-9.
9. McCarthy J, Thurmond AS, Jones MK, Sistrom C, Scanlan RM, Jacobson SL, et al. Circumvallate placenta: sonographic diagnosis. J Ultrasound Med. 1995;14(1):21-6.
10. Oppenheimer L; Maternal Fetal Medicine Committee. Diagnosis and management of placenta previa. J Obstet Gynecol Can. 2007;29(3):261-6.
11. Oyelese Y. Placenta previa: the evolving role of ultrasound. Ultrasound Obstet Gynecol. 2009;34(2):123-6.
12. Ghourab S. Third-trimester transvaginal ultrasonography in placenta previa: does the shape of the lower placental edge predict clinical outcome? Ultrasound Obstet Gynecol. 2001;18(2):103-8.
13. Predanic M, Perni SC, Baergen RN, Jean-Pierre J, Chasen ST. A sonographic assessment of different patterns of placenta previa "migration" in the third trimester of pregnancy. J Ultrasound Med. 2005;24(6):773-80.

14. Ghi T, Contro E, Martina T, Piva M, Morandi R, Orsini LF, et al. Cervical length and risk of antepartum bleeding in women with complete placenta previa. Ultrasound Obstet Gynecol. 2009;33(2):209-12.
15. Saitoh M, Ishihara K, Sekiya T, Araki T. Anticipation of uterine bleeding in placenta previa based on vaginal sonographic evaluation. Gynecol Obstet Invest. 2002;54(1):37-42.
16. Hata K, Hata T, Aoki S, Takamori H, Takamiya O, Kitao M. Succenturiate placenta diagnosed by ultrasound. Gynecol Obstet Invest. 1988;25(4): 273-6.
17. Mazouni C, Gorincour G, Juhan V, Bretelle F. Placenta accreta: a review of current advances in prenatal diagnosis. Placenta. 2006;28(7):599-603.
18. Shih JC, Jaraquemada JMPP, Su YN, Shyu MK, Lin CH, Lin SY, et al. Role of three-dimensional power Doppler in the antenatal diagnosis of placenta accreta: comparison with gray-scale and color Doppler techniques. Ultrasound Obstet Gynecol. 2009;33(2);193-203.
19. Bromley B, Benacerraf BR. Solid masses on the fetal surface of the placenta: differential diagnosis and clinical outcome. J Ultrasound Med. 1994;13(11):883-6.
20. Nagy S, Bush M, Stone J, Lapinski RH, Gardó S. Clinical significance of subchorionic and retroplacental hematomas detected in the first trimester of pregnancy. Obstet Gynecol. 2003;102(1):94-100.
21. Ahmed N, Kale V, Thakkar H, Hanchate V, Dhargalkar P. Sonographic diagnosis of placental teratomas. J Clin Ultrasound. 2004;32(2):98-101.
22. Altman JF, Lowe L, Redman L, Esper P, Schwartz JL, Johnson TM, et al. Placental metastasis of maternal melanoma. J Am Acad Dermatol. 2003;49(6):1150-4.
23. Prapas N, Liang RI, Hunter D, Copel JA, Lu LC, Pazkash V, et al. Color Doppler imaging of placental masses: differential diagnosis and fetal outcome. Ultrasound Onstet Gynecol. 2000;16(6):559-63.
24. Vizza E, Correr S, Goranova V, Heyn R, Angelucci PA, Forleo R, et al. The collagen skeleton of the human umbilical cord at term. A scanning electron microscopy study after 2N-NaOH maceration. Reprod Fertil Dev. 1996;8(5):885-94.
25. Di Naro, Ghezzi F, Raio L, Franchi M, D'Addario V, Lanzillotti G, et al. Umbilical vein flow in fetuses with normal and lean umbilical cord. Ultrasound Obstet Gynecol. 2001;17(3):224-8.
26. Raio L, Ghezzi F, Di Naro E, Franchi M, Maymon E, Mueller MD, et al. Prenatal diagnosis of a lean umbilical cord: a simple marker for the fetus at risk of being small for gestational age at birth. Ultrasound Obstet Gynecol. 1999;13(3):176-80.
27. Ghezzi F, Raio L, Duwe DG, Cromi A, Karousou E, Dürig P. Sonographic umbilical vessel morphometry and perinatal outcome of fetuses with a lean umbilical cord. J Clin Ultrasound. 2005;33(1):18-23.
28. Bruch JF, Sibony O, Benali K, Challier JC, Blot P, Nessmann C. Computerized microscope morphometry of umbilical vessels from pregnancies with intrauterine growth retardation and abnormal umbilical artery Doppler. Hum Pathol. 1997;28(10):1139-45.
29. Cromi A, Ghezzi F, Di Naro E, Siesto G, Bergamini V, Raio L. Large cross-sectional area of the umbilical cord as a predictor of fetal macrosomia. Ultrasound Obstet Gynecol. 2007;30(6):861-6.
30. Weissman A, Jakobi P. Sonographic measurements of the umbilical cord in pregnancies complicated by gestational diabetes. J Ultrasound Med. 1997;16(10):691-4.
31. Persutte WH, Hobbins J. Single umbilical artery: a clinical enigma in modern prenatal diagnosis. Ultrasound Obstet Gynecol. 1995;6(3):216-29.
32. Raio L, Ghezzi F, Di Naro E, Gomez R, Saile G, Brühwiler H. The clinical significance of antenatal detection of discordant umbilical arteries. Obstet Gynecol. 1998;91(1):86-91.

9

CHAPTER

Role of Doppler in IUGR and Pregnancy-induced Hypertension

Sonal Panchal, Chaitanya Nagori

INTRODUCTION

Intrauterine growth restriction (IUGR) or fetal growth restriction (FGR) is one of the major concerns in the fetomaternal health. Fetal growth is influenced by genetic predisposition, parental influence, ethnic differences,[1] environment (altitude), and fetal gender also. IUGR is a very loosely used term. It is very important to clear the concepts of the similar terms used interchangeably. These are low-birth weight (LBW), small for gestational age fetuses (SGA), and IUGR fetuses. Another school classifies these fetuses into normal SGA, abnormal SGA, and IUGR.[2] Though all these terms have been used interchangeably at times, but clearly identify different groups of patients. Low-birth weights are the neonates that are born with a weight of <2,500 g. These LBW fetuses may be due to prematurity or may be constitutional or may be due to circulatory derangements, infections, or genetic diseases in their intrauterine life.

The most common causes for low-birth weight babies are:

- *Maternal*:
  - Pregnancy-induced hypertension
  - Antiphospholipid antibody syndrome/ prothrombotic states
  - Chronic hypertension
  - Severe diabetes mellitus
  - Collagen vascular disease
  - Cardiac or renal disease
  - Smoking and poor nutrition
  - Previous history of IUGR baby
- *Uterine—placental*:
  - Uteroplacental dysfunction
  - Placental infarct
  - Chronic abruption
  - Multiple gestation—twin-to-twin transfusion
  - Confined placental mosaicism
  - Placental bleeding
  - Placental infections
  - Immunological causes
- *Fetal*:
  - Chromosomal abnormalities
  - Confined placental mosaicism
  - Major structural anomalies
  - Skeletal dysplasias
  - Multiple anomaly syndromes
  - Infections
  - Teratogens.

Of all these, if the aneuploidies are excluded, the most common causes of LBW are pregnancy-induced hypertension and uteroplacental vascular dysfunction.

Let us understand a more precise usage of the terms, small for gestational age and IUGR, which is now termed as FGR. Small for gestational age fetuses are those who have a fetal weight of less than 10th centile. Those fetuses that are constitutionally small but have normal fetal and umbilical circulatory parameters and no other cause for restricted growth are normal SGA fetuses. But those that have infections or genetic causes or other causes that may lead to restriction of growth in these fetuses, are abnormal SGA fetuses. Whereas those fetuses that have restricted growth due to circulatory abnormalities are IUGR or FGR fetuses. This means that the fetuses that do not grow to their inherited growth potential due to derangement in their cerebral and/or placental circulation are FGR fetuses.

Another simpler method of differentiating SGA from FGR fetuses is to plot the growth of these fetuses on the nomogram chart. If the growth curve of the fetus follows the curve of the nomogram, may be even lower than the nomogram curve, it is indicative of SGA fetus, but if the fetal growth curve crosses across the nomogram curve, it is indicative of FGR. It is therefore necessary to have serial measurements of biometric parameters at least 2 weeks intervals—to diagnose growth abnormalities of the fetus.[3]

The incidence of FGR varies from 1 to 12%, and the risk is higher in the females who had a history of FGR or PIH or stillbirth in previous pregnancy or have hypertension, are exposed to toxic substances such as alcohol or tobacco, or to infections such as CMV or rubella, etc., or have autoimmune, renal, or vascular diseases.

Approximately, 20–30% of all small for gestational age fetuses are true growth-restricted fetuses,[4] whereas only 10–20% are abnormal SGA fetuses.[5] It is essential to diagnose FGR because these fetuses have lots of immediate and late consequences such as higher perinatal morbidity and mortality, perinatal asphyxia, hypothermia, persistent fetal circulation, hypoglycemia, polycythemia and some neurological deficits, and learning and behavioral problems.[6]

To decide whether the fetus is FGR or not, it is essential to first establish the correct gestational age and to assess the fetal growth by biometric measurements. The gestational age can be established by either last menstrual period (LMP), which has a higher error rate or by first trimester or possibly earliest US (ultrasound—CRL measurement), which has lowest deviations from standard measurements. Crown-rump length (CRL) is measured in the midsagittal plane from top of the head to the end of the rump of the embryo on transvaginal scan.[7]

The fetal age is best decided between 9 and 11 weeks based on CRL. CRL is considered to be more reliable after it reaches 18–22 mm.[8] Provided CRL should be correctly measured. The CRL must be measured in the true midsagittal plane of the fetus (confirmed by nonvisualization of the proximal parts of the limbs in that image plane), with the fetus in neutral position (neither extended, nor flexed, and no rotation of the neck) **(Figs. 1A and B)**. Later in the pregnancy, other biometric parameters such as biparietal diameter, head circumference, femur length, etc. **(Figs. 2A to C)**. Standardized planes/sections are achieved and standard methods are used to achieve correct measurements to assess the fetal age.

The first scan done to assess the fetal age is known as pregnancy dating scan. Even if the dating is done in the second trimester, it is reliable, because acceleration of normal fetal growth does not begin till the third trimester. If the fetus is assessed for the first time in the third trimester, the transcerebellar

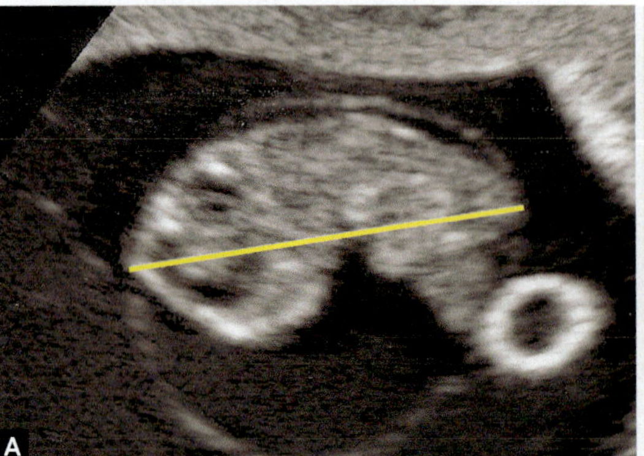

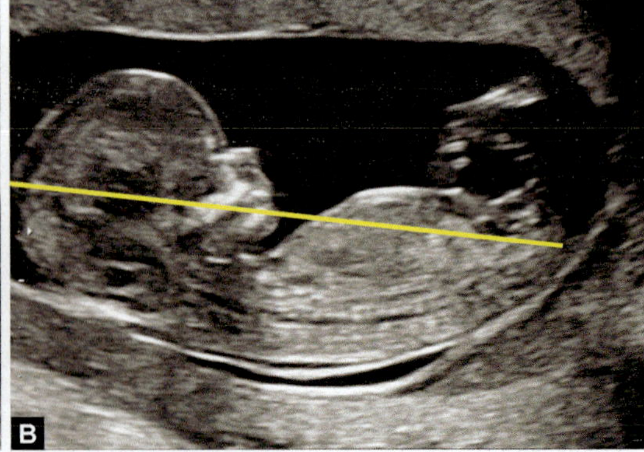

Figs. 1A and B: Measurement of crown-rump length at around 9 weeks (A) and at 11–12 weeks (B).

diameter[9] **(Fig. 3)** and the clavicular length[10] **(Fig. 4)** can be taken to exactly assess the gestational age, because these are the ones which show the gestational age most accurately and are not affected by FGR. When there is a discrepancy of 7 days or more in

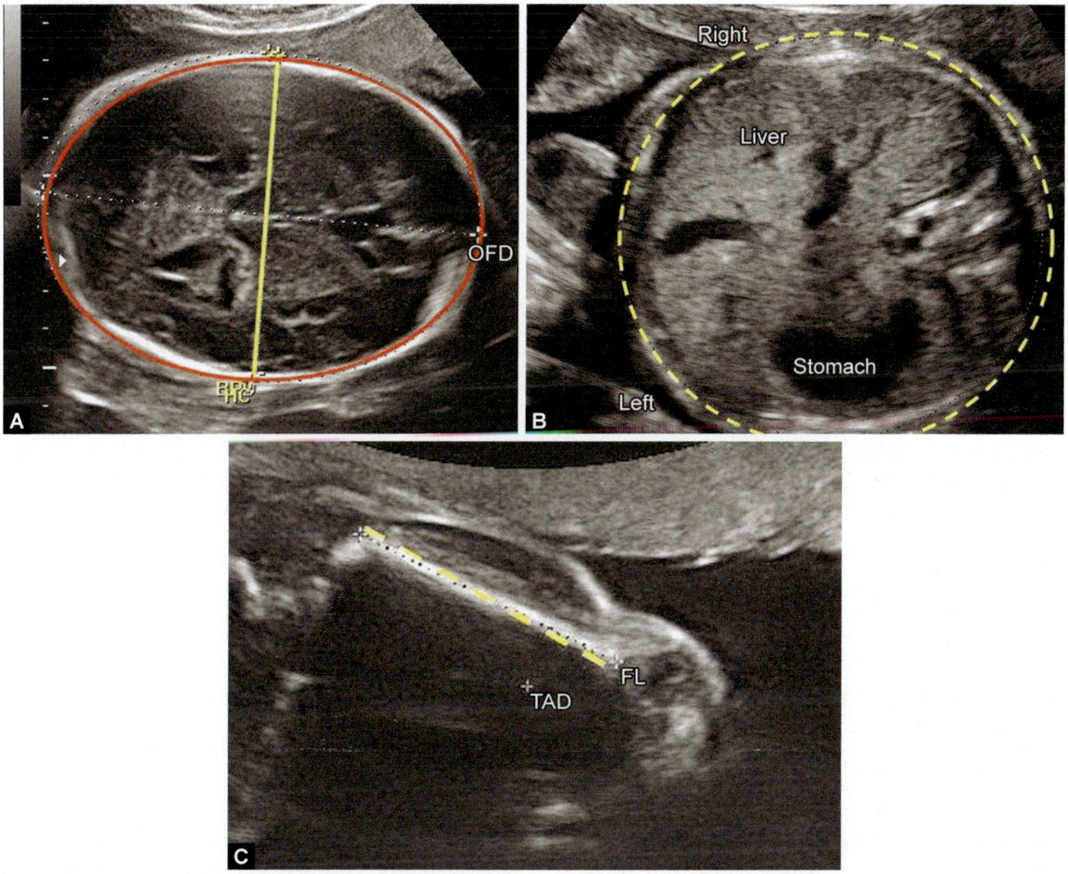

Figs. 2A to C: (A) 2D ultrasound image of the axial section (transthalamic) of the fetal head showing BPD and head circumference measurements; (B) 2D ultrasound image of the axial section of fetal trunk showing abdominal circumference measurement; (C) 2D ultrasound image of femur showing femur length measurement.

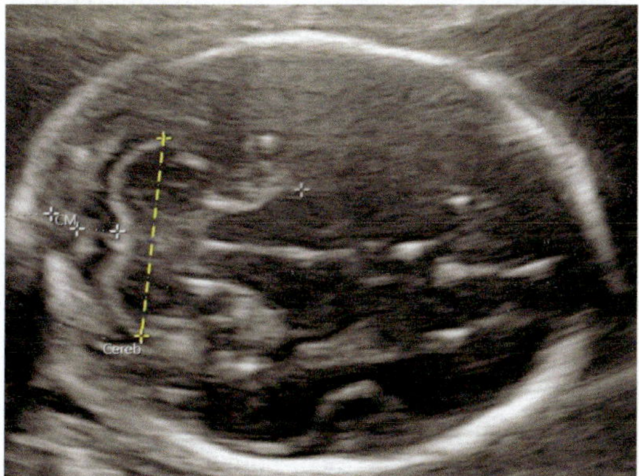

Fig. 3: 2D ultrasound image of the axial section head (transcerebellar section) showing measurement of cerebellar diameter.

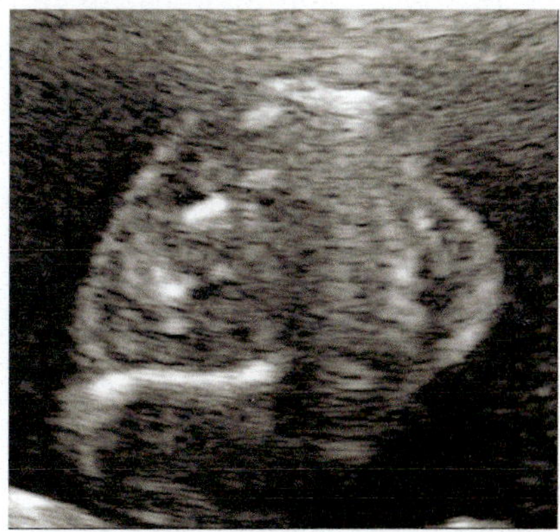

Fig. 4: 2D ultrasound image clavicle showing measurement of clavicle length.

the first trimester between the gestational age calculated by LMP and gestational age calculated by ultrasound, the dates are reassigned. From 14 to 20 weeks of gestational age when the difference between the dates calculated according to LMP and ultrasound assigned gestational age is more than 10 days, the dates are reassigned according to the gestational age assigned by ultrasound. From 20 to 26 weeks, the difference allowed is 14 days. Another method used to decide whether the dates need to be reassigned or not is by following the rule of 8%. Maximum 8% of discrepancy is acceptable during pregnancy between the gestational age calculated by LMP and that calculated by biometric parameters on ultrasound. If the difference between the gestational age calculated by LMP and by ultrasound is more than 8% of the ultrasound calculated age, the dates are reassigned. For example, according to LMP, the gestational age is 149 days and that according to ultrasound is 133 days. The difference between the two is 16 days. The expected margin of error 8% of 133 days is 10.64 days. Since 16 is more than 10.64, the dates will be reassigned according to the gestational age calculated by ultrasound, i.e., 133 days. Dates once assigned have to be followed throughout the pregnancy and have to be taken as a standard to further judge growth derangements. In spite of the fact that for the pregnancy, dating head and long bone biometric parameters are considered more reliable for the birth weight assessment and prediction of IUGR, AC is considered to be more reliable. Estimated fetal weight (EFW) has a more stronger association with birth weight below 10th centile.[11] EFW could be assessed against birth weight and has a random error of 8%.[12]

Apart from the growth discrepancy, uteroplacental circulatory derangement also leads to oligohydramnios. It is therefore essential to assess the amniotic fluid in all the pregnancies that show growth discrepancy or are at a risk for IUGR. It may be measured as a single largest vertical measurement of fluid pouch, free of cord or fetal parts or as a sum of vertical depth of the deepest fluid pocket, free of cord loop or limbs, in all the four quadrants of the uterus, named as amniotic fluid index (AFI) **(Fig. 5)**. When a single pocket is considered, <5 cm is considered abnormal and then AFI should be checked. When AFI is assessed, it normally should be between 15 cm and 25 cm near term, but <10 cm is considered oligohydramnios.

It is in FGR fetuses that Doppler plays an important role for monitoring and management planning. This is so because FGR is due to uteroplacental vascular dysfunction.

UTEROPLACENTAL VASCULAR ANATOMY

On implantation of the embryo in the endometrium and development of the chorionic villi, the high resistance spiral vessels are converted into low-resistance chorionic villous vessels. It is because of this conversion that the placental vessels have a low-resistance flow. The key area in the placenta is intervillous space, filled with maternal blood, in which the tertiary villi are immersed and across these vessel walls, there is exchange of blood and nutrients for the fetal nutrition. Any decrease in the blood supply to the placenta leads to decrease in oxygenated blood in intervillous space and therefore decreased oxygen supply to fetus.

Normal umbilical artery flow velocity waveform (FVW) is the indicator of normal mother to fetus blood supply. Increase in umbilical artery flow velocities and decreased resistance are seen, as the pregnancy advances seen with normally advancing pregnancy are due to:

- Continuous maturation of placental villi
- Widening of placental vessels
- Continuous rise in fetal cardiac output
- Continuous changes in vessel compliance
- Continuous rise in fetal blood pressure.

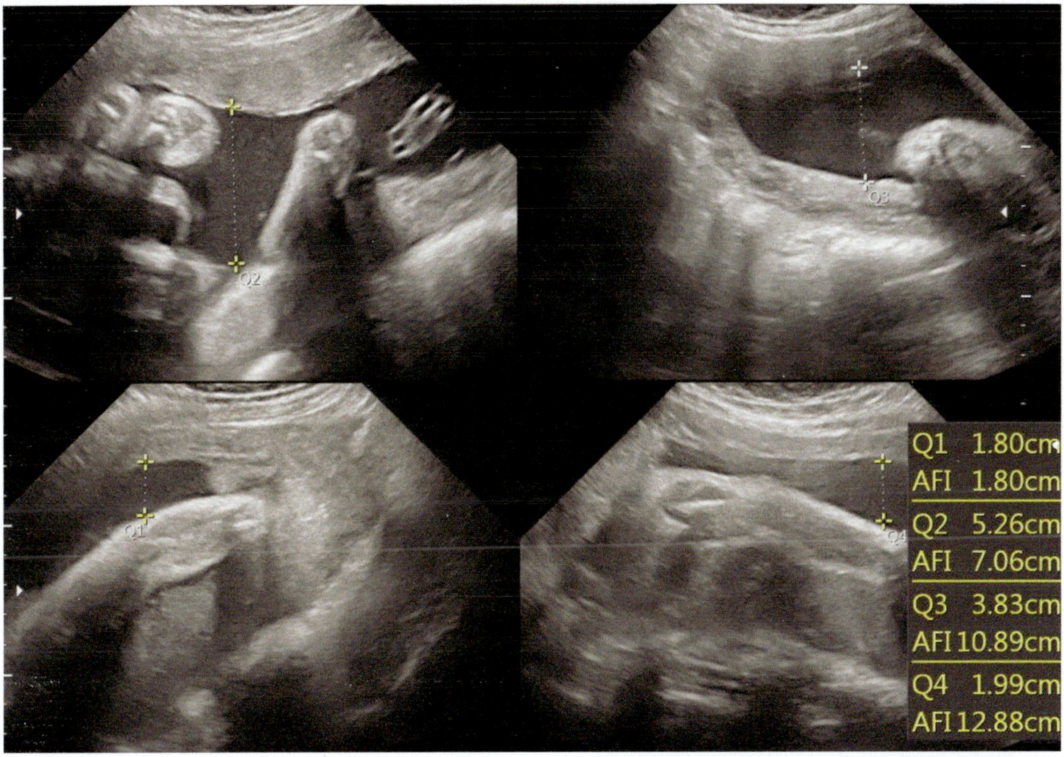

Fig. 5: Measurement of amniotic fluid index.

This conversion chiefly occurs in two phases—at 8–9 weeks of gestation and at 18–20 weeks of gestation. When the conversion of high-resistance system into low-resistance system is inadequate or incomplete **(Fig. 6)**, more pressure is required for the large quantities of blood to be pushed through the high-resistance spiral vessels for fetal support, leading to increased uterine artery resistance and ultimately reduction in the umbilical artery flow. This is inadequate placentation and it leads to pregnancy-induced hypertension (PIH) and/or IUGR.

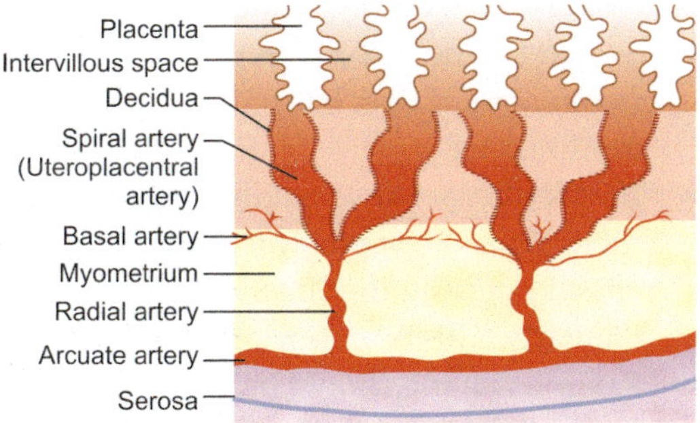

Fig. 6: Diagrammatic presentation of vascular changes occurring during placentation.

Inadequate trophoblastic invasion
↓
Absence of uterine vasodilatation
↓
Reduced placental perfusion
↓
Hampered villous microcirculation
↓
Umbilical hypoxemia
↓
Vascular changes for compensation

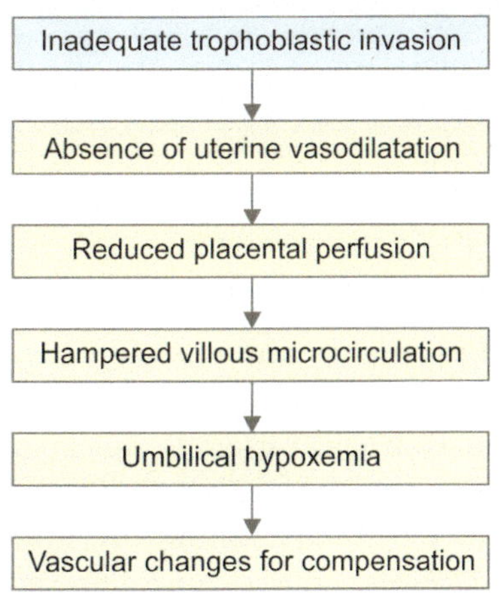

So, primarily the flows in uterine and the umbilical arteries are to be assessed in FGR fetuses. Uterine artery Doppler is the main screening method for prediction of IUGR. Normally, the uterine artery and

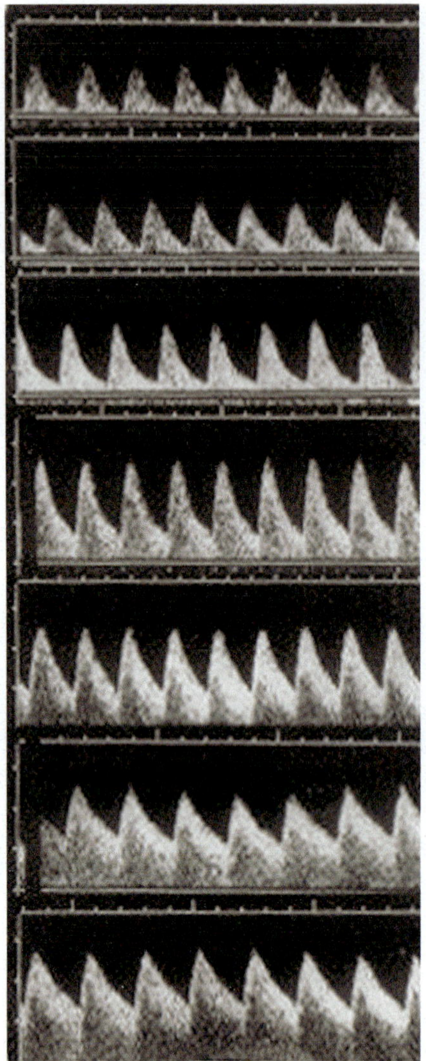

Fig. 7: Serial changes occurring in the umbilical artery flow as pregnancy progresses.

umbilical artery flow velocity increases in the normal pregnancy and resistance decreases as pregnancy advances[13] **(Figs. 7 and 8)**. Abnormal umbilical artery Doppler correlates with histological evidence of placental vascular pathology. Therefore, umbilical artery Doppler indices correlate with the fetal levels of glucose, amino acids, and blood gases.[14] There is also a strong evidence to show that SGA fetuses with abnormal umbilical artery flow are at a higher risk of abnormal perinatal outcome.[15] And perinatal death with normal umbilical artery flow is very uncommon.[16] Decreased umbilical vein flow is also documented in otherwise asymptomatic fetuses with decreased placental volume.[17] But to study the oxygenation status of the fetus, it is essential to also evaluate the fetal vessels, and middle cerebral artery (MCA) is the one that is considered to be representing the fetal oxygenation status because the cerebral cortex reflects to hypoxia and MCA is the vessel that supplies more than 50% of the cerebral cortex.

Hypoxia leads to cellular dysfunction, as the cells lose their ability for oxidative phosphorylation. This changes aerobic metabolism to anaerobic metabolism, accumulation of lactic acid and hydrogen ions, and decreased adenosine triphosphate (ATP) generation. This leads to failure of sodium–potassium pump and cellular edema. Activation of phospholipases also leads to accumulation of free fatty acids. All these lead to cell death and are the bases for neurological deficit in hypoxic fetuses.

TECHNIQUE OF DOPPLER ASSESSMENT

Uterine Artery Doppler

Uterine artery can be best located, as it crosses the internal iliac vessels perpendicular to their path.

- Place the probe on the symphysis pubis and slide it laterally, holding vertically.
- Iliac artery and vein are seen as two easily recognizable vessels in their long axis.
- Switch on the color with pulse repetition frequency (PRF) of 0.6–0.9 and a low-wall motion filter.
- Rotate the probe laterally and angulate medially and Doppler will show a pulsatile vessel crossing the iliac vessels perpendicularly. This is uterine artery **(Fig. 9)**.
- Sample volume should be of 2 mm.
- Switch on the pulse Doppler and align the angle almost parallel to iliac vessels.

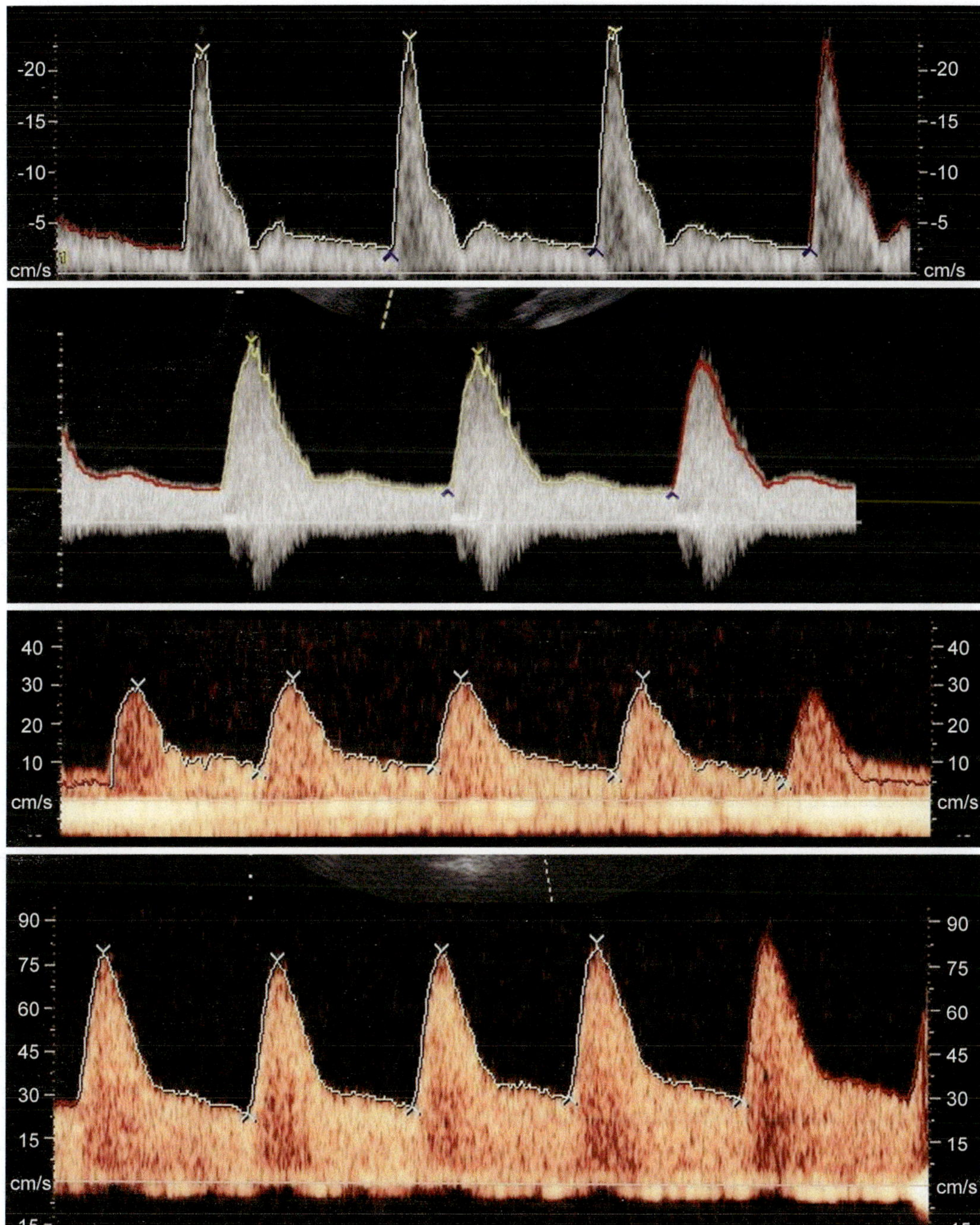

Fig. 8: Serial changes occurring in the uterine artery flow as pregnancy progresses.

- Adjust the PRF to get a complete spectrum on one side of the baseline.
- Calculate pulsatility index (PI) of uterine artery.

Umbilical Artery Doppler (Fig. 10)

- In a free loop of umbilical cord
- On a zoomed image
- Pulsed Doppler sample volume of 1–2 mm

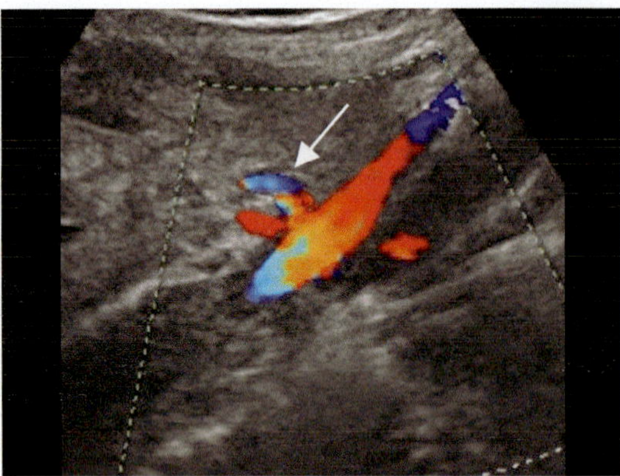

Fig. 9: Color Doppler image showing uterine artery on transabdominal scan.

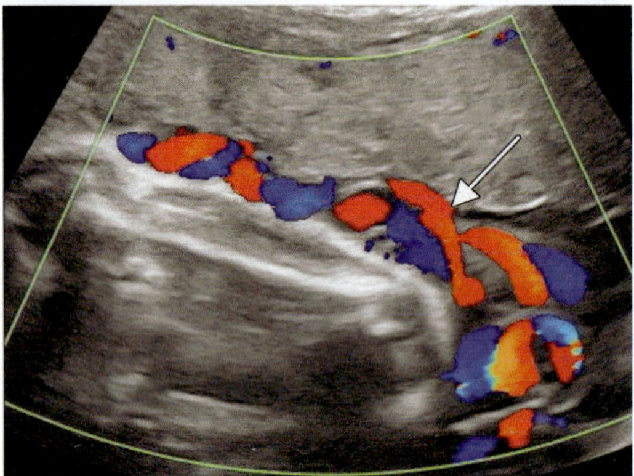

Fig. 10: Color Doppler image showing umbilical artery on transabdominal scan.

- Sample volume on one umbilical artery
- Adjust power Doppler scale for velocity
- Obtain at least five waveforms for measurement of indices
- To be assessed when fetus is not breathing and not moving
- As low as reasonably achievable (ALARA) principle is followed.

Umbilical artery flow assessment is to monitor IUGR fetus but is not reliable screening tool for prediction of IUGR.[18]

Middle Cerebral Artery Doppler

- Locate the MCA closest to the transducer on the circle of Willis section.
- Magnify the image for MCA to occupy >50% of the image.
- Pulse Doppler sample volume of 1–2 mm
- Sample volume is placed close to its origin **(Figs. 11A and B)**.
- Adjust pulse Doppler scale to fit the velocity
- Angle between ultrasound beam and blood flow should be smallest possible.
- Obtain at least five waveforms.
- Ensure no fetal movements or breathing.
- Follow ALARA (as low as reasonably achievable) principle.
- Take at least three traces and use the highest peak systolic velocity (PSV) for clinical care.

SILENT PERIOD OF INCREASED RESISTANCE

Pathophysiology

Till decreased villous microcirculation up to 50%, no change is seen in the umbilical artery flow, if there is no defect in maternal supply.

During this stage, no change is seen in the Doppler parameters of umbilical artery or middle cerebral artery that are the most commonly interrogated vessels in mothers with PIH or fetuses with FGR. If growth parameters of the fetus are normal and umbilical artery waveform is normal, then no other Doppler studies are required.

Stage of Hypoxemia

When the placental circulatory compromise progresses beyond that, fetal hypoxemia starts developing, and fetal partial pressure of oxygen (PO_2) may fall up to 18–19 mm of Hg and pH reaches 7.20–7.25. As primary compensatory mechanism to hypoxemia, there is reopening of the ductus venosus (DV) to divert blood from liver toward the heart **(Figs. 12A and B)** and increase in the MCA flow in the distal segment for better peripheral cerebral circulation **(Fig. 13)**. This leads to decreased MCA PI in sector 2, the distal segment of MCA as compared to the proximal segment of MCA, M1/M2 > 1, and increased velocity and low resistance in DV.

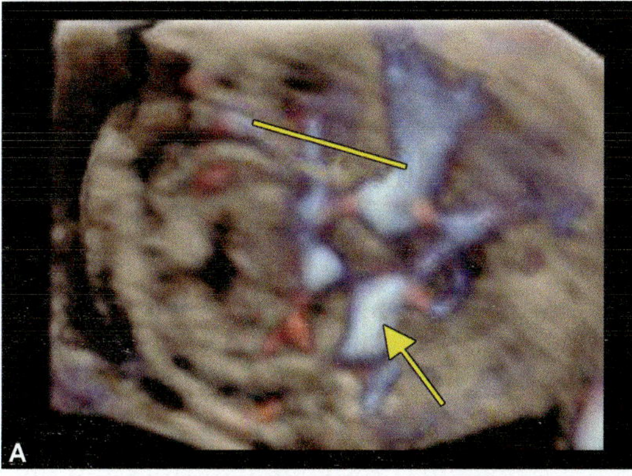

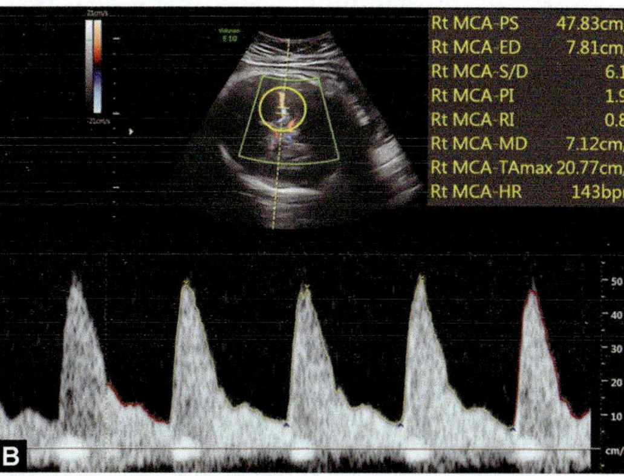

Figs. 11A and B: (A) Color Doppler image showing MCA on transabdominal scan of fetus; (B) Spectral Doppler image showing MCA on transabdominal scan of fetus.

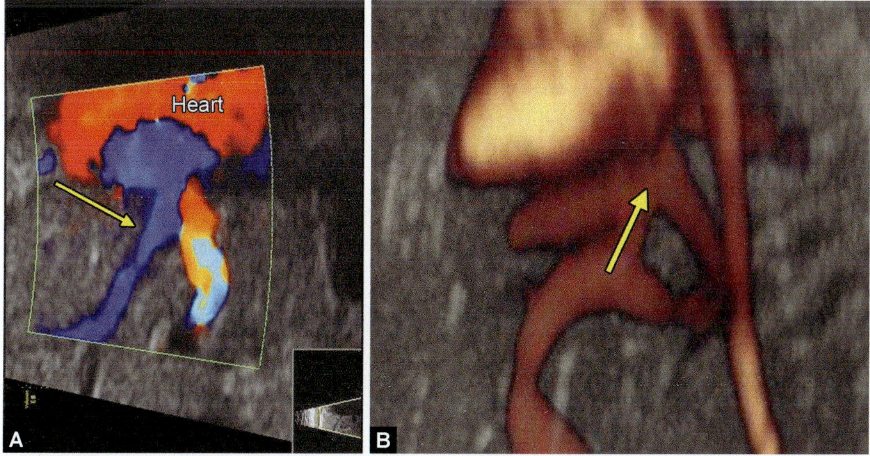

Figs. 12A and B: Color Doppler (A) and power Doppler (B) images showing ductus venosus.

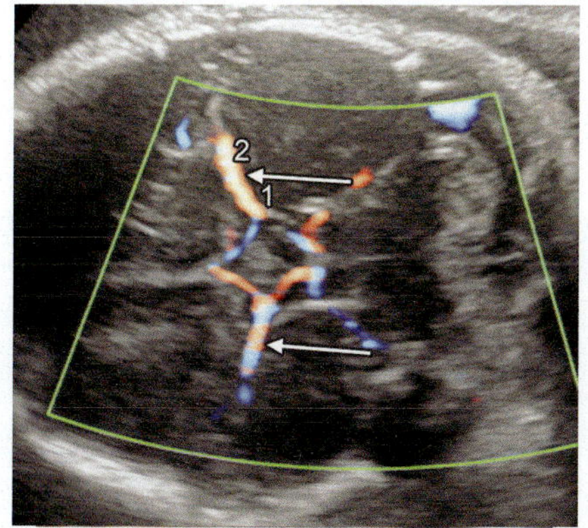

Fig. 13: Color Doppler image showing MCA on transabdominal scan of fetus.

Reduction in circulatory oxygen level is sensed by peripheral chemoreceptors and leads to vagal stimulation of heart with preferential shift of cardiac circulation toward LV leading to increased umbilical artery resistance and lower resistance MCA flow. But aortic and carotid chemoreceptors are mostly not affected. Fetal hypoxemia is reflected by reduced heart rate variation and heart rate decelerations.[19]

Mild increase in umbilical artery PI is the cause of hypoxemia, whereas lower resistance in MCA flow is the indication of the adaptation to hypoxemia.

The third phase is the phase of hypoxia that can be divided into:

1. Initial phase
2. Advanced phase
3. Terminal phase.

1. *Initial phase: Vascular changes during this period are*—rise in umbilical artery PI but still positive flow is seen throughout the cardiac cycle in the umbilical artery **(Fig. 14)**. Due to fall in resistance in the cerebral circulation, presence of end-diastolic flow is seen at 32–34 weeks along with low MCA PI **(Fig. 15)**. Umbilical artery PI/MCA PI ratio [cerebroplacental ratio (CPR)] is the best indicator for fetal hypoxia. Prediction of the adverse outcome is improved using umbilical and cerebral parameters in combined ratio are 70%. CPR is the single most sensitive parameter for assessment of the IUGR and has a single cut off value of one.[20] Biophysical profile may be unaltered at this stage and the biophysical score is usually <7. This phase lasts for 9–60 days, but its length is usually about 2–3 weeks.
   Other progressive changes that occur during this period are reduced fetal respiratory and somatic movements, reduced AFI (5–8 cm), and raised aortic PI. It gives the summation of blood supply information to kidneys, abdominal organs, lower limbs, and placenta. It must be remembered that—fetal aortic flow is a direct reflection of the cardiac output and the peripheral resistance of systemic circulation. It is to divert the blood flow to the heart and brain; that the circulation to the periphery is decreased. This is a compensatory mechanism. Renal artery PI is also raised as a consequence to rise in aortic resistance.
2. *Advanced phase:* When the placental villous circulation is compromised to about 80%, this is an advanced stage of fetal hypoxia. The vascular changes observed on Doppler at this stage are:
   - Absent end-diastolic flow in umbilical artery **(Fig. 16)**. But, it is to be remembered that—although umbilical artery waveform is a good reflector of placental resistance, it does not give any information as to fetus is coping up with the compromised blood supply or not.
   - Absent end-diastolic flow in aorta is seen and this leads to significantly decreased circulation to the abdominal organs thus leading to high risk of necrotizing enterocolitis. Thus increasing the risk of morbidity and mortality.
   - Low MCA PI values **(Fig. 17)** are seen as a compensation to cerebral hypoxia by cerebral vasodilatation. But, it must be kept in mind that prolonged cerebral vasodilatation and low MCA PI cannot be taken as a compensatory mechanism, as in the second phase of vasodilatation, deoxygenated blood floods the brain and can lead to cerebral edema. There is also a higher risk of intracranial hemorrhages in the

Fig. 14: Umbilical artery flow with high resistance flow as seen on pulsed wave Doppler.

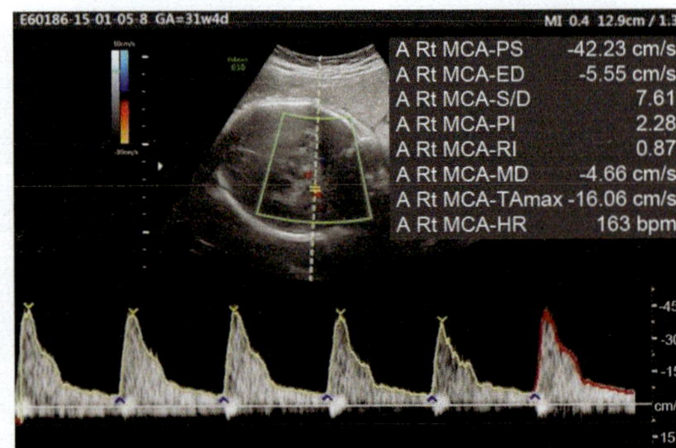

Fig. 15: Spectral Doppler of the MCA flow with diastolic flow.

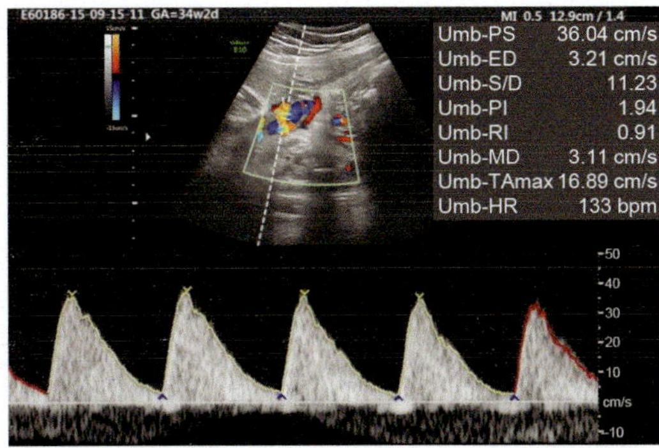

Fig. 16: Umbilical artery flow with high resistance (nearly absent end-diastolic flow) flow as seen on pulsed wave Doppler.

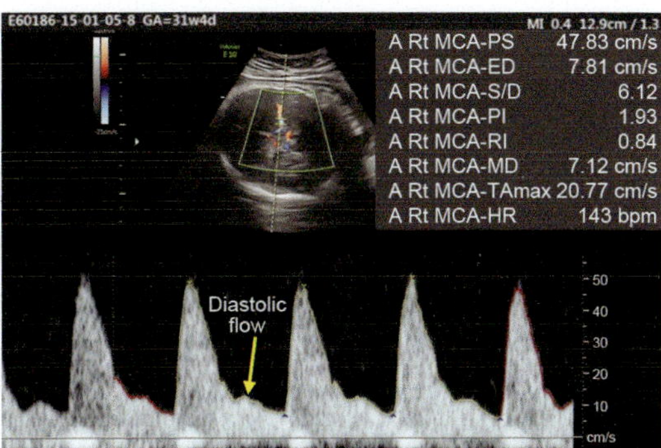

Fig. 17: Spectral Doppler of the MCA flow with low resistance flow.

neonatal life in these cases. Fetus will also show loss of reactivity at this stage due to cerebral hypoxia.

3. *Terminal phase*: This is a phase of acidosis. Doppler shows reversed end-diastolic flow in umbilical artery and aorta **(Fig. 18)**.

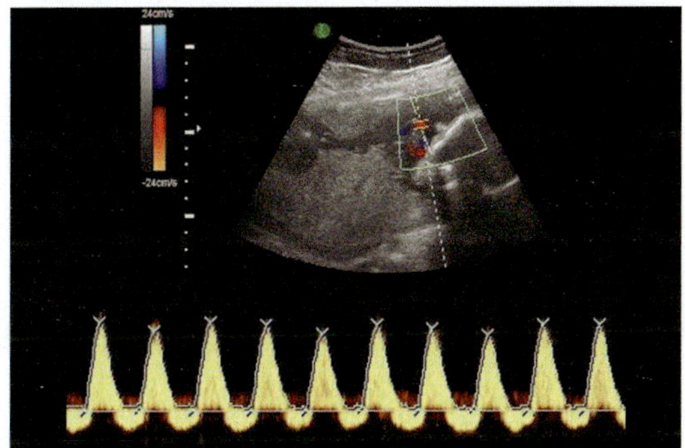

Fig. 18: Spectral Doppler of the umbilical artery with reverse end-diastolic flow.

MCA resistance may start rising due to cerebral edema. Severe hypoxia in the myocardium leads to failing of cardiac muscle and therefore marked reduction in ventricular ejection fraction. This leads to marked reduction in intracardiac flow velocities. To compensate for myocardial hypoxia, there is dilatation of the coronary vessels to the extent that sometimes blood flows in the coronaries may be documented. The dysfunction of the myocardium leads to decreased ventricular compliance, therefore incomplete emptying of the atrium and increasing preload reflecting as reversed flow or decreased telediastolic velocity values **(Fig. 19A)** in DV. But, this stage precedes the stage when there is increase in the ductus venous PI **(Fig. 19B)**. Inferior vena

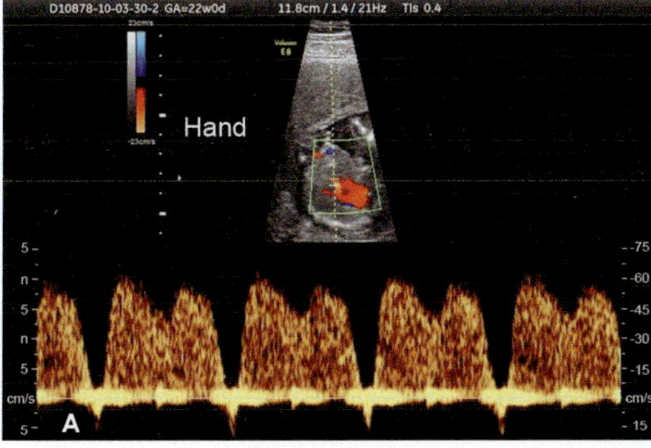

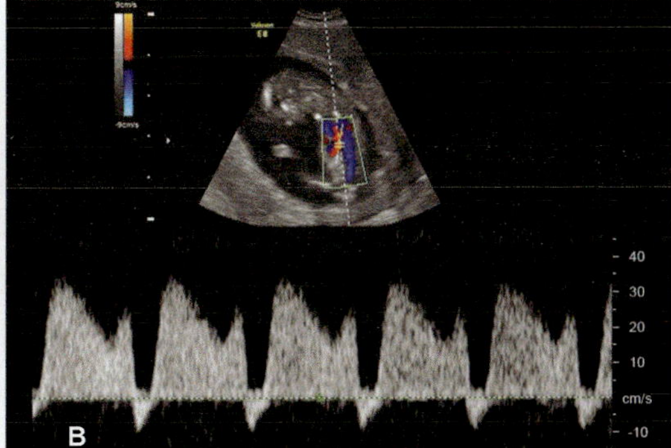

Figs. 19A and B: Spectral Doppler of the ductus venosus showing: (A) Absent A wave; (B) Reversed A wave.

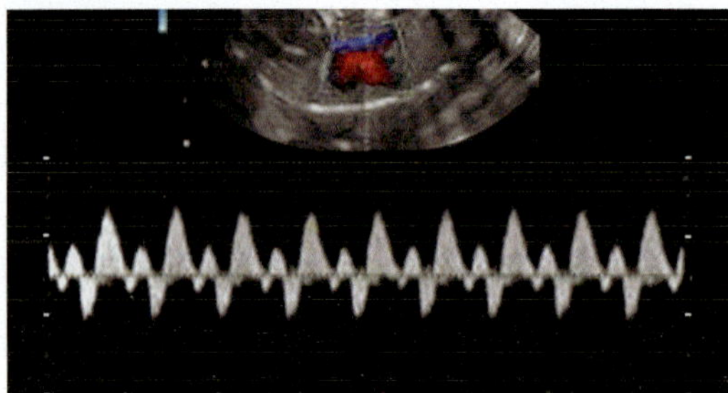

Fig. 20: Spectral Doppler of fetal IVC showing increased reverse flow of A wave.

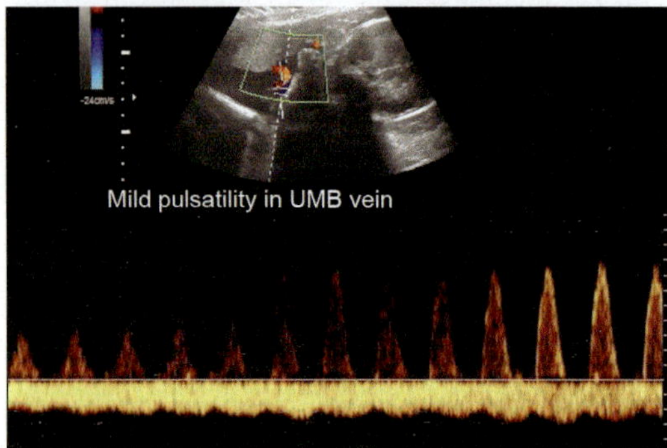

Fig. 21: Spectral Doppler showing absent end-diastolic flow in umbilical artery and pulsatile umbilical venous flow.

cava (IVC) normally also shows negative flow during atrial contraction up to 10% but rises up to 30% in terminal phase of centralization **(Fig. 20)**. Umbilical vein flow may also show pulsatility **(Fig. 21)**. Venous Doppler reflects the physiological status of right ventricle giving specific information regarding the ventricular preload, myocardial compliance, and right ventricular end-diastolic pressure.

These findings with reversed flow in hepatic vein and deceleration in heart rate are indicators of acidosis.

Fetal acidemia reliably presents as very short-term and low-value variations in fetal heart rate (FHR), and precedes intrauterine fetal death.

In about 90% of cases, DV flow also becomes abnormal only 48–72 hours before abnormal biophysical profile.[21] Longitudinal studies have demonstrated that AFI and FHR are the only two parameters that may change a little earlier in fetal compromise.

Abnormal DV flow may be seen as ***(Figs. 22A to D)***:

- Deep "A" nadir (atrial control)
- Reduced second peak (diastole)
- Reduced diastolic flow
- Reversed diastolic flow
- PI 0.5 is normal and >0.9 is very bad.

Progressively increasing umbilical artery PI leads to impaired fetal cardiac performance, increased central venous pressure, and reduced diastolic flow in DV. Vasodilatation of DV diverts flow to the heart, further increasing the arterial pressure and leads to further decrease in DV flow during atrial contraction.

This follows the phase of fetal decompensation.

Severe tissue hypoxia leads to anaerobic metabolism for energy production. This leads to acidemia and then acidosis. In the brain, it leads to lactic acid accumulation and cerebral edema due to altered cell membrane permeability. Severe hypoxemia and hypoxia lead to irreversible interference in the central mechanism of the arterial tone. In severe hypoxemia PO_2 is less than 4 SD of mean, leading to generalized fetal vascular paralysis.

This results in myocardial cell necrosis phenomena and replacement of myocardial tissue with fibrous tissue, affecting myocardial compliance and increase in telediastolic pressure in both the ventricles.

Doppler studies show:

- Reversed end-diastolic flow in umbilical artery **(Fig. 23)**, aorta, and renal artery
- Regaining PI values in MCA with reduced or even absent end-diastolic flow in umbilical artery. This is known as paradoxical reversal of MCA PI **(Figs. 24A and B)**. Porencephaly or ventriculomegaly due to hypoxic necrosis of brain may develop due to severe oxygenation and vascular insult to the cerebral tissue.

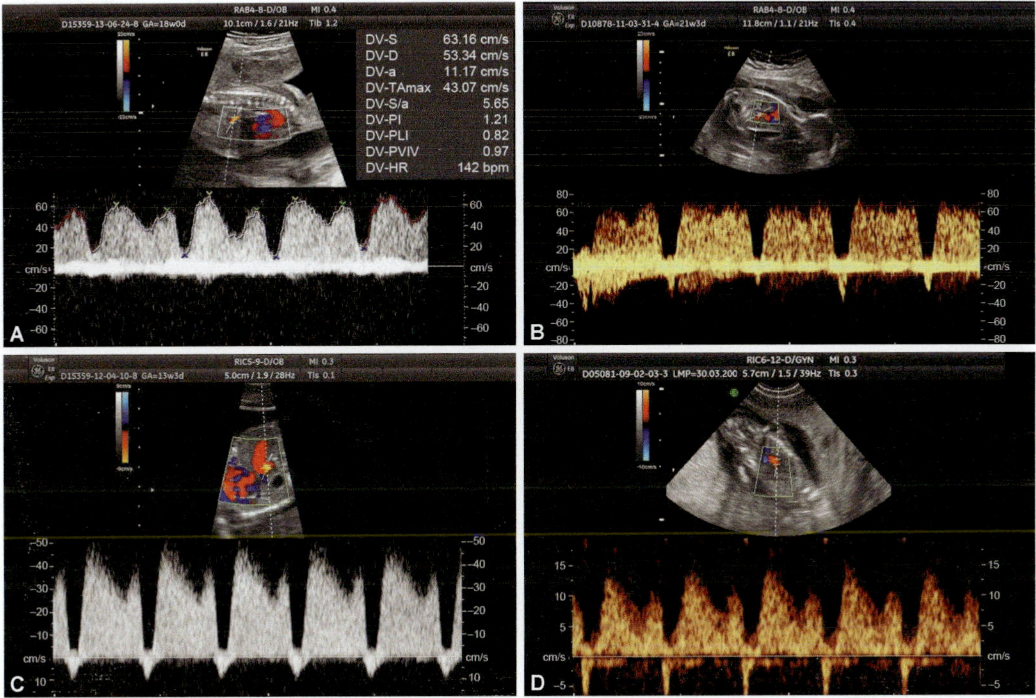

Figs. 22A to D: Spectral Doppler of ductus venosus flow: (A) High DVPI; (B) Absent A wave; (C) Reverse A wave; (D) Marked reversal of A wave.

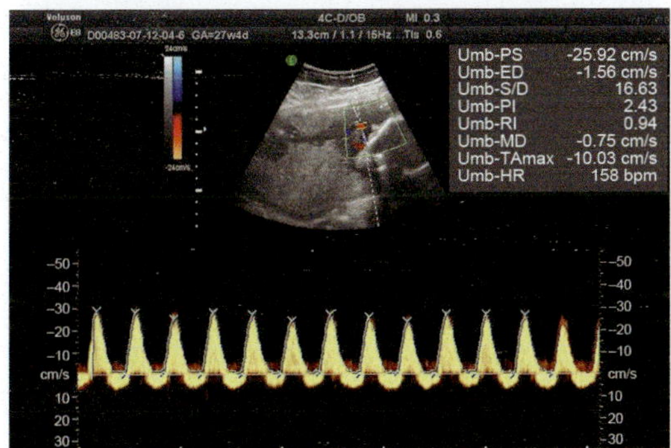

Fig. 23: Reversed end-diastolic flow in umbilical artery on spectral Doppler.

- Fixed fetal cardiac frequency and no alteration in HR even with oxytocin test.

AORTIC ISTHMUS FLOW

Aortic isthmus is the part of aorta, just beyond the origin of brachiocephalic trunk **(Figs. 25A and B)**. The flow in this part of the aorta is usually a continuous positive flow with high velocity. Aortic isthmus flow represents the balance between right and left ventricular outputs. *In systolic phase, forward flow indicates LV output and reverse flow indicates RV output. Whereas in diastole, forward flow indicates upper body resistance and reverse flow indicates lower body resistance.* Retrograde flow in the aortic isthmus represents increased right ventricular afterload and decreased left ventricular afterload. Though a small flow reversal in early diastole is normal in third trimester. Normal peak velocity in aortic isthmus is 30–100 cm/s from 11 weeks to term as compared to ductus arteriosus that is 40–120 cm/s. Low velocities and high resistance in aortic isthmic flow are seen in IUGR fetuses. Abnormality of this flow occurs about a week before the changes of hypoxia are seen in DV.[22]

Abnormal DV flow indicates high morbidity and mortality of the fetus. And therefore, if delivery of the fetus is done after ductus venosus flow becomes abnormal, the chances of fetal survival is very low. But, if the delivery

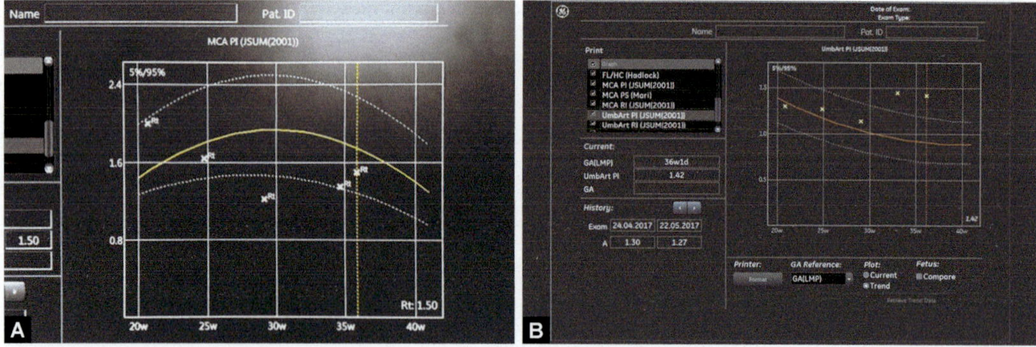

Figs. 24A and B: (A) Graph showing plotting of MCA flows against weeks of gestation with paradoxical reversal of the MCA resistance; (B) Graph showing plotting of umbilical artery flows against weeks of gestation with rising PI values.

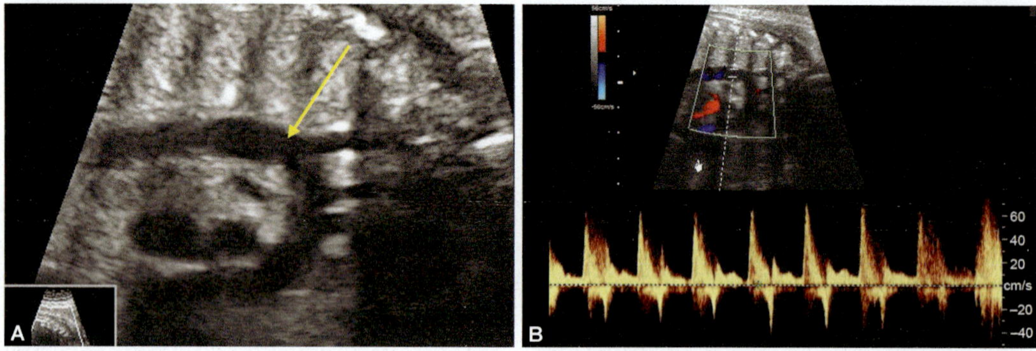

Figs. 25A and B: (A) Aortic isthmus on 2D ultrasound; (B) Spectral Doppler showing aortic isthmic flow.

of the fetus can be done before this stage, fetal survival and chances of its well-being can be improved significantly. The risk of hypoxia needs to be compared with the risk of prematurity. Abnormal aortic isthmic flow impedance is an intermediate step between placental insufficiency-hypoxemia and cardiac decompensation.[23] Abnormality of aortic isthmus flow can be recorded approximately a week before abnormality in the DV flow.[22] Retrograde flow in the aortic isthmus in growth-restricted fetuses correlated strongly with adverse perinatal outcome.[24] Reversed diastolic flow in aortic isthmus clearly indicates poor neurological outcome. Abnormal aortic isthmus flow is a better marker than abnormal ductus venosus flow for predicting bad perinatal outcome, whereas abnormal ductus venosus flow is a better marker for predicting fetal mortality.

The aortic isthmic flow can be quantitatively rated by the isthmic flow index as follows:

- *Type 1*: IFI < 1—antegrade systolic and diastolic flow
- *Type 2*: IFI = 1: Absent diastolic flow
- *Type 3*: IFI = 0–1—predominant systolic but some reversed diastolic flow
- *Type 4*: IFI = 0—some antegrade and some retrograde flow
- *Type 5:* IFI >1—chiefly retrograde flow
- IFI types 3–5 have bad to worst prognosis.

Applying this knowledge for the assessment of fetal well-being:

These tests could be classified as chronic or acute. Chronic tests progressively become abnormal due to increasing hypoxemia and/or hypoxia. Whereas, acute tests correlate with the acute changes occurring in advanced stages of fetal compromise due to severe hypoxia and metabolic acidosis.

UMBILICAL ARTERY

It is known that with the functional damage in the placental villi, the umbilical artery resistance increases. But, the placental histological changes cannot always be correlated with the severity of increased resistance in the umbilical artery. Though when the umbilical artery shows a reverse end-diastolic flow, it is considered that there is a severe placental damage and there is an increased risk of perinatal death. And, this has a sensitivity and specificity of about 60%.[25] Studies have shown that 80% of the fetuses have abnormal umbilical artery flow, 2 weeks before acute deterioration of fetal condition, and therefore this may be considered a chronic marker for fetal non-well-being. The same study has also shown that up to 1 week before fetal death, the umbilical artery diastolic flow may be present.[26] Absent or reversed end-diastolic flow in the umbilical artery respectively has a relative risk of 4 and 10.6 for prediction of fetal morbidity and mortality and is also associated with long-term abnormal neurodevelopment.[27] A multicentric randomized trial on growth restriction intervention (GRIT) has concluded that early delivery for fetuses with reversed end-diastolic flow does not improve the outcome and 24–48 hours of interval after corticosteroids injection for lung maturation and then delivery should be planned.[28]

MIDDLE CEREBRAL ARTERY

In deteriorating FGR, MCA PI progressively becomes abnormal.[29] Up to 80% of fetuses have vasodilatation 2 weeks before acute deterioration according to one study[26] and <50% according to other.[28] Moreover, the paradoxical reversal of the MCA flow that is explained to be due to terminal cerebral edema has also not been documented in few other studies.[29] In near-term SGA fetuses, MCA could be useful to predict adverse outcome, independently of umbilical artery Doppler. But its value in overall SGA population is not proved in another study.[30] Some studies have also shown that MCA vasodilatation may be a protective mechanism against hypoxia, but is associated with suboptimal neurological development[31] and in one study, its association is also shown with impaired visual function and visual motor capabilities at 11 years.[32] Brain-sparing effect can also be considered a chronic marker of FGR.

DUCTUS VENOSUS

Acidemia, acidosis, and abnormal venous Doppler are acute markers. Increasing PI in the ductus venosus may occur early but reversal of A wave represents the terminal changes. In preterm fetuses, a 3SD (standard deviation) cut-off optimizes the sensitivity and specificity.[33] With absent or reversed A wave, perinatal mortality ranges from 60 to 100%.[33] However, its sensitivity for perinatal death is 40–70%. Abnormal venous flow may be ductus venosus or inferior vena cava or hepatic vein identifies about 90% of newborns with acidosis.[34] But in about 90% of cases, a ductus venosus flow shows reverse A wave only 48–72 hours before the biophysical profile shows changes.[21]

Heart rate deceleration or loss of variability in heart rate is not a reliable guide to predict perinatal morbidity or mortality according to one study,[35] but other longitudinal studies have proved its potential role as acute marker.[29]

Fetal growth restriction can be divided into two types depending on the time of initiation of the manifestations. In some patients, FGR sets in as early as 26–28 weeks of pregnancy and this is known as early onset IUGR, whereas when FGR sets in at about 32–33 weeks, it is late onset FGR. It is important to differentiate between the two because the behavior of the fetus and deterioration pattern in the two situations are different. The basic pathophysiology of the two is also different. Where early onset FGR is due to abnormal or inadequate placental vascularization, late onset FGR is due to inadequate perfusion. In the early onset IUGR, the fetal adaptation is better and in spite of redistribution of circulation, or marked circulatory changes, the fetus does survive the situation. But, in late onset FGR, the fetus does not get sufficient time to get adapted to the circulatory derangements and therefore the fetal deterioration is fast. In the early onset FGR cases, therefore, one can wait even with absent umbilical artery diastolic flow and also at times till ductus venosus flow becomes abnormal. Because of fast deterioration in the late onset cases, the entire cascade of vascular changes may not be followed and may result into unexplained fetal death. Unfortunately, 70–80% of FGR fetuses are late onset IUGR.

The management strategies therefore in both the situations have to be different **(Table 1)**.[36,37]

When and how often should these patients be monitored by Doppler?

It is very important to understand that a single Doppler assessment cannot be relied upon for decision making on the fetal oxygenation as well as obstetric management. One has to observe the trend of the vascular resistance in MCA and umbilical artery. Therefore, a baseline Doppler at about 30–32 weeks will be helpful to serve as a guide for further Doppler changes in FGR fetuses. The follow-up would depend on gestational age at the onset of disease, severity of vascular changes at the primary examination, and presence of deterioration on subsequent assessment. The deterioration may be in the form of discrepancy in growth, reducing amount of liquor, abnormal NST (nonreactive stress test), or worsening of Doppler parameters. The monitoring intervals may also vary depending on whether it is an early onset FGR or a late onset IUGR.

For example in an early onset FGR even with umbilical artery flow showing absent end diastolic flow, once a weekly Doppler follow-up may be maintained till the MCA flow and in turn the DV flow becomes abnormal, or fetus reaches 34 weeks or more of gestation or even with reversed end-diastolic flow in umbilical artery and DV PI > 95th centile, time can be bought to give steroids and plan a delivery. Whereas in late onset IUGR, even with umbilical artery PI > 95th centile or MCA PI < 5th centile, monitoring may be required much more often and any new development in Doppler finding is considered an emergency and especially when the fetus has already reached 34 weeks, no unnecessary delay in delivery is advisable. In short, in early onset FGR, the sequential changes that take days, in late onset FGR, the same changes may occur in hours.

TABLE 1: Management strategies of early and late onset fetal growth restriction (FGR).

Early onset FGR	***Late onset FGR***
Problem: Management	Problem: Diagnosis
Severe placental disease (abnormal umbilical artery, associated with preeclampsia)	Mild placental disease (normal umbilical artery Doppler, less associated with preeclampsia)
Hypoxia-systemic cardiovascular adaptation	Hypoxia may or may not be there, cardiovascular adaptation is central
Better fetal tolerance and adaptation to hypoxia	Lower fetal tolerance to hypoxia and poor adaptation
High morbidity and mortality, lower prevalence	Low mortality (but common cause of late stillbirth)

Source: Adapted from Muresan D, Miller DA, Rabello YA, Paul RH. The modified biophysical profile: antepartum testing in the 1990s. Am J Obstet Gynecol. 1996;174(3):812-7.

OBSTETRIC MANAGEMENT DEPENDING ON DOPPLER FINDINGS

1. *FGR with normal hemodynamic profile*: No immediate action and repeat Doppler and BPP every 2 weeks.
2. *FGR with hemodynamic redistribution 32–34 weeks*: Early stage of centralization,

Doppler, and BPP monitoring. With late stage of centralization, termination of pregnancy.

3. If FGR with hemodynamic redistribution is seen between 28 and 32 weeks depending on neonatal intensive care unit (NICU) facilities, termination of pregnancy with advanced and terminal stages of centralization but expectant management with early stage of centralization with Doppler and BPP monitoring every 5 days.
4. Same is true for the gestational age of < 28 weeks. All chances are taken to allow the pregnancy to reach 30 weeks.

It was believed that as long as the fetal growth and the umbilical artery indices are normal, no further hemodynamic study is required. Though there are situations in which, in spite of normal umbilical artery flow, the fetal circulation is affected and reflects as abnormal MCA flow. This is especially common, when the causes for fetal hypoxia are nonplacental. Therefore, as a rule in all high-risk cases for fetal hypoxia, MCA flow must be assessed with umbilical artery flow. Doppler findings must be evaluated in conjunction with gestational age, fetal weight, liquor, biophysical profile, fetal activity, and CTG (cardiotocography). *Delivery must be considered, if one of these parameters is persistently abnormal.*[29]

Role of Biophysical Profile

When used alone, it has 50% false-positive rate and so has a limited value clinically.[38] A meta-analysis has also not shown its significant benefit in high-risk pregnancies. But, both Doppler and biophysical profile effectively stratify FGR into risk categories.[39]

Advances

Computerized CTG myocardial performance index (MPI) is a novel method in fetal medicine that assesses both systolic and diastolic functions by including the measurement of isovolumetric and ejection times and would be useful in assessing the progressive hemodynamic deterioration. It has been reported to be associated with perinatal mortality in very preterm IUGR fetuses.[39]

Prediction of IUGR

If predicted, pregnancies with FGR fetuses can be better managed. Uterine artery Doppler has an effective application for the same. Several workers have published on the importance and efficacy of biochemical markers along with uterine artery Doppler for prediction of FGR. High-uterine artery resistance at 11–14 weeks with low pregnancy-associated plasma protein A (PAPP-A) can provide early assessment of risk for uteroplacental insufficiency.[40] Uterine artery PI and PAPP-A have negative linear correlation. Low PAPP-A in first trimester in euploid fetus with growth restriction at 18–24 weeks predicts high chance of PIH, FGR, and preterm birth.[41] It has been shown that low placental growth factor (PlGF) and high uterine artery PI have a sensitivity of 89.5% and specificity of 95% for prediction of early onset preeclampsia and FGR.[42] According to another study, combination of first-trimester low PP13, high uterine artery PI, and uterine artery notch can be promising signs for prediction of preeclampsia in women with high a priori risk of pulmonary embolism (PE).[43] *One more study shows that* persistent early diastolic notch increases predictive value from 4.3 to 23% for FGR and 68-fold increased risk of developing preeclampsia.[44]

Low PAPP-A (<0.3 MoM), small placental size (<10 cm), and elevated α-fetoprotein (AFP) (>2.0 MoM) even in absence of abnormal uterine artery indices (PI>1.45) identify women with high risk of FGR, extreme preterm delivery, and stillbirth.[45]

At 22–24 weeks, if Doppler shows high resistance in uterine artery, a 24-fold increased chance of preeclampsia and FGR is estimated. It has an overall sensitivity of growth restriction of 16%. But, its sensitivity for preeclampsia related or no preeclampsia growth restriction with risk of requiring delivery before 32 weeks is 93% and 56%, respectively with specificities of 95%.[46] A systematic review with meta-analysis showed that uterine artery Doppler had limited accuracy in predicting FGR and perinatal death.[47]

Combining all together, effective screening for early preeclampsia can be provided by a combination of maternal factors:

- Low PAPP-A
- Low PP13
- High-soluble endoglin
- Low placental growth factor
- Uterine artery resistance
- Uterine artery notch.

SUMMARY

Doppler is an important modality for predicting FGR. It has an important role in deciding the progress and prognosis of the fetuses having FGR and thus has an important role in taking management decisions. For long-term monitoring, it is better than CTG. It warns for the potential of intrauterine oxygen deprivation. Though it is important to understand that definite cut offs that may accurately predict the outcome of the fetus/neonate is still not available. Association of abnormal intrafetal Doppler study and poor fetal outcome does not equate to cause. Our Doppler fetal tests do not measure the potential for damage. Damage to fetus may occur without gross alterations in hemodynamics.[48]

REFERENCES

1. Alexander GR, Kogan MD, Hims JH, Mor JM, Goldenberg R. Racial differences in birth weight for gestational age and infant mortality in extremely low US populations. Pediatr Perinat Epidemiol. 1999;13(2):129-43.
2. Todros T, Plazztta C, Patorin L. Body proportionality of small-for-date fetus: is it related to etiological factors? Early Hum Dev. 1996;45(1-2):1-9.
3. Mongelli M, Ek S, Tambirajya R. Screening for fetal growth restriction: a mathematical model of the effect of time interval and ultrasound error. Obstet Gynecol. 1998;92(6):908-12.
4. Wilcox AJ. Intrauterine growth retardation: beyond birth weight criteria. Early Hum Dev. 1983;8(3-4):189-93.
5. Snijders RJ, Sherrod C, Gosden CM, Nicolaides KH. Fetal growth retardation: associated malformations and chromosomal abnormalities. Am J Obstet Gynecol. 1993;168(2):547-55.
6. Spinillo A, Capuzzo E, Piazzi G, Baltaro F, Stratanati M, Ometto A. Significance of low birth weight for gestational age among very preterm infant. Br J Obstet Gynecol. 1997;104(6):668-73.
7. Illescas T. 11-14 weeks' scan. Donald School Textbook of Power Point Presentations on Advanced Ultrasound in Obstetrics and Gynecology, 1st edition. New Delhi: Jaypee Brothers Medical Publishers; 2015.
8. Honemeyer U, Kurjak A, Monni G. Normal and abnormal early pregnancy. Donald School Textbook of Ultrasound in Obstetrics and Gynecology, 3rd edition. New Delhi: Jaypee Brothers Medical Publishers; 2011.
9. Altman DG, Chitty LS. New charts for ultrasound dating of pregnancy. Ultrasound Obstet Gynecol. 1997;10(3):174-91.
10. Stebbins B, Jaffe R. Fetal biometry and gestational age estimation. In: Jaffe R, Bui TH (Eds). Textbook of Fetal Ultrasound. Nashville, US: Parthenon Publishing; 1999: pp. 47-57.
11. Chang TC, Robson SC, Boys RJ, Spencer JA. Prediction of the small for gestational age infant: which ultrasonic measurement is best? Obstet Gynecol. 1992;80(6):1030-8.
12. Hadlock FP, Harrist RB, Sharman RS, Deter RL, Park SK. Estimation of fetal weight with the use of head, body, and femur measurements—a prospective study. Am J Obstet Gynecol. 1985;151(3):333-7.
13. Wherry KL, Cdubinsky TJ, Waitches GM, Richardson ML, Reed S. Low resistance endometrial arterial flow in the exclusion of ectopic pregnancy revisited. J Ultrasound Med. 2001;20(4):335-42.
14. Nicolaides KH, Bilardo CM, Soothill PW, Campbell S. Absence end diastolic frequencies in umbilical artery: a sign of fetal hypoxia and acidosis. BMJ. 1988;297(6655):1026-7.
15. MoCowan LM, Harding JE, Stewart AW. Customized birth weight centiles predict SGA pregnancies with perinatal morbidity. BJOG. 2005;112(8):1026-33.
16. MoCowan LM, Harding JE, Stewart AW. Umbilical artery Doppler studies in small for gestational age babies reflect disease severity. BJOG. 2000;107(7):916-25.
17. Trudinger BJ, Cook CM, Giles WB, Ng S, Fong E, Connelly A, et al. Fetal umbilical artery velocity

waveforms and subsequent neonatal outcome. Br J Obstet Gynecol. 1991;98(4):378-84.

18. Society for Maternal Fetal Medicine Publications Committee, Berkley E, Chauhan SP, Abuahmad A. Doppler assessment of the fetus with intrauterine growth restriction. AJOG. 2012;206: 300-8.
19. Bekedam DJ, Visser GHA, Mulder EJH, Poelmann-Weesjes G. Heart rate variation and movement incidence in growth retarded fetuses: The significance of antenatal late heart rate decelerations. Am J Obstet Gynecol. 1987;157(1):126-33.
20. Odibo AO, Riddick C, Pare E, Stamilio DM, Macones GA. Cerebroplacental Doppler ratio and adverse perinatal outcomes in intrauterine growth restriction: evaluating the impact of using gestational age-specific reference values. J Ultrasound Med. 2005;24(9):1223-8.
21. Baschat AA, Gembruch U, Harman CR. The sequence of changes in Doppler and biophysical parameters as severe fetal growth restriction worsens. Ultrasound Obstet Gynecol. 2001;18(6):571-7.
22. Figueras F, Benavides A, Del Rio M, Crispi F, Eixarch E, Martinez JM, et al. Monitoring of fetuses with intrauterine growth restriction: longitudinal changes in ductus venosus and aortic isthmus flow. Ultrasound Obstet Gyneol. 2009;33(1):39-43.
23. Bachat AA, Guclu S, Kush ML, Gembruch U, Weiner CP, Harman CR. Venous Doppler in prediction of acid-base status of growth-restricted fetuses with elevated placental blood flow resistance. Am J Obstet Gynecol. 2004;191(1):277-84.
24. Del Rio M, Martinez JM, Figueras F, Bennasar M, Olivella A, Palacio M, et al. Doppler assessment of the aortic isthmus and perinatal outcome in prenatal fetuses with severe intrauterine growth restriction. Ultrasound Obstet Gynecol. 2008;31(1):41-7.
25. Sebire NJ. Umbilical artery Doppler revisited: pathophysiology of changes of intrauterine growth restriction revealed. Ultrasound Obstet Gynecol. 2003;21(5):419-22.
26. Ferrazzi E, Bozzo M, Rigano S, Bellotti M, Morabito A, Pardi G, et al. Temporal sequence of abnormal Doppler changes in the peripheral and central circulatory systems of severely growth-restricted fetus. Ultrasound Obstet Gynecol. 2002;19(2):140-6.
27. Cosmi E, Ambrosini G, D'Antona D, Saccardi C, Mari G. Doppler cardiotocography and biophysical profile changes in growth-restricted fetuses. Obstet Gynecol. 2005;106(6):1240-5.
28. Thornton JG, Hornbuckle J, Vail A, Spiegelhalter DJ, Levene M, GRIT Study Group. Infant wellbeing at 2 years of age in growth restriction intervention trial (GRIT): Multicentred randomized controlled trial. Lancet. 2004;18(6):571-7.
29. Hecher K, Bilardo CM, Stigter RH, Ville Y, Hackelöer BJ, Kok HJ, et al. Monitoring of fetuses with intrauterine growth restriction: a longitudinal study. Ultrasound Obstet Gynecol. 2001;18(6):564-70.
30. To WW, Chan Am, Mok KM. Use of umbilical-cerebral Doppler ratios in predicting fetal growth restriction in near-term fetuses. Aust N Z J Obstet Gynecol. 2005;45(2):130-6.
31. Scherjon S, Briet J, Oosting H, Kok J. The discrepancy between maturation of visual-evoked potentials and cognitive outcome at five years in very pre-term infants with and without hemodynamic signs of fetal brain-sparing. Paediatrics. 2000;105(2):385-91.
32. Kok JH, Prick L, Merckel E, Everhard Y, Verkerk GJQ, Scherjon SA. Visual function at 11 years of age in preterm-born children with and without fetal brain sparing. Paediatrics. 2007;119(6):e1342-50.
33. Bilardo CM, Wolf H, Stigter RH, Ville Y, Baez E, Visser GHA, et al. Relationship between monitoring parameters and perinatal outcome in severe, early intrauterine growth restriction. Ultrasound Obstet Gynecol. 2004;23(2):119-25.
34. Baschat AA, Cosmi E, Bilardo C, Wolf H, Berg C, Rigano S, et al. Predictors of neonatal outcome in early-onset placental dysfunction. Obstet Gynecol. 2007;109(2 Pt 1):253-61.
35. Pattison N, McCowan L. Cardiotocography for antepartum fetal assessment. Cochrane Database Syst Rev. 2000;(2):CD001068.
36. Muresan D, Rotar IC, Stamatian F. The usefulness of fetal Doppler evaluation in early versus late onset intrauterine growth restriction. Review of literature. Med Ultrason. 2016;18(1):103-9.
37. Miller DA, Rabello YA, Paul RH. The modified biophysical profile: antepartum testing in the 1990s. Am J Obstet Gynecol. 1996;174(3):812-7.
38. Baschat AA, Galan HL, Bhide A, Berg C, Kush ML, Oepkes D, et al. Doppler and biophysical assessment in growth restricted fetuses: distribution of test results. Ultrasound Obstet Gynecol. 2006;27(1):41-7.
39. Hernandez-Andrade E, Crispi F, Benavides-Serralde A, Plasencia W, Diesel HF, Eixarch E, et al. Contribution of the modified myocardial performance index and aortic isthmus blood flow index to refine prediction of mortality in pre-term intrauterine growth restricted fetuses. Ultrasound Obstet Gynecol. 2009;34(4):430-6.

40. Pilalis A, Souka AP, Antsaklis P, Daskalakis G, Papantoniou N, Mesogitis S, et al. Screening for pre-eclampsia and fetal growth restriction by uterine artery Doppler and PAPP-A at 11-14 weeks' gestation. Ultrasound Obstet Gynecol. 2007;29(2):135-40.
41. Fox NS, Shalom D, Chasen ST. Second trimester fetal growth as a predictor of poor obstetric and neonatal outcome in patients with low first trimester serum pregnancy associated plasma protein-A and a euploid fetus. Ultrasound Obstet Gynecol. 2009;33:34-8.
42. Crispi F, Llurba E, Dominguez C, Martín-Gallán P, Cabero L, Gratacós E. Predictive value of angiogenic factors and uterine artery Doppler for early-versus late onset preeclampsia and uterine artery growth restriction. Ultrasound Obstet Gynecol. 2008;31:303-9.
43. Khalil A, Cowans NJ, Spencer K, Goichmans S, Meiri H, Hrrington K. First trimester markers for the prediction of pre-eclampsia in women with a-priori high risk. Ultrasound Obstet Gynecol. 2010;35:671-9.
44. Giguere Y, Bujoid E, Charland N, Grenier S, Lafond J, Forest JC, et al. Literature Review. Annales de Biologie Clinique. 2011;69(3):257-71.
45. Proctor LK, Toal M, Keating S, Chitayat D, Okun N, Windrim RC, et al. Placental size and the prediction of severe early-onset intrauterine growth restriction in women with low pregnancy-associated plasma protein-A. Ultrasound Obstet Gynecol. 2009;34:274-82.
46. Papageorghiou AT, Yu CK, Bindra R, Pandis G, Nicolaides KH, Fetal Medicine Foundation Second Trimester Screening Group. Multicenter screening for pre-eclampsia and fetal growth restriction by transvaginal uterine artery Doppler at 23 weeks of gestation. Ultrasound Obstet Gynecol. 2001;18(5):441-9.
47. Chien PF, Amott N, Gordon A, Owen P, Khan KS. How useful is uterine artery Doppler flow velocimetry in the prediction of pre-eclampsia, intrauterine growth retardation and perinatal death? An overview. BJOG. 2000;107(2):196-208.
48. Trudinger B. Doppler: more or less? Ultrasound Obstet Gynecol. 2007;29(3):243-6.

10 CHAPTER

Role of Ultrasound in Medical Disorders in Pregnancy

Darshan Wadekar, Zalak Mehta

CLASSIFICATION (TABLE 1)

Metabolic Disorders

- Hypertension in pregnancy
- Diabetes in pregnancy.

Systemic Disorders Complicating Pregnancy

- Cardiac disease
- Respiratory disorders complicating pregnancy such as asthma and pneumonia
- Disease of gallbladder and pancreas
- Renal disorders in pregnancy
- Seizure disorders in pregnancy
- Venous thromboembolism and pregnancy
- Hematological disorders
- Psychiatric illness
- Substance abuse.

Infections

- TORCH [toxoplasmosis, other (syphilis, varicella-zoster, parvovirus B19), rubella, cytomegalovirus (CMV), and herpes] infection
- Urinary tract infections during pregnancy.

Autoimmune

- Thyroid disorder
- Sjogren's syndrome
- Systemic lupus erythematosus (SLE).

THYROID DISEASE AND PREGNANCY

The second most common endocrine disorder after diabetes mellitus (DM) in women of childbearing age is thyroid dysfunction. Thyroid gland is located in the anterior neck, it is bilobed, which are connected in center by an isthmus. Thyroid glands are composed of follicles. Each follicle is composed of colloid in center and follicular and parafollicular cells in periphery. Now, we will discuss the functioning of thyroid gland. Thyroid gland produces thyroid hormone T3 and T4, which affect each and every cell of the body. Production of hormone is dependent on hypothalamus-pituitary-thyroid axis. Hypothalamus releases thyroid-releasing hormone. Anterior pituitary gland secrets TSH; action of TSH is mainly to increase production of T3 and T4. In plasma, more than 99% of T3 and T4 is bound. Only the free hormones—free T3 and free T4 are biologically active, which is less than 1%.

Fetal thyroid gland develops at 5 weeks of gestation and gradually starts to function at 35–37 weeks and hence radioactive tracer cannot be used for diagnosis or treatment of mother to avoid the risk of exposure to the fetus.

In early pregnancy when the level of human chorionic gonadotropin (hCG) increases, TSH is suppressed, this is due to hCG-stimulating TSH receptors due to common alpha subunit and some beta subunits. Hence, TSH is suppressed and total T4 is increased.

DIABETES AND PREGNANCY

Diabetes mellitus is a group of disorder thereby having hyperglycemia either due to defect in insulin secretion or insulin action or both. It is the most common medical complication of pregnancy. Normal pregnancy is a state of insulin resistance. The placenta produces several hormones to spare glucose for the developing fetus that antagonize insulin.

TABLE 1: Different types of medical disorders of pregnancy and their effect on fetus and mother and management.

Medical disorders of pregnancy	*Causes*	*Effects on fetus during 1st trimester*	*Effects on fetus during 2nd trimester and 3rd trimester*	*Effects on offspring and mother*	*Diagnosis and management*
Hypothyroidism	• Chronic autoimmune thyroiditis (Hashimoto thyroiditis) • Endemic iodine deficiency • History of either ablative radioiodine therapy or thyroidectomy • Secondary hypothyroidism is pituitary in origin. For example, Sheehan syndrome resulting from prior obstetric hemorrhage is characterized by pituitary ischemia and necrosis, with subsequent deficiencies in some or all pituitary responsive hormone	Early pregnancy failure	• Low-birth weight • Stillbirth • Placental abruption • Preeclampsia • Preterm birth and fetal death	• Impaired neurological implications in newborn • Symptoms in mother—fatigue, constipation, cold intolerance, and muscle cramps, insomnia, weight gain, carpal tunnel syndrome, hair loss, voice changes, and intellectual slowness, goiter, periorbital edema, dry skin, and prolonged relaxation phase of deep tendon reflexes	• Elevated serum TSH and a low serum fT4 • If the free thyroxine concentration is low in the presence of a normal or depressed TSH, then pituitary (central) hypothyroidism should be suspected. Reference ranges for serum TSH and fT4 concentration are 0.4–4.5 mIU/L and 0.7–1.8 ng/dL, respectively • During pregnancy, maternal serum chorionic gonadotropin (hCG) peaks at approximately 10 weeks' gestation and has some thyroid-stimulating activity as a result of its structural homology with TSH. This results in a decrease in the maternal serum TSH and a modest increase in fT4 during the first trimester. • *Subclinical hypothyroidism* occurs in asymptomatic women whose thyroid-stimulating hormone (TSH) concentration is above the

Contd...

Contd...

Medical disorders of pregnancy	***Causes***	***Effects on fetus during 1st trimester***	***Effects on fetus during 2nd trimester and 3rd trimester***	***Effects on offspring and mother***	***Diagnosis and management***
					statistically defined upper limit of normal while their serum-free thyroxine (fT4) concentration is within its reference range • *Antithyroid antibodies testing*—thyroid peroxidase antibodies • Levothyroxine sodium is the treatment of choice. Starting doses usually range from 1.6 to 1.8 µg/kg/d. Serum TSH is then measured at 6-week intervals and thyroxine is adjusted
Hyperthyroidism	Graves' disease or autoimmune thyrotoxicosis. Graves' disease is an organ-specific autoimmune process whereby thyroid-stimulating autoantibodies attach receptors.		• Preterm labor • Preeclampsia, fetal growth restriction, and perinatal mortality	• Congestive heart failure, thyroid storm in mother • Symptoms in mother are nervousness, heat intolerance, palpitations, goiter, failure to gain weight or weight loss, and exophthalmos • Infant with fetal or neonatal hyperthyroidism	• *Subclinical hyperthyroidism* defined as a serum TSH concentration below the statistically defined lower limit of normal with a serum concentration of fT4 within the reference range, is typically identified in asymptomatic women. • In women with a depressed serum TSH level (<0.4 mIU/L), clinical hyperthyroidism is confirmed by an elevation in fT4 (>1.8 ng/dL) concentration

Contd...

Contd...

Medical disorders of pregnancy	***Causes***	***Effects on fetus during 1st trimester***	***Effects on fetus during 2nd trimester and 3rd trimester***	***Effects on offspring and mother***	***Diagnosis and management***
					• Thioamide drugs are used for treatment. Initial daily dose of 100–600 mg for propylthiouracil or 10–40 mg for methimazole. Prefer propylthiouracil because it inhibits peripheral conversion of T4 to T3 and it crosses the placenta less readily than methimazole • Ablative radioactive iodine is contraindicated in pregnancy, as it can cause fetal thyroid destruction.
Gestational hypertension—preeclampsia and eclampsia—wide spectrum of patients who may have only mild elevation in blood pressure (BP) or severe hypertension with various organ dysfunctions including hemolysis, elevated liver	Hypertension is the most common medical disorder during pregnancy. The prevalence is 1–5%. Chronic hypertension is blood pressure >140 mm Hg systolic and/or 90 mm Hg diastolic before pregnancy or by hypertension occurring during pregnancy before 20 weeks gestation or by hypertension persisting beyond 12 weeks before		Fetal complications are prematurity, stillbirth, LBW and neonatal death, and FGR	Maternal complications include preeclampsia, stroke and abruption placenta, increased likelihood of cesarean delivery. Preeclampsia: after 20 weeks of gestation, SBP > 140 mm Hg or DBP >90 mm Hg in a previously normotensive women + proteinuria (excretion of >0.3 g protein in 24-h urine collection) or with other systemic manifestation	Gestational hypertension is defined as a systolic BP of at least 140 mm Hg and/or a diastolic BP of at least 90 mm Hg on at least two occasions at least 6 hours apart but not more than 7 days apart after the 20th week of gestation in women known to be normotensive before pregnancy and before 20 weeks' gestation. Gestational hypertension is considered severe, if there are sustained elevations in systolic BP to at least 160 mm Hg and/or in diastolic BP to at least

Contd...

Contd...

Medical disorders of pregnancy	***Causes***	***Effects on fetus during 1st trimester***	***Effects on fetus during 2nd trimester and 3rd trimester***	***Effects on offspring and mother***	***Diagnosis and management***
enzymes, low-platelet count (HELLP) syndrome	delivery. Chronic hypertension with superimposed preeclampsia: New onset of proteinuria in the previously hypertensive pregnant women or increase in proteinuria				110 mm Hg for at least 6 hours. Preeclampsia is primarily defined as gestational hypertension plus proteinuria (≥300 mg/24-hour period)
Seizure disorder in pregnancy	Seizures are the result of disorganized firing of neural cells. Epilepsy is a neurological condition characterized by two or more unprovoked seizures. Causes of seizures could be idiopathic, intracranial tumors, metabolic abnormality, trauma to head, and stroke.	How does epilepsy affect pregnancy? • Fetal heart rate deceleration • Decreased oxygen to the fetus • If there is trauma, fall during a seizure, it can cause—fetal injury, abruption placenta (premature separation of the placenta from the uterus), miscarriage • Preterm labor	Carbamazepine, valproic acid, phenytoin, and phenobarbital are known to cross the placenta and have teratogenic effects. Birth defects, which may increase due to AEDs are cleft lip, cleft palate, neural tube defects, congenital heart disease, and urinary tract defects. Others are ocular hypertelorism and broad nasal bridge Risk increases with higher dose of medication • Multiagent therapy also increases the risk	About 33% of women will have an increase in frequency, whereas rest may have no change or decrease Babies born to mother who have epilepsy also have a slightly higher risk of developing seizures as they get out Long-term neuropsychological consequences of maternal epilepsy and its AEDs are noted in adolescent children A significant decrease in the IQ score of these children exposed to polypharmacy in utero	As a rule, the lesser the frequency of seizures occurring before conception, the less the risk of worsening epilepsy during pregnancy Folic acid helps to prevent neural tube defects and other abnormalities of brain and spinal cord Some AEDs alter the folic acid metabolism and hence the dose of folic acid should be increased. Folic acid supplementation should be started 3 months prior to conception.

Contd...

Contd...

Medical disorders of pregnancy	*Causes*	*Effects on fetus during 1st trimester*	*Effects on fetus during 2nd trimester and 3rd trimester*	*Effects on offspring and mother*	*Diagnosis and management*
Drugs		**Defects**			
Carbamazepine Phenytoin Phenobarbital		Craniofacial defects Fingernail hypoplasia and distal digit hypoplasia Development delay Neural tube defects			
Valproate		Increases the chance of NTDs by ten folds			
Phenobarbital		Coagulopathies in babies due to deficiency of vitamin K-dependent clotting factors			
Alcohol and substance abuse	Consuming many drinks per occasion (i.e., binge drinking, ≥5 drinks) may be more harmful to the developing fetus than the same amount spread over several days, because of higher peak blood alcohol content	Spontaneous abortion	Microcephaly; growth deficiency; CNS dysfunction including mental retardation and behavioral abnormalities; craniofacial abnormalities (i.e., short palpebral fissures, hypoplastic philtrum, flattened maxilla); behavioral abnormalities		Patient counseling and if necessary de-addiction clinic referral.
Cigarette			Preterm birth Placenta previa Placental abruption	No anomalies; reduced birthweight (200 g lighter)	Patient counseling and if necessary de-addiction clinic referral
Opioids		No anomalies; corresponding decrease in birthweight	Spontaneous abortion	Preterm birth Placenta previa Placental abruption	Patient counseling and if necessary de-addiction clinic referral

Contd...

Contd...

Medical disorders of pregnancy	***Causes***	***Effects on fetus during 1st trimester***	***Effects on fetus during 2nd trimester and 3rd trimester***	***Effects on offspring and mother***	***Diagnosis and management***
Sickle cell disease	Sickle hemoglobin S results from the substitution of glutamic acid by valine in the beta-globin chain at position 6. Red blood cells with hemoglobin S undergo sickling under conditions of decreased oxygen tension. This results in hemolysis, increased viscosity, and vaso-occlusion (VOC), and leads to further decreased oxygenation. This VOC leads to local infarction in all major organ systems	Sickle syndromes end in abortion, stillbirth, or neonatal more than one-third of pregnancies in women with death	Pregnancy outcomes in patients with S/S anemia Spontaneous abortion Stillbirth Neonatal death Low birthweight Perinatal mortality	This results in hemolysis, increased viscosity, and vaso-occlusion (VOC), and leads to further decreased oxygenation. This VOC leads to local infarction in all major organ systems. The bone pain represents VOC in the bone marrow. Other changes from sickling include bony abnormalities such as osteonecrosis of the femoral and humeral heads; renal medullary damage; hepatomegaly; ventricular hypertrophy; pulmonary infarctions; pulmonary hypertension; cerebrovascular accidents; leg ulcers; and a propensity to infection and sepsis	Folic acid requirements, however, are considerable as there is an intense shortened red blood cell lifespan. No need for prenatal counseling, as it is a treatable/ manageable cause.
Beta-thalassemia disease	Variable amounts of hemoglobin A are produced depending on the variant of the beta-thalassemia allele inherited in its most usual form, a level of A2 above	The risk of low birthweight, fetal growth restriction, preterm delivery, and preeclampsia are increased.	Spontaneous abortion Stillbirth Neonatal death Low birthweight Perinatal mortality Risk of transmission from parents depending on	Genetic evaluation Amniocentesis or chorionic villous sampling should be offered and polymerase chain reaction (PCR) is utilized to detect abnormal fetal genotypes.	With the increased red cell mass typically required during pregnancy, folate supplementation is important. Pneumonia is common, caused by *Streptococcus pneumoniae*, and the polyvalent pneumococcal vaccine is

Contd...

Contd...

Medical disorders of pregnancy	***Causes***	***Effects on fetus during 1st trimester***	***Effects on fetus during 2nd trimester and 3rd trimester***	***Effects on offspring and mother***	***Diagnosis and management***
	3.5% on hemoglobin electrophoresis is diagnostic.		whether they are minor, major, or normal If both the parents are thalassemia minor/ carrier—chances of normal child is 25%; of diseased child is 25% and child with carrier is 50%.		recommended. Annual inactivated influenza vaccine should be administered. Hepatitis B vaccination is recommended. For patients who have undergone autosplenectomy, vaccination against *Haemophilus influenzae* type B is recommended. Intravenous hydration along with opioid analgesics should be given. Oxygen by nasal cannula will decrease the sickling at the capillary level and improve symptoms.
Combined hemo-globinopathies		Low birthweight, fetal growth restriction, preterm delivery, and preeclampsia	Spontaneous abortion Stillbirth Neonatal death Low birthweight Perinatal mortality	Genetic evaluation with amniocentesis or chorionic villous sampling should be offered and polymerase chain reaction (PCR) utilized to detect abnormal fetal genotypes.	

Contd...

Contd...

Medical disorders of pregnancy	***Causes***	***Effects on fetus during 1st trimester***	***Effects on fetus during 2nd trimester and 3rd trimester***	***Effects on offspring and mother***	***Diagnosis and management***
Cardiac disease in pregnancy	Acquired valvular lesions are typically sequelae of rheumatic fever; however, valvular endocarditis secondary to intravenous drug use is not uncommon	Increased risk of fetal structural cardiac anomalies Paternal cardiac abnormalities also increase the risk of congenital cardiac disease; however, maternal disease poses the greatest risk by up to 3.5 times.	***Table 2*** *showing the risk factor in fetus*	Dysrhythmias and congestive failure resulting in pulmonary edema due to most of the disorders	Therefore, fetal echocardiography is recommended for all patients with a congenital cardiac abnormality.

(AED: antiepileptic drug; FSH: follicle-stimulating hormone; FGR: fetal growth restriction; DBP: diastolic blood pressure; SBP: systolic blood pressure; NTD: neural tube defect; CNS: central nervous system; LBW: low birth weight)

TABLE 2: Risk of fetal congenital cardiac defects (%) in presence of different risk factors (Lupton et al.).

	Cardiac lesion	*Prior sibling affected*	*Father affected*	*Mother affected*	
	Tetralogy of Fallot	2.5	1.5	2.6	
	Aortic coarctation			14.1	
	Atrial septal defect	2.5	1.5	4.6–11	
	Ventricular septal defect	3	2	9.5–15.6	
	Pulmonary stenosis	2	2	6.5	
	Aortic stenosis	2	3	15–17.9	
Renal disease in pregnancy	Proteinuria is defined as total protein excretion of more than 300 mg/24 hours, and usually denotes renal disease.		• Fetal growth restriction • Stillbirth • Preterm delivery • Preeclampsia • Fetal death	Kidney function may worsen during pregnancy	The dietary intake of sodium should be limited to 1.5 g sodium/day. Frequently, bed rest in a lateral recumbent position will suffice to mobilize pre-existing edema by promoting an increase in the excretion of sodium. In general, the use of diuretic agents has been discouraged because of the possibility that reduction of extracellular fluid volume could decrease blood flow to the placenta.

Contd...

Contd...

	Cardiac lesion	***Prior sibling affected***	***Father affected***	***Mother affected***	
Mother on immunosuppressive agents due to renal transplant or any other organ transplant	Prednisone, azathioprine, cyclosporine, or tacrolimus are used because these are safe drugs		• Fetal growth restriction and preterm birth	Possibility of delayed adverse effects in adulthood such as later development of fertility problems, autoimmune disorders, and neoplasia	
Asthma in pregnancy	Asthma severity improves in one-third of women, worsens in one-third of women, and remains unchanged in one-third of women Asthma appears to be more likely to worsen during pregnancy in women with more severe asthma before becoming pregnant			LBW Preterm birth Preeclampsia	
Hepatitis in pregnancy	The typical clinical manifestations of hepatitis include low-grade fever, malaise, poor appetite, right upper quadrant pain and tenderness, jaundice, and alcoholic stools			Infants delivered to seropositive mothers should receive hepatitis B immunoglobulin within 12 hours of birth. Prior to their discharge from the hospital, these infants also should begin the hepatitis B vaccination series.	Hepatitis A: Perinatal transmission virtually never occurs, and therefore the infection does not pose a major risk to either the mother or the baby unless the mother develops fulminant hepatitis and liver failure.

Contd...

Contd...

	Cardiac lesion	***Prior sibling affected***	***Father affected***	***Mother affected***	
	The diagnosis of hepatitis B and C is best confirmed by serologic tests				Hepatitis B and C: The infection also can be transmitted perinatally from an infected mother to her infant depending on mother's viral load.
Parvovirus		• Spontaneous miscarriage	• Fetal anemia, fetal hydrops		
Varicella infection		• Congenital Varicella infection • Highest risk between 13 and 20 weeks	• Preterm birth • IUFD	• If in last 3 weeks before delivery • Neonatal varicella (risk 25–30%)	
Cytomegalovirus	• First child having cold • Risk of transmission 30% in primary infection • 3% in secondary infection	• Spontaneous miscarriage	• 90% asymptomatic • 10% (CNS, e.g., lateral ventriculomegaly, microcephaly, ocular defects, IUGR, preterm birth) Placenta—heterogeneous appearance and thickened (more than gestational age)	• 5–10% may be asymptomatic initially and later develop neurological impairment and sensorineural deafness	
Toxoplasmosis	• Vertical transmission • 15% at 13 weeks • 44% at 26 weeks • 71% at 36 weeks				

Contd...

Contd...

	Cardiac lesion	*Prior sibling affected*	*Father affected*	*Mother affected*	
HIV	Ideally, every pregnant women should undergo HIV testing as a part of their routine antenatal checkup. Options for testing are detection of either antigen from the virus itself, antibodies to portions of the virus, viral nucleic acid, or, less commonly, culture of the virus. The most widely used method [enzyme-linked immunosorbent assay (ELISA) confirmed by Western blot] involves the detection of antibodies to virus in the patient's sera.	• HIV virus can pass through the placenta and infect the fetus. • During labor and delivery, the fetus is exposed to mother's blood.	• Prematurity • Low-birth weight • Neurodevelopmental problems • Stillbirth • SGA	• Bottle-fed a baby instead of breast milk to avoid transmission of virus. • Cesarean delivery is preferred over normal vaginal delivery. • Mother is advised to take ART properly.	Patient should be explained the psychosocial and medical aspect of the disease. They should be counseled about safe sex practices, not sharing razors, about the transmission of infection to fetus, etc. Patient should also be screened for hepatitis B, C, and syphilis. Management—baseline CD4 count and viral load has to be done, appropriate anti-retroviral therapy and cesarean section to prevent mother-to-child transmission. If CD4 count >350 mm/mL^3 and the viral load under 100,000 copies—no need of ART at present.

Contd...

Contd...

	Cardiac lesion	*Prior sibling affected*	*Father affected*	*Mother affected*	
					If CD4 count <350 mm/mL^3 and the viral load >100,000 copies—highly active antiretroviral therapy (HAART) regimen to be started.
Sjogren's syndrome	Chronic inflammatory autoimmune disease in which salivary and lacrimal glands are progressively destroyed	• 96% of the fetus will be normal. • However 4% will have some congenital anomalies out of which 47% have cardiac anomalies	• Increased rate of spontaneous abortion and preterm deliveries	• Worsening of pulmonary hypertension • Infertility	
SLE	Systemic lupus erythematosus (SLE) is a chronic autoimmune disorder. It can follow a relatively benign course, affecting only the skin and musculoskeletal system, or be more aggressive with life-threatening involvement of vital organs such as the kidney and brain.	Affects approximately 1% of pregnancies, however, 99% are normal.	Placentas from women with SLE demonstrate characteristic changes: reduction in size, placental infarctions, intraplacental hemorrhage, deposition of immunoglobulin, and complement and thickening of the trophoblast basement membrane. Hence [e.g., increased rates of preeclampsia, intrauterine growth restriction (IUGR), preterm delivery]	Affects approximately 1% of pregnancies	

Contd...

Contd...

	Cardiac lesion	***Prior sibling affected***	***Father affected***	***Mother affected***	
Antiphospholipid antibody syndrome			Growth restriction and third trimester fetal death, or recurrent pregnancy loss	Fetal loss rates as high as 50–90%	Either unfractionated or low-molecular weight heparin (LMWH) may be used. Severe APS or those who have been refractory to heparin therapy Intravenous immunoglobulin (IVIG) is used. Aspirin therapy can be initiated at the first positive pregnancy test and heparin therapy can be initiated at 5–7 weeks of gestation.
Complications		*Fetal complications due to hyperglycemia*		*Maternal complications*	
Diabetes in pregnancy		• Fetal macrosomia hence likelihood of operative delivery and birth trauma • Metabolic complications in the neonate including hypoglycemia, hypocalcemia, and hyperbilirubinemia • Prematurity and perinatal mortality • Fetal oxygenation problems—sudden fetal demise, chronic fetal hypoxia, and respiratory distress syndrome		• Risk of recurrent pregnancy loss increases • Macrovascular and microvascular complications such as retinopathy, nephropathy, and cardiomyopathy • Preeclampsia and hypertensive disorders • Other complications of diabetes include preterm labor, chorioamnionitis, polyhydramnios, urinary tract infections, and others.	

Contd...

Contd...

	Cardiac lesion	Prior sibling affected	Father affected	Mother affected	
		• Fetal malformations: – *CNS*: Neural tube defects including anencephaly, meningomyelocele, and encephalocele – *CVS*: Transposition of great vessels, ventricular and atrial septal defects, hypoplastic left heart and others – *Skeletal*: Caudal regression syndrome, spinal anomalies – *Renal*: Hydronephrosis, renal agenesis, and cystic kidneys – *Intestinal*: Duodenal atresia, anorectal malformation			

(IUFD: intrauterine fetal death; IUGR: intrauterine growth restriction; SGA: small for gestational age; SLE: systemic lupus erythematosus)

Still, most pregnant women maintain normal blood glucose levels despite the increased insulin resistance through more production and release of insulin by the pancreas. However, in some women, β-cell of pancreas producing insulin cannot keep pace with the resistance to insulin produced by the diabetogenic hormones from the placenta. The prevalence of gestational diabetes mellitus (GDM) in the USA is 2–5%.

- Pregestational or gestational
- Uncomplicated or complicated.

The etiological classification refers to the underlying cause for the glucose intolerance. It can be classified as follows:

- Insulin-dependent or type 1 diabetes
- Insulin-independent or type 2 diabetes
- Gestational diabetes mellitus (GDM)
- *Type A1*: Abnormal oral glucose tolerance test, but normal fasting and postprandial (2 hours after meals) blood glucose levels. Dietary modifications are sufficient to control blood glucose levels.
- *Type A2*: Abnormal oral glucose tolerance test (OGTT) compounded by abnormal glucose levels during fasting and/or after meals. Additional therapy with insulin or other medications are required.
- *Type B*: Onset at age of 20 or older and duration of less than 10 years.
- *Type C*: Onset at age of 10–19 or duration of 10–19 years.
- *Type D*: Onset before age of 10 or duration greater than 20 years.
- *Type E*: Overt diabetes mellitus with calcified pelvic vessels.
- *Type F*: Diabetic nephropathy.
- *Type R*: Proliferative retinopathy.
- *Type RF*: Retinopathy and nephropathy.
- *Type H*: Ischemic heart disease.
- *Type T*: Prior kidney transplant.

GESTATIONAL DIABETES MELLITUS

The definition of gestational diabetes mellitus according to American College of Obstetricians and Gynecologists (ACOG) is—"any degree of glucose intolerance that either commences or is first diagnosed in pregnancy". This definition includes women whose glucose tolerance will return back to normal after pregnancy and also those who will persist with glucose intolerance and develop type 2 diabetes.

Criteria for Avoiding Laboratory Screening for Gestational Diabetes

All criteria must be met for a patient to be considered "low-risk" and glucose testing avoided (from American Diabetes Association):

- Age <25 years
- Not a member of an ethnic group with an increased prevalence of type 2 diabetes mellitus
- Body mass index of ≤25
- No prior history of glucose intolerance [GDM, DM, impaired glucose tolerance (IGT), or impaired fasting glucose (IFG)]
- No prior history of obstetric outcomes associated with GDM (macrosomia, stillbirth, and malformations)
- No known diabetes in a first-degree relative.

Women have to be screened for GDM with the 1-hour 50-g glucose challenge test (GCT)—cut off for positive result is 130 mg/dL.

American Diabetes Association's Fourth International Workshop Conference on Gestational Diabetes

Diagnostic thresholds for gestational diabetes using the 3-hour 100-g glucose tolerance test:

- Fasting—95
- 1-hour—180
- 2-hour—155
- 3-hour—140

If two or more values *meet or exceed* these thresholds, the diagnosis of gestational diabetes is made.

For women at low risk for GDM, screening should occur between 24 and 28 weeks, because insulin resistance during pregnancy increases as a function of increasing gestational age until approximately 32 weeks of gestation.

Women who are at high risk should be tested upon entry to prenatal care.

Therapeutic Modalities in Gestational Diabetes

Medical management of GDM aims to optimize glycemic control to prevent or minimize the complications associated with the disease, while avoiding ketosis and poor nutrition. Diet, exercise, and patient education are needed.

The cornerstone of care of a pregnancy complicated by diabetes is diet. Smaller, more frequent meals lead to better satiety, improved compliance with the diet, and reduced magnitude of postprandial peaks.

Exercise is another key component in diabetic care. Cardiovascular exercise reduces insulin resistance.

Commonly used targets include fasting values below 95 mg/dL and 2-hour postprandial values below 120 mg/dL. Alternatively, 1-hour postprandial values may be used, with a target below 130–140 mg/dL.

One essential component of this regimen is frequent daily reading. Using this intensified approach, rates of macrosomia, shoulder dystocia, cesarean delivery, and neonatal hypoglycemia were reduced.

Ultimately, some women with GDM will not be able to meet glycemic targets with diet therapy alone and will require medical intervention with insulin or a hypoglycemic agent.

This can usually be determined once dietary therapy has been in place for 2 weeks. Insulin dosage is calculated according to body weight, starting in the range of 0.7–1.0 U/kg of current body weight, usually given in the form of short- and intermediate-acting human insulin, in split doses. Two-thirds of the total calculated dose is given with breakfast and one-third in the evening.

HYPERTENSION IN PREGNANCY

Chronic hypertension defined by American College of Obstetricians and Gynecologists as blood pressure >140 mm Hg systolic and/or 90 mm Hg diastolic before pregnancy or by hypertension occurring during pregnancy before 20 weeks of gestation or by hypertension persisting beyond 12 weeks before delivery.

- *Preeclampsia:* After 20 weeks of gestation, systolic blood pressure (SBP) > 140 mm Hg or diastolic blood pressure (DBP) > 90 mm Hg in a previously normotensive women + proteinuria (excretion of >0.3 g protein in 24-hour urine collection) or with other systemic manifestation.
- *Gestational hypertension:* Elevated SBP >140 mm Hg, DBP > 90 mm Hg in a previously normotensive woman.
- *Chronic hypertension with superimposed preeclampsia:* New onset of proteinuria in the previously hypertensive pregnant women or increase in proteinuria.
- *HELLP syndrome:* Hemolysis, elevated liver enzymes, and low platelets.

SEIZURE DISORDERS IN PREGNANCY

Seizures are the result of disorganized firing of neural cells.

Epilepsy is a neurological condition characterized by two or more unprovoked seizures.

Causes of seizures could be idiopathic, intracranial tumors, metabolic abnormality, trauma to head, and stroke.

Epilepsy during pregnancy raises special concerns while most women who have epilepsy deliver healthy babies.

How does epilepsy affect pregnancy?

- Fetal heart rate deceleration
- Decreased oxygen to the fetus
- If there is trauma, there is fall during a seizure, it can cause—fetal injury, abruption placenta (premature separation of the placenta from the uterus), and miscarriage.
- Preterm labor.

Does epilepsy change during pregnancy?

About 33% of women will have an increase in frequency, whereas rest may have no change or decrease.

Causes of increased frequency are:
- Metabolic changes in mother
- Increased steroid hormone levels
- Stress
- Sleep deprivation
- Patient not taking medication in fear of ill effects of drug on fetus.

As a rule, the lesser the frequency of seizures occurring before conception, the less the risk of worsening epilepsy during pregnancy.

In pregnancy, lower total blood levels of antiepileptic drugs are due to:
- Gastrointestinal absorption decreases due to vomiting
- Hepatic and renal clearance increases
- Albumin level decreases, hence, protein binding site decreases.

Effects of Antiepileptic Drugs on Fetus (Table 3)

- Carbamazepine, valproic acid, phenytoin, and phenobarbital are known to cross the placenta and have teratogenic effects.
- Birth defects, which may increase due to antiepileptic drugs (AEDs), are cleft lip, cleft palate, neural tube defects, congenital heart disease, and urinary tract defects. Other are ocular hypertelorism and broad nasal bridge.
- Risk increases with higher dose of medication.
- Multiagent therapy also increases the risk.

TABLE 3: Effect of anti-epileptic drugs on fetus.

Drugs	*Defects*
Carbamazepine Phenytoin Phenobarbital	Craniofacial defects Fingernail hypoplasia and distal digit hypoplasia Development delay NTDs
Valproate	Increases the chance of NTDs by tenfold
Phenobarbital	Coagulopathies in babies due to deficiency of vitamin K-dependent clotting factors

(NTDs: neural tube defects)

Antiepileptic drug syndrome:
- Also knows as fetal hydantoin syndrome
- Growth deficiency
- Microcephaly
- Dysmorphic facial features
- Mental deficiency

How does mother's epilepsy affect baby?

Babies born to mother who have epilepsy also have a slightly higher risk of developing seizures as they get out.

Long-term neuropsychological consequences of maternal epilepsy and its AEDs are noted in adolescent children.

A significant decrease in the IQ score of these children exposed to polypharmacy in utero.

How should the women having epilepsy be prepared for pregnancy?
- Ideally, the women with epilepsy should receive counseling before conception about effects of seizures, anticonvulsants drugs, and neurological effects on babies.
- Evaluate the frequency of seizure episodes in last 1 year.
- If the frequency of seizure is high (one episode or more per month), you may advice the patient to wait to get pregnant until the epilepsy is better controlled.
- Counsel the patient to take anticonvulsant drugs exactly as prescribed. Advise her not to stop or alter the dose on her own. Explain her that uncontrolled seizures pose more risk to the baby than any other medication.

Advise her to have:
- Healthy diet
- Prenatal vitamins and folic acid
- Enough sleep
- Avoid smoking, alcohol, and illegal drugs.

Why do these patients need more folic acid than other pregnant women do?
- Folic acid helps to prevent neural tube defects and other abnormalities of brain and spinal cord.
- Some AEDs alters the folic acid metabolism and hence the dose of folic acid should be increased.

- Folic acid supplementation should be started 3 months prior to conception.

Other Important Points

- It is advisable to patient to have frequent blood tests to monitor her medication level and alter accordingly, if needed.
- Oral vitamins K supplements during the last month of pregnancy help to prevent bleeding problems in the baby after birth.

CARDIAC DISEASE IN PREGNANCY (BOXES 1 AND 2)

The incidence of serious cardiac disease complicating pregnancy is 1% **(Table 4)**.

Dyspnea, fatigue, palpitations, orthopnea, and pedal edema are the symptoms.

The adaptations that occur during normal pregnancy place substantial demands on cardiac function.

Four fundamental alterations are:

1. Increased intravascular volume
2. Decreased systemic vascular resistance
3. Increased cardiac output
4. Hypercoagulability.

HIV INFECTION

Ideally, every pregnant woman should undergo HIV testing as a part of their routine antenatal checkup.

BOX 1: New York Heart Association (NYHA) functional classification system.

- *Class I*: No limitations of physical activity. Ordinary physical activity does not precipitate cardiovascular symptoms such as dyspnea, angina, fatigue, or palpitations
- *Class II*: Slight limitation of physical activity. Ordinary physical activity will precipitate cardiovascular symptoms. Patients are comfortable at rest.
- *Class III*: Less than ordinary physical activity precipitates symptoms that markedly limit activity. Patients are comfortable at rest.
- *Class IV*: Patients have discomfort with any physical activity. Symptoms are present at rest

BOX 2: Maternal mortality associated with pregnancy (Clark).

Group 1—mortality <1%:
- Atrial septal defect
- Ventricular septal defect
- Patent ductus arteriosus
- *Mitral stenosis*: NYHA class I and II
- Pulmonic/tricuspid valve disease
- Corrected tetralogy of Fallot
- Bioprosthetic valve

Group 2—mortality 5–15%:

Group 2A:
- *Mitral stenosis*: NYHA class III and IV
- Aortic stenosis
- Coarctation of aorta without valvular involvement
- Uncorrected tetralogy of Fallot
- Previous myocardial infarction
- Marfan syndrome with normal aorta

Group 2B:
- Mitral stenosis with atrial fibrillation
- Artificial valve

Group 3—mortality 25–50%:
- Pulmonary hypertension
- Eisenmenger
- Coarctation of aorta with valvular involvement
- Marfan syndrome with aortic involvement
- Peripartum cardiomyopathy with persistent left ventricular dysfunction

TABLE 4: Risk of fetal congenital cardiac defects (%) (Lupton, et al.).

Cardiac lesion	*Prior affected sibling*	*Father affected*	*Mother affected*
Tetralogy of Fallot	2.5	1.5	2.6
Aortic coarctation			14.1
Atrial septal defect	2.5	1.5	4.6–11
Ventricular septal defect	3	2	9.5–15.6
Pulmonary stenosis	2	2	6.5
Aortic stenosis	2	3	15–17.9

Options for testing are detection of either antigen from the virus itself, antibodies to portions of the virus, viral nucleic acid, or, less commonly, culture of the virus. The most widely used method [enzyme-linked immunosorbent assay (ELISA) confirmed by Western blot] involves the detection of antibodies to virus in the patient's sera.

POST-TEST COUNSELING OF SEROPOSITIVE WOMEN

Patient should be explained the psychosocial and medical aspect of the disease. They should be counseled about safe sex practices, not sharing razors, about the transmission of infection to fetus, etc.

Patient should also be screened for hepatitis B, C, and syphilis.

Management

Baseline CD4 count and viral load have to be done, appropriate antiretroviral therapy (ART) and cesarean section to prevent mother-to-child transmission.

- If CD4 count > 350 mm/mL^3 and the viral load under 100,000 copies—no need of ART at present.
- If CD4 count < 350 mm/mL^3 and the viral load >100,000 copies—highly active antiretroviral therapy (HAART) regimen to be started.

For example, if a woman's viral load is 2,000 and her CD4 count is 400 mm/mL^3, she would not be a candidate for therapy if she was not pregnant (the usual starting points are CD4 counts <350 mm^3 or a viral load >100,000 copies). However, because of the pregnancy, HAART would be recommended in order to minimize the risk of transmission.

Three classes of antiretroviral therapy [nucleoside reverse transcriptase inhibitors (NRTIs), non-nucleoside reverse transcriptase inhibitors (NNRTIs), and protease inhibitors (PIs)] are commonly used. The most frequently used regimens comprise two NRTIs and either an NNRTI or a PI (sometimes two PIs are used with one acting as a "booster" of the second). If the chosen regimen fails, the possibility of poor adherence, viral resistance, or both must be considered. Resistance testing should be performed before the failing regimen is discontinued.

- If CD4 count < 200 mm/mL^3—risk of developing opportunistic infection, hence start PCP prophylaxis (e.g., Bactrim DS daily)
- If CD4 count <50 mm/mL^3—start *Mycobacterium avium* complex prophylaxis (azithromycin, 1,200 mg/week).

PERINATAL INFECTIONS

- TORCH (toxoplasmosis, rubella, cytomegalovirus, and herpes virus)

Parvovirus B19:

- Erythema infectiosum or Fifth disease
- Severe anemia in the fetus. The line of management depends on the type of infection, its effect on fetus and result of amniocentesis at 18–20 weeks of gestation.

SICKLE CELL DISEASE

Each hemoglobin is made up of two alpha-globin (141 amino acids) and two beta-globin chains. Sickle hemoglobin S results from the substitution of glutamic acid by valine in the beta-globin chain at position 6; and hemoglobin C from substitution of the same amino acid, but by lysine. Approximately 1 in 600 African-American newborns has sickle cell anemia. The overall rate of sickle cell disorders at birth for African-Americans is 1 in 300.

Red blood cells with hemoglobin S undergo sickling under conditions of decreased oxygen tension. This results in hemolysis, increased viscosity, and vaso-occlusion (VOC), and leads to further decreased oxygenation. This VOC leads to local infarction in all major organ systems. The bone pain represents VOC in the bone marrow. Other changes from sickling include bony abnormalities such as osteonecrosis of the femoral and humeral heads, renal medullary damage, hepatomegaly, ventricular hypertrophy, pulmonary infarctions, pulmonary hypertension, cerebrovascular accidents, leg ulcers, and a propensity to infection and sepsis. Folic acid requirements, however, are considerable, as there is an intense shortened red blood cell lifespan. More than one-third of pregnancies in women with sickle syndromes end in abortion, stillbirth, or neonatal death.

Pregnancy outcomes in patients with S/S anemia:

- Spontaneous abortion
- Stillbirth
- Neonatal death
- Low birthweight
- Perinatal mortality.

BETA-THALASSEMIA DISEASE

Variable amounts of hemoglobin A are produced depending on the variant of the beta-thalassemia allele inherited. In its most usual form, a level of A2 above 3.5% on hemoglobin electrophoresis is diagnostic.

MANAGEMENT DURING PREGNANCY

With the increased red cell mass typically required during pregnancy, folate supplementation is important. Frequent (monthly or every trimester) screening urine cultures should be employed to discover asymptomatic bacteriuria and treat before it becomes symptomatic. Acute pyelonephritis can result in the release of endotoxin, which lyses sickle cells and suppresses hematopoiesis resulting in severe anemia and sickle crises. Pneumonia is common, caused by *Streptococcus pneumoniae*, and the polyvalent pneumococcal vaccine is recommended. Annual inactivated influenza vaccine should be administered. Hepatitis B vaccination is recommended. For patients who have undergone autosplenectomy, vaccination against *Haemophilus influenzae* type B is recommended. Intravenous hydration along with opioid analgesics should be given. Oxygen by nasal cannula will decrease the sickling at the capillary level and improve symptoms. Any focus of infection should be discovered and treated, as it may be responsible for the crisis. The risk of low birthweight, fetal growth restriction, preterm delivery, and preeclampsia is increased. Prophylactic red blood cell transfusions may be considered. Hematocrit and hemoglobin electrophoresis are monitored monthly and transfusion affected to keep the hematocrit between 25 and 30% is recommended. Exchange transfusion in the face of crisis, acute chest syndrome, stroke, and infection can be valuable. Labor and delivery management should take into account the degree of underlying dysfunction. Fluid administration should be conservative to avoid circulatory overload and pulmonary edema.

GENETIC EVALUATION

Amniocentesis or chorionic villous sampling should be offered and polymerase chain reaction (PCR) is utilized to detect abnormal fetal genotypes.

SYSTEMIC LUPUS ERYTHEMATOSUS

Systemic lupus erythematosus (SLE) is a chronic autoimmune disorder. It can follow a relatively benign course, affecting only the skin and musculoskeletal system, or be more aggressive with life-threatening involvement of vital organs such as the kidney and brain. It affects approximately 1% of pregnancies, lupus affects women 3–10 times as often as men, increases the risk for thrombosis. Renal damage is secondary to immune complex deposition, complement activation, and inflammation and subsequent fibrosis. Placentas from women with SLE demonstrate characteristic changes—reduction in size, placental infarctions, intraplacental hemorrhage, deposition of immunoglobulin and complement, and thickening of the trophoblast basement membrane. These may result into increased rates of preeclampsia, intrauterine growth restriction (IUGR) and preterm delivery. Women with lupus can develop a number of systemic manifestations including arthralgias, rashes, renal abnormalities, neurologic complications, thromboemboli, myocarditis, and serositis. Lupus is characterized by a variety of autoantibodies. Antinuclear antibody (ANA) is the most common antibody for screening for autoimmune syndromes. Antibodies to double-stranded DNA (dsDNA) and Smith (Sm) are more specific for lupus and anti-dsDNA has been correlated with disease activity (generally renal involvement). Anti-SSA/Ro and anti-SSB/La are more often associated with Sjogren syndrome but are also found in 20–40% of women with SLE and are associated with neonatal lupus syndrome.

A person is classified as having SLE, if any 4 of the 11 criteria are present (serially or simultaneously) during any interval of the evaluation:

1. Malar rash
2. Discoid rash
3. Photosensitivity
4. Oral ulcers
5. Arthritis
6. Serositis
7. Renal disorders such as proteinuria
8. Neurological disorders such as psychosis and seizures
9. Hematological disorders such as leukopenia and lymphopenia
10. Immunologic disorders—(a) anti-DNA antibody *or* (b) anti-Sm antibody
11. Antinuclear antibody.

Symptoms of flares include fatigue, fever, arthralgias/myalgias, weight loss, rash, renal deterioration, serositis, lymphadenopathy, and central nervous system symptoms. The main differential diagnosis for SLE is between other rheumatologic and connective tissue disorders. Many of the manifestations of SLE flare can be similar to preeclampsia (hypertension, proteinuria, and activation of the coagulation cascade) although the treatment for each is very different. The treatment for severe preeclampsia often involves delivery, while lupus flares can be treated and the pregnancy can be allowed to continue. A rising anti-dsDNA titer, active urinary sediment, and low complement levels (C3, C4, and CH50) suggest a lupus flare. Women with SLE are more prone to cardiovascular disease, thromboembolic phenomena, infection, and renal disease.

Systemic Lupus Erythematosus and Pregnancy

Effect of SLE on Pregnancy and Effect of Pregnancy on SLE

- Increased stillbirth rate worsening of renal status, if (25 times baseline) nephropathy present
- Increased risk of preeclampsia [higher rate (20–30%) if active at start of pregnancy]
- Increased growth restriction rate (12–32%)
- Increased preterm delivery rate (50–60%)
- Increased preterm premature rupture of membrane (PPROM) rate
- Neonatal lupus (1–2%, if SSA/SSB present)
- PPROM—preterm premature rupture of membranes

Consequently, the literature data for incidence of lupus flares range from 13 to 74%. It is generally believed that the risk for flare in pregnancy is increased, if women are not in remission prior to becoming pregnant. Lupus nephropathy is the end result of autoimmune-mediated inflammation and renal damage.

Stillbirth rates in women with SLE have been found to be 150 per 1,000 births, 25 times the national average. Much of the effect of SLE on fetal loss rates has been attributed to concomitant antiphospholipid antibody syndrome (APS). In women with stable lupus nephritis and plasma creatinine values <1.5 mg/dL, proteinuria <2 g/24 hours and no hypertension have lower risks of adverse pregnancy outcome. Preeclampsia occurs in 20–30% of women with SLE with higher rates seen in women with underlying hypertension, renal disease, or APS. IUGR has been reported in 12–32% of lupus pregnancies, which were found to be higher than control populations. Preterm birth is increased in SLE pregnancies, with rates as high as 50–60% resulting from preeclampsia, IUGR, abnormal fetal testing, and preterm premature rupture of membranes (PPROM).

Management during Pregnancy

Management of SLE during pregnancy begins with preconceptional counseling. At this time, maternal disease status can be assessed and risks of pregnancy discussed. Evaluation for any pre-existing renal disease is performed with a 24-hour urine collection and serum creatinine to measure proteinuria and creatinine clearance. Remission for 6 months prior to pregnancy reduces adverse outcomes. Early pregnancy assessment should include assessment of maternal disease status including 24-hour urine collection, plasma creatinine, complete blood count, anti-SSA/Ro antibody, anti-SSB/La antibody, anti-dsDNA antibody, lupus anticoagulant, anticardiolipin antibody, C3, and C4 levels. Repeat anti-dsDNA, 24-hour urine, plasma creatinine, C3, and C4 levels to monitor disease status should be performed each trimester. Lupus anticoagulant and anticardiolipin antibodies can be repeated in the second trimester to screen for development of APS. Early genetic risk assessment is important as lupus pregnancies carry increased maternal risk and early diagnosis of genetic abnormalities gives patients the option of termination of a nonviable pregnancy.

- *Glucocorticoids—safe*: Association with growth restriction at high dose, increased risk of preterm rupture of membranes, preterm delivery. Need stress-dose steroids at delivery or for medical illnesses, if chronic use through pregnancy.
- Hydroxychloroquine—generally considered safe: Antimalarial. Reduces disease flares.
- *Nonsteroidal anti-inflammatory agents*: Association with polyhydramnios, and ductus arteriosus closure. Avoid after 28 weeks.
- *Azathioprine*: Risk of fetal growth restriction and immunosuppression.
- *Cyclophosphamide—unsafe*: Skeletal and palate defects, also defects in eyes and limbs.
- *Methotrexate—unsafe*: Folic acid antagonist. Abortifacient and teratogen.

Flares can be managed conservatively with adjustment of medication regimen as outlined above or addition of analgesics such as acetaminophen. Glucocorticoid therapy can be initiated for more severe flares.

Antiphospholipid Antibodies

Antiphospholipid antibodies can be present alone or in conjunction with APS. APS has specific diagnostic criteria and results in thrombosis, adverse pregnancy outcome (including growth restriction and third trimester fetal death), or recurrent pregnancy loss. APS without treatment have shown fetal loss rates as high as 50–90%.

Clinical criteria:

- Vascular thrombosis
- Pregnancy morbidity:
  - Unexplained intrauterine fetal death (IUFD) at ≥10 weeks of a morphologically normal fetus
  - Severe preeclampsia/eclampsia or severe placental insufficiency before 34 weeks
  - Three or more unexplained spontaneous abortions at <10 weeks.

Laboratory criteria:

- Anticardiolipin antibody (IgG or IgM) at moderate or high titer, on two or more occasions at least 6 weeks apart
- Lupus anticoagulant present on two or more occasions at least 6 weeks apart.

Either unfractionated or low molecular weight heparin (LMWH) may be used (pregnancy class B). In severe APS or those who have been refractory to heparin therapy, intravenous immunoglobulin (IVIG) is used. Aspirin therapy can be initiated at the first positive pregnancy test and heparin therapy can be initiated at 5–7 weeks of gestation. As there is no maternal blood flow through the placenta prior to 5–7 weeks, heparin is not necessary before this point and may potentiate implantation bleeding. Heparin therapy can either be therapeutic (i.e., 1 mg/kg enoxaparin every 12 hours with maintenance of anti-Xa levels between 0.5 and 1.0) or prophylactic (i.e., 40 mg/day enoxaparin). A platelet count should be obtained within 2 weeks of initiation of therapy. Because of the 1–2% risk of osteoporosis and fracture with unfractionated heparin anticoagulation in pregnancy, we recommend daily calcium, vitamin D supplementation, and daily weight-bearing exercise as tolerated. At 36 weeks, aspirin can be discontinued and LMWH switched to unfractionated heparin to facilitate anticoagulation management at delivery. Postpartum anticoagulation (if indicated) can be with either warfarin or LMWH. Antepartum complications remain common with elevated rates of preeclampsia, growth restriction, and premature birth.

BIBLIOGRAPHY

1. Alter BP. Prenatal diagnosis of hematologic diseases: 1986 update. Acta Haematol. 1987;78:137-41.
2. Angastiniotic M, Modell B. Global epidemiology of hemoglobin disorders. Ann N Y Acad Sci. 1998;850:251-69.
3. Beicher SJ, Sullivan JB, Freinkel N. Carbohydrate metabolism in pregnancy. V. The interrelations of glucose, insulin and free fatty acids in late pregnancy and postpartum. N Engl J Med. 1964;271:866-72.
4. Charache S, Scott J, Niebyl J, Bonds D. Management of sickle cell disease in pregnant patients. Obstet Gynecol. 1980;55:407-10.
5. Cox JV, Steane E, Cunningham G, Frenkel EP. Risk of alloimmunization and delayed hemolytic transfusion reactions in patients with sickle cell disease. Arch Intern Med. 1988;148:2485-9.
6. Cunningham FG, Pritchard JA, Mason R. Pregnancy and sickle hemoglobinopathy: results with and without prophylactic transfusions. Obstet Gynecol. 1983;62:419-24.
7. Driscoll MC, Hurlet A, Styles L, McKie V, Files B, Olivieri N, et al. Stroke risk in siblings with sickle cell anemia. Blood. 2003;101(6):2401-4.
8. el-Shafei AM, Dhaliwal JK, Sandhu AK. Pregnancy in sickle cell disease in Bahrain. Br J Obstet Gynaecol. 1992;99:101-4.
9. Engelgau MM, Herman WH, Smith PJ, German RR, Aubert RE. The epidemiology of diabetes and pregnancy in the US, 1988. Diabetes Care. 1995;18(7):1029-33.
10. Felig P. Maternal and fetal fuel homeostasis in human pregnancy. Am J Clin Nutr. 1973;26(9):998-1005.
11. Fischer DA, Klein AH. Thyroid development and disorders of thyroid-function in the newborn. N Engl J Med. 1981;304(12):702-12.
12. Garratty G. Severe reactions associated with transfusion of patients with sickle cell disease. Transfusion. 1997;37:357-61.
13. Gladwin MT, Sachdev V, Jison ML, Shizukuda Y, Plehn JF, Minter K, et al. Pulmonary hypertension as a risk factor for death in patients with sickle cell disease. N Engl J Med. 2004;350:886-95.
14. Glinoer D. Pregnancy and iodine. Thyroid 2001;11(5):471-81.
15. Howard RJ, Tuck SM, Pearson TC. Pregnancy in sickle cell disease in the UK: results of a multi-centre survey of the effect of prophylactic blood transfusion on maternal and fetal outcome. Br J Obstet Gynaecol. 1995;102:947-51.
16. Jackson BR, Busch MP, Stramer SL, AuBuchon JP. The cost-effectiveness of NAT for HIV, HCV, and HBV in whole-blood donations. Transfusion. 2003;43:721-9.
17. Koshy M, Burd L, Wallace D, Moawad A, Baron J. Prophylactic red-cell transfusions in pregnant patients with sickle cell disease: a randomized cooperative study. N Engl J Med. 1988;319:1447-52.
18. Miller JM Jr, Horger EO 3rd, Key TC, Walker EM Jr. Management of sickle cell hemoglobinopathies in pregnant patients. Am J Obstet Gynecol. 1981;141:237-41.
19. Milner PF, Jones BR, Dobler J. Outcome of pregnancy in sickle cell anemia and sickle cell-hemoglobin C disease. Am J Obstet Gynecol. 1980;138:239-45.
20. Morrison JC, Schneider JM, Whybrew WD, Bucovaz ET, Menzel DM. Prophylactic transfusions in pregnant patients with sickle cell hemoglobinopathies: benefit versus risk. Obstet Gynecol. 1980;56:274-80.
21. Morrison JC, Wiser WL. The effect of maternal partial exchange transfusion on the infants

of patients with sickle cell anemia. J Pediatr. 1976;89:286-9.

22. Motulsky AG. Frequency of sickling disorders in US Blacks. N Engl J Med. 1973;288:31-3.
23. Poddar D, Maude GH, Plant MJ, Scorer H, Serjeant GR. Pregnancy in Jamaican women with homozygous sickle cell disease: fetal and maternal outcome. Br J Obstet Gynaecol. 1986;93:927-32.
24. Powars D, Weidman JA, Odom-Maryon T, Niland JC, Johnson C. Sickle cell chronic lung disease: prior morbidity and the risk of pulmonary failure. Medicine (Baltimore). 1988;67:66-76.
25. Powars DR, Sandhu M, Niland-Weiss J, Johnson C, Bruce S, Manning PR. Pregnancy in sickle cell disease. Obstet Gynecol. 1986;67:217-28.
26. Rees DC, Olujohungbe AD, Parker NE, Stephens AD, Telfer P, Wright J. Guidelines for the management of the acute painful crisis in sickle cell disease. British Committee for standards in Haematology General Haematology Task Force by the Sickle Cell Working Party.Br J Haematol. 2003;120:744-52.
27. Seoud MA, Cantwell C, Nobles G, Levy DL. Outcome of pregnancies complicated by sickle cell and sickle-C hemoglobinopathies. Am J Perinatol. 1994;11:187-91.
28. Serjeant GR, Loy LL, Crowhter M, Hambleton IR, Thame M. Outcome of pregnancy in homozygous sickle cell disease. Obstet Gynecol. 2004;103:1278-85.
29. Silliman CC, Boshkov LK, Mehdizadehkashi Z, Elzi DJ, Dickey WO, Podlosky L, et al. Transfusion related acute lung injury: epidemiology and a prospective analysis of etiologic factors. Blood. 2003;101:454-62.
30. Smith JA, Espeland M, Bellevue R, Bonds D, Brown AK, Koshy M. Pregnancy in sickle cell disease: experience of the cooperative study of sickle cell disease. Obstet Gynecol. 1996;87:199-204.
31. Sun PM, Wilburn W, Raynor BD, Jamieson D. Sickle cell disease in pregnancy: twenty years of experience at Grady Memorial Hospital, Atlanta, Georgia. Am J Obstet Gynecol. 2001;184:1127-30.
32. Vichinsky EP, Neumayr LD, Earles AN, Williams R, Lennette ET, Dean D, et al. Causes and outcomes of the acute chest syndrome in sickle cell disease. N Engl J Med. 2000;342:1855-65.
33. Weatherall DJ, Provan AB. Red cell I: Inherited anaemias. Lancet. 2000;355:1169-75.

11 CHAPTER

Fetal Thoracic Abnormalities

Khurshid Alam, Rafat Jamal

ANATOMY OF THORACIC CAGE

Stages of Human Lung Development (Fig. 1)

The fetal lung development and maturation occur in five stages—embryonic, pseudoglandular, canalicular, saccular, and alveolar **(Fig. 2)**. The timings of these stages are approximate and have significant overlapping with each other. For successful first neonatal breath, the fetal lungs undergo functional and structural maturation process.

Normal Sonographic Appearance of Fetal Thorax

The prenatal diagnosis of fetal abnormalities originating from the lung is dependent upon the sonographic appearance of intrathoracic space-occupying lesions **(Figs. 3A to D)**.

The fetal lungs are identified as homogeneously echogenic tissue surrounding the heart, separated by the hypoechoic, dome-shaped diaphragm from the abdominal organs. Lung echogenicity varies with gestational age, in general increasing echogenicity as lung development progresses **(Figs. 4A to D)**.

The fetal ribs are highly echogenic, curved bony structures arising near the spine and extending anteriorly to encompass more than half the thoracic circumference.

Fetal Lung Lesions

With development in both fetal ultrasonography and magnetic resonance

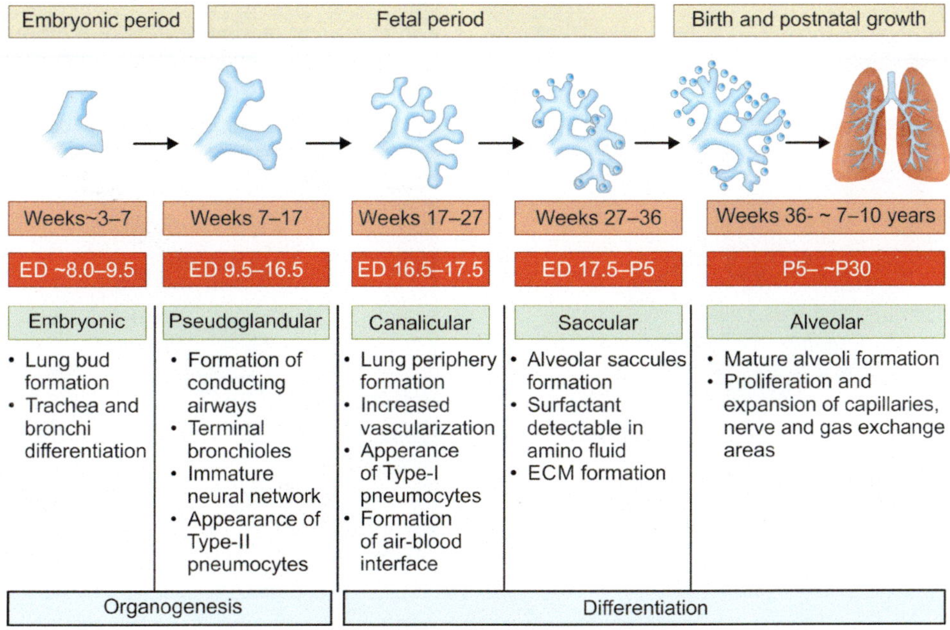

Fig. 1: Stages of human lung development. (ECM: extracellular matrix)

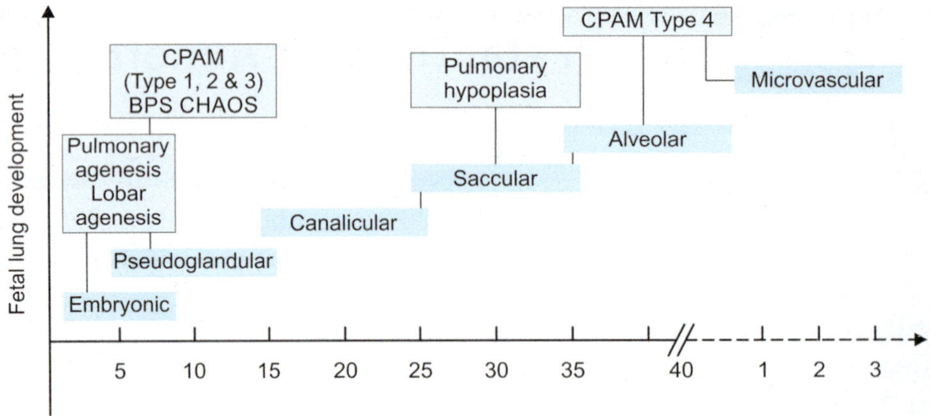

Fig. 2: Fetal lung development and maturation.
(CPAM: congenital pulmonary airway malformation; BPS: bronchopulmonary sequestration; CHAOS: congenital high airway obstruction syndrome)

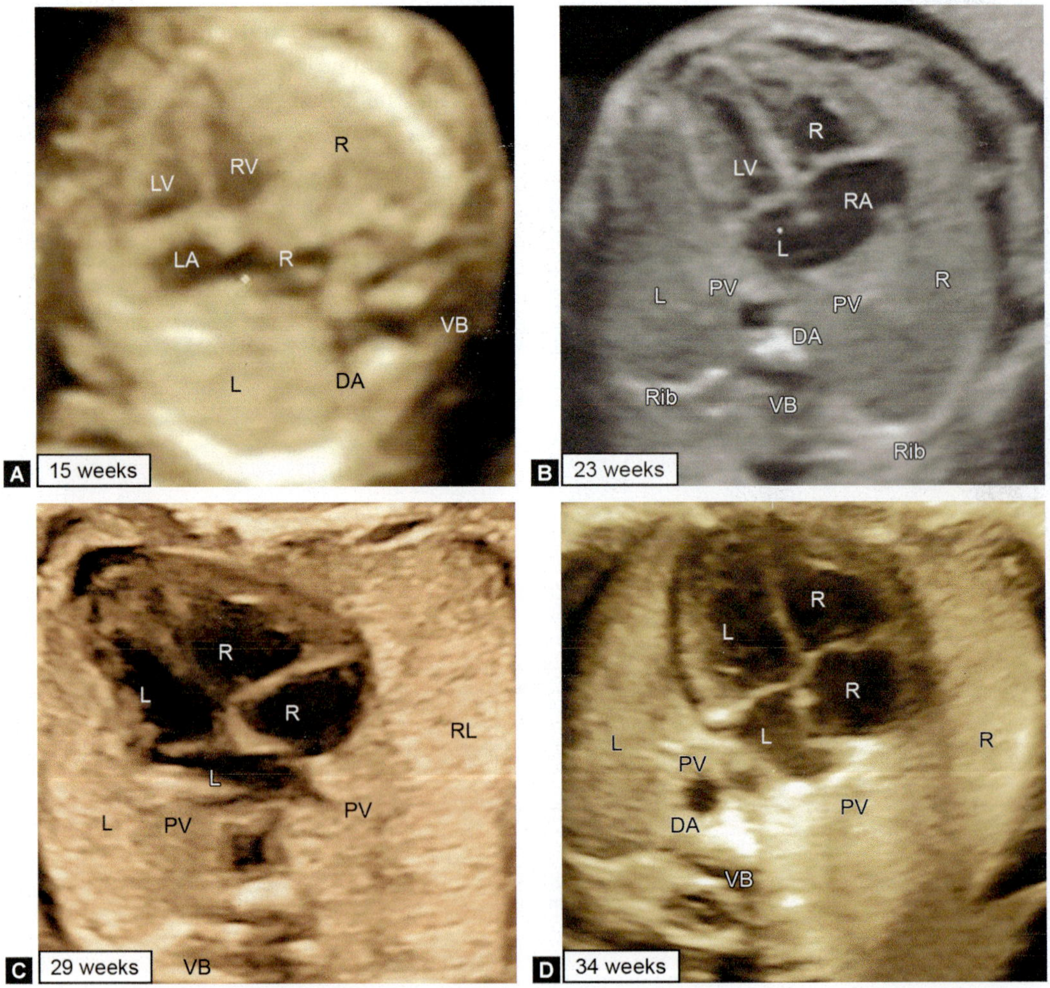

Figs. 3A to D: Sonographic appearance of intrathoracic space-occupying lesions.
(LL: left lung; RL: right lung; R: right; L: left; RA: right atrium; RV: right ventricle; LA: left atrium; LV: left ventricle; DA: descending aorta; PV: pulmonary vein; VB: vertebral body; IVC: inferior vena cava; SVC: superior vena cava)

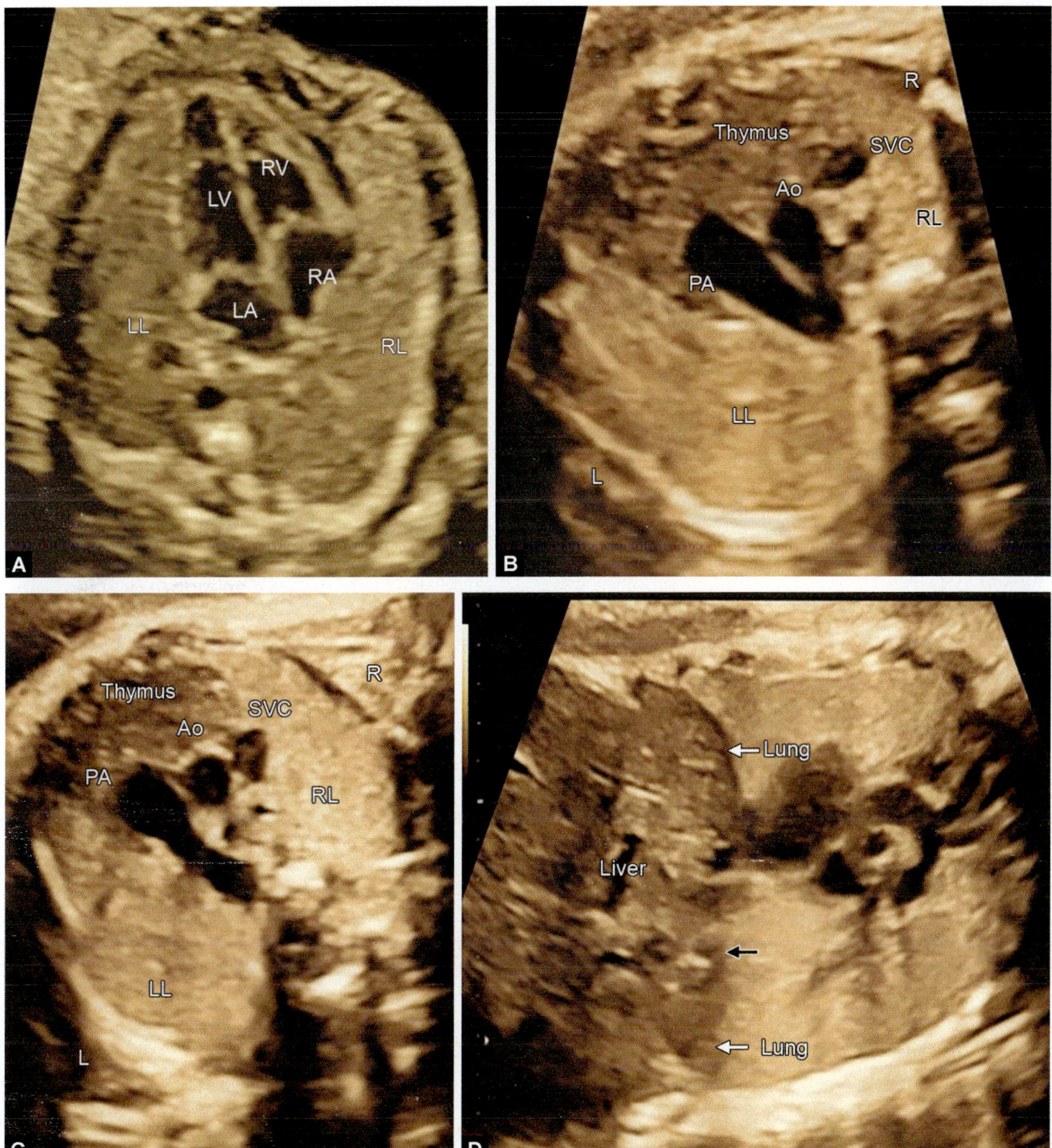

Figs. 4A to D: Different views of the fetal thorax: (A) Transverse view of the thorax in apical four-chamber view shows right lung (RL) and left lung (LL) on either side of the four-chamber heart; (B) Three-vessel trachea view shows confluence of transverse aortic arch and ductal arch to the left of the trachea, thymus is seen superiorly; (C) Three-vessel view shows pulmonary artery (PA), aorta (Ao), and superior vena cava (SVC) arranged from left (L) to right (R), thymus, and both lungs are also seen; (D) Left parasagittal view shows echogenic lungs separated from liver by diaphragm, black arrow showing diaphragm.
(LA: left atrium; RA: right atrium; LV: left ventricle; RV: right ventricle)

imaging, thoracic lesions are increasingly being identified antenatally, allowing obstetricians, radiologist, and pediatricians to—(a) anticipate management issues at the time of delivery or later in neonatal life, and (b) help parents comprehend the prognosis. Few indirect sonographic patterns, which indicate lung lesion, are **(Flowchart 1)**:

- Abnormal collection of fluid in or around lung

Flowchart 1: Classification of lung lesion.

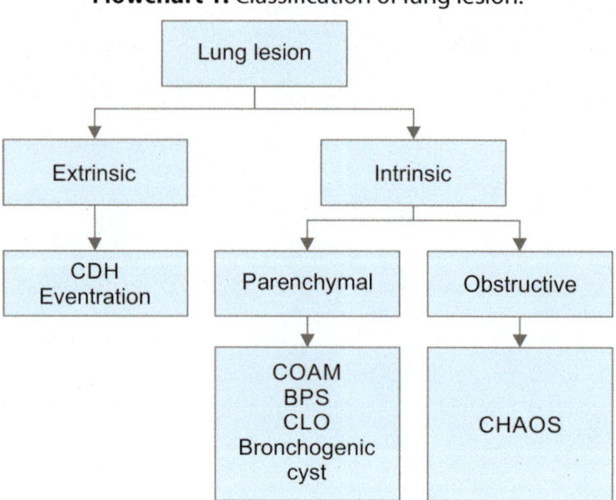

(CPAM: congenital pulmonary airway malformation; BPS: bronchopulmonary sequestration; CLO: congenital lobar overinflation; CHAOS: congenital high airway obstruction syndrome; CDH: congenital diaphragmatic hernia)

- Echogenic focus in lung
- Mediastinal shift of the heart.

The four-chamber view of the heart is an important landmark in the fetal chest and should be visualized in all fetuses during the 2nd and 3rd trimester as part of routine obstetric imaging. Few extracardiac signs, which prompt for detailed sonographic evaluation of lungs, include volume changes in amniotic fluid; doubtful fetal malformation or hydrops.

The current section is aimed at exploration of few fetal thoracic lesions, which are identifiable in antenatal period, their management (antenatal and intrapartum), and prognosis. The correct identification of these conditions not only gives us an opportunity to intervene in antenatal period itself but also provides us with opportunity to prepare and plan for postnatal management.

BRONCHOPULMONARY SEQUESTRATION

Bronchopulmonary sequestration (BPS) is an anomaly in which nonfunctioning pulmonary tissue is not in normal continuity with the native tracheobronchial tree and has a blood supply from the systemic circulation

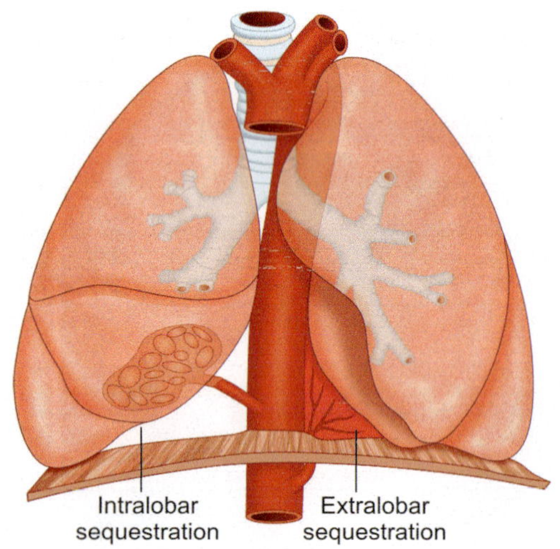

Fig. 5: Bronchopulmonary sequestration (BPS).

(Fig. 5). Sequestrations account for up to 6% of congenital lung malformations.

Etiopathogenesis

The etiology is unknown. Due to frequent occurrence of congenital pulmonary airway malformation (CPAM) in association with BPS, they might share the same pathogenesis.

There are two main types of sequestration—intralobar and extralobar. It is not possible to

TABLE 1: Difference between intralobar and extralobar sequestration.

	Intralobar sequestration	***Extralobar sequestration***
Incidence	75% (postnatal series)	25% (postnatal series)
Pleura	Shares the visceral pleura	Supernumerary lung bud invested by its own pleura
Location	Lower lobes and slightly more often on the left	Left posterior costodiaphragmatic sulcus between the lower lobe and the hemidiaphragm (80%); below the diaphragm in suprarenal locations in 10–15% of cases
Blood supply	Systemic arterial supply within the normal lung	Splanchnic vessels surrounding the foregut
Venous drainage	Pulmonary veins although connect to the vena cava, azygous vein, or right atrium	Systemic venous drainage into the azygous, hemiazygos, and/or the vena cava system
Prognosis	Relatively good	Relatively poor

differentiate intralobar BPS from extralobar BPS in prenatal life **(Table 1)**.

Other types are:

- Hybrid CPAM and BPS lesion (having connection with both the pulmonary and the systemic arterial supply)
- Bronchopulmonary foregut malformation [sequestrated lung tissue is connected with gastrointestinal tract (GIT)]

Genetics

The risk of associated chromosomal anomalies and nonchromosomal syndromes is very low. Microarray is recommended prior to initiating fetal therapy or if associated with additional anomalies or non-immune hydrops.

Counseling session should include—possible course of the BPS during pregnancy (decrease/increase in size, potential for hydrops), options for prenatal intervention (e.g., thoracoamniotic shunt, laser ablation), and postnatal issues (clinical manifestations, postnatal evaluation, postnatal management, potential complications, prognosis of associated anomalies, and range of outcomes).

Imaging

Typically, a sequestration appears as a well-defined, homogeneous, echogenic wedge-shaped pulmonary mass in the lower lobe adjacent to the hemidiaphragm **(Figs. 6A to F)**. Sequestration can be distinguished from other congenital lung masses by identifying on Doppler systemic arterial supply.

Checklist (prenatal ultrasound) for imaging:

- Size and location of the BPS
- Assess caudal extension of the lesion
- Detection and characterization of subdiaphragmatic extralobar sequestration
- Sliding sign—unique feature of extralobar BPS (nonsynchronized movement of the echogenic mass with respect to adjacent organs on respiration or forced excursion)
- Recognition of the feeding artery branching off the descending aorta
- Detect possible association such as ipsilateral hydrothorax, frank hydrops, or other thoracic malformations.

Differential Diagnosis

- Congenital pulmonary airway malformation
- Congenital lobar emphysema
- Congenital diaphragmatic hernia
- Neuroblastoma (late onset, poorly defined margin, complex echogenic mass with cysts, and/or calcification, avid vascularity on color Doppler)

- Adrenal hemorrhage (echotexture changes longitudinally over the period of time).

Magnetic resonance imaging (MRI) can help to confirm the diagnosis and location of the mass (above, within, or below the diaphragm).

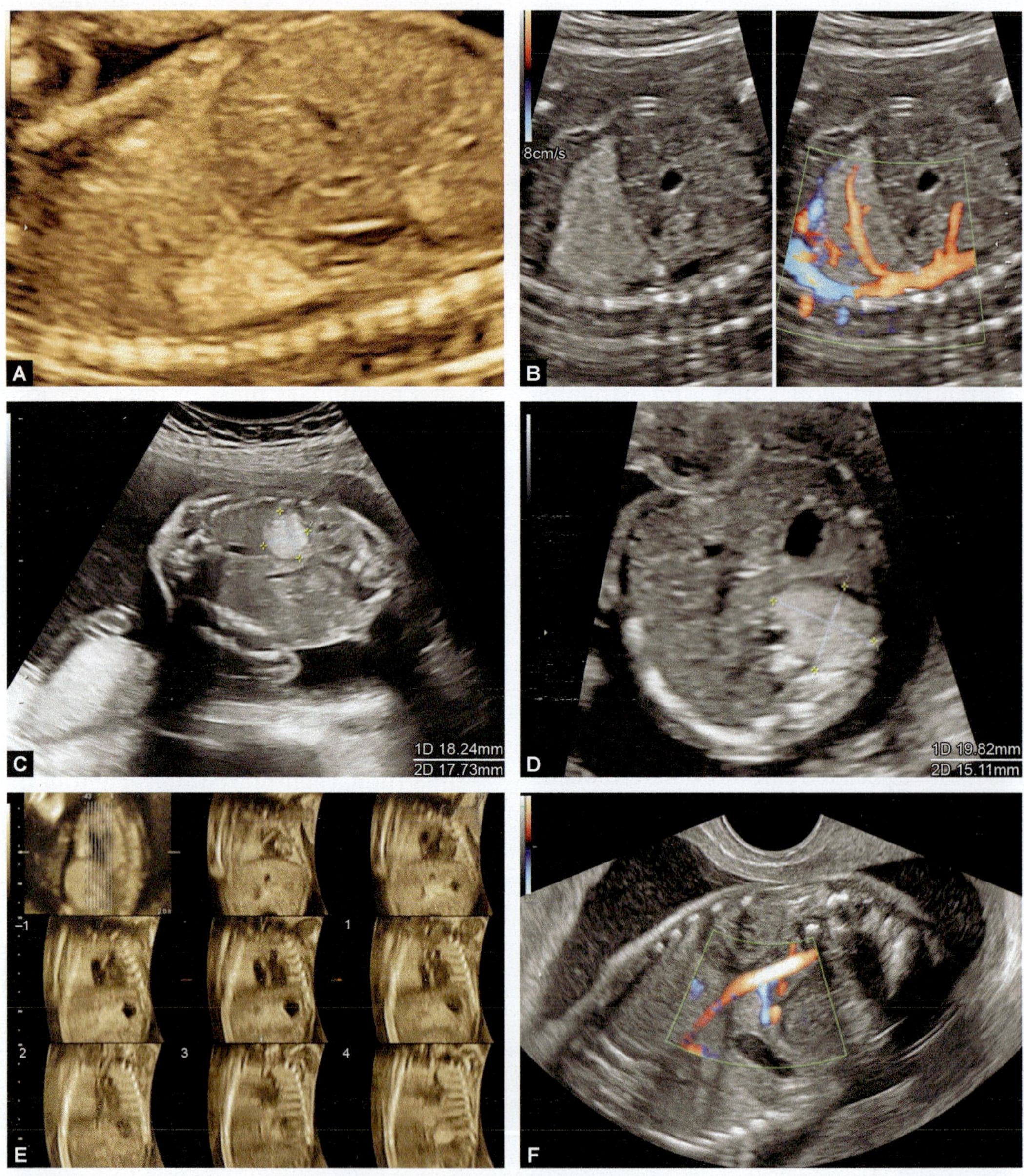

Figs. 6A to F: (A) Parasagittal view of the thorax shows wedge-shaped echogenic mass in relation to right costodiaphragmatic sulcus/posterobasal segment; (B) On color Doppler, the echogenic lung lesion shows vascular feeder arising directly from aorta (systemic arterial supply); (C and D) Coronal and axial view of the abdomen shows well-circumscribed echogenic mass in relation to left adrenal region; (E) Multiplanar tomographic ultrasound imaging (TUI) reconstruction demonstrates the infradiaphragmatic echogenic lesion in left suprarenal region; (F) Color Doppler demonstrates systemic arterial supply (extrathoracic intraabdominal extralobar bronchopulmonary sequestration (BPS).

The mass is high signal on T2-weighted images. A feeding vessel may be noted as a low-signal line coursing from the aorta to the mass.

Natural History of the Disease

In 30% of cases, there is a tendency to regress and even disappear during the 3rd trimester as reported in some case series. The apparent resolution has been attributed to decompression into the normal lung, outgrowth of the systemic circulation, or torsion around vascular pedicle.

Hence, the possibility of spontaneous regression and a good outcome even in cases complicated by hydrops (after placement of thoracoamniotic shunt) should be communicated to parents during prenatal counseling.

Prognosis

Small sequestrations with minimal mediastinal shift have a benign clinical course.

Large sequestrations can be complicated by pleural effusions and with hydrops, these can lead to increased prenatal mortality. Hydrops is rare but can occur secondary to shunting of the systemic arterial feeder or mass effect from the sequestration itself with associated mediastinal shift and compression of the heart or inferior vena cava. Compression of esophagus may lead to polyhydramnios.

Like prognostication of CPAM, CPAM volume ratio (CVR) can be used in pulmonary sequestration as well. CVR is obtained by multiplying height, length, and width of the lung lesion and dividing by the head circumference. A CVR >1.6 is associated with a higher risk for development of hydrops but has poor predictive value; hence, it can be used only as a proxy to triage high-risk fetuses who need close follow-up (Zhang H, et al., Pediatr Surg Int. 2014;30:47).

Prognosis is excellent in the absence of hydrops. Mortality rate is as high as 80%, if hydrops is present. Masses that appear to resolve in utero are typically still present on postnatal CT scans.

Management

Fetal intervention is needed in cases with hydrops or pleural effusion. Thoracoamniotic shunting for coexisting pleural effusion, interstitial laser of systemic feeder vessel supplying BPS. In absence of pleural effusion, the likelihood of spontaneous regression of BPS is high. In cases of massive pleural effusion, treatment with interstitial laser ablation of the feeding vessel seems to be more effective than pleuroamniotic shunting, with fewer complications. It might also reduce the need for postnatal surgery (Mallamann MR et al., UOG. 2014). There is progressive decrease in CVR and increment in size of both lungs after full laser ablation of feeding artery (Martinez et al., 2017).

Delivery planning should include input from the neonatologist and pediatric surgeon. If hydrops develops after 32 weeks of gestation, early delivery is recommended, possibly with use of the EXIT procedure.

In cases of hybrid lesion, course of antenatal betamethasone (two doses of 12 mg intramuscularly 24 hours apart) and cyst drainage are options, as with CPAM.

Postdelivery, all babies should undergo chest radiography or preferably computed tomography (CT) of the chest along with CT angiography (CTA) to trace the vascular feeder. Surgical or endoscopic removal of mass or selective embolization of feeding vessel under catheterization is the method available for postnatal management of lesion. Long-term outcome depends on the degree of pulmonary hypoplasia.

CONGENITAL PULMONARY AIRWAY MALFORMATION

Congenital pulmonary airway malformation is a congenital hamartomatous lung lesion that communicates with the bronchial

TABLE 2: Revised histopathological classification of postnatal congenital pulmonary airway malformation (CPAM) (Stockers, et al., 2002).

Types	*Percentage*	*Location in the airways*	*Description*	*Prognosis*	*Comments*
Type 0	1–3%	From trachea/ bronchi and involves the entire lung	Solid, lungs are small and firm	Incompatible with life	
Type 1	60–70%	From distal bronchi or proximal bronchioles	*One large cyst* 2–10 cm, may present late	Most common—*good* prognosis	Rarely associated with malignancy BAC
Type 2	15–20%	Bronchiolar	*Multiple small cysts* 0.5–2 cm Neonatal period	*Poor*	Associated with other anomalies
Type 3	5–10%	Alveolar	*Solid appearance*—small cystic area with solid tissue	Respiratory distress in newborn/death	*Life threatening*
Type 4	10–15%	Acinar	Thin-walled large/ air-filled cysts up to 10 cm	*Good*	*Associated with pneumothorax*

Note: Earlier terminology congenital cystic adenomatoid malformation (CCAM) is replaced by CPAM because only 3 out of 5 lesions are cystic and 1 lesion is adenomatoid.

tree through an abnormal communication and has normal pulmonary blood supply and venous drainage into the pulmonary veins.

Congenital pulmonary airway malformation accounts for about 25% of congenital lung masses, with an incidence of 1 in 8,300–35,000 live births. It is comprised of pulmonary tissue with abnormal bronchial proliferation that may involve either lung or any lobe. In 85–95% of cases, CPAM is limited to one lobe or segment.

Pathogenesis

- It is hamartomatous proliferation of abnormal bronchioles at the expense of normal alveolar development.
- It communicates with the proximal airways, albeit via a minute tortuous passage.
- Most derive blood supply from the pulmonary circulation

Classification

There are different classification schemes for CPAMs depending on histology or on prenatal sonographic appearance **(Tables 2 and 3, and Figs. 7 and 8)**.

Prenatal sonographic classification system: The three main types are shown in **Figures 7A to C**.

Congenital pulmonary airway malformation may appear as a solid echogenic lung mass (microcystic) or as a mixed, cystic, and solid mass. Color Doppler ultrasound may demonstrate vascular flow to the lesion from branches of the pulmonary artery. The lesions with microcysts appear solid and echogenic, whereas the macrocystic CPAMs have demonstrable cysts. Occasionally, only a single large cyst is visualized.

TABLE 3: Prenatal classification of congenital pulmonary airway malformation (CPAM) (Wilson, et al.).

Microcystic	*Macrocystic*
Less than 5 mm diameter cyst	More than 5 mm diameter cyst
Appears as solid hyperechogenic mass	Seen on USG as cysts of variable sizes

(USG: ultrasonography)

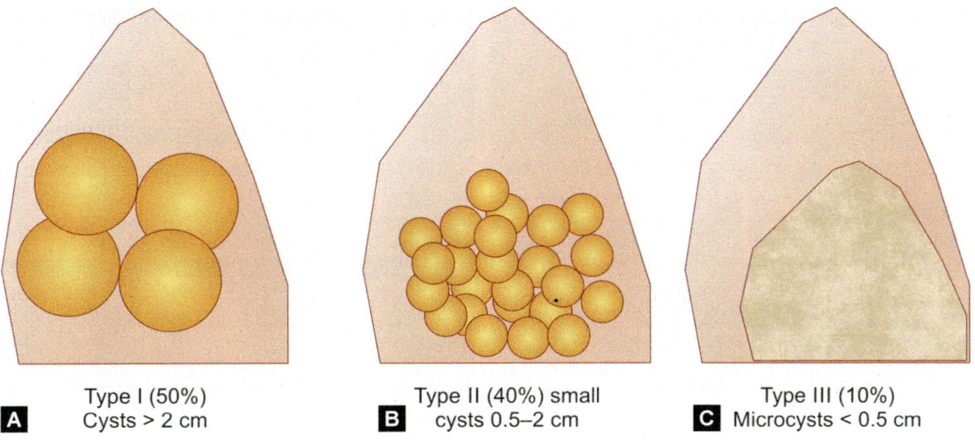

Figs. 7A to C: Prenatal sonographic classification system.

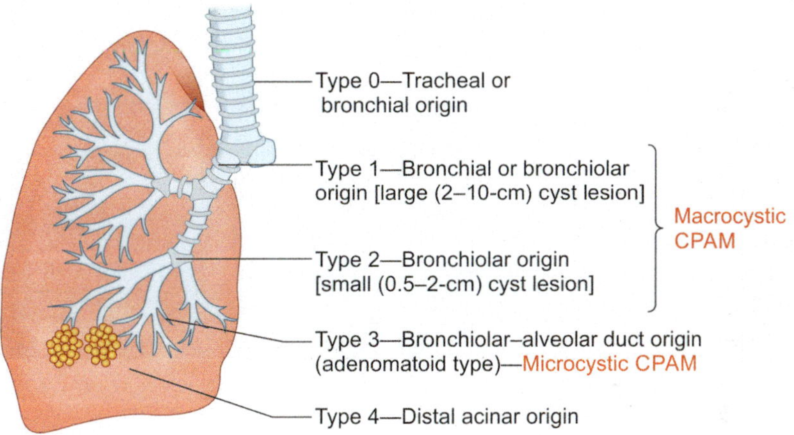

Fig. 8: Microcystic and macrocystic congenital pulmonary airway malformation (CPAM).

Typically, there is no systemic feeding vessel. However, in hybrids, a CPAM can occur in concert with sequestration.

Imaging (Prenatal Ultrasound) Checklist (Figs. 9A to G)

- Size and location of the CPAM
- Size of the cysts within the lesion
- Color flow Doppler to demonstrate or exclude systemic blood supply
- Evidence of mediastinal shift
- Subtle signs of hydrops
- Fetal ECHO—increased incidence of cardiac anomalies, especially truncus and tetralogy of Fallot (TOF).

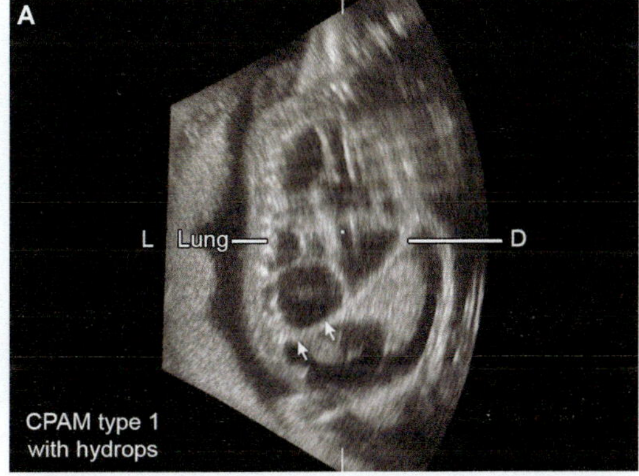

Fig. 9A: Coronal section of the fetal thorax demonstrating multiple medium to large size confluent cysts with mass effect on the mediastinum, inversion of the diaphragm, mild ascites, and pleural effusion (type 1 CPAM with hydrops).
(CPAM: congenital pulmonary airway malformation)

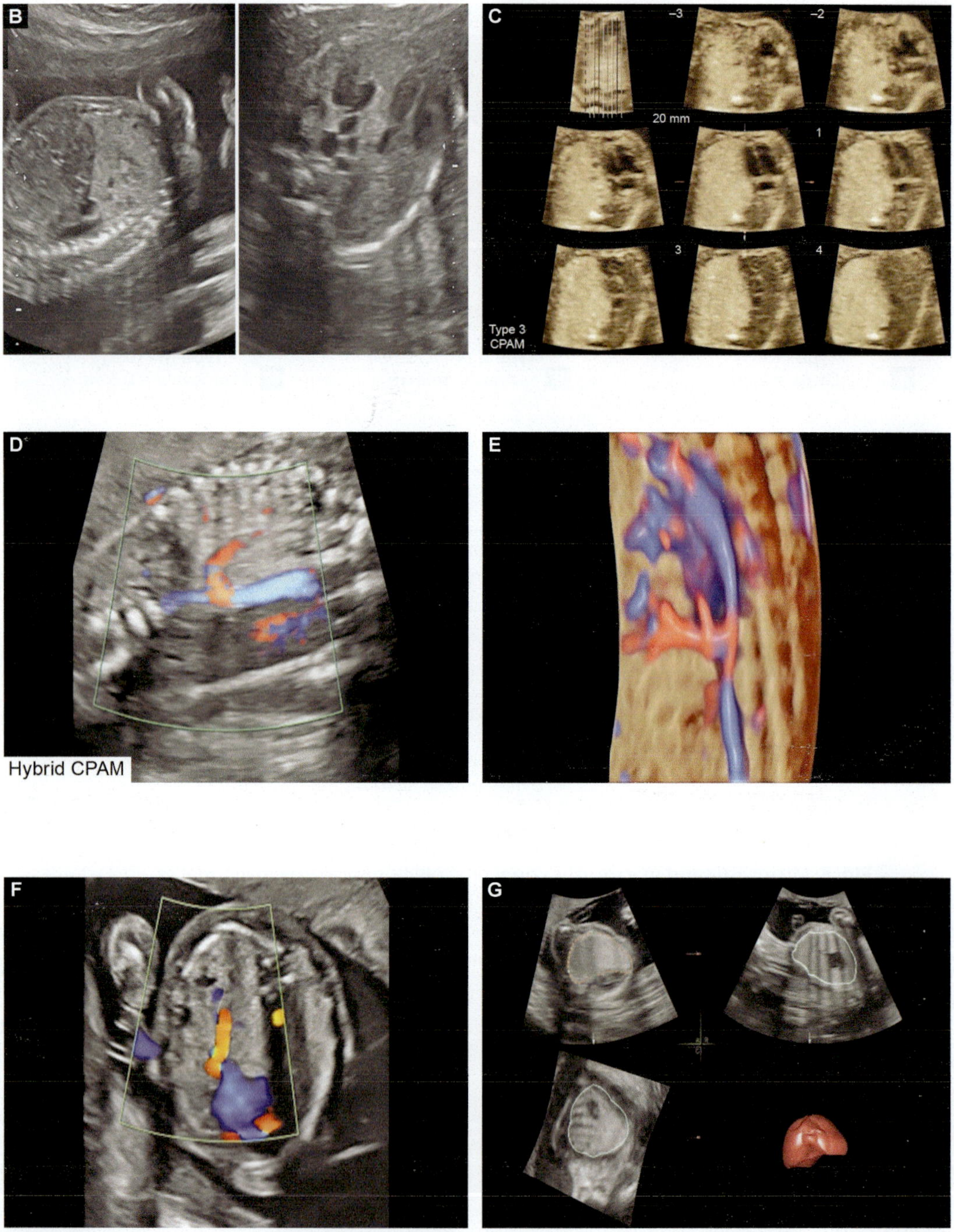

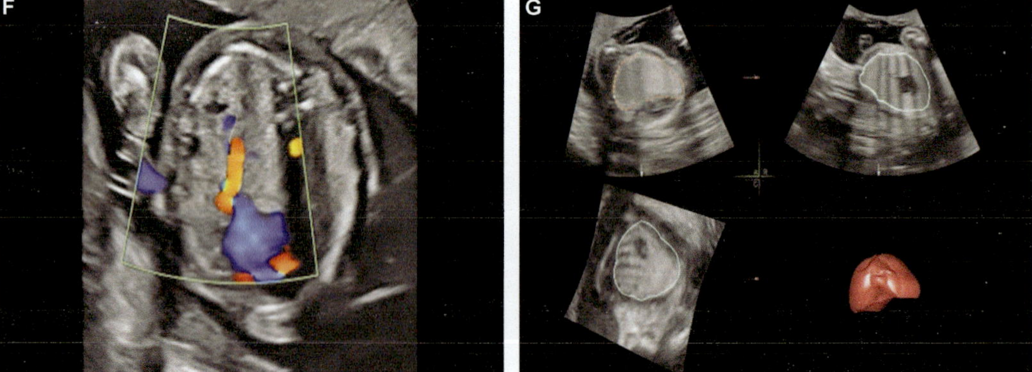

Figs. 9B to G: (B) Right parasagittal and axial view at 24 weeks shows echogenic lung lesion with multiple small-sized cysts and mediastinal shift; (C) TUI of fetal thorax at 25 weeks shows large well-defined echogenic lung lesion on right side with contralateral cardiomediastinal displacement (type 3 CPAM); (D and E) Coronal view demonstrating echogenic lung lesion with systemic arterial supply and 3D power Doppler angiography demonstrating feeder vessel originating from aorta (hybrid CPAM); (F) Color Doppler of the thorax showing echogenic lung lesion fed by branch pulmonary artery; (G) Volume of the CPAM calculated by 3D VOCAL technique.

(CPAM: congenital pulmonary airway malformation; TUI: tomographic ultrasound imaging)

Role of MRI

MRI has become a useful adjunct in the evaluation and management of CPAM to better delineate abnormal and normal anatomy when the entire lung is involved by the mass, in the presence of hydrops or bilateral lesions, and when the diagnosis is uncertain (Hubbard AM et al., Radiology. 1999).

At fetal MR imaging, large cyst CPAMs manifest as hyperintense unilocular or multilocular lesions with discrete walls on T2-weighted images.

Genetics of CPAM

It does not increase the baseline risk for aneuploidy and almost always is a sporadic developmental disorder.

Counseling session should include possible course of the CPAM during pregnancy, options for prenatal intervention, differential diagnosis of prenatally suspected CPAM, postnatal follow-up, and management options.

Natural History of CPAM

Longitudinal studies of fetal CPAM have reported that most have rapid progressive growth within 20–26 weeks of gestation approximately, peaking at 25 weeks and then growth plateaus by 26–28 weeks often followed by regression (Kunisaki SM et al., J Pediatr Surg. 2007).

As masses decrease in size, their echogenicity can become similar to that of surrounding normal lung because of an increase in normal lung echogenicity and decrease in echogenicity of the CPAM. Thus, they may become difficult to visualize late in gestation, with residual mass effect being the main finding on ultrasound.

Prognosis

- Macrocystic lesions usually have a more favorable prognosis.
- *Mediastinal shift*: Large CPAMs can result in cardiac and vena cava compression, leading to altered hemodynamics and hydrops as a result of elevated central venous pressure.
- *Hydrops*: It is single best predictor of poor outcome/impending fetal demise, which in turn depends on volume rather than size. In the absence of hydrops, the prognosis is good, with reported live birth rates of 95% and higher.
- *Polyhydramnios* may develop due to compression on esophagus.

Quantitative assessment: There are various quantitative methods such as mass-to-thorax ratio (MTR), fetal MRI-derived lung mass volume ratio (LMVR), lesion-to-lung volume ratio (LLV); however, the most popular, reproducible, and robust method of choice is CPAM volume ratio (CVR) for prognostication.

It is the size of the CPAM rather than the size of the cysts that determines whether or not the fetus develops *hydrops*.

- The CPAM volume ratio (CVR), a measurement initially described by ultrasound, should be measured to assess prognosis and risk of hydrops.

  CVR = Volume of lung mass divided by head circumference

  Volume of lung mass = (Height × Anteroposterior diameter × Transverse diameter) of lung mass × 0.52

A CVR < 1.6 indicates 14% risk of developing hydrops for fetuses with macrocystic lesions and 3% for those with microcystic lesions. If the CVR > 1.6, the risk is increased. Close surveillance of the growth of these lesions is recommended throughout the second trimester particularly if the CVR is higher than 1.6 (Crombleholme TM et al., J Pediatr Surg. 2002).

The CPAM volume ratio may help to predict the risk of neonatal respiratory problems **(Figs. 10A and B)**.

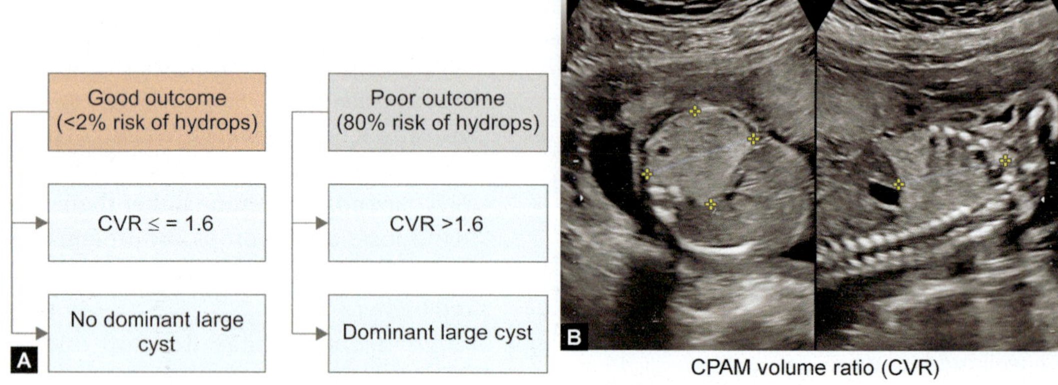

Figs. 10A and B: The CPAM volume ratio (CVR) and its outcomes.
(CPAM: congenital pulmonary airway malformation)

Work-up

- Appropriate counseling
- *Karyotyping/chromosomal microarray (KT/CMA)*:
  - Chromosomal anomaly is < 1%
  - May be offered in cases where fetal therapy is planned
- *Prenatal consultation*: Pediatric surgeon, neonatologist, and pediatric cardiologist
- *Associated life-threatening anomalies*: The family may choose not to continue the pregnancy.
- Maternal "mirror syndrome" warrants immediate delivery.

Differential Diagnosis

- Bronchopulmonary sequestration (BPS)
- Congenital lobar emphysema (CLO)
- Bronchogenic cyst
- Congenital diaphragmatic hernia (CDH)
- Laryngeal or tracheal occlusion
- Neuroenteric/enteric cysts
- Mediastinal teratomas.

Follow-up and Management

- *Careful serial antenatal observation*: Actual frequency will depend on CVR and associated sequelae
  - CVR > 1.6 (2–3 times/week), CVR 1.2–1.6 (twice/week), CVR <1.2 (weekly), CVR <0.9 (monthly follow-up)
  - CVR may predict the risk of neonatal respiratory problems. In a retrospective study, a final CVR > 1.0 in nonhydropic fetuses was predictive of respiratory symptoms at birth and perinatal resection (Zamora IJ et al., J Pediatr Surg. 2014).
- Initial surveillance for 3 weeks or till 28 weeks of gestation
- Monitor the progression of volume/development of hydropic changes
- Monitor the liquor volume, cardiac function, mediastinal shift, placental thickness, and ductus venosus (DV) Doppler.
- Associated anomalies, most often renal, intestinal, and cardiac, are present in up to 26% of cases, more frequently when CPAM is bilateral. Therefore, a complete fetal anatomic survey is indicated.

Fetal Intervention (Flowchart 2 and Fig. 11)

Steroids have been used in an attempt to prevent the development of hydrops or help to speed the regression of the lesion, particularly with microcystic CPAM. It is the only medical fetal intervention. With macrocystic CPAM, steroid therapy appears to be less helpful.

Course of antenatal betamethasone (two doses of 12 mg intramuscularly 24 hours apart) and cyst drainage are options. One or two additional doses of steroids may be

Flowchart 2: Algorithm for antenatal management in a prenatally suspected congenital pulmonary airway malformation (CPAM).

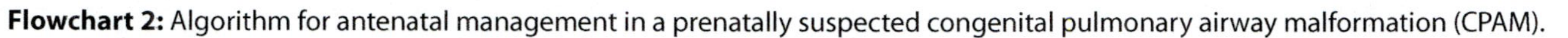

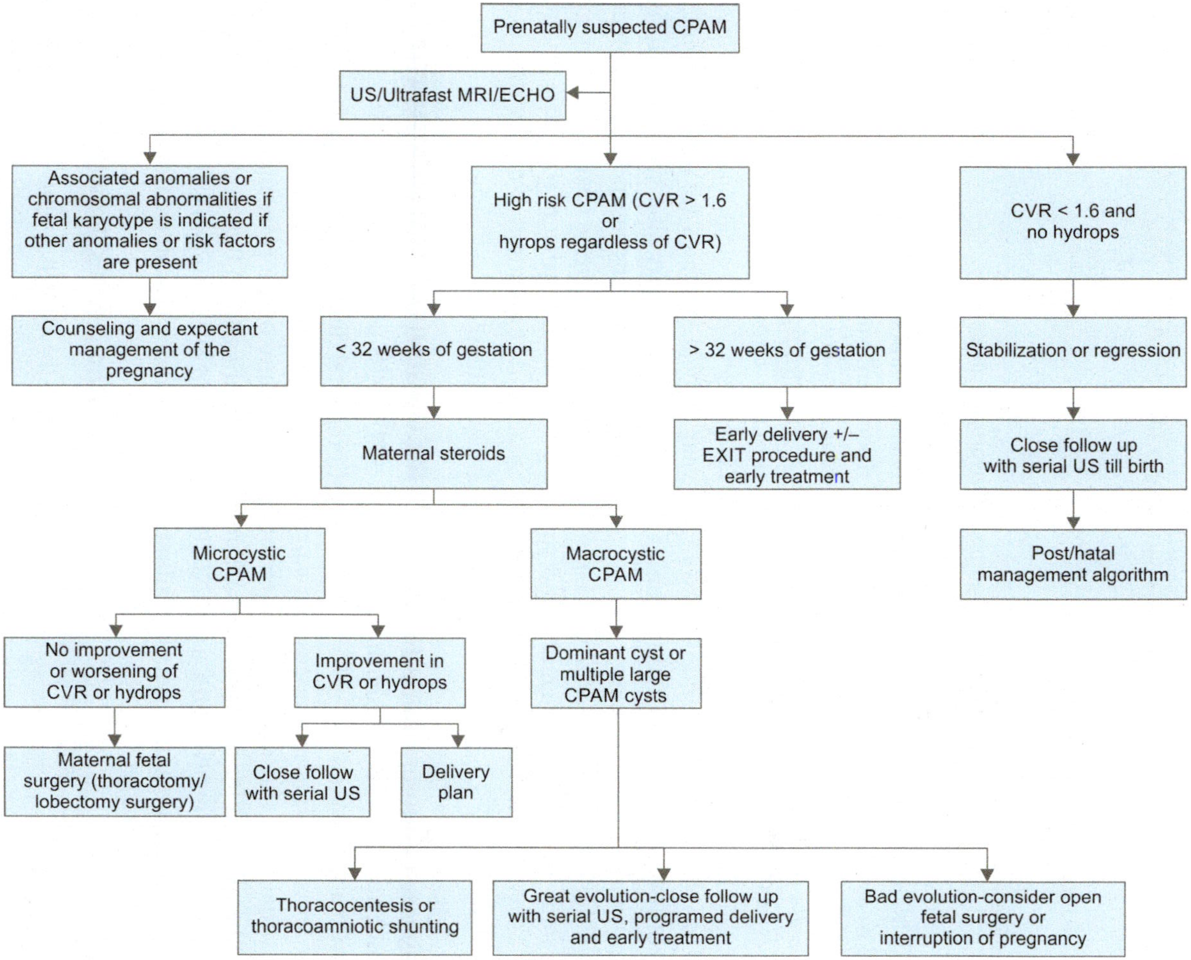

(CVR: CPAM volume ratio)

Source: David M, et al., Neonatology. 2016.

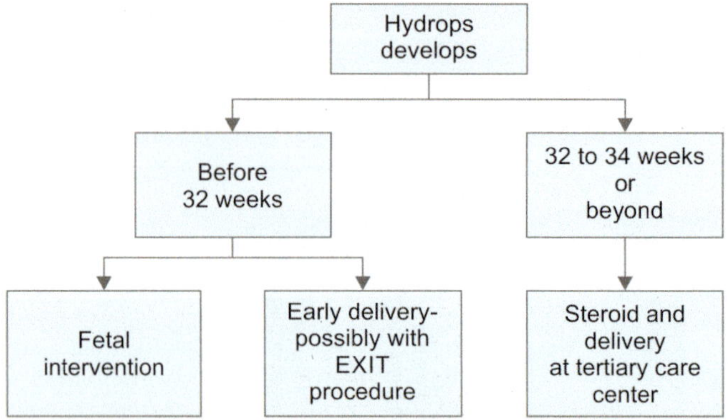

Fig. 11: Management of hydrops in pregnancy.

administered at least 1 week after previous steroid treatment in case of persistently high CVR, lesion growth, or persistent hydrops.

- *Invasive fetal intervention*:
  - CPAMs with a large, dominant cyst respond favorably to the placement of a *thoracoamniotic shunt* → Average of 70% reduction in CPAM volume → Overall 74% survival rate
  - Simple thoracocentesis/cyst aspiration—ineffective as a definitive therapy, as cyst fluid will usually rapidly reaccumulate to 75%
  - Surgical resection.

Delivery planning should be made in conjunction with the neonatology and/or pediatric surgery teams.

For fetuses with large masses that cause mediastinal shift and/or hydrops, delivery should be planned for a tertiary care center with neonatal intensive care unit (NICU) capable of providing extracorporeal membrane oxygenation (ECMO).

Postnatal Follow-up (Flowchart 3)

- Chest X-ray
- Computed tomography (CT) of chest

In asymptomatic neonates, the lesion may not be seen on chest radiography after birth. In these cases, postnatal CT/MRI is recommended. Postnatal removal of asymptomatic masses is recommended because of potential secondary infection, and risk of carcinomas arising in CPAM. (Ruano R et al., Prenat Diagn. 2012)

The timing of surgical resection of CPAM remains controversial, but most centers favor elective surgical resection in the 1st year of life. Outcomes are worse for patients undergoing surgery after symptoms develop compared with those undergoing elective surgery. Most experts also agree that some patients can be observed, if the lesion is small and the patient remains completely asymptomatic.

CONGENITAL DIAPHRAGMATIC HERNIA

Congenital diaphragmatic hernia (CDH) is a defect in closure of the diaphragm resulting from failure of the pleuroperitoneal canal to close (during 4th to 10th week postfertilization) at the end of organogenesis. The incidence of CDH is about 1 in 3,000 births **(Fig. 12)**.

Etiopathogenesis (Flowchart 4)

There is no known definite etiology. "Dual-hit" hypothesis suggests that the defect arises in the embryologic period (first hit), and during further gestation, lung development is impaired (second hit). Genetic and/or environmental factors may disrupt the differentiation of mesenchymal cell during formation of diaphragm.

Flowchart 3: Algorithm for postnatal management of a prenatally diagnosed case of congenital pulmonary airway malformation (CPAM).

Prenatal diagnosis of CPAM

Asymptomatic

Simple chest radiograph at birth

Low risk, defined as:
1. Small or no lesion
2. No PPB risk factors

Advanced thoracic imaging within 6 months#

Confirms low risk:
1. Small or no lesion
2. No PPB risk factors
3. Patient remains completely asymptomatic

Observation:
1. Monitor for symptoms
2. Annual imaging

Early surgical resection by 12 months

Any symptoms or high-risk characteristics

Early surgical resection

High risk, defined as:
1. Large lesion (> 20% of the hemithorax) or
2. PPB risk factors

Immediate advanced thoracic imaging#

Symptomatic*

Immediate advanced thoracic imaging#

Early surgical resection (during index hospitalization)

*Symptoms may consist of respiratory distress, tachypnea, and/or failure to thrive.

#Either CT or MRI may be used for advanced thoracic imaging. PPB risk factors include bilateral or multifocal cysts, pneumothorax, or family history of PPB-associated conditions, including lung cysts, spontaneous pneumothorax, and several specific childhood cancers or dysplasias.

(PPB: pleuropulmonary blastoma)

Source: David M, et al. Neonatology, 2016.

Flowchart 4: Etiopathogenesis of congenital diaphragmatic hernia.

Mass effect (Lungs)

↓

Compression of developing lung

↓

Reduction in bronchiolar branching | Changes in pulmonary vascular bed | Loss of pulmonary mass | Surfactant system dysfunction

The defect in the diaphragm allows herniation of viscera into the chest with increase in intra-abdominal pressure. Mass effect from visceral organs in the chest has an adverse impact on the normal development of the fetal cardiac and pulmonary systems. Thus, CDH is associated with substantial morbidity and mortality.

Congenital diaphragmatic hernias can be classified based on location; types include:

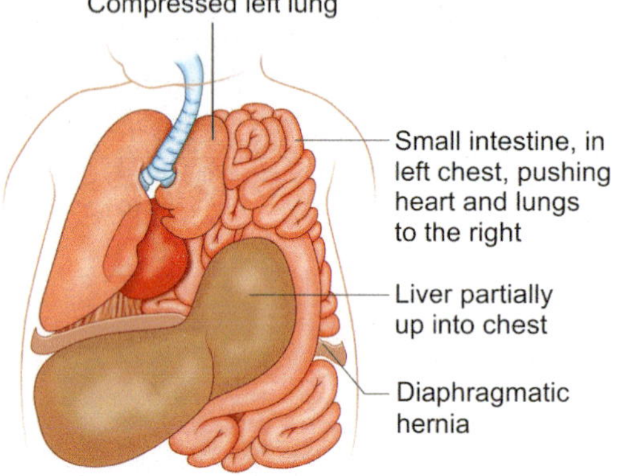

Fig. 12: Congenital diaphragmatic hernia.

- Posterolateral Bochdalek hernia (70–75%)
- Anterior Morgagni hernia (23–28%)
- Central defects (2–7%)
- Most CDHs (85–90%) are left sided, 10–15% are right sided, and only 2% are bilateral.

Genetics

Majority of CDH reported occur sporadically. In more than 30–50% of the cases, there is associated anomalies, which may be syndromic, chromosomal, single gene disorder, or major structural abnormalities **(Fig. 13; Table 4)**.

Fryns syndrome is autosomal recessive with facial dysmorphism, short limbs, diaphragmatic hernia, and CNS anomalies.

Nonsyndromic, non-chromosomal associations: In many cases, CDH is seen in association with abnormalities of other systems:

- *Cardiovascular system*: Septal defect, conotruncal anomalies
- *Central nervous system*: Neural tube defects, ventriculomegaly

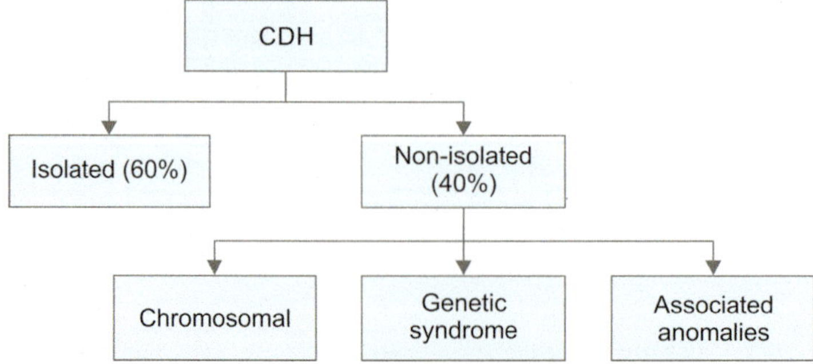

Fig. 13: Genetics of congenital diaphragmatic hernia.

TABLE 4: Chromosomal and syndromic abnormalities.

Chromosomal abnormalities	***Syndromic abnormalities***
Trisomy 18 (Edwards syndrome)	Denys–Drash syndrome
Tetrasomy 12p (Pallister–Killian syndrome)	Donnai–Barrow syndrome
Trisomy 21 (Down syndrome)	Fryns syndrome
Deletion 4p (Wolf–Hirschhorn syndrome)	Jarcho–Levin syndrome
Deletion 15q	Simpson–Golabi–Bechtel syndrome Matthew–Wood syndrome Goldenhar syndrome Poland syndrome Pentalogy of Cantrell Beckwith–Wiedemann syndrome

- *Musculoskeletal and limb defects*: Absence defect, polydactyly, syndactyly, rib, and vertebral anomalies
- *Genitourinary defects*: Cryptorchidism, ectopic kidney, and horseshoe kidney
- *Environmental*: CDH has been reported in cases with vitamin A deficiency or exposure to drugs such as thalidomide, anticonvulsants, and quinine.

Diagnosis

Fetal CDH is diagnosed most commonly as an incidental finding during routine ultrasound screening. Ultrasound findings of CDH include presence of stomach bubble, gallbladder or bowel within the thoracic cavity, deviation of the heart and mediastinum, herniated liver, abnormal position of the umbilical and hepatic veins, pleural effusion, and polyhydramnios **(Fig. 14)**. Small and large bowel as well as the liver, spleen, and kidney can herniate into the thorax. Occasionally, only small bowel may be herniated into thorax, while stomach and

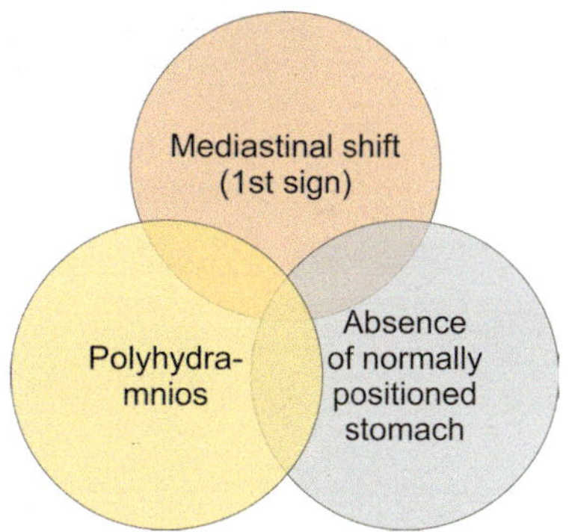

Fig. 14: Classical triad of congenital diaphragmatic hernia.

bladder appear in close juxtaposition below the diaphragm. Gastrocardiac angle >54.5° is highly predictive of liver herniation with accuracy of >97% (Vivek K. UOG, 2018).

In some cases, it is diagnosed during work-up for *polyhydramnios*. Compression of the heart, impaired swallowing, and partial obstruction of the gastrointestinal tract lead to polyhydramnios, which is present in up to 69% of cases, particularly late in gestation (by the third trimester). Rarely, excessive polyhydramnios may lead to premature rupture of membrane and preterm labor.

The abdominal circumference is often small, secondary to displacement of viscera into the chest.

Left-sided CDH is most often diagnosed when the stomach is in the chest near the left atrium, with absence of the normal stomach below the diaphragm. In cases where identification of herniated liver lobe is technically difficult, examination of the course of the portal and hepatic veins is helpful to demonstrate hepatic vessels extending into the chest.

In a right-sided hernia, the liver herniates into the chest, and mediastinal shift is to the left. Liver echogenicity can appear similar to the lung, so visualization of gallbladder and hepatic vessels in the thorax is helpful in confirming the diagnosis **(Fig. 15)**.

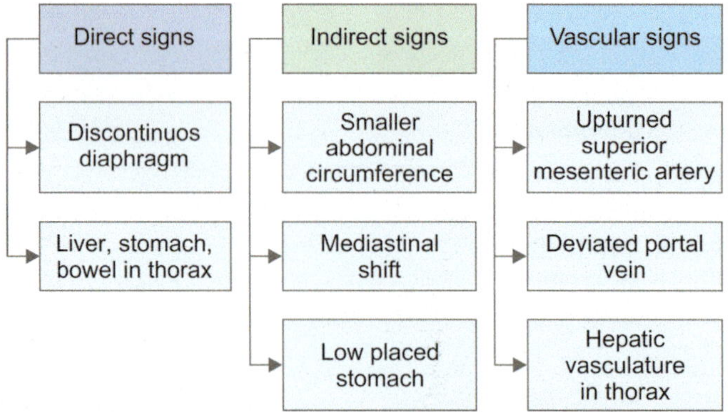

Fig. 15: Sonographic signs of congenital diaphragmatic hernia (CDH).

Postdiagnosis Fetal Evaluation (Figs. 16A to F)

Complete anatomic examination should be performed to assess for presence of associated anomalies (25–75%).

Echocardiography is indicated because congenital cardiac defects occur in 10–35% of cases.

MRI is a useful adjuvant for confirming the diagnosis of a CDH and determines total lung volume. It is also useful for assessing additional associated abnormalities.

Chromosomal microarray should be offered to all patients, as it helps in prognostic counseling and guides in decision for management of labor and the plan for neonatal resuscitation.

TABLE 5: Favorable and poor prognostic features of congenital diaphragmatic hernia.

Favorable features	*Poor prognostic features*
• Liver in abdomen (70–80% survival) • O/E LHR > 45% • Appropriate abdominal circumference • No polyhydramnios • Gestational age at diagnosis > 25 weeks	• Chromosomal anomaly/associated malformation • Early diagnosis < 20 weeks • Intrathoracic liver (30–50% survival) • O/E LHR < 25% • Observed LHR < 1 • Abdominal circumference < 5th percentile • Associated left ventricular hypoplasia

(LHR: lung-to-head circumference ratio; O/E: observed/expected)

Prognosis (Table 5)

Prognosis varies depending on the side of the herniation, the position of the liver, associated abnormalities, and gestation age at diagnosis. The severity of lung hypoplasia and pulmonary hypertension are major determinants in mortality and morbidity rates.

By ultrasound, the *lung-to-head circumference ratio* (LHR) has been used as a predictor of outcome for left-sided CDH. The measurement of fetal LHR has been used for the prediction of pulmonary hypoplasia and/or hypertension in the neonatal period.

Pitfalls: Postnatal survival is related not only to the degree of fetal lung development but also to the expertise of the neonatal center caring for the affected infant. Consequently, it is necessary to adjust the observed/expected (O/E) LHR according to the level of neonatal care (Nicolaides KH. UOG, 2007, 2009, 2012).

The LHR appears to be most reliable between 24 and 34 weeks of gestation.

Three techniques to calculate the LHR using ultrasound have been described ***(Figs. 17A to C)****:*

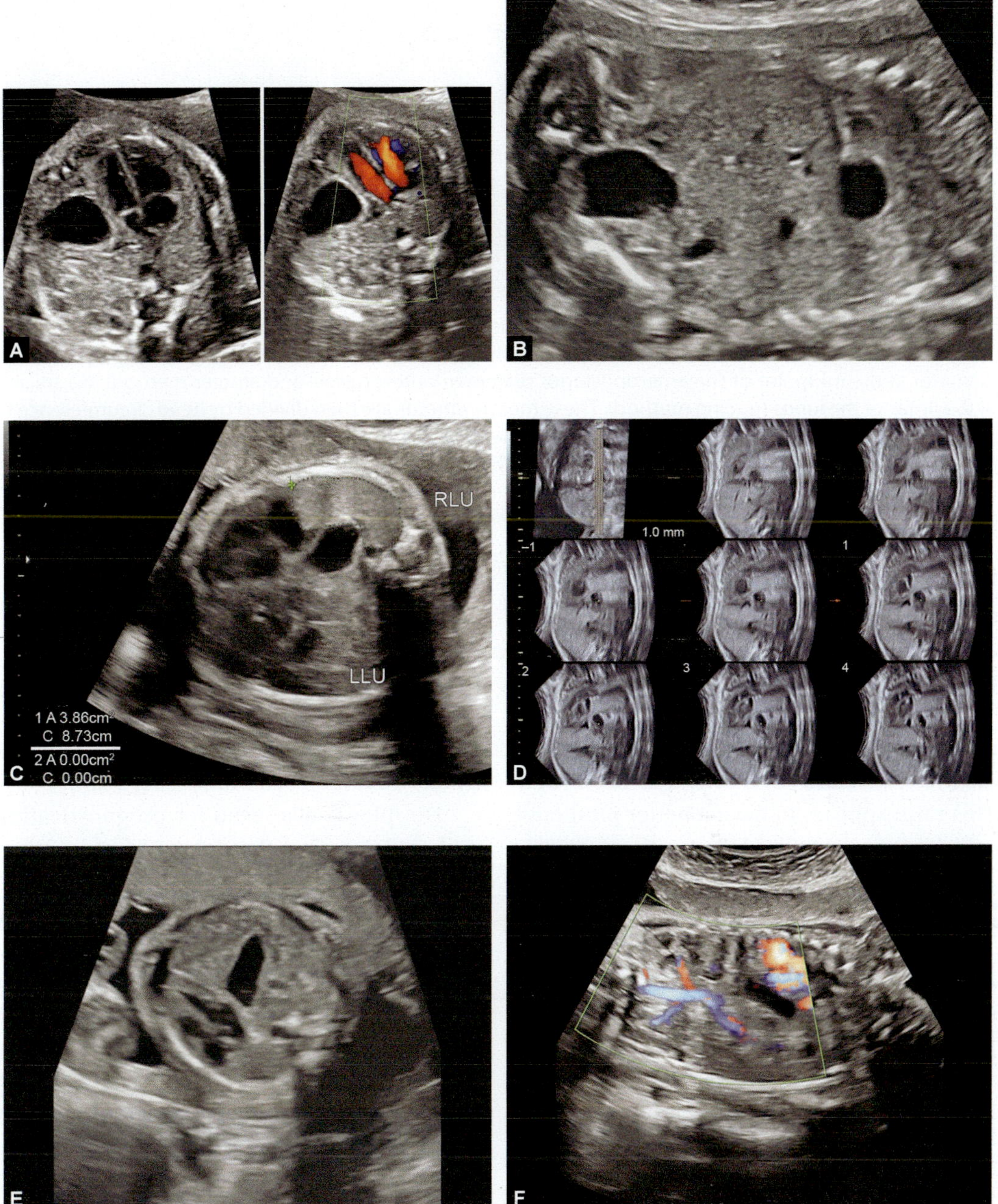

Figs. 16A to F: (A) Transverse view of the thorax shows stomach and small bowel occupying left hemithorax with contralateral shift of the mediastinum, apical four-chamber view in gray scale and color Doppler appears normal; (B) Coronal view shows stomach bubble migrated into thorax with indistinct diaphragmatic outline; (C) Right lung measured by area trace method (to calculated LHR) in left diaphragmatic hernia; (D) Multiplanar reconstruction (TUI) shows herniated small bowel and stomach content into left hemithorax; (E) Transverse view of the thorax shows stomach bubble migrated into hemithorax and forms an angle with lateral border of the heart (gastrocardiac angle) indicative of liver herniation; (F) Color Doppler in coronal view shows upturned superior mesenteric artery (SMA) to supply herniated small bowel.
(LHR: lung-to-head circumference ratio)

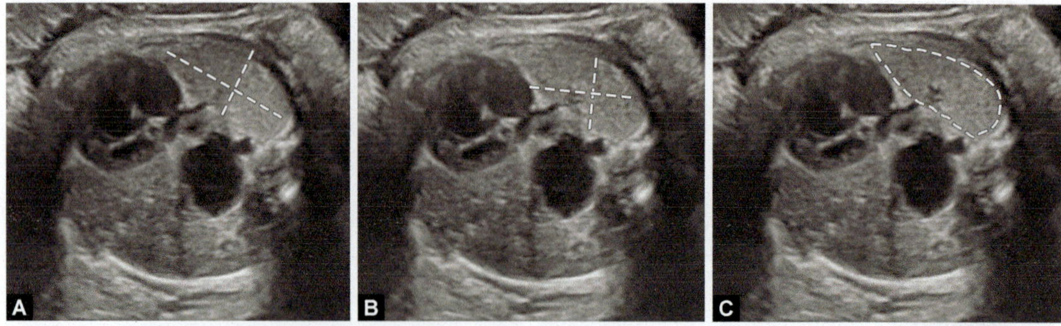

Figs. 17A to C: (A) Multiplication of the longest diameter of the lung by its longest perpendicular diameter (longest diameter method); (B) Multiplication of the anteroposterior diameter of the lung by the perpendicular diameter at the midpoint of the anteroposterior diameter (anteroposterior diameter method); (C) Tracing of the limits of the lungs (tracing method). These measurements are then divided by head circumference to get lung to head ratio (LHR). This observed LHR is then divided by expected mean LHR for the gestational age to get observed/expected lung to head ratio (O/E LHR).
Source: Nicolaides KH, et al. UOG. 2012.

The tracing method has been shown to be the most accurate in predicting survival in some centers. Generally, an LHR < 1 suggests a poor outcome, with a survival rate of 45% **(Fig. 18)**.

To improve outcome assessment, another ultrasound measure, *the observed-to-expected lung-to-head ratio (O/E LHR)* has been used. This ratio appears to have a better predictive value compared with LHR. A ratio of <25% is associated with lower survival rates (JM Biard, 2010).

Magnetic resonance imaging provides more accurate measurement of lung volumes than does sonographic assessment by LHR. Measurements obtained by MRI are easier to standardize and allow assessment of both lungs (Jani J, Nicholaides KH, et al. UOG, 2008).

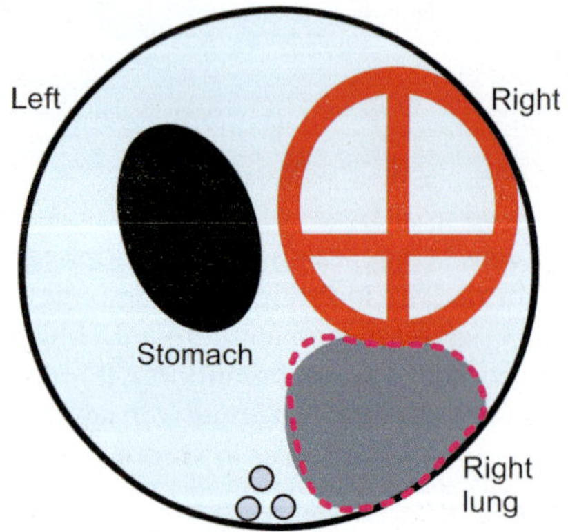

Fig. 18: The outline of the right lung is traced in millimeters—this is the most accurate method.

Lung-to-liver signal intensity ratio (LLSIR) has been found to be related to lung maturity in T2-weighted MRI, and appears to be associated with prognosis in CDH patients (Akiko Yokoi A, et al. Transl Ped, 2018).

Doppler is also used for prognostication and to determine the degree of pulmonary hypoplasia **(Fig. 19)**. Measuring the main right and left pulmonary artery and comparing with normal via an observed-to-expected ratio show a reduction in values in fetuses with CDH and pulmonary hypoplasia. In fetuses having pulmonary hypoplasia along with altered pulmonary vasculature, there is high risk of developing persistent pulmonary hypertension (PPHN).

- Significant Discrepancy between branch pulmonary arteries/progressively small ipsilateral branch pulmonary artery carries poor prognosis
- *McGoon index*

$$= \frac{\text{RPA diameter + LPA diameter}}{\text{AORTA diameter}}$$

  - >1.7—favorable prognosis
  - <1.3—very high mortality

Fetal stomach position in left CDH is a useful adjunct in antenatal prognosis **(Fig. 19)**.

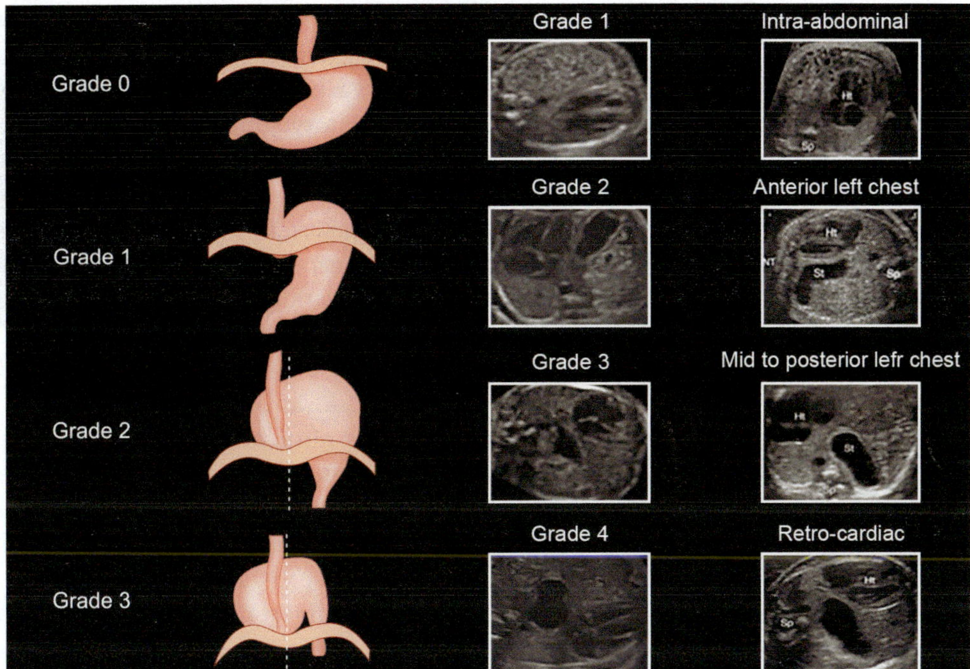

Fig. 19: Antenatal sonographic fetal stomach positions and its prognosis in left CDH. Grade 1: Intraabdominal; Grade 2: Close contact with anterior chest wall; Grade 3: Mid-to-posterior left chest; Grade 4: Retrocardiac; Grade 1 and 2 have better prognosis compared to grade 3 and 4.
Source: Oluyomi Obi TF, Benediktson I, Abbasi N, Ryan G. Fetal stomach position for prognostication in left congenital diaphragmatic hernia (CDH): a systematic review and meta-analysis. UOG. 2018;52(S1):5-5.

Predictors of Decreased Survival in CDH

- Ultrasound LHR < 1, O/E LHR < 25% (most preferred method)
- Three-dimensional ultrasound total functional lung volume (TFLV) < 35% (still an experimental tool)
- Lower McGoon index (it is not universally accepted due to significant interobserver variability)
- MRI O/E total fetal lung volume TFLV <25% (more reliable and reproducible but limited)
- Lung to liver signal intensity ratio (LLSIR) < 2 (novel MRI-based risk stratification technique).

Clinical Presentation

Often, postnatally, CDH is diagnosed by the attending obstetrician and neonatologist when confronted with a neonate having severe respiratory distress and a scaphoid abdomen. Breath sound is reduced on the side of the hernia. Chest radiograph confirms the diagnosis.

Pregnancy Management

Fetal Surgery

- Expectant management (favorable)
- *Open surgery*: Fetal tracheal occlusion.

Fetal Endoscopic Tracheal Occlusion

The goal of in utero therapy in severe CDH is to prevent or reverse pulmonary hypoplasia and restore adequate lung growth for neonatal survival. Prenatal fetal endoscopic tracheal occlusion (FETO) obstructs the normal egress of lung fluid during pulmonary development, thereby increasing transpulmonic pressure and resulting in large fluid-filled lungs. It appears to be effective but increases the risk of preterm delivery. It is not widely available and fails in half of cases.

Criteria for FETO are isolated left CDH, observed/expected lung area to head circumference ratio (O/E LHR) <25%, normal microarray, singleton pregnancy, absence of short cervical length, and gestational age 27^{+0} to 29^{+6} weeks at the time of the procedure.

Ideally, the occlusion is reversed at 34 weeks, usually by fetoscopy or ultrasound-guided puncture.

Prenatal Care

- *Serial ultrasound examination and biophysical profile*: The risk of intrauterine fetal demise is 2–8% and even higher depending on the presence of associated abnormalities. The cause of this increased risk of demise is unknown. Hence, serial ultrasound examination to be done every 4 weeks to measure fetal growth and amniotic fluid index. Weekly biophysical profile to be done beginning from 32 to 34 weeks.
- *Polyhydramnios*: Polyhydramnios usually develops at 28–32 weeks. Amnioreduction may be done to relieve maternal discomfort. Early delivery is planned in case of severe polyhydramnios with risk for preterm labor or cord prolapse with rupture of membrane.
- Antenatal glucocorticoids are given to reduce the morbidity and mortality associated with preterm labor, as per standard protocol.

Delivery

Delivery is recommended in tertiary care center, preferably, with ECMO facility. The timing and mode of delivery is uncertain. Cesarean section should be performed for standard obstetrics indications.

Postnatal Management

The major issues at birth are respiratory insufficiency secondary to pulmonary hypoplasia and persistent pulmonary hypertension due to change in pulmonary vascular bed.

Supportive medical management consists of reducing lung compression, cardiovascular support with fluids and inotropic agents, and ventilatory support using conventional or high-frequency ventilation (HFV). ECMO is used in severe cases of patients who are not responsive to the supportive medical interventions.

A nasogastric tube connected to continuous suction is placed in the stomach so as to decompress abdominal contents and reduce lung compression.

Inhaled nitric oxide (iNO) administration was associated with improved oxygenation and a decrease in ECMO for infants with normal left ventricular function.

Gentle ventilation or spontaneous breathing with planned delayed surgical repair of the diaphragm is the preferred strategy. Repair is done usually in 1st week of life after stabilizing the baby.

After discharge from neonatal intensive care unit, long-term multidisciplinary follow-up is required, as baby with CDH may have bronchopulmonary dysplasias, gastroesophageal reflux, failure to thrive, nutritional disorders, neurodevelopmental delay, and musculoskeletal problems.

BRONCHOGENIC CYST

Bronchogenic cysts are rare anomalies that result from abnormal budding or branching of the tracheobronchial tree, derived from an abnormal budding of the ventricular diverticulum of the foregut. They are most often located in the mediastinum in the subcarinal region (85%), in lung parenchyma (15%).

Most cysts are asymptomatic and missed in prenatal scans. They are diagnosed in children and adults during routine chest radiograph and ultrasonography.

Prenatally, clinical manifestations will depend on the size, presence of bronchial obstruction or mediastinal shift, and location. If the cyst does not cause mass effect, it typically will not cause a problem in utero.

However, if the cyst compresses the airway, it can lead to airway obstruction at birth.

Diagnosis (Figs. 20A to C)

On prenatal ultrasound, they usually appear as anechoic, unilocular, intrathoracic cysts within the lung parenchyma or mediastinum. The cyst can be mediastinal or parenchymal. Mediastinal lesions are typically unilocular, located midline in the subcarinal region (75%). Parenchymal lesions are usually simple unilocular cysts located along the tracheobronchial tree. Visualization of small mediastinal cysts can be challenging because of difficult differentiation from other structures, so they should be suspected in the presence of mediastinal enlargement without a clear mass.

Fetal MRI can be helpful in cases with an unclear diagnosis.

Differential Diagnosis (Table 6)

- CPAM
- Bronchopulmonary sequestration
- Neuroenteric cyst
- Duplication cyst.

Prognosis

Risk of chromosomal anomalies and nonchromosomal syndrome is extremely low (KT is not indicated).

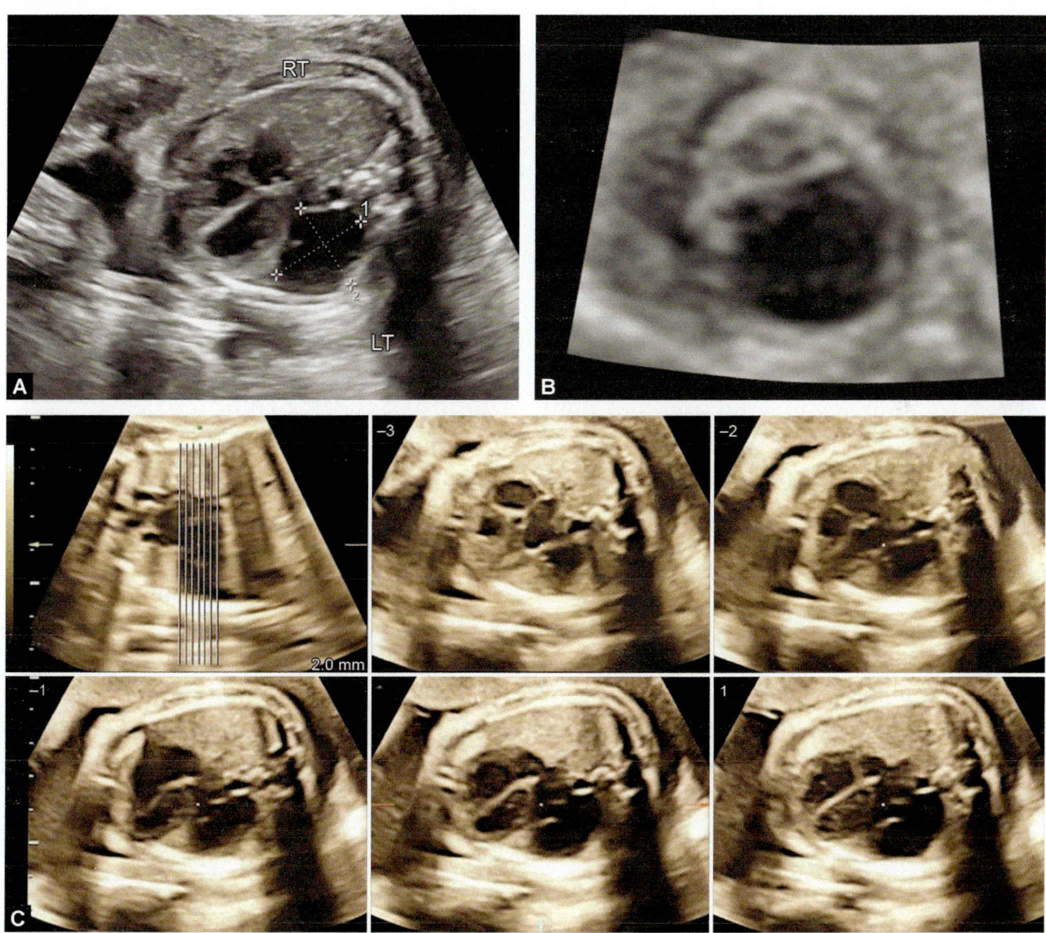

Figs. 20A to C: (A) Transverse view of the thorax shows a well-defined unilocular cystic mass in left lung displacing the heart toward the right; (B) Zoomed view of the left lung cyst; (C) Multiplanar reconstruction (TUI) image demonstrates spatial relationship of the left lung cyst with respect to mediastinal structures. (TUI: tomographic ultrasound imaging)

TABLE 6: Differential diagnosis of cysts.

Features	***Bronchogenic cyst***	***Enteric duplication cyst***	***Neuroenteric cyst***
Embryology	Portion of lung bud gets separated from tracheo-bronchial tree to form cyst	Aberration of posterior division of embryonic foregut	Incomplete separation of notochord from foregut
Location	Middle mediastinum adjacent to distal trachea and mainstem bronchi	Posterior mediastinum	Posterior mediastinum, connected to meninges and spinal cord by narrow stalk
Characters	Unilocular fluid-filled cyst not communicating to tracheobronchial tree	May or may not communicate to gastrointestinal tract	May extend to spinal canal through vertebral defect/ spinal anomalies

They have generally benign outcome, though if large may compress the venous structure or cause tracheobronchial obstruction.

Management

The risk of chromosomal anomalies and non-chromosomal syndromes is extremely low; hence, karyotyping is recommended only in special cases.

Prenatal

Only massive cyst producing mediastinal shift necessitates prenatal intervention. In utero pulmonary drainage may be tried but fluid may reaccumulate. EXIT with cyst resection by thoracotomy has been recently described to prevent acute respiratory distress at birth.

Postnatal

Bronchogenic cysts tend to grow constantly after birth, hence surgical resection is recommended before 2 years of age to prevent recurrent respiratory infections. Prenatally diagnosed large cyst requires urgent removal post-delivery.

BRONCHIAL ATRESIA

Congenital bronchial atresia is a relatively rare lesion characterized by localized atresia or stenosis of a segmental bronchus. Bronchial atresia can involve lobar, segmental, or mainstem bronchi. Prenatally diagnosed congenital lobar overinflation can be caused by lobar bronchial atresia.

Etiopathogenesis

The most accepted pathogenetic mechanism is disruption of blood supply to a segment of bronchus during embryogenetic phase of development leading to impaired growth and bronchial atresia. The risk of associated chromosomal anomalies and non-chromosomal syndrome is extremely rare.

Diagnosis (Figs. 21A and B)

Prenatal ultrasound findings of bronchial atresia demonstrate an extremely large, massively overexpanded unilateral lung or lung segment. The mass effect will typically result in mediastinal shift, with compression of chest structures and often with eversion of the ipsilateral hemidiaphragm. Branching fluid-filled structures may be seen within the enlarged echogenic lung, representing dilated airways peripheral to the central obstructed bronchus.

Ultrasonographic differentiation between bronchial atresia and CPAM may be challenging, as the large echogenic lung appears very similar to microcystic (type 3) CPAM. In bronchial atresia, part of the distal bronchi is seen as sonolucent area.

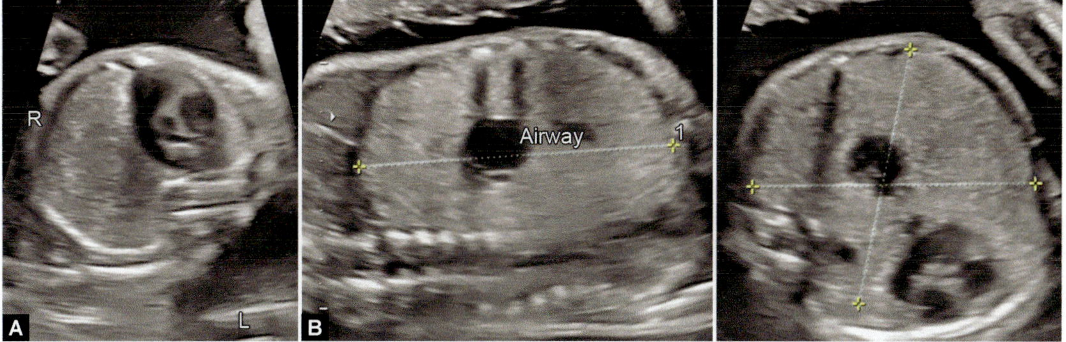

Figs. 21A and B: (A) On transverse section of the thorax (at the level of short axis view) a large echogenic mass with contralateral mass effect is seen; (B) Right parasagittal and axial view shows grossly echogenic and enlarged right lung mass with dilatation of the distal bronchi and indentation of the diaphragm.

Prognosis

The risk of hydrops is increased with larger lesions, but the ability to prognosticate, based on lesion size at the time of initial diagnosis, is limited. Distal bronchial atresia has better prognosis compared to mainstream bronchial atresia, which is associated with concurrent hydrops and perinatal mortality.

Presence of ascites is poor prognostic indicator, as it signifies central venous compression.

Risk of chromosomal anomalies and nonchromosomal syndrome is extremely low (KT is not indicated).

Management

Delivery should be planned in a tertiary care center, as the baby may need immediate postnatal resuscitation. Prenatal fetoscopic approach for decompression via tracheobronchial endoscopy of bronchial atresia has been recently applied with success.

If not symptomatic at birth, it may remain asymptomatic throughout life. However, dyspnea, pneumonia, and bronchial asthma have been reported in some.

CONGENITAL HIGH AIRWAY OBSTRUCTION

Congenital high airway obstruction syndrome (CHAOS) is a spectrum of conditions characterized by incomplete or complete obstruction of the upper fetal airway. Any fetal abnormality that obstructs the larynx or trachea, causing intrinsic atresia or extrinsic compression, can result in CHAOS.

Intrinsic lesion can be either agenesis of glottis, agenesis of larynx, or agenesis of both. Extrinsic causes may be cervical teratoma, lymphatic malformation, and vascular rings such as double aortic arch.

Etiopathogenesis

Majority of cases are sporadic with unknown incidence. CHAOS may be associated with congenital anomalies, especially of the skeletal system **(Fig. 22)**. **Flowchart 5** shows sequence of events following CHAOS.

Genetics

Laryngeal atresia, most commonly, can occur as part of *Fraser syndrome* (tracheal or laryngeal atresia, renal agenesis, microphthalmia, and syndactyly or polydactyly) with autosomal recessive inheritance. Other reported syndromes are VACTERL, TACRD (tracheal atresia, cardiac, radial ray defect, and duodenal atresia), Cri-du-chat syndrome, velocardiofacial syndrome, and short-rib polydactyly syndrome. It may be associated with bronchoesophageal/tracheoesophageal atresia. All patients with CHAOS need

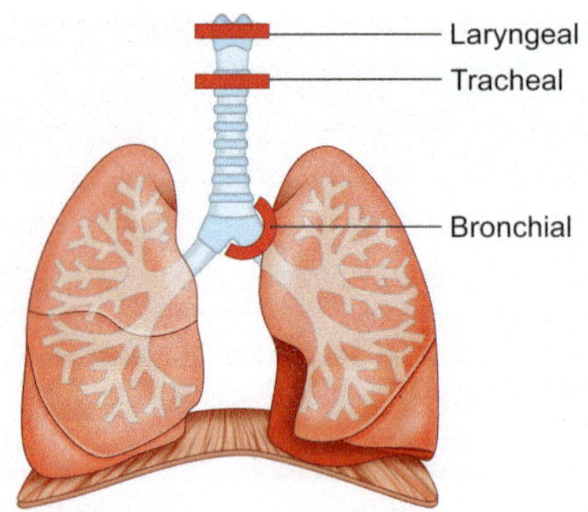

Fig. 22: Causes of congenital high airway obstruction syndrome (CHAOS).

detailed evaluation to avoid inheritance in future pregnancies.

Diagnosis (Figs. 23A to D)

Radiological findings include bilateral symmetrically enlarged echogenic lungs, dilated fluid-filled trachea and central bronchi, and flattened or everted diaphragms.

The heart usually assumes a more central and anterior position than normal and is often compressed, as the size of the lungs increases. Due to hyperinflated lungs, mass effect on the heart leads to increased distance between descending aorta and left atrium.

Frequently, there are associated findings of ascites and other signs of hydrops. The mechanism of ascites may be from compression of the heart and great vessels by the enlarged lungs. Either polyhydramnios or oligohydramnios may be present.

MRI can be used to identify the region of obstruction and assist in patient's selection regarding in utero intervention and intrapartum procedures.

Management

If untreated, laryngeal and tracheal atresia can lead to death either in utero from hydrops or within minutes after birth from respiratory compromise. Even though chances of survival

Flowchart 5: Progression of congenital high airway obstruction syndrome (CHAOS).

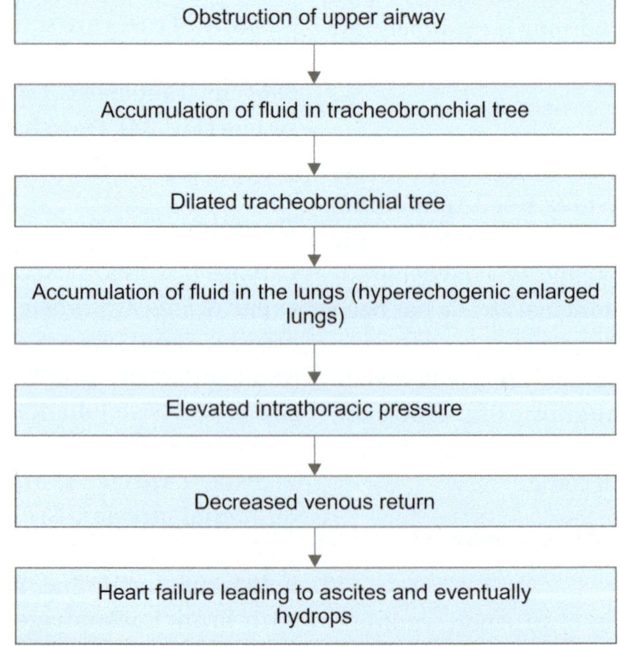

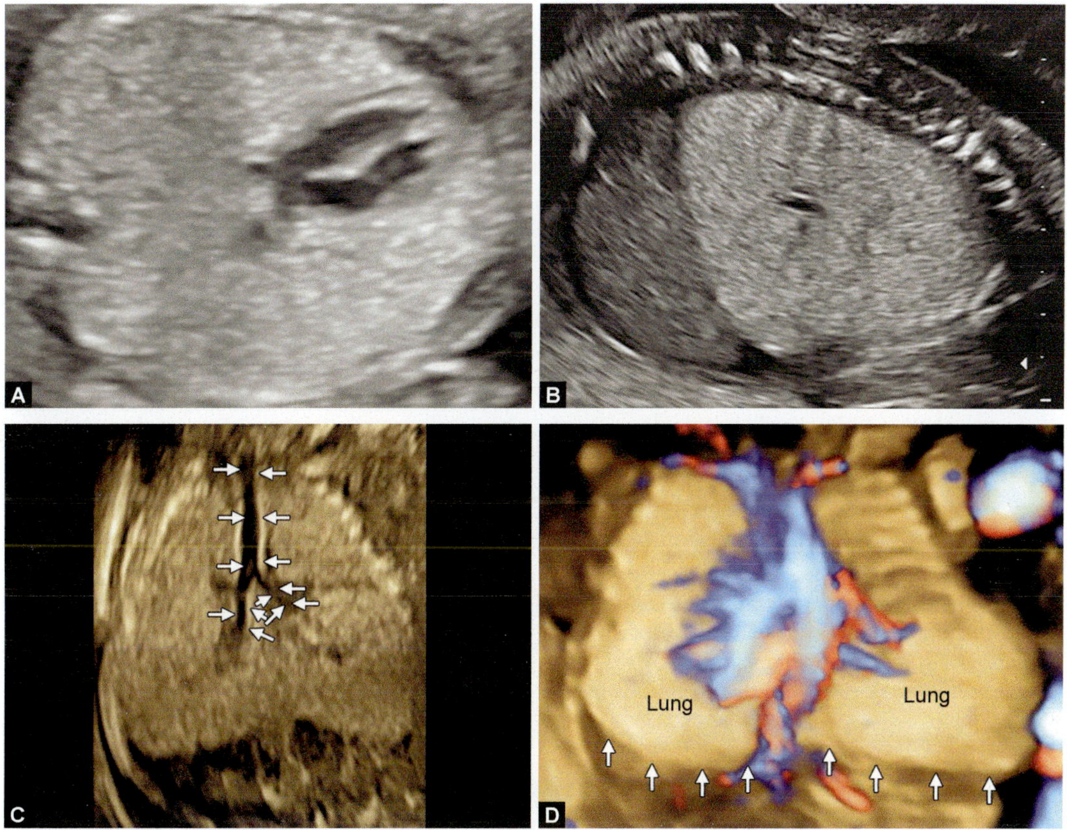

Figs. 23A to D: (A) On axial four-chamber view, lungs appears to be enlarged and hyperechogenic. The heart appears to be squeezed and mesocardiac is seen; (B) Right parasagittal view shows eversion of diaphragm due to massively enlarged lung and mild ascites; (C and D) Coronal view shows bilateral enlarged lung with fluid-filled trachea and right and left mainstem bronchus.

may arise after treatments such as fetoscopic procedures and EXIT, CHAOS results in high morbidity-mortality rates.

PLEURAL EFFUSION

Any fluid in the pleural space is abnormal. It may be unilateral or bilateral, or may be primary or secondary.

Etiopathogenesis

Primary Pleural Effusion

It is most often caused by chylothorax, which results from defective development of the lymphatic system. Primary pleural effusion is suspected when the effusion is unilateral or is much larger on one side than the other, and when no other signs of hydrops are present.

Primary chylothorax is associated with mosaicism and aneuploidy in 2–6% of cases.

Secondary Pleural Effusion

It usually occurs as a part of complex disease. In **Table 7** common causes of secondary pleural effusion has been put together.

These syndromes typically present with bilateral pleural effusions (particularly in fetuses with hydrops) but occasionally with unilateral effusion.

If sufficiently large, pleural effusion may result in mass effect, leading to compression of

TABLE 7: Association of secondary pleural effusion with different diseases.

Alloimmunization:	*Infectious:*
Pulmonary:	• Parvovirus
Lung malformation:	• TORCH
• CPAM	*Chromosomal:*
• BPS	• Turner syndrome
• CDH	• Trisomy 21
Cardiac:	*Metabolic:*
• Structural defects	• Lysosomal storage
• Tumors	• Glycogen storage
• Cardiomyopathy	*Genetic syndromes:*
• Arrhythmias	Noonan syndrome
Anomalies of umbilical cord and placenta	Fetal akinesia

[CPAM: congenital pulmonary airway malformation; BPS: bronchopulmonary sequestration; CDH: congenital diaphragmatic hernia; TORCH: toxoplasmosis, other (syphilis, varicella-zoster, and parvovirus B19), rubella, cytomegalovirus (CMV), and herpes infections]

the heart and hydrops as well as compression of the lungs, resulting in pulmonary hypoplasia. Compression of esophagus may lead to polyhydramnios.

Diagnosis (Figs. 24A to H)

Pleural effusions appear on prenatal ultrasound as anechoic fluid collections in the pleural space, leading to the appearance of the lung floating in the fluid, surrounded by the chest wall and diaphragm.

Larger unilateral effusions result in mass effect, causing mediastinal shift and flattening or eversion of the diaphragm. Prenatal pleural effusion has a variable natural course ranging from spontaneous resolution to progressive development of hydrops and polyhydramnios with high risk for perinatal morbidity and mortality.

Fetal assessment for associated anomalies, including echocardiography, diagnostic

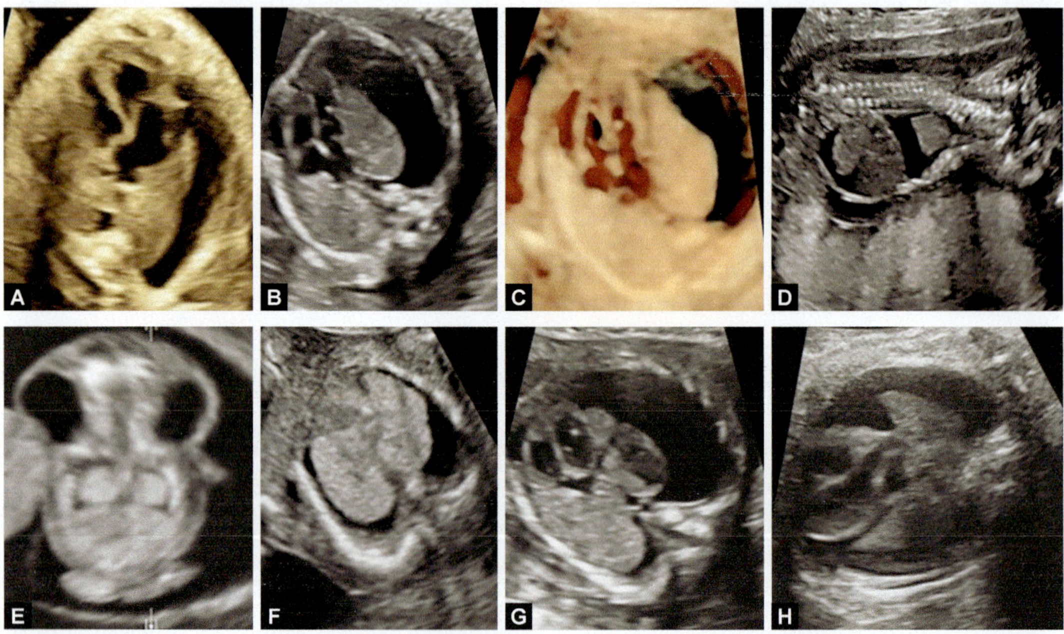

Figs. 24A to H: (A) Mild right-sided pleural effusion with no significant mediastinal shift; (B and C) Moderate to gross left-sided pleural effusion with contralateral mediastinal displacement leading to dextroposition of the heart due to mass effect, 3D HD live demonstrating the same; (D) Parasagittal view shows fluid collection in both pleural and peritoneal space; (E and F) Bilateral pleural effusion with dilated jugular lymphatic sac, cystic hygroma and subcutaneous edema (hydrops) in first trimester; (G) Gross pleural effusion on left side and mild on right side with mediastinal shift; (H) Bilateral moderate pleural effusion.

thoracocentesis to test for cell count, differential count and viral markers (PCR for parvovirus, CMV), Noonan syndrome testing, and fetal karyotyping (5% association with Down syndrome) should be performed. *Maternal assessment* includes complete blood count, blood group and antibody screening, hemoglobin electrophoresis, serology for infections, parvovirus, and TORCH.

Prognosis

Prognosis depends on the—(1) presence of associated structural/chromosomal abnormalities, (2) whether it is unilateral or bilateral, (3) the size of hydrothorax, and (4) severity of mediastinal shift (tension hydrothorax).

Progression from unilateral to bilateral effusions is associated with impending hydrops. Secondary hydrothorax has a worse outcome. The mortality rate in these cases can be up to 98% depending on size, progression to hydrops, and underlying cause. The prognosis improves from 50% survival to more than 90% survival with treatment after ruling out secondary causes, in isolated fetal hydrothorax.

Management (Flowchart 6)

Prenatal

Prenatal evolution of fetal hydrothorax is variable with 10–20% undergoing spontaneous resolution with good postnatal outcome. Those with mild and moderate effusion, that remained stable throughout pregnancy, have a good outcome, in fair proportion of patient, with postnatal treatment.

Invasive fetal therapy is considered only in severe cases. Typically, a pleural effusion is drained with a single stick procedure (thoracocentesis). This allows proper visualization of heart and evaluation of the ability of lungs to reinflate. If effusion recurs, placement of a thoracoamniotic shunt is an option.

Indications of invasive fetal therapy:

- Severe isolated cases of hydrothorax (tension hydrothorax)
- Asymmetrical effusion, without additional anomalies, with significant mediastinal shift or with other signs of hydrops already present.

Flowchart 6: Algorithm for the management of pleural effusion.

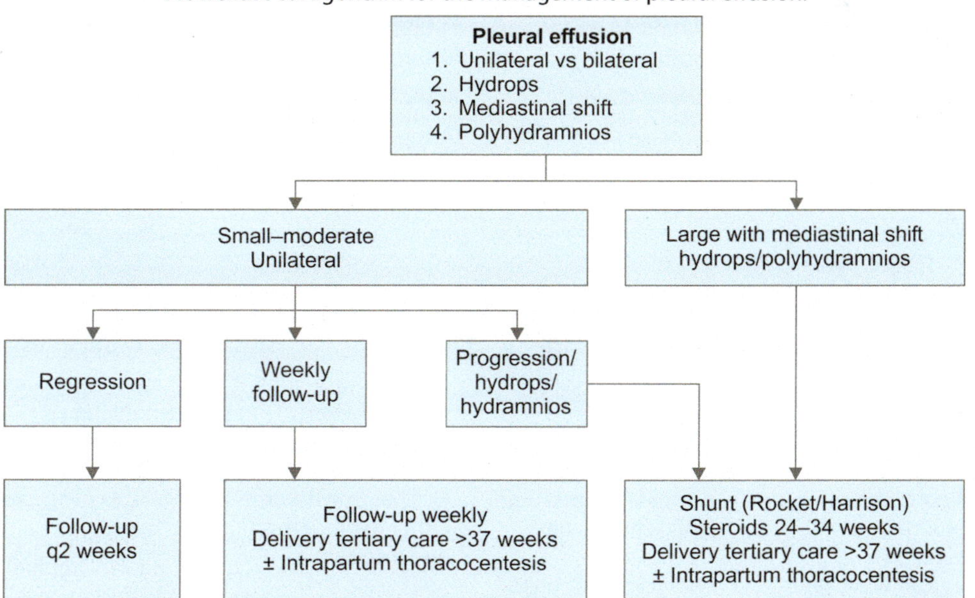

Source: Abbasi N, Ryan G. 2019.

Postprocedure complications are shunt failure leading to reaccumulation (15%), shunt migration, preterm pre-labor rupture of membrane (PPROM) (5%), preterm birth (15–20%), maternal hemorrhage, chorioamnionitis, etc.

Postnatal

Severe hydrothorax needs immediate postnatal care, hence should be delivered in tertiary care hospital. In cases treated with pleuroamniotic shunt, clamping of shunt should be done immediately after fetal extraction to avoid risk of neonatal pneumothorax at birth.

Postnatal confirmation and evaluation of the effusion is to be done to determine the evolution of the disease.

PULMONARY HYPOPLASIA

Pulmonary underdevelopment has been classified into three categories—pulmonary agenesis, pulmonary aplasia, and pulmonary hypoplasia **(Table 8)**. Lung agenesis is usually unilateral and it occurs at approximately 4 weeks of gestation, when the primitive lung is forming. The contralateral lung is normal in structure but has compensatory hypertrophy.

Pulmonary hypoplasia may be primary or secondary. Secondary pulmonary hypoplasia is much more commonly diagnosed.

Developing fetus must have appropriate fluid in the air spaces, normal intrauterine breathing movement and appropriate space to facilitate normal lung development, and transition to extrauterine environment. Any aberration in these prerequisites may cause pulmonary hypoplasia as illustrated in **Table 9**.

The most common cause of pulmonary hypoplasia is congenital diaphragmatic hernia. The most common extrathoracic cause of pulmonary hypoplasia is severe oligohydramnios, due to either—(1) fetal genitourinary anomalies or (2) prolonged rupture of membrane. Thoracic compression syndrome is most destructive to lung growth during canalicular stage of lung development, after 16–26 weeks of gestation.

TABLE 8: Pulmonary underdevelopment.

	Bronchus	***Vasculature***	***Parenchyma***
Pulmonary agenesis	Absent	Absent	Absent
Pulmonary aplasia	Rudimentary	Absent	Absent
Pulmonary hypoplasia	Decrease size and number	Decrease size and number	Decrease size and number

TABLE 9: Causes of pulmonary hypoplasia.

Thoracic compression	***Decreased intrathoracic space***	***Decreased fetal breathing***	***Other entities***
• Renal agenesis (Potter syndrome) • Urinary tract outflow obstruction • Oligohydramnios before 28 weeks' gestation • Extra amniotic fetal development	• Diaphragmatic hernia • Agenesis of diaphragm • Pleural effusions • Abdominal distension sufficient to limit chest volume • Thoracic dystrophies	• Intrauterine central nervous system damage • Fetal Werdnig-Hoffmann syndrome • Other neuropathies and myopathies	• Primary pulmonary hypoplasia • Trisomy 21 (abnormal breathing) • Multiple congenital anomalies • Erythroblastosis fetalis

Diagnosis (Figs. 25A to C)

Antenatally, thoracic circumference measurements are obtained in an axial plane at the level of the four-chamber view of the heart. Normograms have been published that illustrate the relationship between thoracic circumference and gestational age. A thoracic circumference below the 5th percentile for gestational age indicates pulmonary hypoplasia.

First hint toward diagnosis of renal agenesis is significant mediastinal shift without any identifiable mass effect from contralateral side. Color Doppler may be used to detect the concurrent absence of the ipsilateral pulmonary artery branch. Computed tomography (CT) helps to confirm the absence of the lung parenchyma, bronchus, and pulmonary artery on the involved side.

Differential Diagnosis

Refer **Figures 26A and B**.

Management

There is no need for karyotyping, due to the very low risk of association with chromosomal abnormalities. Delivery should be planned in a referral center, because early neonatal intubation may be needed. Right lung agenesis has poorer prognosis as compared to left lung agenesis because of a greater degree of heart and mediastinum displacement, with corresponding distortion of blood vessels and bronchi.

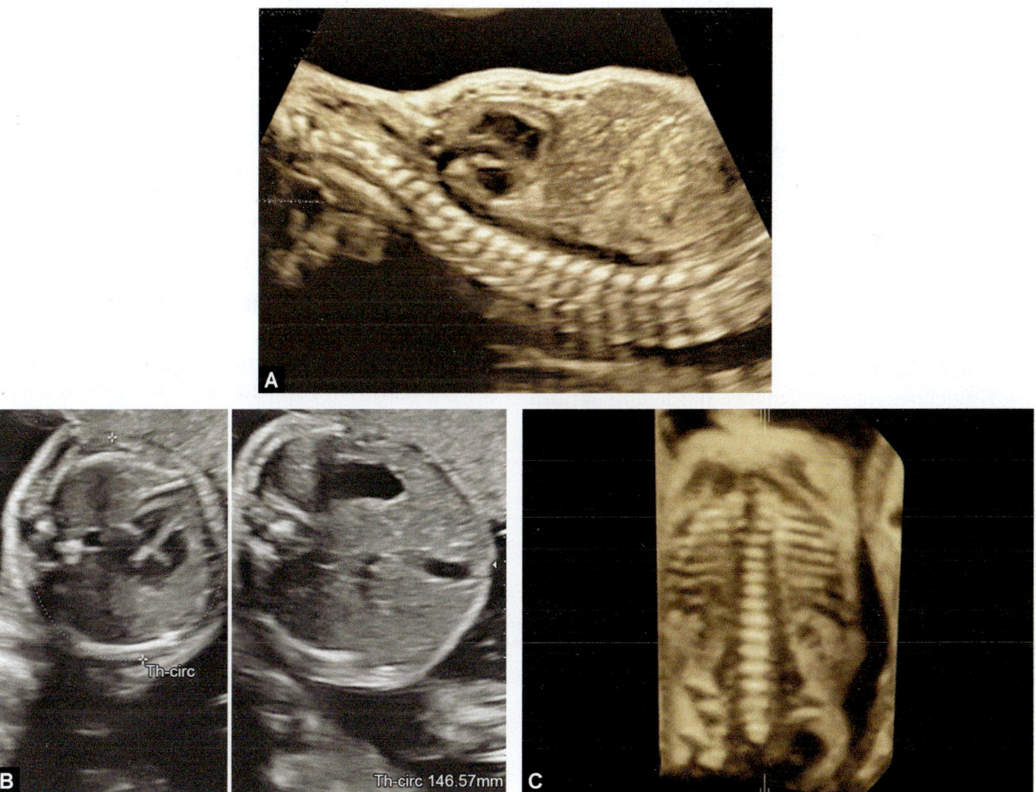

Figs. 25A to C: (A) Left parasagittal view shows relatively bell-shaped thorax indicative of narrow thorax; (B) Transverse view, if thorax and abdomen to demonstrate subjectively thoracic hypoplasia where thoracic circumference was less than 5th percentile for the period of gestation; (C) 3D skeletal mode shows normal appearance of the ribs and vertebral bodies.

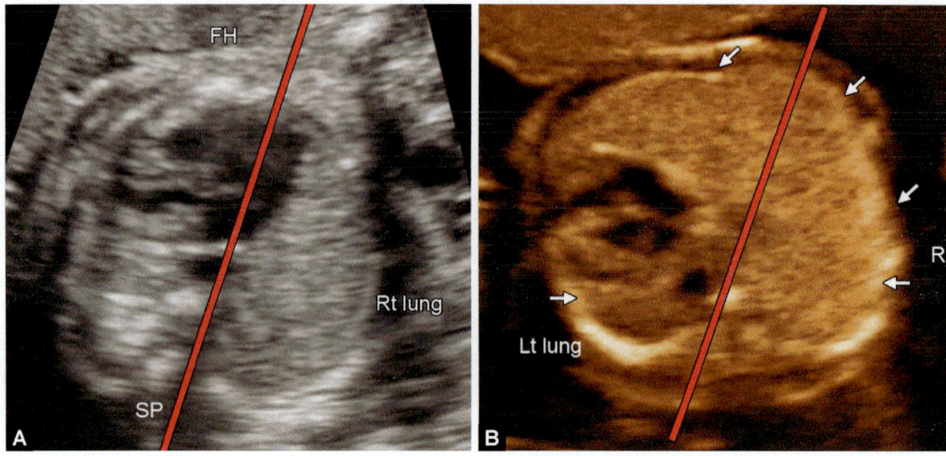

Figs. 26A and B: (A) Lung hypoplasia: Normal lung not crossing midline; (B) Echogenic lung lesion: Lung lesion crossing the midline. (SP: spine, FH: fetal heart)

BIBLIOGRAPHY

1. Abbey P, Das CJ, Pangtey GS, Seith A, Dutta R, Kumar A. Imaging in bronchopulmonary sequestration. J Med Imaging Radiat Oncol. 2009;53(1):22-31.
2. Abramov A, Fan W, Hernan R, Zenilman AL, Wynn J, Aspelund G, et al. Comparative outcomes of right versus left congenital diaphragmatic hernia: A multicenter analysis. J Pediatr Surg. 2020;55(1):33-8.
3. Adzick NS, Harrison MR, Glick PL, Golbus MS, Anderson RL, Mahony BS, et al. Fetal cystic adenomatoid malformation: prenatal diagnosis and natural history. J Pediatr Surg. 1985;20(5):483-8.
4. American Institute of Ultrasound in Medicine. Guidelines for performance of the antepartum obstetrical ultrasound examination. J Ultrasound Med. 1996;15:185-7.
5. Avni EF, Vanderelst A, Van Gansbeke D, Schils J, Rodesch F. Antenatal diagnosis of pulmonary tumors: report of two cases. Pediatr Radiol. 1986;16(3):190-2.
6. Azizkhan RG, Crombleholme TM. Congenital cystic lung disease: contemporary antenatal and postnatal management. Pediatr Surg Int. 2008;24(6):643-57.
7. Azizkhan RG, Crombleholme TM. Congenital cystic lung disease: contemporary antenatal and postnatal management. Pediatr Surg Int. 2008;24(6):643-57.
8. Benachi A, Cordier AG, Cannie M, Jani J. Advances in prenatal diagnosis of congenital diaphragmatic hernia. Semin Fetal Neonatal Med. 2014;19(6):331-7.
9. Berrocal T, Madrid C, Novo S, Gutiérrez J, Arjonilla A, Gómez-León N. Congenital anomalies of the tracheobronchial tree, lung, and mediastinum: embryology, radiology, and pathology. RadioGraphics. 2004;24(1):e17.
10. Biyyam DR, Chapman T, Ferguson MR, Deutsch G, Dighe MK. Congenital lung abnormalities: Embryologic features, prenatal diagnosis, and postnatal radiologic-pathologic correlation. RadioGraphics. 2010;30(6):1722-4.
11. Bulas D. Fetal magnetic resonance imaging as a complement to fetal ultrasonography. Ultrasound Q. 2007;23(1):3-22.
12. Burgos CM, Frenckner B, Luco M, Harting MT, Lally PA, Lally KP. Prenatally diagnosed congenital diaphragmatic hernia: optimal mode of delivery? J Perinatol. 2017;37(2):134-8.
13. Bush A, Hogg J, Chitty LS. Cystic lung lesions-prenatal diagnosis and management. Prenat Diagn. 2008;28(7):604-11.
14. Chitkara U, Rosenberg J, Chervenak FA, Berkowitz GS, Levine R, Fagerstrom RM, et al. Prenatal sonographic assessment of the fetal thorax: normal values. Am J Obstet Gynecol. 1987;156(5):1069-74.
15. Costanzo S, Filisetti C, Vella C, Rustico M, Fontana P, Lista G, et al. Pulmonary Malformations: Predictors of Neonatal Respiratory Distress and Early Surgery. J Neonatal Surg. 2016;5(3):27.
16. Crombleholme TM, Coleman B, Hedrick H, Liechty K, Howell L, Flake AW, et al. Cystic adenomatoid malformation volume ratio predicts outcome in prenatally diagnosed cystic adenomatoid malformation of the lung. J Pediatr Surg. 2002;37(3):331-8.

17. Crombleholme TM, Sylvester K, Flake AW, Adzick NS. Salvage of a fetus with congenital high airway obstruction syndrome by ex utero intrapartum treatment (EXIT) procedure. Fetal Diagn Ther. 2000;15(5):280-2.
18. Cruz MR, Cruz LM, Gratacós E. Congenital Cystic Adenomatoid Malformation of the Lung. [online] Available from https://praenatal-zuerich.ch/wp-content/uploads/2017/05/Obstetric_Imaging_2nd_ed-ch-002.pdf. [Last accessed September, 2021].
19. Daltro P, Werner H, Gasparetto TD, Domingues RC, Rodrigues L, Marchiori E, et al. Congenital chest malformations: a multimodality approach with emphasis on fetal MR imaging. Radiographics. 2010;30(2):385-95.
20. Daltro P, Werner H, Gasparetto TD, Domingues RC, Rodrigues L, Marchiori E, et al. Congenital chest malformations: a multimodality approach with emphasis on fetal MR imaging. RadioGraphics. 2010;30(2):385-95.
21. Davenport M, Warne SA, Cacciaguerra S, Patel S, Greenough A, Nicolaides K. Current outcome of antenatally diagnosed cystic lung disease. J Pediatr Surg. 2004;39(4):549-56.
22. Deprest J, Gratacos E, Nicolaides KH, FETO Task Group. Fetoscopic tracheal occlusion (FETO) for severe congenital diaphragmatic hernia: evolution of a technique and preliminary results. Ultrasound Obstet Gynecol. 2004;24(2):121-6.
23. Deprest J, Jani J, Van Schoubroeck D, Cannie M, Gallot D, Dymarkowski S, et al. Current consequences of prenatal diagnosis of congenital diaphragmatic hernia. J Pediatr Surg. 2006;41(2):423-30.
24. Derderian SC, Coleman AM, Jeanty C, Lim FY, Shaaban AM, Farrell JA, et al. Favorable outcomes in high-risk congenital pulmonary airway malformations treated with multiple courses of maternal betamethasone. J Pediatr Surg. 2015;50(4):515-8.
25. De Santis M, Masini L, Noia G, Cavaliere AF, Oliva N, Caruso A. Congenital cystic adenomatoid malformation of the lung: antenatal ultrasound findings and fetal-neonatal outcome—fifteen years of experience. Fetal Diagn Ther. 2000;15(4):246-50.
26. Deurloo KL, Devlieger R, Lopriore E, Klumper FJ, Oepkes D. Isolated fetal hydrothorax with hydrops: a systematic review of prenatal treatment options. Prenat Diagn. 2007;27(10):893-9.
27. Epelman M, Kreiger PA, Servaes S, Victoria T, Hellinger JC. Current imaging of prenatally diagnosed congenital lung lesions. Semin Ultrasound CT MR. 2010;31(2):141-57.
28. Goldstein RB. A practical approach to fetal chest masses. Ultrasound Q. 2006;22(3):177-94.
29. Gorincour G, Bouvenot J, Mourot MG, Sonigo P, Chaumoitre K, Garel C, et al. Prenatal prognosis of congenital diaphragmatic hernia using magnetic resonance imaging measurement of fetal lung volume. Ultrasound Obstet Gynecol. 2005;26(7):738-44.
30. Gornall AS, Budd JL, Draper ES, Konje JC, Kurinczuk JJ. Congenital cystic adenomatoid malformation: accuracy of prenatal diagnosis, prevalence and outcome in a general population. Prenat Diagn. 2003;23(12):997-1002.
31. Houdael M, Ahmed Z, Amine K, Amina BS, Raja F, Chiraz H. Antenatal diagnosis of extralobar pulmonary sequestration. Pan Afr Med J. 2014;19:54.
32. Hubbard AM, Adzick NS, Crombleholme TM, Coleman BG, Howell LJ, Haselgrove JC, et al. Congenital chest lesions: diagnosis and characterization with prenatal MR imaging. Radiology. 1999;212(1):43-8.
33. Jani J, Nicolaides KH, Keller RL, Benachi A, Peralta CFA, Favre R, et al. Observed to expected lung area to head circumference ratio in the prediction of survival in fetuses with isolated diaphragmatic hernia. Ultrasound Obstet Gynecol. 2007;30(1):67-71.
34. Jani JC, Benachi A, Nicolaides KH, Allegaert K, Gratacós E, Mazkereth R, et al. Prenatal prediction of neonatal morbidity in survivors with congenital diaphragmatic hernia: a multicenter study. Ultrasound Obstet Gynecol. 2009;33(1):64-9.
35. Jani JC, Cannie M, Peralta CF, Deprest JA, Nicolaides KH, Dymarkowski S. Lung volumes in fetuses with congenital diaphragmatic hernia: comparison of 3D US and MR imaging assessments. Radiology. 2007;244(2):575-82.
36. Jani JC, Peralta CF, Nicolaides KH. Lung-to-head ratio: a need to unify the technique. Ultrasound Obstet Gynecol. 2012;39(1):2-6.
37. Jobe AH, Kamath-Rayne BD. Fetal lung development and surfactant. Scientific Basis of Perinatal, 7th edition. 2014;15:175-77.
38. Kane SC, Ancona E, Reidy KL, Palma-Dias R. The Utility of the Congenital Pulmonary Airway Malformation-Volume Ratio in the Assessment of Fetal Echogenic Lung Lesions: A Systematic Review. Fetal Diagn Ther. 2020;47:171-81.
39. Keller RL, Glidden DV, Paek BW, Goldstein RB, Feldstein VA, Callen PW, et al. The lung-to-head ratio and fetoscopic temporary tracheal occlusion: prediction of survival in severe left congenital diaphragmatic hernia. Ultrasound Obstet Gynecol. 2003;21(3):244-9.
40. Kohl T, Van de Vondel P, Stressig R, Wartenberg HC, Heep A, Keiner S, et al. Percutaneous fetoscopic laser decompression of congenital high airway obstruction syndrome (CHAOS)

from laryngeal atresia via a single trocar current technical constraints and potential solutions for future interventions. Fetal Diagn Ther. 2009;25(1):67-71.

41. Kunisaki SM, Barnewolt CE, Estroff JA, Ward VL, Nemes LP, Fauza DO, et al. Large fetal congenital cystic adenomatoid malformations: growth trends and patient survival. J Pediatr Surg. 2007;42(2):404-10.
42. Lawrence KM, Monos S, Adams S, Herkert L, Peranteau WH, Munson DA, et al. Inhaled nitric oxide is associated with improved oxygenation in a subpopulation of infants with congenital diaphragmatic hernia and pulmonary hypertension. J Pediatr. 2020;219:167-72.
43. Levine D, Jennings R, Barnewolt C, Mehta T, Wilson J, Wong G. Progressive fetal bronchial obstruction caused by a bronchogenic cyst diagnosed using prenatal MR imaging. AJR. 2001;176(1):49-52.
44. Liggins GC. Growth of the fetal lung. J Dev Physiol. 1984;6(3):237-48.
45. Logan JW, Rice HE, Goldberg RN, Cotton CM. Congenital diaphragmatic hernia: a systematic review and summary of best-evidence practice strategies. J Perinatol. 2007;27(9):535-49.
46. Maki E, Oh K, Rogers S, Sohaey R. Imaging and differential diagnosis of suprarenal masses in the fetus. J Ultrasound Med. 2014;33(5): 895-904.
47. Mallmann MR, Geipel A, Bludau M, Matil K, Gottschalk I, Hoopmann M, et al. Bronchopulmonary sequestration with massive pleural effusion: pleuroamniotic shunting vs intrafetal vascular laser ablation. Ultrasound Obstet Gynecol. 2014;44(4):441-6.
48. Martínez JM, Prat J, Gómez O, Crispi F, Bennasar M, Puerto B, et al. Decompression through tracheobronchial endoscopy of bronchial atresia presenting as massive pulmonary tumor: a new indication for fetoscopic surgery. Fetal Diagn Ther. 2013;33(1):69-74.
49. Maurin S, Hery G, Bourliere B, Potier A, Guys JM, De Lagausie P. Bronchogenic cyst: Clinical course from antenatal diagnosis to postnatal thoracoscopic resection. J Minim Access Surg. 2013;9(1):25-8.
50. Mon RA, Johnson KN, Ladino-Torres M, Heider A, Mychaliska GB, Treadwell MC, et al. Diagnostic accuracy of imaging studies in congenital lung malformations. Arch Dis Child Fetal Neonatal Ed. 2019;104(4):F372-7.
51. Moore KL, Persaud TVN. The developing human: clinically oriented embryology, 7th edition. Philadelphia, PA: Saunders; 2002.
52. Paladini D, Volpe P. Ultrasound of Congenital Fetal Anomalies: Differential Diagnosis and Prognostic Indicators, 2nd edition. Boca Raton, IL, USA: Taylor and Francis; 2007.
53. Peranteau WH, Boelig MM, Khalek N, Moldenhauer JS, Martinez-Poyer J, Hedrick HL, et al. Effect of single and multiple courses of maternal betamethasone on prenatal congenital lung lesion growth and fetal survival. J Pediatr Surg. 2016;51(1):28-32.
54. Priest JR, Williams GM, Hill DA, Dehner LP, Jaffé A. Pulmonary cysts in early childhood and the risk of malignancy. Pediatr Pulmonol. 2009;44(1):14-30.
55. Riley JS, Urwin JW, Oliver ER, Coleman BG, Khalek N, Moldenhauer JS, et al. Prenatal growth characteristics and pre/postnatal management of bronchopulmonary sequestrations. J Pediatr Surg. 2018;53(2):265-9.
56. Roybal JL, Liechty KW, Hedrick HL, Bebbington MW, Johnson MP, Coleman BG, et al. Predicting the severity of congenital high airway obstruction syndrome. J Pediatr Surg. 2010;45(8): 1633-9.
57. Ruano R, da Silva MM, Salustiano EM, Kilby MD, Tannuri U, Zugaib M. Percutaneous laser ablation under ultrasound guidance for fetal hyperechogenic microcystic lung lesions with hydrops: a single center cohort and a literature review. Prenat Diagn. 2012;32(12): 1127-32.
58. Ruano R, Joubin L, Sonigo P, Benachi A, Aubry MC, Thalabard JC, et al. Fetal lung volume estimated by 3-dimensional ultrasonography and magnetic resonance imaging in cases with isolated congenital diaphragmatic hernia. J Ultrasound Med. 2004;23(3):353-8.
59. Ruano R, Ramalho AS, Cardoso AK, Moise K Jr, Zugaib M. Prenatal diagnosis and natural history of fetuses presenting with pleural effusion. Prenat Diagn. 2011;31(5):496-9.
60. Saadai P, Jelin EB, Nijagal A, Schecter SC, Hirose S, MacKenzie TC. Long-term outcomes after fetal therapy for congenital high-airway obstructive syndrome. J Pediatr Surg. 2012;47(6):1095-100.
61. Sepulveda W. Perinatal imaging in bronchopulmonary sequestration. J Ultrasound Med. 2009;28(1):89-94.
62. Skandalakis JE, Gray SW, Symbas P. The trachea and the lung. In: Skandalakis JE, Gray SW (Eds). Embryology for Surgeons, 3rd edition. Baltimore, Md: Williams & Wilkins; 1994. pp. 414-50.
63. Stocker JT. Congenital pulmonary airway malformation: a new name for and an expanded classification of congenital cystic adenomatoid malformation of the lung. Symposium 24: non-neoplastic lung disease. Histopathology. 2002;41(suppl 2):424-30.

64. Victoria T, Bebbington MW, Danzer E, Flake AW, Johnson MP, Dinan D, et al. Use of magnetic resonance imaging in prenatal prognosis of the fetus with isolated left congenital diaphragmatic hernia. Prenat Diagn. 2012;32(8): 715-23.
65. Vijayaraghavan SB, Rao PS, Selvarasu CD, Rao TM. Prenatal sonographic features of intralobar bronchopulmonary sequestration. J Ultrasound Med. 2003;22(5):541-4.
66. Vogel M, Mc Elhinney DB, Marcus E, Morash D, Jennings RW, Tworetzky W. Significance and outcome of left heart hypoplasia in fetal congenital diaphragmatic hernia. Ultrasound Obstet Gynecol. 2010;35(3):310-7.
67. Vu L, Tsao KJ, Lee H, Nobuhara K, Farmer D, Harrison M, et al. Characteristics of congenital cystic adenomatoid malformations associated with nonimmune hydrops and outcome. J Pediatr Surg. 2007;42(8):1351-6.
68. Yancey MK, Richards DS. Antenatal sonographic findings associated with unilateral pulmonary agenesis. Obstet Gynecol. 1993;81(5 pt 2):847-9.
69. Yinon Y, Kelly E, Ryan G. Fetal pleural effusions. Best Pract Res Clin Obstet Gynaecol. 2008;22(1):77-96.
70. Zamora IJ, Sheikh F, Cassady CI, Olutoye OO, Mehollin-Ray AR, Ruano R, et al. Fetal MRI lung volumes are predictive of perinatal outcomes in fetuses with congenital lung masses. J Pediatr Surg. 2014;49(6):853-8.
71. Zeidan S, Gorincour G, Potier A, Ughetto F, Dubus JC, Chrestian MA, et al. Congenital lung malformation: evaluation of prenatal and postnatal radiological findings. Respirology. 2009;14(7):1005-11.

12
CHAPTER

Abnormalities of Cardiovascular System

Binodini M Chauhan

INTRODUCTION

Fetal heart is the most common organ affected by anomalous development with an incidence of 8–9 per 1,000 live births. The term "congenital heart disease (CHD)" refers primarily to anatomical malformations of the heart, which arise during cardiac embryogenesis prior to 8 weeks postconception. Cardiac anomalies are the most common cause of death from an anomaly in the neonatal period. Despite its obvious importance, the fetal cardiac evaluation remains an area of weakness in obstetric ultrasound examination. Efforts should be directed toward enhancing the prenatal detection of CHD. Targeted education and training have shown to improve the detection of CHD. High level of suspicion for the presence of CHD and attention to anatomic details is vital for improving the detection and thereby reducing the neonatal morbidity and mortality.

To increase the detection of cardiac anomalies, an organized approach for defining the anatomy of the heart is essential and evaluation of heart in sequential fashion, beginning from below the diaphragm and ending at the thoracic inlet.

EMBRYOLOGY OF THE HUMAN HEART

Cardiovascular system is the first system to develop due to the ever-increasing metabolic demands of the growing embryo. It is active by the beginning of the 4th week—when the placenta is unable to meet the requirements of the growing embryo.

Primitive Heart Tube (Figs. 1 and 2)

The development of the heart begins with the formation of the *primitive heart tube* following the folding of the embryo during the end of the 3rd week. Firstly, *lateral folding* creates the heart tube by bringing together two precursor regions, then cephalocaudal folding positions the heart tube in the future thorax. The cephalic portion of the tube bends ventrally, caudally, and to the right. The atrial (caudal) portion shifts dorsocranially and to the left. This bending creates the cardiac loop and is completed by day 28. The atrial portion initially a paired structure outside the pericardial cavity forms a common atrium and is incorporated into the pericardial cavity. The atrioventricular junction remains narrow and forms the atrioventricular canal. This atrioventricular canal connects the common atrium and the early embryonic ventricle.

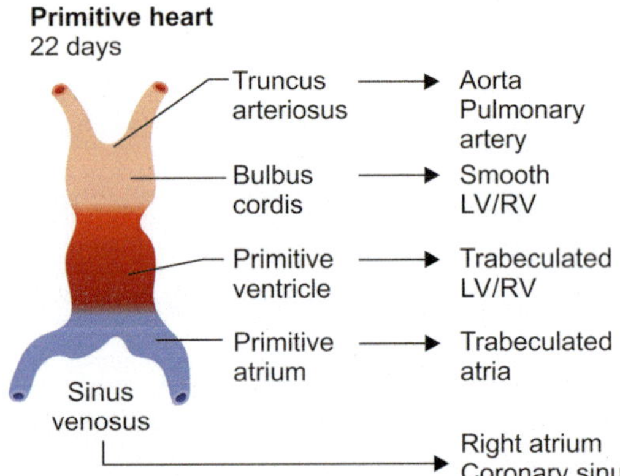

Fig. 1: Formation of a single heart tube from two paired tubular structures. Ventral view at approximately 22 days showing almost complete fusion.

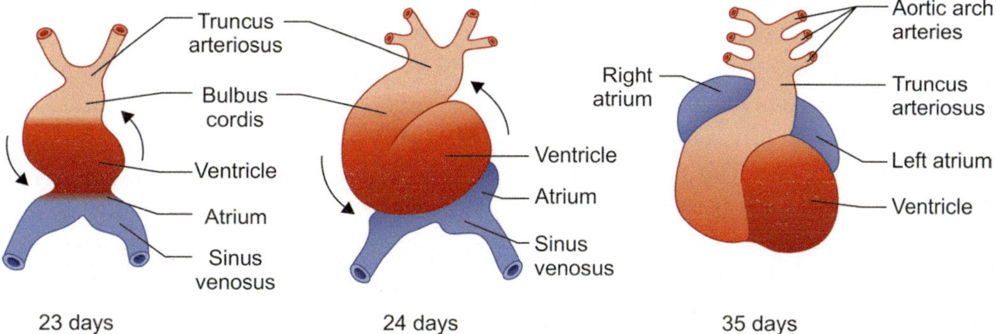

Fig. 2: Formation of atrioventriculobulbar loop at approximately 23–24 days. As this loop is formed, a common atrium is formed and enters the pericardial cavity.

The heart tube consists of three layers:

1. The endocardium, forming the internal endothelial lining of the heart
2. The myocardium, forming the muscular wall
3. The epicardium or visceral pericardium, covering the outside of the tube. This outer layer is responsible for the formation of the coronary arteries.

From superior to inferior, the primitive heart tube is comprised of *six regions*:

1. Aortic roots (arterial poles)
2. Truncus arteriosus
3. Bulbus cordis
4. Ventricle
5. Atrium
6. *Sinus venosus (venous poles)*:
   - The heart tube continues to elongate, and begins *looping* at around day 23 of development and produces a shape that is much closer to the developed heart.
   - Atria
   - At the 4th week, the *sinus venosus* receives venous blood from the right and left sinus horns and empties into the primitive atrium. As the venous return shifts to the right side of the heart, the left sinus horn recedes and forms the coronary sinus (responsible for the drainage of venous blood from the heart itself). The enlarged *right sinus horn* is absorbed by the growing right atrium and eventually forms part of the inferior vena cava.
   - In the left atrium, the four pulmonary veins are incorporated into the left atrium, forming the smooth inflow portion of the left atrium.
   - Aortic arches will form the major vessels that exit the heart.

Septation of the Heart

Septation of the heart occurs when endocardial cushion that develops in the atrioventricular region expands to divide the heart.

Atrial Septum

The septation of the primitive atrium involves the formation of two septa—the septum primum and septum secundum and three "holes", ostium primum, ostium secundum, and foramen ovale.

Ventricular Septum

The *interventricular septum* has two components—muscular and membranous.

The *muscular portion* forms much of the septum and grows up from the floor of the ventricles toward the fused endocardial cushions, but a small gap, the primary interventricular foramen, remains.

This gap is filled by the membranous portion of the interventricular septum, which is comprised of connective tissue derived from endocardial cushions.

The bulbus cordis is narrow except for its proximal third, which forms the trabeculated part of right ventricle. The mid portion—the conus cordis—will form the outflow tracts of both ventricles. The distal part of bulbus cordis—the truncus arteriosus—will form the roots and proximal portion of aorta.

The high-risk conditions where the incidence of congenital cardiac defect is high and expert fetal cardiac evaluation and fetal echo should be done:

- *Fetal*:
  - Abnormal four-chamber view
  - Intrauterine growth restriction (IUGR)
  - Extracardiac abnormality
  - NIH
  - Increased nuchal translucency (NT)
  - In vitro fertilization (IVF)/intracytoplasmic sperm injection (ICSI)
  - Rhythm abnormality
  - Abnormal cardiac axis
  - Monochorionic twin pregnancy
- *Maternal:*
  - Advanced maternal age
  - Maternal obesity
  - Diabetes mellitus
  - Maternal CHD
  - Systemic lupus erythematosus (SLE)
  - Infection
  - Teratogenic drugs exposure [lithium, hydantoin, valproic acid, isotretinoin, angiotensin-converting enzyme (ACE) inhibitors, ethanol, indomethacin, selective serotonin reuptake inhibitors (SSRIs)]
- *Familial:*
  - Paternal/sibling/family h/o CHD
  - Genetic
  - Chromosomal

International Society of Ultrasound in Obstetrics and Gynecology (ISUOG) protocol—the transverse sweep—caudal to cranial.

Situs → four chamber → outflows (LVOT and RVOT) → 3VV → 3V trachea view.

TIMINGS

The cardiac screening examination is performed optimally between 18 and 22 weeks menstrual age. Some anomalies may be identified during the late 1st and early 2nd trimesters of pregnancy, especially when increased nuchal translucency thickness is identified.

TECHNICAL FACTORS

Ultrasound Transducer

Higher-frequency probes will improve the likelihood of detecting subtle defects, at the expense of reduced acoustic penetration. The highest possible transducer frequency should be used for all examinations. Harmonic imaging may provide improved images, especially for patients with increased maternal abdominal wall thickness.

Zoom and Cine-loop

Images should be magnified until the heart fills at least one-third to one-half of the screen. The cine- loop feature should be used to assist the real-time evaluation of normal cardiac structures, for example, to confirm movement of heart valve leaflets throughout the cardiac cycle. Image magnification and use of cine-loop may help in identifying abnormalities.

The step-by-step analysis is crucial for fetal cardiac examination:

- Identification of the fetal position
- Position of the heart in relation to the body
- Number of chambers and their connections
- Rhythm.

Cardiac Position (Figs. 3A and B)

In fetal thoracic cavity, sternum lies anteriorly, vertebra posteriorly, and ribs on the lateral

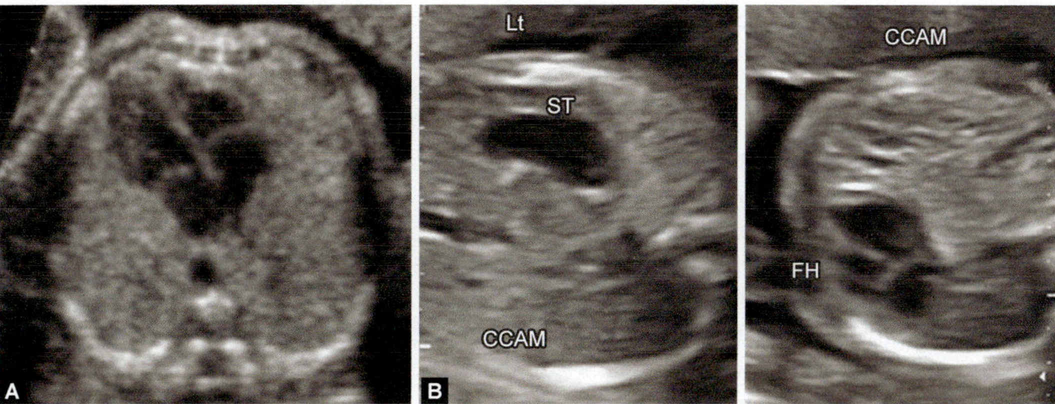

Figs. 3A and B: *Cardiac position:* (A) Transverse image through fetal chest showing the normal orientation of the fetal heart (FH), with the apex pointing to the left. The bulk of the heart occupies the left side of the chest; (B) Dextroposition due to left-sided congenital pulmonary adenomatoid malformation (CPAM) of the lung. The stomach (ST) is seen normally located in the abdomen (to differentiate from left-sided congenital diaphragmatic hernia).
(CCAM: congenital cystic adenomatoid malformation)

side. Heart occupies central region with bilateral lungs occupying most of the thoracic cavity. Two-thirds of the heart along with apex lies on the left of midline and one-third of heart including the base lies on the right of the midline. Mediastinal shift occurs when there is any space-occupying lesion or pathology in one hemithorax such as congenital pulmonary airway malformation (CPAM), pleural effusion, CDH, etc. Unilateral pulmonary aplasia/hypoplasia can cause ipsilateral shift in mediastinum. This shift of heart is known as dextrocardia, if the shift is toward the right side of mediastinum and similarly levocardia, if shift is toward left of mediastinum. Cardiac position in middle of the mediastinum is known as mesocardia. And, if the heart is found to be outside the thoracic cavity, it is known as ectopia cordis. It should be noted that above-mentioned abnormalities are independent of cardia axis, situs, cardiac anatomy, or chamber organization and, therefore, they should be reported separately from position.

Situs (Figs. 4A and B)

Cardiac situs is first critical step in fetal echocardiography. It could identify a cardiac defect ranging from simple ventricular septal

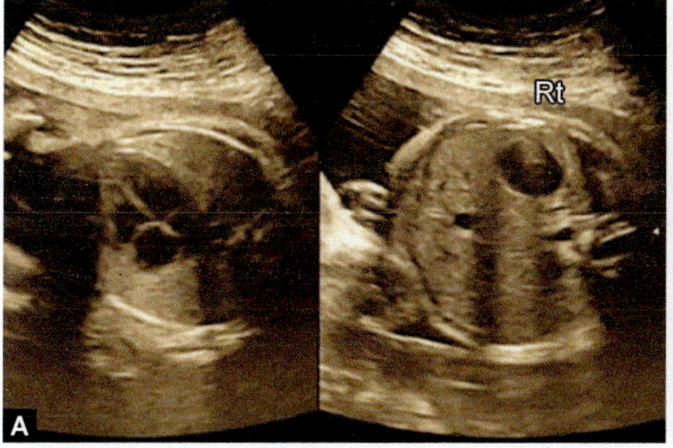

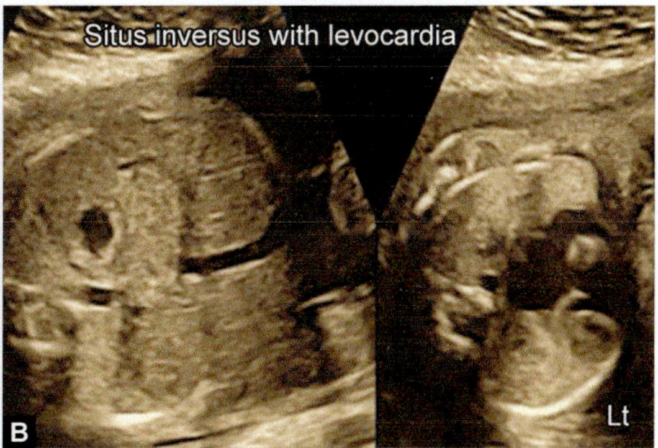

Figs. 4A and B: *Cardiac situs: Normal cardiac Situs*: (A) Levocardia with situs solitus. Apex of the heart is to the left, stomach is on the left; (B) Situs inversus with levocardia. Heart is located in normal position in the chest and is anomalous, abdominal situs is opposite. The stomach is seen on the right side.

defect (VSD) to a complex cardiac defect. An abnormal situs is associated with a higher incidence of congenital heart defects.

Several methods for determining fetal situs during the ultrasound examination have been described. Cordes, et al., described a technique that involves orienting the transducer in a standardized way so that the fetal head is on the right side of the screen in a fetal sagittal plane as a starting point and then rotating the transducer 90° in clockwise to obtain the caudocranial transverse views.

Another method reported by Bronshtein, et al., is referred to as the right-hand rule for abdominal scanning and the left-hand rule for transvaginal scanning. The palm of the hand corresponds to the face of the fetus, and the examiner holds the hand according to the side of the fetal face; the fetal heart and stomach are shown by the examiner's thumb.

The upper abdominal transverse section (AC) is a compulsory view in assessment of situs and cardiac abnormalities. Liver to right, stomach to the left, descending aorta to the left, and inferior vena cava (IVC) to the right and anterior to the aorta are the normal spatial arrangements in this view. Comparing this AC view with 4C view in thoracic chamber will give idea regarding spatial rearrangements if any. Position of stomach can be confusing sometimes, so it is generally agreed that the positions of the aorta and inferior vena cava below the diaphragm are more reliable criteria for the determination of right or left isomerism than the location of the stomach in the abdomen.

Abnormalities recognized in this section are:

- *Situs inversus totalis*: Mirror image arrangement.
- *Heterotaxy*: Stomach to the right (heart and stomach on opposite sides), close to spine, midline large liver, and absence of spleen. Occasionally, the stomach is found in the midline in heterotaxy.
- *Right atrial isomerism*: Juxtaposed IVC (IVC anterior and on the same side of the aorta) is seen.
- *Left atrial isomerism*: Absent or interrupted IVC is seen along with azygos prominence.

On Ultrasound

Ultrasound features are described in **Table 1**.

Cardiac Axis (Figs. 5A and B)

Fetal cardiac axis is examined in normal four-chamber view.

A line is drawn from the spine to the anterior chest wall dividing the chest into equal halves. The cardiac axis is the angle that the interventricular septum makes with this line.

The normal cardiac axis is 45° ± 20° left to the midline at any gestational age.

Left axis rotation is associated with outflow tract anomalies (tetralogy of Fallot), as also in Ebstein anomaly and coarctation of aorta most

TABLE 1: Ultrasound features in situs abnormalities.

Situs	*Right side*	*Left side*
Solitus (normal)	Morphologic right atrium Major hepatic lobe	Morphologic left atrium Stomach
	Inferior vena cava	Descending aorta
	Trilobed lung	Bilobed lung
	Short eparterial bronchus	Long hyparterial bronchus
Inversus	Morphologic left atrium	Morphologic right atrium
	Stomach	Major hepatic lobe
	Descending aorta	Inferior vena cava
	Bilobed lung	Trilobed lung
	Long hyparterial bronchus	Short eparterial bronchus
Ambiguous (heterotaxy)	Variable	Variable

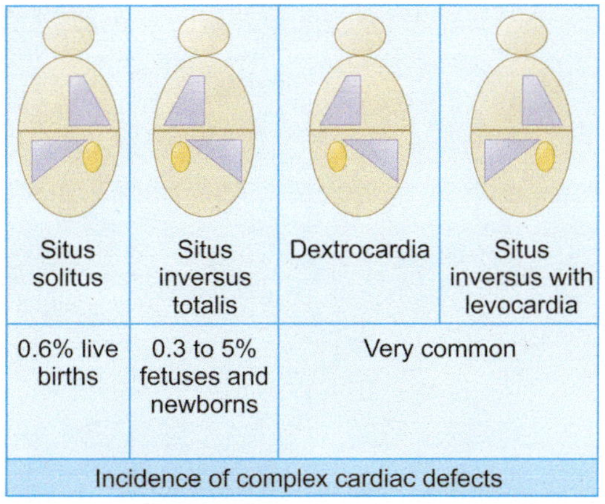

commonly. Whereas right axis deviation is associated more commonly with double outlet right ventricle (DORV) and atrioventricular septal defect (AVSD). Fetuses with large abdominal wall defects are also observed to be having cardiac axis deviations such as large omphalocele and gastroschisis.

Cardiac Size (Figs. 6A and B)

Cardiac size is most often assessed subjectively. Objective assessment may be done by the cardiothoracic (CT) ratio. Area CT ratio >35% and perimeter CT ratio >50% indicate cardiomegaly. Cardiomegaly could occur in valvular regurgitation (e.g., Ebstein anomaly), dilated cardiomyopathy, cardiac failure due to fetal acidemia, anemia, or arrhythmia.

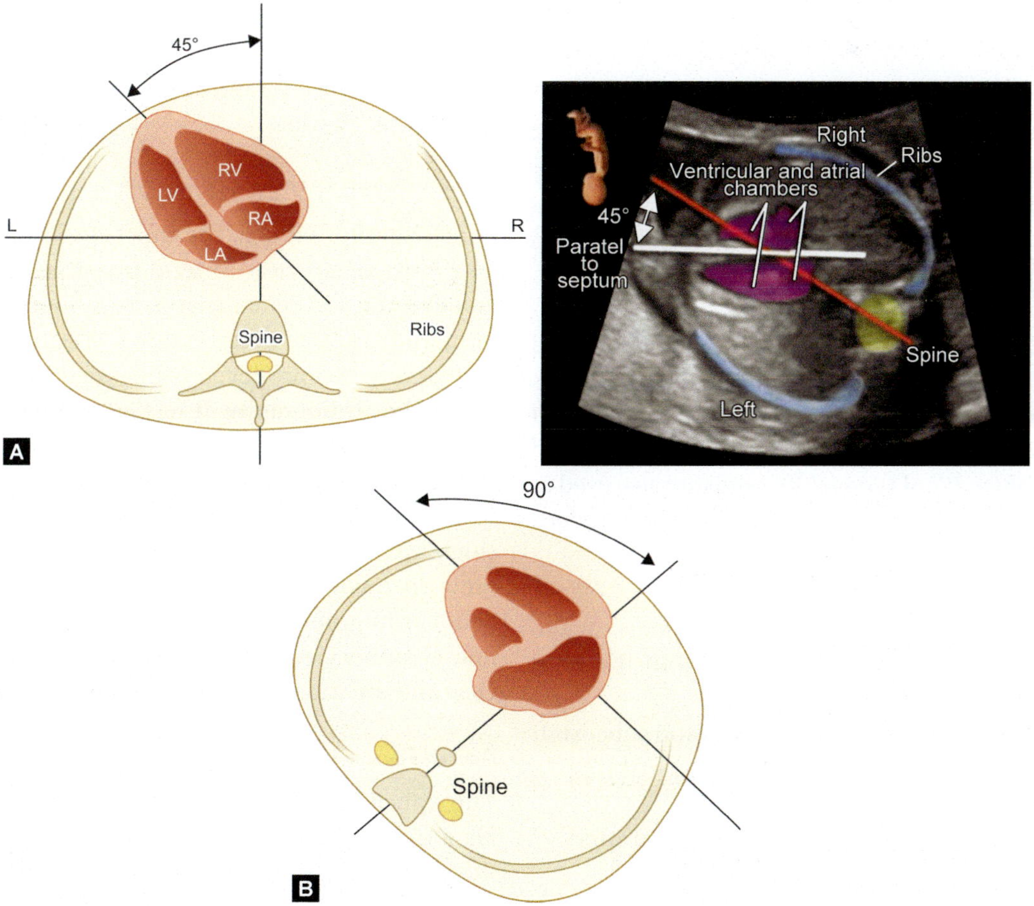

Figs. 5A and B: *Cardiac axis*: (A) Normal heart with cardiac axis of 45°. Measurement of the cardiac axis from a four-chamber view plane of the fetal chest with the corresponding plane on ultrasound; (B) Left axis deviation, abnormal cardiac axis (nearly 90°) in a case of cardiac anomaly.

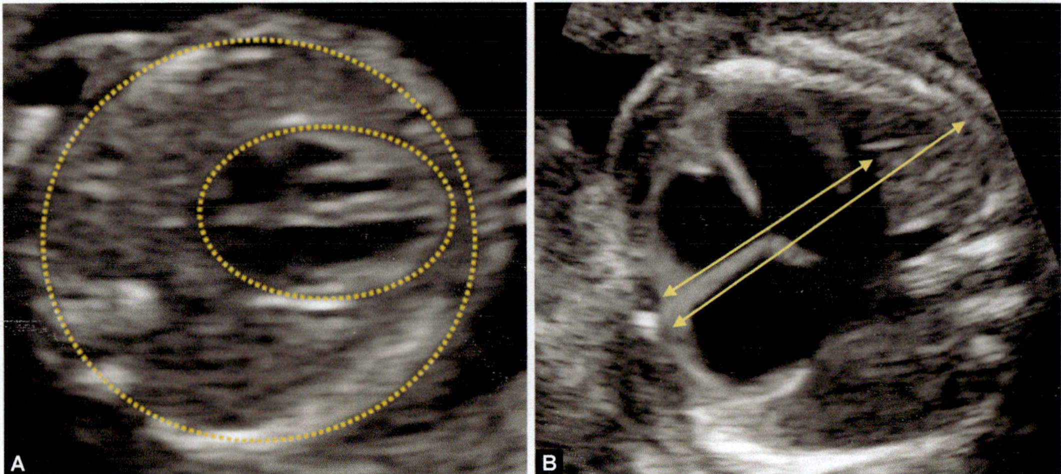

Figs. 6A and B: *Cardiac size*: Figure A shows normal cardiac size occupying one-third of the thoracic cavity. Fetal cardiothoracic circumference is obtained as a ratio of cardiac to chest circumference at the level of four-chamber view. Figure B shows cardiomegaly.

Cardiac Symmetry

Abnormal size of cardiac chambers as well as outlets is early indicator in abnormal cardiac development. The size and growth rate of fetal cardiac structures are evaluated with the help of normal percentile growth curves, which are based on menstrual health.

Now, Z-scores are also available for fetal echocardiography based on FL or GA. This allows better quantification of individual measurements above or below expected values. PA:AO and LV:RV ratios are also used as screening tests for congenital cardiac anomaly.

CARDIAC EXAMINATION

The echocardiographic views necessary to perform complete evaluation of the fetal cardiac system includes:

- *Four-chamber view*: Apical and subcostal/lateral
- Long axis view of the aorta
- Long axis view of the pulmonary artery
- Short axis view of the ventricles
- Short axis view of great arteries
- View of arch of aorta
- View of ductal arch
- View of superior and inferior vena cava
- Three-vessel view and three-vessel trachea view.

Four-chamber Views (Figs. 7A and B)

Four-chamber view is the most important and most basic view of fetal heart, which has maintained its consistency to identify numerous cardiac abnormalities. It was the first view to be introduced while establishing fetal echocardiography. It has advantage of getting information about atria, ventricles, arteriovenous connections, and interatrial septum as well as interventricular septum in single view. Because of this, it is an essential view in basic as well as advanced fetal echocardiography. There are two different four-chamber views—the apical four-chamber view and the subcostal four-chamber view.

Apical Four-Chamber View

The apical four-chamber view is obtained via a transverse view of the fetal chest, with the apex of the heart pointing directly toward or away from the transducer. In the apical four-chamber view, the interventricular and interatrial septa are parallel to the transducer. From this projection, all four heart chambers

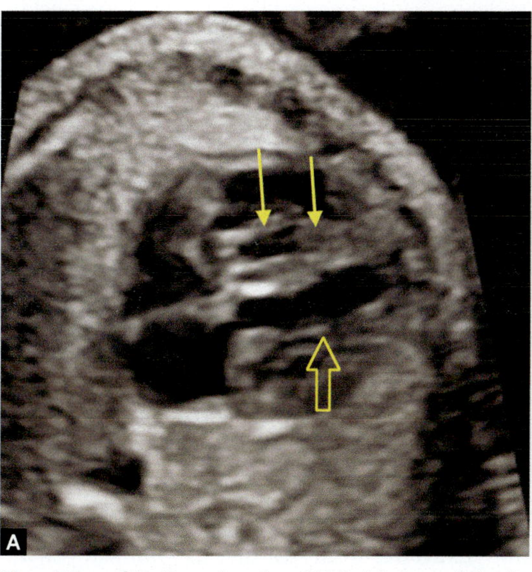
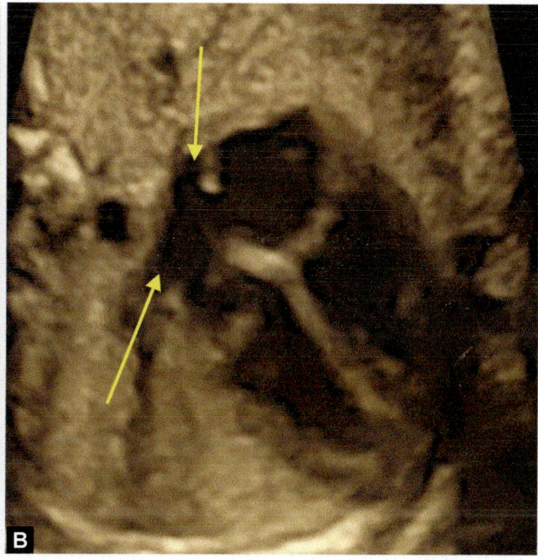

Figs. 7A and B: *Four chamber*: (A) Axial view of the fetal heart at the level of four-chamber view. Note in the right ventricle (RV), the apical insertion of chordate tendineae of the tricuspid valve (TV) to the RV wall and the apex of the heart (two solid arrows). Open arrow in LV points to the free wall attachment of the papillary muscle of the mitral valve (MV); (B) Basal view of the fetal heart showing the right atrium (RA), left atrium (LA), right ventricle (RV), left ventricle (LV), and interventricular septum. The right and left inferior pulmonary veins (solid arrows) can be seen entering the LA posteriorly on either side of descending aorta.

BOX 1: Assessment of fetal situs/laterality and the four-chamber view.

Situs and general aspects:
- Fetal laterality (identify right and left sides of fetus): Stomach and heart on left
- Heart occupies a third of thoracic area: Majority of heart in left chest
- Cardiac axis (apex) points to left by 45°±20°: Four chambers present
- Regular cardiac rhythm: No pericardial effusion

Atrial chambers:
- Two atria, approximately equal in size
- Foramen ovale flap in left atrium
- Atrial septum primum present (near to crux)
- Pulmonary veins entering left atrium

Ventricular chambers:
- Two ventricles, approximately equal in size
- No ventricular wall hypertrophy
- Moderator band at right ventricular apex
- Ventricular septum intact (apex to crux)

Atrioventricular junction and valves ***(Fig. 8)***:
- Intact cardiac crux
- Two atrioventricular valves open and move freely
- Differential offsetting: Tricuspid valve leaflet inserts on ventricular septum closer to cardiac apex than does mitral valve

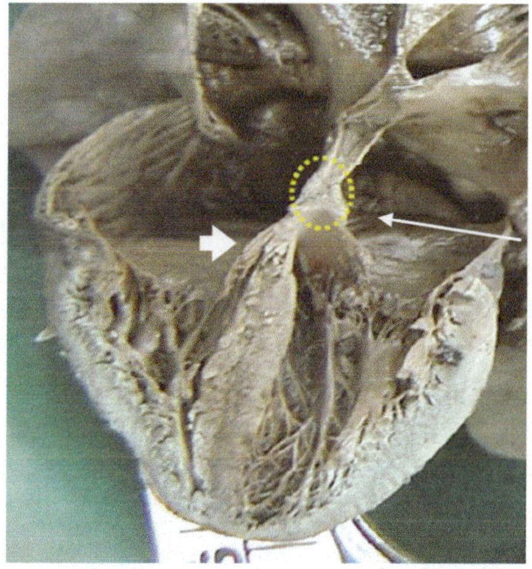

Fig. 8: It is the pathologic specimen image showing the crux of the heart (circle). The crux (center) of the heart is point at which the atrial septum meets the ventricular septum and at which the atrioventricular valves also insert. Note the more apical insertion of tricuspid valve (short arrow) resulting in an offset.

can be visualized. The apical four-chamber view is not optimal for interrogating the interventricular septum. The IVS is parallel to the ultrasound beam, and this may result in an artifactual dropout of echoes at the level of the membranous IVS simulating a "pseudo" septal defect. The mitral and tricuspid valves are evaluated optimally in this view because the angle of insonation of the sound beam is perpendicular to the AV valves.

Subcostal Four-chamber View

The subcostal four-chamber view is obtained by imaging the fetal chest in a transverse projection from the anterior chest wall and angling the transducer slightly cephalad. In this view, the interventricular septum is perpendicular to the transducer and is the best view to evaluate the Interventricular septum for septal defect. As with the apical four-chamber view, this view also allows identification and comparison of both atria and ventricles. M-mode measurements of the ventricles can be obtained in this view by placing the M-mode cursor perpendicular to the septum at the level of AV valves. It is also possible to evaluate an arrhythmia by placing the M-mode cursor through an atrial wall and a ventricular wall simultaneously.

The "crux" or center of the heart is the point at which the atrial septum meets the ventricular septum and at which the atrioventricular valves also insert. The septal leaflet of the tricuspid valve is attached to the septum slightly more apically than the mitral (so-called differential insertion) creating an offset on the right side. This appearance is more readily appreciated in the apical than in the lateral or subcostal four-chamber view.

Long Axis View of Aorta: Left Ventricular Outflow Tract (Figs. 9A to D)

A slight angulation from the subcostal four-chamber view toward the fetal right shoulder will result in visualization of a long axis view of proximal aorta. In this view, septoaortic continuity, i.e., continuity of the anterior wall of aorta with the interventricular septum and the posterior wall of aorta with the anterior leaflet of mitral valve can be ascertained. The aorta at this level normally courses anteriorly and the aortic root can be measured in this view at the level of the valve.

Uses for Long Axis View of the Aorta

- Evaluate continuity of anterior aortic root with interventricular septum
- Evaluate continuity of posterior aortic root with anterior leaflet of mitral valve
- Evaluate interventricular septum for ventricular septal defect
- Evaluate aortic valve above and below valve (if Doppler angle is appropriate)
- Evaluate arrhythmias by placing pulsed Doppler sample volume between aortic valve and mitral valve
- Evaluate arrhythmias by placing M-mode cursor through right ventricle and left atrium.

Long Axis View of Pulmonary Artery: Right Ventricular Outflow Tract

The right ventricular outflow tract (RVOT) can be visualized by rotating the transducer further in the direction of the fetal right shoulder. In the normal fetus, this view demonstrates the pulmonary artery coursing cephalad, leftward and posteriorly from the right ventricle. BY angling the transducer from the long axis view of the aorta to the long axis view of the pulmonary artery, the great vessels should "criss-cross", if they are oriented correctly.

Uses for Long Axis View of Pulmonary Artery

- Evaluate the continuity of pulmonary artery with right ventricle
- Doppler imaging of pulmonic valve above and below valve (proximally for pulmonary insufficiency and distally for pulmonary stenosis).

Short Axis View of the Ventricles

A further rightward rotation of the transducer results in a sagittal view of fetal thorax and

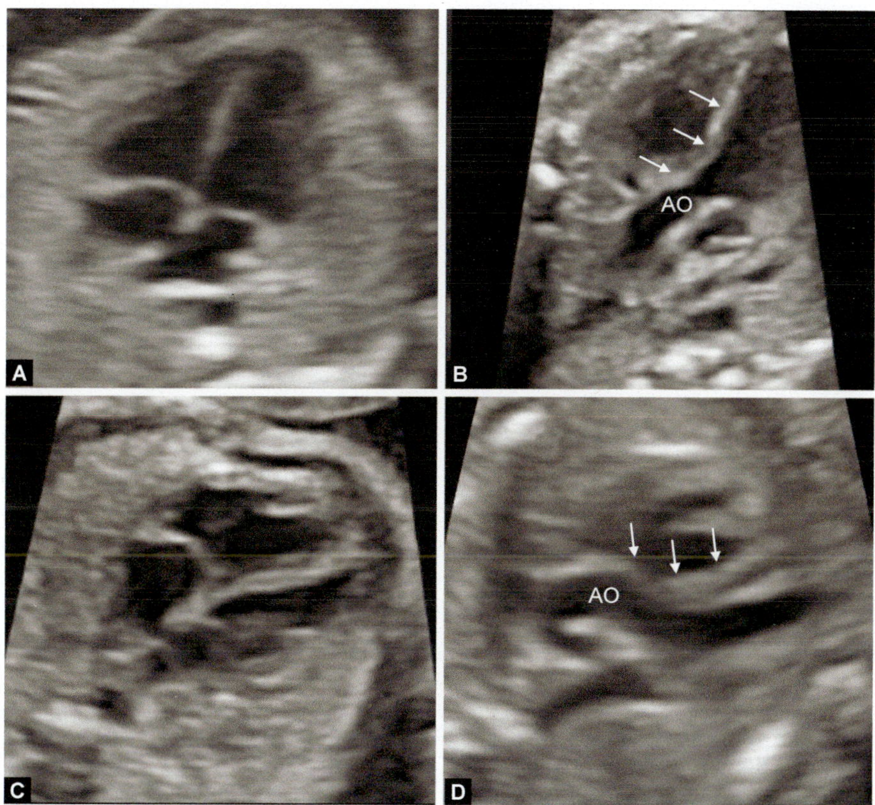

Figs. 9A to D: *Left ventricular outflow tract (LVOT) (five-chamber view)*: (A and B) Parasternal long-axis view of the mid-section of the heart showing the left ventricular outflow tract in apical four chamber (septoaortic continuity seen long arrow); (C and D) Lateral four-chamber and the left ventricular outflow tract. Note the septoaortic continuity (arrows).

a short axis view through the ventricles. The more echogenic moderator band should be apparent near the apex to help identify the right ventricle. The short axis view of the ventricles is useful for obtaining measurements of the ventricular-free walls, interventricular septum for defects, and the chamber size. It is also useful to evaluate the heart wall contractility with M-mode.

Short Axis View of the Great Vessels (Fig. 10)

From the short axis view of the ventricles, the short axis view of the great vessels is obtained by angling the transducer slightly toward the fetal left shoulder. This view is also referred as "circle sausage" view, because the aorta appears as a circular structure and the

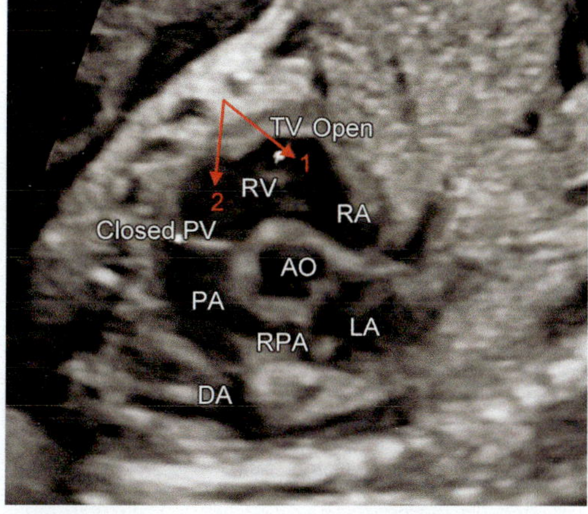

Fig. 10: *Right ventricular outflow tract (RVOT) view*: Figure shows the circle sausage view, RV inflow (1), and outflow (2) are seen in the same plane. The pulmonary artery (PA) is seen, as it crosses over aorta and divides into right pulmonary artery and ductus arteriosus (DA).

pulmonary artery coursing over it. The aortic, pulmonic, and tricuspid valves are usually well visualized in this view. The main pulmonary artery is seen bifurcating into the ductus arteriosus and the right pulmonary artery.

In the normal heart, this short axis view confirms the perpendicular relationship of aorta to pulmonary artery, thereby excluding certain defects such as transposition of great arteries (TGA) and truncus arteriosus (common arterial trunk).

Uses for Short Axis View of the Great Vessels

- Evaluate relationship of aorta to pulmonary artery
- Measure the aortic and pulmonic valve size
- Doppler imaging of pulmonic valve proximal and distal to valve
- Doppler imaging of tricuspid valve above and below the valve
- Evaluate arrhythmia by placing M-mode cursor through aorta and left atrium.

View of the Aortic Arch (Figs. 11A and B)

The aortic arch view is obtained from the longitudinal plane of the fetal torso, with the transducer angled from the left shoulder to the right hemithorax. The aortic arch can be differentiated from the ductal arch by identifying the three head and neck vessels arising from its superior aspect (brachiocephalic artery, left common carotid artery, and left subclavian artery). The aortic arch has a rounded "candy cane" appearance.

Uses for Aortic Arch View

- Asses diameter of arch for areas of narrowing
- Doppler imaging of aortic arch from aortic valve to descending aorta for coarctation. Of particular importance is the section of the arch between the origin of left subclavian artery and the insertion of ductus arteriosus called "isthmus", which is the most common site for coarctation to occur
- Confirm antegrade flow.

View of the Ductal Arch (Figs. 12A and B)

The ductal arch view is obtained by returning to a more anteroposterior axis of the thorax. The appearance of the ductal arch is flatter than that of aortic arch and is often referred to as a "hockey stick" appearance. The ductal arch is composed of—pulmonary artery, ductus arteriosus, and descending aorta.

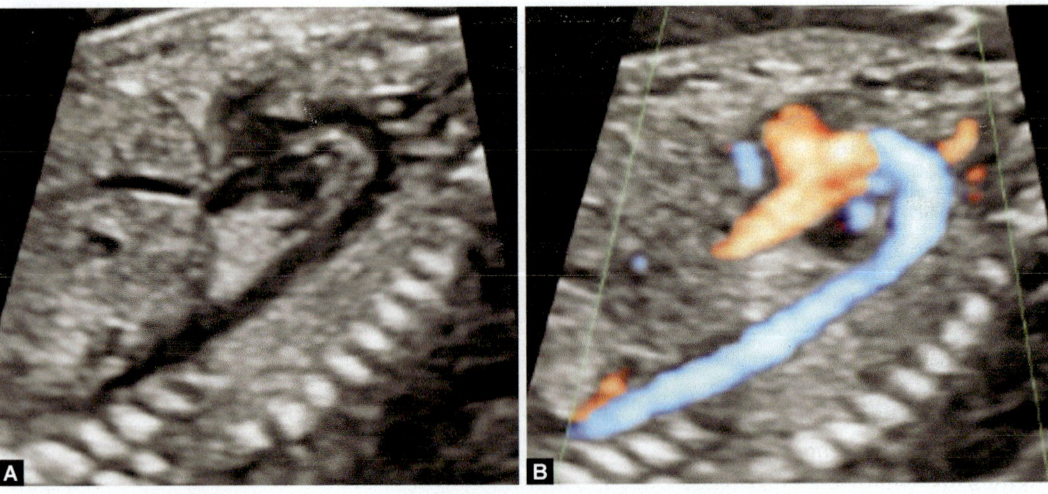

Figs. 11A and B: *The aortic arch (AoA) view*: (A) Aorta arising from the central portion of the chest with an acute circular curvature. The three neck vessels are also seen; (B) AoA view in color Doppler flow with neck vessels.

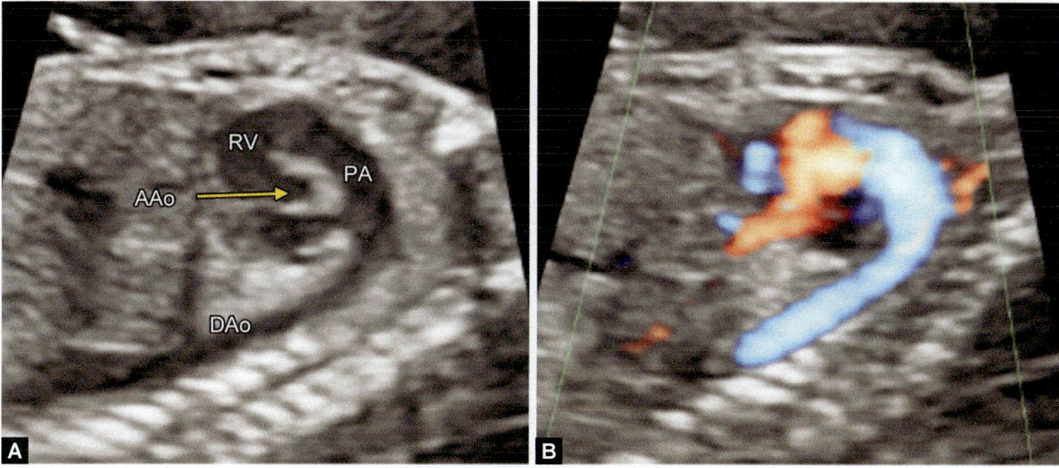

Figs. 12A and B: *The ductal arch view (sagittal approach)*: (A) Ductal arch (DA) view, with spine posterior, the ascending aorta (AAo) (arrow) is seen in the oblique section centrally and the descending aorta (DAo) is seen in its entirety; (B) Ductal arch view in color flow Doppler.

Uses for Ductal Arch View

- Doppler imaging of ductal arch from pulmonary artery to descending aorta
- Confirm antegrade flow
- Quantitative peak systolic velocity (>1.4 m/s) used for diagnosis of ductal constriction.

View of the Inferior Vena Cava and Superior Vena Cava (Figs. 13A and B)

An inferior vena cava and superior vena cava view or right atrial inflow view can be obtained by acquiring an aortic arch view and then sliding the transducer from the left parasagittal chest to the right parasagittal chest. In this view, the inferior vena cava (IVC) and superior vena cava (SVC) can be seen entering the right atrium.

Three-vessel View and Three-vessel Trachea View (Figs. 14A to C)

The three-vessel view is very useful to access the great vessels. It is obtained by acquiring an apical four-chamber view and then sliding the transducer cephalad. In this view, the pulmonary artery at the level of ductus

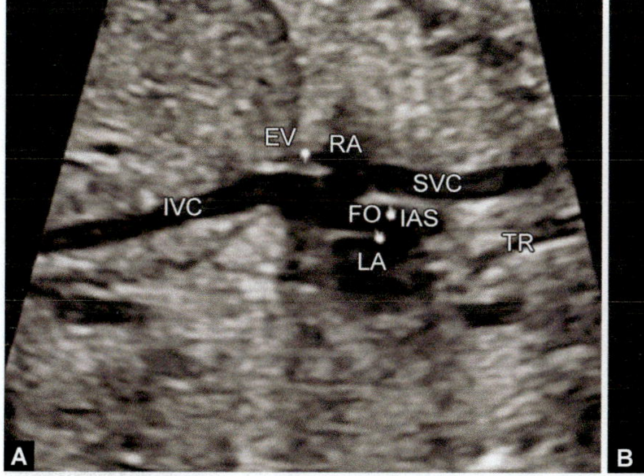

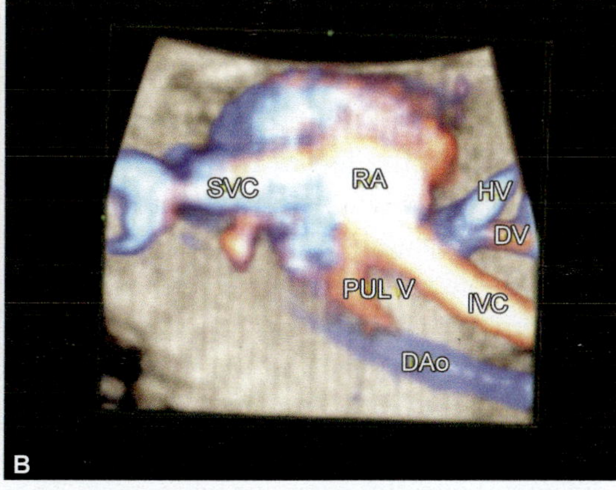

Figs. 13A and B: *Superior vena cava (SVC) and inferior vena cava (IVC):* (A) Para-sagittal view of right atrium showing the Hammock view of inferior and superior vena cava; (B) The SVC and IVC are seen in color Doppler. (RA: right atrium; LA: left atrium; FO: fossa ovalis; IAS: interatrial septum; EV: eustachian valve; TR: tricuspid regurgitation; HV: hepatic vein; DV: ductus venosus; DAo: descending aorta)

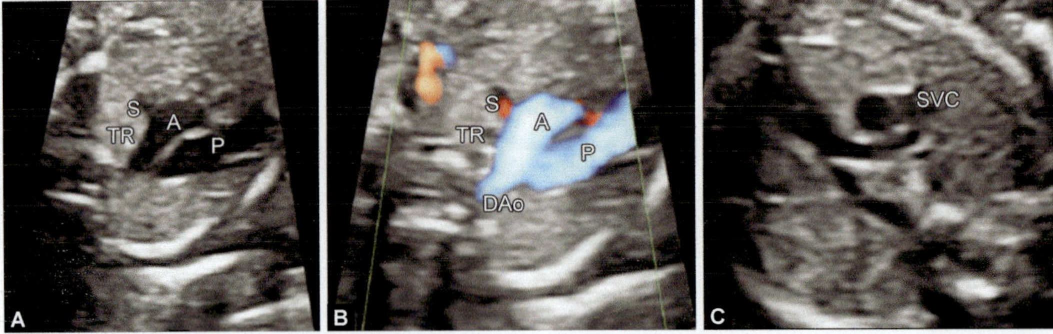

Figs. 14A to C: *Three-vessel trachea (3VT) view:* (A) The 3VT view demonstrating the aortic arch (A) and ductal arch (P) merging together into the descending aorta (DAo). The superior vena cava (SVC) (S) is seen on the right of aortic arch; (B) The 3VT view in color flow with forward color in both great arteries; (C) Three-vessel view of the fetal heart demonstrating the pulmonary artery (PA) with bifurcation, the ascending aorta (AAo) and the SVC in the upper chest arranged in the oblique line, with PA most anterior, SVC most posterior, and ascending aorta in-between. Note the right pulmonary artery (RPA) originates at a right angle and runs behind the AAo and the SVC.

arteriosus, the aortic arch, and the superior vena cava are seen in the same plane from left to right. This allows identification of the two great vessels and a side-by-side comparison of size. Color Doppler imaging in this view will confirm antegrade flow through both outflow tracts in a normal heart. In the normal heart, the pulmonary artery and the aorta lay in a "V" formation, in this plane with the confluence of the V pointing to the posterior thorax.

By moving the transducer even more cephalad, the trachea can also be visualized between aorta and SVC and can be used to determine the situs of aorta. The trachea is usually identified as a hyperechogenic ring surrounding a small fluid-filled space. In normal heart, both the aortic and ductal arches are on the left of trachea. The 3VT view is likely to enable detection of lesions such as coarctation of the aorta, right aortic arch, double aortic arch, and vascular rings. Abnormalities in the number of vessels, orientation of vessels, and the size of vessels can be diagnosed in this view. From left to right, the vessels are the pulmonary artery, the aorta, and the superior vena cava. The pulmonary artery is the most anterior vessel and the superior vena cava is the most posterior. Their relative diameters decrease from left to right, with the pulmonary artery being larger than the aorta, and the aorta larger than the superior vena cava. Typically, certain abnormalities associated with a normal four-chamber view, such as complete transposition of the great arteries, tetralogy of Fallot (TOF), and pulmonary atresia with a ventricular septal defect, are likely to have an abnormal 3V view. The thymus can also be evaluated in this view.

Uses for Three-vessel View

- Identify presence of three vessels, the pulmonary artery, aorta, and SVC from left to right and from anterior to posterior
- Identify "V" configuration of pulmonary artery and aorta
- Identify PA and AO to the left of trachea
- Subjective comparison of size of both great vessels
- Color Doppler imaging will confirm same direction flow in both great arteries.

Identification of Chambers

Left Atrium

- Posterior and close to spine
- Descending aorta lies between left atrium and spine
- Flap valve of foramen ovale opens in left atrium

- Four pulmonary veins open in left atrium
- Left atrium (LA) appendage is narrow, finger-like
- Anterior and posterior portions are smooth.

Right Atrium

- Right atrium (RA) is seen on the right and anterior of LA
- RA appendage is pyramidal with broad base
- SVC, IVC, and coronary sinus open in right atrium
- Eustachian valve is also seen in RA
- Post-wall of RA is smooth and anterior is trabeculated.

Ventricles

- RV to LV ratio—1 in mid-pregnancy
- RV increases with advancing gestation 1.3:1
- Ventricles are inferior and to the left of atria
- Left ventricle is posterior
- Right ventricle is anterior.

Anatomic Characteristic of Right Ventricle

- Inlet and apical regions are heavily trabeculated
- Most anterior chamber, located below sternum
- Outlet (infundibulum) is smooth
- Moderator band located in apical region
- Tricuspid atrioventricular valve
- TV is more apically inserted on the septum than MV
- Ventricular wall receives direct chordae insertions
- Three papillary muscles.

Anatomic Characteristics of Left Ventricle (Fig. 15)

- Conical in shape, posterolateral location with smooth inlet
- Bicuspid atrioventricular (mitral) valve
- Close anatomic relationship of the inlet and outlet (mitral and aortic valves)
- Two prominent papillary muscles that insert into the free ventricular wall
- No moderator band
- Ventricular wall receives no direct chordae tendineae insertions.

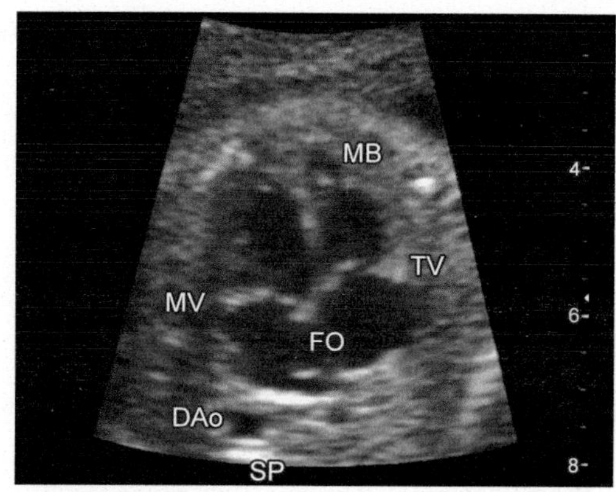

Fig. 15: Apical four-chamber of the fetal heart with left atrium (LA), right atrium (RA), left ventricle (LV), and right ventricle (RV). At the apex of the heart in right ventricle, the typical thickened moderator band (MB) is recognized. Between both atria, the inter-atrial septum is seen formed but septum primum and secundum. Foramen ovale (FO) is an opening in the midportion of the septum secundum. Note the more apical insertion of the tricuspid valve (TV) in relation to mitral valve (MV).

Limitations of Four-chamber View

- Allows display of only the AV connections
- Does not allow recognition of aorta and pulmonary artery
- Will not define complexes of TGA, TOF, DORV, and truncus arteriosus
- Does not pass through the outlet part of IVS and will not define outlet VSDs and malaligned VSD
- The arterial valve anatomy is not defined, so aortic stenosis and pulmonic stenosis cannot be detected
- Abnormalities of aortic arch, as interrupted aortic arch and coarctation will not be identified.

Abnormalities identified on four-chamber view are:

- Mitral/aortic atresia
- Tricuspid/pulmonary atresia
- Ebstein anomaly/tricuspid valve dysplasia
- Atrioventricular septal defect
- Large ventricular septal defects
- Single ventricle (double inlet)
- Severe aortic/pulmonary stenosis
- Severe coarctation of the aorta
- Total anomalous venous connection
- Cardiomyopathies/heart tumors.

Abnormalities with normal four-chamber view:
- Tetralogy of Fallot
- Transposition of great arteries
- Double-outlet right ventricle
- Small ventricular septal defects
- Common arterial trunk
- Mild semilunar valves stenosis
- Aortic arch abnormalities.

SPECIFIC CARDIAC ABNORMALITIES

Segmental examination of the connections of the heart will allow detection of abnormalities at the atrioventricular, ventriculoarterial, and venoatrial junctions.

Connection Abnormalities at Atrioventricular Junction

Atrioventricular Septal Defect (Figs. 16A to D)

In the atrioventricular septal defects, there is a common atrioventricular valve and a common atrioventricular junction. There are two types of AVSD. In complete form, there is a defect in the lower part of atrial septum (primum defect) and the upper part of ventricular

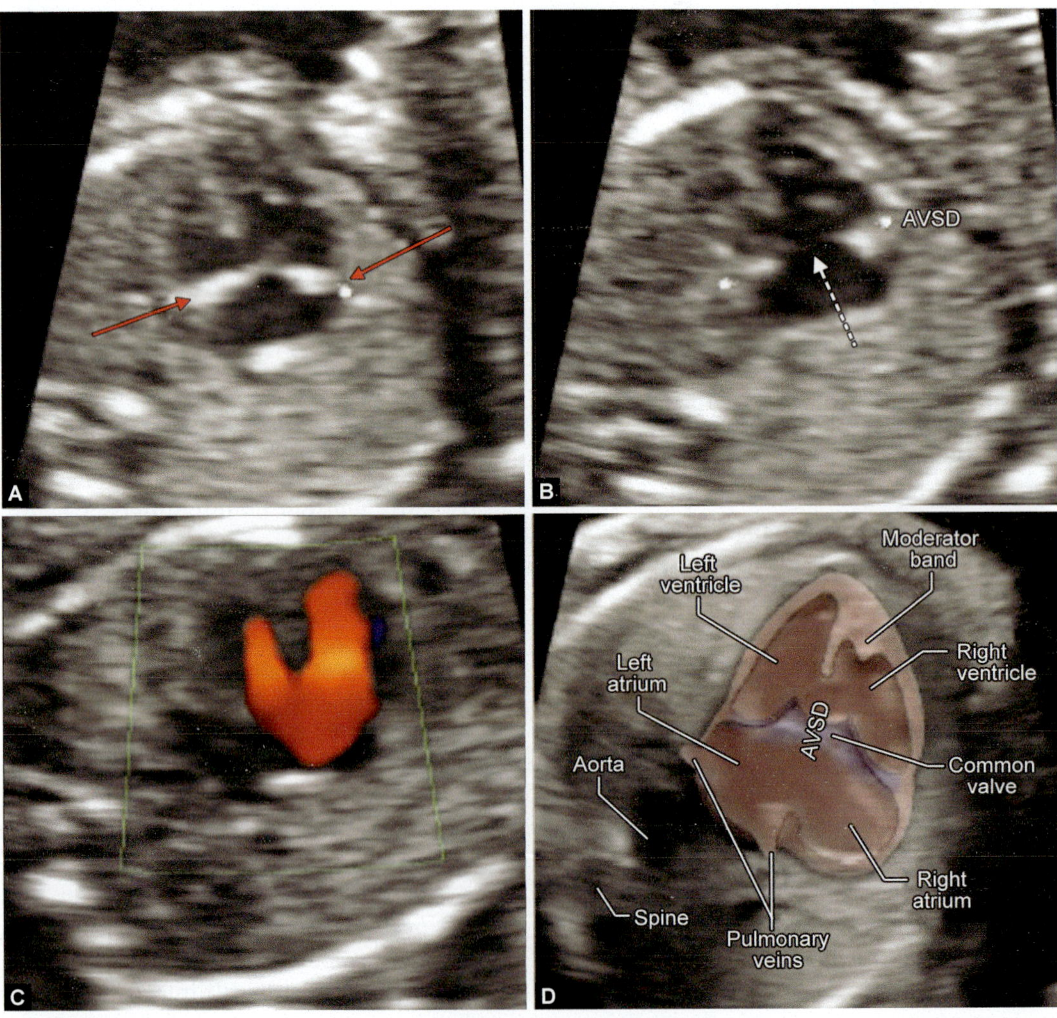

Figs. 16A to D: *Atrioventricular septal defect (AVSD)*: (A) Four-chamber view in systole. Note the linear insertion of the common AV valves when closed (solid arrows); (B) Four-chamber view in diastole. The center of the heart—crux is absent (dotted arrow); (C) Color Doppler of four-chamber in diastole. Note the central channel of ventricular filling is seen; (D) Shows a super-imposed sketch image on the ultrasonographic image of AVSD. All the ultrasound features of AVSD can be seen clearly.

septum, at the crux of the heart. The size of both atrial and ventricular component can be variable. In the partial form, there is a primum atrial septal defect with a common AV valve, but no ventricular component to the defect.

In the four-chamber view, there is a defect in the center of the heart (crux) with loss of normal offset of the two AV valves. This is due to the common AV valve with resulting loss of the normal differential insertion of the two AV valves on the interventricular septum. This gives an echocardiographic appearance of a single valve opening into both ventricular chambers. The defect can be best appreciated in diastole when the valve is open.

Atrioventricular septal defects are one of the most common forms of heart disease in prenatal life and are commonly associated with chromosomal anomalies, particularly with trisomy 21. It is also frequently found associated with isomerism of the atrial appendages known as heterotaxy syndrome.

Summary of echocardiographic features:

- No offset cross at crux due to loss of differential insertion
- Common atrioventricular junction
- Atrial and ventricular component of varying sizes (balanced and unbalanced AVSD)
- Color flow will demonstrate single inflow from the center of the heart.

Tricuspid Atresia (Figs. 17A to D)

In tricuspid atresia, there is no connection between the right atrium and right ventricle. The four-chamber view in the fetus will be abnormal, as a patent tricuspid valve is not seen and the right ventricular chamber is

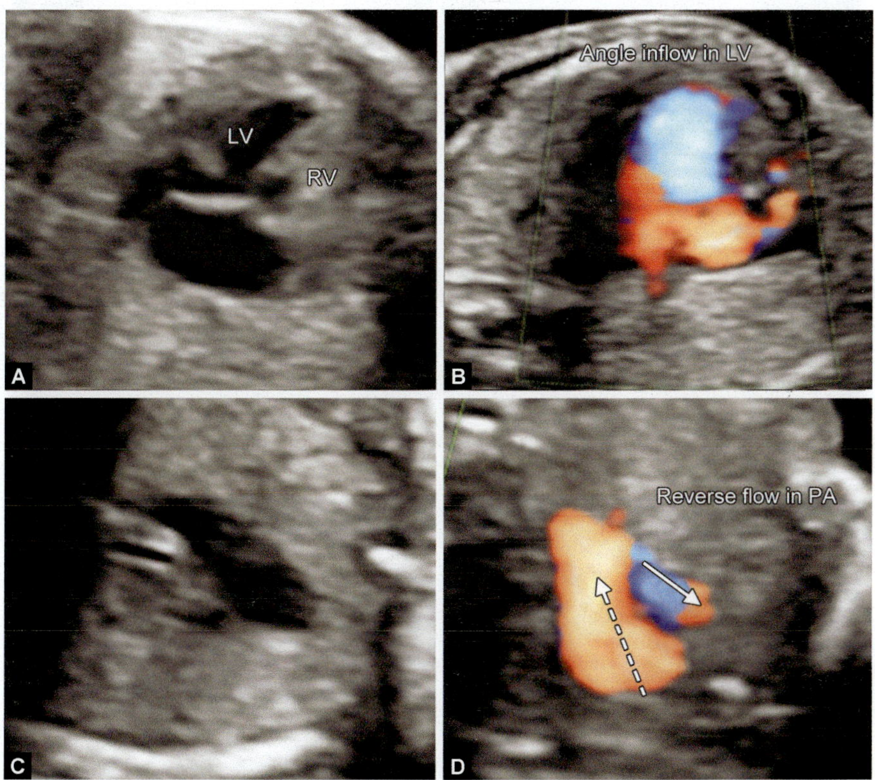

Figs. 17A to D: *Tricuspid atresia (HRHS—hypoplastic right heart syndrome) or pulmonary atresia with intact ventricular septum*: (A) Apical four-chamber showing hypoplastic right ventricle; (B) Four-chamber view in color Doppler showing no perfusion in right ventricle (RV) across dysplastic tricuspid valve; (C) 3VV in gray scale showing two vessels—aorta and superior vena cava (SVC); (D) 3VV in color Doppler showing antegrade flow in transverse aorta (dotted arrow) and retrograde flow (solid arrow) in the small pulmonary artery.

hypoplastic. Ventricular septal defect when present can be of variable size and will influence the size of right ventricular cavity. There is no flow detected across tricuspid valve on color Doppler. Tricuspid atresia is rarely associated with extracardiac abnormalities.

Summary of echocardiographic features:

- Small right ventricle
- No opening tricuspid valve
- No flow from right atrium to right ventricle
- Associated ventricular septal defect.

Mitral Atresia (Figs. 18A to D)

In mitral atresia, there is no connection between the left atrium and left ventricle. The four-chamber view in the fetus will be abnormal, as a patent mitral valve is not seen and the left ventricular chamber is hypoplastic. There is no demonstrable flow from left atrium to left ventricle on color flow examination. Mitral atresia can occur in three settings. It most commonly occurs in association with aortic atresia in the setting of hypoplastic left heart syndrome. Alternatively, mitral atresia can occur with ventricular septal defect with either a normally connected but patent aorta or with DORV. In this setting, the aorta is often malpositioned anterior to the pulmonary artery. In fetal life, mitral atresia has a significant association with chromosomal

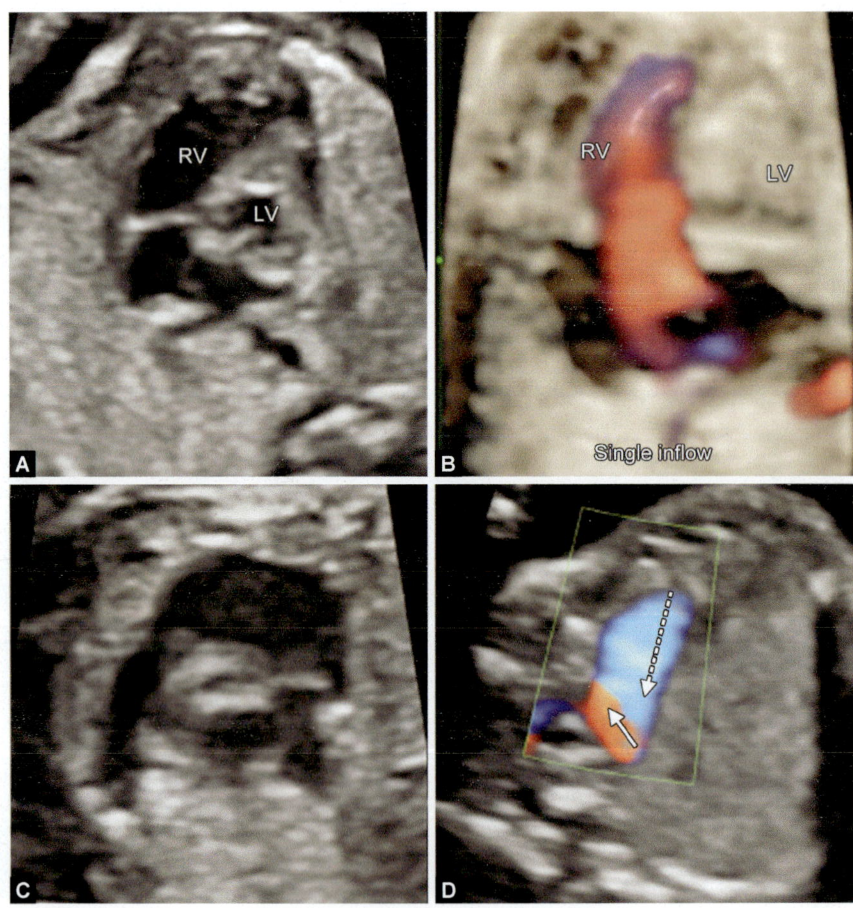

Figs. 18A to D: *Mitral atresia/HLHS (hypoplastic left heart syndrome)*: (A) an apical view with small/diminutive left ventricle (LV) with wall hypertrophy; (B) Apical four-chamber in color Doppler showing no filling in LV; (C) The circle sausage view with small aorta; (D) Color Doppler in 3VV, with retrograde flow in aortic arch (solid arrow) and antegrade flow in pulmonary artery (dotted arrow).

anomalies (18%), usually trisomy 18 but 13, 21 and translocation/deletion syndrome are also possible.

Summary of echocardiographic features:

- Small left ventricle
- No opening of the mitral valve
- No flow from left atrium to left ventricle
- Ventricular septal defect
- With aortic atresia, it forms hypoplastic left heart syndrome.

Double Inlet Ventricle (Figs. 19A to D)

In double-inlet connection, both atrioventricular valves drain predominantly to one ventricle. In most cases, there is one dominant ventricle and one rudimentary chamber. The four-chamber view will be abnormal as no ventricular septum is seen dividing the ventricles equally between the two atrioventricular valves. The flow from both AV valves drains into the same ventricular chamber, which is usually of left ventricular morphology. The great arteries are frequently transposed and arise in parallel orientation with aorta arising from the rudimentary chamber (usually an anterosuperior morphologically right ventricle), which communicates with the

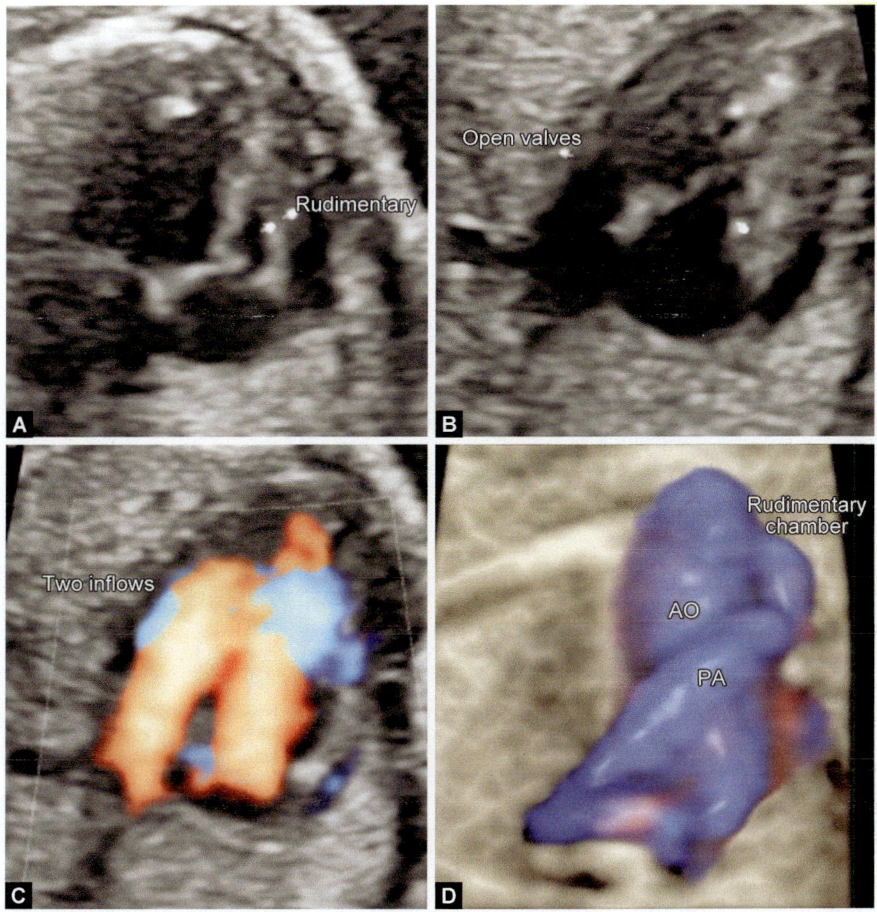

Figs. 19A to D: *Double inlet ventricle (DIV)*: (A and B) Apical four-chamber in systole and diastole. Both the atria are seen draining through two atrioventricular valves into a single ventricle; (C) Apical four-chamber with color Doppler demonstrating blood flow during diastole from both atria into a single ventricle; (D) Long axis view in color Doppler showing the remnant ventricle as small outlet chamber giving rise to pulmonary artery.

main chamber via a ventricular septal defect. Double-inlet ventricle is rarely associated with extracardiac syndromes.

Summary of echocardiographic features:

- Both AV valves drain predominantly into one ventricle
- Usually drain into the dominant ventricle (mostly left) with second ventricle being rudimentary
- Great arteries are frequently transposed.

Ebstein's Malformation (Figs. 20A to E)

In Ebstein's malformation, the attachment of the septal and mural leaflets of the tricuspid valve are displaced downward into the right ventricle also referred as atrialization of right ventricle. The right atrium appears big due to atrialization of right ventricle. The degree of displacement is variable.

There is variable degree of tricuspid incompetence and a variable degree of right atrial enlargement, resulting in an increased cardiothoracic ratio. Obstruction to the right ventricular outflow tract is common. Ebstein malformation is rarely associated with extracardiac anomalies.

Summary of echocardiographic features:

- Displacement of septal and mural leaflet
- Long anterior leaflet
- Right atrial enlargement
- Tricuspid incompetence
- Increased cardiothoracic ratio.

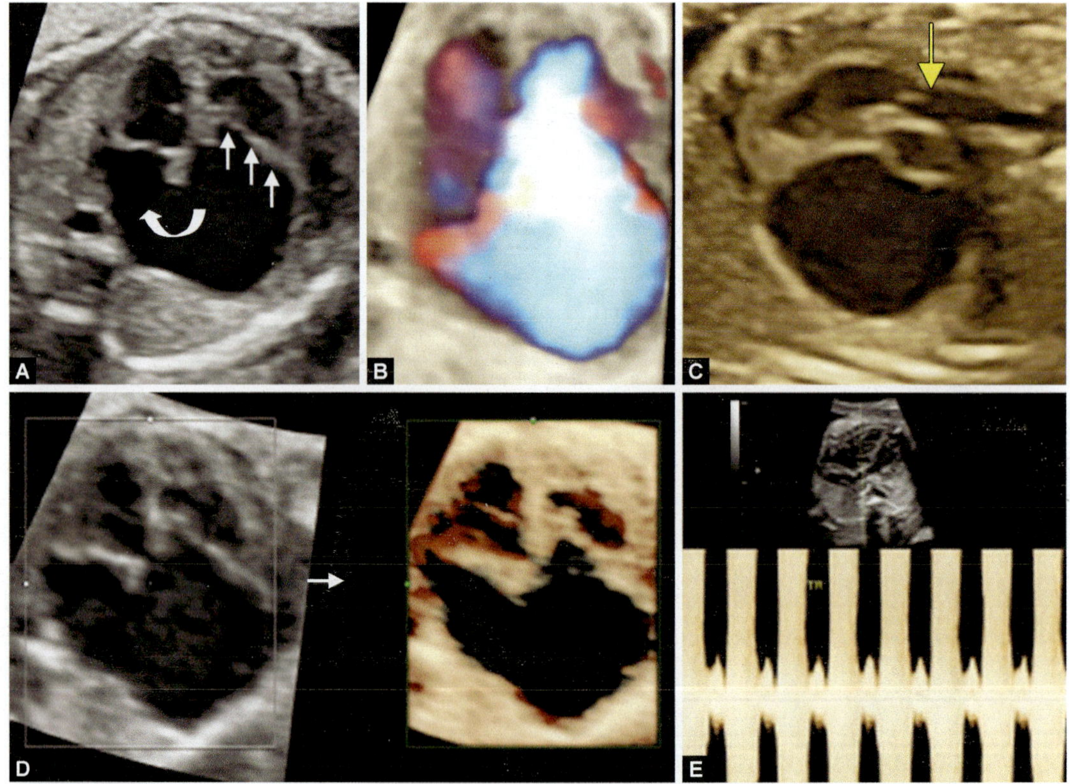

Figs. 20A to E: *Ebstein anomaly*: (A and B) Four-chamber view demonstrating the typical apical displacement of the tricuspid valve (solid arrows). The right atrium is dilated due to severe tricuspid regurgitation (seen in color Doppler image). The Foramen ovale is wide open (curved arrow) due to increased right-to-left shunting of blood; (C) Right ventricular outflow tract (RVOT)—circle sausage view showing small pulmonary artery (open arrow) and dilated right atrium; (D) 4D reconstructed image showing the displaced tricuspid valve; (E) Pulse Doppler in Ebstein anomaly showing holosystolic duration of regurgitant jet with very high velocity.

Tricuspid Valve Dysplasia (Figs. 21A to D)

In tricuspid valve dysplasia, the attachments of the tricuspid valve leaflets are normal but the leaflets are dysplastic resulting in an incompetent tricuspid valve. The four-chamber view is abnormal due to associated cardiomegaly, which is due to right atrial and ventricular enlargement. Tricuspid valve appears thick and nodular and there is variable degree of tricuspid regurgitation. Secondary lung hypoplasia as a result of long-standing compression from severe cardiomegaly can be life-threatening. Obstruction to the right ventricular outflow tract is commonly manifested as pulmonary stenosis or atresia, which depends on the severity of tricuspid regurgitation. Tricuspid dysplasia can be difficult to distinguish from Ebstein's malformation; however, the differentiation is not important in fetal life, as the prognosis is similar when diagnosed in utero. Tricuspid dysplasia is not commonly associated with extracardiac lesions but chromosomal anomalies can occur.

Summary of echocardiographic features:

- Dysplastic but normally positioned tricuspid valve leaflets
- Right atrial enlargement
- Right ventricular enlargement
- Tricuspid incompetence
- Increased cardiothoracic ratio.

Connection Abnormalities at Ventricular–Arterial Junction

Pulmonary Atresia with Intact Ventricular Septum

In this anomaly, there is complete obstruction to forward flow from right ventricle to

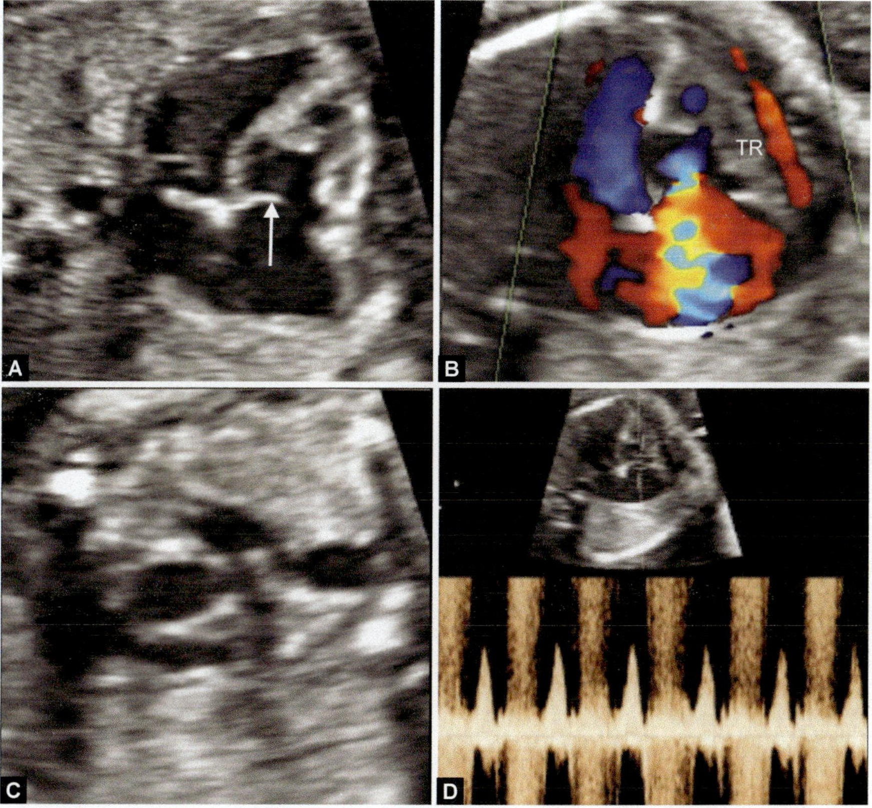

Figs. 21A to D: *Tricuspid valve (TV) dysplasia*: (A) Four-chamber view showing thickened dysplastic TV, attached at their normal anatomic location; (B) Color Doppler shows the regurgitant jet from normally placed TV; (C) Narrow pulmonary artery; (D) Pulse Doppler shows pansystolic regurgitation with high-peak velocity.

pulmonary trunk and the interventricular septum is intact. The four-chamber view will be abnormal. The right ventricle is hypoplastic, hypertrophied with poor contractility. The tricuspid valve movement is restricted and there may be a jet of tricuspid regurgitation at high velocity. The three-vessel view will show a smaller pulmonary artery and will demonstrate reverse flow in pulmonary artery from the arterial duct. This condition is not commonly associated with extracardiac malformations (**Figs. 17A to D**).

Summary of echocardiographic features:

- Hypoplastic right ventricle
- Hypertrophied right ventricle
- Poorly contracting right ventricle
- Small atretic tricuspid valve
- Tricuspid regurgitation (high velocity)
- Small pulmonary artery
- No forward flow in pulmonary artery
- Reverse flow in arterial duct.

Aortic Atresia (Hypoplastic Left Heart Syndrome)

The four-chamber view will be abnormal with small left ventricle. The size of left ventricle can vary from small to slit like and indiscernible, with no detectable flow in the cavity. The left atrium will also be small with left to right shunt across foramen ovale at atrial level. The aortic valve is atretic and the ascending aorta is hypoplastic. In the three-vessel view, there is reverse flow in aortic arch via arterial duct. The hypoplastic left heart syndrome (HLHS) can occasionally be associated with chromosomal anomalies, particularly Turner's syndrome, trisomy 18 and 13, and also partial deletion of 11q has been implicated in few cases **(Figs. 18A to D)**.

Summary of echocardiographic features:

- Hypoplastic left ventricle
- Echogenic left ventricle with patent mitral valve
- Hypoplastic aorta
- No forward flow across aortic valve
- Retrograde flow in aortic arch.

Simple Transposition of Great Arteries (Figs. 22A to D)

The term "transposed great arteries" means that the aorta (vessel that forms an arch) arises from right ventricle and the pulmonary artery (vessel that branches) from left ventricle. It constitutes 5–7% of all CHD. The four-chamber view is normal. The diagnosis is made in the outflow tract views. The two great arteries are parallel at origin instead of criss-cross. Since the aorta arises from the anterior chamber–right ventricle, the aortic arch will form wide-sweeping arch instead of normal tight-hooked arch. Aorta assumes a right convex shape termed as "I" sign. Circle sausage view is not possible to obtain. In simple transposition, the interventricular septum is intact and it is rarely associated with extracardiac lesions **(Figs. 22A to D)**.

In transposition of great arteries with ventricular septal defect, there is an associated ventricular septal defect of variable size. This condition can be associated with either pulmonary stenosis or coarctation of aorta. This condition can be mistaken for double outlet right ventricle with subpulmonary ventricular septal defect. Prognosis is good.

Summary of echocardiographic features:

- Normal four-chamber view
- Parallel arrangement of great arteries
- Artery forming arch and giving rise to head and neck vessels (aorta) arises from right ventricle
- Branching artery (pulmonary artery) arises from left ventricle
- 3VV will show two vessels, aorta, and SVC (PA is not visible as its posterior).

Congenitally Corrected Transposition of Great Arteries (Figs. 23A to D)

In this anomaly, there is discordant atrio-ventricular connection and discordant ventriculoarterial connection. The right atrium is connected to the left ventricle, which in turn gives rise to pulmonary artery. The left atrium

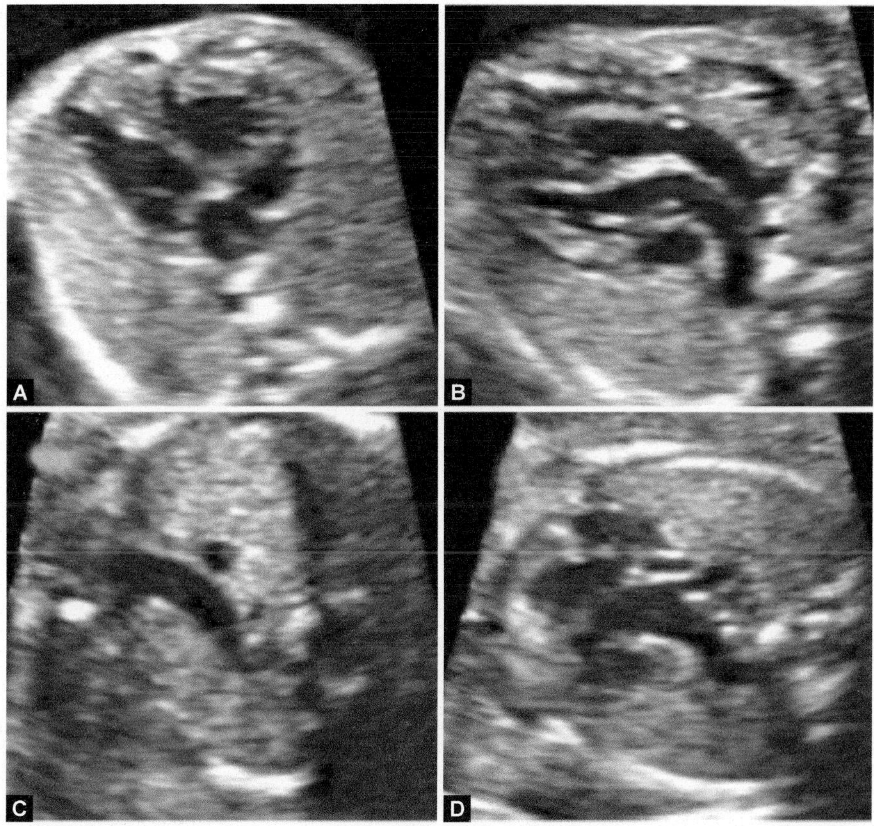

Figs. 22A to D: *Simple transposition of great artery (TGA) [TGA without ventricular septal defect (VSD)]*: (A) The four-chamber view, which is normal; (B) The parallel origin of the great vessels; (C) The 3VV in gray scale demonstrating the aorta as a single large vessel with the SVC to its right; (D) The pulmonary artery (vessel which bifurcates) arising from the posterior chamber (left ventricle).

is connected to the right ventricle, which gives rise to the aorta, so that the circulation is anatomically "corrected" even though the ventricular anatomy is inverted.

The heart often lies with the interventricular septum in a more anteroposterior position than normal. On the four-chamber view, the atrioventricular offset is on the left (instead of right). The more apically attached tricuspid valve and the moderator band, which are features of the morphological right ventricle, are seen on the left side. The great arteries arise in parallel orientation, with the aorta (vessel that forms an arch), these arise from the left-sided morphologically right ventricle and the pulmonary artery (vessel that branches) from the right-sided morphologically left ventricle. It is commonly associated with other cardiac lesions, such as ventricular septal defect, pulmonary stenosis, and complete heart block. Extracardiac malformations are uncommon.

Summary of echocardiographic features ***(Figs. 24A to D)***:
- Centrally positioned heart
- "Reversed" offset of atrioventricular valves
- Moderator band in left ventricle
- Parallel great arteries
- Aorta arises from right ventricle and to the left of pulmonary artery.

Tetralogy of Fallot ***(Figs. 25A to D):*** This is the most common cyanotic congenital heart disease. It has four components—over-riding and anteriorly displaced aorta, malaligned ventricular septal defect, infundibular

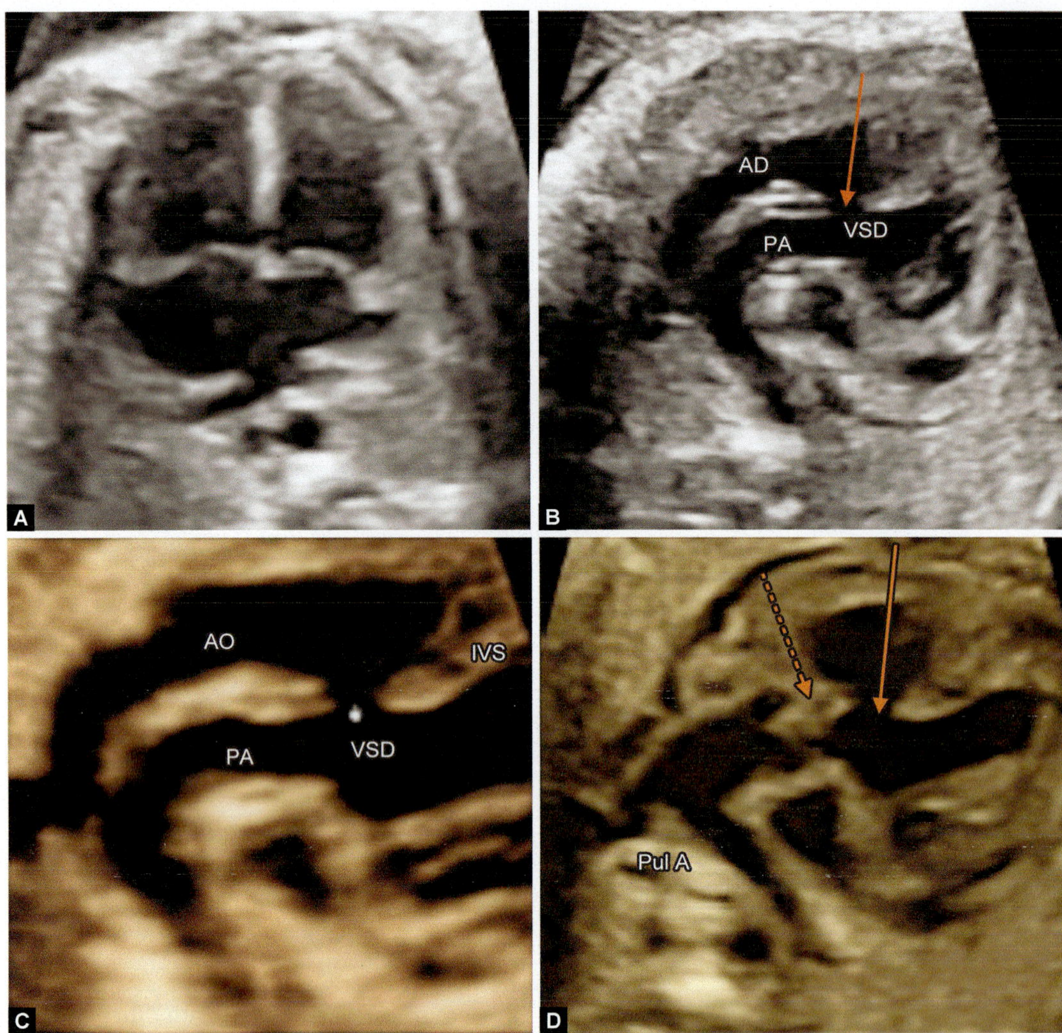

Figs. 23A to D: *Transposition of great artery (TGA) with ventricular septal defect (VSD) (subpulmonic)*: (A) A normal apical four chamber; (B) Parallel outflows with VSD (arrow); (C) A 4D reconstructed image of parallel arrangement of great arteries with VSD; (D) The bifurcating vessel (pulmonary artery) is arising from posterior (left) ventricle and the VSD (subpulmonic VSD, solid arrow) is close to pulmonic valve (dotted arrow).

pulmonary stenosis, and right ventricular hypertrophy. The four-chamber view is essentially normal. In the five-chamber view, the malaligned ventricular septal defect and the over-riding aorta are seen. The pulmonary artery is usually smaller than aorta indicating some degree of right ventricular outflow tract obstruction and is best appreciated in 3VV. The right ventricular hypertrophy may not be evident in the fetus. TOF is associated with increased nuchal translucency in 1st trimester. Cardiac and extracardiac abnormalities are common. Chromosomal abnormalities are found in 30%, microdeletion of 22q11 in 10–15%, right aortic arch in 25%, and left superior vena cava in 11%.

Poor prognostic signs are decreasing size of PA, cessation of forward flow in PA, reverse flow in PA from DA and associated extracardiac malformation and chromosomal anomalies.

Summary of echocardiographic features:

- Normal four-chamber view (often)
- Ventricular septal defect

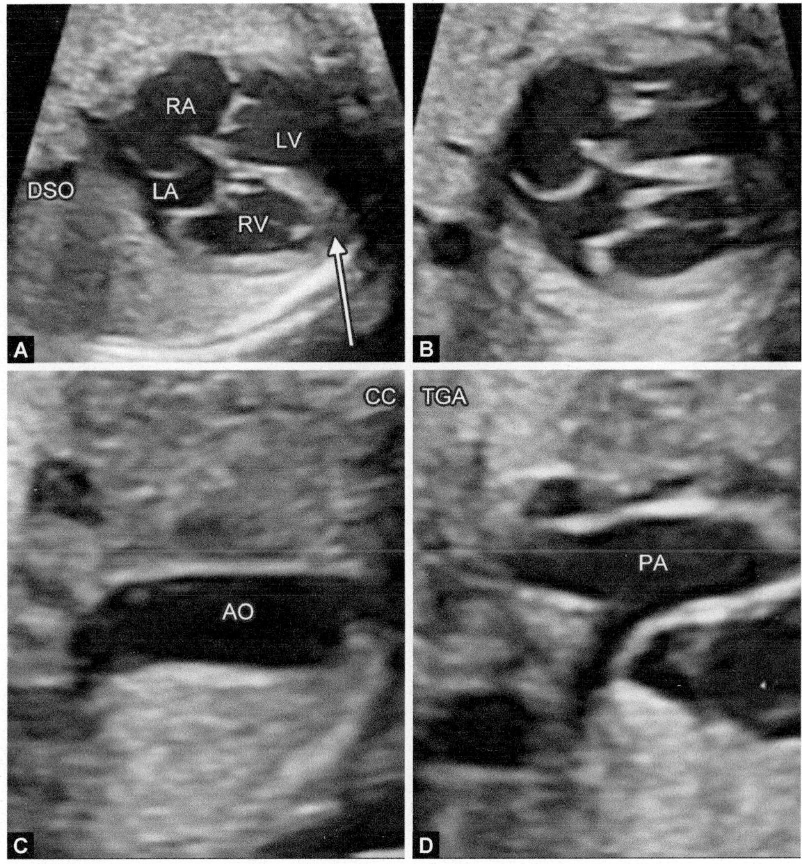

Figs. 24A to D: *CC-TGA*: (A and B) Abnormal four-chamber view showing discordance in atrioventricular connections. The atria are in normal positions but the left ventricle (LV) and mitral valve are on the right side connected to right atrium. The more apically inserted tricuspid valve and right ventricle (RV) are on the left side connected to left atrium (LA). Apex of the heart is formed by the right-sided LV (solid arrow); (C) Aorta arising from posterior chamber, which is morphological right ventricle connected to left atrium; (D) The bifurcating artery (pulmonary artery) arising from the anterior chamber, which is morphological left ventricle connected to right atrium.

- Aortic override
- Small pulmonary artery.

Pulmonary Atresia with Ventricular Septal Defect (Figs. 26A to D)

This condition is a spectrum of tetralogy of Fallot and is also referred as severe tetralogy of Fallot. It constitutes 20% of all TOF and 2% of CHD. Here, the pulmonary artery is atretic and there is no patent connection between the right ventricle and the main pulmonary artery. There may be multiple aortopulmonary collateral arteries (MAPCAs) arising directly from the aorta and supplying the lungs. The four-chamber view of heart may be normal. The long axis of aorta view will show a ventricular septal defect with aortic override. Usually, no main pulmonary artery can be identified, but branch pulmonary arteries are sometimes found.

The pulmonary blood supply is either retrogradely from the arterial duct or from collaterals. It is more common in fetuses of diabetic mothers. 22q11 microdeletion is seen in 20%, right aortic arch is seen in 20–50%, and secundum atrial septal defect or patent foramen ovale postnatally is also common.

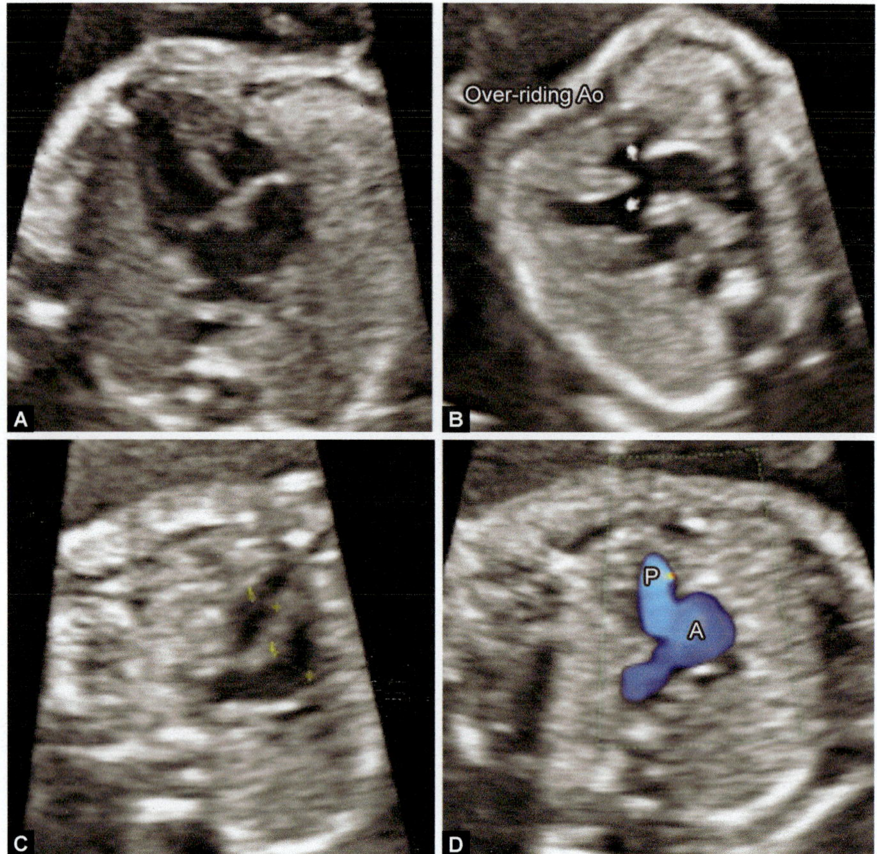

Figs. 25A to D: *Tetralogy of Fallot*: (A) A normal four-chamber view; (B) A five-chamber view with ventricular septal defect (VSD) and an over-riding aorta; (C) 3VV in 2D showing a small pulmonary artery; (D) Color Doppler in 3VV demonstrating a small pulmonary artery with forward flow.

Chromosomal aberrations are in 8% and extracardiac malformations are in 46% of fetuses. Prognosis is poor.

Summary of echocardiographic features:

- Normal four-chamber view (often)
- Ventricular septal defect
- Aortic override
- Difficult to identify main pulmonary artery
- Hypoplastic branch pulmonary arteries
- Retrograde flow in arterial duct
- Multiple aortopulmonary collateral arteries (MAPCAs).

Common Arterial Trunk (Figs. 27A to D)

This anomaly is characterized by a single great artery arising from the heart, which gives rise to the systemic, pulmonary, and coronary circulation. There is a ventricular septal defect with great artery override. It constitutes 1.6% of CHD and is common in diabetic mothers.

Truncal valve is often thickened and dysplastic. It can be tricuspid (69%), quadricuspid (22%), and bicuspid (9%) and there may be truncal valve regurgitation. This condition can be associated with chromosomal defects and has been associated with 22q phenotypes (DiGeorge and Shprintzen syndromes).

Subtypes are based on origin of pulmonary arteries:

- *Type I*: Short pulmonary trunk arises from CAT, which divides into right and left PAs (most common)

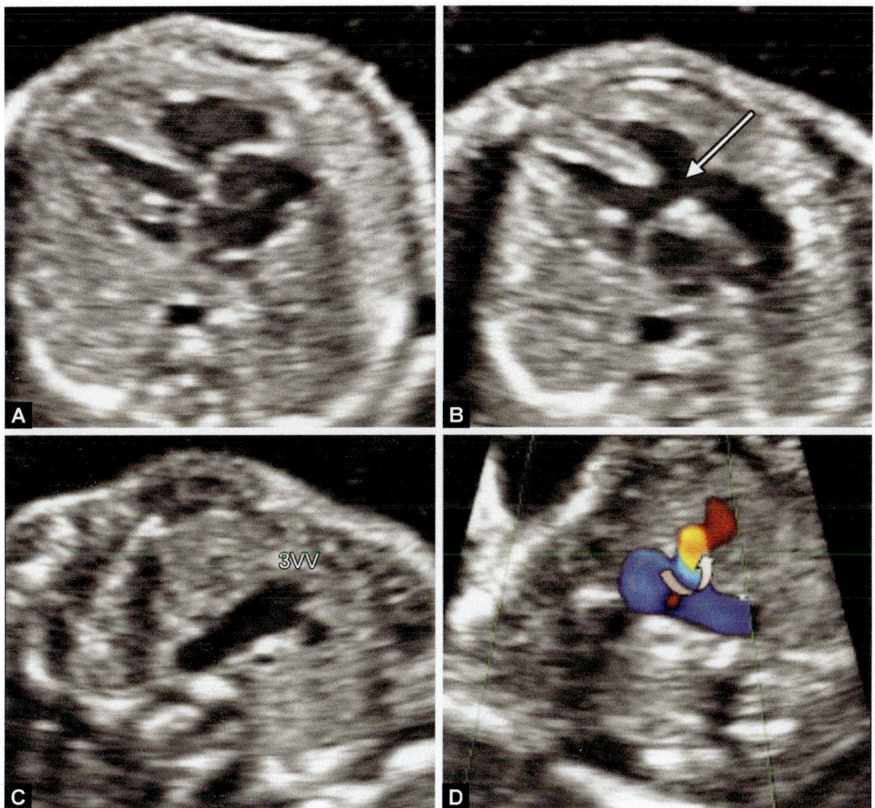

Figs. 26A to D: *Pulmonary atresia with ventricular septal defect (VSD)*: (A) The normal four-chamber view; (B) The five-chamber view showing VSD with large over-riding aorta (solid arrow); (C) The 3VV, where PA is absent, aorta and superior vena cava (SVC) are seen; (D) The 3VV in color Doppler shows retrograde drainage into the pulmonary artery via ductus arteriosus (curved arrow).

- *Type II and III*: Both pulmonary arteries arise separately from CAT, either close (type II) or at some distance from one another (type III)
- *Type IV*: Pulmonary arteries arise from aortic arch or descending aorta (Dao) (is now reclassified as PA atresia with VSD).

Ultrasonography findings:

- Four-chamber appears normal
- Five-chamber large malaligned VSD with overriding large vessel, thick echogenic (dysplastic) valve is seen
  - Separate PA is absent
  - Diagnosis is confirmed by identifying PA arising from CAT
  - *3VT view*: Single large vessel, with absent DA and PA
  - Thymus may be absent in the anterior thorax
  - Color flow will show increase velocity across overriding CAT and truncal regurgitation.

Double Outlet Right Ventricle (Figs. 28A to D)

- DORV comprises of complex cardiac malformations where both great arteries arise primarily from morphologic right ventricle. Incidence is 1–1.5% of CHD. Various types of DORV are on the basis of:
  - Spatial relationship of great arteries
  - Location of VSD
  - +nce/–nce of pulmonary and rarely aortic outflow obstruction.

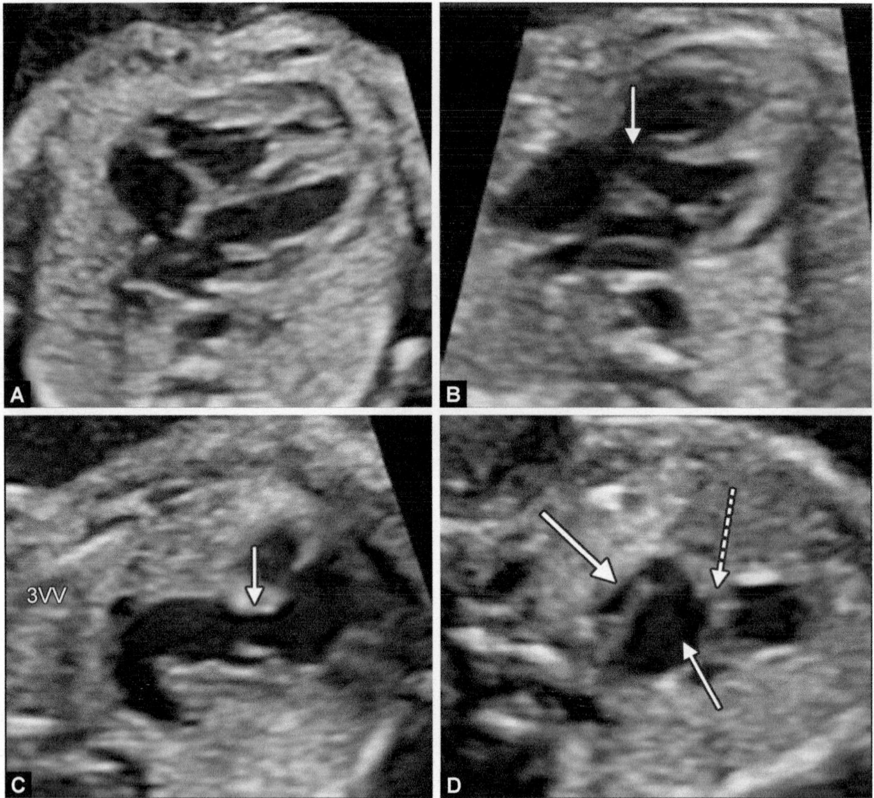

Figs. 27A to D: *Common arterial trunk*: (A) A normal four-chamber view; (B) The transverse view at the level of five-chamber view demonstrating a large common trunk (solid arrow); (C) A thickened truncal valve (solid arrow); (D) The large common arterial trunk bifurcating into pulmonary artery (notched arrow) and aorta (solid arrow). Note the thickened dysplastic truncal valve (dotted arrow).

Transposition of great arteries with VSD is also a close differential diagnosis. Aorta and pulmonary artery arise entirely or predominantly from morphologic RV. Relation of great arteries, location of VSD, and presence or absence of pulmonary stenosis and less commonly aortic stenosis will decide the subtypes of DORV.

Ultrasonography findings:

- Normal four chamber till 2nd trimester, later the LV becomes diminutive hence four chamber in 3rd trimester may be abnormal
- Five chamber is abnormal. VSD and both vessels arising from anterior chamber or right ventricle
- Position of VSD should be ascertained
- 3VV—variable depending on the arrangement of great vessels
- Outflow obstruction is assessed by size discrepancy; pulmonary stenosis is more common.

Associated cardiac findings are common in 70%. Extracardiac malformations are also common. Chromosomal abnormalities are seen, especially trisomies when DORV is present with AVSD, 22q11 deletions is common when associated with conotruncal anomaly. Association with heterotaxy rules out chromosomal abnormalities.

Absent Pulmonary Valve Syndrome (Figs. 29A to D)

This term is a misnomer because there is a tissue seen in the position of the pulmonary

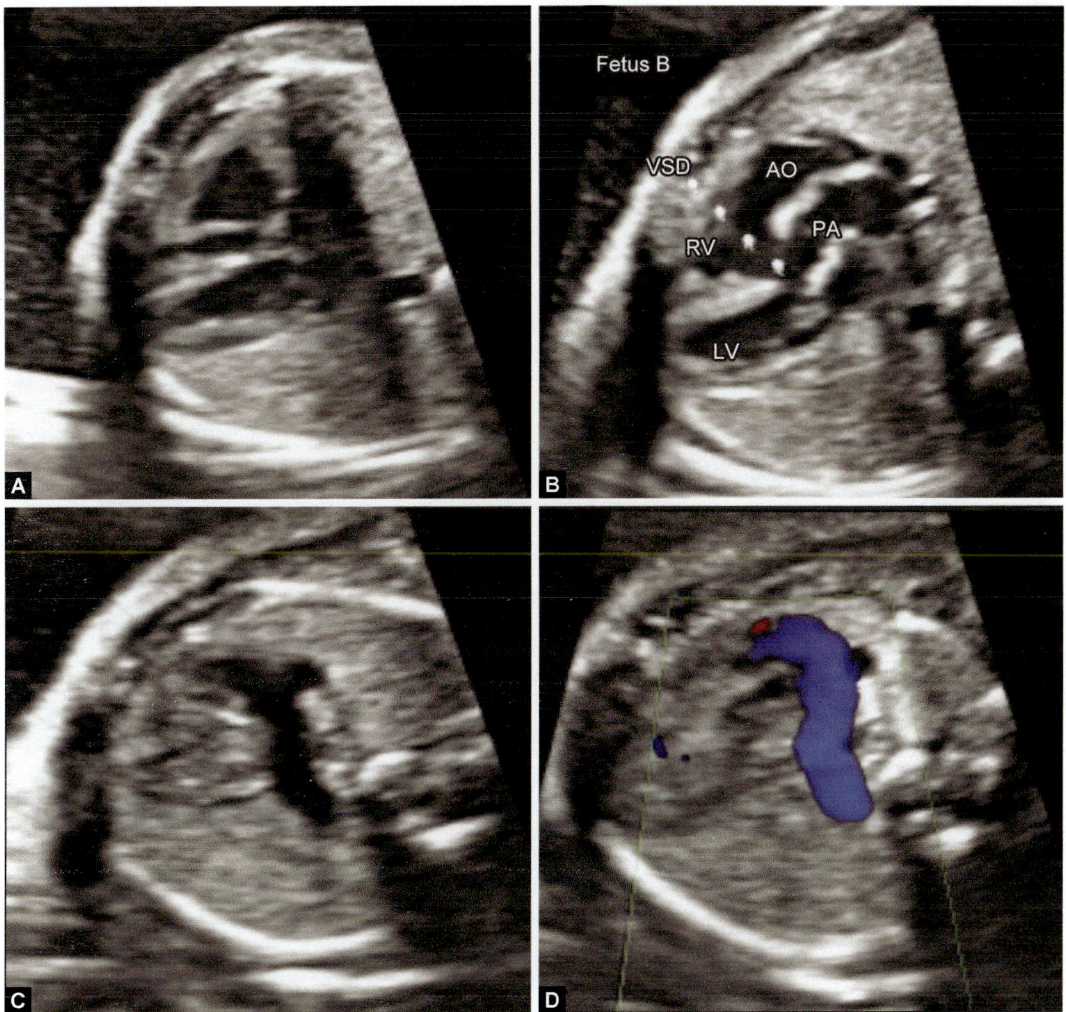

Figs. 28A to D: *Double outlet right ventricle*: (A) A 2D gray scale image of lateral four chamber with slightly small left ventricle (LV); (B) A five-chamber view with VSD and parallel outflows. The PA is posterior and aorta is anterior. Both the great arteries are seen arising from right ventricle (RV); (C and D) A single vessel in 3VV in 2D and color flow. Note the single vessel is aorta arising from anterior chamber right ventricle. PA is not seen due to its posterior position.

valve both echocardiographically and anatomically. It is the most severe form in TOF spectrum. It constitutes 3–6% of TOF and 0.2–0.4% of CHD. Pulmonary valve is either absent or severely dysplastic resulting in free pulmonary regurgitation, with malaligned VSD and aortic override. It is associated with absent DA. There is massive dilatation of branch pulmonary arteries. Bronchomalacia with airway abnormalities is common. Rarely, in case of pulmonary valve stenosis with intact septum, a little less dilated PA and presence of DA is also seen.

Ultrasonography findings: Four-chamber view is abnormal as the right ventricle is dilated. Five-chamber view shows VSD and overriding aorta (classic dilatation of aortic root as seen in TOF is missing), 3 VV will show dilated branch pulmonary arteries (normal 2–6 mm, can increase to 10–18 mm), and absent ductus

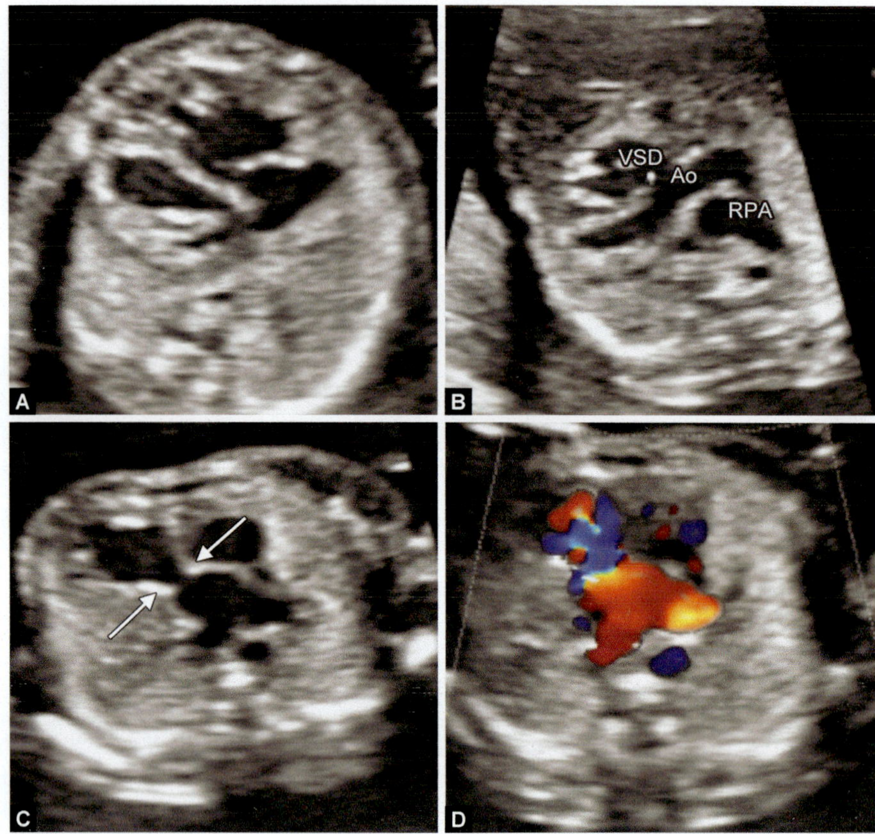

Figs. 29A to D: *Absent pulmonary valve syndrome*: (A) A 2D gray scale image of 4 chamber with enlarged RV (due to volume overload from insufficient pulmonary valve); (B) The five-chamber view in 2D gray scale showing an over-riding aorta over mal-aligned ventricular septal defect (VSD); (C) A 2D gray scale image of right ventricular outflow tract (RVOT) with dilated branch pulmonary arteries and remnant of pulmonary valve (solid arrow); (D) The 2D gray scale image with color Doppler showing turbulent to and fro flow in PA.

arteriosus. Color Doppler will show to and fro flow in pulmonary artery, high-velocity flow across pulmonary artery annulus (up to 200–250 cm/s).

Coarctation of Aorta and Aortic Arch Anomalies (Figs. 30A to D)

Formation of the great vessels of the heart and their branches is an early event during the embryogenesis. These structures originally come from paired aortic arches. The final aortic arch is created by parts left from the primitive aortic arches; its initial part comes from truncus arteriosus, ascendant part from the aortic sac, transverse arch from the left fourth aortic arch, and descending aorta comes from the left dorsal aorta. Ductus arteriosus normally comes from the left sixth aortic arch.

This anomaly constitutes 8% of cardiac defects—0.2–0.62 per 1,000 live births with males affected more than females—1.27–1.74. The isthmic region is typically involved (between left subclavian and ductus). The recurrence is high 2–6%. It is associated with chromosomal (Turners most common) and extracardiac anomalies.

There are two types—simple and complex [commonly associated anomalies—VSD, persistent left superior vena cava (PLSVC),

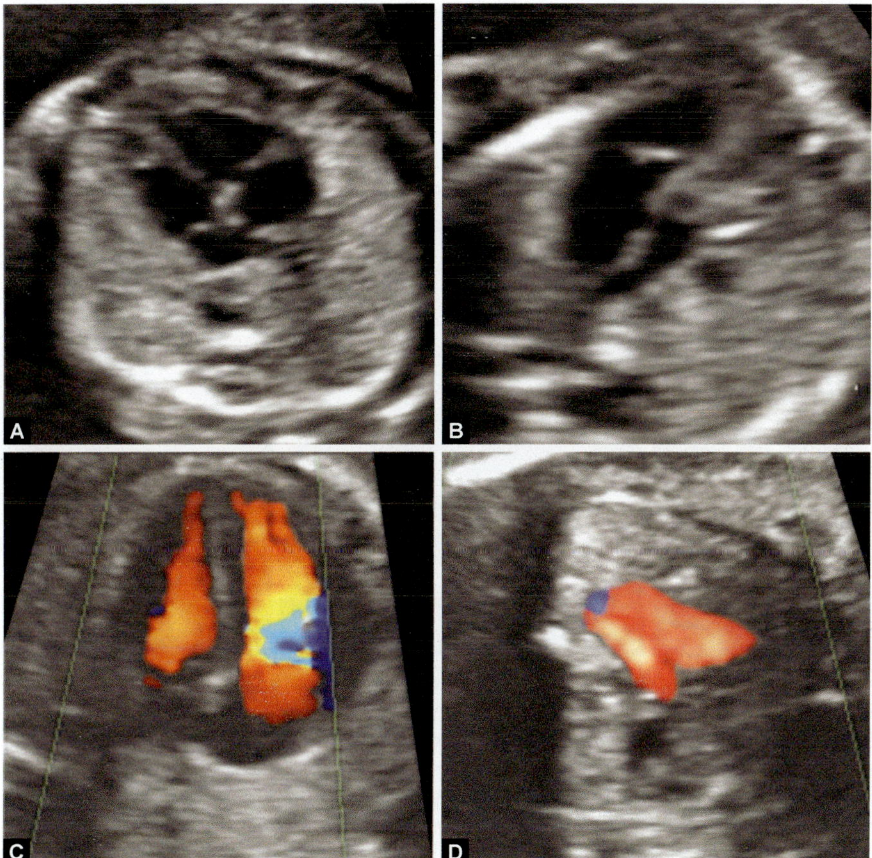

Figs. 30A to D: *Coarctation of aorta*: (A) Typical ventricular disproportion in four-chamber view with slightly small left ventricle (LV); (B) The disproportion of great vessels in 3VV with small transverse arch when compared to the size of pulmonary artery; (C) The apical four-chamber in color Doppler shows the disproportion in the size of ventricles with small LV; (D) The same disproportion in the 3 VV with small transverse in color Doppler (note the forward flow in seen is both great arteries).

and bicuspid aortic valve] (can be associated with unbalanced AVSD, DORV, HLHS, corrected TGA, etc.). The prenatal diagnosis is challenging.

The ultrasound findings raise strong suspicion:

- *Ventricular disproportion* in four-chamber view is the leading clue (RV:LV 1:19 normal, 1:69)
- *3VT view* will show great vessel disproportion
- *Longitudinal view*: Arch appears narrow and tortuous. There is appearance of "contraductal shelf" (represents residual fibrous tissue derived from the ductus arteriosus).

Color Doppler findings will show:

- *In the four-chamber view*, left ventricular filling in diastole differentiates from HLHS
- Five-chamber or left ventricular outflow tract (LVOT) view will show forward flow in aorta and associated perimembranous VSD, if present.
- 3VT view will show narrow transverse arch, which becomes progressively smaller toward isthmus.
- Longitudinal/sagittal view will show the "shelf sign" at junction between DA and DAo.

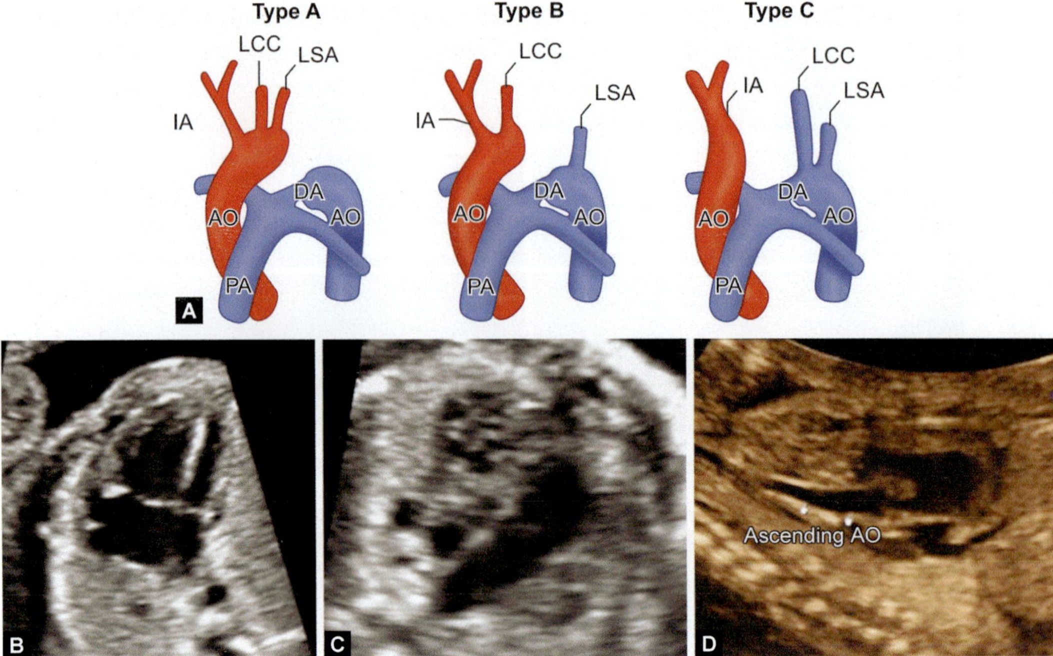

Figs. 31A to D: *Interrupted aortic arch*: (A) Four different types of interrupted aortic arches. Type A—interruption is distal to left subclavian artery (LSA). Type B—interruption is between left common carotid (LCC) and the LSA. Type C—interruption is between the brachiocephalic and LCC; (B) An apical four-chamber with a classical small LV; (C) The 3VV in 2D gray scale, where it is not possible to get "V" of 3VV; (D) The ascending aorta is straight and does not show the normal "candy cane"-shaped curvature.
(IA: innominate artery; AO: aorta; PA: pulmonary artery; DA: ductus arteriosus)

Interrupted Aortic Arch (Figs. 31A to D)

Interrupted aortic arch (IAA) is a rare and severe form of CHD, characterized by a discontinuity between the ascending and descending thoracic aorta. It accounts for <1% of all congenital heart diseases. It can be subdivided into three groups according to the site of interruption:

- Type A, (30%) interruption distal to the left subclavian artery; rarely associated with 22q11 deletion
- Type B, (65%) interruption between the left carotid and left subclavian arteries; is associated with 22q11 deletion and other extracardiac features in 50–80% of cases
- Type C, (5%) interruption between the innominate artery and the left carotid artery, is the least common.

Ultrasound diagnosis:

- In the four-chamber view, there is a LV/RV size discrepancy
- Size discrepancy between the great arteries. To check the continuity of the aortic arch is vital.

In Type B, the ascending aorta runs a straight course to the innominate and left carotid arteries (the typical V shape); type B is also associated with malaligned VSD in 90%.

In type A, there is a slight curvature after the origin of the innominate artery (the typical W shape). The identification of IAA on a prenatal echocardiogram can be challenging. A low aortopulmonary diameter ratio in the absence of a ventricular size discrepancy should prompt consideration of this diagnosis. It is possible to distinguish between IAA and coarctation of the aorta at ultrasound examination. In IAA, the ascending aorta runs with a straight course to its branches, unlike in coarctation, which has a normal aortic curvature and continuity with the descending aorta.

Right Aortic Arch (Figs. 32A to D)

"The left or right sidedness of the aortic arch refers to the position of the aortic arch relative to the trachea. It does not refer to which side of the midline the aorta ascends." The right-sided aortic arch is the most common arch anomaly with incidence of 1 in 1,000 in a low-risk population. It is due to an abnormal development of the fourth branchial arch. Normally, the aortic arch is formed by the left fourth aortic arch and the left dorsal aorta (if the right dorsal aorta persists and the distal left aorta disappears, then we have a right aortic arch). When the RAA is identified, fetal karyotype analysis (including the integrity of chromosome 22) is warranted.

Connection Abnormalities at Venoatrial Junction

Anomalous Pulmonary Venous Connection (Figs. 33A to C)

One or more pulmonary veins drain anomalously to one or three different sites. These are intracardiac to the coronary sinus, supracardiac to either innominate vein or superior vena cava, or infracardiac to the hepatic venous system and inferior vena cava. The diagnosis of total or partial anomalous pulmonary venous connection is difficult in the antenatal period. However, there will be no pulmonary veins seen entering the left atrium in the four-chamber view. The left atrium will be small and there will be right atrial and right ventricular dominance, giving an abnormal appearance of the four-chamber view. A confluence can sometimes be seen behind the left atrium, into which the pulmonary veins drain. The coronary sinus may appear prominent, if the anomalous drainage is intracardiac variety. The degree of right ventricular overload will depend upon the degree of obstruction to drainage; hence, in some cases, the four-chamber view may appear normal. The infracardiac form is usually obstructed and right ventricular overload is not a feature.

Summary of echocardiographic features:

- Pulmonary veins not seen draining to left atrium
- Sometimes right heart dominance
- Dilated/prominent coronary sinus
- Confluent vein behind left atrium.

CARDIAC EXAMINATION IN 1ST TRIMESTER (FIGS. 34A TO C)

The prenatal diagnosis of cardiac malformations has been traditionally limited to the mid-2nd trimesters of pregnancy. The ability to image the fetal heart in early gestation with sufficient clarity to make a diagnosis of a cardiac malformation was made possible by the advent of high-resolution transvaginal and transabdominal probes. The widespread adoption of 1st trimester risk assessment with nuchal translucency and other 1st trimester ultrasound markers have increased the interest in early fetal echocardiography. A targeted cardiac examination is performed in the first and early 2nd trimester window (10–16 weeks) as early echocardiography. Fetal cardiac imaging performed by the transvaginal approach is achievable and reliable in most cases between 12 and 13 weeks (crown-rump length 60–70 mm).

INDICATIONS FOR EARLY FETAL ECHOCARDIOGRAPHY

- An enlarged nuchal translucency
- A positive family history of a previous child with severe cardiac malformation
- The presence of a major extracardiac abnormality detected in 1st trimester

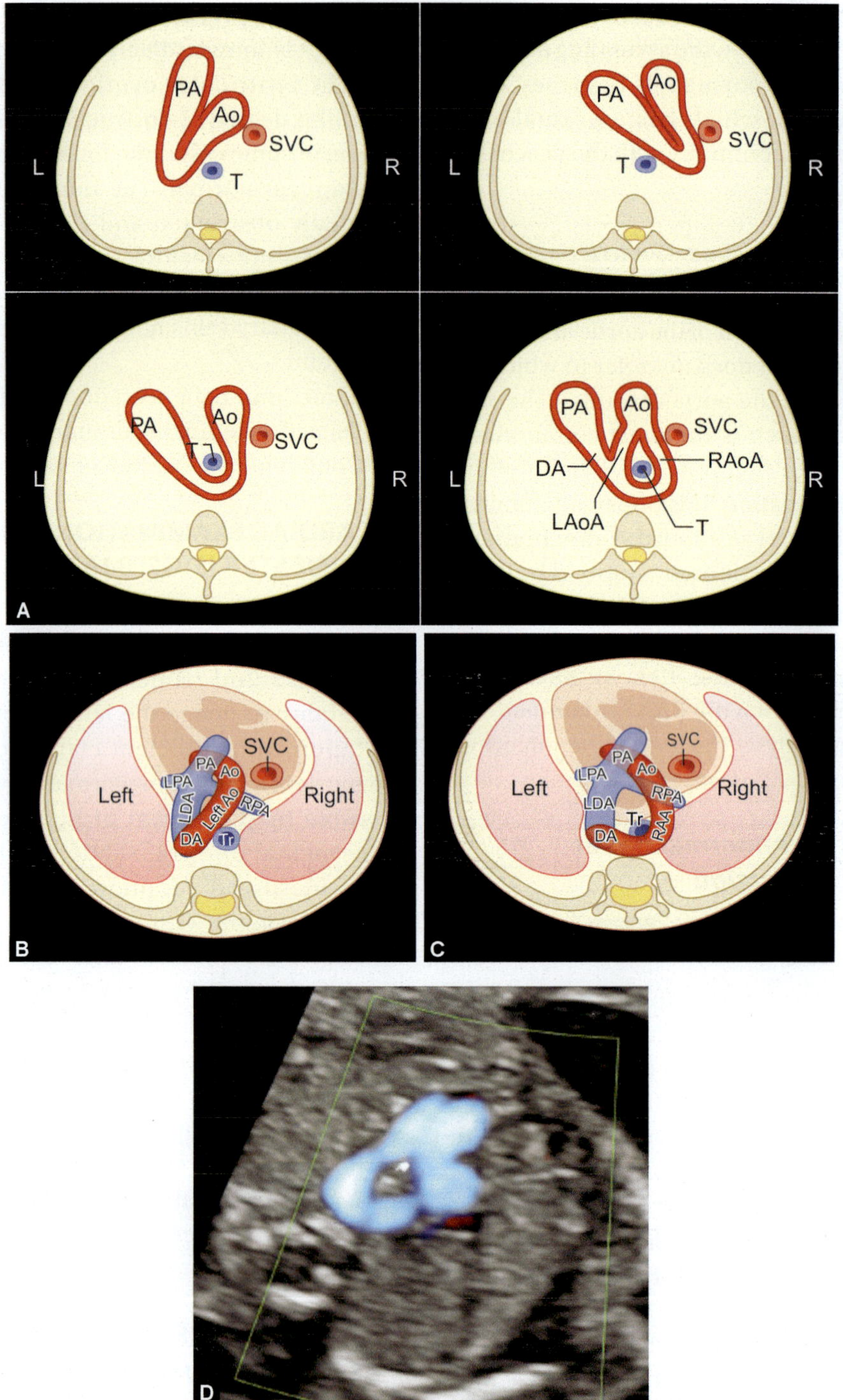

Figs. 32A to D: *Right aortic arch*: (A) Different types of aortic arches; (B) Normal left-sided aortic arch with left-sided ductus arteriosus; (C) Right aortic arch with left-sided ductus, the typical "U" configuration of 3VV; (D) Right-sided aortic arch with left ductus and trachea between the "U" of 3VV in color Doppler.
(Ao: aorta; DA: descending aorta; LAoA: left aortic arch; RAoA: right aortic arch; PA: pulmonary artery; LPA: left pulmonary artery; RPA: right pulmonary artery; RAA: right aortic arch; SVC: superior vena cava)

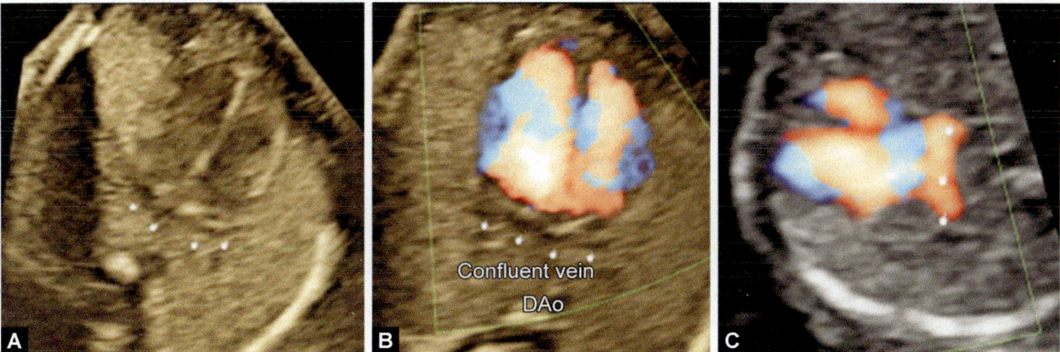

Figs. 33A to C: *Total anomalous pulmonary venous connection (TAPVC)*: (A) An apical four-chamber in TAPVC where the posterior region of the left atrium is enlarged and there is a pulmonary confluence behind atria; (B) An apical view in color Doppler showing normal filling of both ventricles and the pulmonary veins are not seen entering the left atrium. The upper border of left atrium (LA) is smooth and is not interrupted by pulmonary veins; (C) The lateral four-chamber view in color Doppler showing the confluent vein (note the direction of flow is not toward heart).
(DAo: descending aorta)

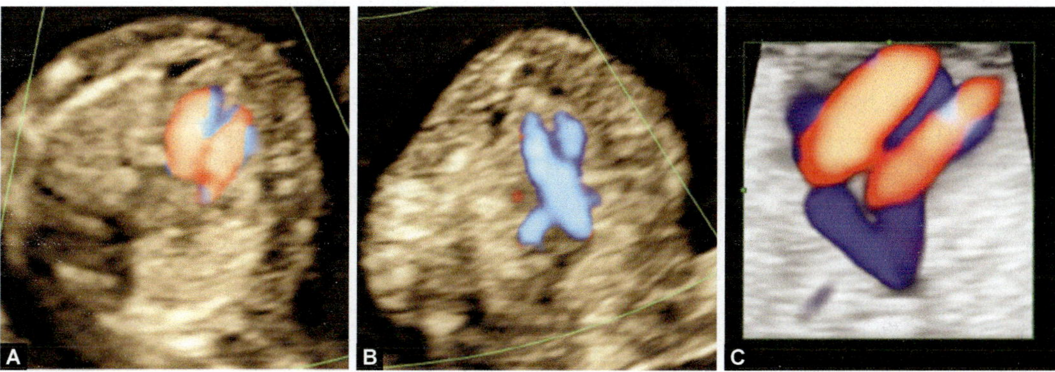

Figs. 34A to C: *Early pregnancy*: (A) Color Doppler of an apical four-chamber view demonstrating two inflows; (B) Color Doppler of outflows in criss-cross pattern; (C) A 4D color Doppler image showing the two inflows (in red) and "V" of 3VV (outflows in blue).

- The presence of reverse flow in ductus venosus
- Detection of tricuspid regurgitation during NT scan.

Basic heart examination at 11–14 weeks should include a good four-chamber view with situs and three-vessel trachea view. Cardiac axis deviation is the strong indicator of cardiac abnormality. Cardiac axis deviation is a more predictive of CHD than NT alone, TR alone, or DV alone or any combination of all three. Color flow examination of the heart is imperative along with a good two-dimensional examination. Power, pulse repetition frequency (PRF), and gain will have to be adjusted for optimal color setting. Complex cardiac defects, which can be diagnosed in early fetal echo (11–14 weeks), are AVSD, HLHS, hypoplastic right heart syndrome (HRHS), Ebstein anomaly, PA with intact IVS, tetralogy of Fallot with pulmonary atresia/stenosis, common arterial trunk, and transposition of great artery.

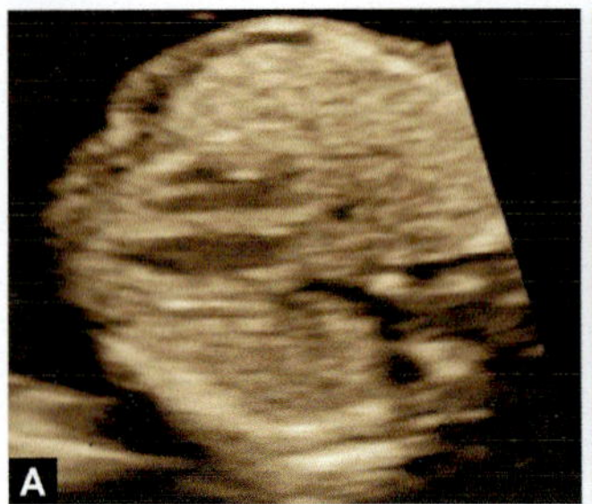

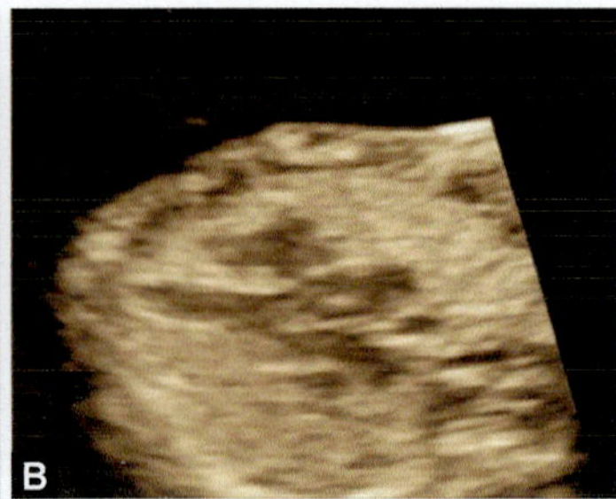

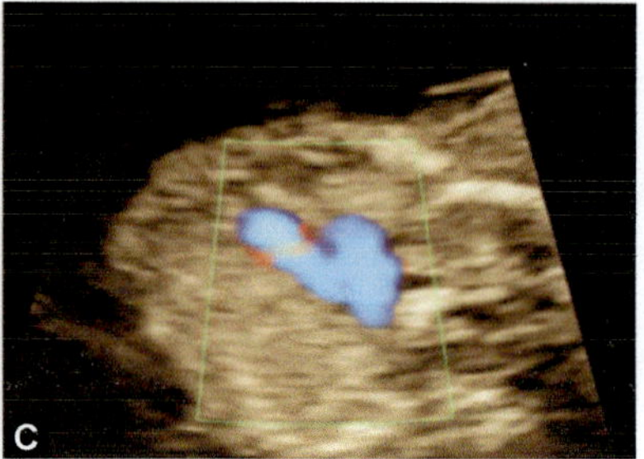

Figs. 35A to C: *Early pregnancy*: (A) Lateral four-chamber view in 2D gray scale; (B) Left ventricular outflow tract or long axis view of aorta in 2D gray scale; (C) 2D view in color Doppler showing three-vessel view with forward flow in both great arteries.

BENEFITS AND DISADVANTAGES OF EARLY FETAL ECHOCARDIOGRAPHY (FIGS. 35A TO C)

The cardiac defects diagnosed in 1st trimester are more complex and have higher association with chromosomal abnormalities than those seen in the second and 3rd trimesters of pregnancy. Early fetal echocardiography provides some benefits to patients such as early reassurance of a normal heart in patients with high risk for cardiac defects. And when a major cardiac malformation is diagnosed, the option for 1st trimester termination is available, which carries a significantly lower risk of morbidity than 2nd trimester termination.

Disadvantages of early fetal echocardiography include the need for a highly skilled and experienced examiner, the need for repeat cardiac examination in early 2nd trimester for confirmation, as several cardiac malformations are more visible at a later gestation, and it is time consuming, as it requires a combined transabdominal and transvaginal approach. There may be chances of false-positive diagnosis in mild anomalies especially in less experienced hands. For safety reasons, early fetal echocardiography should be performed only when there is a valid medical indication, and the lowest possible ultrasound exposure setting should be used under the ALARA (as low as reasonably achievable) principle. The duration of examination, especially power Doppler, should be limited thereby abiding by the safety principles of ultrasound.

BIBLIOGRAPHY

1. Abuhamad AZ. A Practical Guide to Fetal Echocardiography. Philadelphia: Wolters Kluwer; 1997. p. 35.
2. Achiron R, Rotstein Z, Lipitz S, Mashiach S, Hegesh J. First trimester diagnosis of fetal congenital heart disease by transvaginal ultrasonography. Obstet Gynecol. 1994;84(1):69-72.
3. Allan LD, Chita SK, Sharland K, Fagg NLK, Anderson RH, Crawford DC. The accuracy of fetal echocardiography in the diagnosis of congenital heart disease. Int J cardiol. 1989;25:279-88.
4. Calcagni G, Digilio CM, Sarkozy A, Dallapiccola B, Marino B. Familial recurrence of congenital heart disease: an overview and review of literature. Eur J Pediatr. 2007;166:111-6.
5. Chaoui R, Bollmann R. Fetal color Doppler echocardiography. Part 2: Abnormalities of the heart and great vessels. Ultraschall Med. 1994;15:105-111.
6. Copel JA, Pilo G, Green J, Hobbins JC, Kleinman CS. Fetal Echocardiographic screening for congenital heart disease: the importance of the four-chamber view. Am J Obstet Gynecol. 1897;157:648-55.
7. Hoffman JI, Kaplan S. The incidence of congenital heart disease. Cir Res. 2004;94:1890-900.
8. Homberger LK, Sahn DJ, Kleinman CS, Copel J, Silverman NH. Antenatal diagnosis of coarctation of aorta: a multicentric experience. J Am Coll Cardiol. 1994;23:417-23.
9. International Society of Ultrasound in Obstetrics & Gynecology. Cardiac screening examination of

the fetus: guidelines for performing the 'basic' and 'extended basic' cardiac scan. Ultrasound Obstet Gynecol. 2006;27(1):107-13.
10. Allan LD, Cook AC, Huggon IC. Fetal Echocardiography: A Practical Guide. Cambridge, UK: Cambridge University Press; 2009.
11. Machlitt A, Heling KS, Chaoui R. Increased cardiac atrial-to-ventricular length ratio in the fetal four-chamber view: a new marker for atrioventricular septal defects. Ultrasound Obstet Gynecol. 2004;24(6):618-22.
12. Paladini D, Rustico M, Todros T, Palmieri S, Gaglioti P, Benettoni A, et al. Conotruncal anomalies in prenatal life. Ultrasound Obstet Gynecol. 1996;8(4):241-6.
13. Twinning P, McHugo JM, Pilling DW. Textbook of Fetal Abnormalities. London, United Kingdom: Churchill Livingstone; 2007.
14. Poon LCY, Huggun IC, Zidere V, Allan LD. Tetralogy of Fallot in the fetus in current era. Ultrasound Obstet Gynecol. 2007;29(6):625-7.
15. Volpe P, Paladini D, Marasini M, Buonadonna AL, Russo MG, Caruso G, et al. Common arterial trunk in the fetus: associations and outcome in a multicentric series of 23 cases. Heart. 2003;89:1437-41.

13 CHAPTER

Fetal Urinary Tract Anomalies

KV Sridevi, Binodini M Chauhan

INTRODUCTION

Congenital anomalies of the kidney and urinary tract (CAKUT) constitute 20% of all congenital malformations occurring in one in 500 live births. CAKUT is responsible for 40–50% of pediatric and 7% of adult end-stage renal disease. High-resolution ultrasound equipment increasingly provides the opportunity to identify congenital anomalies of the urinary tract with a detection rate of approximately 89%. Prenatal diagnosis requires a systemic assessment of fetal kidneys, urinary bladder, amniotic fluid, and associated anomalies; however, family history and genetic tests provide information to improve the ability to make an accurate prenatal diagnosis of CAKUT.[1]

ULTRASOUND IMAGING OF FETAL URINARY TRACT

First Trimester Ultrasound Appearance of Fetal Urinary Tract

Visualization of the fetal urinary tract in the first trimester is performed by the identification of the bladder and then the kidneys. The fetal bladder appears as an anechoic structure in the anterior lower pelvis. The bladder is easily seen in the sagittal view of the fetus **(Fig. 1A)** in the same plane used for the crown-rump length (CRL) measurement. The axial plane of the fetal pelvis also demonstrates the fetal bladder in a central-anterior location surrounding umbilical arteries. The longitudinal length of the normal bladder should be <7 mm in the first trimester **(Fig. 1B)**. The fetal bladder is

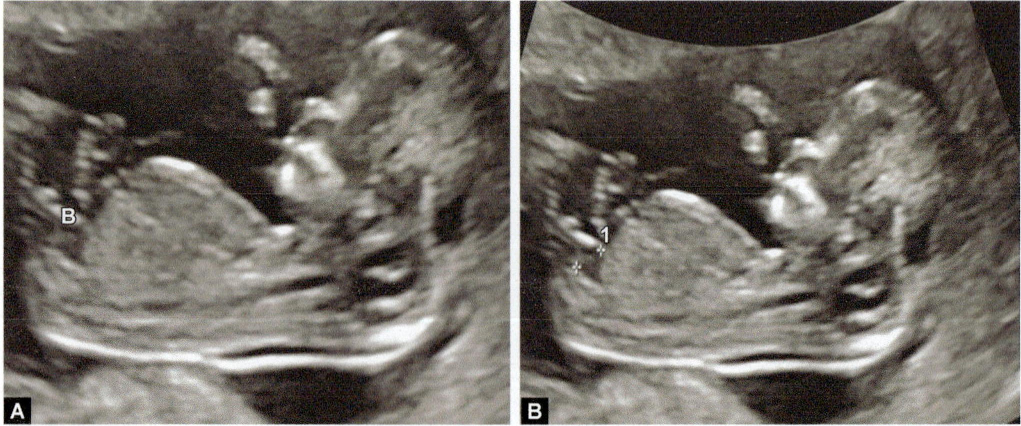

Figs. 1A and B: (A) Sagittal view of the fetus [crown-rump length (CRL) plane] bladder is easily seen as hypoechoic structure in the anterior lower pelvis and bladder; (B) Midsagittal view of the fetus showing longitudinal measurement of the bladder (<7 mm normal).

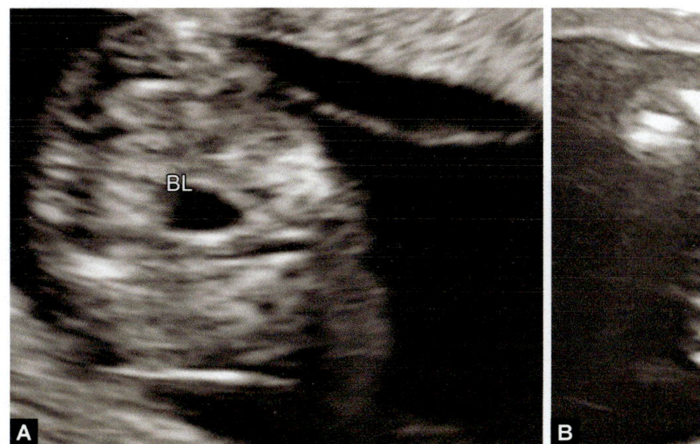

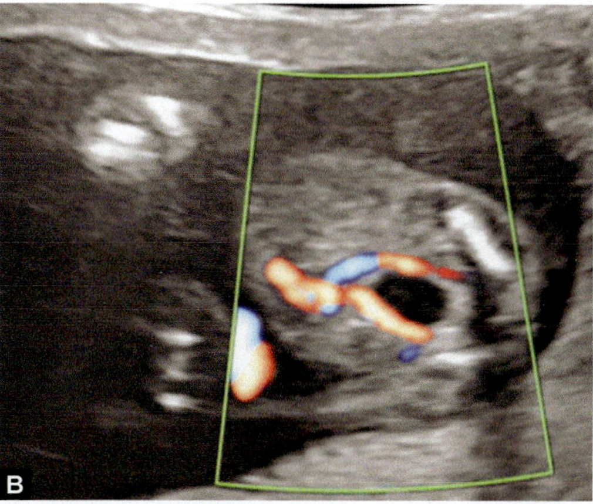

Figs. 2A and B: (A) Transverse two-dimensional (2D) view of 12 weeks fetal lower pelvis showing bladder as central anechoic area surrounding umbilical arteries on either side of the bladder (BL); (B) Color Doppler showing umbilical arteries on either side of the bladder.

seen on ultrasound in about 88% of fetuses at 12 weeks of gestation and in 92–100% of fetuses at 13 weeks of gestation **(Figs. 2A and B)**. With transabdominal ultrasound, the fetal kidneys are generally difficult to visualize and differentiate from the surrounding bowel; therefore, transvaginal scanning in the first trimester improves visualization. The fetal kidneys appear in the first trimester as rounded, slightly bright structures in the posterior abdomen lateral to the spine, with the renal pelvis noted as anechoic circles, centrally within the renal tissue. Visualization of the fetal kidneys in the first trimester can be achieved in the coronal, sagittal, or axial planes of the fetal abdomen **(Fig. 3A)**. The coronal plane of the fetal abdomen is the optimal plane for first trimester imaging of the kidneys **(Fig. 3B)**. Color Doppler can also be added to demonstrate the right and left renal arteries arising from the descending aorta **(Fig. 3C)**. The fetal kidneys can be identified in 86–99% of fetuses at 12 weeks of gestation and in 92–99% of fetuses at 13 weeks of gestation.[2]

Second and Third Trimester Normal Ultrasound Appearance of Urinary Tract (Box 1)

The kidneys gradually become hypoechoic compared with the adjacent bowel and liver. It is recommended that the kidneys are seen

BOX 1: Ultrasound imaging of fetal urinary tract.

- Always asses the kidneys in two planes to avoid fallacies
- Identify kidneys by means of renal pelvis
- Color Doppler—renal arteries seen arising from the aorta
- Urinary bladder is identified as anechoic structure in the fetal pelvis surrounded by two umbilical arteries

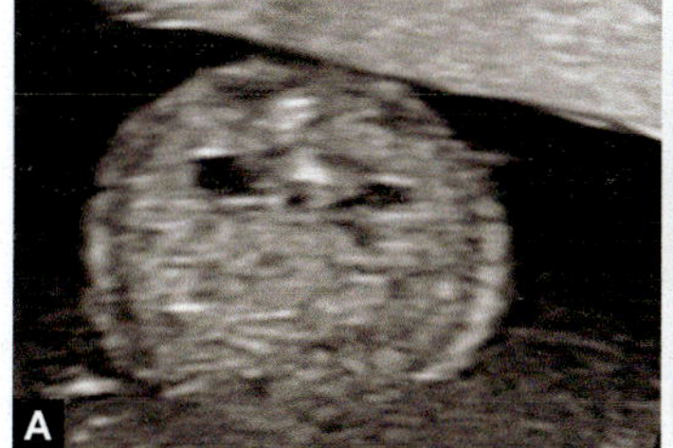

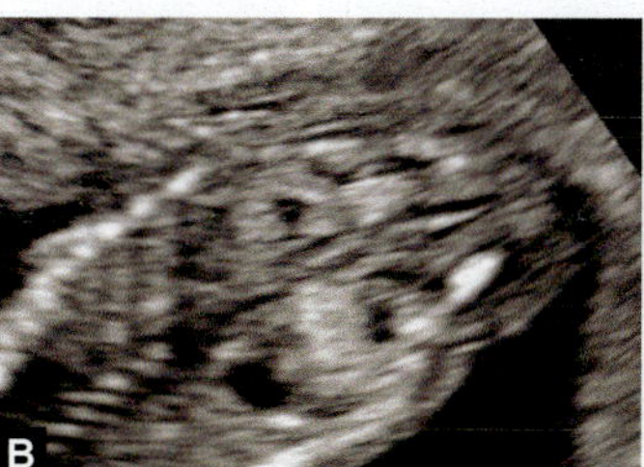

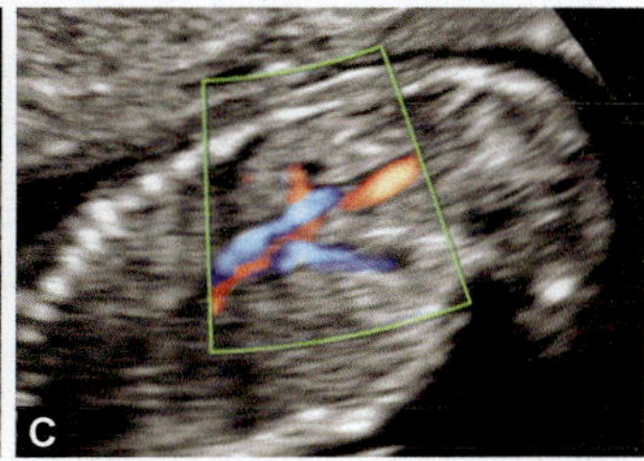

Figs. 3A to C: (A) Transverse view of 13 weeks fetus with normal appearing kidneys and axial view of fetal kidneys; (B) Coronal view showing echogenic kidneys on either side of the spine; (C) Color Doppler showing bilateral renal arteries arising from aorta.

in axial, sagittal, and coronal planes. The renal cortex appears echogenic compared with the medulla and the renal pelvises are seen as anechoic spaces in the medial aspect in the transverse sections **(Figs. 4A and B)**. In the third trimester, the pyramids can be differentiated from the cortex as it appears more hypoechoic **(Fig. 4C)**. The kidneys grow

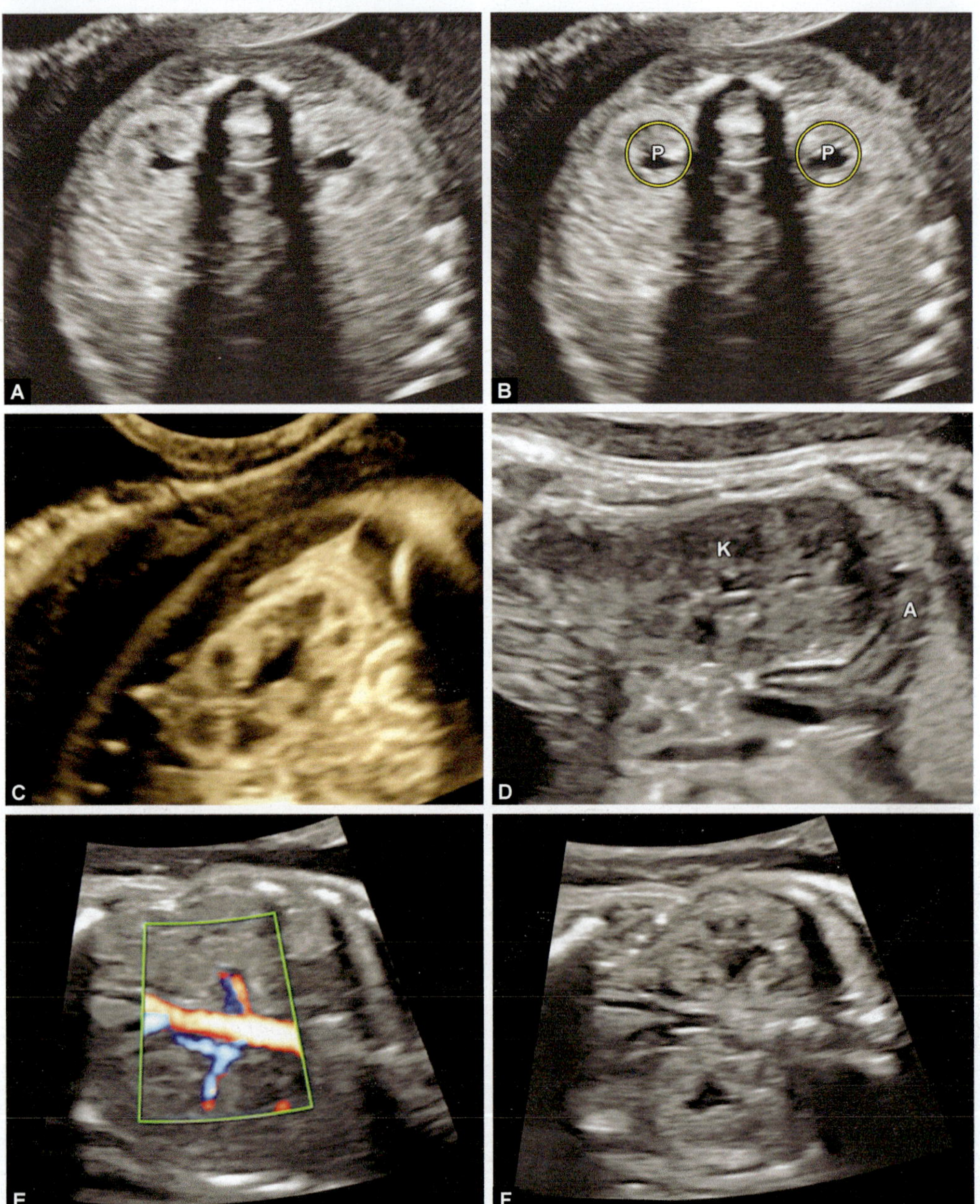

Figs. 4A to F: (A) Axial view of normal kidneys and spine at 12 o'clock position; (B) Axial view of fetal kidneys with spine at 12 o'clock position and hypoechoic central renal pelvis (p); (C) Longitudinal scan shows good corticomedullary differentiation with hyperechoic cortex and hypoechoic triangular pyramids on the inner side of the kidney; (D) Sagittal view shows slightly curved adrenal gland that is seen on the superior border of the kidney (K) and adrenal gland (A); (E) Bilateral renal arteries seen arising from the descending aorta; (F) Coronal scan showing bilateral bean-shaped kidneys.

as long as the pregnancy continues and the size is directly proportional to the gestational age. Adrenal glands can be seen on the superior pole of the kidney **(Fig. 4D)**. Kidneys may also be seen in coronal planes and Doppler may be used to demonstrate both the renal arteries **(Figs. 4E and F)**. Fetal ureters are not usually visible antenatally unless they are dilated. The fetal bladder can be visualized in the pelvis from 10 weeks of gestation, the urinary bladder can be identified as an anechoic structure in the fetal pelvis surrounded by two umbilical arteries, and persistent absence of the bladder should be considered as abnormal from 15 weeks[2] **(Figs. 5A to D)**.

RENAL AGENESIS

Bilateral Renal Agenesis

Bilateral renal agenesis is defined as complete absence of both kidneys and ureters resulting from their failure to form. Incidence of bilateral renal agenesis is 1:240 stillbirths and about 1:3,000 live births.[3,4]

Ultrasound Diagnosis

Kidneys and the bladder are not visualized **(Fig. 6A)** and severe oligohydramnios after the 16th weeks of gestation. Adrenal glands sometimes appear merely rounder than normal and fill the renal fossa[5] in what has

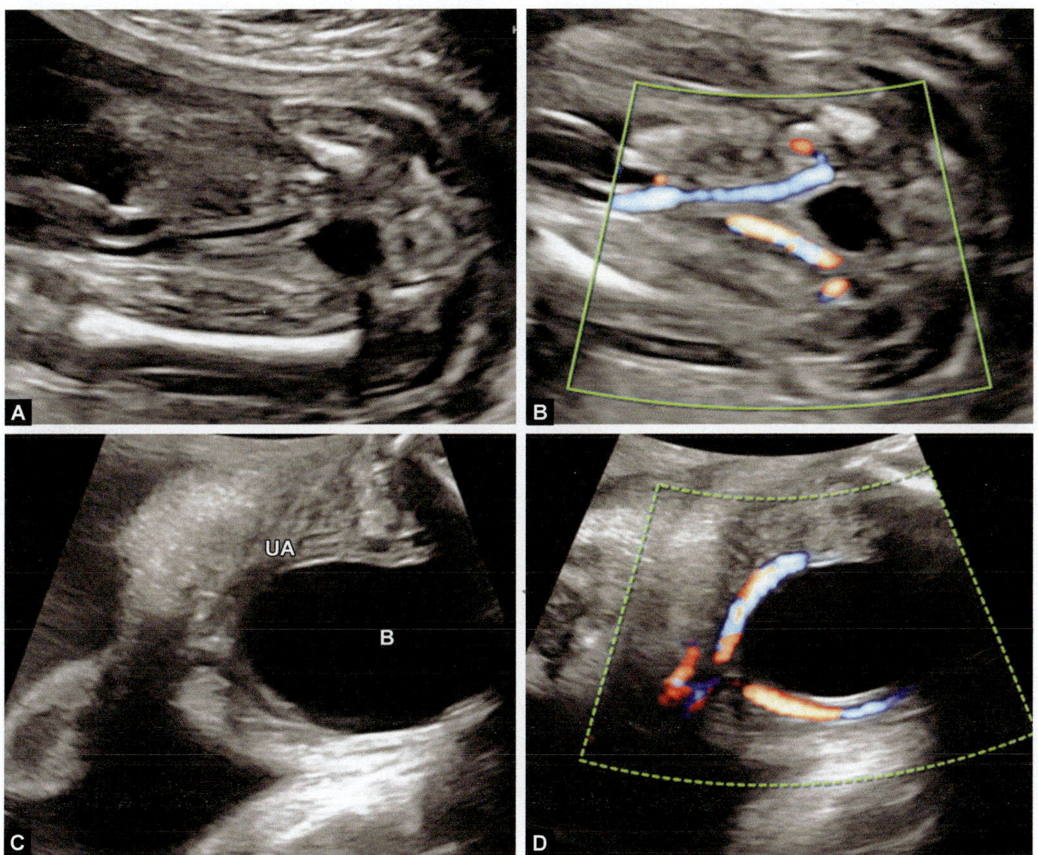

Figs. 5A to D: (A) Transverse two-dimensional (2D) view of the 20 weeks fetal lower pelvis showing bladder as central anechoic area surrounding umbilical arteries on either side of the bladder; (B) Color Doppler showing umbilical arteries on either side of the bladder; (C) Transverse 2D view of the 33 weeks fetal lower pelvis showing bladder as central anechoic area surrounding umbilical arteries on either side of the bladder and the umbilical cord entry into the fetal abdomen is also seen [bladder (B) and umbilical artery (UA)]; (D) Color Doppler in the same fetus showing umbilical arteries on either side of the bladder.

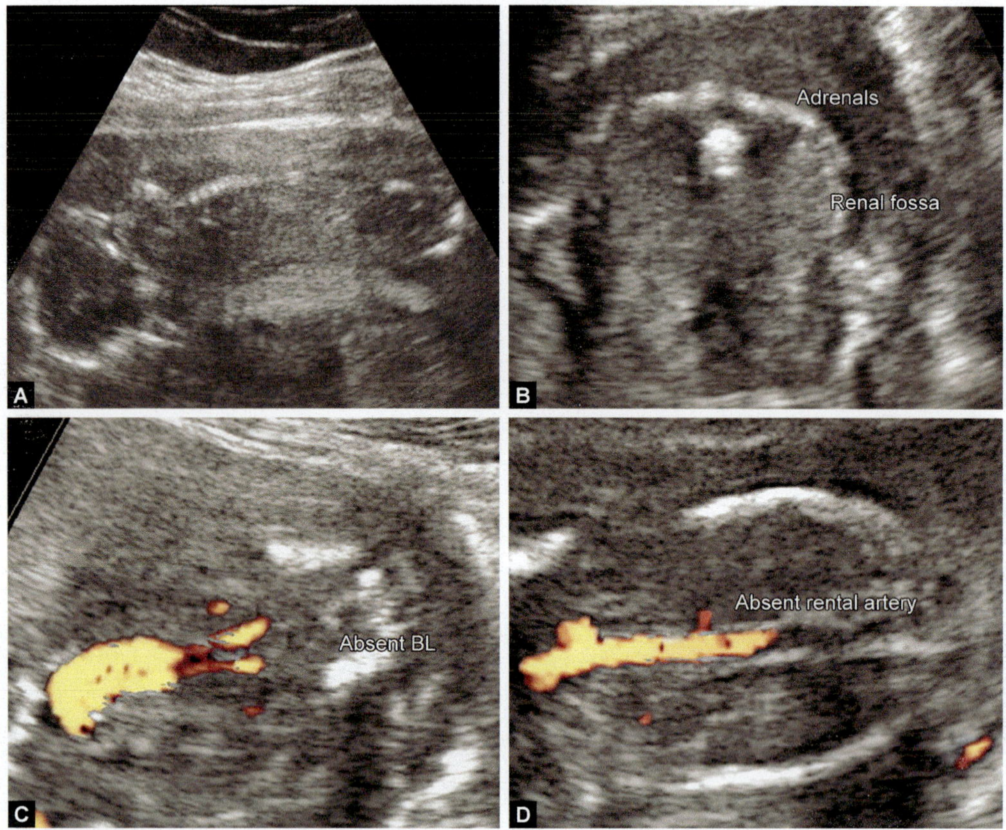

Figs. 6A to D: (A) Lack of urine leads to complete anhydramnios by 16 weeks; (B) Transverse scan showing absence of both kidneys and prominent adrenal gland on one side; (C) Color Doppler—both umbilical arteries are separate; however, there is absence of bladder; (D) Absence of the renal arteries noted while the aorta is clearly seen.

been termed as the "lying down" adrenal sign **(Fig. 6B)**. Color/power Doppler is to confirm the absence of the renal arteries. In first trimester screening **(Fig. 6C)** when the amniotic fluid would still be normal in case of bilateral renal agenesis, the routine visualization of the fetal bladder could help to exclude this malformation **(Fig. 6D)**.[6,7]

Prognosis

The outcome of bilateral renal agenesis is uniformly fatal due to the associated severe pulmonary hypoplasia.

Recurrence

X-linked and autosomal dominant and recessive inheritance have been reported for renal agenesis. If renal agenesis is isolated, the empiric risk of recurrence is 3–4%, whereas if it is one sign of a syndrome, the risk of recurrence is obviously the risk associated with the underlying syndrome.[5,8,9]

Unilateral Renal Agenesis (Figs. 7A and B)

Unilateral renal agenesis (URA) is defined as complete absence of one kidney and ipsilateral ureter. URA occurs in 1–2/1,000 births.

Ultrasound Diagnosis

There is absence of kidney in the renal fossae. The bladder and amount of amniotic fluid are normal. Adrenal gland appears rounder than normal and fills the renal fossa in what has been termed as the "lying down" adrenal **(Fig. 8)**. It mimics kidney; therefore, unilateral renal agenesis escapes prenatal diagnosis many

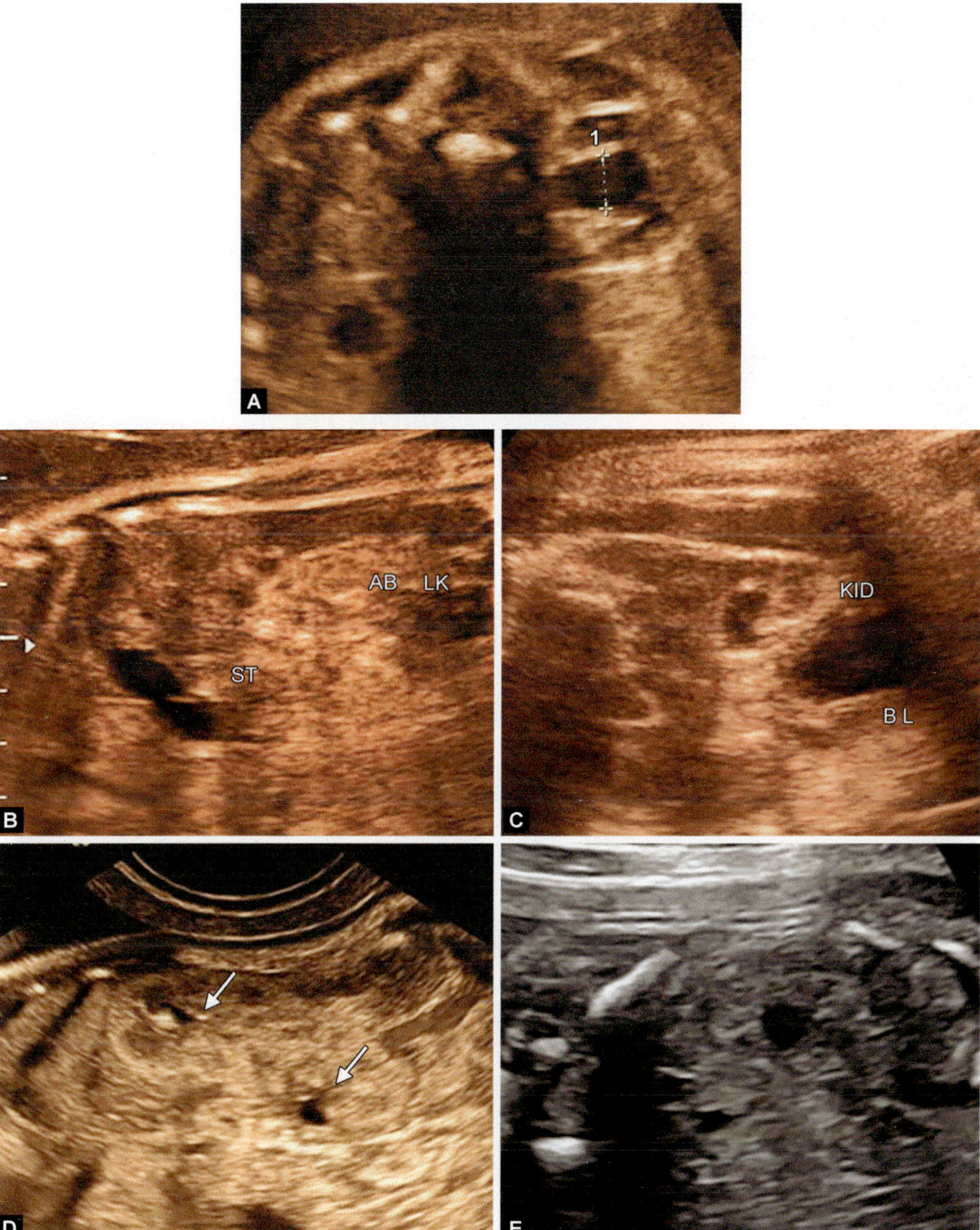

Figs. 7A to E: (A) Axial scan revealing the kidney in one renal fossae and nonvisualized kidney on the opposite side; (B) Unilateral renal agenesis; (C) Kidney seen in the pelvis above the fetal bladder—ectopic pelvic kidney; (D) Horseshoe kidney (coronal) in which lower poles of both kidneys are fused; (E) Bilobed kidney—crossed renal ectopia.

times.[8] Color/power Doppler can be used in cases that are uncertain to confirm the absence of the ipsilateral renal artery **(Figs. 9A to D)**.

Prognosis

Unilateral renal agenesis is isolated and the prognosis is good.[5,8]

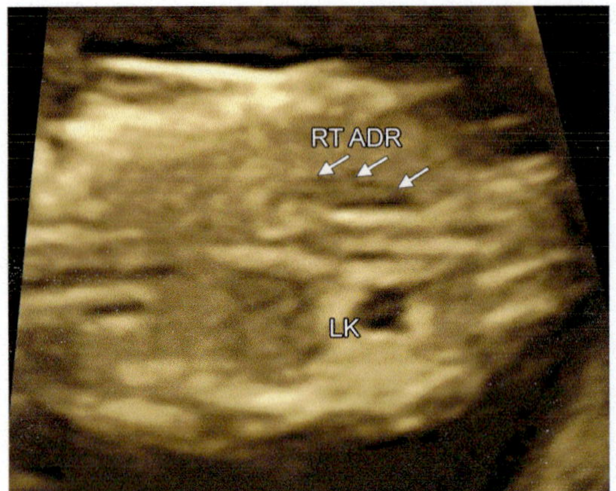

Fig. 8: Coronal plane of 13 weeks fetus demonstrates empty renal fossae on the right side and the adrenal gland has become vertical (the lying down adrenal sign) confirms that the renal fossa is empty and kidney is absent.
(RT ADR: right adrenal; LK: left kidney)

Recurrence Risk

X-linked and autosomal dominant and recessive inheritance have been reported for renal agenesis. If renal agenesis is isolated, the empiric risk of recurrence is 3–6%. The finding of a renal agenesis in one of the parents increases the recurrence risk to 15–20%. In particular, in cases of autosomal dominant inheritance pattern, the recurrence risk could be up to 50%, while in recessive ones, it is 25%.[10-12]

ECTOPIC KIDNEY (FIGS. 7C, AND 10A AND B)

Horseshoe Kidney (Fig. 7D)

Horseshoe kidney is a fusion of the lower poles of both kidneys. Incidence is 1:400 live births and more common in boys.

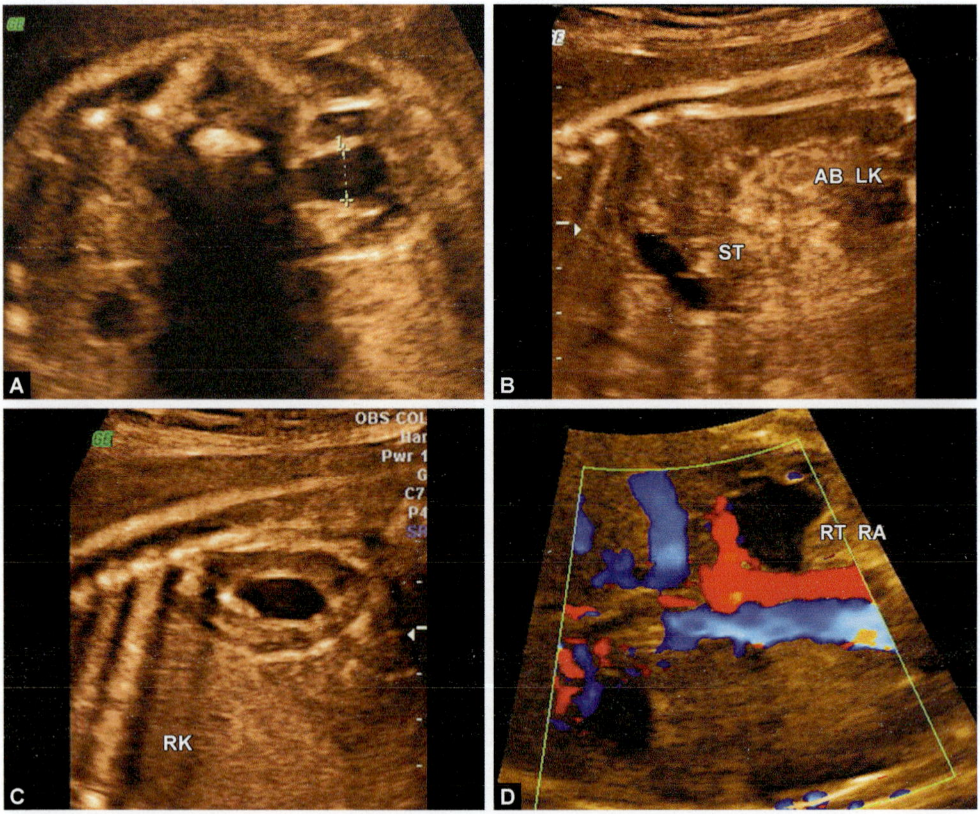

Figs. 9A to D: (A) Transverse view—one kidney is not seen in the renal fossae with prominent renal pelvis in the other kidney; (B) Sagittal view—stomach is seen and the left kidney is absent; (C) Right kidney is seen in the right renal fossae with prominent renal pelvis; (D) Color flow image demonstrates a single renal artery indicating unilateral agenesis.
(ST: stomach; AB: absent; LK: left kidney; RT: right; RA: renal artery)

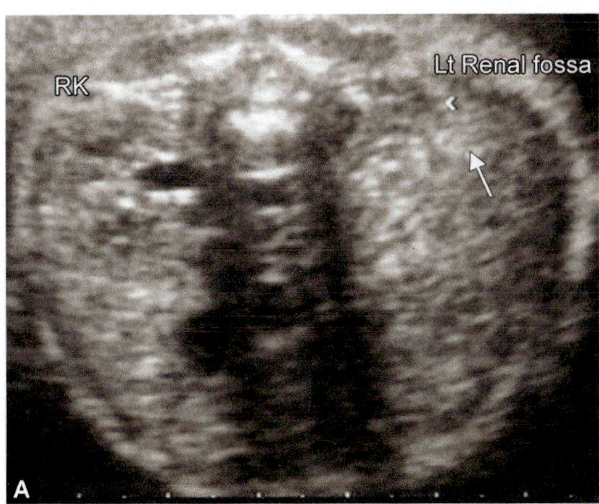

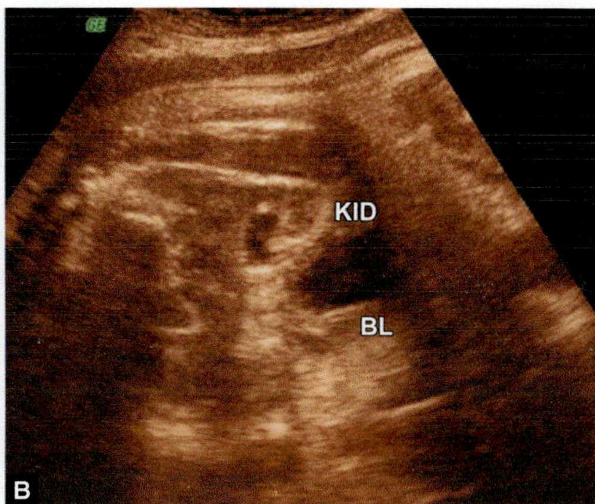

Figs. 10A and B: (A) Transverse view isolated 20 weeks fetus—empty left renal fossae seen on the left side; (B) Left kidney (KID) is seen in the pelvis just above the bladder (BL) indicating ectopic pelvic kidney.

Ultrasound Diagnosis

It involves fusion of the lower poles of both kidneys in front of the descending aorta. Horseshoe kidney is best demonstrated on the coronal and transverse scans when renal tissue will be seen crossing the midline **(Fig. 11)**. Normal bladder and amniotic fluid volume are present.

Chromosomal Abnormalities

Horseshoe kidney is found in 30% of cases of Turner syndrome and in 20% of trisomy 18. Associated syndromes are found in 15% of cases. Other defects include hydronephrosis and genital anomalies, central nervous system (CNS), cardiac, or skeletal is found in 30% of cases. In isolated forms, the prognosis is good **(Figs. 12A and B)**. Postnatal follow-up is advised because of significant risk of infections, hydronephrosis, and nephrolithiasis (70%). Ultrasound scans every 4 weeks during pregnancy to detect possible late-onset hydronephrosis. Isolated or part of Turner syndrome causes no increased risk. Part of trisomy 18: 1%.[2]

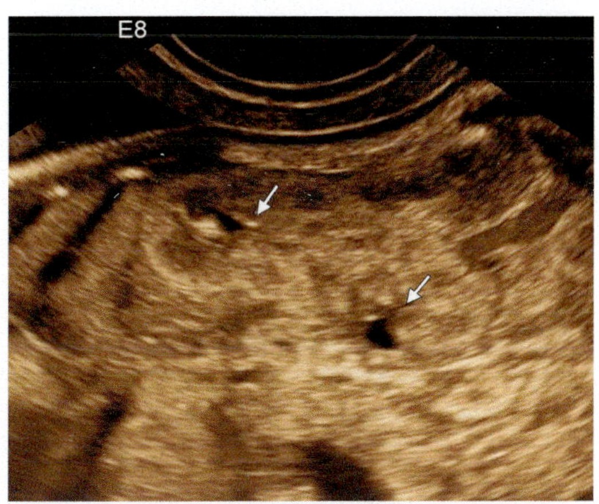

Fig. 11: Horseshoe kidney (coronal) and lower poles of both kidneys are fused.

Crossed Fused Kidneys (Fig. 7E)

In crossed renal ectopia, the ectopic kidney lies entirely on the opposite side of the abdomen relative to its ureteral insertion into the bladder and crossed kidney fuses with its partner. Incidence 1:7,000. In ultrasound diagnosis, one renal fossa is empty and an enlarged bilobed kidney is seen **(Figs. 13A and B)**. Associated anomalies are sacral agenesis, anal atresia, and myelomeningocele. Prognosis is good in isolated cases and postnatal follow-up is probably indicated due to higher incidence of vesicoureteric reflux.[2,8]

URINARY TRACT DILATATION

Urinary tract dilatation (UTD) is one of the most common anomalies seen prenatally in around 1–2% of all pregnancies. UTD

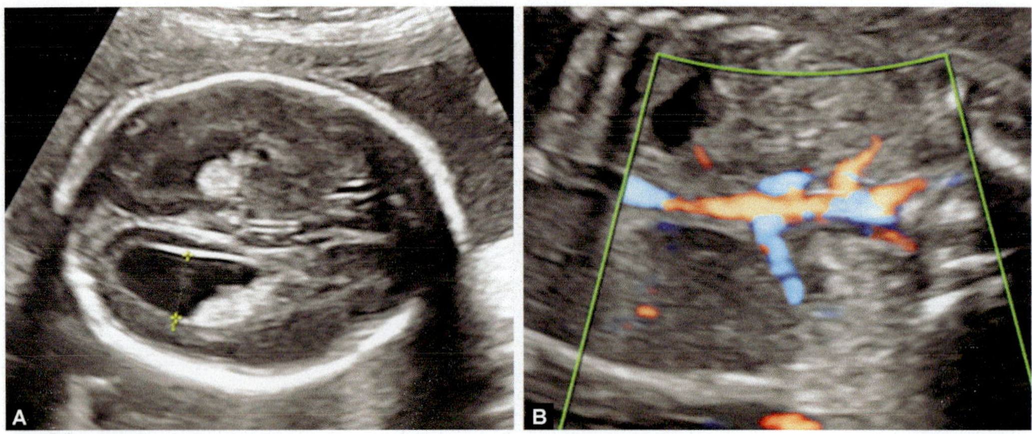

Figs. 12A and B: (A) Axial view 22 weeks fetal head showing teardrop ventricle with absence of cavum septum pellucidum (CSP); (B) Coronal view showing one kidney in the pelvis and the other one normally placed. Color Doppler also shows renal arteries at different levels.

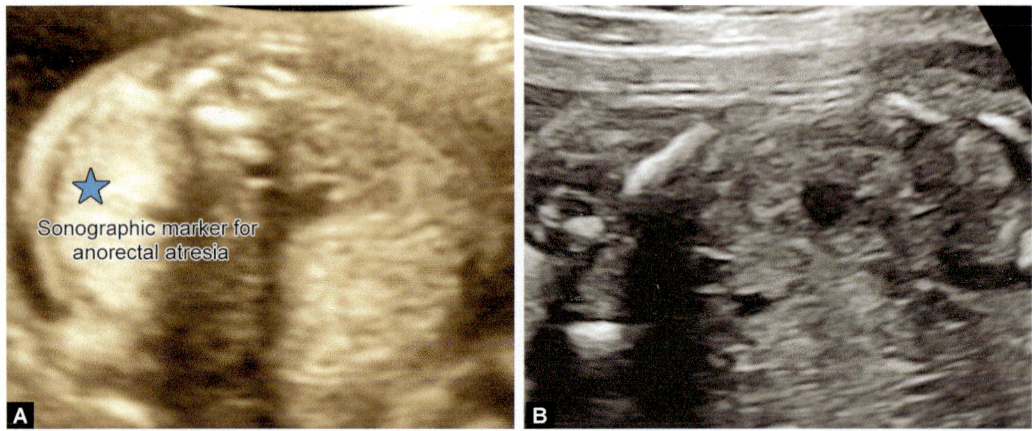

Figs. 13A and B: (A) Unilateral empty renal fossa; (B) Bilobed kidney—crossed renal ectopia.

presents as a spectrum of severity. In most of the cases (50–70%), the UTD is transient or physiologic without any clinical significance. In the rest, posterior urethral valves (1–5%), pelviureteric junction obstruction (10–30%), and vesicoureteric reflux (10–40%) are present. The less common causes are duplex collecting system and ectopic ureter.[12,13]

Urinary tract dilatation classification system is a proposed unified classification of UTD for prenatal and postnatal care. This system is designed to be used in cases of isolated UTD and not applied to unique situations or anomalous kidneys.[12-14]

Anterior-posterior renal pelvis diameter (APRPD) measurements are done with spine at 12 or 6 o'clock position and maximum diameter of the intrarenal pelvis is measured **(Figs. 14A and B)**.[15] The renal pelvis is considered normal if the APRPD is <4 mm at <28 weeks of gestation, <7 mm at >28 weeks of gestation, and <10 mm postnatally without calyceal dilatation, normal parenchyma, nonvisualized ureter, and normal urinary bladder. Above these threshold measurements, it is diagnosed as UTD. In antenatal period, the UTD is classified into two groups—a low-risk group of UTD A1 with low risk for postnatal

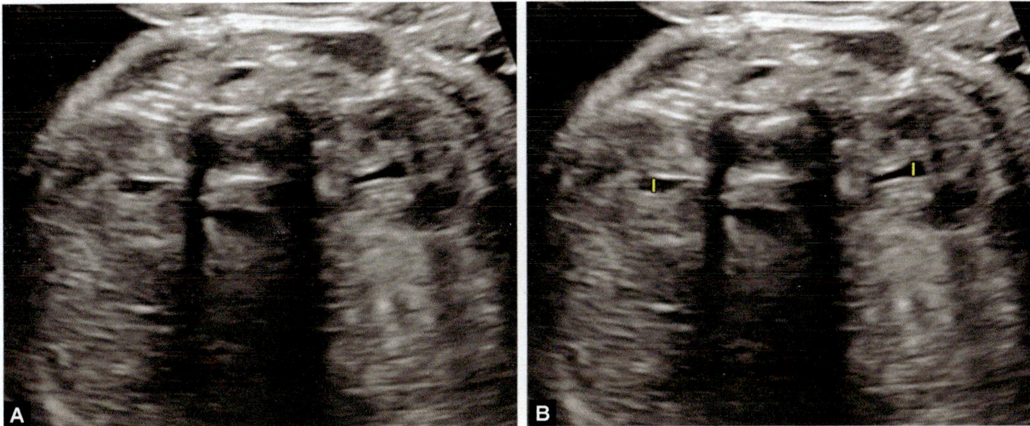

Figs. 14A and B: Anterior-posterior renal pelvis diameter (APRPD) measurement technique. (A) Axial scan of fetal abdomen demonstrates the fetal spine at 12 o'clock position; (B) Yellow bar represents placement of calipers for the measurement.

uropathy and an increased risk group of UTD A2-A3 with increased risk for postnatal uropathy. Prenatally classification is applicable after 16 weeks of gestation.

The UTD classification system uses six ultrasound findings to describe the urinary tracts.

1. Anterior-posterior renal pelvic diameter
2. Calyceal dilation with distinction between central and peripheral calyces postnatally
3. Renal parenchymal thickness
4. Renal parenchymal appearance
5. Bladder abnormalities
6. Ureteral abnormalities

UTD A1—low risk for postnatal uropathy:

- *Anteroposterior renal pelvic diameter* ***(Fig. 15)***:
  - *16–27 weeks*: 4 mm to <7 mm
  - *≥28 weeks*: 7 mm to <10 mm
- With or without central calyceal dilatation

UTD A2-A3-increased risk for postnatal uropathy:

- *Anteroposterior renal pelvic diameter* ***(Figs. 16A to C)***:
  - *16–27 weeks*: ≥7 mm
  - *≥28 weeks*: ≥10 mm
- Peripheral calyceal dilatation, abnormal parenchyma thickness or appearance, abnormal ureter or bladder, and unexplained oligohydramnios.

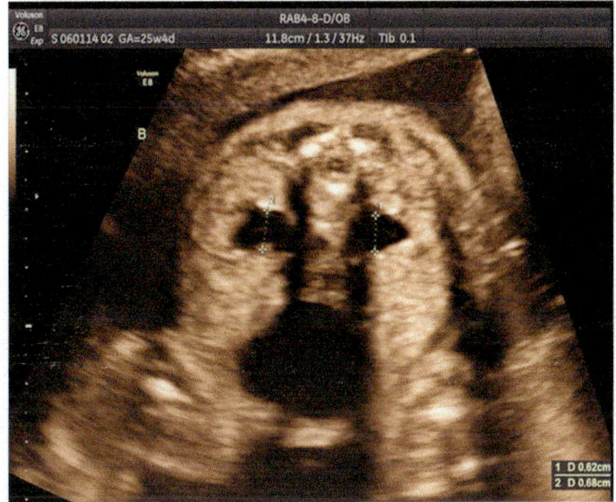

Fig. 15: Ultrasound appearance of urinary tract dilatation (UTD) A1—fetal kidney at 29 weeks of gestation: Transverse scan showing anterior-posterior renal pelvic diameter (APRPD) measuring 6 mm and no calyceal dilatation which is within UTD A1 range.

Based on the UTD classification system, a follow-up management scheme has been proposed. For UTD A1 diagnosed before 32 weeks, a follow-up prenatal ultrasound is recommended at >32 weeks. If the ultrasound at >32 weeks reveals resolution of the UTD with normal renal parenchyma, bladder, and ureters, no further prenatal of postnatal follow-up is necessary. If there is persistent UTD A1 or UTD A2-A3, evaluation after

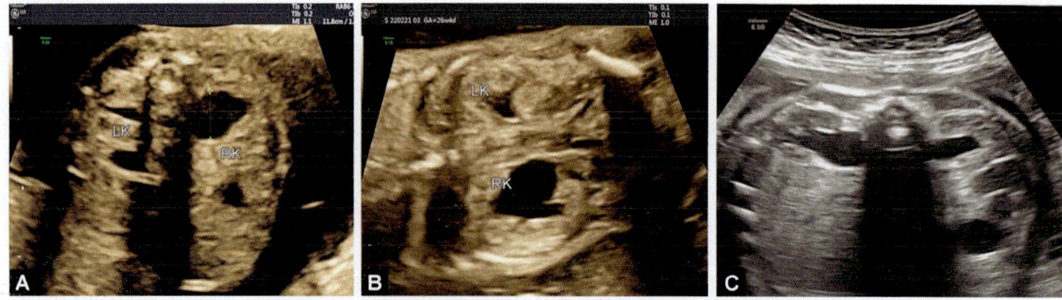

Figs. 16A to C: Ultrasound appearance of UTD A2-A3—fetal kidney at 29 weeks of gestation: (A) Transverse scan showing anterior-posterior right renal pelvic diameter (APRPD) measuring 12 mm and left renal anterior-posterior diameter measuring 3 mm, which is normal; (B) Right minimal calyceal dilatation noted within UTD A2-A3 range; (C) Fetal kidney at 30 weeks of gestation: Transverse scan showing APRPD measuring 13 mm and left renal anterior-posterior diameter measuring 9 mm which is within UTD A2-A3.

birth is recommended. Postnatal evaluation should include two ultrasound evaluations: the first at >48 hours but <1 month after birth and the second 1–6 months later. In fetuses considered at increased risk for postnatal uropathy (UTD A2-A3), a follow-up prenatal ultrasound is recommended within 4–6 weeks of the initial diagnosis of UTD. Where there is substantial risk for surgery or renal dysfunction, prenatal consultation with a specialist is recommended. UTD is most often transient and associated with an increased risk of trisomy 21 warranting a detailed ultrasound and correlation with aneuploidy screening protocols. Likelihood ratio of pyelectasis for Tr-21 is 1.9 and anteroposterior diameter of renal pelvis ^{3} 4 mm between 16 and 20 weeks is considered as marker.

FETAL PELVIURETERIC JUNCTION OBSTRUCTION

In pelviureteric junction (PUJ) obstruction, there is dilatation of fetal renal pelvis and calyces. Most cases of PUJ obstruction are functional than anatomic lesions. Its prevalence is 0.6–5.4% with male predominance.

Ultrasound Features

Anterior-posterior right renal pelvic diameter > 10 mm is present with calyceal dilatation. In coronal scan, the peripheral dilated calyces communicate with the medial larger renal pelvis. The ureter and bladder are not dilated. Prognosis is dependent on uni-/bilateral involvement **(Figs. 17 and 18)**, degree of renal pelvis dilatation, and parenchymal involvement. Ultrasound scans every 4 weeks to monitor the evolution of hydronephrosis and assess amniotic fluid volume.[2]

URETEROVESICAL JUNCTION OBSTRUCTION

Presence of hydroureter and hydronephrosis with normal bladder is present **(Figs. 19A and B)**. The dilated ureter is tortuous **(Figs. 20A to C)** and appears as a collection of cysts of variable size localized between the dilated renal pelvis and the bladder. The etiology is diverse including ureteric stricture or atresia, vascular obstruction, diverticulum, or ureterocele. Ureteroceles (visible as a thin-walled and fluid-filled small circular area inside the bladder) are usually found in association with a duplex kidney and collecting system **(Figs. 21A and B)**. The upper pole characteristically obstructs and the lower one refluxes. The incidence of chromosomal abnormalities and genetic syndromes is not increased. Ultrasound scans every 4 weeks to monitor the evolution of hydronephrosis and assess amniotic fluid volume. Postnatal intervention is indicated

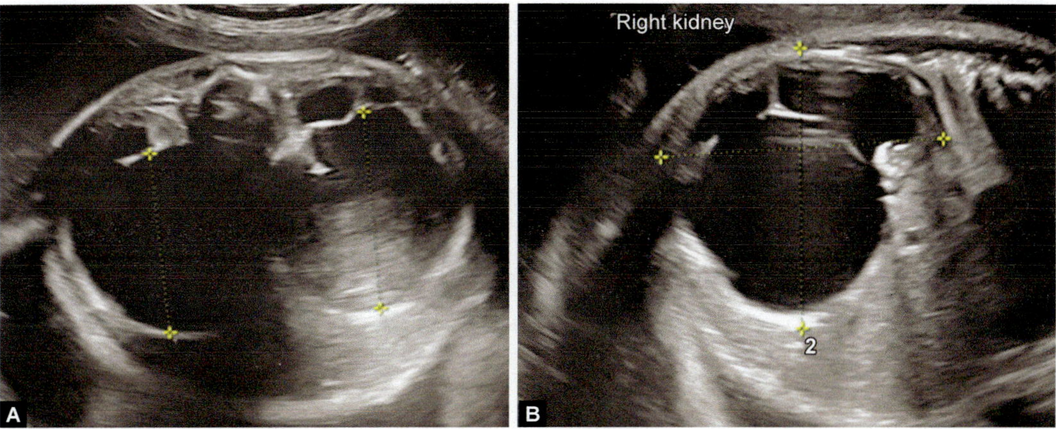

Figs. 17A and B: Bilateral pelviureteric junction (PUJ) obstruction. (A) Axial scan at 30 weeks fetal kidneys shows marked dilatation of renal pelvis and calyces; (B) Oblique scan shows peripheral dilated calyces communicating with dilated medial pelvis, thin parenchyma, ureters are not dilated, and bladder is small.

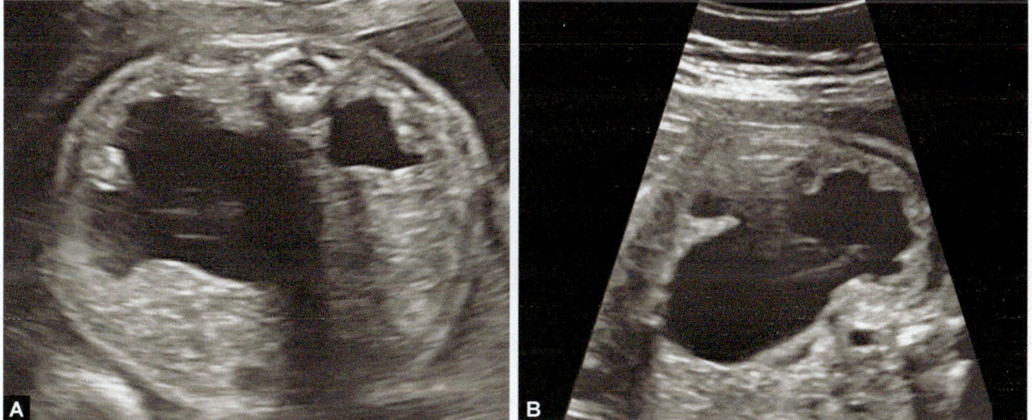

Figs. 18A and B: Unilateral pelviureteric junction (PUJ) obstruction. (A) Axial scan at 26 weeks fetal right kidney shows marked dilatation of renal pelvis and calyces; (B) Oblique scan shows peripheral symmetrical dilated calyces communicating with dilated medial pelvis and ureters are not dilated.

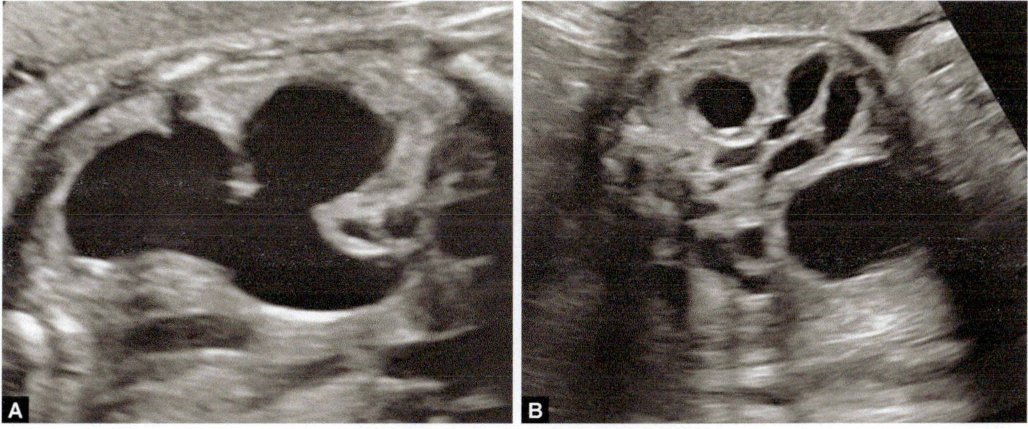

Figs. 19A and B: (A) Coronal scan of 28 weeks fetus showing unilateral pelvicalyceal dilatation; (B) Dilatation of ureter also noted and bladder is normal.

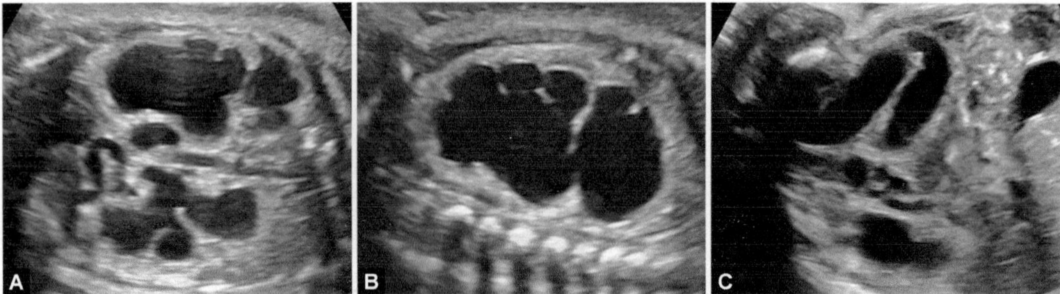

Figs. 20A to C: (A) Coronal scan 26 weeks fetus with bilateral pelvicalyceal dilatation; (B) Coronal scan shows peripheral symmetrical dilated calyces communicating with dilated medial pelvis; (C) Ureteric dilatation is noted and normal bladder and liquor are noted.

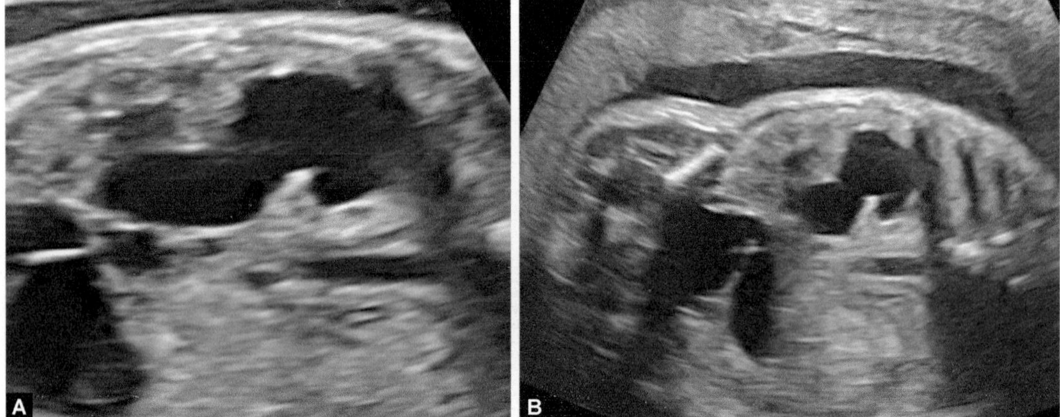

Figs. 21A and B: Duplex collecting system. (A) Longitudinal scan of the kidney shows duplex collecting system with hydroureteronephrosis of upper moiety and normal lower moiety; (B) Coronal scan showing duplex collecting system with hydroureteronephrosis of upper moiety.

if the vesicoureteric reflux is associated with abnormal renal function. No increased risk of recurrence.[2]

URETHRAL OBSTRUCTION

Urethral obstruction can be caused by urethral agenesis, persistence of the cloaca, urethral stricture, or posterior urethral valves. With posterior urethral valves **(Figs. 22A and B)**, there is usually incomplete or intermittent obstruction of the urethra resulting in an enlarged and hypertrophied bladder with varying degrees of hydroureters, hydronephrosis, a spectrum of renal dysplasia (echogenic renal parenchyma with peripherally placed cysts), oligohydramnios, and pulmonary hypoplasia. In some cases, there is associated urinary ascites from rupture of the bladder **(Figs. 23A and B)**. Reduced amount of the amniotic fluid is >17 weeks of gestation. In the first trimester, the condition presents as megacystis (longitudinal bladder diameter of ≥7 mm). If the bladder diameter is 7–15 mm, there is spontaneous resolution of the megacystis in about 90% of cases. If the bladder diameter is ≥15 mm **(Figs. 24A and B)**, the condition is invariably associated with progressive obstructive uropathy leading to hydronephrosis and dysplastic kidneys **(Figs. 25A to C)**. Associated abnormalities—chromosomal defects, mainly trisomies 21, 18, or 13, are found in about 10% of cases. Other defects mainly cardiac and gastrointestinal are found in

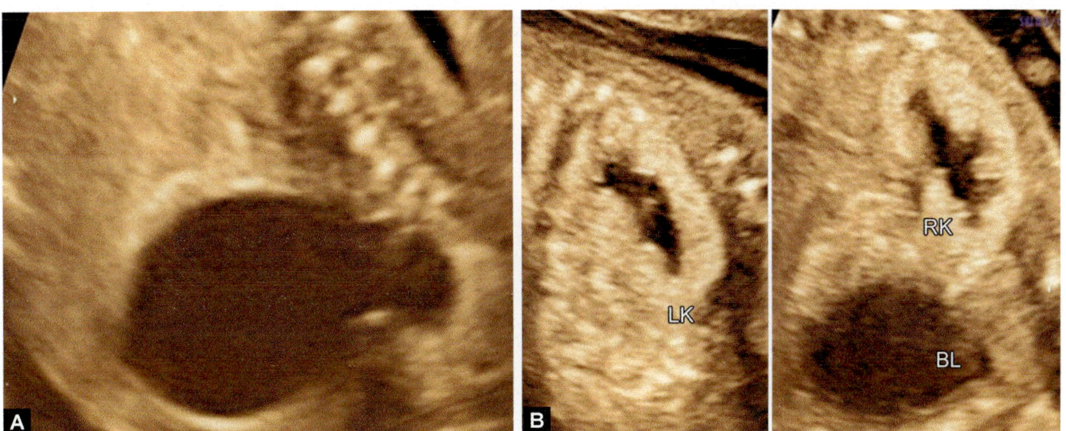

Figs. 22A and B: Posterior urethral valves. (A) Oblique scan of 16 weeks fetal pelvis shows the keyhole appearance of dilated thickened urinary bladder is noted; (B) Coronal scan shows bilateral echogenic kidneys and with prominent renal pelvis.
(BL: bladder; LK: left kidney; RK: right kidney)

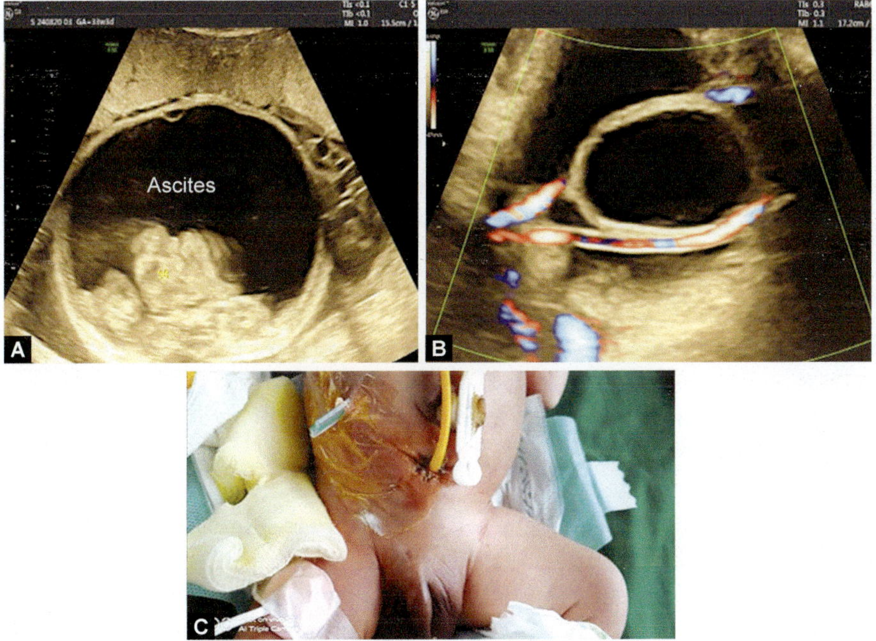

Figs. 23A to C: (A) Urinary ascites; (B) Urinary ascites and bladder with umbilical arteries on either side; (C) Postnatal suprapubic catheter.

up to 40% of cases. Investigations—detailed ultrasound examination. Amniocentesis is done for karyotyping or analysis of cfDNA from maternal blood. If pregnancy continues, ultrasound scans every 4 weeks to monitor the evolution of the condition and assess amniotic fluid volume. Antenatal evaluation of renal function relies on a combination of ultrasonographic findings and analysis of fetal urine obtained by urodochocentesis. Severe cases of high perinatal mortality are due to pulmonary hypoplasia secondary to severe oligohydramnios. Even in those that survive, about 30% develop renal failure necessitating

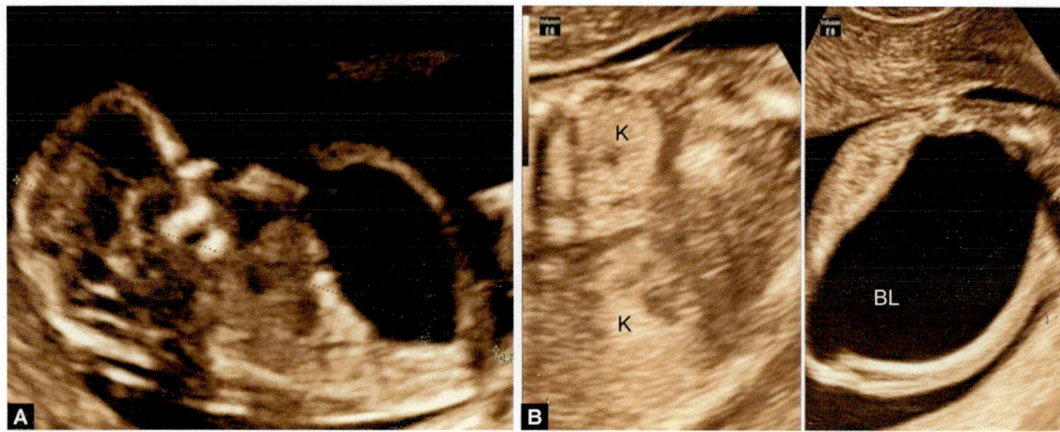

Figs. 24A and B: Megacystis. (A) Midsagittal plane of the 13 weeks fetus showing a dilated bladder (megacystis) with a bladder longitudinal diameter of >15 mm. The presence of megacystis with bladder longitudinal diameter of >15 mm is associated with fetal aneuploidy and renal abnormalities along with distension of the anterior abdominal wall; (B) Axial plane at the level of the pelvis showing the presence of a keyhole sign and echogenic kidneys.

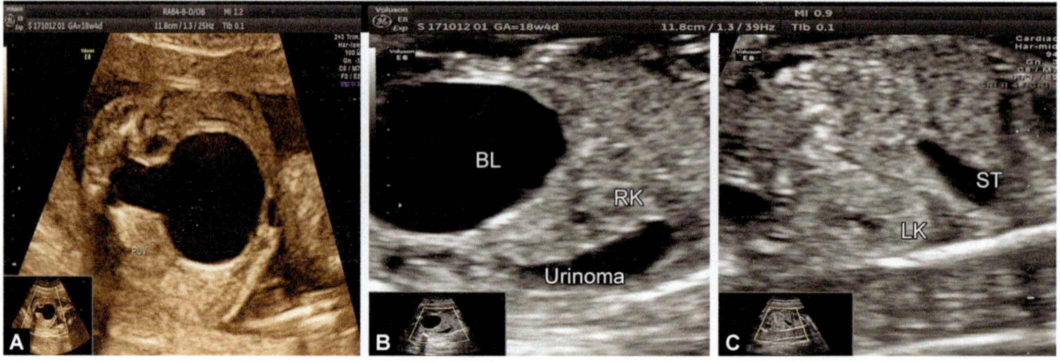

Figs. 25A to C: Posterior urethral valves. (A) Axial scan of 18 weeks fetal pelvis shows the keyhole appearance of dilated urinary bladder (BL) and thickened bladder wall is noted; (B) Coronal scan shows bilateral echogenic kidneys and right perinephric urinoma; (C) Echogenic left kidney (LK).
(RK: right kidney)

dialysis and/or transplantation before the age of 5 years. Recurrence isolated: no increased risk of recurrence. Part of trisomies: 1%.[2,5]

CYSTIC RENAL DISEASE

The renal cystic disease has two sonographic patterns: (1) cysts and (2) renal hyperechogenicity. The cysts can be of varying size, can occur anywhere in the kidney, and uni-/bilateral involvement is seen. Renal hyperechogenicity can be visualized in the entire kidney, only in the cortex or only in the medulla; hyperechogenicity is related to the numerous interfaces created by microscopic cysts and dilated tubules. Some degree of interstitial fibrosis and inflammation contributed to ultrasound appearance. There are no objective criteria for comparison of echogenicity up to 32 weeks and later echogenicity is compared to liver and spleen.

A decision tree approach was postulated depending on sonographic evaluation of the kidney, clinical data, and the family history **(Flowchart 1)**. Ultrasound features are: (1) Renal size; (2) Cortex—hypoechoic, isoechoic, and hyperechoic; (3) Medulla—hyperechoic and hypoechoic; (4) Corticomedullary

Flowchart 1: Decision tree approach to renal cystic diseases.

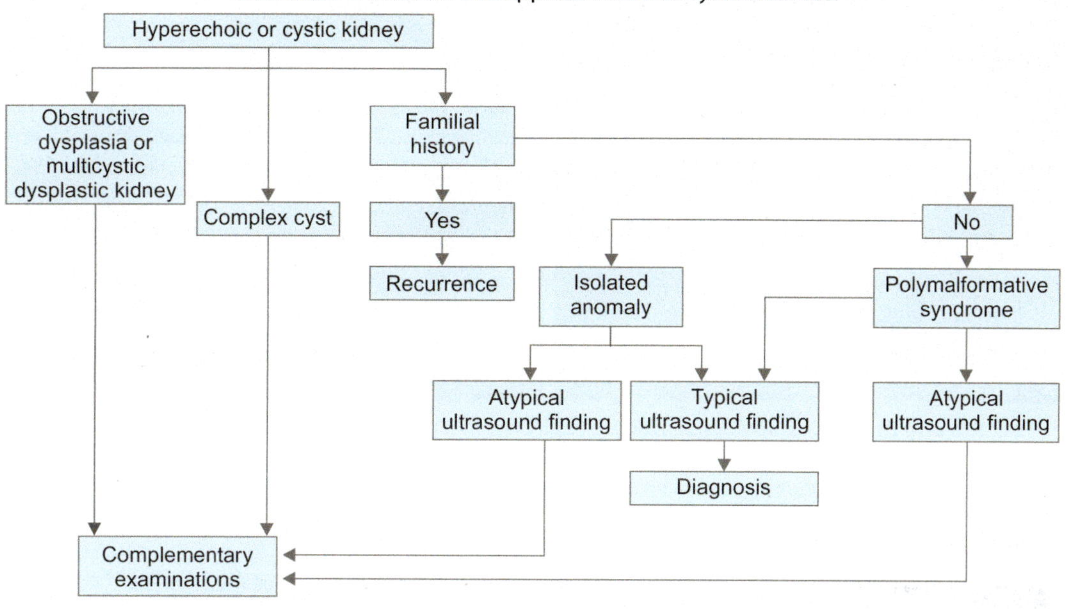

differentiation (CMD)—preserved, absent, and reversed; (5) Cysts—number, size, and location; (6) Calcifications; and (7) Pelvicalyceal system. Sonographic examination of the parents/grandparents is useful to check for unknown familial disease.

The first step is to rule out dysplasia associated with obstructive uropathy in which there is often dilatation of the collecting system. Obstructive dysplasia is the most common cause of hyperechoic cortex with or without cysts. It can be unilateral or bilateral. The affected kidneys are of variable size, the cortex is usually hyperechoic, thinned, and irregular, and the CMD is absent.

The multicystic dysplastic kidney (MCDK) is the second diagnosis to consider. Its sonographic pattern is usually straightforward: enlarged kidney whose parenchyma is replaced by multiple, noncommunicating cysts of variable size and number. The ipsilateral ureter is usually atretic and the normal functioning renal parenchyma is commonly scarce or even absent. It is seen in 1/1,000–5,000 live births and unilateral in approximately 75–80% of cases.

Synonyms—Potter type II, multicystic dysplasia, and multicystic kidney.

Ultrasound Features (Figs. 26 and 27)

It shows multiple noncommunicating cysts of variable size, cysts that do not communicate with a renal pelvis, and could even alter the normal renal shape with hyperechogenic parenchyma. The dimensions of the kidney are often significantly increased. The bladder and quantity of amniotic fluid are usually normal in unilateral MCDK. Bilateral multicystic kidneys and bladder are small, not imaged, and liquor anhydramnios is seen. In bilateral forms, the prognosis is unfavorable[16] due to the presence of the oligohydramnios related to the complete renal insufficiency, which may result in the Potter sequence and death from lethal pulmonary hypoplasia. If MCKD is not isolated, the prognosis depends on the associated abnormality.[16-18]

Renal anomalies with typical ultrasound pattern are seen as isolated findings.

AUTOSOMAL RECESSIVE POLYCYSTIC DISEASE

The condition is characterized by symmetric enlargement of both kidneys secondary to renal collecting tubule dilatation. Incidence:

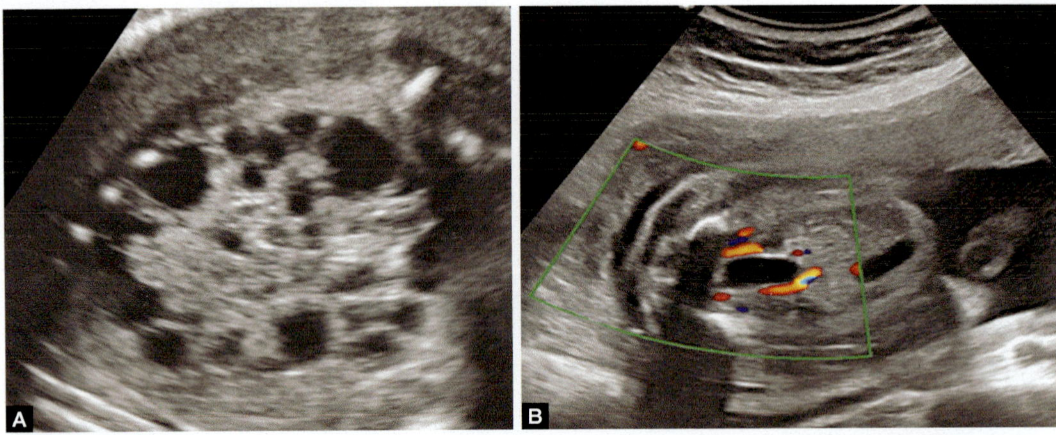

Figs. 26A and B: (A) Multicystic dysplastic kidney in one kidney—multiple noncommunicating cysts of various sizes; (B) Normal bladder.

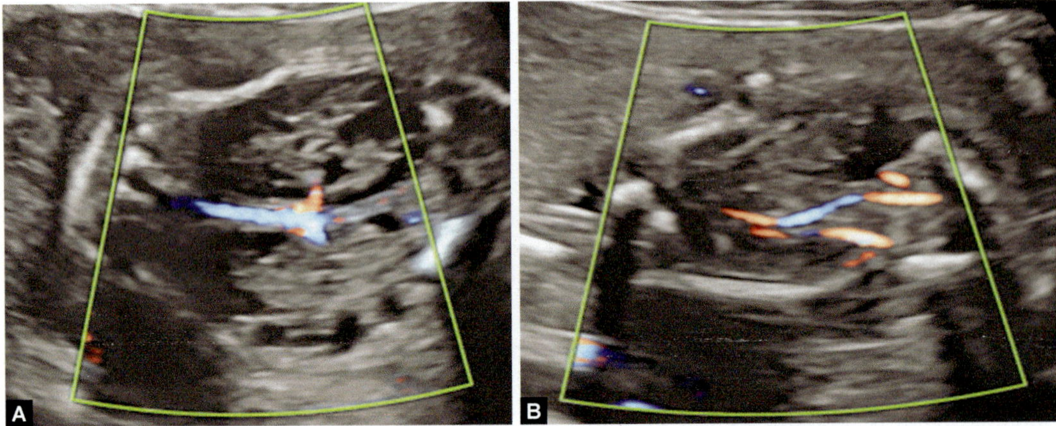

Figs. 27A and B: (A) Bilateral multicystic dysplastic kidneys and multiple noncommunicating cysts of various sizes are seen; (B) Fetal lower abdomen showing umbilical cord entry, absent bladder, and anhydramnios.

1:40,000–50,000 live birth. The disease has a wide spectrum of renal and hepatic involvement and it is subdivided into perinatal, neonatal, infantile, and juvenile types on the basis of the age of onset of the clinical presentation.[2]

Ultrasound Diagnosis

It shows bilaterally enlarged and homogeneously hyperechogenic kidneys. CMD is lost and usually found >24 weeks of gestation. Renal pelvises cannot be visualized **(Figs. 28A to E)**. Small or absent bladder and liquor—oligohydramnios/anhydramnios are present. Some cases of sonographic features may not be prevent until third trimester; therefore, follow-up scan in later pregnancy can be planned for patients at risk. Transvaginal sonography (TVS) at 12–14 weeks—enlarged, hyperechogenic kidneys may be seen.

Prognosis

The prenatal type is lethal either in utero or in the neonatal period due to pulmonary hypoplasia. The infantile and juvenile types result in chronic renal failure, hepatic fibrosis, and portal hypertension; many cases survive into their teens and require renal

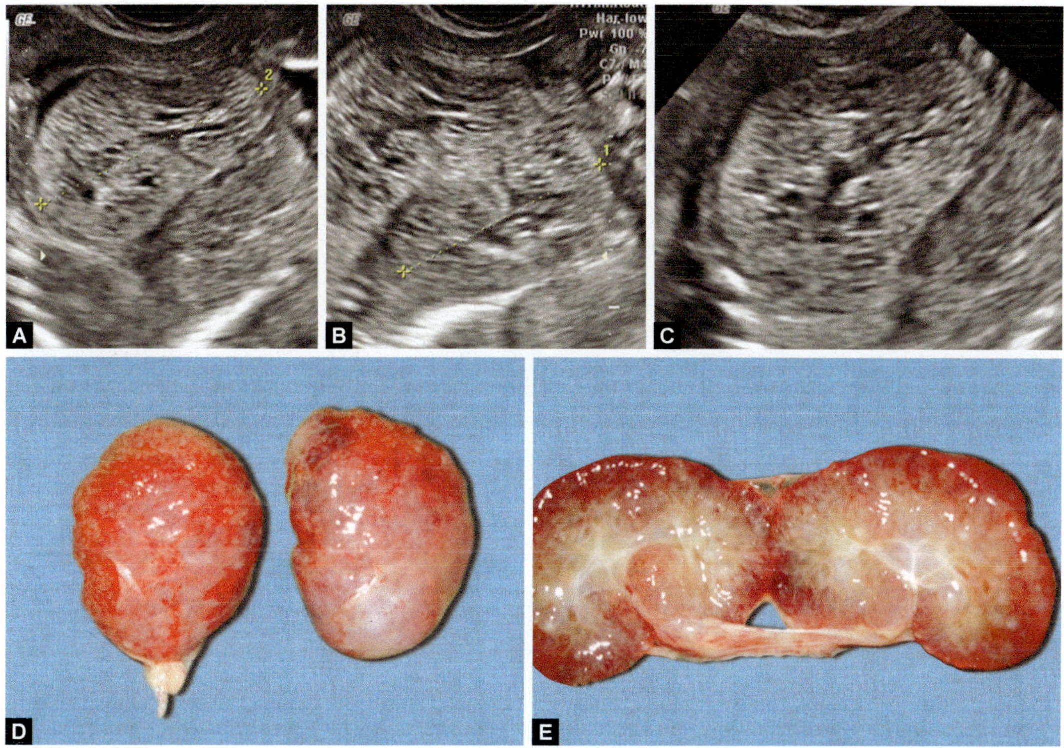

Figs. 28A to E: Autosomal recessive polycystic kidney. (A) Bilateral markedly enlarged hyperechoic kidneys; (B) Hyperechogenic kidney with tiny cysts and loss of corticomedullary differentiation noted; (C) Gross specimen of bilateral enlarged echogenic kidneys; (D and E) Cut section shows loss of corticomedullary differentiation.

transplant. Recurrence risk—25%. Family history with enlarged echogenic kidneys with oligohydramnios and the outlook is likely to be very poor.[2] The presence of other anomalies should prompt karyotype.

AUTOSOMAL DOMINANT POLYCYSTIC KIDNEY DISEASE

Both kidneys show cystic dilatation of the nephrons. In the established adult disease, the kidneys are enlarged and contain multiple cysts of varying size. Incidence: 1:1,000 live birth. Autosomal dominant polycystic kidney disease (ADPKD) is a systemic disorder characterized by cyst formation in ductal organs, kidneys, liver, spleen, pancreas, and CNS.[2]

Ultrasound Diagnosis

It shows bilateral symmetrically enlarged echogenic kidneys and increased CMD. Bladder is normal **(Figs. 29A and B)**. Liquor volume is normal. Kidneys may look normal in the second trimester in few cases and follow-up scans are essential in the high-risk cases. 90% of cases are linked to *PKD1* gene on short arm of chromosome 16 and 5% of cases are linked to *PK2* gene on chromosome 4. Prenatal diagnosis is possible by mutation analysis. The condition is often asymptomatic and usually presents in the fifth decade with hypertension and end-stage renal failures. The parents may not be aware that one or the other may have the condition **(Figs. 30A and B)**. The diagnosis of their condition requires

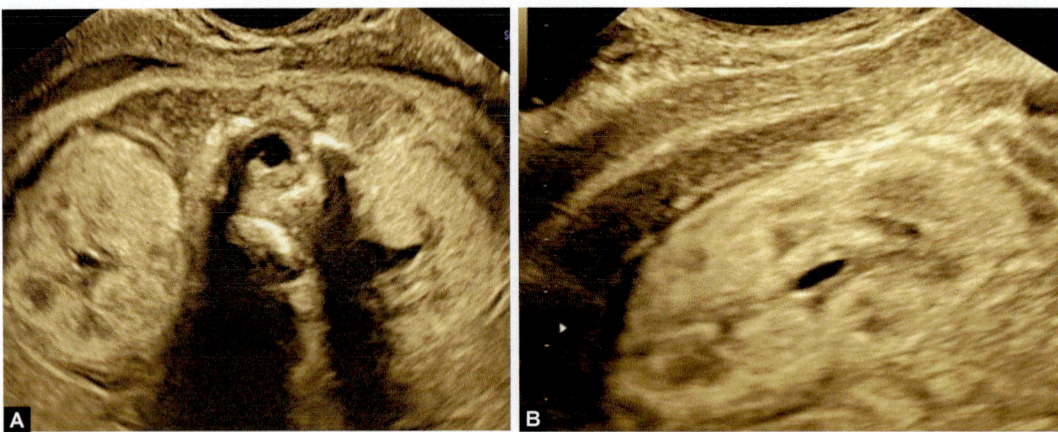

Figs. 29A and B: (A) Axial scan of 29 weeks fetus shows bilaterally enlarged echogenic kidney and normal liquor is noted; (B) Longitudinal scan of unilateral enlarged echogenic kidney, hyperechogenic cortex, and increased corticomedullary differentiation.

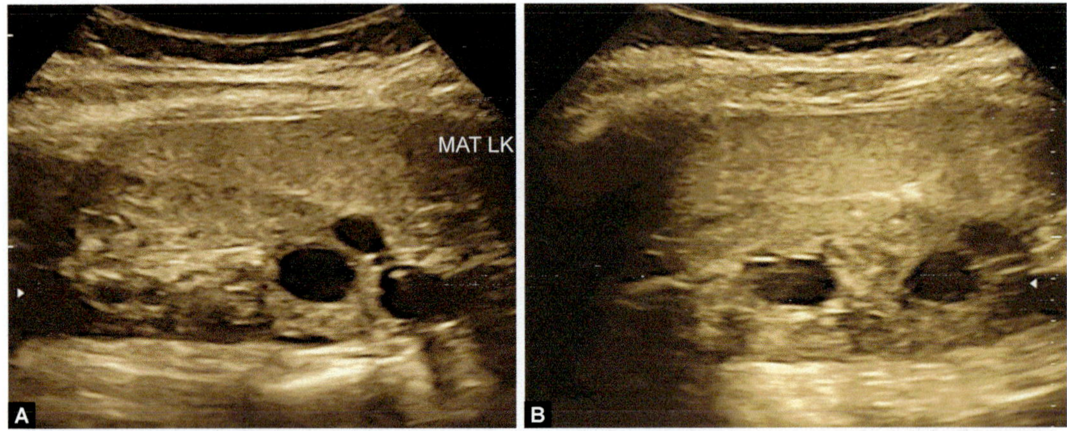

Figs. 30A and B: Ultrasound screening of the pregnant mother shows cysts in the kidney, although mother was affected and disease was unknown in the family.

very careful counseling and evaluation of the family members. Recurrence risk—50%.[2]

GLOMERULOCYSTIC KIDNEY DISEASE

This is an autosomal dominant disease. Fetus shows diffusely hyperechoic and enlarged kidneys without CMD, but with multiple subcapsular cysts and additional cortical cysts. The cysts develop in utero or postnatally. The same pattern can be seen in *HNF1B/TCF2* gene mutation. Mutation of gene expresses various renal anomalies (renal agenesis, hypoplasia, and cystic dysplasia). Cysts of varying size and location can develop in utero or after birth. TCF2 mutation can be confirmed only with knowledge of a familial history or results of genetic studies.

NEPHRONOPHTHISIS

These are group of autosomal recessive condition diagnosed at any age. Ultrasound features—hyperechoic normal sized or small kidneys without CMD with cysts at CMD.

NONVISUALIZED URINARY BLADDER

When urinary bladder is not visualized, scan should be repeated multiple times at 30 minutes interval and it may be physiological due to emptying cycles of fetal micturition. Ultrasound features—narrow space between the umbilical arteries on color Doppler study, amniotic fluid volume is to be assessed, oligohydramnios/anhydramnios may be secondary to bilateral renal agenesis, and bilateral cystic renal disease. The urinary bladder persistently nonvisualized with normal liquor is seen in exstrophy of bladder.[2]

Bladder Exstrophy

Bladder exstrophy consists of externalization of the bladder onto the anterior abdominal wall. Incidence: 1 in 30,000 live birth. Bladder exstrophy results from rupture of the cloacal membrane after completion of the caudal growth of the urorectal septum. The umbilicus is low lying and there is separation of the pubic bones. Diagnosis involves absence of bladder, a lower abdominal bulge representing the atrophied bladder, low insertion of the umbilical cord, and abnormal widening of the iliac crests. Color flow Doppler imaging was useful in demonstrating absence of the bladder **(Figs. 31A to D)**. The kidneys and liquor volume are usually normal. Prognosis after initial bladder closure, major reconstructive surgery is required. Despite multiple operations, urinary leakage and deviant genitalia are seen. Recurrence risk is 1:275 for siblings. Children of parents with bladder exstrophy have a much higher incidence of 1:70 live birth.[8]

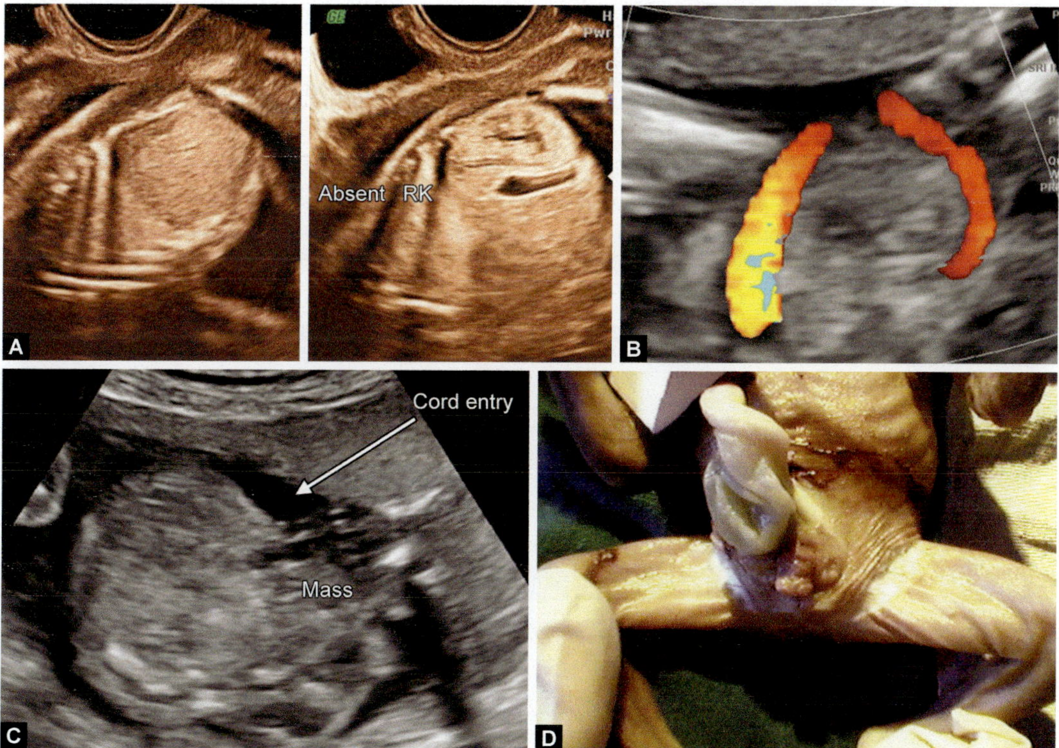

Figs. 31A to D: (A) Unilateral absent kidney; (B) Absent urinary bladder and two umbilical arteries as well as a wide-set umbilical cord; (C) Transverse view of the fetal abdomen and pelvis showing a low-set umbilical cord insertion and an anterior abdominal wall mass; (D) Postabortal specimen showing bladder exstrophy.

RENAL ANOMALIES WITH SYNDROMES

Meckel–Gruber Syndrome

Classically, it is characterized by the triad of:

- *Renal cystic dysplasia*: Multiple renal cysts (present in most of the cases)
- Occipital encephalocele/holoprosencephaly (~70%)
- *Postaxial polydactyly*: Usually hexadactyly (~65%) **(Figs. 32 to 34)**

The incidence is estimated to be 1:30,000. It is inherited as an autosomal recessive fashion and the risk of the condition affecting a subsequent child is, therefore, 25%.[1] There is genetic heterogeneity with at least three genes (*MKS1*, *MKS2*, and *MKS3*) having been identified.

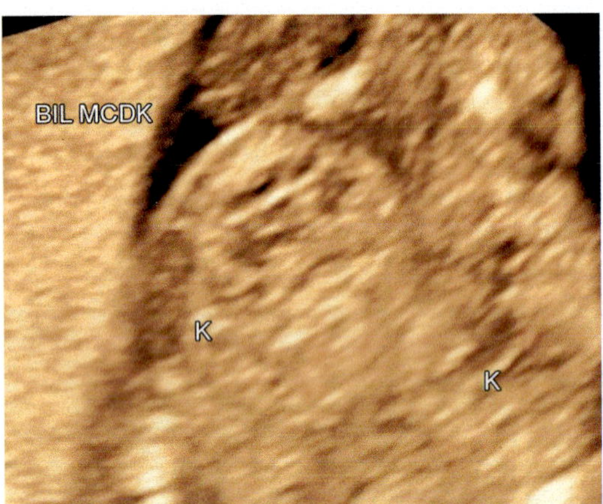

Fig. 32: Coronal scan of 13 weeks fetus showing bilateral enlarged echogenic kidney.

Ultrasound Features

It shows occipital encephalocele, multiple renal cysts and polydactyly, liquor, oligohydramnios (or anhydramnios in severe cases), and microcephaly. In utero (and early neonatal life) multicystic renal disease is usually evident as enlarged echogenic kidneys **(Fig. 32)** and physical cysts within the kidneys are seen in minority of cases. The condition is almost always fetal at birth either because of pulmonary hypoplasia or neonatal renal failure. Parent can be counseled appropriately that the subsequent risk is 25%.[2,8,13]

Trisomy 13/Patau Syndrome

The incidence of trisomy 13 live births has been reported to range from 1/5,000 to 1/30,000. Prenatal ultrasound has been extensively applied in the assessment of fetal chromosomal aneuploidy. Clinically, two types of sonographic markers suggestive of

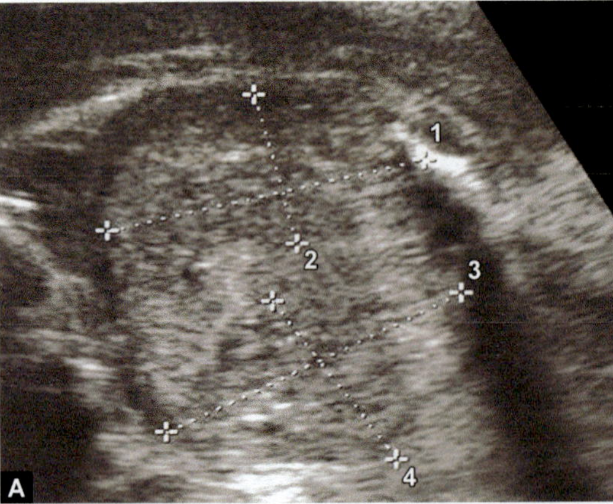

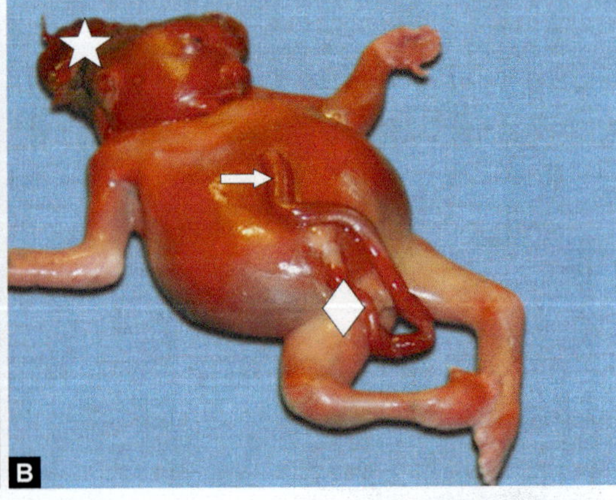

Figs. 33A and B: Case of dichorionic diamniotic twin pregnancy with one twin normal and other twin had Meckel–Gruber syndrome. (A) Bilateral coronal scan through fetal abdomen shows enlarged echogenic kidney with loss of corticomedullary differentiation; (B) Postnatal specimen showing occipital encephalocele, distended abdomen due to enlarged kidneys, and postaxial polydactyly.

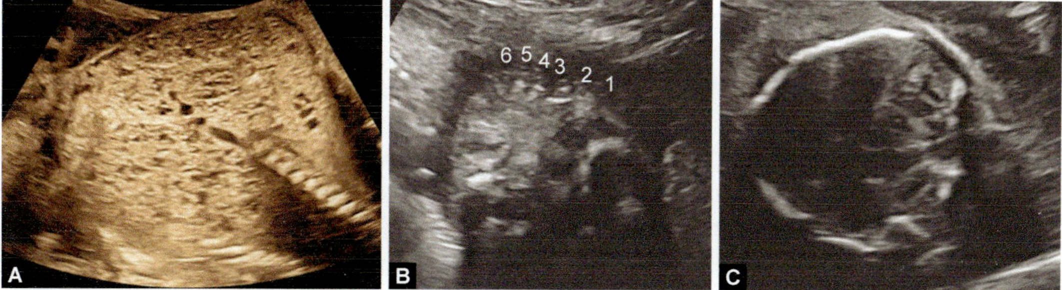

Figs. 34A to C: Singleton pregnancy—Meckel–Gruber syndrome. (A) Coronal scan showing bilateral echogenic enlarged kidneys with loss of corticomedullary differentiation and small tiny cysts are seen; (B) Polydactyly; (C) Intracranial anatomy is distorted and occipital encephalocele is not seen clearly due to oligohydramnios.

aneuploidy are used. Type I markers represent major fetal structural abnormalities and type II markers, also called soft markers, are characterized by nonspecific and often transient fetal abnormalities.

- Type I markers—major structural anomalies of brain, face, heart, genitourinary tract, limb anomalies, and anterior abdominal wall defects **(Figs. 35B to D)**
- Type II markers—soft markers

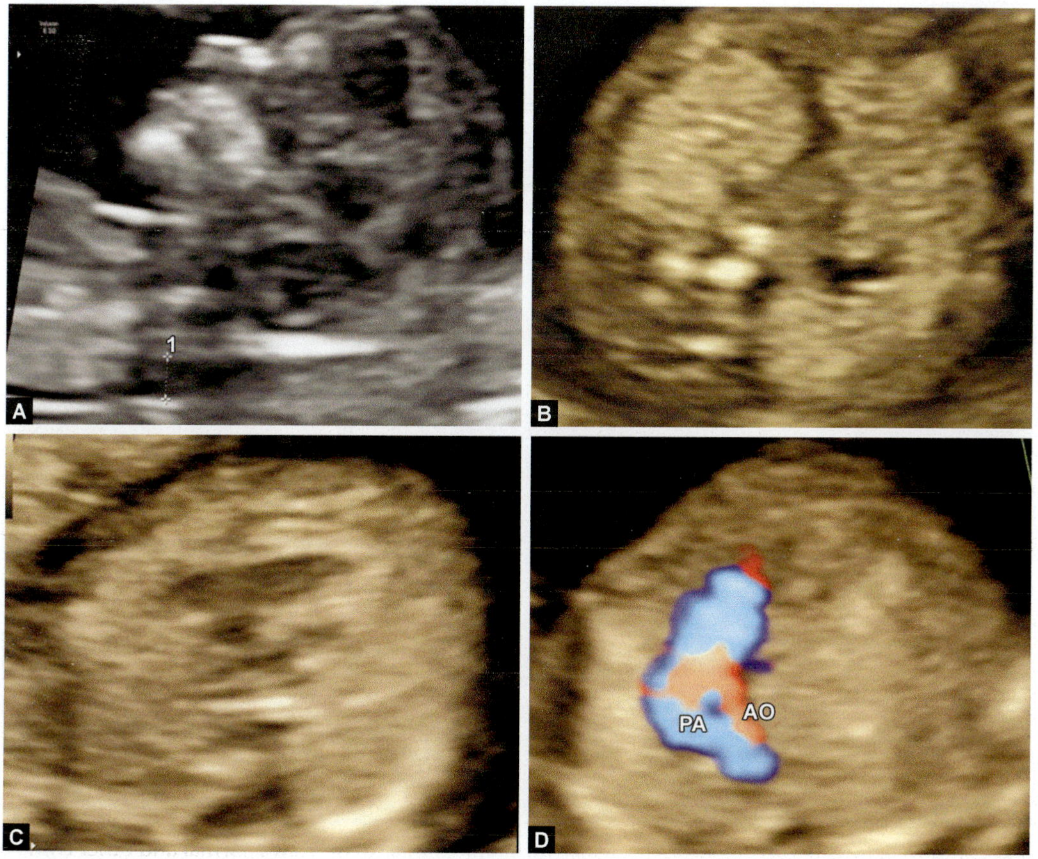

Figs. 35A to D: Case of trisomy 13. (A) Increased nuchal thickness (NT)—3 mm; (B) Echogenic kidneys; (C) Asymmetry of cardiac chambers and left ventricle is smaller as compared to the right ventricle; (D) Three-vessel view aorta narrow as compared to the pulmonary artery karyotype of the fetus revealed trisomy 13.

It also shows increased nuchal translucency thickness **(Fig. 35A)**, echogenic intracardiac focus, fetal tachycardia, and megacystis.[8]

VACTERL SYNDROME

Vertebral defects, anal atresia, cardiac defects, tracheoesophageal fistula, renal anomalies, and limb abnormalities (VACTERL) syndrome is considered as a congenital defect, which affects multiple organ structures. Abnormality in any three involved body parts, i.e., thorax, lower abdomen or pelvis, and limbs with the probable presence of two or more anomalies represent VACTERL syndrome[2,8] **(Figs. 36A to E)**.

Sirenomelia

Sirenomelia is a rare congenital malformation and its prevalence is estimated to vary between 1/600,000 and 100,000,019.

Sirenomelia is characterized by the fusion of the lower extremities and renal agenesis, absent urinary tract and genitalia, imperforate anus, oligohydramnios, and a single umbilical artery **(Figs. 37 and 38)**. Sirenomelia is definitely a serious threat to fetal survival due to the associated severe malformations. More than 50% of sirenomelia cases result in stillbirths and the live neonates with sirenomelia often die within 1–2 days after birth.[4] Chromosomal abnormality of the fetus with sirenomelia is unlikely.

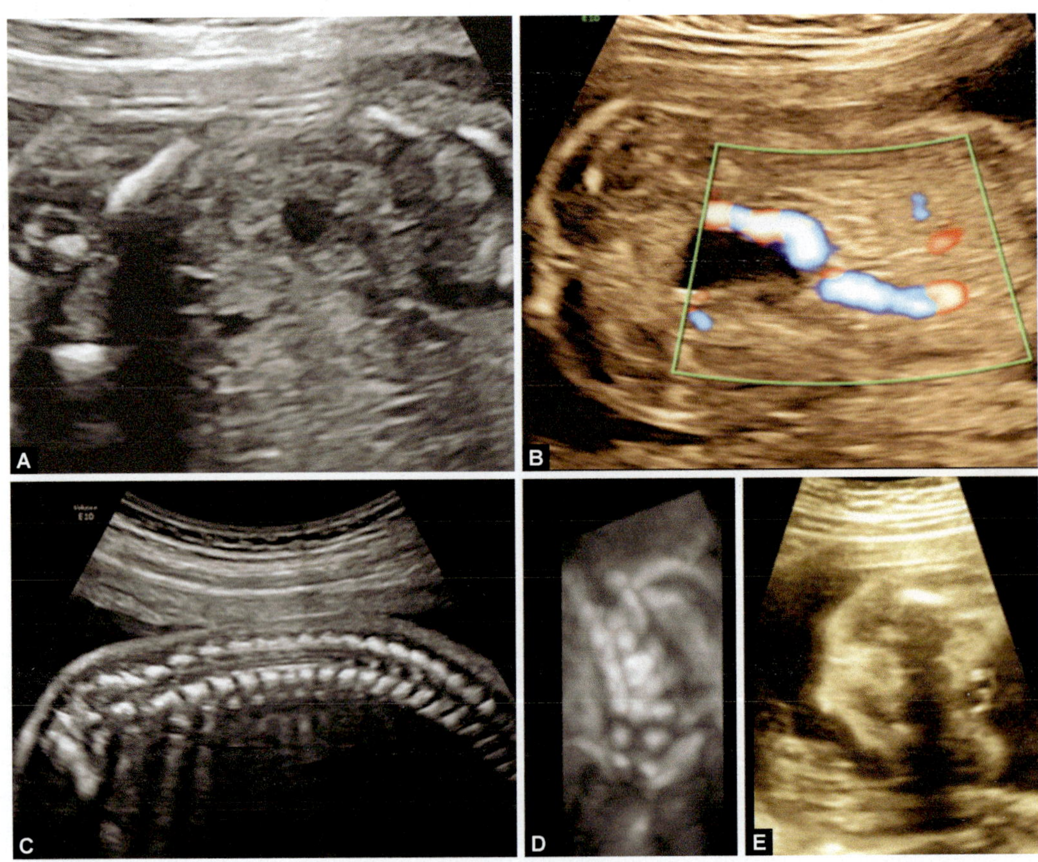

Figs. 36A to E: (A) Crossed fused renal ectopia; (B) Single umbilical artery; (C) Sacral agenesis; (D) 3D—hemivertebrae; (E) Absence of perianal muscle complex, which is a feature of anal atresia.
(3D: three-dimensional; VSD: ventricular septal defect)

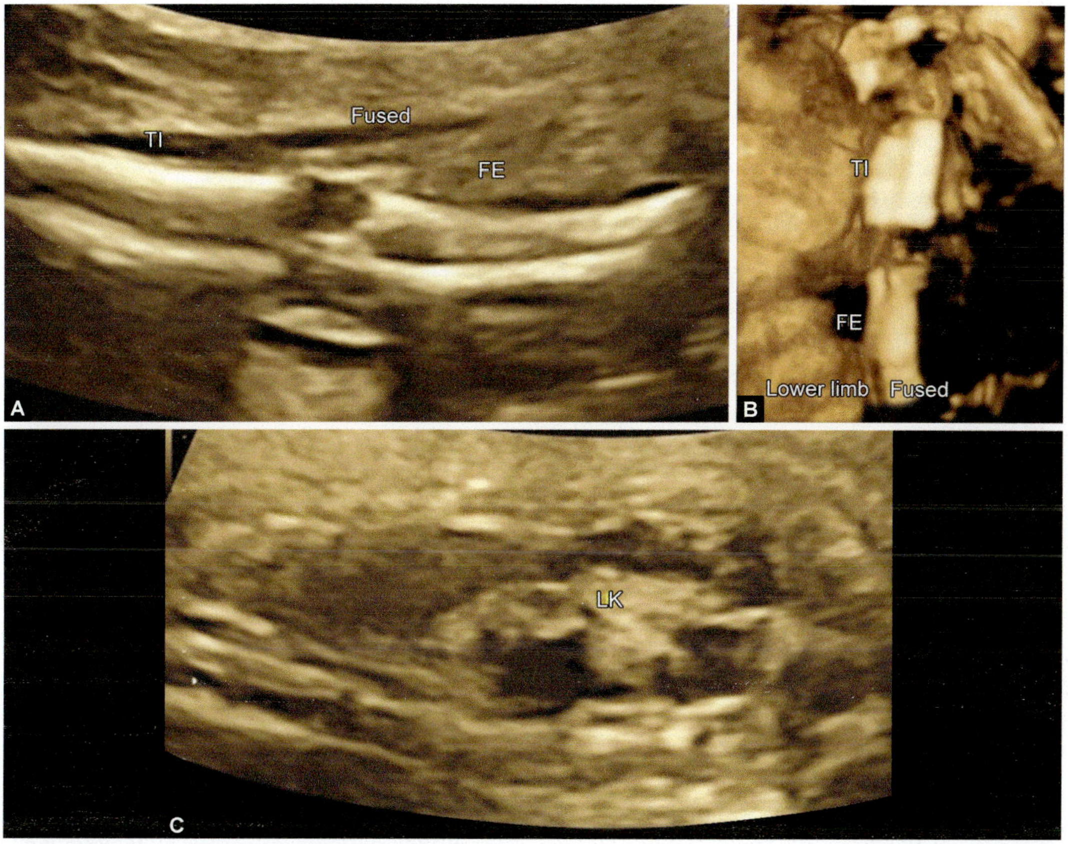

Figs. 37A to C: (A) 2D—fused lower limbs; (B) 3D—fused lower limbs; (C) Absence of bladder is noted. (2D: two-dimensional; 3D: three-dimensional)

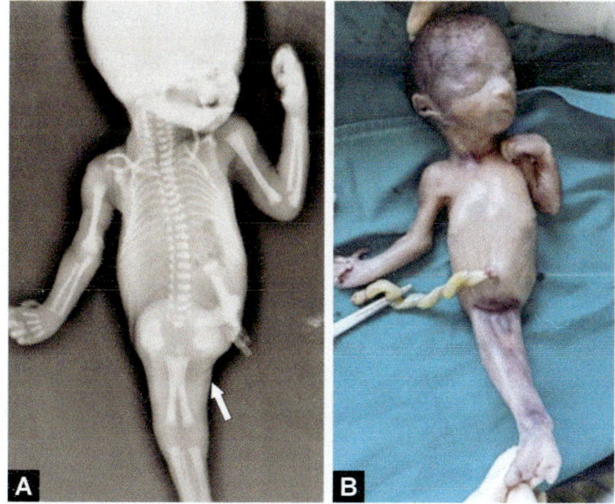

Figs. 38A and B: (A) Postnatal X-ray—single fused lower limb; (B) Postnatal specimen—single fused lower limb.

The risk factors of sirenomelia include maternal diabetes mellitus, exposure to teratogenic drugs or agent (such as retinoic acid, cyclophosphamide, or cadmium), and a maternal age < 20 years or >40 years. There are two hypotheses commonly regarding the pathogenesis. The vascular steal hypothesis proposes that sirenomelia arises from a deformed blood vessel that originates from the high abdominal aorta, which performs the function of the umbilical artery and transports a large amount of blood from the umbilical cord to the placenta and the blood perfusion to the abdominal aorta is insufficient, eventually leading to severe malformations of the spine, lower limbs, and genitourinary system. The other hypothesis is the defective blastogenesis hypothesis, which proposes that damage to the caudal mesoderm of the embryo between 13 and 22 days in early life may result in the merging, malrotation, and dysgenesis of the lower extremities.[2,19,20]

REFERENCES

1. Kohl S, Habbig S, Weber LT, Liebau MC. Molecular causes of congenital anomalies of kidney and urinary tract (CAKUT). Springer Open. Molecular and cellular Pediatrics 8, article number: 2 (February 2021).
2. Diagnostic Imaging of Fetal Anomalies. Philadelphia: Lippincott Williams and Wilkins; 2003.
3. Cardwell MS. Bilateral renal agenesis: clinical implications. South Med J. 1988;81:327-8.
4. Potter EL. Normal and Abnormal Development of the Kidney. Chicago: Yearbook Medical Publishers; 1972.
5. Droste S, Fitzsimmons J, Pascoe-Mason J, Shepard TH, Mack LA. Size of the fetal adrenal in bilateral renal agenesis. Obstet Gynecol. 1990;76:206-9.
6. Hoffman CK, Filly RA, Callen PW. The "lying down" adrenal sign: a sonographic indicator of renal agenesis or ectopia in fetuses and neonates. J Ultrasound Med. 1992;11:533-6.
7. Twining P. Genitourinary malformation. In: Nyberg DA, McGahan JP, Pretorius DH, Pilu G (Eds). Diagnostic Imaging of Fetal Anomalies. Philadelphia: Lippincott Williams & Wilkins; 2003. pp. 610-14.
8. Evans JA. Urinary tract. In: Stevenson RE, Hall JG (Eds). Human Malformations and Related Anomalies, 2nd edition. Oxford: Oxford University Press; 2006. pp. 1161-90.
9. Paladini D, Volpe P. Ultrasound of congenital fetal anomalies. London: Informa Healthcare; 2007.
10. Roodhooft AM, Birnholz JC, Holmes LB. Familial nature of congenital absence and severe dysgenesis of both kidneys. N Engl J Med. 1984;310:1341-5.
11. Pallotta R, Bucci I, Celentano C, Liberati M, Bellati U. The "skipped generation phenomenon" in a family with renal agenesis. Ultrasound Obstet Gynecol. 2004;24:586-7.
12. Sinha A, Bagga A, Krishna A, Bajpai M, Srinivas M, Uppal R, et al. Revised guidelines on management of antenatal hydronephrosis. Indian J Nephrol. 2013;23:83-97.
13. Benjamin T, Amodeo RR, Patil AS, Robinson BK. The impact of gestational age at delivery on urologic outcomes for the fetus with hydronephrosis. Fetal Pediatr Pathol. 2016;35:359-68.
14. Ismaili K, Hall M, Donner C, Thomas D, Vermeylen D, Avni FE. Results of systematic screening for minor degrees of fetal renal pelvis dilatation in an unselected population. Am J Obstet Gynecol. 2003;188:242-6.
15. Yiee J, Wilcox D. Management of fetal hydronephrosis. Pediatr Nephrol. 2008;23:347-53.
16. Atiyeh B, Husmann D, Baum M. Contralateral renal abnormalities in patients with renal agenesis and noncystic renal dysplasia. Pediatrics. 1993;91:812-5.
17. Mir S, Rapola J, Koskimies O. Renal cysts in pediatric autopsy material. Nephron. 1983;33:189-95.
18. Kuwertz-Broeking E, Brinkmann OA, Von Lengerke HJ, Sciuk J, Fruend S, Bulla M, et al. Unilateral multicystic dysplastic kidney: experience in children. BJU Int. 2004;93:388-92.
19. Fetal Medicine Foundation (FMF). (2021). Fetal abnormalities. [online] Available from https://fetalmedicine.org/education/fetal-abnormalities. [Last accessed on September, 2021].
20. International Society of Ultrasound in Obstetrics and Gynecology (ISUOG). (2021). Renal system. [online] Available from https://www.isuog.org/clinical-resources/patient-information-series/patient-information-pregnancy-conditions/renal-system.html. [Last accessed on September, 2021].

14
CHAPTER

Gastrointestinal Tract Abnormalities

Darshan Wadekar, Zalak Mehta

GASTROINTESTINAL TRACT

Abdomen is called a magic box for a physician and it holds true for the fetal medicine consultants too. They are difficult to identify as they evolve over months (second to third trimester). Although fetal magnetic resonance imaging (MRI) is useful, it has its own limitations. Most of the times, differential diagnosis is given during the fetal period and postnatal evaluation is done using ultrasound and MRI for confirmation of diagnosis.

NORMAL EMBRYOLOGIC DEVELOPMENT

The primitive gut forms at the end of the fifth menstrual week (20 days postfertilization), when the dorsal part of the yolk sac invaginates into the growing embryonic disc.[1] It has three parts: foregut (derivatives—pharynx, respiratory tract, esophagus, stomach, proximal duodenum, liver, and pancreas), midgut (derivatives—small bowel and proximal large bowel), and hindgut (derivatives—distal colon, rectum, and portions of vagina and urinary bladder).

Intestinal peristalsis begins by 11 menstrual weeks and fetal swallowing begins shortly thereafter.[2] The stomach must be visible by 12 weeks of gestation. Meconium gets accumulated in the large bowel until term. The peristalsis is important for gastrointestinal tract development.

NORMAL SONOGRAPHIC APPEARANCE (TABLES 1 AND 2)

Just as for a clinician, abdomen is a magic box, in fetal medicine, also the abdominal abnormalities can be detected over a period of time, mostly in the third trimester. Liver occupies the upper abdomen and spleen occupies the space behind the fetal stomach.

Sonographic appearance varies with gestational age of the fetus. As the swallowing begins by 11 weeks of gestation, the stomach should be visualized by 12 weeks. In case of nonvisualization of the stomach, review after a few hours/days. The stomach should be on the same side as the axis of the heart to be situs solitus. Situs inversus is most frequently seen with polysplenia/asplenia syndromes. During the second trimester, the small bowel located more in mid and lower abdomen appears hyperechoic, while the large bowel located in the periphery of the abdomen has more hypoechoic meconium.

The large bowel slowly enlarges with meconium throughout the pregnancy, measuring 3–5 mm at 20 weeks to 23 mm by term. While small bowel does not normally exceed 5–7 mm in diameter.

ABNORMALITIES OF GASTROINTESTINAL TRACT (TABLE 3)

Esophageal Atresia

Esophageal atresia (EA) results from incomplete division of foregut into the ventral respiratory and dorsal digestive portion by tracheoesophageal septum. Hence, EA is associated with tracheoesophageal fistula (TEF) in >90% of cases.[3,4]

- *Incidence*: 1 in 2,500 to 4,000 births[5]
- *Associated with*: Trisomies 18 and 21 and VACTERL (vertebral anomalies, anal atresia, cardiac malformations,

TABLE 1: Normal anatomy and physiology.

Liver	***Left lobe of liver is larger than the right***	***Because of more blood supply***
By 11 weeks	Visualization of stomach may begin	Due to swallowing of fluid by fetus
By 14 weeks	Stomach should is seen	In all normal fetus
In first and second trimesters	Stomach and bowel are seen	
Large bowel	Measures 3–5 mm at 20 weeks	23 mm near term
Large bowel	Located in periphery and more dilated	Filled with hypoechoic meconium
Small bowel	Located in center and less dilated (does not exceed 7 mm in diameter)	More echogenic than large bowel

TABLE 2: Milestones in development of gastrointestinal tract.

Primitive gut	Forms by 5 weeks	When dorsal part of yolk sac invaginates into embryonic disk
Three parts		Foregut, midgut, and hindgut
Intestinal peristalsis	Begins by 11 weeks	
Fetal swallowing	By 11 weeks	
Meconium	By 20 weeks	Begins to accumulated

tracheoesophageal fistula, renal anomalies, limb abnormalities) anomalies.

- *Ultrasound findings*:
  - Small or "absent" stomach in the presence of polyhydramnios >25 weeks of gestation.[6,7]
  - Polyhydramnios combined with intrauterine growth restriction (IUGR) (though generally IUGR is associated with oligohydramnios).[8-10]
  - EA may be suspected prenatally in only about 40% of cases because if there is an associated TEF (found in >90% of cases).
  - The stomach may look normal.
  - Non-visualization of stomach at times.

Management

- Look for other anomalies. Direct testing to rule out chromosomal abnormalities
- Ultrasound scans every 2–3 weeks to monitor growth and assess amniotic fluid volume. Amniodrainage may be necessary if there is polyhydramnios and cervical shortening.
- Delivery at hospital with neonatal intensive care and pediatric surgery
- *Time:* 38 weeks
- *Method:* Induction of labor aiming for vaginal delivery

Duodenal Atresia

- Atresia (closure) of first part of small intestine, i.e., duodenum
- *Incidence*: 1 in 5,000 births
- *Associated anomalies*: Trisomy 21,[11,12] cardiac, renal, vertebral abnormalities[13]
- *Ultrasound finding*: "Double bubble" sign as a result of an enlarged stomach and duodenal cap. Usually found >24 weeks of gestation.[14,15] Polyhydramnios >24 weeks of gestation in 50% of cases.

Management

- Direct testing to rule out chromosomal anomalies
- Amniodrainage may be necessary if there is polyhydramnios and cervical shortening.
- *Delivery place*: Hospital with neonatal intensive care and pediatric surgery
- *Time*: 38 weeks
- *Method*: Induction of labor aiming for vaginal delivery

TABLE 3: Gastrointestinal tract abnormalities.

Anomaly	*Cause and associations*	*Ultrasound findings*	*Differential diagnosis and management*
Esophageal atresia	• 1 in 2,500 to 4,000 births[5] • Trisomies 18 and 21 • VACTERL anomalies Results from incomplete division of foregut into the ventral respiratory and dorsal digestive portion by tracheoesophageal septum. Hence, EA associated with: • TEF in >90% of cases[20,21]	• Small or "absent" stomach in the presence of polyhydramnios >25 weeks of gestation[6,7] • Polyhydramnios combined with IUGR[8-10] • Esophageal atresia may be suspected prenatally in only about 40% of cases because if there is an associated tracheoesophageal fistula (found in >90% of cases), the stomach may look normal	• Nonvisualization of stomach can be due to facial clefts and CNS abnormalities • Ultrasound scans every 2–3 weeks to monitor growth and assess amniotic fluid volume. Amniodrainage may be necessary if there is polyhydramnios and cervical shortening • Delivery at hospital with neonatal intensive care and pediatric surgery. *Time:* 38 weeks • *Method*: Induction of labor aiming for vaginal delivery
Duodenal atresia	• 1 in 5,000 births • Trisomy 21[11,12] • Cardiac, renal, and vertebral abnormalities[13]	• "Double bubble" sign as a result of an enlarged stomach and duodenal cap. Usually found >24 weeks of gestation[14,15] • Polyhydramnios >24 weeks of gestation in 50% of cases	• Amniodrainage may be necessary if there is polyhydramnios and cervical shortening *Delivery:* • *Place*: Hospital with neonatal intensive care and pediatric surgery • *Time*: 38 weeks • *Method*: Induction of labor aiming for vaginal delivery
Anorectal atresia	• 1 in 2,000 births • It can be supralevator or infralevator • Trisomies 21 and 18 • Urogenital malformations • VACTERL association	• Overdistension of the rectum and sigmoid colon in the third trimester • Occasionally, intraluminal calcifications (meconium) can be visualized	*Delivery:* • *Place*: Hospital with neonatal intensive care and pediatric surgery • *Time*: 38 weeks • *Method*: Induction of labor aiming for vaginal delivery

Contd...

Contd...

Anomaly	***Cause and associations***	***Ultrasound findings***	***Differential diagnosis and management***
Abdominal cysts	The most common causes are renal tract anomalies or dilated bowel, other causes are the cyst arising from the biliary tree, ovaries, mesentery or uterus. The most likely diagnosis is usually suggested by the position of the cyst, its relationship with other structures and the normality of other organs	*Choledochal cysts*: Cystic dilatation of the common biliary duct *Location:* Upper right side of the fetal abdomen Absence of polyhydramnios or peristalsis may help to differentiate the condition from bowel disorders *Mesenteric or omental cysts*: Obstructed lymphatic drainage. *Location:* Usually midline	*Hepatic cysts*: • Located in liver *Intestinal duplication cysts*: Thickness of the muscular wall of the cysts and presence of peristalsis • *Splenic cyst*: Located in the spleen • *Ovarian cyst*: Located in pelvis
Hirschsprung disease	1 in 10,000–20,000[21] associated with trisomy 21[22-32]	The condition is characterized by congenital absence of intramural parasympathetic nerve ganglia in a segment of the colon. The aganglionic segment is unable to transmit a peristaltic wave, and therefore meconium accumulates and causes dilatation of the lumen of the bowel.[16-20] Polyhydramnios and dilatation of the loops of intestine	Amniocentesis for karyotyping or analysis of cfDNA in maternal blood. Amniodrainage may be necessary if there is polyhydramnios and cervical shortening. Surgical removal of the affected segment
GB duplication	1 in 4,000[24,25]	Two GB can be seen	Differential diagnosis: GB fold, choledochal, hepatic, mesenteric cyst
Agenesis of the GB	Occurs in 20 % of patient with biliary atresia[26,27] Trisomy 21	GB not visualizes By about 24–32 weeks, in 95% of cases, GB should be visualized	

Contd...

Contd...

Anomaly	***Cause and associations***	***Ultrasound findings***	***Differential diagnosis and management***
Meconium peritonitis	• 1 in 3,000 births • Associated with cystic fibrosis • Amniocentesis: DNA studies for cystic fibrosis if both parents are carriers	• Presence of intra-abdominal hyperechogenic areas (peritoneal calcifications). Results from intrauterine perforation of the bowel which leads to a local sterile chemical peritonitis • *Additionally:* Dilated bowel loops, ascites and meconium pseudocyst	Bowel resection and primary anastomosis[28]
Hiatal hernia	It is the sliding of the stomach into the chest so that the gastroesophageal junction is above the diaphragm. Types are sliding, rolling, and mixed	Dilated esophagus Stomach bubble is not there at its normal location	Surgical repair[29]
Small bowel obstruction	• 1 in 5,000 births • Malrotation, gastroschisis, duplication, and meconium ileus are associated anomalies	• Multiple fluid-filled loops of the bowel in the abdomen >7 mm in diameter presenting >25 weeks of gestation[30,31] • Distension of the abdomen with active peristalsis • Polyhydramnios >25 weeks of gestation, especially in proximal obstructions[32]	• Amniodrainage may be necessary if there is polyhydramnios and cervical shortening *Delivery:* • *Place*: Hospital with neonatal intensive care and pediatric surgery • *Time*: 38 weeks • *Method*: Induction of labor aiming for vaginal delivery

(CNS: central nervous system; DNA: deoxyribonucleic acid; DD: differential diagnosis; EA: esophageal atresia; GB: gallbladder; TEF: tracheoesophageal fistula; VACTERL: vertebral anomalies, anal atresia, cardiac malformations, tracheoesophageal fistula, renal anomalies, limb abnormalities)

Anorectal Atresia

- *Occurrence*: 1 in 2,000
- It can present as supralevator or infralevator. It may be simple like membranous atresia (imperforate anus) to complex like persistent cloaca (rectum, vagina, and anus communicate with perineum with single opening)
- Associated with trisomies 21 and 18. It is frequently associated with VACTERL syndrome.
- *Diagnosis*: Overdistension of the rectum and sigmoid colon in third trimester with intraluminal calcification (meconium) visualized

Management

The prognosis is poor. Direct testing to rule out chromosomal abnormalities. Delivery at a hospital with neonatal intensive care unit (ICU) and pediatric surgery department for better care. Induction of labor for obstetric delivery.

Abdominal Cysts

The most common causes are renal tract anomalies or dilated bowel, other causes are the cyst arising from the biliary tree, ovaries, mesentery, or uterus. The most likely diagnosis is usually suggested by the position of the cyst, its relationship with other structures, and the normality of other organs. The various differentials in the abdominal cysts are described below.

Choledochal Cysts

- Cystic dilatation of the common biliary duct
- Location—upper right side of the fetal abdomen
- Absence of polyhydramnios or peristalsis may help to differentiate the condition from bowel disorders.

Mesenteric or Omental Cysts

- Obstructed lymphatic drainage
- Location—usually midline

Hepatic Cyst

Located in liver

Intestinal Duplication Cysts

Thickness of the muscular wall of the cysts and presence of peristalsis

Splenic Cyst

Located in the spleen

Ovarian Cyst

Anechoic cystic structure located in pelvis (female fetus).

Hirschsprung Disease

The condition is characterized by congenital absence of intramural parasympathetic nerve ganglia in a segment of the colon. The aganglionic segment is unable to transmit a peristaltic wave, and therefore meconium accumulates and causes dilatation of the lumen of the bowel.[16-20]

- *Incidence*: 1 in 10,000–20,000[21]
- *Associated anomalies*: Trisomy 21[22,23]
- *Ultrasound findings*: Polyhydramnios and dilatation of the loops of intestine

Management

- Amniocentesis for karyotyping or analysis of cell-free deoxyribonucleic acid (cfDNA) in maternal blood
- Amniodrainage may be necessary if there is polyhydramnios and cervical shortening.
- *Treatment:* Surgical removal of the affected segment postnatally

GALLBLADDER DUPLICATION

- Two gallbladders seen in the liver
- *Incidence*: 1 in 4,000[24,25]
- *Differential*: Gallbladder (GB fold), choledochal, hepatic, mesenteric cyst

Agenesis of the Gallbladder

- Occurs in 20% of patients with biliary atresia[26,27]

- *Associated anomalies*: Trisomy 21
- *Ultrasound findings*:
  - GB not visualized
  - By about 24–32 weeks, in 95% of cases, GB should be visualized.

Meconium Peritonitis

Meconium peritonitis is the presence of intra-abdominal hyperechogenic areas (peritoneal calcifications). It results from intrauterine perforation of the bowel which leads to a local sterile chemical peritonitis.

- *Incidence*: 1 in 3,000 births
- *Associated anomalies*: Associated with cystic fibrosis

Management

- *Amniocentesis*: DNA studies for cystic fibrosis if both parents are carriers.
- *Postnatal management*: Bowel resection and primary anastomiosis[28]

Hiatal Hernia

Hiatal hernia is the sliding of the stomach into the chest so that the gastroesophageal junction is above the diaphragm.

- Types are sliding, rolling and mixed.
- *Ultrasound findings*: Dilated esophagus and stomach bubble is not there at its normal location
- *Management*: Surgical repair[29]

Small Bowel Obstruction

- *Incidence:* 1 in 5,000 births
- *Associated anomalies*: Malrotation, gastroschisis, duplication, and meconium ileus
- *Ultrasound findings*: Multiple fluid-filled loops of the bowel in the abdomen >7 mm in diameter presenting >25 weeks of gestation.[30,31] There may be distension of the abdomen with active peristalsis. Polyhydramnios >25 weeks of gestation is noted especially in proximal obstructions.[32]
- *Management*: Amniodrainage may be necessary if there is polyhydramnios and cervical shortening.
- *Delivery place*: Hospital with neonatal intensive care and pediatric surgery
- *Time*: 38 weeks
- *Method*: Induction of labor aiming for vaginal delivery.

REFERENCES

1. Moore KL. The developing human, 4th edition. Philadelphia: WB Saunders; 1988. pp. 217-45.
2. Grelin ES. Functional anatomy of the newborn. New Haven: Yale University Press; 1973. pp. 54-60.
3. Gray SW, Skandalakis JE. Embryology for Surgeons. The Embryological Basis for the Treatment of Congenital Anomalies, 2nd Edition. Philadelphia: WB Saunders; 1972. pp. 63-100.
4. Waterson DJ, Bonham CRE, Aaberdeen E. Oesophageal atresia: tracheo-oesophgeal fistula. A study of survival in 218 infants. Lancet. 1962;21(7234):819-22.
5. Depaepe A, Dolk H, Lechat MF. The epidemiology of trachea-oesophageal fistula and oesophageal atresia in Europe. EURO-CAT Working Group. Arch Dis Child. 1993;68(6):743-8.
6. Pretorius DH, Drose JA, Dennis MA, Manchester DK, Manco-Johnson ML. Tracheoesophageal fistula in utero. J Ultrasound Med. 1987;6(9): 509-13.
7. Weinberg B, Diakoumakis EE. Three complex cases of foregut atresia: Prenatal sonographic diagnosis with rediographic correlation. J Clin Ultrasound. 1985;13(7):481-4.
8. Pretorius DH, Merier PR, Johnson ML. Diagnosis of esophageal atresia in utero. J Ultrasound Med. 1983;2(10):475-6.
9. Sparey C, Jawaheer G, Barrett AM, Robson SC. Esophageal atresia in the Northern region Congenital Anomaly Survey, 1985-1997: Prenatal diagnosis and outcome. Am J Obstet Gynecol. 2000;182(2):427-31.
10. Stringer MD, McKenna KM, Goldstein RB, Filly RA, Adzick NS, Harrison MR. Prenatal diagnosis of esophageal atresia. J Pediatr Surg. 1995;30(9):1258-63.
11. Nyberg DA, Resta R, Luthy DA, Hickok DE, Mahony BS, Hirsch JH. Prenatal sonographic finding of Down syndrome: review of 94 cases. Obstet Gynecol. 1990;76(3 Pt 1):370-7.
12. Murshed R, Nichoolls G Spitz L. Intrinsic duodenal obstruction: trends in management

and outcome over 45 years (1951-1995) with relevance to prenatal counselling. Br J Obstet Gynaecol. 1999;106(11):1197-9.

13. Fonkalsrud EW, deLorimier AA, Hays DM. Congenital atresia and stenosis of the duodenum. A review compiled from the members of the surgical section of the American Academy of Pediatrics. Pediatrics. 1969;43(1): 79-83.
14. Loveday BJ, Barr JA, Aitken J. The intrauterine demonstration of duodenal atresia by ultrasound. Br J Radiol. 1975;48(576):1031-2.
15. Petrikovsky BM. First-trimester diagnosis of duodenal atresia. Am J Obstet Gynecol. 1994;171(2):569-70.
16. Ikeda K, Goto S. Diagnosis and treatment of Hirschsprung disease: In Japan: an analysis of 1628 patients. Ann Surg. 1984;199(4):400-5.
17. Jarmas AL, Weaver DD, Padilla LM, Stecker E, Bender HA. Hirschsprung disease: etiologic implications of unsuccessful prenatal diagnosis. Am J Med Genet. 1983;16(2):163-7.
18. Wrobleski D, Wesselhoeft. Ultrasonic diagnosis of prenatal interstinal obstruction. J Pediatr Surg. 1979;14(5):598-600.
19. Vermish M, Mayden KL, Confino E, Giglia RV, Gleicher N. Prenatal sonographic diagnosis of Hirschsprung disease. J Ultrasound Med. 1986;5(1):37-9.
20. Eliyahu S, Yanai N, Blondheim O, Reich D, Siplovich L, Shalev E. Sonographic presentation of Hrischprung's disease. A case of an entirely aganglionic colon and ileum. Prenat Diagn. 1994;14(12):1170-2.
21. Gray SW, Skandalakis JE. The colon and rectum. In: Embryology for Surgeons. Philadelphia: WB Saunders; 1972. pp. 187-216.
22. Blisard KS, Kleinman R. Hirschsprungs disease: a clinical and pathologic overview. Hum Pathol. 1986;17(12):1189-91.
23. Buyse ML. Birth defects encyclopedia. Cambridge: Blackwell Science; 1990. pp. 427-8.
24. Boyden EA. The accessory gallbladder. Am J Anat. 1926;38:177-231.
25. Gross RE. Congenital anomalies of the gallbladder: A review of 148 cases with a report of double gallbladder. Arch Surg. 1936;32(1):131-62.
26. Bronshtein M, Weiner Z, Abramovici H, Filmar S, Erlik Y, Blumenfeld Z. Prenatal diagnosis of gall bladder anomalies - report of 17 cases. Prenat Diagn. 1993:13(9):851-61.
27. Duchatel F, Muller F, Oury JF, Mennesson B, Boue J, Boue A. Prenatal diagnosis of cystic fibrosis: ultrasonography of the gallbladder at 17-19 weeks of gestation. Fetal Diagn Ther. 1993:8(1):28-36.
28. Rescorla FJ, Grosfeld JL. Contemporary management of meconium ileus. World J Surg. 1993;17(3):318-25.
29. Jawad AJ, al-samarrai AI, al-mofada S, al-Howasi M, Hawass NE, al-Beiruti Z. Congenital paraoesophageal hiatal hernia in infancy. Pediatr Surg Int. 1998;13(2-3):91-4.
30. Petrikovsky BM, Nochimson DJ, Campbell WA, Vintzileos AM. Fetal jejunoileal atresia with persistent omphalomesenteric duct. Am J Obstet Gynecol. 1988;158(1):173-5.
31. Skoll AM, Marquette GP, Hamilton EF. Prenatal ultrasonic diagnosis of multiple bowel atresias. Am J Obstet Gynecol. 1987;156;472-3.
32. Cheng W, Mya GH, Saing H. Does the amniotic fluid protein absorption contribute significantly to the fetal weight? J Paediatr Child Health. 1996;32(1):39-41.

15

CHAPTER

Skeletal Dysplasia: Abnormalities of Skeletal System

Binodini M Chauhan, Kairavi Desai

INTRODUCTION

The osteochondrodysplasias and dysostoses comprise a group of more than 350 disorders of the skeleton. By definition, the osteochondrodysplasia or skeletal dysplasia refers to disorders with generalized abnormalities of the skeleton, whereas the dysostoses are those disorders that have a single or group of abnormal bones. However, as more is known about all of these disorders, the distinction between osteochondrodysplasias and dysostoses has become blurred. In most osteochondrodysplasias, there is a generalized abnormality in linear skeletal growth and in some disorders there are concomitant abnormalities in organ systems other than the skeleton. The skeletal dysplasias can be inherited as autosomal dominant, autosomal recessive, or X-linked disorders, and some disorders that result from imprinting errors, somatic mosaicism, and teratogen exposure. There has been substantial progress in identification of the molecular defects responsible for the osteochondrodysplasias, and the genetic defects have been identified for approximately 160 of the 350 well-recognized disorders. Many of these discoveries have led to availability of DNA diagnostics for both molecular confirmation of ultrasound and postmortem findings, as well as invasive prenatal diagnosis for at-risk families.

The fetal skeleton develops relatively early in the fetal period and, thus, prenatal diagnosis of these disorders is possible. The appendicular and the axial skeleton undergo a programmed pattern of endochondral ossification, whereas the calvarium and portions of the clavicle and pubis ossify via membranous ossification. Ossification occurs at relatively early human gestational ages: clavicle and mandible at 8 weeks; the appendicular skeleton, ileum, and scapula by 12 weeks; and the metacarpals and metatarsals are ossified by 12–16 weeks. Secondary (epiphyseal) ossification centers are seen by radiographs at approximately 20 weeks gestation and at a similar time period by ultrasound.

ULTRASOUND EVALUATION

Second trimester ultrasound evaluation of the fetus for detection of congenital anomalies has become standard of care in many communities. The fetal skeleton is readily visualized by two-dimensional (2D) ultrasound by 14 weeks, and measurements of the fetal femora and humeri are considered part of any basic midtrimester ultrasound evaluation. Any fetus showing femora or humeri length measurements less than 5th centile or –2 SD from the mean in the second trimester (<24 weeks) should be evaluated in a center that has expertise in evaluating the entire fetal skeleton and has the ability to provide genetic counseling.

The following fetal ultrasound parameters must be visualized and plotted against normative values when a fetus manifesting a skeletal dysplasia is suspected; fetal cranium (biparietal diameter, occipital-frontal diameter, and head circumference), abdominal circumference, mandible, clavicle, scapula, chest circumference, and all fetal long bones. Comparison of the relative length of all the long bones and against normative values will determine whether there is primarily rhizomelia, mesomelia, or that both segments are involved. One helpful ratio is the femur to foot ratio, which approaches 1.0 throughout gestation. In addition to evaluation of the long bones, there are other ultrasound parameters that should be evaluated and can be helpful in these differentiating disorders. These include the fetal facial profile (glabellar bossing, flattened nasal bridge, micrognathia), presence and shape of the vertebral bodies, and relative appearance of the hands and feet (extra, missing, or malformed digits). Fetuses with long bone measurements more than 3D below the mean should be strongly suspected of having a skeletal dysplasia, especially if the head circumference is greater than the 75th centile. Most prenatal-onset skeletal dysplasias present with relative disproportion of the skeletal measurements when compared with those of the cranium. In addition, close attention should be paid to the shape and mineralization pattern of the fetal calvarium and fetal skeleton (poor or ectopic mineralization).

One of the most important determinations that must be made by ultrasound is that of neonatal or infantile lethality. Lethality occurring in most skeletal dysplasias is a result of a small chest circumference and resultant pulmonary hypoplasia. However, not all skeletal dysplasias associated with small thoracic circumferences are associated with immediate lethality. By using ultrasound criteria for lethality, chest-to-abdominal circumference ratio of <0.6 and femur length-to-abdominal circumference ratios of <0.16 are strongly suggestive of lethality. When concomitant abnormalities in other organ systems are visualized, there is increased morbidity and mortality in these disorders. The accuracy of prenatal diagnosis of the skeletal dysplasias using routine ultrasound approaches 40%. All fetuses suspected of having a skeletal dysplasia should have the diagnosis confirmed by postdelivery clinical and radiologic evaluation. Postdelivery and/or postmortem evaluation includes anterior-posterior radiographs of the appendicular skeleton including hands and feet, and anterior-posterior and lateral radiographs of the cranium and spine (vertebral column). In all appropriate cases, photographs should be taken and autopsies should be offered and encouraged, because it provides the most useful information for accurate diagnosis. Pathologists should collect cartilage and bone, ideally femora and humeri for histomorphic analysis. Tissue (fibroblasts, cartilage, and bone) and/or DNA should be saved for molecular analysis whenever possible, because many skeletal disorders are associated with a significant recurrence risk.

For fetuses suspected as having a skeletal dysplasia delivered at a viable gestational age, predelivery consultations and management plan should be initiated between the obstetrical, neonatal, anesthesia, and genetics consultants.

NOMENCLATURE OF THE BONE DEFECTS

Abnormal Shapes of the Skull

- *Cloverleaf skull*: It is due to very early closure of lambdoid, coronal, and sagittal sutures, parietal bones are most severely affected. It is typical of thanatophoric dysplasia. It is best appreciated on coronal view.
- *Acrocephaly or turricephaly*: It can be simply explained as pointed head or a tower head. It has increased craniocaudal diameter due to early closure of all structures.
- *Brachycephaly*: Early closure of the two coronal sutures leading to short anterior-posterior diameter of the skull.
- *Scaphocephaly*: Premature closure of sagittal suture leads to long occipitofrontal diameter of the skull.
- *Plagiocephaly*: Unilateral premature closure of coronal and lambdoid suture leads to asymmetrical skull but is usually not seen antenatally.

Flowchart 1: Evaluation and causes of short femur in each trimester. We can see how the cause of short femur will vary in different trimesters.

Evaluation of short femur

Stage	Causes
1st trimester NT scan	• Wrong dates • Delayed conception • Skeletal dysplasia
Anomaly scan (2nd trimester)	• Skeletal dysplasia • Trisomy 21 • Early IUGR • Isolated femur hypoplasia • Constitutional shortening
3rd trimester	• Constitutionally small (SGA) • IUGR • Achondroplasias

(IUGR: intrauterine growth restriction; SGA: small for gestational age; NT: nuchal translucency)

- *Trigonocephaly*: Triangular shape of the upper most part of the skull, due to closure of metopic suture.
- *Abnormal spine*
- *Platyspondyly*: Flattened vertebral bodies and decreased distance between the end plates (**Flowcharts 1 and 2**).

First trimester ultrasound findings in skeletal dysplasia (**Figs. 1A to D**):

- Thickened nuchal translucency
- Abnormality of ductus venosus flow
- *Femur*: Short, bowed, broken, absent
- *Arms and legs*: Short, abnormal shape, asymmetric
- *Thorax*: Small, narrow, short ribs, broken ribs
- *Skull ossification*: Decreased or increased
- *Abnormal hands*: Polydactyly, oligodactyly, hitchhiker thumb, radius aplasia, club hand, cleft hand, absent hand
- *Abnormal feet*: Clubfoot, polydactyly, oligodactyly, absent foot, cleft foot
- *Spine*: Reduced ossification, abnormal shape, convex angle.

Making a diagnosis in the first trimester of a specific type of skeletal dysplasia is challenging. In general, the main leading sign for the presence of a skeletal abnormality in the first trimester is short limbs or short femur(s). Despite all these anatomic markers, a detailed ultrasound examination in the early second trimester along with fetal echocardiogram is indicated when a skeletal dysplasia is suspected in the first trimester, because additional anatomic findings can become more apparent with the growth of the fetus.

Diagnosed by 14 weeks of gestation:

- Achondrogenesis I and II
- Ellis-van Creveld syndrome
- Osteogenesis imperfecta II
- Thanatophoric dysplasia
- Campomelic dysplasia

Flowchart 2: Papageorghiou et al., reported outcome of antenatally diagnosed short femur, where they reviewed 129 cases of short femur (FL <5%) between gestational age of 18–24 weeks. They divided all the cases of short femur according to their causes as follows.[16]

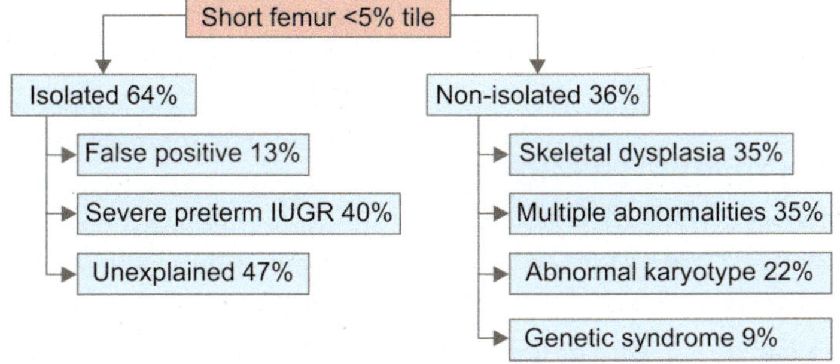

(IUGR: intrauterine growth restriction)

Source: Papageorghiou AT, Fratelli N, Leslie K, Bhide A, Thilaganathan B. Outcome of Fetuses with Antenatally Diagnosed Short Femur. Obstetrical and Gynecological Survey. 2008;63(7);425-6.

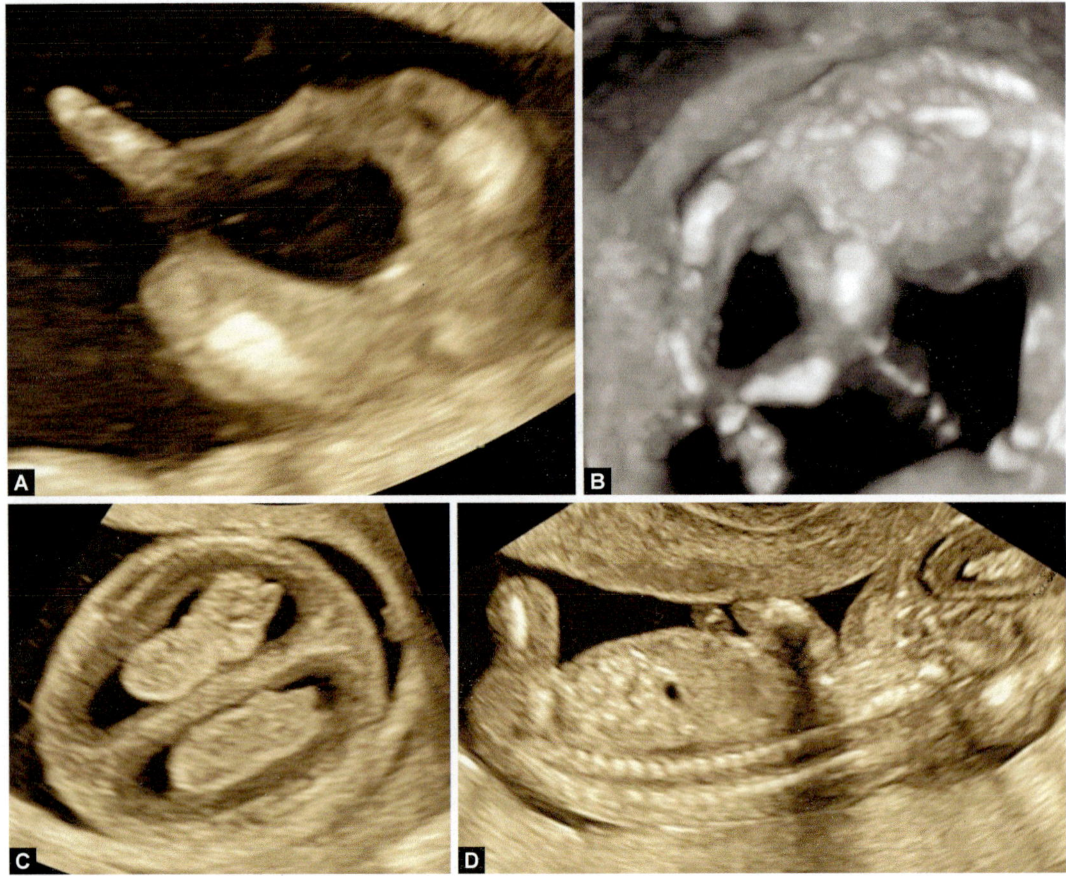

Figs. 1A to D: First trimester skeletal dysplasia: (A and B) Short and curved femurs; (C) Normal mineralization of skull; (D) Normal mineralization of spine. These findings collectively indicate diagnosis of lethal first trimester skeletal dysplasia, most likely thanatophoric dysplasia.

- Diastrophic dysplasia
- Congenital hypophosphatasia
- Jeune syndrome or asphyxiating thoracic dysplasia
- Short-rib polydactyly syndromes
- Roberts syndrome
- Cleidocranial dysplasia

CAUSE OF 2ND TRIMESTER SHORT FEMUR: INTRAUTERINE GROWTH RESTRICTION AND SMALL FOR GESTATIONAL AGE

A fetus is considered to be small for gestational age (SGA) when its size (biometric evaluation) falls below a predefined threshold for its gestational age. The most common definition of SGA is estimated fetal weight or abdominal circumference below the 10th percentile of given reference ranges. Fetal growth restriction (FGR) is defined as the fetal weight <10 percentile on ultrasound, that, because of a pathologic process, fails to reach its genetically predetermined growth potential. The main distinction between SGA and FGR is that a SGA fetus may be small but not at increased risk of adverse perinatal outcome, while a fetus with size above the 10th percentile may be FGR and at increased risk of adverse perinatal and long-term outcome. **Table 1** shows the salient differentiating points between low growth profile or SGA and fetal growth restriction.

TABLE 1: Key differentiating characteristics between low growth profile fetus and fetal growth restriction.

Low growth profile	*Fetal growth restriction*
Constitutionally small	May be associated with syndrome/anomaly/aneuploidy
Growth curve parallel to nomogram	Curve drops off
Anatomy normal	Anatomy normal/abnormal
Biophysical profile, liquor normal	Normal/abnormal
Doppler normal	Normal/abnormal
No management required	Karyotype, infection profile, markers of aneuploidy as per requirement
Placenta—normal	Abnormal placental histology and/or morphology
Good outcome	Poorer outcome

COUNSELING FOR SHORT FEMUR IN SECOND TRIMESTERS

- *Constitutional*: Good prognosis. No management is required.
- *Trisomy 21*: Short femur alone is not a strong soft marker (isolated LR 1.6)
- If isolated, further investigations are not essential. If associated with other soft markers, karyotyping is essential to rule out aneuploidy.
- Pregnancies in which there is a suspected fetal skeletal dysplasia should be referred to appropriate high-risk maternal fetal medicine/perinatal medicine specialists for management or recommendations for management.
- Prenatal next-generation skeletal panel gene sequencing or whole exome/genome testing should be offered to increase diagnostic yield in suspected skeletal dysplasia and should be interpreted by qualified expert.
- If the dysplasia is suspected to be nonlethal, then counseling of that couple should also include a discussion of possible therapies and new treatments that may be available to the child.
- These fetuses should be delivered in departments with specialized pediatric teams, and some cases may require pulmonary, orthopedic, and neurological specialists.
- Regardless of any previous diagnosis or indicator of prognosis, all infants with suspected skeletal dysplasia who deliver at term should be reevaluated as soon as possible after delivery.
- If possible, instrumentation during delivery should be avoided when fetal skeletal dysplasia is suspected due to increased risk of intracranial and cervical spine complications.
- *Fetal growth restriction:* Monitoring should be scheduled based on the severity of FGR and alterations in UA Doppler.

COUNSELING FOR SHORT FEMUR IN THIRD TRIMESTER

- Fetal growth restriction has to be managed accordingly.
- Small for gestational age does not require any management. Good prognosis.
- *Achondroplasia:* Management of delivery by C-section.
- Autosomal dominant inheritance—*de novo* pathogenic variant. Such parents have a very low-risk of having another child with achondroplasia.
- An individual with achondroplasia who has a reproductive partner with average stature is at 50% risk in each pregnancy of having a child with achondroplasia.
- When both parents have achondroplasia, the risk to their offspring of having average stature is 25%; of having achondroplasia, 50%; and of having homozygous achondroplasia (a lethal condition), 25%.

ASSESSMENT OF LONG BONES

- *Shortening* of the extremities can involve the entire limb (micromelia), the humerus or femur (rhizomelia), the radius, ulna, tibia or fibula (mesomelia), or the hands and feet (acromelia). The femur is abnormally short even in mesomelic dwarfism and, therefore, in routine fetal abnormality screening the femur is measured and compared subjectively to all long bones. Severe limb reductions, as in thanatophoric dwarfism and achondrogenesis can be detected from 16 weeks' gestation, whereas in achondroplasia limb shortening becomes obvious >22 weeks.

- *Abnormal shape:* In some conditions there is pronounced bowing (e.g., campomelic dysplasia, thanatophoric dwarfism), and in others fractures and callus formation may also be detected [e.g., osteogenesis imperfecta (OI), achondrogenesis, and hypophosphatasia].
- *Reduced echogenicity* of bones due to hypomineralization is seen in some disorders (e.g., hypophosphatasia, OI, and achondrogenesis). Virtual absence of ossification of the spine in achondrogenesis may lead to the erroneous diagnosis of complete spinal agenesis. Poor mineralization of the skull in hypophosphatasia may result in the misdiagnosis of hydrocephalus.
- *Absence of extremities*, such as amelia (complete absence of extremities), acheiria (absence of the hand), phocomelia (seal limb) or aplasia–hypoplasia of the radius or ulna, are often inherited as part of a genetic syndrome (Holt–Oram syndrome, thrombocytopenia with absent radii syndrome). Another cause of focal limb loss is the amniotic band syndrome.

EVALUATION OF HANDS AND FEET

Several skeletal dysplasias are associated with alterations of the hands and feet.

- *Polydactyly*: Presence of more than five digits. It is classified as postaxial if the extra digits are on the ulnar or fibular side and preaxial if they are located on the radial or tibial side.
- *Syndactyly*: Soft tissue or bony fusion of adjacent digits.
- *Clinodactyly*: Deviation of a finger(s).
- *Disproportion* between hands and feet and the other parts of the extremity may also be a sign of a skeletal dysplasia.

Examination of fetal movements: Arthrogryposis and multiple pterygium syndrome are characterized by limitation of flexion or extension of the limbs.

Evaluation of the fetal thorax: Several skeletal dysplasias are associated with a small thorax, which leads to pulmonary hypoplasia and neonatal death. The diagnosis of a small thorax can be made by examining the thoracic-to-abdominal circumference ratio or the thoracic-to-head circumference ratio. The thoracic circumference is measured at the level of the four-chamber view of the heart.

Evaluation of the fetal head: Several skeletal dysplasias are associated with reduced ossification of the skull bones. The face should also be examined for the diagnosis of hypertelorism, micrognathia, short upper lip, and abnormalities of the ears.

Diagnostic tests complementary to sonography: Prenatal or postnatal evaluation includes DNA analysis for an increasing number of skeletal dysplasia. Some can now be diagnosed by cfDNA testing of maternal blood. Postnatally, examination of skeletal radiographs is of particular importance, since the classification of skeletal dysplasias is largely based on radiographic findings.

TERMINOLOGY

Abnormalities of the Limbs

- Shortening of the proximal portion of the limbs (femur and humerus) is rhizomelia
- Shortening of middle portion of the limbs (forearm and leg bones) is mesomelia
- Shortening of hand and feet bones is acromelia
- Severe shortening of all portions of the limbs is called micromelia

- Absent limb: Amelia
- Absence or deformity of distal part of limb/limbs: Peromelia
- Absence of distal portion of one limb: Hemimelia (type of peromelia)
- Partial absence of a limb: Meromelia
- Poor development of proximal portions of limbs when hands and feet are directly attached to trunk: Phocomelia
- Hypoplasia of long bones of limb: Ectromelia
- Fused lower extremities: Sirenomelia.

Abnormalities of Extremities

- *Pathological contracture of ankle*: Clubfoot
- *Pathological contracture of the hand*: Ulnar deviation of the hand
- *Inwards bent of heel and foot*: Varus
- *Outwards bent of heel and foot*: Valgus
- *Abnormal hyperextension of the foot*: Equinus
- *Polydactyly*: An extradigit. It is called postaxial if the sixth digit is on the ulnar or fibular side (after fifth digit), and it is called preaxial, if it is on radial or tibial side (before thumb or toe), respectively, in upper limb and lower limb
- *Split hand/foot malformation:* Ectrodactyly
- *Fused fingers*: Syndactyly
- *Absence of one or both hands*: Acheiria
- *Absence of one or both feet*: Apodia
- *Absence of hands and feet*: Achieropodia
- *Absence of fingers or toes*: Adactyly
- *Subnormal number of fingers or toes*: Oligodactyly
- *Short fingers or toes*: Brachydactyly
- *Permanent medial or lateral deflections of one or more fingers*: Clinodactyly
- *Permanent flexion of fingers and toes*: Camptodactyly

Table 2 shows common lethal and non-lethal skeletal dysplasias.

TABLE 2: Common lethal and non-lethal skeletal dysplasias.

Lethal	***Nonlethal***
Thanatophoric dysplasia (most common lethal)	Achondroplasia (most common non-lethal)
Achondrogenesis	Club and rocker-bottom feet (vertical talus)
Campomelic dysplasia	Diastrophic dysplasia
Osteogenesis imperfecta type II	Osteogenesis imperfecta type I, III, and VI
Jeune's thoracic dystrophy	Radial ray aplasia/hypoplasia

THANATOPHORIC DYSPLASIA

This most common lethal skeletal dysplasia can be of two types, both caused by gene mutation with autosomal dominant inheritance.

The gene affected is FGGR3. Its incidence is 0.69/10,000 live births. It can be classified into two types: type 1 which is more common and is characterized by curved femur, and type 2 which is characterized by straight femur but cloverleaf skull. It is severe rhizomelic micromelia.

- All limbs are affected and all are short.
- Bones are bowed especially in type 1 with metaphyseal cupping of femur and humerus (French telephone receiver deformity).
- Bone mineralization is normal.
- Ribs are short and on mid sagittal view, a dip typical of severe thoracic dysplasia can be seen at the level of thoraco-abdominal junction. This also leads to pulmonary dysplasia and that makes this pathology lethal.
- Skull is large—macrocrania with frontal bossing and depressed nasal bridge. In type 2, there is premature closure of cranial sutures giving it a cloverleaf configuration and appears trilobed on coronal section. It is often associated with renal, cardiac, and central nervous system anomalies. Polyhydramnios is seen in about 50% of cases.

Tips to Differential Diagnosis

- *Achondrogenesis*: Micrognathia and severe hypomineralization

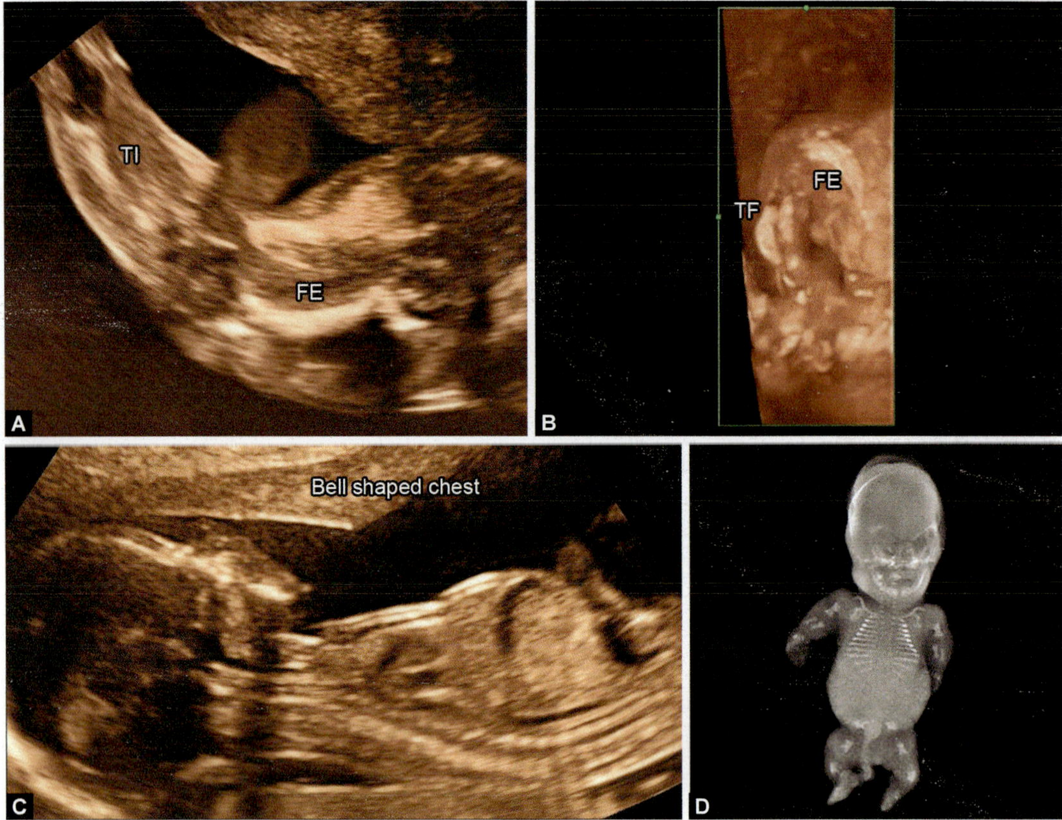

Figs. 2A to D: Thanatophoric dysplasia type 1: (A) Short and curved femur and tibia; (B) 3D rendered image showing short and curved femur and tibia; (C) Narrow bell-shaped thorax with normal mineralization of skull and spine; (D) Postabortal X-ray showing narrow thorax, short ribs, and short long bones. These findings collectively suggest a diagnosis of thanatophoric dysplasia type 1.

- *Hypophosphatasia*: Generalized hypomineralization
- *Osteogenesis imperfecta type 2*: Fractures
- Cloverleaf skull may be present in Pfeiffer syndrome that has different skeletal anomalies and Crouzon's syndrome that has no limb shortening.

Prognosis, survival, and quality of life: Thanatophoric dysplasia is always lethal due to the severe pulmonary and thoracic hypoplasia.

Recurrence risk: Both types are due to de novo mutations. Therefore, the recurrence risk is trivial. **Figures 2 and 3** show cases of thanatophoric dysplasia type 1 and 2 respectively.

ACHONDROGENESIS

It is a lethal osteochondrodysplasia with severe micromelia where long bones are very small and are curved. There are various subtypes of achondrogenesis that differ in inheritance pattern, genetics, and phenotype; however, the classification is continuously evolving and is not completely clear.

Achondrogenesis is of two types:

- *Type 1: Parenti-Fraccaro type*: Cranium looks disproportionately large due to soft tissue edema, lack of ossification of the skull and spine with short bones, and thin ribs with rib fractures. It has autosomal

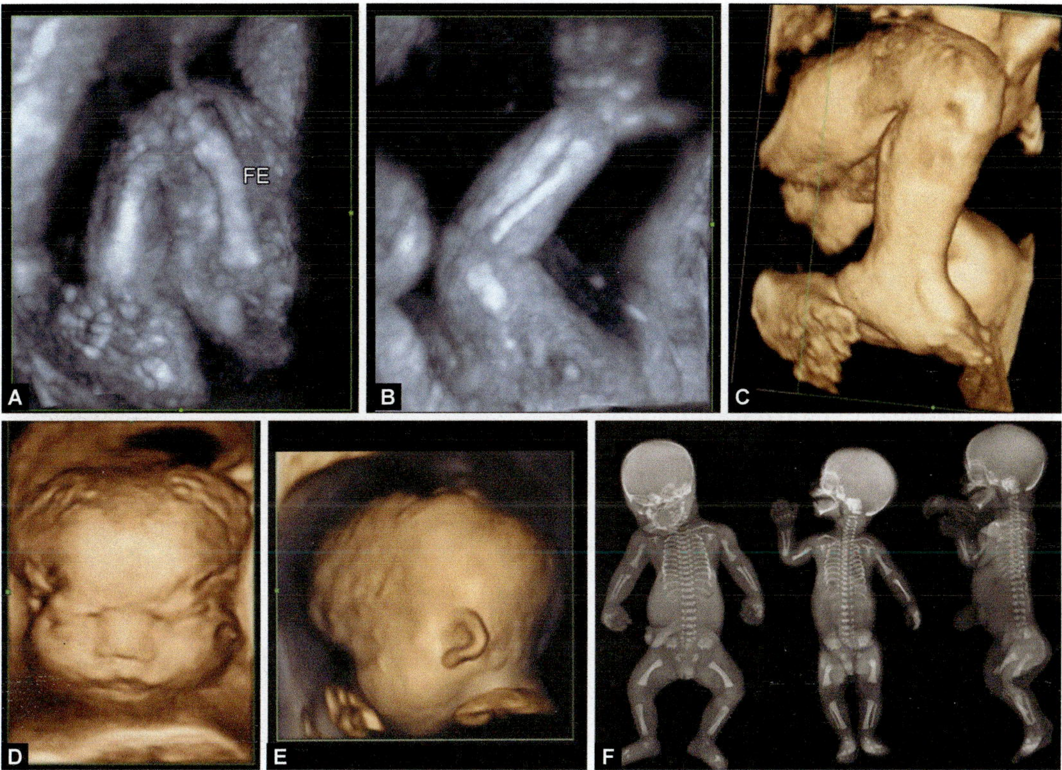

Figs. 3A to F: Thanatophoric dysplasia type II: (A) Normal length and curvature of femur; (B) Normal bones of upper limb; (C) Normal lower limb length and structure; (D) Classic cloverleaf shape of skull; (E) Frontal towering of fetal head; (F) Postabortal X-ray showing narrow thorax and short ribs, with normal shape of long bones. These findings collectively suggest a diagnosis of thanatophoric dysplasia type 2.

recessive inheritance and is seen in about 25% of cases of achondrogenesis.

- *Type 2: Langer-Saldino type*: It is due to de novo mutations with autosomal dominant inheritance pattern. In some cases, it is mutation in COL2A1 gene coding for collagen type 2. It is characterized by virtual absence of ossification in spine and pubic bones. But normal skull ossification and no rib fractures are seen. Outcome is fatal in neonatal life.

Ultrasound Diagnosis

The ultrasound diagnosis is based on the recognition of micromelia, thoracic hypoplasia, hypomineralization, and micrognathia. In particular, the long bones appear curved and barely visible and the thorax extremely hypoplastic due to the underdeveloped ribs. The hypomineralization predominantly involves the spine, pelvis, and calvarium. Micrognathia is almost always seen. If the condition is recognized at 12–14 weeks of gestation, which is likely, hydrops and diffuse subcutaneous edema (spaceman's suit) may also be seen.

Associated gastrointestinal abnormalities and polyhydramnios may be a feature.

Tips to differential diagnosis:

- *Thanatophoric dysplasia*: No hypomineralization
- *Hypophosphatasia*: No micrognathia
- *Osteogenesis imperfecta type 2*: Constant occurrence of fractures.

Prognosis and Management

Achondrogenesis is always lethal, due to the severity of the skeletal underdevelopment. Termination of pregnancy can be offered before viability. Standard prenatal care is not altered when continuation of pregnancy is opted. Confirmation of diagnosis after birth is important for genetic counseling.

Recurrence Risk

Achondrogenesis is autosomal recessive (type I) and dominant (type II). Because there are lethal disorders, type II autosomal dominant involves a new mutation. It therefore carries a much lower recurrence risk than the 25% risk of type I (**Figs. 4A to E**).

CAMPOMELIC DYSPLASIA

This is an extremely rare, always lethal disease, always a result of a de novo mutation (SOX9 allele that codes for SRY—box 9 protein, expressed in testis and skeleton). Sex reversal in affected male is characteristic with bifid scrotum and micropenis or ambiguous genitalia.

Ultrasound Diagnosis

Ultrasound shows bones with abnormal curvature, especially of the lower limbs (femur and tibia), bell shaped narrow chest with eleven pairs of ribs, hypoplasia of mid-thoracic vertebrae and scapulae, scoliosis, tracheobronchomalacia, flat and small face, high forehead with prominent occiput, low nasal bridge, micrognathia, low set and malformed ears, hypertelorism, and ambiguous genitalia.

It may be associated with hydronephrosis, hydrocephalus, and cardiac anomalies, sometimes even fibular hypoplasia may be seen.

Though in most cases, it is fatal in neonatal life or infancy because of trachea-broncho-malacia and respiratory complications.

Tips to Differential Diagnosis

Osteogenesis imperfect types 1, 3, 4: Calvarial hypomineralization is the differentiating point.

Prognosis and Management

Campomelic dysplasia is almost always lethal, because of the severity of the ubiquitous laryngotracheomalacia. In very rare instances, survival until adolescence has been reported, but mild-to-moderate developmental delay is present in the majority of these cases.

Recurrence Risk

Most cases are new mutations. Very rare cases of autosomal recessive inheritance have been found. **Figures 5A and B** show a case of campomelic dysplasia.

OSTEOGENESIS IMPERFECTA

It is a genetic disorder that affects type 1 collagen. It is generally caused by a new gene mutation with an autosomal dominant inheritance. It is characterized by severe bone fragility, prenatal growth deficiency, and blue sclera. Osteogenesis imperfecta (OI) can be classifies into four types. Of these, type 1 and 4 are not seen in fetus because the associated fractures occur only after birth. Type 3 can sometimes be recognized in the third trimester. Type 2 (Vrolich type) is the most severe form and can be diagnosed by antenatal scans. This type 2 OI is micromelic type. It is uniformly lethal. This is believed to be due to pulmonary hypoplasia as a consequence of multiple rib fractures leading to thoracic hypoplasia.

Incidence including all types of OI is 0.4/10,000 live births, and approximately one-half (0.19 per 10,000) represents type II.

Etiology and Pathogenesis

Osteogenesis imperfecta is due to a mutation in one of the two genes involved in the production of collagen type I (COLIA1 and COLIA2). Because this type of collagen is present in bones,

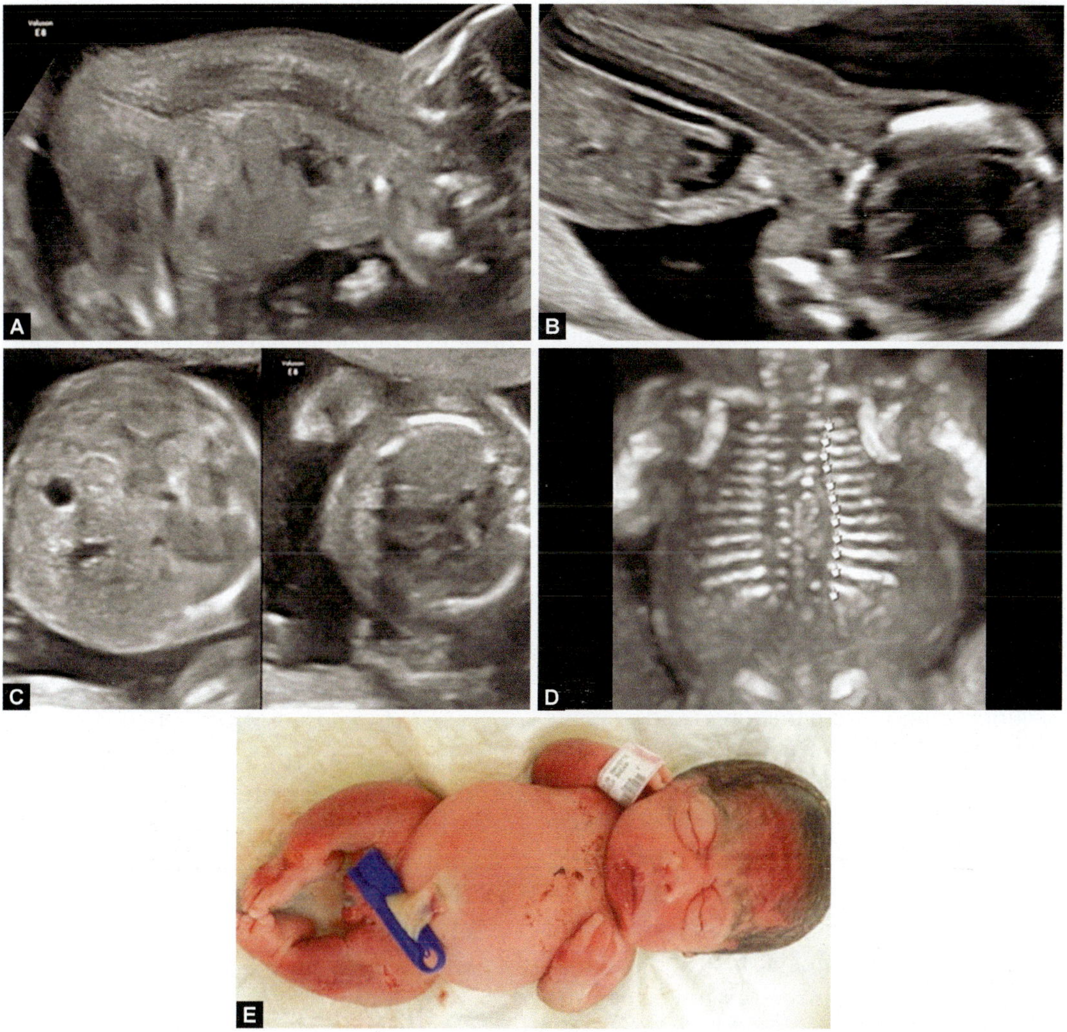

Figs. 4A to E: Achondrogenesis: (A and B) Sagittal view of spine showing poor mineralization; (C) Narrow thoracic circumference compared to abdominal circumference. Ribs appear short; (D) 3D rendered image showing narrow thorax, short ribs, and poor mineralization of spine. Rest of the skeleton shows normal mineralization; (E) Postabortal picture showing short long bones and narrow thorax.

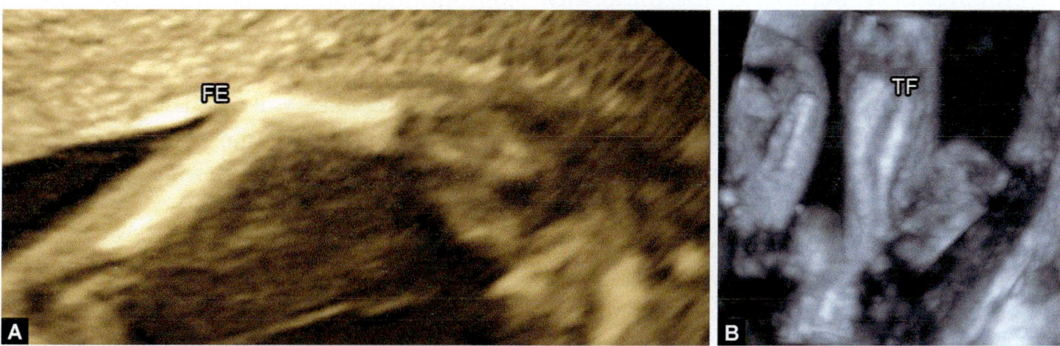

Figs. 5A and B: Campomelic dysplasia: (A) Short and angulated femur; (B) Short and angulated tibia and fibula.

tendons, tooth enamel, and sclera, the anomaly in collagen I is the cause of all expressions of the disease in the various subtypes.

Ultrasound Diagnosis

Severe bone fragility due to defective ossification leads to multiple fractures, leading to bone angulations (*severe bone hypomineralization*). Because of the bone fragility, there may also be skull damage and cerebral hemorrhage. Type 3 shows multiple fractures and kyphosis in third trimester or after birth.

Tips to Differential Diagnosis

- *Achondrogenesis*: Micrognathia and no fractures
- *Hypophosphatasia*: Clavicle sparing hypomineralization.

Prognosis: Type II is invariablely lethal. OI type III shows motor disability of variable severity (kyphosis and fractures) and worsens with age, due to the extreme fragility of the bones. Though these patients survive till adult age, they have bad quality of life due to walking disability, fragile bones, otosclerosis, and dentition problems. Types I and IV, which cannot be detected in the fetus, are associated with a better prognosis. In the nonlethal variants, promising results have recently been obtained with oral bisphosphonates (alendronate and pamidronate). Stem cells have proved to be effective in experimental cases.

Management: Because of the uniformly fatal outcome, termination of pregnancy could be offered when type II is diagnosed. For other forms, if continuing the pregnancy is opted, standard prenatal care should not be altered.

Recurrence risk: In OI type I and IV, an autosomal dominant pattern is involved. Type II is a de novo mutation, and type III is either autosomal recessive or dominant. In general, the recurrence risk for OI type II ranges from 2% to 6%. **Figures 6A to E** show a case of osteogenesis imperfecta.

ASPHYXIATING THORACIC DYSTROPHY (JEUNE'S SYNDROME)

It is a rare disorder with the locus on 15q13 genetically. It is diagnosed by thoracic hypoplasia with moderate rhizomelia and renal anomalies.

Ultrasound Diagnosis

The most striking ultrasound finding is the presence of a very narrow chest with short limbs (moderate rhizomelia). The additional findings, which are not always present, include renal anomalies and postaxial polydactyly.

If the anomaly is not severe, it is nonlethal, and in that case, it may also be missed antenatally. Neonatal mortality is 60%.

Tips for Differential Diagnosis

- *Chondroectodermal dysplasia*: Which may have cardiac defect and polydactyly.
- All other disorders with thoracic hypoplasia, such as thanatophoric dysplasia, osteogenesis imperfecta type-2, achondrogenesis, and hypophosphatasia, also need consideration.
- However, all of these disorders are also characterized by severe micromelia, which is absent in asphyxiating thoracic dystrophy.

Prognosis and Management

Neonatal mortality is 60%. Not all newborns are asphyxiated, and some patients have a fairly normal outcome after corrective surgery of the chest. Confirmation of diagnosis after birth is important for genetic counseling. Surviving neonates will have short stature and renal and cardiovascular problems, always related to the degree of thoracic hypoplasia. Intelligence is normal.

Recurrence Risk

Asphyxiating thoracic dystrophy has an autosomal recessive inheritance pattern, with a 25% recurrence rate. Therefore, in the case

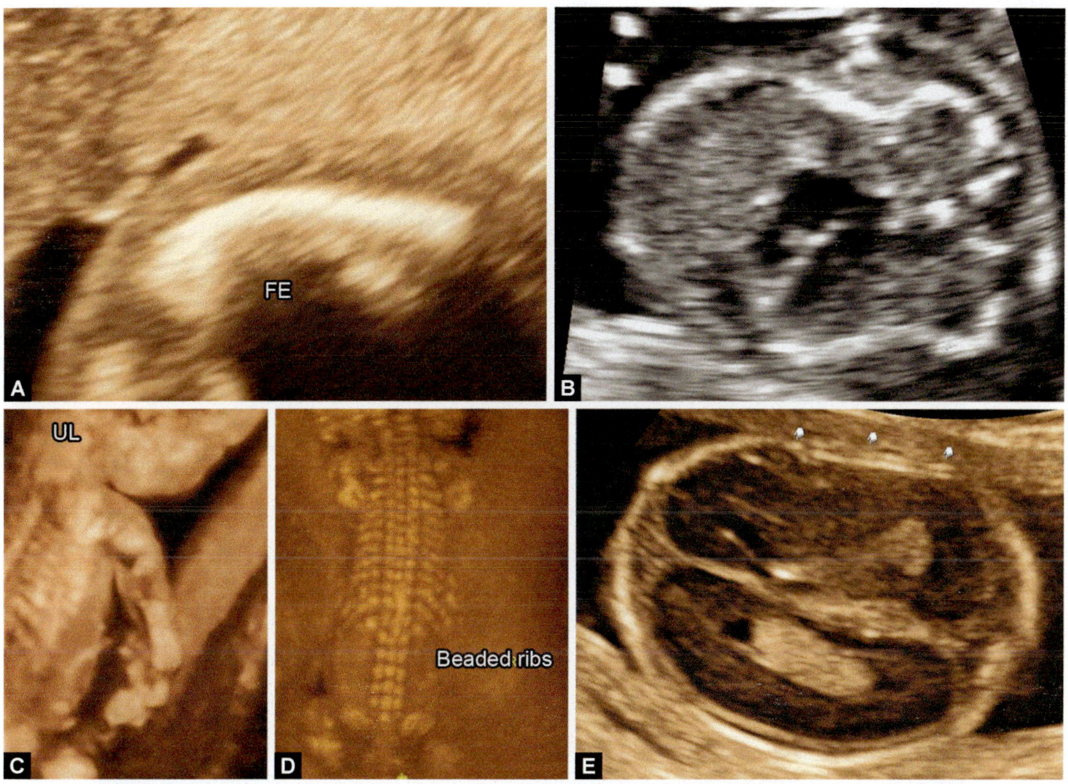

Figs. 6A to E: Osteogenesis imperfecta: (A) Bent and curved femur; (B) Short and angulated ribs showing multiple fractures; (C) 3D rendered image showing short long bones with rib fractures; (D) Ribs showing beaded appearance, suggestive of fractures; (E) Poor mineralization of skull.

of termination of pregnancy, a confirmation of the ultrasound diagnosis by autopsy is of the utmost importance for correct counseling and for advising early ultrasound monitoring of the next pregnancy.

ACHONDROPLASIA (FIGS. 7A TO D)

Achondroplasia is one of the best known and most common types of non-lethal skeletal chondrodysplasia. The incidence is about one in 10,000–30,000. It is one of the most common forms of short limb dwarfism. It is usually suspected on third trimester routine ultrasound because of very shortened long bones.

Conventional 2D ultrasound alone is extremely challenging for diagnosing achondroplasia. Boulet et al. identified a new *prenatal ultrasound* finding of "collar hoop" sign at the proximal end of the femur in fetuses with achondroplasia. "Collar hoop" sign is an overrounded metaphyseal–epiphyseal interface at the femur ends with wide angle 143.55° while connecting to diaphysis. "Collar hoop" sign.

This is a rhizomelic micromelia. It may be homozygous or heterozygous type. The heterozygous type is usually due to new mutations and therefore carries a low recurrence risk, but with homozygous type (one/both parents affected) the recurrence risk is as high as 50–75%. The gene that undergoes mutation is the fibroblast growth factor receptor (FGFR3) at 4p16.3. This mutation prevents binding of FGF to its receptors and in turn impairs bone growth.

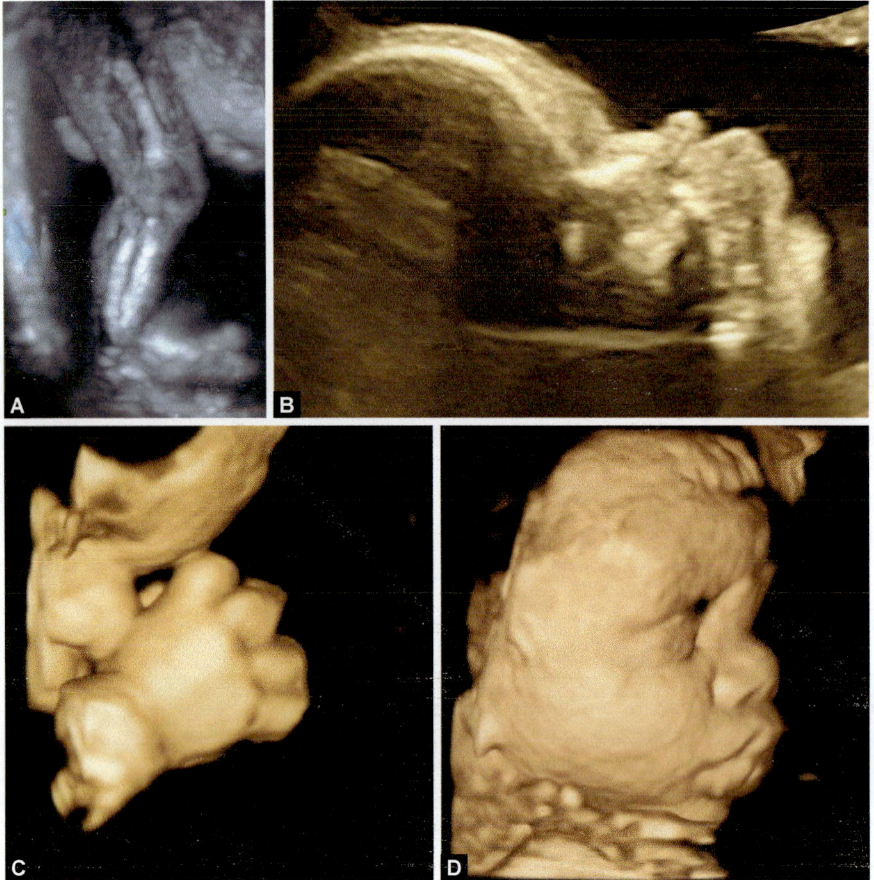

Figs. 7A to D: Achondroplasia: (A) 3D rendered image showing short femur at 31st weeks of GA; (B) Frontal bossing and depressed nasal bridge; (C) Trident hand; (D) 3D rendered image showing frontal bossing and depressed nasal bridge.

Ultrasound Features

This is typically a late onset rhizomelia appearing at around 26–28 weeks of gestation. Normal bone mineralization and morphology with short femur and humerus (1–5 centile of the growth chart matching the ethnicity). Macrocrania and frontal bossing may be seen. This can be appreciated by abnormal HC/FL (head circumference/femoral length) ratio or abnormal BPD/FL (biparietal diameter/femoral length) ratio. The nasal bridge may be flat. Thorax is typically normal.

Trident hand (increased space between 3rd and 4th digit) may be present. Lack of widening of lumbar canal may be found in some cases. This during life may be a cause of peripheral neurological deficits.

TIPS TO DIFFERENTIAL DIAGNOSIS (SHORT LONG BONES)

- *Trisomy 21*: Nuchal fold thickness, and abnormal karyotype.
- *Campomelic dysplasia*: Bowed long bones and micrognathia.
- *Chondroectodermal dysplasia* (*Ellis van Creveld syndrome*): Marked thoracic hypoplasia, polydactyly, and congenital heart disease.
- *Osteogenesis imperfecta*: Fractures and bowed long bones.

DIASTROPHIC DYSPLASIA

Diastrophic dysplasia is a type of osteochondrodysplasia caused by homozygous mutation in *diastrophic dysplasia sulfate transporter gene*. Abnormalities occurring particularly in the skeletal and cartilaginous system are typical of the disease, which has an incidence of 1 in 100,000 live births.

Diastrophic dwarfism is a skeletal dysplasia that can be identified by ultrasound usually during the second trimester of pregnancy. This severe but nonlethal disorder of the cartilage can be diagnosed earlier using transvaginal sonography.

An obstetric ultrasound scan produced in second trimester reveals characteristic findings of rhizomelia of the lower and upper limbs (shortening of the proximal portions) and mesomelia (shortening of the intermediate portions). Both upper limbs show marked curvature, with the first finger of the upper limbs in abduction referred to as "hitchhiker thumb" and clinodactyly of the fifth finger. There may be associated abnormalities: micrognathia, cleft palate, and thickened deformed "cauliflower" ears.

Prognosis: This disease is not lethal and neurodevelopment is normal. Long-term medical problems include short stature, progressive scoliosis, and joint deformities making it difficult to walk.

Recurrence: Autosomal recessive inheritance: 25%.

RADIAL RAY ANOMALY

Radial ray anomalies comprise of a large spectrum of upper limb anomalies which range from partial (radial hypoplasia) to a complete (radial aplasia) deficiency of the radius with or without accompanying deficiency of the thumb bones.

Subtypes

Radial ray anomalies can be classified into four main subtypes depending upon the extent of severity:

1. *Type I*: Radius is slightly (>2 mm) short and the hand bends sideways at the wrist (often associated with a hypoplastic thumb); proximal radius is usually unaffected.
2. *Type II*: The radius bone is very short and the ulna curves sideways and supports the wrist poorly.
3. *Type III*: Partial absence of radius.
4. *Type IV*: Complete absence of radius.

Radial aplasia with or without ectrodactyly may also be seen in trisomy 18 (multiple anomalies + micrognathia), thrombocytopenia with absent radius syndrome, also shows absent thumb, Holt-Oram syndrome (with syndactyly), and Robert's syndrome (phocomelia + cleft lip/palate). Unlike radial aplasia, all these also present with congenital heart disease. Nager syndrome and VACTERL association may also present with radial aplasia, wherein Nager syndrome has micrognathia and external ear anomalies, and VACTERL association also present with vertebral and renal abnormalities and tracheoesophageal fistula.

Ultrasound Findings

The typical finding on ultrasound imaging is of a single forearm bone and radial deviation of the hand, as seen in **Figures 8A and B**.

This diagnosis should be suspected in the presence of absent or hypoplastic radius and abnormal hand position (radial deviation that is fixed on prolonged scanning). Thumb may or may not be present, and other anomalies present may suggest a syndromic cause.

Genetic Evaluation

Many syndromes are associated with radial ray malformations; they can be sporadic, autosomal dominant, autosomal recessive, or X-linked. If there are additional anomalies, consanguinity, or a family history of a specific condition, gene panel testing or exome sequencing may be useful because chromosomal microarray (CMA) does not detect single-gene (Mendelian) disorders.

Prognosis

The prognosis in isolated cases includes functional limitations that result from the skeletal deformity. Reconstructive surgery

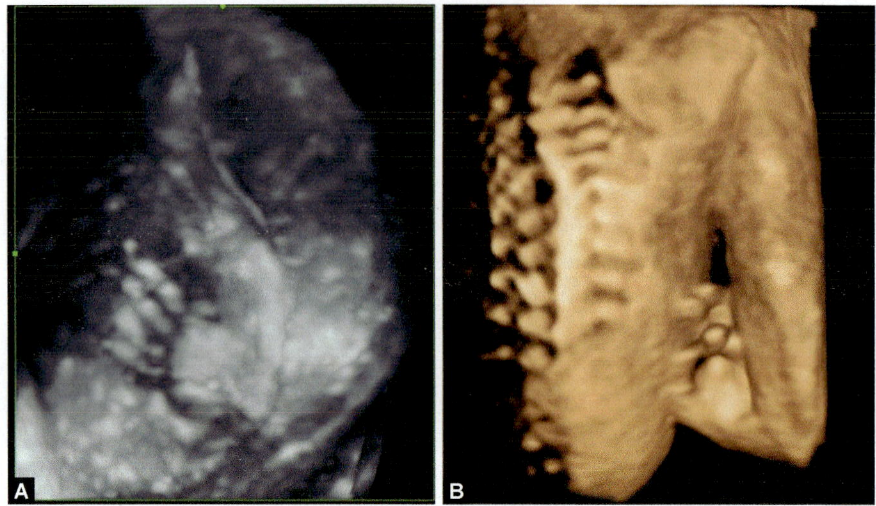

Figs. 8A and B: Radial ray defect: (A and B) 3D rendered image showing absent radius with medial rotation of hand.

may improve the mobility of the affected limb. Prognosis also depends on the severity of associated abnormalities, underlying causes, and potential association with genetic syndromes. Isolated findings are usually sporadic, with a low recurrence risk. Recurrence of syndromic cases depends on the underlying cause.

JARCHO-LEVIN SYNDROME/ SPONDYLOCOSTAL DYSPLASIA

Spondylocostal dysplasia or Jarcho-Levin syndrome is a rare genetic disorder characterized by defects of the bones of the spine (vertebrae), abnormalities of the ribs, *respiratory* insufficiency, and/or other abnormalities. The term Jarcho-Levin syndrome is used as an "umbrella" term to describe a broad range of conditions associated with spinal and rib defects.

Individuals with Jarcho-Levin typically appear to have a short trunk and neck, with arms appearing relatively long in comparison, and a slightly protuberant abdomen. The bones of the spine (vertebrae) may be fused together or misshapen. Sometimes, they are underdeveloped and wedge-shaped (hemivertebrae). Multiple vertebrae are always affected. The ribs may be fused together, misaligned, broadened, split or forked (bifid), and sometimes some of the ribs are missing.

Diagnosis

Sonographic criteria for Jarcho-Levin syndrome include costovertebral segmentation defect, indistinct or fused posterior ribs, irregularly shortened spine, and short trunk and neck, found alongside normal amniotic fluid, limb length, and biparietal diameter. **Figures 9A to C** show the images of a case of Jarco-Levin syndrome.

Inheritance: Spondylocostal dysplasia is inherited in an autosomal recessive manner and is caused by a change (mutation) in one of four genes, *DLL3, MESP2, LFNG, and HES7.* Rarely, spondylocostal dysplasia can be inherited in an autosomal dominant manner. One gene, *TBX6,* is known to cause autosomal dominant spondylocostal dysplasia.

There are numerous disorders that have malformations of the spine and ribs, which are similar to those seen in spondylocostal dysplasia. A partial list of these disorders includes Alagille syndrome, camptomelic dysplasia, oculo-auriculo-vertebral spectrum, Klippel–Feil syndrome, Robinow syndrome,

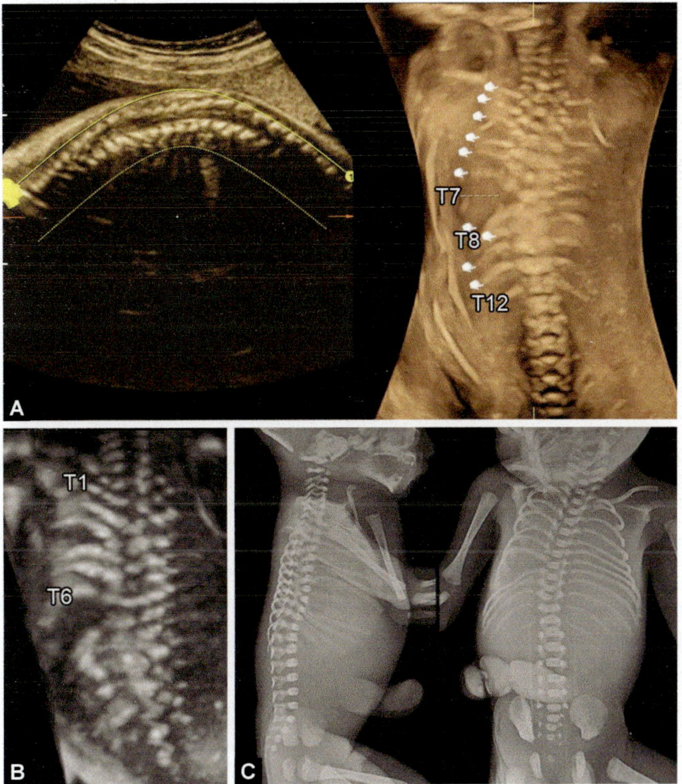

Figs. 9A to C: Jarco-Levin syndrome: (A and B) 3D rendered image of spine shows absent 7th rib with abnormal curvature of spine; (C) Postabortal X-ray showing absent 7th rib and abnormal curvature of spine, thereby confirming the antenatal findings.

multiple pterygium syndrome, sirenomelia, and VACTERL syndrome. Casamassima-Morton-Nance syndrome is characterized by the spinal and rib malformations of spondylocostal dysplasia combined with urogenital abnormalities. Urogenital refers to both the urinary and genital organs.

CHONDROECTODERMAL DYSPLASIA

It affects the cartilaginous layer between diaphysis and epiphysis and dysplasia of ectodermal tissues (nails and teeth). But these cannot be identified on antenatal ultrasound. It is rare abnormality (1 in 60,000 live births) due to mutation in chromosome 4p16. It has 50% infant mortality. It has an autosomal recessive inheritance and therefore 25% recurrence risk after an affected pregnancy.

Ultrasound shows acromesomelia, short ribs and moderate thoracic hypoplasia, postaxial polydactyly (always in hand and at times in feet). Congenital cardiac anomaly may be associated, but the most common is arterial septal defect, which may be difficult to diagnose antenatally.

Tips to Differential Diagnosis

- Asphyxiating thoracic dystrophy (Jeune's syndrome) has significantly more thoracic hypoplasia, and there is no polydactyly or micromelia.
- Short-rib polydactyly syndrome also has more severe thoracic hypoplasia.

HYPOPHOSPHATASIA

This also is a rare disorder and detected antenatally only if severe. It occurs because of defect in serum and tissue alkaline phosphatase. The genetic basis is defect of tissue nonspecific alkaline phosphatase gene mapping on 1p36.1-p34 chromosome. Malfunction of the bone isoform correlated with the severity of phenotypic expression.

Severe micromelia, severe thoracic hypoplasia, diffuse mineralization (except clavicles), hydrops, and subcutaneous edema are the diagnostic features on ultrasound.

Differential diagnosis from most other skeletal dysplasias is difficult.

SHORT RIB POLYDACTYLY SYNDROME

This is a skeletal dysplasia with autosomal recessive inheritance and 25% recurrence risk and is invariably lethal. This syndrome also has four subtypes: (1) Saldino-Noonan type; (2) Majewski type; (3) Verma-Naumoff type; (4) Beemer-Langer type. These are all characterized by micromelia, thoracic hypoplasia, and postaxial polydactyly.

There may be associated cleft lip (in type 2 and 4), congenital heart disease (transposition of great arteries), renal dysplasia (polycystic kidneys), and anophthalmia. These are the diagnostic features on ultrasound also. It is always lethal.

Tips to differential diagnosis:

- Achondrogenesis
- Thanatophoric dysplasia
- Hypophosphatasia
- Osteogenenesis imperfecta type 2
- Postaxial polydactyly present and hypomineralization is almost always absent in post rib polydactyly syndrome
- Chondroectodermal dysplasia has similar features but much less severe.

Figures 10A to F show ultrasound and post-abortal images of a case of short rib polydactyly syndrome.

REDUCTION DEFECTS

It is a heterogeneous group of anomalies. There may be absence of any portion of the limb. According to EUROCAT definition, an intercalary reduction defect is represented by usually severe underdevelopment of one mesomelic bone segment only, whereas terminal transverse reduction defect is complete absence of terminal part of one limb (upper/lower). Transverse defects are congenital or acquired in utero.

These may be:

- Terminal defects
- Phocomelias
- Proximal focal femoral deficiency
- Split hand/split foot syndromes

In at least half of the cases, there are isolated defects affecting only one limb and in another 25%, there may be more than one limb affected, but in the rest there are other structural defects also and may also show features of genetic syndrome. The outcome depends on the amount of compromise and the postnatal surgical outcome.

Figures 11A to C show ultrasound and post-abortal images of a case of limb reduction defects.

PROXIMAL FEMORAL FOCAL DEFICIENCY (FIGS. 12A TO D)

Congenital short femur refers to a group of disorders encompassing a wide range of congenital developmental anomalies of the femur. Femoral focal deficiency syndrome is considered a sporadic condition, but a familial form has been described. Except in bilateral proximal focal deficiency, the diagnosis is usually suspected when there is unilateral short femur, in the absence of other anomalies.

If the defect is unilateral, it may correspond to the femur–fibula–ulna or femur–tibia–radius complex. These two syndromes have different implications for genetic counseling: the former is nonfamilial, whereas the second has a strong genetic component.

Five groups:

1. Simple hypoplasia of the femur
2. Short femur with angulated shaft

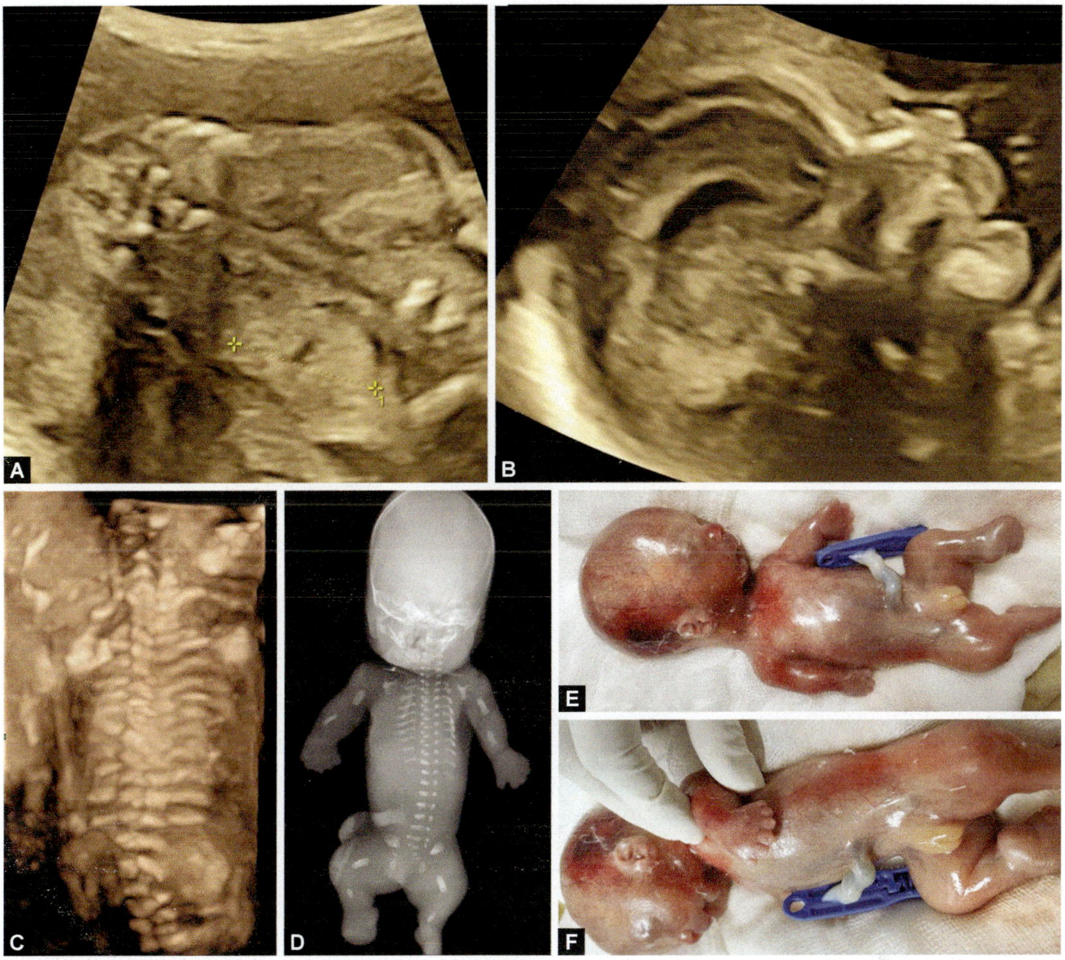

Figs. 10A to F: Short rib polydactyly syndrome: (A) Narrow bell shaped thorax with short ribs; (B) Thickened upper lip; (C) 3D rendered image showing normal mineralization of spine with short ribs; (D) Postabortal X-ray showing short ribs, normal skeletal mineralization, and short long bones; (E) Postabortal image showing short limbs and micrognathia; (F) Postabortal image showing postaxial polydactyly.

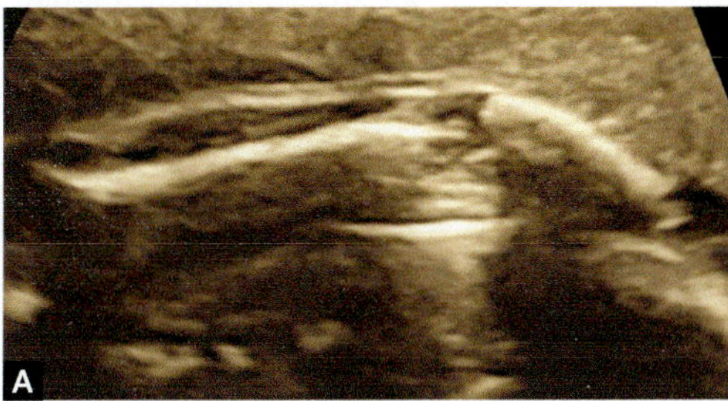

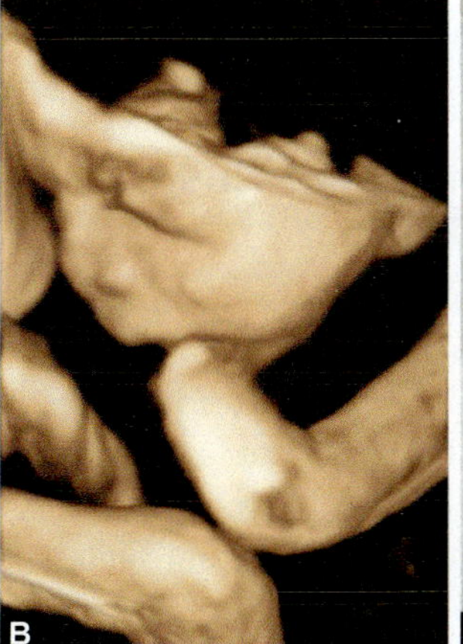

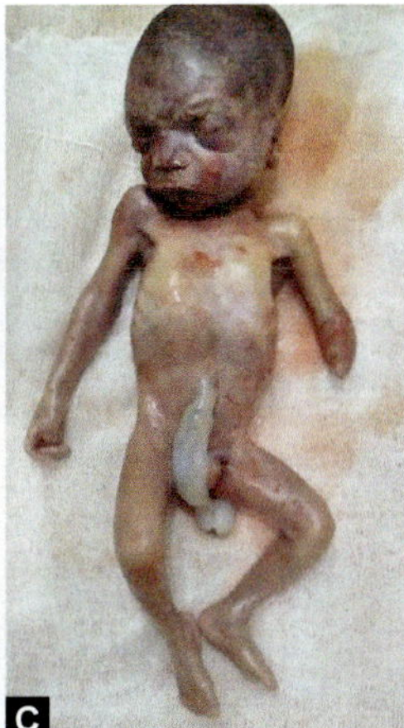

Figs. 11A to C: Transverse limb reduction defect: (A) 2D image of left hand showing short forearm bones with abrupt end and absence of hand; (B) 3D rendered image confirming the 2D findings; (C) Postabortal image showing transverse limb reduction defect of left hand.

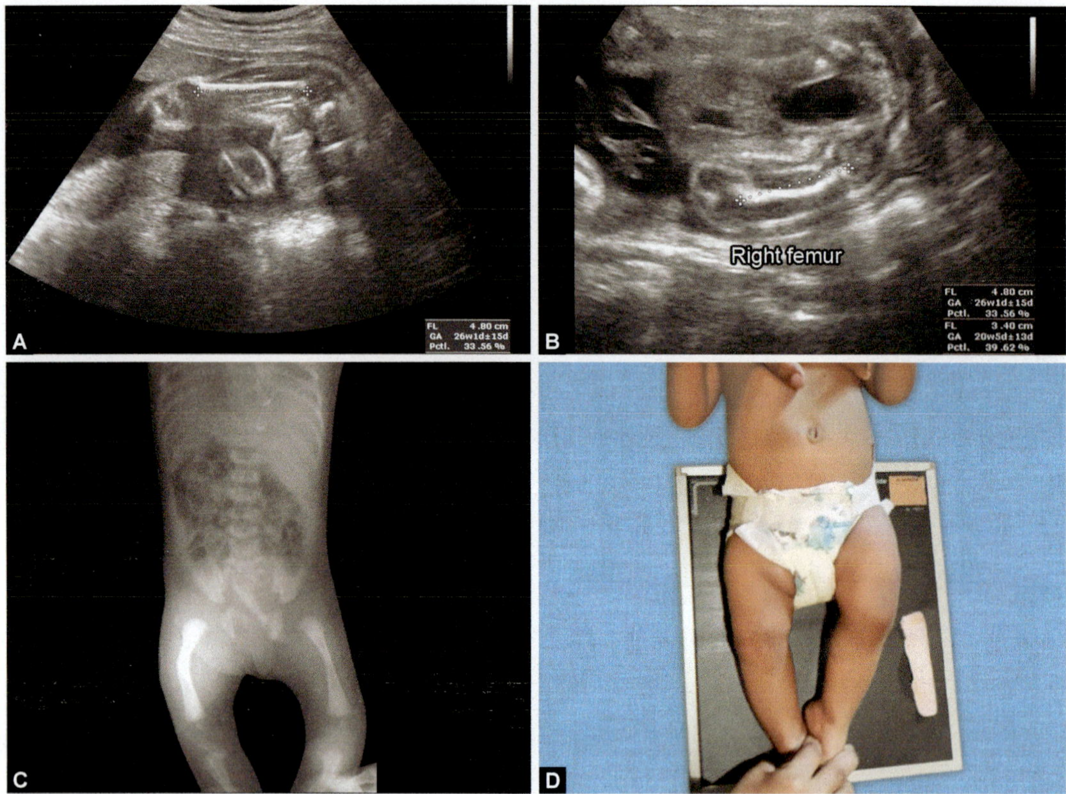

Figs. 12A to D: Focal femoral hypoplasia: (A) Normal femur of right leg; (B) Short and curved femur of left leg; (C) Postnatal X-ray showing curved and short femur of left leg; (D) Postnatal image confirming the antenatal findings.

3. Short femur with coxa vara (most common)
4. Absent or defective proximal femur
5. Absent or rudimentary femur

One or both femora can be affected, although the right femur is more frequently involved. Anomalies of the upper limbs can also be present and do not exclude the diagnosis.

FEMORAL HYPOPLASIA-UNUSUAL FACIES SYNDROME

The definition of femoral hypoplasia-unusual facies syndrome is based upon two major signs: (1) focal femoral hypoplasia and (2) the characteristic unusual face, characterized by a small nose, possible cleft lip and palate, and micrognathia. It is also called femoral-facial syndrome. Incidence: Extremely rare.

Etiology: Unknown. The syndrome is often associated with maternal insulin-dependent diabetes mellitus.

Ultrasound diagnosis: Focal femoral hypoplasia, uni- or bilateral, possibly associated with fibular hypoplasia; micrognathia; cleft lip and palate; and mandibular asymmetry.

Outcome: Normal survival and intelligence. Motor disabilities due to the femoral hypoplasia.

Recurrence risk: Sporadic.

SPLIT HAND AND SPLIT FOOT MALFORMATION (ECTRODACTYLY)

Ectrodactyly is an autosomal dominant ectodermal dysplasia presenting as bilateral congenital malformed hands and feet. It affects about 1 in 90,000 births with males and females are equally likely to be affected.

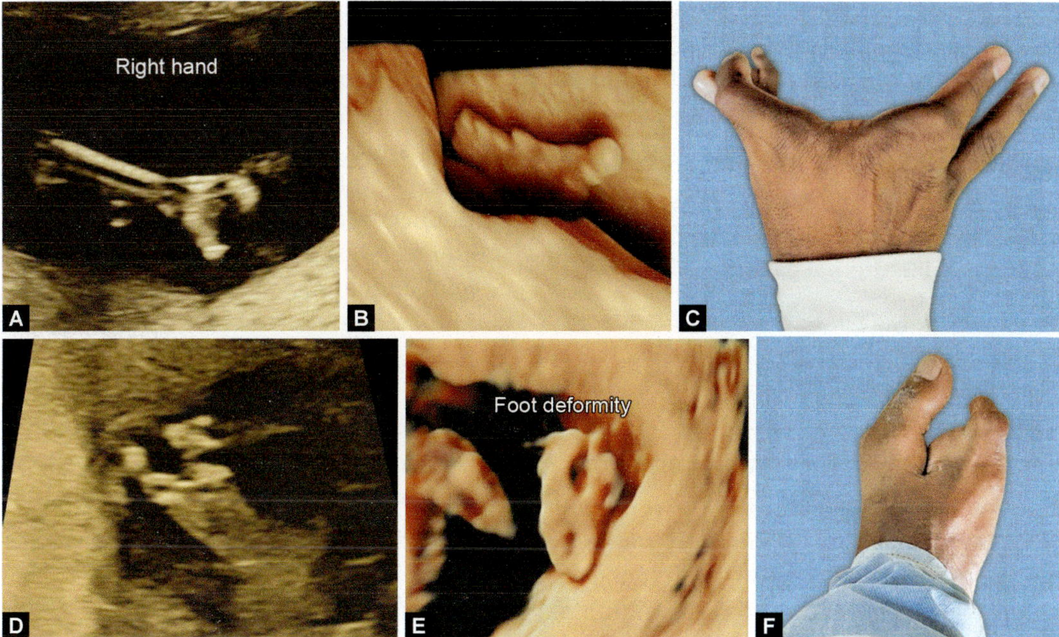

Figs. 13A to F: Ectrodactyly: (A and B) Right hand deformity showing ectrodactyly; (C) Right hand of parent (father) showing the same defect; (D and E) Showing ectrodactyly in foot; (F) Same defect is seen in father.

Ectrodactyly, also known as split hand/foot malformation, is a rare developmental abnormality of the limbs that consists of absent central digits, a deep median cleft, and fusion of the remaining lateral digits, ultimately producing claw-like extremities. The EEC syndrome is a genetic anomaly characterized by the triad: ectodermal dysplasia (development of anomalies of the structures derived from the embryonic ectodermal layer), ectrodactyly (extremities, hands, and feet malformations) and cleft lip and/or palate; these malformations can be seen together or in isolation.

The prenatal diagnosis is usually confirmed by two-dimensional ultrasonography (2DUS), that demonstrates the classic extremity malformations, such as the lobster-claw hands and face (cleft lip and/or palate), frequently associated with urinary tract malformations.

The EEC syndrome should be differentiated from the other syndromes that have ectodermal dysplasia and facial clefts such as: Rapp-Hodgkin syndrome, the Hay-Wells syndrome, ankyloblepharon ectodermal and harelip facial cleft; the split-hand and foot malformation syndrome, syndactyly—median clefts of hands and feet—and aplasia/hypoplasia of the phalanges, metacarpals, and metatarsals.

The EEC syndrome has been linked to two genetic locations. The form of EEC syndrome designated EEC1 has been linked to chromosome 7q11.2-q21.3. The second and most common form of this disorder, designated EEC3, is caused by a mutation in the TP63 gene. EEC2 does not exist. The precise prenatal diagnosis is possible by DNA extraction by chorionic villus sample done between the 11th and 14th week of pregnancy.

Figures 13A to F show the ultrasound images of a fetus with ectrodactyly and similar deformity in parent (father).

Associated Abnormalities

Chromosomal abnormalities: found in trisomy 18. High incidence of genetic syndromes. The most common are:

Roberts syndrome: Autosomal recessive; ectrodactyly, phocomelia, facial cleft.

Ectrodactyly-ectodermal dysplasia (EEC): Autosomal dominant; deformities of all four extremities but more severe in the hands, and ectodermal defects (dry skin, sparse hair, dental defects, and defects of the tear ducts).

Nager syndrome: Autosomal dominant but in most cases de novo mutations; ectrodactyly, micrognathia, external ear anomalies.

Split hand and foot malformation: Ectrodactyly presenting as "lobster claw" anomaly.

ABNORMALITIES OF JOINTS

Fetal Akinesia Deformation Sequence

The fetal akinesia deformation sequence (FADS) includes a large group of syndromic conditions characterized by fixed joint contractures, e.g., arthrogryposis multiplex congenital and Pena Shokeir syndrome, Neu-Laxova syndrome, multiple pterygium syndrome, etc. The basic defect in FADS is the presence of severe and progressive contractures virtually involving all muscles. The FADS refers to a clinically and genetically heterogeneous constellation of features including fetal akinesia, intrauterine growth retardation, arthrogryposis, and developmental anomalies, including lung hypoplasia, cleft palate, and cryptorchidism.

Sonographically: The lower limbs are in fixed extension and crossed, since the quadriceps (extensors) are more powerful than the femoral biceps (flexors). There is often bilateral talipes. On the contrary the upper limbs show flexion deformities and appear adducted on the thorax, because of the prevalence of the flexors (biceps) over extensors (triceps). The hands often show ulnar deviation, and clenched and overlapping fingers.

Possible causes for decreased fetal movement which may contribute to the features of FADS may include:

- Neurologic abnormalities such as cerebral and cerebellar dysgenesis (abnormal development); spinal tract, myelin, and end plate disturbances; and ischemia (deficient blood supply) with secondary loss of neuron function.
- Myopathic (muscle-related) abnormalities such as dystrophies and dysplasias.
- Connective tissue abnormalities including chondrodysplasias, restrictive skin, and joint limitation or laxity.
- Fetal edema for a variety of reasons (storage, metabolic, heart failure, lymphatic dysplasia, etc.).
- Maternal illness, drugs, and antibodies (including maternal myasthenia gravis).
- Ischemic changes during embryonic/fetal development, which may be due to developmental vascular abnormalities, trauma, hypotension, drugs, infections, and maternal illness or thrombophilia.

Figures 14A and B show ultrasound and post-abortal images of a case of fetal akinesia deformation sequence.

Inheritance: FADS may be inherited in an autosomal recessive manner in some cases and may sometimes be caused by mutations in the *RAPSN* or *DOK7* genes.

SACRAL DYSGENESIS/CAUDAL REGRESSION SYNDROME

Caudal regression syndrome (CRS) is a rare complex congenital anomaly which is characterized by agenesis of the sacral and lumbar spine. Pelvis, lower extremity, genitourinary, cardiac anomalies, and lower extremity neurological and motor development deficits may be accompanied. The exact etiology is unclear but the maternal insulin-dependent diabetes mellitus (hyperglycemia during embryogenesis seems to act as a teratogen), genetic factors, vascular hypoperfusion may play a role in the etiology.

Sacral agenesis is a less severe variant of CRS and in the presence of normal amniotic fluid, the diagnosis can be made by demonstrating

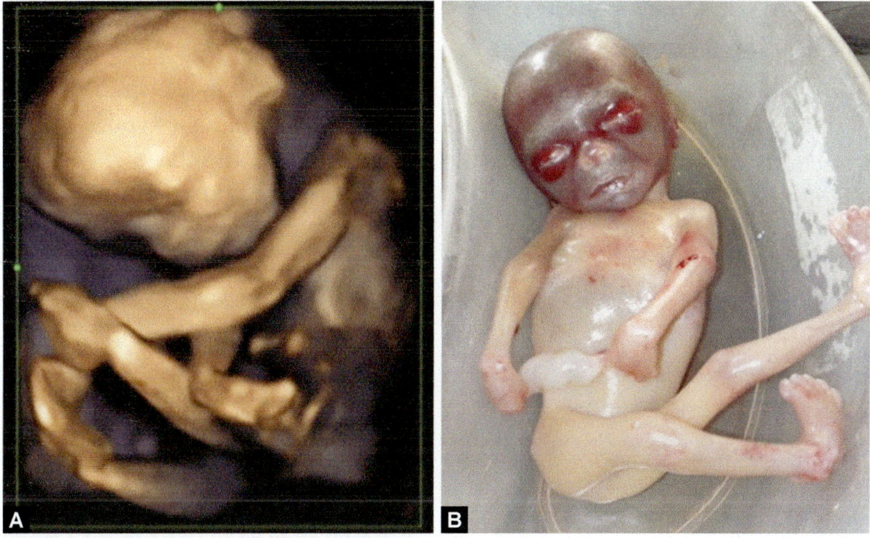

Figs. 14A and B: Fetal akinesia deformation sequence (FADS): (A) 3D rendered image showing abnormal position of upper and lower limbs, wrists are persistently flexed and foot shows talipes; (B) Postabortal image confirming the antenatal findings.

the termination of lumbar spine and small and abnormal lower extremities.

Fetal MRI makes it possible to confirm the diagnosis and to determine the level of the terminal medullary cone, which will be a major prognostic factor. The spinal cord is usually dysplastic and the terminal cone is too high.

The abnormal development of the caudal region of the spine can cause additional abnormalities affecting the spinal cord and lower limbs. In some patients, disruption or damage to the lower portion of the spinal cord may occur causing a variety of neurological abnormalities including defective bladder and bowel control, increased urinary frequency, and failure of the bladder to empty completely (neurogenic bladder). Damage to the nerves can also cause abnormalities of the lower limbs. Such abnormalities may include flexion contractures of the knee and hip.

Infants with CRS may have a wide variety of additional physical findings including kidney abnormalities, abnormalities of the upper vertebrae, facial anomalies, such as cleft lip, cleft palate, and anal atresia or imperforate anus.

Figures 15A to C show the ultrasound images of a case of caudal regression syndrome.

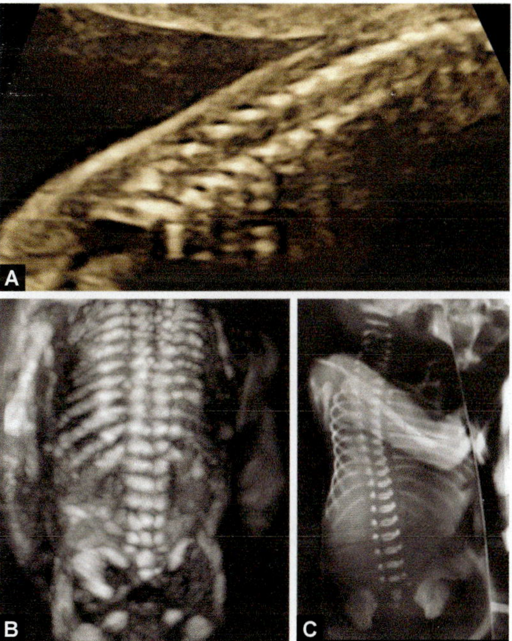

Figs. 15A to C: Caudal regression syndrome (sacral agenesis): (A) Absence of sacral tapering; (B) 3D rendered image showing no vertebrae after iliac bones s/o sacral agenesis; (C) Postnatal X-ray confirms the antenatal findings.

SKELETAL DYSPLASIAS (SHORTCUT TO DIAGNOSIS)

Due to some overlapping features in different skeletal dysplasias, it is often confusing and difficult to reach a definitive diagnosis. This can be simplified if we consider certain distinct features as landmarks and then considering the differential diagnosis.

Severe Micromelia

- *Thanatophoric dysplasia type 2*: Thoracic hypoplasia +/- cloverleaf skull
- *Osteogenesis imperfecta type 2*: Ubiquitous fractures + hypomineralization
- *Achondrogenesis*: Thoracic hypoplasia +/- hypomineralization
- *Hypophosphatasia*: Severe ubiquitous hypomineralization except clavicle
- *Short-rib polydactyly syndrome*: Thoracic hypoplasia +/- hypomineralization + congenital heart disease + polydactyly.

Rhizomelia

- *Achondroplasia*: Frontal bossing +/- mild macrocrania
- *Asphyxiating thoracic dystrophy (Jeune's syndrome)*: Thoracic hypoplasia +/- polydactyly +/- renal anomalies
- *Diastrophic dysplasia*: Postural deformities + Hitchhiker's thumb + micrognathia.

Thoracic Hypoplasia

- Thanatophoric dysplasia Type 2
- Asphyxiating thoracic dystrophy (Jeune's syndrome)
- Achondrogenesis
- Hypophosphatasia
- Short-rib polydactyl syndrome.

Hypomineralization

- Osteogenesis imperfecta type 2
- Hypophosphatasia
- Achondrogenesis
- Short-rib polydactyly syndrome.

Micrognathia

- Achondrogenesis
- *Campomelic dysplasia*: Bowed tibia and femur + clubfoot + hypoplastic scapula
- Diastrophic dysplasia
- *Fetal akinesia deformation sequence*: Arthrogryposis + clubfoot +/- hydrops
- *Cerebro-oculo-facio-skeletal syndrome*: Arthrogryposis (lower limbs) + microphthalmia
- *Femoral hypoplasia-abnormal facies syndrome*: Focal femoral hypoplasia + clubfoot.

DIFFERENTIAL DIAGNOSIS: ABNORMALITIES OF EXTREMITIES

Polydactyly

- Short-rib polydactyly syndrome
- Trisomy 13
- Asphyxiating thoracic dysplasia
- *Meckel–Gruber syndrome*: Polycystic kidney + cephalocele
- Chondroectodermal dysplasia (Ellis-van Creveld syndrome): Congenital heart disease + acromesomelia.

Ectrodactyly

- *Robert's syndrome*: Phocomelia + cleft lip/palate
- *Trisomy 18*: Radial aplasia + micrognathia + multiple anomalies
- *Ectrodactyly + ectodermal dysplasia (EEC)*: Cleft lip/palate or malar hypoplasia
- *Nager syndrome*: Micrognathia + external ear abnormality
- Split hand-split foot syndrome.

DIFFERENTIAL DIAGNOSIS OF JOINT ABNORMALITIES

Arthrogryposis

- Cerebro-occulo-facial skeletal syndrome
- *Trisomy 18*: Arthrogryposis (lower limbs) + congenital heart disease + exomphalos + cleft lip/palate + holoprosencephaly, etc.

- *Neu-Laxova syndrome*: Upper and lower limbs both involved + microcephaly + agnesis of corpus callosum + cerebellar hypoplasia + cataract + syndactyly
- *The fetal akinesia deformation sequence*: Upper and lower limbs both involved + micrognathia + hydrops
- *Multiple pterygium syndrome*: Upper and lower limbs both involved + clubfoot + micrognathia + hydrops + pterygia

Clubfoot

- *Lower spine neural tube defects*: Neural tube defects
- Campomelic dysplasia
- *Femoral hypoplasia-abnormal facies syndrome*: Focal femoral hypoplasia + micrognathia
- Multiple pterygium syndrome
- The fetal akinesia deformation sequence.

These anomalies are present with involvement of different parts of fetal body and therefore for the simultaneous demonstration of all 3D ultrasound may be a more effective imaging tool. 3D ultrasound is also a preferred imaging modality for the assessment of the cranial sutures and also for the assessment of the joint contractures and anomalies. Even for assessment of shortened limbs or limb parts is more evidently demonstrated by 3D ultrasound in relation to other body parts.

BIBLIOGRAPHY

1. Baker ER, Goldberg MJ. Diagnosis and management of skeletal dysplasias. Semin Perinatol. 1994;18(4):283-91.
2. Cassart M. Suspected fetal skeletal malformations or bone diseases: How to explore. Pediatr Radiol. 2010;40(6):1046-51.
3. Dighe M, Fligner C, Cheng E, Warren B, Dubinsky T. Fetal skeletal dysplasia: An approach to diagnosis with illustrative cases.
4. Dighe M, Fligner C, Cheng E, Warren B, Dubinsky T. Radiographics. 2008;28(4):1061-77.
5. Gaffney G, Manning N, Boyd PA, Rai V, Gould S, Chamberlain P. Prenatal sonographic diagnosis of skeletal dysplasias—a report of the diagnostic and prognostic accuracy in 35 cases. Prenat Diagn.1998;18(4):357-62.
6. Glanc P, Chitayat D. Approach to prenatal diagnosis of the lethal skeletal dysplasias. [Online] Available from www. https://www.uptodate.com/contents/approach-to-prenatal-diagnosis-of-the-lethal-skeletal-dysplasias.com [Last accessed Sep., 2021]
7. Krakow D, Lachman RS, Rimoin DL. Guidelines for the prenatal diagnosis of fetal skeletal dysplasias. Genet Med. 2009;11(2):127-33.
8. Milks KS, Hill LM, Hosseinzadeh K. Evaluating skeletal dysplasias on prenatal ultrasound: An emphasis on predicting lethality. Pediatr Radiol. 2017;47(2):134-45.
9. Nelson DB, Dashe JS, McIntire DD, Twickler DM. Fetal skeletal dysplasias: Sonographic indices associated with adverse outcomes. J Ultrasound Med. 2014;33:1085.
10. OMIM (Online Mendelian Inheritance in Man). [Online] Available from www. https://www.ncbi.nlm.nih.gov/omim.com [Last accessed Sep., 2021].
11. Schramm T, Gloning KP, Minderer S, Daumer-Haas C, Hörtnagel K, Nerlich A, et al. Prenatal sonographic diagnosis of skeletal dysplasias. Ultrasound Obstet Gynecol. 2009;34(2):160-70.
12. Stembalska A, Dudarewicz L, Śmigiel R. Lethal and life-limiting skeletal dysplasias: Selected prenatal issues. Adv Clin Exp Med. 2021;30(6):641-7.
13. Victoria T, Zhu X, Lachman R, Epelman M. Oliver ER, Adzick NS, Biko DM. What is new in prenatal skeletal dysplasias? AJR Am J Roentgenol. 2018;210(5):1022-33.
14. Witters I, Moerman Ph, Fryns JP. Skeletal dysplasias: 38 prenatal cases. Genet Couns. 2008;19(3):267-75.
15. Yeh P, Saeed F, Paramasivam G, Wyatt-Ashmead J, Kumar S. Accuracy of prenatal diagnosis and prediction of lethality for fetal skeletal dysplasias. Prenat Diagn. 2011;31:515-8.

16

CHAPTER

Fetal Hydrops

KV Sridevi

INTRODUCTION

Fetal hydrops is defined as excessive fluid present in two of the body cavities (i.e., pleural, pericardial, and peritoneal) or in one of the body cavities, in the presence of skin and subcutaneous thickening, due to edema (fluid collection).[1]

Hydrops fetalis is thus a descriptive term used for abnormal fluid collection in different body cavities and compartments. Hydrops can be because of severe causes but these are chiefly divided as hydrops due to immune causes and hydrops due to nonimmune causes.

IMMUNE HYDROPS

Maternal Rh alloimmunization occurs when a pregnant woman develops an immunological response to a paternally derived red blood cell antigen (D) that is foreign to the mother and is inherited by the fetus from the father.

PATHOPHYSIOLOGY

The incidence of RhD negative blood group varies worldwide. Approximately 5% of Indian population is RhD negative.[2] The RhD polypeptide is an integral membrane protein expressed exclusively on erythrocytes.[3] Individuals with Rh factor are "Rh positive"; others who lack it are "Rh negative". Rh factor is inherited and the Rh gene is located on the short arm of chromosome 1. Only two genes are identified, an *RhD* gene and an Rh CE.[3] The D antigen is the most potent among the Rh antigens and is clinically the most important. Individuals who are homozygous dominant (DD) or heterozygous (Dd) are "Rh positive". Those who are homozygous recessive (dd) are "Rh negative" (i.e., they do not have the D Rh antigen).

A heterozygous father has 50% chance of passing one Rh negative gene to the offspring, in such a case the child of an Rh negative mother has 50% chance of being Rh negative and therefore being unaffected by any immune response (**Figs. 1A and B**).

Paternal and fetal genotyping is performed when anti-D antibodies are detected in the maternal circulation. Fetal genotype can be determined by using (1) cell-free fetal DNA from maternal blood,[4] (2) amniocentesis, or (3) fetal blood sampling.

ISOIMMUNIZATION

Isoimmunization has been defined as the process in which antibodies are produced in an individual in response to the injection of antigen (that is foreign to the recipient) from another individual of the same species.[5] Because this antigen belongs to the same

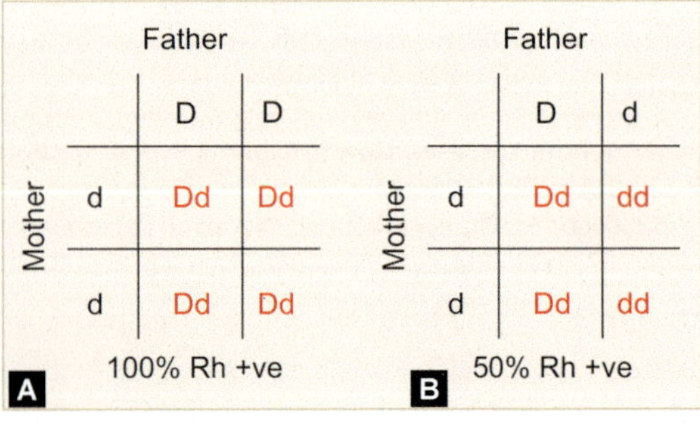

Figs. 1A and B: (A) 100% Rh +ve; (B) 50% Rh +ve genotype. Diagrammatic explanation of Rh inheritance.

species it is called "iso"-immunization. There are two possible methods by which isoimmunization can occur; the first one is by transfusion of blood that has nonmatching antigens. The second is when an Rh-negative mother is carrying Rh-positive fetus.

When the blood of an Rh-negative mother comes in contact with blood from an Rh-positive fetus, the Rh-negative mother produces antibodies against the Rh factor. A person with RhD negative blood group who makes anti-RhD antibodies is called *"Rh sensitized"*.

During pregnancy small volumes of fetal red cells continually get into the maternal circulation. This trafficking of fetal red cells increases as gestation progresses. Bowman et al. showed at least 0.01 mL of fetal cells in 3%, 12%, and 14% of women in each trimester.[6] This load of RhD antigen on fetal erythrocytes does not stimulate the mothers immune system because fetal red cells are rapidly cleared by reticuloendothelial system. However, in certain sensitizing events, such as bleeding during pregnancy or interventions, when a large volume of fetal blood enters the maternal circulation, her immune system is stimulated and anti-D antibodies are produced leading to Rh isoimmunization.[7]

The initial immunoglobulin M (IgM) anti-D immunoglobulin response is short lived with a rapid switch over to immunoglobulin G (IgG) production. Unlike IgM, IgG antibodies cross the placenta and destroy fetal erythrocytes. This represents the basic pathogenetic mechanism responsible for Rh hemolytic disease of fetus and newborn. In the fetus in response to immunological fetal red cell destruction, extramedullary erythropoiesis takes place in the liver leading to hepatic dysfunction, portal and umbilical venous hypertension resulting in ascites and placental edema. Amino acid synthesis and transfer are impaired due to liver dysfunction and placental edema that leads to generalized edema and anasarca.

Many different antibodies (anti-D, anti-Kell, anti-C, anti-E, etc.) can cause hemolytic disease of the fetus/neonate; this chapter covers the management of pregnancies affected with RhD alloimmunization. The principles of management are similar regardless of the type of antibody involved, although care needs to be taken with pregnancies complicated by Kell alloimmunization, where antibody concentration does not always correlate with the severity of the disease.[8,9]

MANAGEMENT OF THE FIRST ALLOIMMUNIZED PREGNANCY

A woman's first pregnancy complicated by RhD alloimmunization shows low anti-D titers at the beginning of the pregnancy. Severe fetal anemia may not develop or develop in the late second trimester or the third trimester. In subsequent affected pregnancies, fetal anemia usually is more severe and develops earlier in gestation.

Finding out which fetus is at risk is the first step. An RhD negative fetus is not risk for complications from RhD alloimmunization. Therefore, when a pregnant woman is found to be RhD negative, it is important to know the Rh status of the partner. If he is RhD negative, no further investigations are required. If the partner is RhD positive, then his genotype needs to be assessed, the maternal serum should be tested for presence of anti-RhD antibodies and the level (titer) should be determined. The presence of red-cell antibodies in the mother signifies that alloimmunization has occurred as a result of a previous pregnancy or a previous blood transfusion (**Flowchart 1**). Maternal cell-free fetal DNA testing—noninvasive assessment of fetal RhD using cell-free DNA can be used to know the fetal status.

Estimation of maternal anti-D antibody titers is done by indirect Coombs test (ICT).

A "critical titer" is one at which there is a significant risk of fetal hydrops, typically between 1:8 and 1:32 dilutions which vary

Flowchart 1: Algorithm for the management of red-cell alloimmunization.[10]

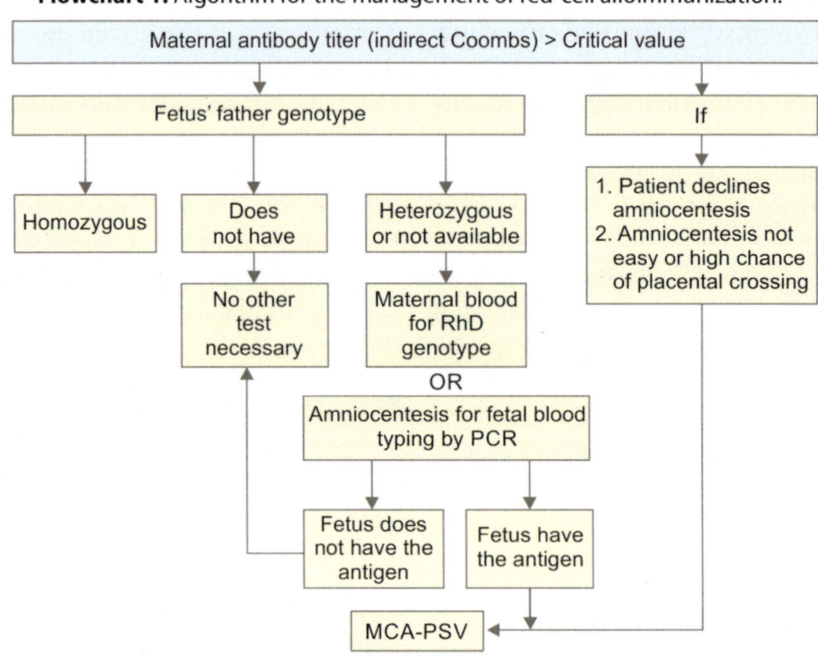

(MCA-PSV: middle cerebral artery peak systolic velocity; PCR: polymerase chain reaction; RhD: rhesus D)

in different laboratories (as it is a semi-quantitative visual test). Maternal antibody titers are screening tests and do not accurately predict the severity of fetal anemia. These have value only till a critical titer is reached. Beyond that serial middle cerebral artery peak systolic velocity is assessed to estimate the severity of fetal anemia.

Anti-D levels if not detected at the initial visit a repeat assessment should be done at 28 weeks.[11,12] Once detected, anti-D levels should be measured every 4 weeks up to 28 weeks of gestation and then every 2 weeks then until delivery.[8,11]

Once there are rising antibody titers, or if the titers are above a specific threshold, or if ultrasound features suggestive of critical fetal anemia, the fetuses are opted for definitive treatment and specialized care. Traditional technique of serial amniocentesis for delta OD 450 has now been superseded by Doppler velocimetry of middle cerebral artery peak systolic velocity (MCA-PSV). A fall in the fetal hemoglobin leads to increased cardiac output and decreased blood viscosity. As a consequence, MCA-PSV increases as the fetal hemoglobin falls. In the year 2009, systematic reviews and many studies showed that Doppler of MCA-PSV performs well as a screening tool for severe fetal anemia of any etiology and sensitivity and specificity reached 75.5 and 90.8%. Sensitivity of increased MCA-PSV (above 1.5 MoMs) for the prediction of moderate to severe anemia was 100%, either in presence or absence of hydrops, with a false positive rate of 12%, positive predictive value of 53% and negative predictive value of 98% (**Table 1**).[8,13-15]

Steps for correct measurement of MCA-PSV:[15]

- Axial section of the head is obtained at the sphenoid bones.
- Color Doppler identifies the circle of Willis.
- Color box is placed around the MCA.
- The MCA is zoomed.
- Middle cerebral artery flow velocity waveforms are displayed and the highest point of the waveform (PSV) is measured.

TABLE 1: Reference range of fetal middle cerebral artery peak systolic velocity (MCA-PSV) median and 1.5 multiples of the median (MoM) values during pregnancy.[13]

GA (weeks)	MCA-PSV (cm/s)	
	Median	1.5 MoM
14	19.3	28.9
15	20.2	30.3
16	21.1	31.7
17	22.1	33.2
18	23.2	34.8
19	24.3	36.5
20	25.5	38.2
21	26.7	40.0
22	27.9	41.9
23	29.3	43.9
24	30.7	46.0
25	32.1	48.2
26	33.6	50.4
27	35.2	52.8
28	36.9	55.4
29	38.7	58.0
30	40.5	60.7
31	42.4	63.6
32	44.4	66.6
33	46.5	69.8
34	48.7	73.1
35	51.1	76.6
36	53.5	80.2
37	56.0	84.0
38	58.7	88.0
39	61.5	92.2
40	64.4	96.6

(GA: gestational age)

The waveforms should be all similar. The above sequence is repeated at least three times in each fetus.

Middle cerebral artery peak systolic velocity should be sampled at its proximal point, soon after its origin from the internal carotid artery, avoiding the need for angle correction, because measurement at this point is associated with lowest intra- or interobserver variability. Sample volume should be placed at the center of the vessel.

Why MCA and not any other vessel?

Middle cerebral artery supplies more than half of the cerebrum and so is most representative of the cerebral circulation. Moreover, studying the MCA-PSV is that it is easy to obtain an angle of 0° between the ultrasound beam and the direction of blood flow (**Figs. 2 and 3**).[16]

The MCA-PSV is found to have a good correlation with fetal anemia. MCA-PSV diagnoses fetal anemia, even in cases of Kell sensitization in which the problem is not hemolysis but the suppression of erythroid precursor cells in the bone marrow.[17]

Middle Cerebral Artery Peak Systolic Velocity-based Management

Middle cerebral artery peak systolic velocity is measured at 1–2 weeks intervals, once the diagnosis of fetal anemia is confirmed. The frequency is increased if indicated by (MoM) approaching 1.5. MCA-PSV ≤ 1.5 MoM for gestational age is consistent with absence of moderate to severe anemia. If MCA-PSV remains at this level, delivery at 37–38 weeks should be planned (**Fig. 4**).[18]

MCA-PSV > 1.5 MoM for the gestational age, fetal blood by cordocentesis is taken for assessing the hemoglobin levels and intrauterine fetal transfusion is recommended if fetal hemoglobin is two standard deviation below the mean (**Flowchart 2**).[8]

Intrauterine transfusion is generally limited to pregnancies 18–35 weeks, after 35 weeks intrauterine transfusion is considered more risky than delivery followed by postnatal transfusion. At a gestational age of >35 weeks with MCA-PSV > 1.5 MoM, delivery of the fetus should be planned.

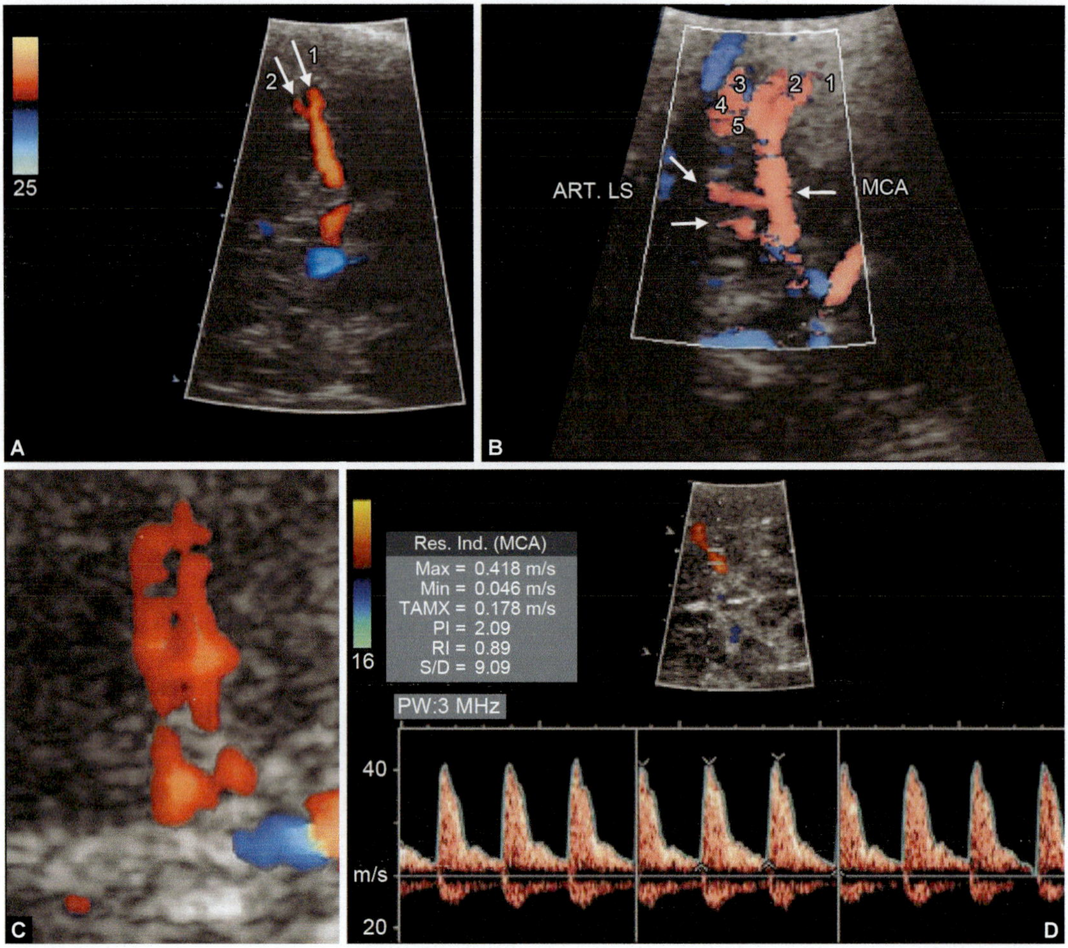

Figs. 2A to D: Color Doppler ultrasound image showing the middle cerebral artery (MCA). (A) The main trunk divides into two terminal branches (indicated by arrows 1 and 2); (B) It divides into five terminal branches (1 to 5); (C) double MCA (normal variant); (D) Color Doppler of the MCA (top); flow velocity waveforms of the MCA (above the baseline) and lenticulostriates arteries (ART-LS) (below the baseline).

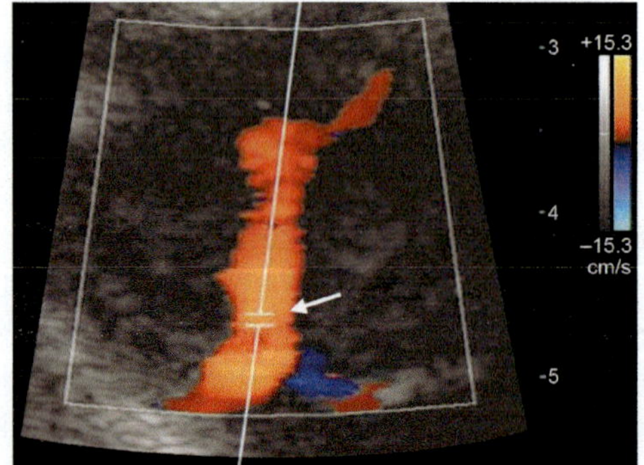

Fig. 3: Color Doppler ultrasound image showing the middle cerebral artery. The sample volume (arrow) is placed in the center of the vessel after its origin from the internal carotid artery.

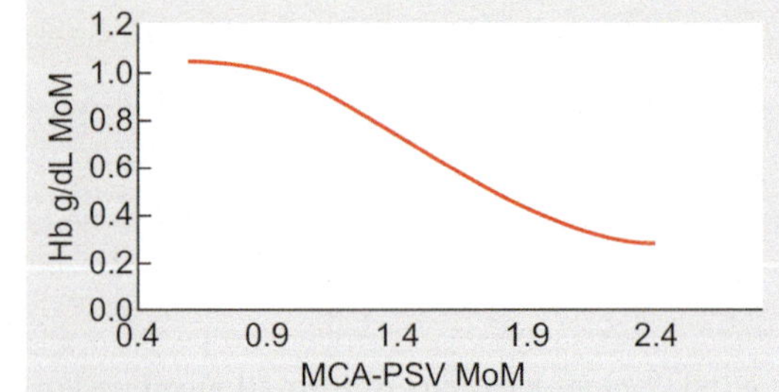

Fig. 4: Cubic function describing the relationship between middle cerebral artery peak systolic velocity (MCA-PSV) and fetal hemoglobin (Hb). The values are expressed as multiples of the median (MoM). y = 0.6835 + MCA-PSV MoM × 1.2794 – 1.2885 MCA-PSV2 + 0.2861 × MCA-PSV.[18]

Flowchart 2: Middle cerebral artery peak systolic velocity (MCA-PSV)—safely used for timing cordocentesis and fetal transfusion if indicated.

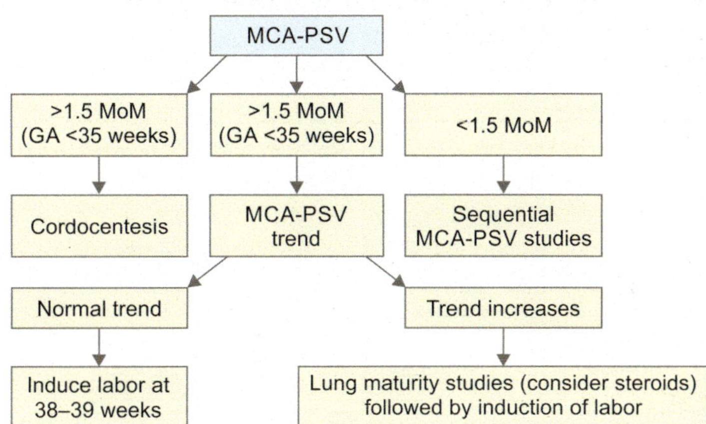

(GA: gestational age; MoM: multiples of the median)

MANAGEMENT OF WOMEN WITH ALLOIMMUNIZATION IN SUBSEQUENT PREGNANCY

A woman who had a history of hydrops fetalis, intrauterine fetal transfusion or neonatal exchange transfusion for the previous child, is considered a high-risk patient for development of fetal anemia in the following pregnancy. Development of severe fetal anemia is anticipated in subsequent pregnancies in these patients especially with an RhD positive fetus and severe anemia may occur earlier than in the previous gestation.

- Determine fetal RhD status using cell-free DNA assessment from the mother's blood.
- Baseline maternal titer early in gestation would be a useful guide for further comparison. Subsequent maternal titers are not informative as they may not be predictive of onset of fetal anemia.
- Middle cerebral artery peak systolic velocity monitoring of RhD-positive fetus is initiated at 16–18 weeks of gestation. MCA-PSV assessment is done in the same way as described above for first alloimmunized pregnancies, but measurement of MCA-PSV is usually done weekly for a closer follow-up.[14]

A MCA-PSV is a better test for detection of fetal anemia than amniocentesis and is considered the standard of care in red cell alloimmunization cases.[19,20] MCA-PSV can be safely used for timing cordocentesis and fetal transfusion if indicated (**Flowchart 2**).[10]

Timing of delivery of women with red-cell antibodies will depend on the RhD antibody titers, rate of rise of antibody titers, and also whether any fetal therapy was required during pregnancy. The mode and timing and place of delivery are otherwise dependent on standard obstetric grounds.

The severity of fetal hemolysis can be predicted by:

- Detailed history of previously affected pregnancies
- Maternal anti-D antibody titers
- Doppler study of fetal circulation which can detect changes in the flow velocity of waveforms
- Altered morphometry of the fetus and placenta
- Presence of pathological fetal heart rate patterns

Ultrasound features of fetal hydrops—ascites, pericardial and pleural effusions, subcutaneous and scalp edema, polyhydramnios, and placentomegaly (**Figs. 5A and B**).

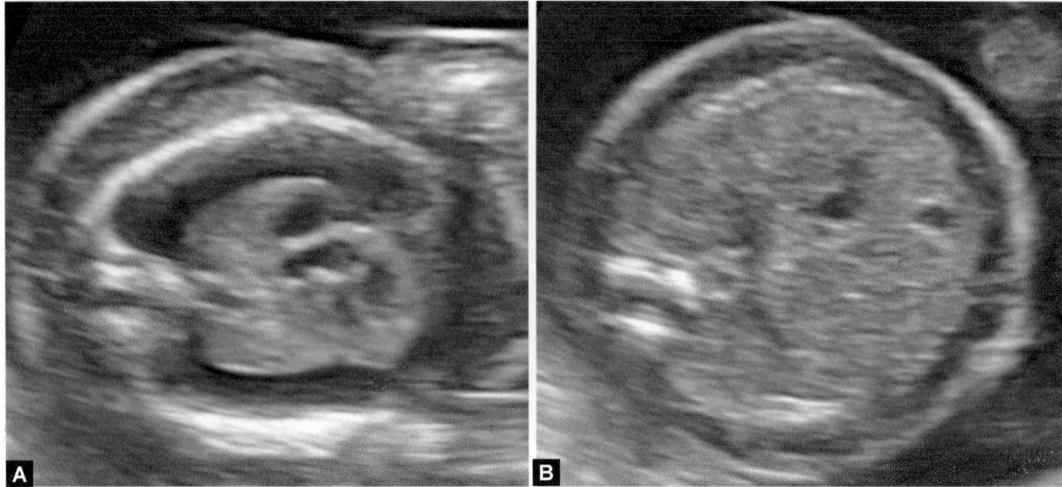

Figs. 5A and B: (a) skin edema with pleural effusion also noted; (b) skin edema noted.

PREVENTION OF AN AFFECTED FETUS

Each subsequent pregnancy after the first affected pregnancy is likely to manifest more severe hemolytic disease at an earlier gestational age can be prevented by avoiding conception of an RhD positive fetus in an RhD negative mother.

- *In vitro fertilization (IVF) with preimplantation genetic diagnosis (PGD)*: If biological father is heterozygous positive for RhD. IVF with PGD can be used to identify RhD-negative embryos and only those are considered to transfer.
- *Gestational surrogate*: If the biological father is homozygous for RhD, parents can conceive by IVF and embryos can be carried by gestational surrogate.
- *Donor sperm*: Sperm of RhD-negative donor can be used for intrauterine insemination.

SPECIAL ISSUES

Assisted reproductive technology (ART) does not increase sensitivity of Rh isoimmunization, though in third party reproduction technology, care should be taken while selecting donor eggs for Rh-negative pregnant women.

Twins (Dichorionic Diamniotic Twins)

Maternal blood test for fetal genotyping will not differentiate between the twins. Noninvasive individual monitoring of each fetus by Doppler ultrasound (MCA-PSV) is the preferable method of monitoring.

Prevention of Rh Isoimmunization by Anti-D Prophylaxis

Anti-D immunoglobulin, when given to a nonsensitized Rh-negative person, it targets and coats any Rh-positive cells in the bloodstream and prevents the production of Rh antibodies.[21]

Anti-D is not useful if the woman is already Rh sensitized.

Indications for anti-D prophylaxis:

- As part of routine antenatal anti-D prophylaxis (RAADP)
- In the occurrence of potential sensitizing events
- Postnatal anti-D prophylaxis

Routine antenatal anti-D prophylaxis: RAADP is administered as two doses of 500 IU; one at 28 weeks and 34 weeks or a single dose of 1,500 IU at 28–30 weeks given IM in the deltoid.

(1,500 IU = 300 μg)

BOX 1: Potential sensitizing events in pregnancy.[22]

- Amniocentesis, chorionic villus biopsy and cordocentesis
- Antepartum hemorrhage/uterine (PV) bleeding in pregnancy
- External cephalic version
- Abdominal trauma (sharp/blunt, open/closed)
- Ectopic pregnancy
- Evacuation of molar pregnancy
- Intrauterine death and stillbirth
- In-utero therapeutic interventions (transfusion, surgery, insertion of shunts, laser)
- Miscarriage, threatened miscarriage
- Therapeutic termination of pregnancy
- Delivery—normal, instrumental or cesarean section
- Intraoperative cell salvage

Potential sensitizing events in pregnancy has been shown in **Box 1**.[22]

The dose of anti-D required to prevent Rh sensitization in an Rh-negative woman when a sensitizing event has occurred depends on the amount of fetomaternal hemorrhage that has occurred and this can be estimated by Kleihauer–Betke test.

No test for fetomaternal hemorrhage (FMH) is required before 20 weeks of gestation.

Postnatal anti-D prophylaxis: 1,500 IU is given IM within 72 hours of delivery. In case this deadline could not be met, some protection may still be got by giving it up to 10 days after delivery, this is in addition to any anti-D given in antenatal period. **Table 2**[23] gives summary of dose administration.

Anti-D Administration Checklist[23]

The overall survival in pregnancies complicated by red-cell antibodies causing fetal anemia following treatment was reported to be 84%, with nonhydropic fetuses having better survival (94%) than hydropic fetuses (74%).[24]

SUMMARY POINTS

- The incidence of RhD alloimmunization is decreasing.
- Genotyping of fetuses can now be done noninvasively, using maternal plasma (cfDNA).
- Serial amniocentesis to assess progression of fetal anemia is no longer necessary.
- Fetal anemia can be monitored noninvasively by using Doppler of the middle cerebral artery peak systolic velocity (MCA-PSV).
- Good neurodevelopmental outcome can be expected in treated fetuses.
- Immunotherapy may be of benefit in selected cases.

Nonimmune Hydrops Fetalis

Nonimmune hydrops fetalis (NIHF) is defined as two or more serous body cavity effusions or one effusion plus anasarca, in a fetus immunologically compatible with the mother. The prevalence of NIHF ranges from 1/1,500 to 1/3,800.[25]

Pathogenesis: Dysregulation of the net fluid movement between the vascular and interstitial spaces leading to NIHF can be caused by various fetal disorders. Fetal disorders associated with NIHF are typically grouped into etiologic categories. Chromosomal, hematologic, cardiothoracic, neoplastic, infections, structural abnormalities, complete list is beyond the scope of this chapter. However, the following discussion will focus on the common ones.

The proportion of hydrops cases attributable to each etiologic category depends on the gestational age at presentation. NIHF prior to 24 weeks of gestation is usually related to aneuploidy, while cardiac, infections and other etiologies account for the majority of cases after 24 weeks.

Edema can be attributed to one of six principal factors (**Figs. 5 and 6**):

1. Primary myocardial failure
2. High output cardiac failure
3. Decreased plasma oncotic pressure
4. Increased capillary permeability

TABLE 2: Summary of dose administration.

Always confirm • The woman's identity • That the woman is RhD negative using the latest laboratory report • That the woman does not have immune anti-D using the latest laboratory report • That informed consent for administration of anti-D Ig is recorded in notes	
Potentially Sensitizing Events (PSEs) during pregnancy	
Gestation <12 weeks	
Vaginal bleeding associated with severe pain ERPC/instrumentation of uterus Medical or surgical termination of pregnancy Ectopic/molar pregnancy	Administer at least **250 IU** anti-D Ig within 72 hours of event. Confirm product/dose/expiry and patient ID preadministration
Gestation 12 to 20 weeks	
For any potentially sensitizing event (PSE)	Administer at least **250 IU** anti-D Ig within 72 hours of event Confirm product/dose/expiry and patient ID preadministration
Gestation 20 weeks to term	
For any potentially sensitizing event (PSE) (**Irrespective** of whether RAADP has been given)	Request a Kleihauer Test (FMH Test) and immediately administer at least **500 IU** anti-D Ig within 72 hours of event Confirm product/dose/expiry and patient ID preadministration
Does the Kleihauer/FMH test indicate that further anti-D Ig is required?	Administer more anti-D Ig following discussion with laboratory
For continuous vaginal bleeding at least **500 IU** anti-D Ig should be administered at a minimum of 6-weekly intervals, irrespective of the presence of detectable anti-D, and a Kleihauer/FMH test requested every 2 weeks in case more anti-D is needed	
Routine Antenatal Anti-D Prophylaxis (RAADP)	
For RAADP (**Irrespective** of whether anti-D Ig already given for PSE)	Take a blood sample to confirm group and check antibody screen—do not wait for results before administering anti-D Ig
	Administer **1500 IU** anti-D Ig at **28–30** weeks
	OR
	Administer at least **500 IU** anti-D Ig at **28** weeks and then administer at least **500 IU** anti-D at **34** weeks
	Confirm product/dose/expiry and patient ID preadministration
At Delivery (or on diagnosis of Intrauterine Death >20 weeks)	
	Request a Kleihauer Test (FMH test)
Is the baby's group oonfirmed as RhD positive ? OR Are cord samples not available?	Administer at least **500 IU** anti-D Ig within **72** hours of delivery Confirm product/dose/expiry and patient ID preadministration
Does the Kleihauer/FMH test indicate that further anti-D Ig is required?	Administer more anti-D following discussion with laboratory

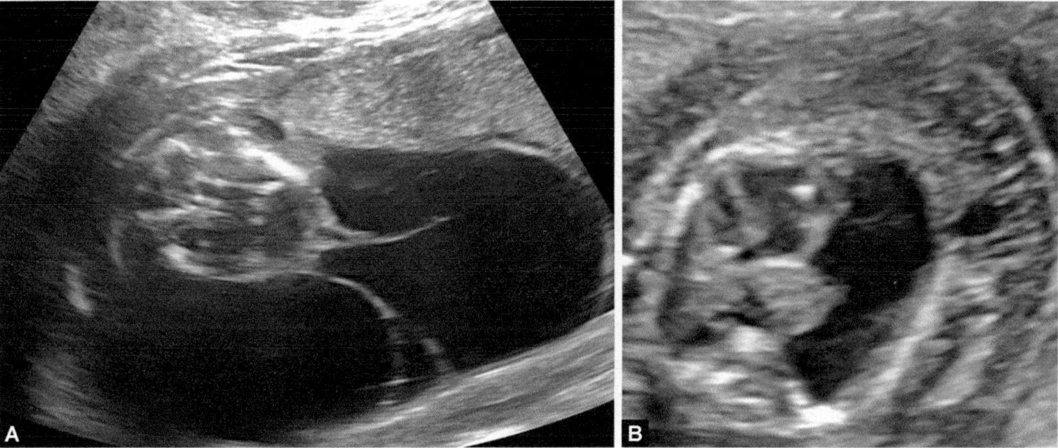

Figs. 6A and B: (A) Cystic hygroma with hydrops, transverse veiw of the fetal head shows large cystic hygroma with multiple internal septations; (b) axial view of fetal thorax showing plueral effusion.

5. Obstruction of venous return
6. Obstruction of lymphatic flow

FETAL STRUCTURAL ANOMALIES

Cardiovascular Abnormalities

Fetal structural cardiac anomalies and fetal arrhythmias represent 40% cases of nonimmune hydrops fetalis (NIHF).[26] The most common cardiac lesions associated with hydrops are atrioventricular septal defects (AVSD), hypoplastic left or right heart syndrome, Ebstein's anomaly, cardiomyopathy, etc. Many of these lesions are also associated with aneuploidy. Most of these lesions are not amenable to intrauterine therapy and in the setting of early onset hydrops prognosis is poor with a mortality rate close to 100%.[27] Genetic counseling should be offered, as the recurrence risk is 2–5%.[28] Isolated congenital heart block is associated with maternal antinuclear antibodies (ANA), anti-SSA (Ro) antibodies and anti-SSB (La) antibodies and tends to have good outcomes.[29]

Thoracic and Lymphatic Abnormalities

These account for up to 10% of hydrops. Those lesions which increase intrathoracic pressure may obstruct venous return to the heart leading to peripheral venous congestion or may obstruct the lymphatic duct resulting in lymphedema. Interference with fluid exchange between the lung and amniotic cavity may also contribute to polyhydramnios.

Congenital cystic adenomatoid malformation (CCAM) occurs when there is an abnormal overgrowth of terminal respiratory bronchioles prior to 7 weeks. CCAM is divided into two groups: Macrocystic tumors containing cysts of at least 5 mm appear cystic on ultrasound. These are not usually associated with NIH and have favorable prognosis. Microcystic tumors contain cysts < 5 mm, appearing solid ultrasonographically and are commonly associated with NIH. The perinatal survival rate of CCAM without hydrops approaches 100%, while the combination of CCAM and NIH and no fetal therapy is almost invariably fatal.[30]

Pulmonary sequestration (PS) is a mass of nonaerated lung tissue that receives its systemic circulation from the aorta. It is either lobar (within the pleura of the normal lung) or extra lobar (outside the pleura of the normal lung). The perinatal survival rate in pure PS with or without NIH is 80–100% respectively, and is significantly reduced by presence of other anomalies.[31]

Pleural effusion may be isolated or associated with NIH which confers worse prognosis. Persistent pleural effusion before 20 weeks of gestation can compromise lung growth and function. Thus, a poor prognostic sign, the degree of pulmonary hypoplasia cannot be reliably determined sonographically.

Needle aspiration of pleural effusion is not recommended as the fluid reaccumulates, in fetus with large pleural effusion placement of pleuroamniotic shunt may alleviate the increased intrathoracic pressure, thereby reducing the risk of pulmonary hypoplasia.

Aneuploidy

Aneuploidy is responsible for 7–16% of NIHF cases.[32] The most common aneuploidy associated with NIHF is monosomy X (Turner syndrome), which accounts for 42–67% of cases.[33] Other aneuploidies associated with hydrops include trisomy 21 (23–30% of cases); Trisomies 13, 18, and 12 (10% of cases); tetraploidy; triploidy; and, rarely, deletions, and duplications.[26,33] The mechanism for fluid accumulation in these fetuses may involve obstruction or incomplete formation of the lymphatic system in the neck or abdomen, leading to lymphatic dysplasia (**Figs. 6 and 7**). Other mechanisms include cardiac failure related to congenital heart disease (present in 15–25% of aneuploid fetuses)[28] and transient abnormal myelopoiesis, a congenital leukemia associated with Down syndrome.[34] The prognosis is poor, with a mortality rate approaching 100% (**Figs. 7A and B**).[28]

Infections

Infections are responsible for 5–10% of NIHF.[32,35] Parvovirus B19 is the most common infection associated with hydrops, followed by cytomegalovirus, toxoplasmosis, and syphilis. The following infections have been associated with NIHF. Not all fetuses with these infections develop hydrops and causation has not been proven for all of the infections. In some cases, a causative organism may not be identified:

Parvovirus B19, TORCH pathogens [toxoplasmosis, cytomegalovirus, rubella, herpes virus (human herpesvirus 6 and 7, herpes simplex type1)], syphilis, varicella, adenovirus, coxsackie virus, leptospirosis, *Trypanosoma cruzi* (Chagas disease), listeria, respiratory syncytial virus, and congenital lymphocytic choriomeningitis virus.

Sonographic signs (in addition to hydrops) that suggest in utero infection include calcifications of the brain, liver, or pericardium; microcephaly; cerebral ventriculomegaly; hepatosplenomegaly; and growth restriction. The pathogenesis for hydrops related to infection is not well understood in most cases; Parvovirus B_{19} is an exception. This

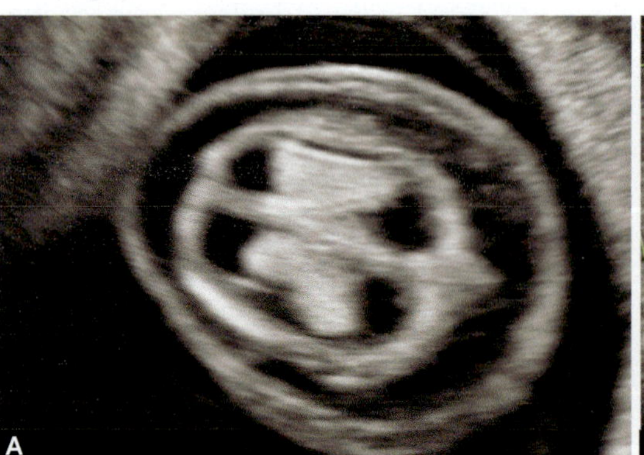

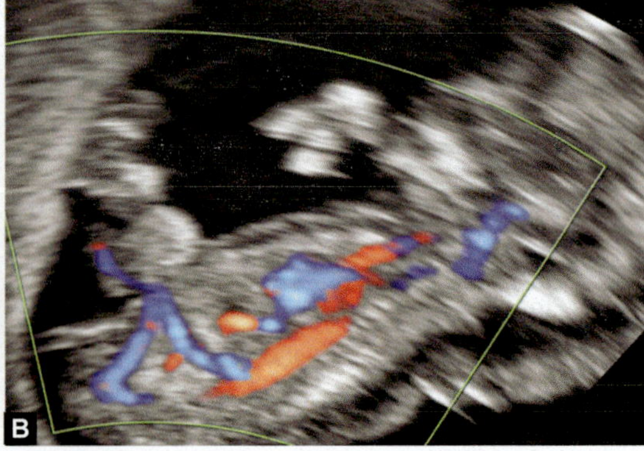

Figs. 7A and B: (A) Transverse view of fetal head showing scalp edema; (B) Sagittal view of the fetus shows edema around the fetus and omphalocele in a case of TR-18.

virus attacks red blood cells, hepatocytes, and myocardial cells causing transient aplastic crisis, hepatitis, and myocarditis.[35-38] Since these processes are selflimited, the prognosis is generally good if the fetus is supported by intrauterine fetal transfusions until the disease remits. Platelet concentrates should also be available since some fetuses may also be profoundly thrombocytopenic. In contrast, the development of hydrops in fetuses with most other infections reflects multisystem failure (e.g., myocarditis leading to heart failure, liver involvement leading to hypoalbuminemia) and is a poor prognostic sign. Therapy, if available, is directed against the infectious agent.

Fetal Tumors

Fetal tumors and lesions that have been associated with NIHF include sacrococcygeal, mediastinal or pharyngeal teratoma; neuroblastoma; and large hemangiomas.

NIHF has also been associated with fetal tuberous sclerosis. Fetal tumors invade and obstruct the vena cava, portal vein, or femoral vessels leading to cardiac failure, hepatic failure, resulting in NIHF.

Placental chorioangiomas occur in 1% of pregnancies. Tumors of >5 cm function as high volume arteriovenous shunts which predispose the fetus to heart failure and/or microangiopathic hemolytic anemia.[39]

Hematological Disorders

Severe fetal anemia accounts for 10–27% of hydrops.[26] It may be due to a variety of causes, including hemorrhage, hemolysis, defective red cell production, and production of abnormal hemoglobins. Hydrops is observed when the fetal hemoglobin is less than half the median value for gestational age.[13] In general terms, fetal anemia is most likely to result in hydrops when the hemoglobin concentration is ≤5 g/dL, which approximates a hematocrit <30%. A presumptive diagnosis of fetal anemia is made by Doppler assessment of the fetal middle cerebral artery (MCA) peak systolic velocity (PSV) ≥ 1.5 multiples of the median (MoM), (sensitivity and specificity for severe anemia 75.5 and 90.8%, respectively), and can be confirmed by cordocentesis. Decision on whether to perform cordocentesis, follow MCAPSV serially, transfuse in utero, or deliver the fetus depends on the gestational age and cause of anemia. Alphathalassemia major is the most common cause of NIHF among Southeast Asians. It is an autosomal recessive condition characterized by a mutation or deletion of the hemoglobin alpha gene. Because there is no alpha globin chain production, affected fetuses cannot synthesize a functional hemoglobin molecule. Gamma chains accumulate and form gamma4 tetramers (hemoglobin Bart's); hemoglobin Bart's binds oxygen, but cannot release it to tissues because its affinity for oxygen is much greater than that of hemoglobin A. Hemoglobin electrophoresis will show greater than 80% hemoglobin of Bart's type, while the remaining hemoglobin will be of embryonic origin, with a small component of hemoglobin H (beta4 tetramers).[40] The fetus may be severely anemic, and a peripheral blood smear will show nucleated red cells and target cells. Profound hypoxia, acidosis, and hydrops develop early in the mid-trimester, followed by intrauterine fetal demise unless the fetus is serially transfused.

Anemia secondary to massive fetomaternal transfusion, as is seen in abruptio placenta, placenta previa, trauma, twin-to-twin transfusion syndrome, is diagnosed by Kleihauer-Betke smear or flow cytometry. Transfusion or delivery can be lifesaving.

Inborn Errors of Metabolism

Inborn errors of metabolism comprise a heterogeneous group of autosomal recessive disorders that may present in the fetal period as NIHF. These account for 1–2%.[32] These rare genetic disorders are due to lack of specific enzymes necessary to process various metabolites within the lysosome in organs such as the brain, heart, liver, and kidneys. The pathogenesis of hydrops is likely related to congestion of abdominal viscera from accumulation of these metabolites.[41] Laboratory investigations for testing for some causes of storage disorders are available. An attempt at prenatal diagnosis is an option with cases of recurrence within a family or when NIHF occurs in a structurally normal fetus and no cause has been identified after a standard workup.[32,42,43] There is no specific therapy in the antenatal period. In utero, death usually occurs. It is important to make an accurate diagnosis postnatally and offer genetic counseling, as the risk of recurrence in a future pregnancy is as high as 1 in 4.

Twin Gestation

Monochorionic twin gestations are at risk for hydrops due to two disorders unique to these twin pregnancies:

Twin-twin transfusion syndrome (TTTS) and twin reversed arterial perfusion (TRAP). (Explain both the pathologies in short.) Polyhydramnios/oligohydramnios sequence is the defining characteristic of TTTS. One or both twins may develop NIHF, but usually the recipient twin is affected because of hypervolemia and increased central venous pressure. In TRAP, the hydropic twin has no apparent cardiac structures. Treatment of both TTTS and TRAP involves an in-utero ablation procedure. (Explain treatment also in short.)

In both monochromic and dichorionic twins, hydrops may develop in one or both twins from any of the etiologies that affect singleton pregnancies described above.

Placental and Umbilical Cord Lesions

Fetal/placental vascular tumors can lead to NIHF due to high output heart failure from arteriovenous shunting.

Chorioangiomas of the placenta > 4–5 cm in diameter may lead to NIHF by this mechanism and can be difficult to treat. Intrauterine endoscopic laser coagulation of the feeding vessels has been successful, but complications such as fetal bleeding, exsanguination, and death have also occurred.[44]

Cord lesions associated with NIHF include angiomyxoma, aneurysm, venous thrombosis, umbilical vein torsion or true knots.[32]

Ultrasound findings: NIHF may be discovered incidentally during prenatal ultrasound performed for standard obstetric indications, during a workup for decreased fetal activity or abnormal antepartum fetal test results, during a work-up for uterine size greater than dates, or during monitoring of fetuses with, or at risk for disorders associated with hydrops.

Fetal findings: Two or more of the following findings should be present on ultrasound examination:

- *Ascites*: In its early stage, fetal ascites appear as a rim of echoluscent fluid just inside the abdominal wall or surrounding the bladder or liver.
- *Pericardial fluid*: Fluid >2 mm thick that increases on serial examinations suggests a pathologic etiology.
- *Skin edema*: Skin edema is a late sign of fetal hydrops. Pathologic skin edema has been defined as subcutaneous tissue thickness on the chest or scalp > 5 mm. Fat under the scalp or in the posterior nuchal region should not be mistaken for skin edema **(Fig. 8)**.

NIHF may be associated with polyhydramnios and placental thickening. Polyhydramnios is generally defined as an amniotic fluid index > 24 cm or a maximum vertical pocket > 8 cm. It is present in up to 75% of pregnancies complicated by NIHF. The placenta may appear thickened due to intravillous edema. In general, a placental thickness ≥ 4 cm in the second trimester and ≥6 cm in the third trimester is considered abnormal and should prompt further investigation.[40,45]

Prognosis: NIHF is associated with an overall perinatal mortality rate of 50–98%.[46-51] Despite advances in fetal diagnosis and therapy, the

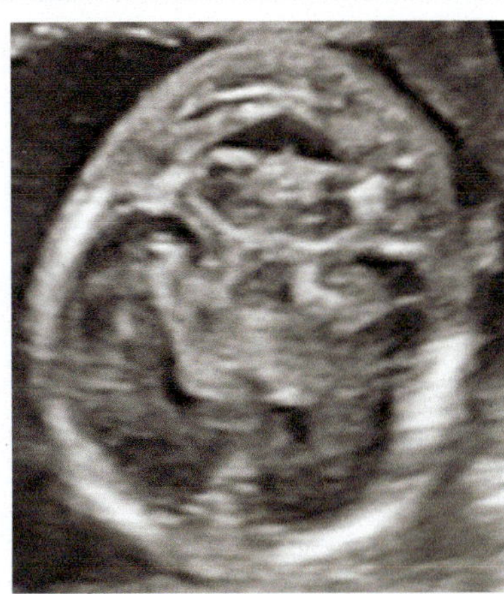

Fig. 8: Axial section of the head showing nuchal fat.

mortality rate has not changed substantially over the past 15 years. Prognosis depends upon the etiology, the gestational age at onset, the gestational age at delivery, and whether pleural effusion is present. In general, the earlier hydrops occurs, the poorer the prognosis. In particular, pleural effusions and polyhydramnios prior to 20 weeks of gestation are poor prognostic signs because of increased risk of pulmonary hypoplasia and preterm premature rupture of membranes, preterm delivery, respectively. On the other hand, absence of aneuploidy and absence of major structural abnormalities confer a better prognosis (**Table 3**).[52,53]

FETAL THERAPY

Maternal administration of medications for selected fetal infections and arrhythmias may help. Invasive procedures include—thoracoamniotic shunting to alleviate compression of fetal lungs, blood transfusion fetal anemia, close fetal monitoring is indicated as there is high incidence of fetal demise.

The timing of delivery depends on the associated conditions, gestational age, and fetal growth. The mode of delivery depends on maternal condition, fetal size, and fetal tolerance to labor. Fetus with NIH may benefit from a multidisciplinary approach.

Stillborns and neonates: We recommend autopsy in all cases of fetal or neonatal death or pregnancy termination associated with NIHF. Consultation with a medical geneticist is also advisable. Storage of amniotic fluid and/or fetal cells has been suggested for future genetic testing.[54]

Recurrence risk: The risk of recurrent NIHF depends upon the underlying etiology; therefore, every effort should be made to determine the cause. If hydrops was related to an anatomical variant the recurrence risk is minimal. Hydrops related to a specific viral exposure should not recur because the mother will develop immunity.

In contrast, the risk of recurrent NIHF can be high when hydrops has a genetic basis. Many of the times the clinician cannot always determine the etiology of fetal hydrops. Genetics consultation can be useful in these cases as the quality of information from genetic testing continues to evolve. In cases where no cause is found, the likelihood of recurrent hydrops is low.[55-57] Since the risk of recurrence is not zero, a mid trimester sonogram in subsequent gestations is reasonable.

SUMMARY AND RECOMMENDATIONS

- Hydrops fetalis refers to abnormal fluid collections in fetal soft tissues and serous cavities. Nonimmune hydrops fetalis (NIHF) comprises the subgroup of cases not caused by red cell alloimmunization [e.g., Rh(D), Kell].
- Women carrying a hydropic fetus may have uterine size large for dates and may notice decreased fetal movement. Although hydrops is a fetal condition, in many cases there are associated maternal findings, such as generalized edema with or without pre-eclampsia (i.e., mirror syndrome).
- The causes of nonimmune hydrops are heterogeneous and include aneuploidy, structural abnormalities, metabolic

TABLE 3: Diagnostic steps in the prenatal evaluation of nonimmune hydrops fetalis (NIHF).

Levels of diagnosis/ invasiveness	***Diagnostic test***	***Possible etiology***
Maternal noninvasive	Complete blood cell count and indices hemoglobin electrophoresis, blood chemistry (e.g., maternal G6 PD, pyruvate kinase carrier status) *Kleihauer–Betke test* • Viral titers (coxsackievirus, parvovirus) syphilis (VDRL) and TORCH titers • Ultrasonography • Fetal echocardiography • Oral glucose tolerance test • Fetal karyotype	Hematologic disorders Alpha thalassemia Possibility of fetal red blood cell enzyme deficiency • Fetal maternal transfusion • Fetal infection • Assessment of NIHF and its progression, exclude multiple pregnancy and congenital malformations • Congenital heart defects • Rhythm disturbances of the fetal heart
Amniocentesis	• Amniotic fluid culture • Alpha-fetoprotein • Specific metabolic tests • Restriction endonuclease tests • Rapid karyotype and metabolic tests • Hemoglobin chain analysis	• Maternal diabetes mellitus • Chromosomal abnormalities • Cytomegalovirus • Congenital nephrosis, sacrococcygeal teratoma • Gaucher disease, Tay–Sachs, GM gangliosidosis, etc. • Alpha thalassemia
Fetal blood aspiration	• Fetal plasma analysis for specific IgM • Fetal plasma albumin • Complete blood cell count	• Chromosomal of metabolic abnormalities • Thalassemias • Intrauterine infection • Hypoalbuminemia • Fetal anemia

[TORCH: toxoplasmosis, other (syphilis), rubella, cytomegalovirus, herpes simplex virus; VDRL: venereal disease research laboratory]

disorders, anemia, genetic causes, and infection.

- Several etiologies can be confirmed or excluded based upon ultrasound findings.
- The cause of hydrops can be determined prenatally or postnatally in 60–85% of cases.
- Management and intervention are dictated by the underlying disease process and the gestational age at detection.
- Fetal anemia, fetal arrhythmias, and complications of monochorionic twin pregnancy are amenable to in-utero intervention.
- In the absence of a lethal etiology of NIHF, weekly nonstress testing or biophysical profile testing delivery if there is evidence of fetal decompensation at a viable gestational age should be the strategy.
- Maternalfetal medicine specialists and neonatologists should be involved in the management of these pregnancies.
- The risk of recurrent NIHF depends upon the underlying etiology.

REFERENCES

1. Chervenak FA, Kurjak A, Papp Z. The Fetus as a Patient: The Evolving Challenge, 1st edition. United States: CRC Press; 2002.

2. Cunningham FG, Gant NF, Leveno KJ, Larry C. Williams Obstetrics, 21st edition. United States: McGraw Hill Medical Publishing Division; 2001. pp. 1059.
3. Colin Y, Cherif-Zahar B, Le Van Kin C, Raynal V, Van Huffel V, Cartron JP. Genetic Basis of the RhD-positive and RhD-negative blood group polymorphism as determined by Southern analysis. Blood. 1991;78(10):2747-52.
4. Moise KJ Jr, Boring NH, O'Shaughnessy R, Simpson LL, Wolfe HM, Baxter JK, et al. Circulating cell-free fetal DNA for the detection of RHD status and sex using reflex fetal identifiers. Prenat Diagn. 2013;33:95.
5. Misra R. Ian Donald's Practical Obstetric Problems, 6th edition. New Delhi: BI Publications Pvt Ltd; 2007. pp. 377.
6. Bowman JM, Pollock JM, Penston LE. Feto-maternal transplacental hemorrhage during pregnancy and after delivery. Vox Sang. 1986;51: 117-21.
7. Kumar S, Regan F. Clinical review: management of pregnancies with RhD alloimmunisation. BMJ. 2005;330(7502):1255-8.
8. Royal College of Obstetricians and Gynaecologists. (2014). Red Cell Antibodies during Pregnancy, The Management of Women with (Green-top Guideline No. 65). [online] Available from https://www.rcog.org.uk/en/guidelines-research-services/guidelines/gtg65/. [Last Accessed September, 2021].
9. Ahaded A, Brossard Y, Debbia M, Lambin P. Quantitative determination of anti-K (KEL1) IgG and IgG subclasses in the serum of severely alloimmunized pregnant women by ELISA. Transfusion. 2000;40:1239-45.
10. Mari G. Opinion, middle cerebral artery peak systolic velocity for the diagnosis of fetal anaemia: the untold story. Ultrasound Obstet Gynecol. 2005;25:323-30.
11. Gooch A, Parker J, Wray J, Qureshi H. Guideline for blood grouping and antibody testing in pregnancy, British Committee for Standards in Haematology, pp. 1-6.
12. NICE Guideline NG201. (2008). Antenatal care for uncomplicated pregnancies. Clinical Guideline [CG62]. [online] Available from guidance.nice.org.uk/cg62 [Last Accessed September, 2021].
13. Mari G, Deter RL, Carpenter RL, Rahman F, Zimmerman R, Moise KJ Jr, et al. Noninvasive diagnosis by Doppler ultrasound of fetal anaemia due to maternal red cell alloimmunisation. Collaborative Group for Doppler Assessment of the Blood Velocity in Anemic Fetuses. N Engl J Med. 2000;342:9-14.
14. Society for Maternal-Fetal Medicine (SMFM). Electronic address: pubs@smfm.org, Mari G, Norton ME, et al. Society for Maternal-Fetal Medicine (SMFM) Clinical Guideline #8: the fetus at risk for anemia—diagnosis and management. Am J Obstet Gynecol. 2015;212:697-710.
15. Mari G, Abuhamad AZ, Cosmi E, Segata M, Altaye M, Akiyama M. Middle cerebral artery peak systolic velocity: technique and variability. J Ultrasound Med. 2005;24:425-30.
16. Van Dongen H, Klumfer FJCM, Sikkkel E, Vanden Bussche FPHA, Oepkes D. Non-invasive tests to predict fetal anaemia in Kell-alloimmunized pregnancies. Ultrasound Obstet Gynecol. 2005;25;341-5.
17. Daniels G, Hadley A, Green CA. Causes of fetal anemia in hemolytic disease due to anti-K [letter]. Transfusion. 2003;43:115-6.
18. Abdel-Fattah SA, Soothill PW, Carroll SG, Kyle PM. Noninvasive diagnosis of anemia in hydrops fetalis with the use of middle cerebral artery Doppler velocity. Am J Obstet Gynecol. 2001;185:1411-5.
19. Mari G, Penson C, Sbracia M, Kern L, Levi D'Ancona R, Copel J. Delta OD450 and Doppler velocimetry of the middle cerebral artery peak velocity in the evaluation of fetal alloimmune haemolytic disease, which is best? Am J Obstet Gynecol. 1997;180(Suppl A):18.
20. Periera L, Jenkins TM, Berghella V. Conventional management of maternal red cell alloimmunisation compared with management of Doppler of MCA-PSV. Am J Obstet Gynecol. 2003;189;1002-6.
21. Finn R, Clarke CA, Donohoe WT, McConnell RB, Sheppard PM, Lehane D, et al. Experimental studies on the prevention of Rh haemolytic disease. Br Med J. 1961;5238:1486-90.
22. Qureshi H, Massey E, Kirwan D, Davies T, Robson S, White J, et al. BCSH guideline for the use of anti-D immunoglobulin for the prevention of haemolytic disease of the fetus and newborn (Table 1). Transfusion Med. 2014;24:8-20.
23. Qureshi H, Massey E, Kirwan D, Davies T, Robson S, White J, et al. BCSH guideline for the use of anti-D immunoglobulin for the prevention of haemolytic disease of the fetus and newborn (Appendix 2). Transfusion Med. 2014;24:8-20.;
24. Schumacher B, Moise KJ Jr. Fetal transfusion for red blood cell alloimmunization in pregnancy. Obstet Gynecol. 1996;88:137-50.
25. Sohan K, Carroll SG, De La Fuente S, Soothill P, Kyle P. Analysis of outcome in hydrops fetalis in relation to gestational age at diagnosis, cause and treatment. Acta Obstet Gynecol Scand. 2001;80:726-30.
26. Forouzan I. Hydrops fetalis: recent advances. Obstet Gynecol Surv. 1997;52:130-8.
27. Crawford DC, Chita SK, Allan LD. Prenatal detection of congenital heart disease: factors

affecting obstetric management and survival. Am J Obstet Gynecol. 1988;159:352-6.
28. Hess DB, Hess LW. Fetal Echocardiography. Stamford, CT: Appleton and Lange; 1999.
29. Adzick NS, Harrison MR, Glick PL, Golbus MS, Anderson RL, Mahony BS, et al. Fetal cystic adenomatoid malformation of the lung: classification and morphology. J Pead Surg. 1985;20;483-8.
30. De santis M, Masini L, Noia G. Congenital cystic adenomatoid malformation of the lung: antenatal ultrasound findings and fetal neonatal outcome. Fetal diag ther. 2000;15:246-50.
31. Adzick NS, Harrison, Flake AW. Management and outcome. A m j obstet gynecol. 1998;179:884-9.
32. Society for Maternal-Fetal Medicine (SMFM), Norton ME, Chauhan SP, Dashe JS. Society for maternal-fetal medicine (SMFM) clinical guideline #7: nonimmune hydrops fetalis. Am J Obstet Gynecol. 2015;212:127-39.
33. Machin GA. Hydrops revisited: literature review of 1,414 cases published in the 1980s. Am J Med Genet. 1989;34:366-90.
34. Malin GL, Kilby MD, Velangi M. Transient abnormal myelopoiesis associated with Down syndrome presenting as severe hydrops fetalis: a case report. Fetal Diagn Ther. 2010;27:171-3.
35. Xu J, Raff TC, Muallem NS, Neubert AG. Hydrops fetalis secondary to parvovirus B19 infections. J Am Board Fam Pract. 2003;16:63-8.
36. Callen P. Ultrasonography in Obstetrics and Gynecology, 4th edition. Philadelphia: WB Saunders; 2000.
37. Barron SD, Pass RF. Infectious causes of hydrops fetalis. Semin Perinatol. 1995;19:493-501.
38. von Kaisenberg CS, Jonat W. Fetal parvovirus B19 infection. Ultrasound Obstet Gynecol. 2001;18:280-8.
39. Woodward PJ, Sohaey R, Kennedy A, Koeller KK. A comprehensive review of fetal tumours with pathology correlation. Radiographics. 2005;25(1):215-42.
40. Arcasoy MO, Gallagher PG. Hematologic disorders and nonimmune hydrops fetalis. Semin Perinatol. 1995;19:502-15.
41. Molyneux AJ, Blair E, Coleman N, Daish P. Mucopolysaccharidosis type VII associated with hydrops fetalis: histopathological and ultrastructural features with genetic implications. J Clin Pathol. 1997;50:252-4.
42. Gort L, Granell MR, Fernández G, Carreto P, Sanchez A, Coll MJ. Fast protocol for the diagnosis of lysosomal diseases in nonimmune hydrops fetalis. Prenat Diagn. 2012;32:1139-42.
43. Gimovsky AC, Luzi P, Berghella V. Lysosomal storage disease as an etiology of nonimmune hydrops. Am J Obstet Gynecol. 2015;212:281-90.
44. Sepulveda W, Wong AE, Herrera L, Dezerega V, Devoto JC. Endoscopic laser coagulation of feeding vessels in large placental chorioangiomas: report of three cases and review of invasive treatment options. Prenat Diagn. 2009;29:201-6.
45. Chitkara U, Wilkins I, Lynch L, Mehalek K, Berkowitz RL. The role of sonography in assessing severity of fetal anemia in Rh- and Kell-isoimmunized pregnancies. Obstet Gynecol. 1988;71:393-8.
46. Carlson DE, Platt LD, Medearis AL, Horenstein J. Prognostic indicators of the resolution of nonimmune hydrops fetalis and survival of the fetus. Am J Obstet Gynecol. 1990;163:1785-7.
47. Castillo RA, Devoe LD, Hadi HA, Martin S, Geist D. Nonimmune hydrops fetalis: clinical experience and factors related to a poor outcome. Am J Obstet Gynecol. 1986;155:812-6.
48. Ismail KM, Martin WL, Ghosh S, Whittle MJ, Kilby MD. Etiology and outcome of hydrops fetalis. J Matern Fetal Med. 2001;10:175-81.
49. Heinonen S, Ryynänen M, Kirkinen P. Etiology and outcome of second trimester non-immunologic fetal hydrops. Acta Obstet Gynecol Scand. 2000;79:15-8.
50. Wy CA, Sajous CH, Loberiza F, Weiss MG. Outcome of infants with a diagnosis of hydrops fetalis in the 1990s. Am J Perinatol. 1999;16: 561-7.
51. Santo S, Mansour S, Thilaganathan B, Homfray T, Papageorghiou A, Calvert S, et al. Prenatal diagnosis of non-immune hydrops fetalis: what do we tell the parents? Prenat Diagn. 2011;31:186-95.
52. McCoy MC, Katz VL, Gould N, Kuller JA. Non-immune hydrops after 20 weeks' gestation: review of 10 years' experience with suggestions for management. Obstet Gynecol. 1995;85: 578-82.
53. Iskaros J, Jauniaux E, Rodeck C. Outcome of nonimmune hydrops fetalis diagnosed during the first half of pregnancy. Obstet Gynecol. 1997;90:321-5.
54. Désilets V, Audibert F, Society of Obstetrician and Gynaecologists of Canada. Investigation and management of non-immune fetal hydrops. J Obstet Gynaecol Can. 2013;35:923-38.
55. Schwartz SM, Viseskul C, Laxova R, McPherson EW, Gilbert EF. Idiopathic hydrops fetalis report of 4 patients including 2 affected sibs. Am J Med Genet. 1981;8:59-66.
56. Cumming DC. Recurrent nonimmune hydrops fetalis. Obstet Gynecol. 1979;54:124-6.
57. Etches PC, Lemons JA. Nonimmune hydrops fetalis: report of 22 cases including three siblings. Pediatrics. 1979;64:326-32.

17

CHAPTER

Fetal Central Nervous System Abnormalities

KV Sridevi

INTRODUCTION

Central nervous system (CNS) malformations are some of the most common of all congenital abnormalities. Neural tube defects are the most frequent CNS malformations and amount to about one to two cases per 1,000 births.[1] The incidence of intracranial abnormalities with an intact neural tube is uncertain.

Ultrasound has been used as the main modality to help diagnose fetal CNS anomalies. Technical aspects of an optimized approach to the evaluation of the fetal brain in surveys of fetal anatomy are referred as a basic examination. Basic examinations of the fetal CNS are described in this chapter, which are usually performed around 19–20 weeks of gestation. Sensitivity of detection of CNS abnormalities by transabdominal ultrasound in low-risk patients undergoing basic examination is 80%.[2-4]

GESTATIONAL AGE

The appearance of the brain and spine changes throughout gestation. To avoid diagnostic errors, it is important to be familiar with normal CNS appearances at different gestational ages. Some abnormalities may be visible in the first and early second trimesters,[5-11] they usually are severe, and early examination requires special skills; however, basic examination is done at 19–20 weeks.

ULTRASOUND TRANSDUCERS

Most basic examinations are performed with 3–5 MHz transabdominal transducer and transvaginal examinations that are usually conveniently performed with transducers between 5 and 10 MHz.[12,13] Three-dimensional (3D) ultrasound may facilitate the examination of the fetal brain and spine.[14,15]

IMAGING PARAMETERS

The examination is mostly performed with grayscale bidimensional ultrasound. Harmonic imaging may enhance visualization. Color and power Doppler may be used mainly to identify cerebral vessels. Proper adjustment of pulse repetition frequency (main cerebral arteries have velocities in the range of 20–40 cm/s during intrauterine life)[16] and signal persistence enhances visualization of small vessels.

BASIC EXAMINATION

Transabdominal sonography is the technique of choice.

The examination should include the evaluation of the fetal head and spine.

Three axial sections are used to study fetal brain are: (1) *transventricular plane*, (2) *transcerebellar plane*, and (3) *transthalamic plane.*

Axial Transventricular Plane

11–14 Weeks

- The shape of the calvarium is oval
- The calvarial bones are ossified and are seen as echogenic rim
- The midline echogenic line is falx and it divides cranium into two symmetrical halves

- Choroid plexus is hyperechoic, prominent, and fills the lateral ventricles
- The ventricular cerebrospinal fluid (CSF) is seen anterior to the choroid plexus in the region of anterior horn
- The midline falx and choroid plexus form the butterfly sign (**Fig. 1**)
- The cerebral mantle is thin.

18–22 Weeks

In the standard transventricular plane only, the hemisphere on the far side of the transducer is usually clearly visualized, as the hemisphere close to the transducer is frequently obscured by reverberation artifacts.

- The anterior and posterior portions of the lateral ventricles are seen
- The atrium of lateral ventricle is characterized by presence of echogenic choroid plexus filling the lumen **(Fig. 2)**
- Lateral ventricles are measured at the atrium at the level of parieto-occipital sulcus. The image setting (focal zone) is to be optimized and calipers are placed on the inner aspect of the medial and lateral walls. Measurement should be perpendicular to the wall of the atrium. Near lateral ventricle should be visualized in all cases. Normal lateral ventricular measurement is <10 mm **(Figs. 3A and B)**.
- The cavum septum pellucidum (CSP) is a rectangular fluid-filled cavity seen anteriorly in the midline. The CSP becomes visible around 16 weeks and undergoes obliteration near-term gestation. With transabdominal ultrasound, it should always be visualized between 18 and 37 weeks or with a biparietal diameter of 44–88 mm.[17] Conversely, failure to demonstrate the CSP prior to 16 weeks or later than 37 weeks is a normal finding.

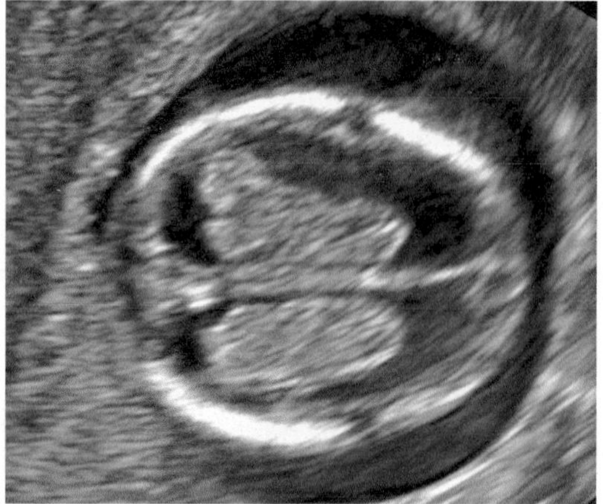

Fig. 1: Calvarial bones ossified seen as echogenic rim, midline falx, and choroid plexus filling the lateral ventricles that form butterfly sign.

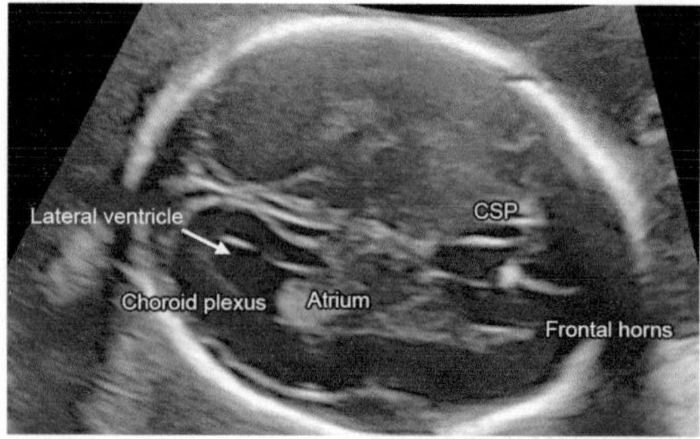

Fig. 2: Transventricular plane—cavum septum pellucidum (CSP), frontal horns, atrium, and choroid plexus of the far side posterior lateral ventricle.

Transcerebellar Plane (Fig. 4)

This plane is obtained at a slightly lower level than that of the transventricular plane and with a slight posterior tilting and includes visualization of the frontal horns of the lateral ventricles, CSP, thalami, cerebellum, and cisterna magna.

- The cerebellum appears as a butterfly-shaped structure formed by the round cerebellar hemispheres joined in the middle by the slightly more echogenic cerebellar vermis.
- The cisterna magna or cerebellomedullaris cistern is a fluid-filled space posterior to the cerebellum. It contains thin septations that are normal structures and should not be confused with vascular structures or cystic abnormalities. In the second half of

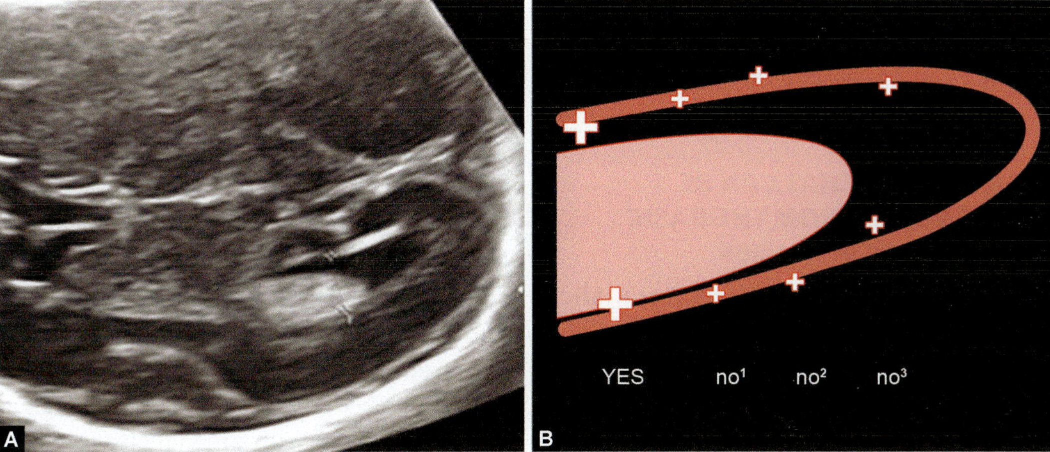

Figs. 3A and B: (A) Measurement of the atrium of the lateral ventricles. The calipers are positioned at the level of the glomus of the choroid plexus inside the echoes generated by the ventricular walls; (B) Diagram to illustrate correct caliper placement for ventricular measurement. Calipers are correctly placed touching the inner edge of the ventricle wall at its widest part and aligned perpendicular to the long axis of the ventricle (YES). Incorrect placements include middle–middle (no[1]), outer–outer (no[2]), and placement that are too posterior in the narrower part of the ventricle or not perpendicular to the ventricle axis (no[3]).

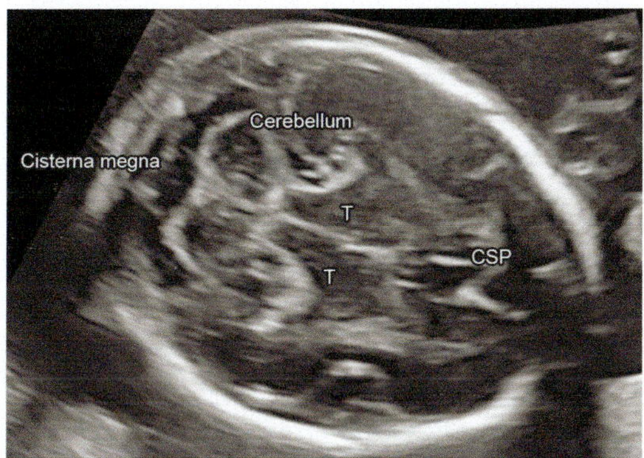

Fig. 4: Transcerebellar plane—dumbbell-shaped cerebellum and cisterna magna.
(CSP: cavum septum pellucidum)

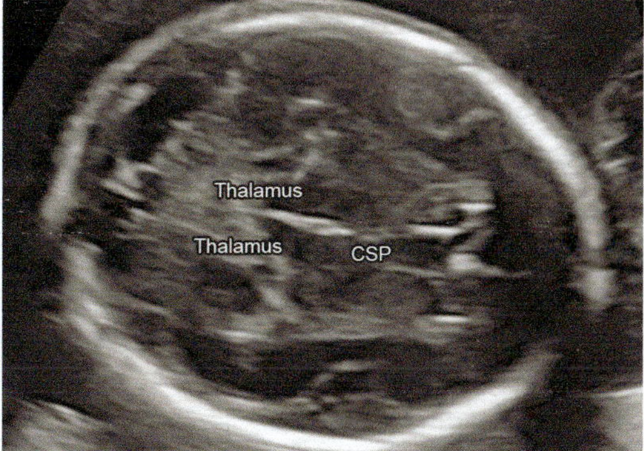

Fig. 5: Transthalamic plane—cavum septum pellucidum (CSP) and both thalamus.

gestation, the depth of the cisterna magna is stable and should be 2–10 mm.[18]

Transthalamic Plane (Fig. 5)

It is obtained at an intermediate level, is also frequently used in the sonographic assessment of the fetal head, and is commonly referred to as the *transthalamic plane* or *biparietal diameter plane*. The anatomic landmarks include from anterior to posterior:

- Frontal horns of the lateral ventricles
- Cavum septi pellucidi
- Thalami
- Third ventricle may be seen as a thin slit between the thalami.

Fetal Spine

The detailed examination of the fetal spine requires expertise and meticulous scanning and the results are heavily dependent upon the fetal position. Longitudinal section of the spine from about 14 weeks of gestation demonstrates the three ossification centers of the vertebrae that surround the neural canal and that appear as either two or three parallel lines depending upon the orientation of the sound beam, intactness of the skin overlying the spine should be seen.[18]

ANOMALIES THAT CAN BE DIAGNOSED FROM THE BASIC EXAMINATION PLANES

Axial Transventricular Plane Anomalies

Ventriculomegaly and Hydrocephalus (Figs. 6A and B)

Hydrocephalus and ventriculomegaly are both the terms used to describe dilatation of the lateral ventricles. However, those two should be distinguished from each other. Hydrocephalus signifies dilated lateral ventricles that resulted from increased amount of CSF inside the ventricles and increased intracranial pressure, while ventriculomegaly is dilatation of lateral ventricles without an increased intracranial pressure due to cerebral hypoplasia or CNS anomaly.[17,19] Ventriculomegaly can sometimes change into hydrocephalic state. Obliterated subarachnoid space and dangling choroid plexus are observed in hydrocephalus, in contrast to ventriculomegaly in which both these are well preserved. Atrial width of cerebral lateral ventricles of 10.0–15 mm—mild ventriculomegaly and >15 mm—severe ventriculomegaly.[20]

Mild ventriculomegaly is defined as isolated if there is no sonographic evidence of associated malformation or markers of aneuploidy at the time of the initial presentation.[20,21] Isolated mild ventriculomegaly represents a considerable diagnostic dilemma, as it can be an apparently benign finding, but can also be associated with abnormalities such as congenital infection, vascular abnormalities, and hemorrhagic causes. Several studies have reported an incidence of associated anomalies (neural and extraneural) as high as 50%. For women with pregnancies in which mild ventriculomegaly is suspected, detailed neurosonographic evaluation should be performed by an expert.[20] Congenital infections can cause mild ventriculomegaly and possible pathogens include *Toxoplasma*, rubella, and cytomegalovirus (CMV).[21-23] CMV infection is of particular concern because of the poor prognosis. Incidence of CMV as a cause of mild ventriculomegaly varies from 0 to 5%.[24,25] On the other hand, cerebral CMV is one of the common prenatal ultrasound abnormalities in fetuses with proven intrauterine transmission of CMV present in around 18% of cases. Poor prognosis in affected children, the potential for treatment, and the simplicity of the screening test should prompt maternal serum studies to be considered. Isolated ventriculomegaly has been

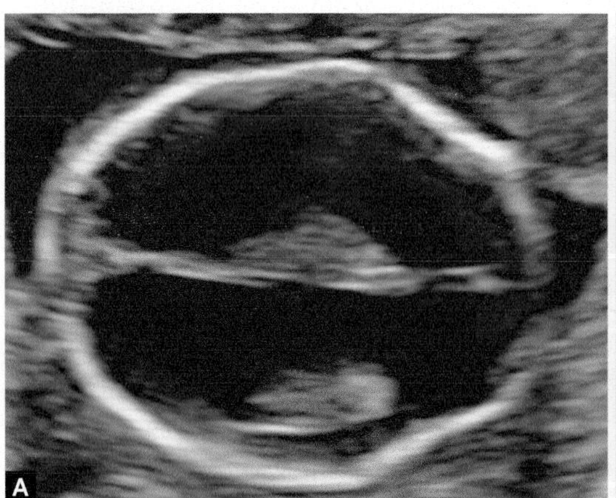

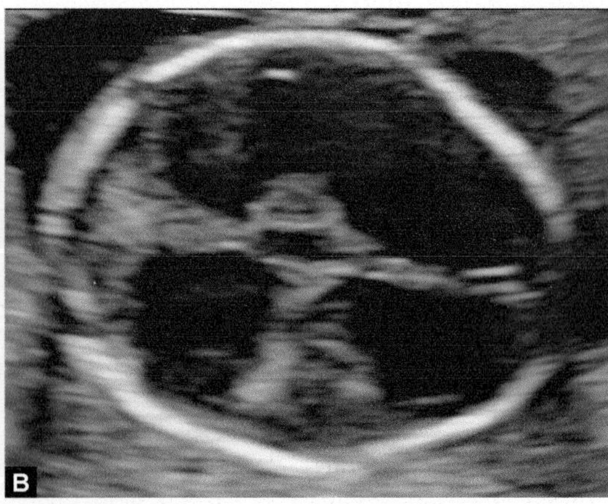

Figs. 6A and B: (A) Bilateral dilated lateral ventricles and dangling choroid plexus; (B) Dilatation of the third ventricle.

associated with chromosomal abnormalities, mainly 1.4% in trisomy 21 fetuses, providing a likelihood ratio of 9 for the risk of aneuploidy. Investigation for aneuploidy in the presence of the finding, therefore, is appropriate.[26] Follow-up USG examination should be performed suggested time interval being 2 weeks.[27] The risks of progression of ventricular dilatation is about 11% (increase in the ventricular measurement of >3 mm is considered as progression). Abnormalities not seen at the initial scan can also be identified later; therefore, one additional detailed ultrasound examination of the fetus should be performed between 28 and 34 weeks in order to search for cerebral and extracerebral abnormalities. There is no solid data to suggest an increased frequency of neurological/neuropsychiatric disorders in infants with prenatal diagnosis of isolated mild ventriculomegaly.[28] Fetal MRI may add important information in 6–10% of cases.

The factors that influence the prognosis of fetus with isolated mild ventriculomegaly are:

- Fetal sex (there is a male preponderance)
- Gestational age at diagnosis
- Bilateral versus unilateral
- Symmetrical versus asymmetrical
- Finally the progression (cases with progression seem to be worse than those with no progression).

Moderate-to-severe ventriculomegaly (atrial width of >15 mm): The term "hydrocephalus" does not signify a specific disease, but is a pathological condition because of abnormal circulation of CSF. Congenital hydrocephalus is classified into three categories based on the causes, which disturb the CSF circulation pathway: (1) Simple hydrocephalus, (2) Dysgenetic hydrocephalus, and (3) Secondary hydrocephalus.[19]

1. *Simple hydrocephalus*: Simple hydrocephalus, caused by developmental abnormality, which is localized within CSF circulation pathway, includes aqueductal stenosis, atresia of foramen of Monro, and maldevelopment of arachnoid granulations type of hydrocephalus due to various sites of obstruction to CSF flow.
2. *Dysgenetic hydrocephalus*: Dysgenetic hydrocephalus indicates hydrocephalus as a result of cerebral developmental disorder and includes hydranencephaly, holoprosencephaly, porencephaly, schizencephaly, Dandy–Walker malformation, spinal dysraphism, and Chiari malformation.
3. *Secondary hydrocephalus*: Secondary hydrocephalus is caused by intracranial pathologic condition such as brain tumor, intracranial infection, and intracranial hemorrhage.

In cases with progressive hydrocephalus, there may be seven stages of progression:

1. Increased fluid collection of lateral ventricles.
2. Increased intracranial pressure.
3. Dangling choroid plexus.
4. Disappearance of subarachnoid space.
5. Excessive extension of the dura and superior sagittal sinus.
6. Disappearance of venous pulsation.
7. Enlarged skull.

To evaluate enlarged ventricles, examiners should carefully observe the structure below and specify the cause of hydrocephalus:

- Choroid plexus, dangling or not
- Subarachnoid space, obliterated or not
- Ventricles, symmetry or asymmetry
- Visibility of third ventricle
- Pulsation of dural sinuses
- Ventricular size (3D volume calculation, if possible)

Cavum Septum Pellucidum

Absent septum pellucidum (Figs. 7A to D): Absence of the septum pellucidum is either primary as part of ventricular induction disorder or secondary to a disruptive process[29] with or without associated anomalies. Isolated absent septum pellucidum is rare but can occur. Absent CSP may be associated with

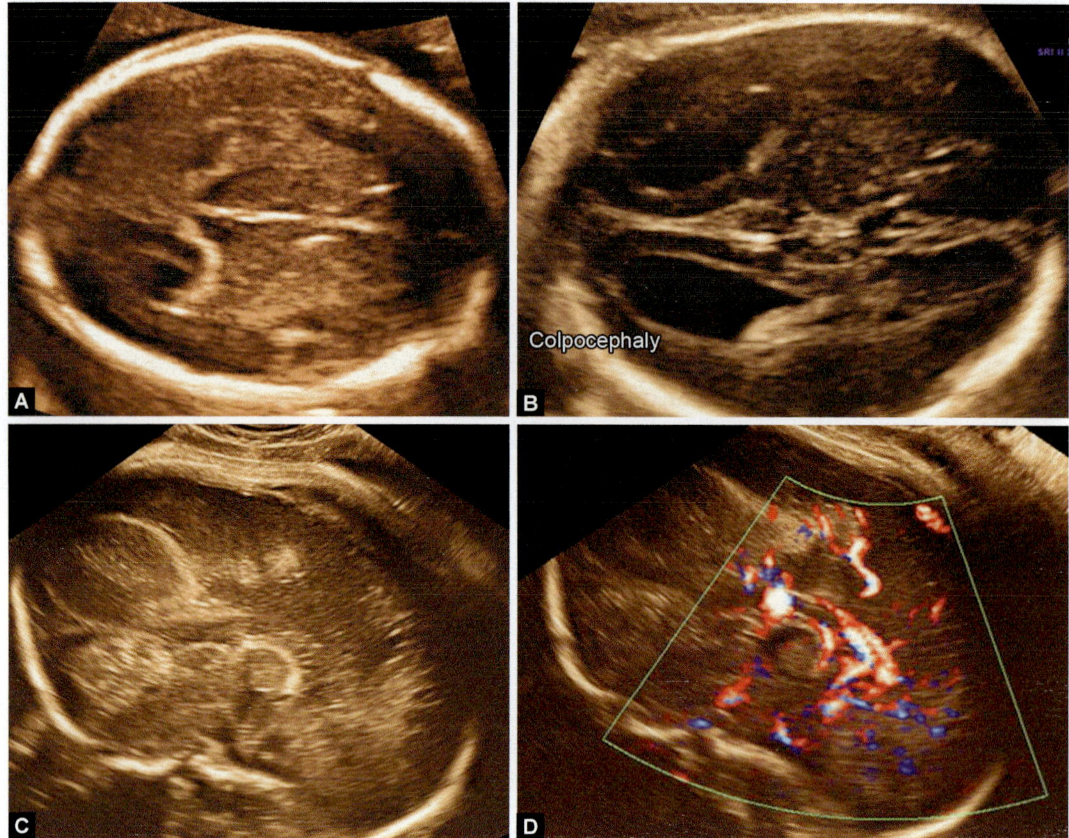

Figs. 7A to D: Transventricular scan of the fetal brain showing: (A) Absent cavum septum pellucidum (CSP); (B) Mild dilatation of lateral ventricle (colpocephaly) while the anterior part is normal; (C) Sagittal view—typical radial sulcus formation; (D) 3D power Doppler shows normal callosomarginal artery that does not exist.

various congenital brain malformations such as holoprosencephaly, septo-optic dysplasia, agenesis of the corpus callosum (ACC), and schizencephaly.

Ultrasound features for differentiation between hydrocephalus and holoprosencephaly are seen in **Table 1**.

Flowchart 1 illustrates differential diagnosis of fetuses with absent septum pellucidum.

Incidence—extremely rare (2–3:100,000).

Etiology—maternal drug abuse such as valproic acid and cocaine. Autosomal recessive, HESX 1 homeodomain gene mutation.[20]

Differential diagnosis—dysgenesis of the corpus callosum and lobar holoprosencephaly.

Prenatal diagnosis—transventricular, transthalamic, and transcerebellar views show absent CSP.

Prognosis—depends upon the associated anomalies, degree of mental deficit, and presence of multiple endocrine dysfunctions. Absence of septum pellucidum in most of the cases is associated with developmental abnormalities. If isolated, the prognosis may be good.

Recurrence risk—unknown.

Management—endocrine dysfunction should be investigated and corrected. Shunt procedure is advised in cases of progressive ventriculomegaly and genetic counseling.

Agenesis of the Corpus Callosum

Complete agenesis: Complete absence of corpus callosum.

Partial agenesis: Absence of splenium of posterior portion in various degrees.

TABLE 1: Major differences between hydrocephalus and holoprosencephaly.

	Hydrocephalus	*Holoprosencephaly*
1	Anterior portion of the lateral ventricles is separated by the falx	The communication begins at the anterior portion of the lateral ventricles
2	The communication between the ventricles is only in the medial portion	The communication between the ventricles is always anteroposterior
3	Normal cleavage of the hemispheres	Noncleavage of the hemispheres
4	Separated thalami	Noncleavage of the thalamus
5	Normal corpus callosum	Agenesis of the corpus callosum
6	Both choroid plexus in the same side	No choroid plexus
7	Normal face	Extreme hypotelorism

Incidence: 0.3–0.7/1,000.

Etiology—variable environmental factors such as alcohol abuse, infections, ischemia, maternal phenylketonuria, and genetic factors.

Prenatal diagnosis—corpus callosum is detected by ultrasound after 18 weeks of gestation. Diagnosis is difficult prior to 18 weeks of gestation even in expert hands.

Complete agenesis—absence of corpus callosum-CSP complex in sagittal and coronal planes. Axial planes usually do not allow diagnosis with certainty, but reveal important clues such as:

- Absent CSP
- Ventriculomegaly (teardrop configuration of the lateral ventricles—colpocephaly)
- Upward displacement of third ventricle
- Abnormal midline lesions, cysts, and lipomas.

Partial agenesis—affects the most posterior portion and is usually associated with less degree of distortion.

Flowchart 1: Differential diagnosis of fetuses with absent septum pellucidum.

Absent septum pellucidum

Communication at the level of the foremost anterior portion of the lateral ventricles

Alobar, semilobar of lobar HPE

Associated confirmatory findings:
Noncleavage of cortex and basal ganglia
Facial anomalies
Agenesis of the corpus callosum

Separated anterior portion of the lateral ventricles

Noncleavage of cortex or basal ganglia

MHV

Normal cleavage

Septal remnants

Absent

Present

Hydrocephalus-associated confirmatory findings

Cortical malformations

Absent

Present

Schizencephaly
Isolated agenesis

SOD

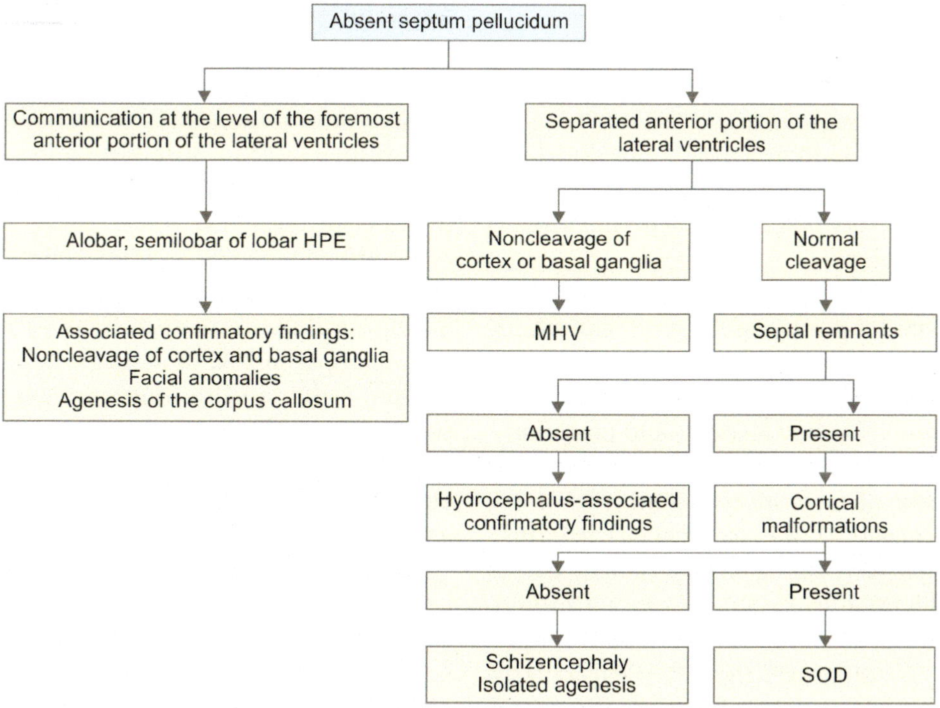

(HPE: holoprosencephaly; SOD: septo-optic dysplasia)

Color Doppler examination—in complete agenesis, semicircular loop of the pericallosal artery is lost. With partial agenesis, it is much shortened.

Three-dimensional ultrasound is useful. MRI may be more informative.

Associated anomalies—chromosomal anomalies (trisomy 18, 13, and 8) are seen in 20% of cases. Neural anomalies are seen in 85% of cases and extraneural anomalies are seen in 62% of cases.

Prognosis—depends upon associated anomalies. Cases of isolated ACC are asymptomatic and neurological prognosis is good. Complete ACC has a worse prognosis than partial agenesis. Epilepsy, intellectual impairment, and psychiatric disorders are noted.

Recurrence risk—depends upon etiology.

Management—chromosomal evaluation is offered and standard obstetric care is recommended.

Transthalamic View Anomalies

Holoprosencephaly

Classification—holoprosencephaly is classified into three varieties:

1. *Alobar type*: A single cerebral structure with a single common ventricle, posterior large cyst of third ventricle (dorsal sac), absence of olfactory bulbs and tracts, and a single optic nerve.
2. *Semilobar type*: With formation of a posterior portion of the interhemispheric fissure.
3. *Lobar type*: With formation of interhemispheric fissure anteriorly and posteriorly, but not in the midhemispheric region. The fusion of the fornices is seen.

Incidence—1 in 15,000–20,000 live births.

Etiology—heterogeneous. Genetic causes are identified in 15–50% of cases. Chromosomes 2, 3, 7, 13, 18, and 21 have been implicated in holoprosencephaly.[23] Particularly, trisomies 13 and 18 have most commonly been observed. An association with several teratogens has been suggested including maternal diabetes, alcohol, and retinoic acid consumption.

Pathogenesis—failure of the prechordal mesenchyme to induce cleavage of the forebrain and midfacial development is thought to result in a combination of cerebral and facial defects.

Associated anomalies—facial abnormalities such as cyclopia, cebocephaly, flat nose, cleft lip and palate are invariably associated with holoprosencephaly (**Figs. 8A and B**). Extracerebral abnormalities are also invariably associated due to a very early derangement of embryogenesis such as renal and cardiac anomalies and omphalocele.

Prenatal diagnosis—in typical cases of alobar holoprosencephaly, sonographic diagnosis is straightforward and has been reported as early as 9 weeks of gestation. There are no midline structures in the anterior part of the brain. The boomerang-shaped ventricle is outlined anteriorly by a rim of cortex and posteriorly by the bulb-shaped thalami. Severe facial anomalies including cyclopia, hypotelorism, proboscis, and median cleft lip are seen commonly.[9,30] Many anatomical variations result in different sonographic appearances such as the pancake, the cup, and the ball types.[31]

Alobar and semilobar varieties have similar appearances and are difficult to differentiate. Sonographic clue is visualization of the hippocampal fornix. In alobar type, hippocampal fornix and rudimentary gyrus are separated from the brainstem (**Figs. 9A to C**). In semilobar type, the hippocampus is seen close to the thalami forming the echogenic ambient cistern.

Specific diagnosis of lobar holoprosencephaly is difficult at times. Sonography will show some degree of enlargement of lateral ventricles, absence of the septum pellucidum, and a wide communication between the fron-

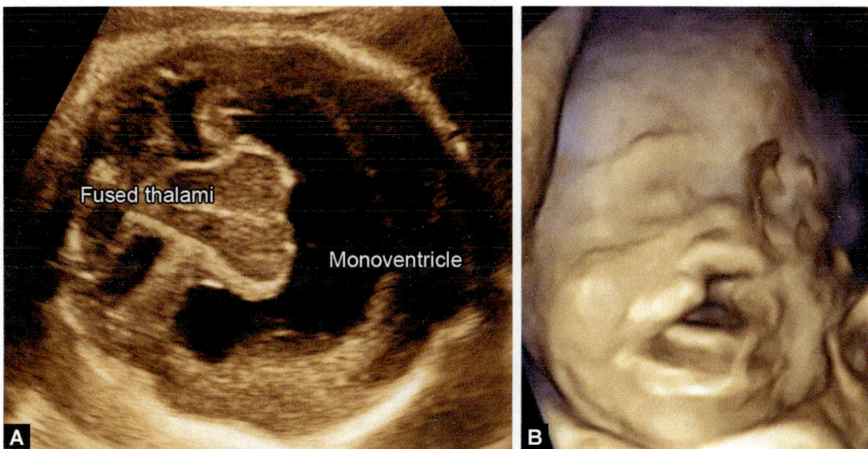

Figs. 8A and B: (A) Alobar holoprosencephaly: Axial scan at the level of the thalamus showing the single ventricle, absence of midline structures, and fused thalamus; (B) Median cleft lip palate—semilobar holoprosencephaly.

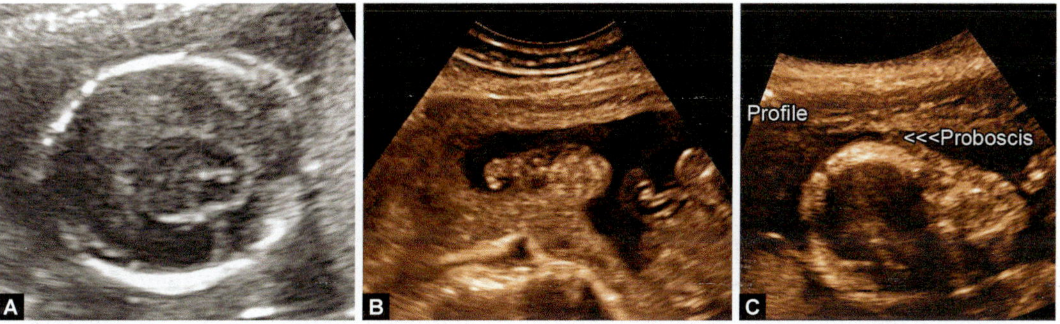

Figs. 9A to C: (A and B) Alobar holoprosencephaly: Axial scan at the level of the thalamus showing the single ventricle, absence of midline structures, and fused thalamus and (C) face—proboscis.

tal horns and the inferior third ventricle (**Figs. 10A and B**). Differentiation of disruption of the septum pellucidum, lobar holoprosencephaly, and hydrocephalus are sometimes difficult. Some of the differences between hydrocephalus and holoprosencephaly are given in **Table 1**.

Differential diagnosis—hydrocephalus and hydranencephaly.

Prognosis—alobar holoprosencephaly is considered a lethal condition. Semilobar holoprosencephaly is associated with extremely severe neurologic compromise.

Recurrence risk—6% but much lower in sporadic or trisomy cases and much higher in genetic cases.

Management—chromosomal evaluation and genetic consultation are to be offered. Severe forms are almost always associated with poor prognosis; therefore, termination of pregnancy should be discussed with the couple (according to the law of the particular country).

Transcerebellar Anomalies

Posterior Fossa Anomaly

The algorithm for the main abnormalities of the posterior fossa that can be depicted on routine ultrasound (axial plane) is seen below:

- *Increased cisterna magna*: Increased fluid-filled space of the posterior fossa
- Abnormal transcerebellar diameter

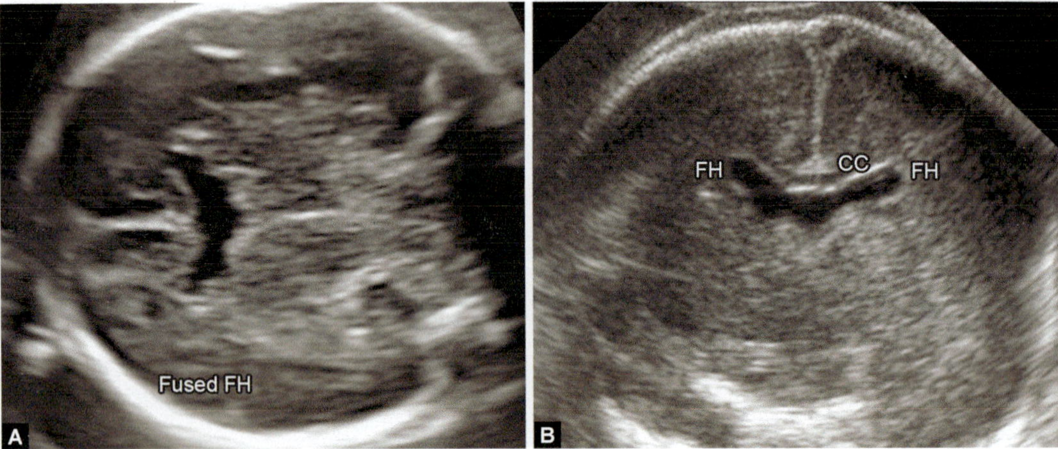

Figs. 10A and B: Lobar holoprosencephaly: Ultrasound image showing the interhemispheric fissure anteriorly with fusion of the frontal horns (FHs).

- Abnormal cerebellar anatomy
- *Increased fluid-filled space of the posterior fossa*: The main anatomic landmark is the position of the cerebellar tentorium and torcular. In case of ascent of the torcular, the increased fluid-filled retro- or pericerebellar space is related to an expansion of the fourth ventricle and this is characteristic of Dandy-Walker malformation. In case of normal positioning of the torcular, the main criterion on which to base the diagnosis is anatomy and biometry of cerebellum. If the cerebellum is biometrically and anatomically normal, the increased fluid-filled space is related either to a rotation of normal vermis with or without Blake's pouch cyst or to an arachnoid cyst or a mega cisterna magna.
- *Abnormal transcerebellar diameter*: Decreased cerebellar biometry can be associated with either normal or abnormal cerebellar anatomy. Decreased cerebellar biometry with normal anatomy can be either focal or global (**Fig. 11A**). Global decrease needs focus on brainstem to differentiate cerebellar hypoplasia from pontocerebellar hypoplasia. Decreased cerebellar biometry can also be focal.
- *Abnormal cerebellar anatomy*: Abnormal cerebellar anatomy (banana sign) and the nonidentification of obliterated cisterna magna are seen in Chiari II malformation.

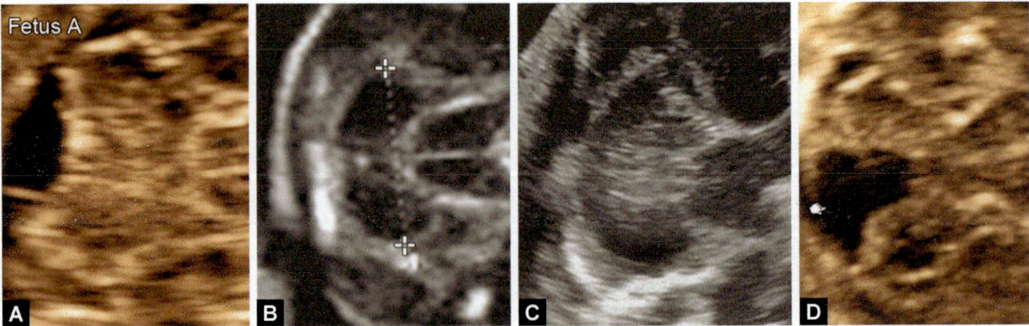

Figs. 11A to D: (A) Normal dumbbell-shaped cerebellum and cisterna magna; (B) Disappearance of cisterna magna and banana-shaped cerebellum—Chiari malformation; (C) Fused cerebellum with absent vermis—rhombencephalosynapsis; (D) Abnormal dilatation of fourth ventricle cyst communication with cisterna magna—Dandy-Walker malformation.

Analysis of vermian fissures, cerebellar hemispheres, and identification of fourth ventricle are important to differentiate rhombencephalosynapsis from partial and complete agenesis[32-34] of vermis (**Fig. 11C**). In this chapter, Chiari malformation and Dandy-Walker malformation are discussed in detail.

Chiari Malformation (Fig. 11B)

Cerebellar herniation into the spinal canal is classified into three types based on the contents of herniated tissue.

1. Type 1—lip of cerebellum.
2. Type 2—part of cerebellum, fourth ventricle, medulla oblongata, and pons.
3. Type 3—large herniation of the posterior fossa.

Incidence—1:1,000.

Synonyms—Arnold-Chiari malformation.

Etiology—Depends on the types.

Pathogenesis—Chiari malformation occurs due to: (1) inferior displacement of the medulla and the fourth ventricle into the upper cervical canal, (2) elongation and thinning of the upper medulla and lower pons and persistence of the embryonic flexure of these structures, (3) inferior displacement of the lower cerebellum through the foramen magnum into the upper cervical region, and (4) a variety of bony defects of the foramen magnum, occiput, and upper cervical vertebrae.

Associated anomalies—88% of fetuses with open spina bifida develop ventriculomegaly and the majority do so by 21 weeks of gestation. Other CNS abnormalities and foot and other system anomalies may be associated with it.

Prenatal diagnosis—lemon and banana signs are evidences of Chiari malformation, which are easily demonstrated in the second trimester. Lemon sign indicates deformity of the frontal bone; banana sign indicates abnormal shape of cerebellum without cisterna magna space (**Figs. 12A and B**).

Prognosis—feeding disturbances, laryngeal stridor, or apneic episodes are found in approximately 9-30% of cases. Prognosis is often poor.

Recurrence risk—depends on the type of malformation.

Dandy-Walker Malformation, Dandy-Walker Variant, and Mega Cisterna Magna

The term Dandy-Walker complex is used to indicate a spectrum of anomalies of the posterior fossa. Dandy-Walker malformation, Dandy-Walker variant, and mega cisterna magna seem to represent a continuum of

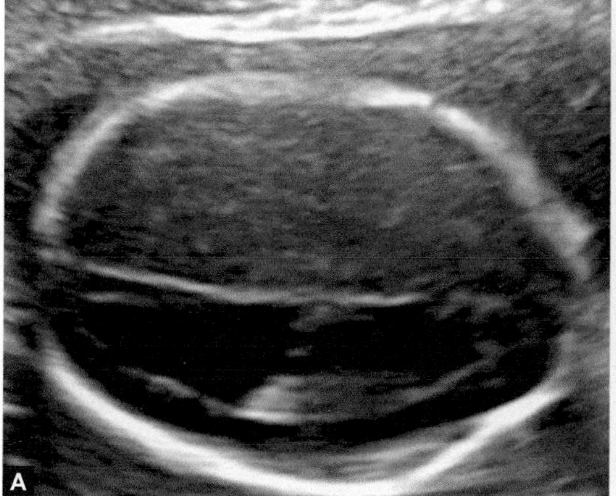

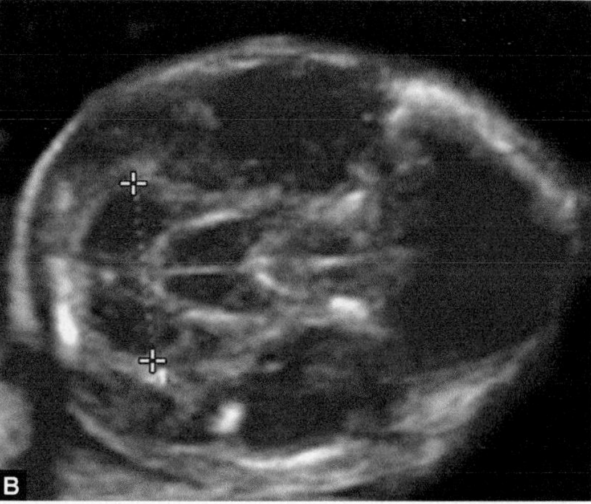

Figs. 12A and B: (A) Dilatation of the lateral cerebral ventricles and "lemon sign" are clearly seen; (B) Disappearance of cisterna magna and banana-shaped cerebellum.

developmental anomalies of the posterior fossa.[35]

Classification:

- *Dandy-Walker malformation (classic)*: Cystic dilation of fourth ventricle, enlarged posterior fossa, elevated tentorium, and complete or partial agenesis of the cerebellar vermis (**Figs. 11D and 13A to C**).
- *Dandy-Walker variant*: Variable hypoplasia of the cerebellar vermis with or without enlargement of the posterior fossa.
- *Mega cisterna magna*: Enlarged cisterna magna with integrity of both cerebellar vermis and fourth ventricle.

Incidence of Dandy-Walker malformation (classic): About 1:30,000 births.

Incidence of Dandy-Walker variant and mega cisterna magna is unknown.

Etiology: Chromosomal aberrations such as partial monosomy/trisomy, viral infections, and diabetes.

Pathogenesis: During development of roof of the fourth ventricle, there is a delay or total failure of the foramen of Magendie to open, allowing a buildup of CSF and development of the cystic dilation of the fourth ventricle. Despite the subsequent opening of the foramina of Luschka, cystic dilation of the fourth ventricle persists and CSF flow is impaired.

Associated anomalies of Dandy-Walker malformation: Cranial abnormalities such as hydrocephalus, ACC, holoprosencephaly, and occipital encephalocele. Extracranial abnormalities such as congenital heart diseases, neural tube defects, and cleft lip/palate.

Prenatal diagnosis: Increased fluid-filled space of the posterior fossa, an ascent of the torcular, and the increased fluid-filled retro- or pericerebellar space are related to an expansion of the fourth ventricle and this is characteristic of Dandy-Walker malformation (perhaps this should be simplified).

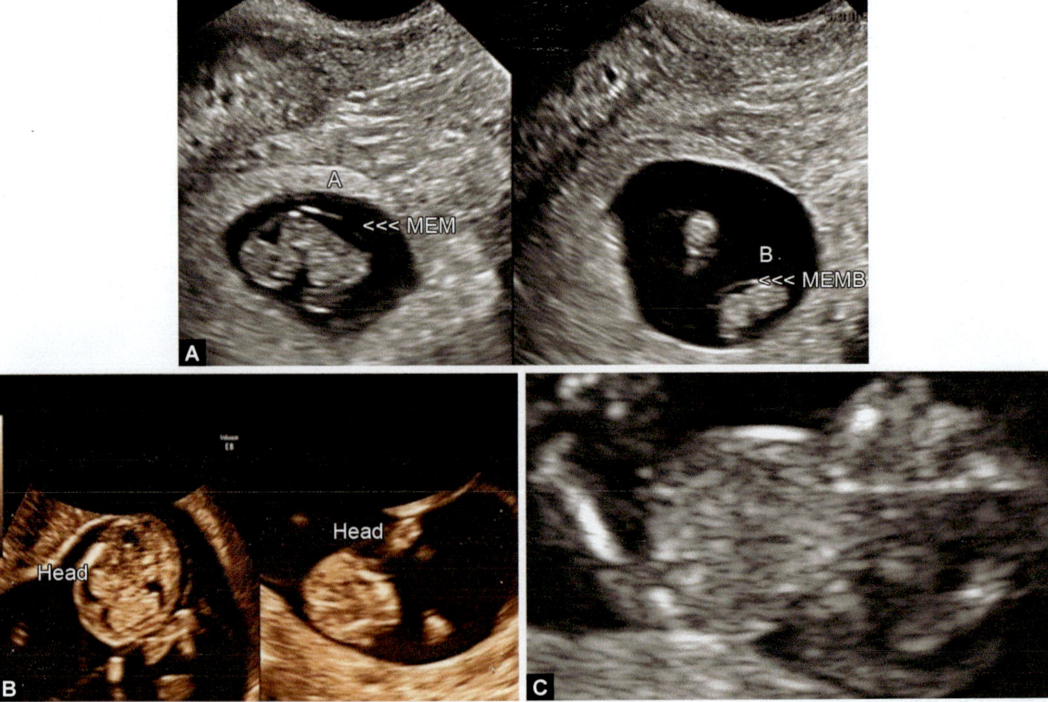

Figs. 13A to C: (A) Monochorionic diamniotic twins at 8 weeks difference in the crown-rump length (CRL); (B) Cranial vault is absent in one twin at 10 weeks; (C) Figure of the same fetus at 14 weeks.

Differential diagnosis: Infratentorial arachnoid cyst, other intracranial cystic tumors, hydrocephalus, and cerebellar dysplasia.

Prognosis: Outcome is generally poor. Nearly 40% of affected fetuses die and 75% of survivors exhibit cognitive deficits.

Recurrence risk: It depends on etiology. Generally, it is 1–5% (Dandy-Walker malformation).

Management: Standard obstetric care and shunting procedures after birth.

NEURAL TUBE DEFECTS

Neural tube gives rise to the brain and the spinal cord. Total or partial closure of the neural groove results in neural tube defects. These include: (1) Anencephaly, (2) Sacral spina bifida, (3) Encephalocele, (4) Open spina bifida, and (5) Craniorachischisis.

Anencephaly (Figs. 14A to C)

Prenatal ultrasound detection of acrania is absence of calvaria above the bony orbits. Exencephaly shows absence of calvaria cephalad to the orbits, but with relatively normal amount of brain tissue.

11–14 weeks of gestational age well-formed brain without calvarium is seen. Brain is not confined by echogenic calvarium and it appears broad and bilobed, as disintegration sites in cystic spaces may be seen.

Base of the skull and face is seen, loose spongy, floating, echogenic glial tissue is seen in the amniotic fluid, and orbits are prominent with frog facies (**Figs. 13 and 15**).[35]

Cephalocele

Herniation of intracranial structures through a calvarial bony defect is termed as a cephalocele (**Figs. 16A and B**). Herniation of meninges alone is meningocele, meninges and part of brain lobe—encepholocele, and ventricles herniation with the brain—encephalocystocele. Depending on the site of the defect, an encephalocele could be occipital, frontal, temporal, or parietal.[35]

Spinal Defects

Failure of closure of the neural tube results in defective fusion of the bony posterior vertebral arch. The defect is classified as open if there is discontinuity in the skin and subcutaneous layer over the defect (85–90%). The defect is classified as closed if the defect is covered with skin (10–15%). In open spina bifida, CSF leaks through the defect into the amniotic cavity, which leads to herniation of the vermis, cerebellar tonsil, and medulla oblongata through the foramen magnum and is termed as Chiari II malformation (**Figs. 17 and 18**). In closed spina bifida (**Figs. 19A to C**), there is no CSF leak into the amniotic cavity and the intracranium is normal.[35]

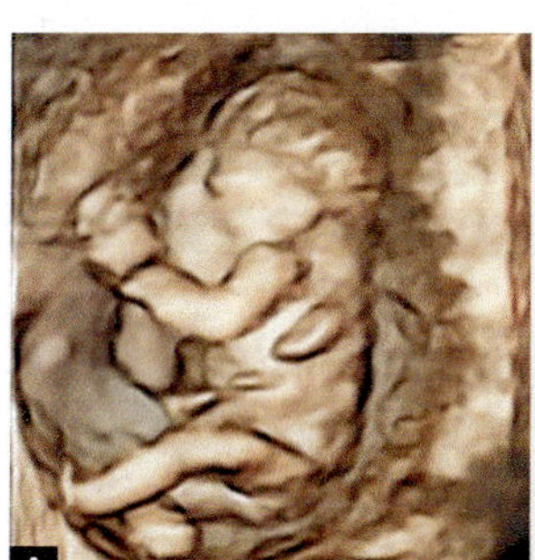

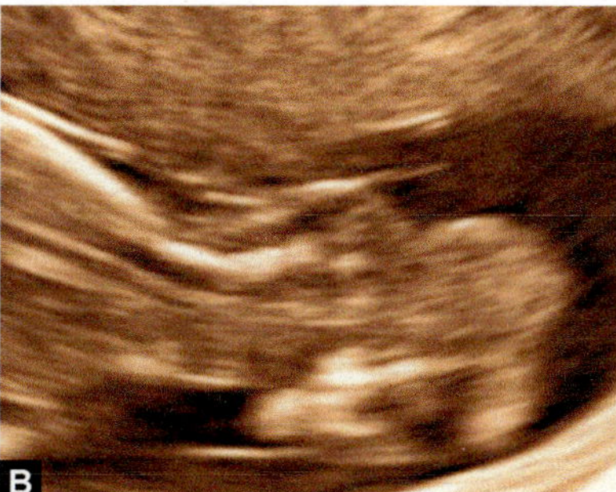

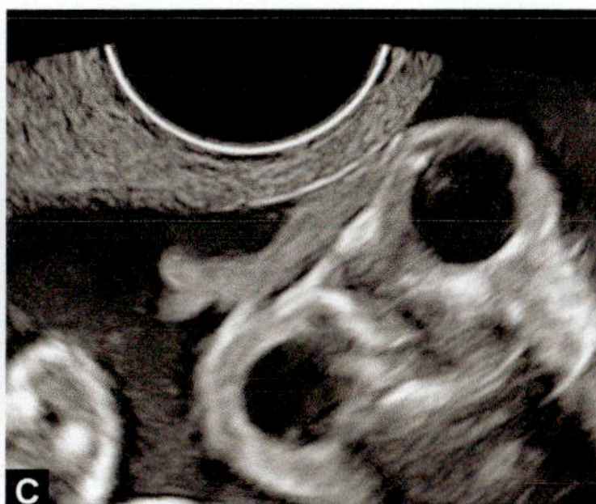

Figs. 14A to C: (A) 13 weeks fetus brain structures are seen covered by membrane; (B) Sagittal section of the fetus and cranial region—absent calvarial bones and spongy neuroglial tissue are seen at 15 weeks; (C) Prominent orbits—frog facies and loose spongy floating glial tissue are seen at 18 weeks.

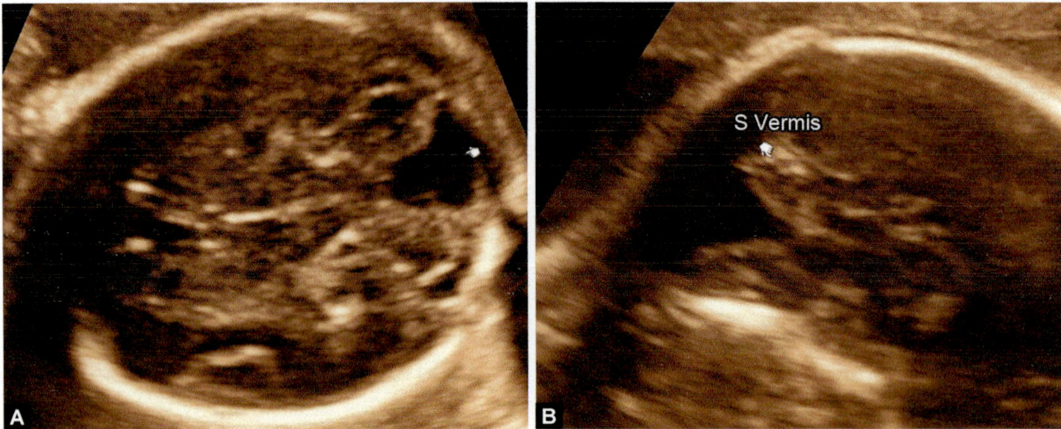

Figs. 15A and B: (A) Vermian hypoplasia with posterior fossa cyst; (B) Ascent of the torcular and the increased fluid-filled retro- or pericerebellar space are related to an expansion of the fourth ventricle and this is characteristic of Dandy–Walker malformation.

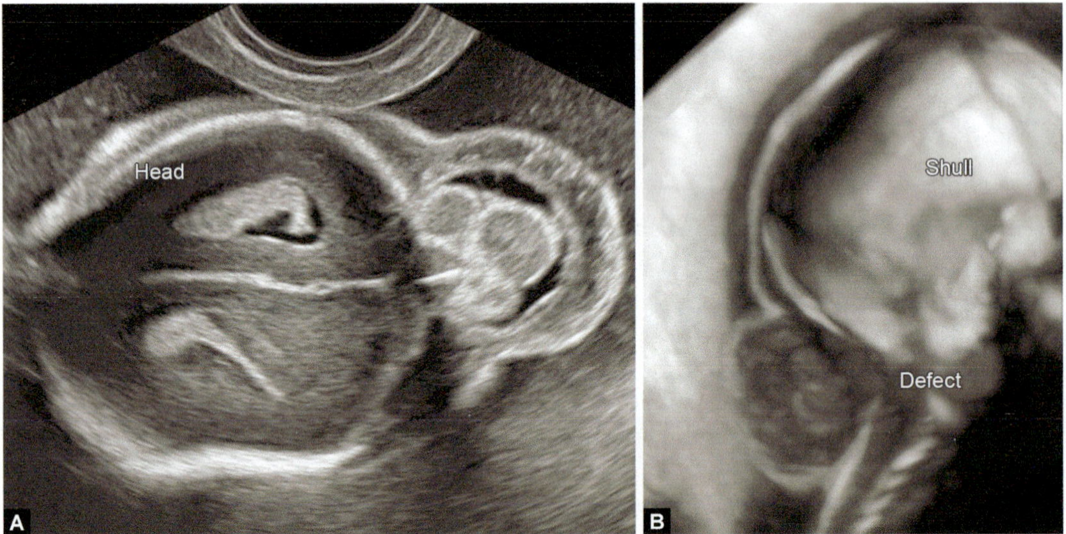

Figs. 16A and B: (A) Axial view of occipital encepholocele is seen; (B) Three-dimensional (3D) picture of the same fetus with the defect at the occipital region.

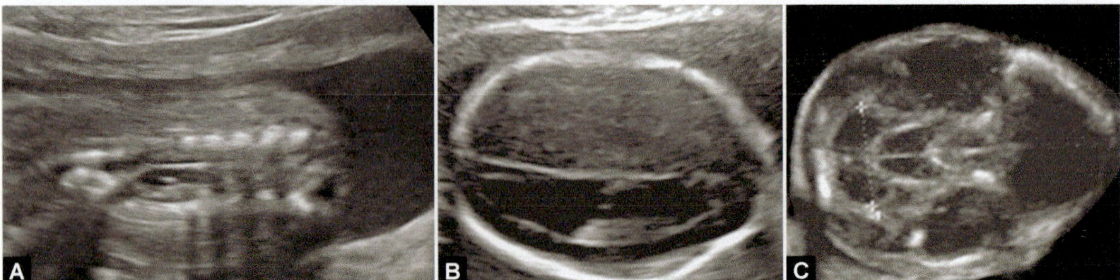

Figs. 17A to C: (A) Open spina bifida—lack of skin continuity over the lesion; (B) Chiari II malformation, lateral ventricular dilatation, and scalloping of the frontal bones (lemon sign); (C) Deformed cerebellum with obliteration of cisterna magna (banana sign).

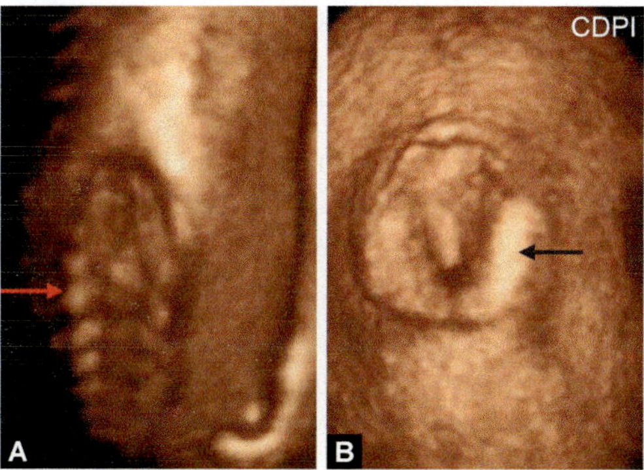

Figs. 18A and B: Three-dimensional (3D) rendering showing open spina bifida (red and black arrows).

EFFECTIVENESS OF ULTRASOUND EXAMINATION OF THE FETAL NEURAL AXIS

In a low-risk pregnancy around midgestation, if the transventricular plane and the transcerebellar plane are satisfactorily obtained, the head measurements (head circumference in particular) are within normal limits for gestational age, the atrial width is <10.0 mm, and the cisterna magna width is between 2 and 10 mm, many cerebral malformations are excluded, the risk of a CNS anomaly is exceedingly low, and further examinations are not indicated.[18] Low-risk patients undergoing basic examinations have reported sensitivities in excess of 80%.

Diagnostic limitations of prenatal ultrasound are well documented and occur for a number of reasons. The brain continues to develop in the second half of gestation and into the neonatal period thus, limiting the detection of anomalies of neuronal proliferation (such as microcephaly, tumors, and cortical malformations). Also, some cerebral lesions are consequence of acquired prenatal or perinatal insults. Detailed evaluation of the fetal CNS (*fetal neurosonogram*) is also possible, but requires specific expertise and

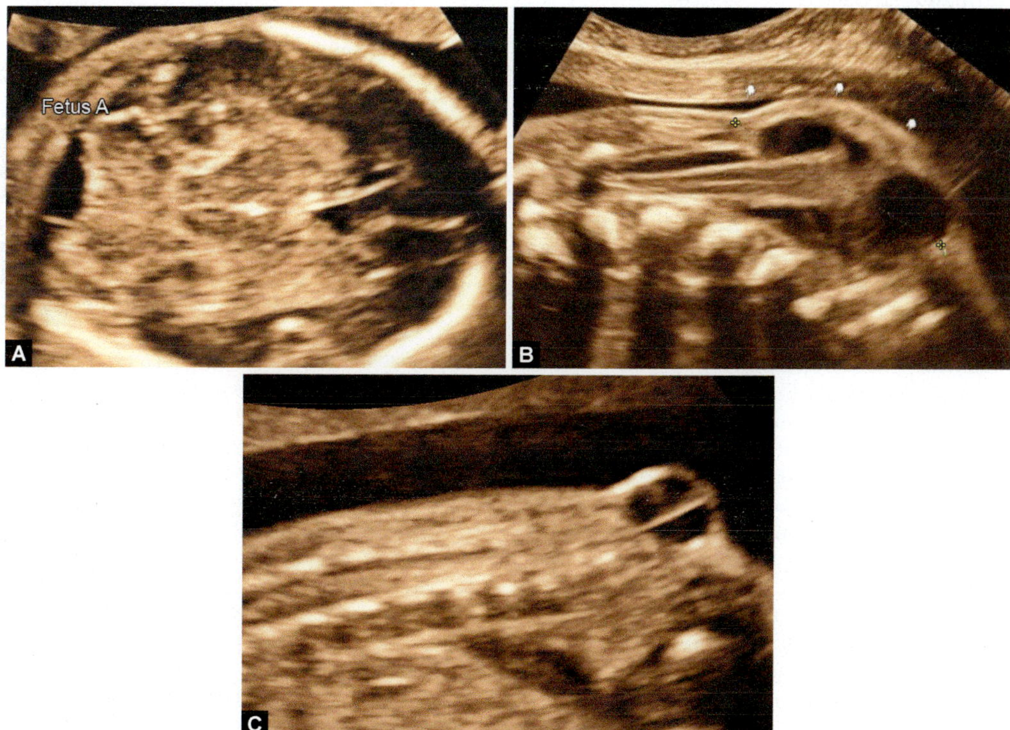

Figs. 19A to C: (A) Normal intracranial anatomy; (B) Closed spina bifida; (C) Sacral closed spina bifida with meningocele.

sophisticated ultrasound machines. This type of examination, at times complemented by 3D ultrasound, is indicated in pregnancies at increased risk of CNS anomalies.

REFERENCES

1. Myrianthopoulos NC. Epidemiology of central nervous system malformations. In: Vinken PJ, Bruyn GW (Eds). Handbook of Clinical Neurology. Elsevier: Amsterdam; 1977. pp. 139-71.
2. Levine D, Barnes PD, Robertson RR, Wong G, Mehta TS. Fast MR imaging of fetal central nervous system abnormalities. Radiology. 2003;229:51-61.
3. Griffiths PD, Paley MN, Widjaja E, Taylor C, Whitby EH. In utero magnetic resonance imaging for brain and spinal abnormalities in fetuses. BMJ. 2005;331:562-5.
4. Malinger G, Ben-Sira L, Lev D, Ben-Aroya Z, Kidron D, Lerman-Sagie T. Fetal brain imaging: a comparison between magnetic resonance imaging and dedicated neurosonography. Ultrasound Obstet Gynecol. 2004;23:333-40.
5. Malinger G, Lev D, Lerman-Sagie T. Is fetal magnetic resonance imaging superior to neurosonography for detection of brain anomalies? Ultrasound Obstet Gynecol. 2002;20:317-21.
6. Ghi T, Pilu G, Savelli L, Segata M, Bovicelli L. Sonographic diagnosis of congenital anomalies during the first trimester. Placenta. 2003;24:S84-7.
7. Monteagudo A, Timor-Tritsch IE. First trimester anatomy scan: pushing the limits. What can we see now? Curr Opin Obstet Gynecol. 2003;15:131-41.
8. Bronshtein M, Ornoy A. Acrania: anencephaly resulting from secondary degeneration of a closed neural tube: two cases in the same family. J Clin Ultrasound. 1991;19:230-4.
9. Blaas HG, Eik-Nes SH, Vainio T, Isaksen CV. Alobar holoprosencephaly at 9 weeks gestational age visualized by two- and three-dimensional ultrasound. Ultrasound Obstet Gynecol. 2000;15:62-5.
10. Blaas HG, Eik-Nes SH, Isaksen CV. The detection of spina bifida before 10 gestational weeks using two- and three-dimensional ultrasound. Ultrasound Obstet Gynecol. 2000;16:25-9.
11. Johnson SP, Sebire NJ, Snijders RJ, Tunkel S, Nicolaides KH. Ultrasound screening for anencephaly at 10–14 weeks of gestation. Ultrasound Obstet Gynecol. 1997;9:14-6.
12. Timor-Tritsch IE, Monteagudo A. Transvaginal fetal neurosonography: standardization of the planes and sections by anatomic landmarks. Ultrasound Obstet Gynecol. 1996;8:42-7.
13. Malinger G, Katz A, Zakut H. Transvaginal fetal neurosonography. Supratentorial structures. Isr J Obstet Gynecol. 1993;4:1-5.
14. Pilu G, Segata M, Ghi T, Carletti A, Perolo A, Santini D, et al. Diagnosis of midline anomalies of the fetal brain with the three-dimensional median view. Ultrasound Obstet Gynecol. 2006;27:522-9.
15. Monteagudo A, Timor-Tritsch IE, Mayberry P. Three-dimensional transvaginal neurosonography of the fetal brain: 'navigating' in the volume scan. Ultrasound Obstet Gynecol. 2000;16:307-13.
16. van den Wijngaard JA, Groenenberg IA, Wladimiroff JW, Hop WC. Cerebral Doppler ultrasound of the human fetus. Br J Obstet Gynaecol. 1989;96:845-9.
17. International Society of Ultrasound in Obstetrics and Gynecology Education Committee. Sonographic examination of the fetal central nervous system: guidelines for performing the 'basic examination' and the 'fetal neurosonogram'. Ultrasound Obstet Gynecol. 2007;29:109-16.
18. Pooh RK, Maeda K, Pooh KH, Kurjak A. Sonographic assessment of the fetal brain morphology. Prenatal Neonat Med. 1999;4:18-38.
19. Pooh RK, Maeda K, Pooh KH. An Atlas of Fetal Central Nervous System Disease: Diagnosis and Management. London: CRC Press; 2003.
20. Vergani P , Locatelli A, Strobelt N, Cavallone M, Ceruti P, Paterlini G, et al. Clinical outcome of mild fetal ventriculomegaly. Am J Obstet Gynecol. 1998;178:218-22.
21. Pilu G, Falco P, Gabrielli S, Perolo A, Sandri F, Bovicelli L. The clinical significance of fetal isolated review cerebral borderline ventriculomegaly: report of 31 cases and review of the literature. Ultrasound Obstet Gynecol. 1999;14:320-6.
22. Senat MV, Bernard JP, Schwarzler P, Britten J, Ville Y. Prenatal diagnosis and follow-up of 14 cases of unilateral ventriculomegaly. Ultrasound Obset Gynecol. 1999;14:327-32.
23. Beke A, Csabay L, Rigo J, Harmath A, Papp Z. Follow-up studies of newborn babies with congenital ventriculomegaly. J Perinant Med. 1999;27:495-505.
24. Greco P, Vimercati A, De Cosmo L, Laforgia N, Mautone A, Selvaggi L. Mild ventriculomegaly as a counseling challenge. Fetal Diagn Ther. 2001;16:398-401.
25. Graham E, Duhl A, Ural S, Allen M, Blkaemore K, Witter F. The degree of antenatal ventriculomegaly is related to pediatric neurological morbidity. J Matern Fetal Med. 2001;10:258-63.

26. Hof MCV, Wilson RD, Diagnostic Imaging Committee, Society of Obstetricians and Gynaecologists of Canada, Genetics Committee, Society of Obstetricians and Gynaecologists of Canada. Fetal soft markers in obstetric ultrasound. J Obstet Gynaecol Can. 2005;27: 592-636.
27. French recommendation of the High Authority of Health regarding the management of fetal cerebral ventriculomegaly.
28. Volpe JJ. Brain tumors and vein of Galen malformation. Neurology of the Newborn, 4th edition. Philadelphia; WB Saunders; 2001. pp. 41-56.
29. Barkovich AJ, Norman D. Absence of the septum pellucidum: a useful sign in the diagnosis of congenital brain malformations. AJR Am J Roentgenol. 1989;152:353-60.
30. Blaas HG, Eriksson AG, Salvesen KA, Isaksen CV, Christensen B, Mollerlokken G, et al. Brains and faces in holoprosencephaly: pre- and postnatal description of 30 cases. Ultrasound Obset Gynecol. 2002;19:24-38.
31. Cohen MM. Holoprosencephaly: clinical, anatomic, and molecular dimensions. Birth Defects Res A Clin Mol Teratol. 2006;76:658-73.
32. Pilu G, Sandri F, Perolo A, Giangaspero F, Giangaspero F, Cocchi G, et al. Prenatal diagnosis of lobar holoprosencephaly. Ultrasound Obstet Gynecol. 1992;2:88-94.
33. Guibaud L, des Portes V. Plea for an anatomical approach to abnormalities of the posterior fossa in prenatal diagnosis. Ultrasound Obstet Gynecol. 2006;27:477-81.
34. Laing F, Frates M, Brown DL, Benson CB, Di Salvo DN, Doubilet PM. Sonography of the fetal posterior fossa: false appearance of mega cisterna magna and Dandy-Walker variant. Radiology. 1994;192:247-51.
35. Rama Murthy BS. Imaging of Fetal Brain and Spine: An Atlas and Guide, 1st edition. Singapore: Springer; 2019.

18

CHAPTER

Fetal Behavior in Normal Pregnancy and Diabetic Pregnancy

Asim Kurjak, Sonal Panchal

INTRODUCTION

Ultrasound has been a modality of choice for assessment of the development of the embryo and fetus in the womb. Three-dimensional (3D) ultrasound has made the study of the fetal anatomy even more accurate and understandable. But the fetal development is not only the development of the structures, it is also their functionality. The functionality of the kidneys, for example, can be confirmed by urine production and filling of the bladder, the functionality of the bladder by its periodical emptying and filling and that of the heart by fetal circulation. The function of the nervous system is the most complex, and this can be studied by fetal movements and fetal expressions. The development of fetal motor behaviors can be studied by real-time ultrasound.[1] The fetal activity observed or recorded with ultrasound equipment is fetal behavior.[2]

Study of the fetal movements has been found to be more correlating with the fetal central nervous system (CNS) development. Studies have shown that the development and maturation of the fetal nervous system is reflected by quality and quantity of fetal movements.[3,4] On comparing the fetal movements with morphological studies, it was found that the fetal behavioral patterns directly reflected the development and maturation of fetal CNS. Therefore, assessment of fetal behavior in different periods of gestation can help distinguish normal brain from abnormal during different phases of development.[5] It also helps to make the diagnosis of functional and structural abnormalities earlier.[6]

B-mode or in a two-dimensional (2D) ultrasound, it is impossible to understand the complexity of these movements and so till the invent of four-dimensional (4D) ultrasound it was not possible to correctly evaluate the fetal movements, especially fetal expressions. The details of fetal face and hands studied by 4D ultrasound has potential to generate information regarding fetal movement and behavior.[7] There is a specific fetal behavioral pattern that corresponds to each week or trimester of fetal life and this pattern reflects the steps of human brain development and maturation.[8-10]

UNDERSTANDING THE NORMAL FETAL ACTIVITY

Spontaneous fetal movements can be observed using 2D ultrasound around 8th gestational week, but 4D ultrasound may show of fetal motility at 7th week of gestation on transvaginal scans.[11,12] From 10 weeks onwards the frequency of fetal movements increase and are maximum between 14 and 19 weeks.[12] The longest interval between movements at this age is 5–6 minutes. Between 9 and 14 weeks of fetal age, mostly general movements are observed.[13]

Using 4D sonography, Kurjak et al. found that from 13th gestational weeks onwards, a "goal orientation" of hand movements **(Figs. 1A to C)** appears and a target point can be recognized for each hand movement. At 15 weeks, 15 different types of movements have been recorded.[14,15]. But according to a study by Kurjak et al., 16 different types of movements can be observed at 15 weeks of gestation.[16]

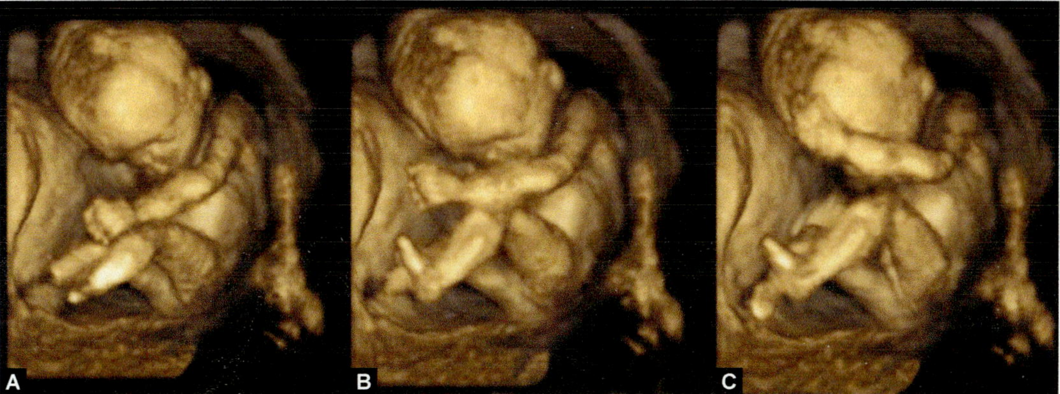

Figs. 1A to C: This series of three pictures show three different positions of hand as three instances of the entire movement of hand to face.

Eye movements are detectable at 16–18 weeks, organized complex movements at 20 weeks, and facial expressions also start at 20 weeks.[17] Facial expressions like smiling, yawning, eyelid movement, mouthing, grimacing, tongue expulsion/swallowing, and sucking were observed during 2nd and 3rd trimester. Mouthing was the most frequent facial movement during early third trimester, where as scowling and sucking were the least frequent.[15,18] In the second half of pregnancy, the frequency of general movements gradually decreases, particularly during the last 10 weeks of pregnancy.[19] In the last trimester of gestation, the range of hand and face movements is the widest.[19] Fetal neuromuscular development is due to alternate periods of increased and decreased movements, though the exact functional significance of the same is still not understood.[20,21]

The movements in an unstimulated fetus is the result of spontaneous behavior without sensory stimulation and is the best method to assess its CNS capacity,[5] and can be used as a marker for fetal brain status.[23] Any fetal brain insult will interfere with endogenous motor activity of the fetus. Genetic factors, external stimuli, pathological conditions, or even environmental changes can affect the fetal human brain up to a degree that may be difficult to assess, especially prenatally. Most times the neurological damage and its effects are difficult to predict.[22,23]

Establishment of neural connections as a developmental process leads to development of new movement patterns of fetus or transformation of existing patterns.[24]

Integrity of the fetal CNS can be assessed by behavioral states of the fetus viz. movement of individual organs like head, trunk, or limbs in an unstimulated but awake fetus and also by qualitative assessment of general movements.[25] When fetal behavior is studied by 4D ultrasound, the altered movement pattern can diagnose abnormal brain development and assist early diagnosis of various abnormalities.[26-28]

The centers in the cerebellum impose controls on the unrestricted movements induced by the lower centers of the brain.[19] The movements also become more complex as pregnancy advances that represent the cerebral maturation. Inhibition is a marker of neurological development (especially cortical centers) and most longitudinal studies have also proved that the fetus becomes less active as gestation advances.[29]

Movements observed and analyzed in 2nd and 3rd trimester are described in **Table 1**.

The spinothalamic tract is established at the 20th week and myelinized by 29th weeks of gestation and the thalamocortical

TABLE 1: Types of hand and facial movements in fetus.[28]

Hand and head movements	*Facial expression*
Head retroflexion	Isolated eye blinking
Head rotation	Mouthing
Head anteflexion	Yawning
Hand to head direction	Tongue expulsion
Hand to eye	Grimacing
Hand to mouth	Swallowing
Hand to face	
Hand to ear	

connections penetrate the cortical plate at 24–26 weeks.[16] Evoked potentials can be detected from the cortex at the 29th week, indicating that the functional connection between periphery and cortex operates from that time onwards.[30,31] This is because of maturation process in the brainstem.[32] Facial expressions are representation of the maturation of the brain. Expressions like grimacing, tongue expulsion, and eye-lid movements **(Figs. 2A and B)** are similar to emotional expressions in adults and can be seen by 4D ultrasound.[17]

General movements (GMs) or Gestalt perception[33] involves the whole body in a variable sequence of arm, leg, neck, and trunk movements. The movements increase and decrease in intensity, but are fluent and elegant, complex and variable. These are called fetal or preterm from 28 to 36 to 38 weeks of postmenstrual age. GMs are considered to be a better predictor of postnatal neurological disability than clinical neurological examination alone.[33]

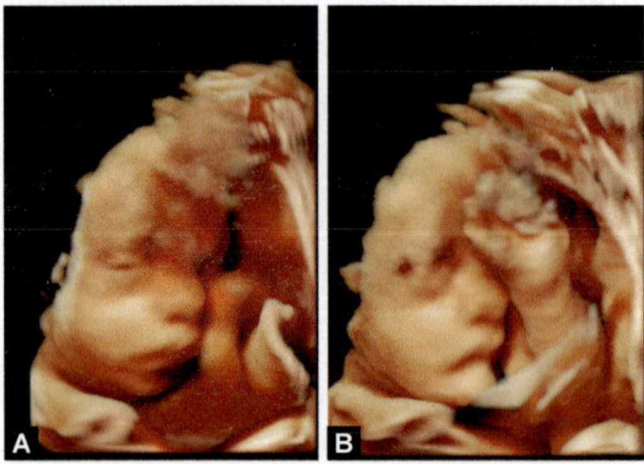

Figs. 2A and B: Eyelid and lip movements: (A) The eye is open and mouth closed; (B) The eye is closed and the mouth is open in the same fetus.

Normal general movements are complex but fluent and involve neck, trunk, and limb movements. Moreover, these should also increase and decrease in their intensity.[34] General movements are complex and fluent and also are not repetitive.[35] If that is not the case, they are considered abnormal.[15,35] Slow, monotonous repetitive movements mimicking cramps are abnormal movements. Even when the movements are occurring with generalized simultaneous muscle contractions and relaxations, it is considered abnormal pattern.[5,23] These also may show variability in strength and the amplitude of movements.[23] These are often seen in the fetuses of mothers with diabetes mellitus, and also other pregnancies at risk like intrauterine growth retardation (IUGR), pregnancy-induced hypertension (PIH), and prematurity.[15] Both term and preterm newborns, who had cerebral insult of any type during their prenatal period may also show abnormal general movement.[11] The identification of fetal CNS depression is based on precompetencies (opening of eyes, variety of facial expressions) also along with the primary reflexes (rhythmical bursts in the sucking pattern) and quality of general movements.[5,36]

Evaluation of general movements must be done on video recordings, may it be prenatal or postnatal. These must be evaluated with "gestalt perception," which could be described as overall impression of GMs with standardized procedure. It is important to recognize, document, and classify the movement pattern and then their complexity, variability, and fluency.[37] These can be classified as normal-optimal, normal-suboptimal, mildly abnormal, and definitely abnormal.[5,11] Quality of neurological movement is more important than the quantity. They can better predict neurodevelopmental outcome than classical neurologic examination alone.

WHY DO FETUSES OF DIABETIC MOTHERS HAVE HIGHER RISK OF NEUROLOGICAL DERANGEMENTS?

Gestational diabetes mellitus with it carries multiple risk factors for the developing fetus, and each have independent effects on neurodevelopment that may impact mnemonic behavior.[38] These risk factors are: (1) chronic hypoxia,[39] (2) hyperglycemia/reactive hypoglycemia, and (3) iron deficiency.[40] On the basis of animal models, these factors selectively affect regions of the fetal brain that are involved in explicit memory (e.g., the hippocampus).[41-43]

Women with diabetic vascular disease have the highest malformation rates, leading to the belief that vascular disease and hypoxia are teratogenic.[43]

Maternal ketonuria in diabetic mothers is associated with reduced intelligence quotient (IQ) in their infants,[43-45] as ketones may interfere with normal development of fetal brain.[43] Abnormal protein synthesis might also result from a lack of glucogenic amino acids or an overabundance of branched-chain amino acids as is seen in poorly controlled diabetes.[43,46] Jovanovic and co-workers (1980) were able to study the pregnancy in diabetic women before the tenth week of gestation. Women with uncontrolled diabetes had estradiol, prolactin, and human chorionic gonadotropin levels below the range associated with normal pregnancy.[43,47]

When these risk factors co-occur, oxygen consumption of the fetus increases and causes fetal hypoxia,[42,48] that can ultimately result in brain iron deficiency through shifting of available fetal iron away from the brain and into the expanding red cell mass.[40,42] Prenatal hypoxia and hyperglycemia/reactive hypoglycemia cause poor behavioral and neurologic outcomes presenting as motor and cognitive deficits in humans[44] and damage to memory areas such as the cerebral cortex, striatum, and hippocampus in animal models.[42,49] These factors together lead to altered normal maturation of the behavioral states in fetuses with IUGR, maternal diabetes mellitus, or alcohol consumption.[50]

WHAT TO OBSERVE FOR?

Assessment of Neurological Function

Even when these movements were documented by 4D ultrasound, it was a very difficult task to classify these movements and based on these to judge the neurological developmental status of fetus. For the first time, a test was structured to assess the fetal CNS integrity and was named as KANET (Kurjak's antenatal neurodevelopmental test).[52] KANET is the first test that is based on 4D ultrasound, with an original scoring system and has been standardized, so it can be implemented in everyday practice, overcoming the practical difficulties and covering the gaps of methods that were used in the past for the evaluation of fetal behavior.[51-53] Improvement of 4D USG technology enabled introduction of KANET, which is a powerful tool in the assessment of fetal behavior and a guide to predict cerebral palsy.[54] After experimental use for 10 years, a consensus was passed in Bucharest concluding that KANET test can be used in everyday clinical practice for follow up of fetuses at neurological risk with strong recommendations for strict and reliable multidisciplinary postnatal follow up for at least 3 years. It has acceptable sensitivity, specificity, positive and negative predictive value for neurodevelopmental anomalies.[55]

The test is of more significance than the morphological studies of the brain. Analysis of the fetal behavior compared with morphological studies has concluded that fetal behavioral patterns are direct reflection of developmental and maturational processes of fetal CNS.[56]

The parameters that have been incorporated in the KANET test are isolated head anteflexion, overlapping cranial sutures, head circumference, isolated eye blinking, facial alterations, mouth opening (yawning or mouthing), isolated hand and leg movements and thumb position, Gestalt perception of general movements.[43,58]

Based on multicentric studies over several years, and on the theory of central pattern generators for general movements, certain fetal movements were chosen as parameters to assess neurological development.[57,58] It is to be performed between 28 and 38 weeks, when fetus is awake. Fetus is observed for 15–20 minutes. If fetus is asleep, the scan is repeated after 30 minutes or after 14–16 hours. Each movement depending on its frequency is given a score of 0, 1, 2 for 9 parameters. A score of 0–5 is abnormal, a score of 6–13 is borderline, and a score of >14 is normal.[59] If the test is abnormal or borderline, it is to be repeated every 2 weeks, till delivery (**Table 2**).[58]

TABLE 2: Score chart of fetal movements according to KANET's.[56]

	Score			
Sign	***0***	***1***	***2***	***Sign Score***
Isolated head anteflexion	Abrupt	Small range (0–3 times of movements)	Variable in full range, many alternation (> 3 times of movements)	
Cranial sutures and head circumference	Overlapping of cranial suttures	Normal cranial sutures with measurement of HC below or above the normal limit (–2 SD) according to GA	Normal cranial sutures with normal measurement of HC according to GA	
Isolated eye blinking	Not present	Not fluent (1–5 times of blinking)	Fluency (> 5 times of blinking)	
Facial alteration (grimace or tongue expulsion) or Mouth opening (yawning or mouthing)	Not present	Not fluent (1–5 times of alteration)	Fluency (> 5 times of alteration)	

Contd...

Contd...

Sign	Score 0	1	2	Sign Score
Isolated leg movement	Cramped	Poor repertoire or small in range (0–5 times of movement)	Variable in full range, many alternation (> 5 times of movements)	
Isolated hand movement or Hand to face movements	Cramped or abrupt	Poor repertoire or small in range (0–5 times of movement)	Variable in full range, many alternation (> 5 times of movements)	
Fingers movements	Unilateral or bilateral clenched fist, (neurological thumb)	Cramped invariable finger movements	Smooth and complex, variable finger movements	
Gestalt perception of GMs	Definitely abnormal	Borderline	Normal	
			Total score	

NEUROLOGICAL FUNCTION IN FETUS OF A DIABETIC FEMALE

The results of a study by Edelberg et al. (1987) and Robertson et al. have shown that it is actually the changing maternal blood glucose level that affects the cyclicity and frequency of fetal motor activity, rather than persistently high blood glucose levels.[21,60]

Schulte et al.[61] studied the neurological development of infants of diabetic mothers, and found longer rapid eye movement sleep in newborn infants of diabetic mothers.

There is evidence that it is the concurrent maternal blood glucose levels according to which the fetal movements may be affected in diabetic and nondiabetic pregnancies, but different studies have mixed results. Some studies have reported increased and some have shown decreased fetal movement with elevated blood glucose levels.[21,62-67]

Some have reported decreased fetal movement,[68-70] and others have reported no effects.[71-75] An increased rate of minor neurological dysfunction was found in a group of 32 children born to mothers with gestational diabetes, including some fine and gross motor deficits, compared with a group of control children.[76,77]

Abnormalities in the fetal motor activity may consists of a delayed first emergence of specific movements, quantitative changes, and an abnormal quality of movements (i.e., changes in execution of movement patterns) and abnormal development of fetal behavioral states.[49,55,56] Qualitative and quantitative assessment of fetal movements can be used for the recognition of cerebral dysfunctions and probably neuromuscular ailments. Alteration in the normal movement pattern in terms of frequency and strength is seen in IUGR, the pathophysiology of which is fetal hypoxia. In the fetuses of diabetic mothers, fetal hypoxia is the main pathophysiological factor and so similar changes in fetal movements can be observed. A study on diabetes-related influence on fetal motor activity revealed 1–2 week delayed appearance of almost all fetal behavioral patterns in first 12 weeks of pregnancy except the fetal breathing movements.[15,49]

Fetal breathing pattern is considered to be one of the important parameters of fetal well-being in late diabetic pregnancies. It is not affected by Braxton-Hicks contractions. This means that the fetal neural control of fetal breathing like movements differ in diabetic pregnancy, than is normal.[15,78]

CYCLIC MOTILITY

Other aspects of fetal neurobehavioral organization are influenced by the altered metabolic environment.[79-90] In spite of good clinical control of diabetes, the infants of these mothers have a risk of compromised neurological developmental outcome.[21,91-99]

Spontaneous fetal movement in the last trimester of human gestation is dominated by irregular oscillations on a scale of minutes (cyclic motility, CM).[21] The movement pattern increased and decreased movements in cyclicity in normal females is steady but is altered in mothers with increased blood glucose levels.[21] Early in the third trimester, changes in the rate of oscillation in fetal CM between the two periods of activity were inversely related to changes in maternal blood glucose levels.[21] It is seen that relatively short-term fluctuations in maternal glucose metabolism, rather than chronically elevated blood glucose, per se, is the effective perturbation of the intrinsic cyclic patterns in spontaneous fetal motor activity in diabetic pregnancies. The results revealed that fetal CM is more sensitive to fluctuations in maternal blood glucose levels during the early part of the third trimester of gestation than during the middle or end of the third trimester. The results suggest that disruption of the temporal organization of spontaneous fetal motor activity in diabetic pregnancies represents an acute response to fluctuations in the metabolic environment rather than alteration of CM development.[100,101]

But according to other studies, the transient abnormality maternal glucose metabolism may affect fetal CM but does not cause any increased risk of poor general developmental outcome in children of diabetic mothers.[21,100] The effects are similar in the fetuses of mothers with type I or gestational diabetes, and no difference when fetuses later classified as appropriate for large for gestational age were considered separately ($p > 0.05$).[21,100]

EFFECT DURING INFANCY AND CHILDHOOD

When gross motor functions were studied in children of diabetic mothers the Bruininks–Oseretsky test of motor proficiency, it was observed that these children were weak performers as compared to the controls.[76] Maternal diabetes adversely affects some fine neurological functions in children at school age, but not their cognitive scores.[76] These effects are not correlated with the degree of glycemic control.[102] Developmental delay, learning difficulties at school, and a high rate of attention and hyperactivity disorders are more often seen in the children born after high-risk pregnancies.[76,103] These children in their early school age have more soft neurological signs (signs of mild, nonspecific brain damage), and lower gross and fine motor achievements than pair matched control children born to nondiabetic mothers.[76,104,105] Variability in muscle tone (hypertonicity or hypotonicity) may cause delayed or abnormal motor development (Miyahara M, Department of Kinesiology, UCLA; unpublished observations).

Children born to the mothers having infants of diabetic mothers (IDM) had a risk of shorter gestational age (mean 38 weeks, SD 2), greater standardized birth weight scores (mean 3,797 g, SD 947), and lower iron stores (mean ferritin concentration 87 µg/L, SD 68) in comparison with the control group.[42]

Children born to the mothers whose diabetes was diagnosed late in pregnancy, had lower cognitive scores and verbal performance compared with controls.[76,106,107]

CAN KANET PREDICT THESE ABNORMALITIES

KANET can be useful for early diagnosis of neurological disorders that become manifest in perinatal and postnatal period.[50] The authors observed that a low KANET score is predictive of both intrauterine or neonatal death.[52] The study demonstrated the evaluated and accepted KANET to detect and discriminate normal and abnormal fetal behavior in normal and in high-risk pregnancies.[108] Except for higher incidence in the abnormal group, there was no marked difference in the different motor patterns studied.[109,110]

Analysis of sick preterm infants revealed a "reduction of elegance and fluency, variability, fluctuation in intensity and speed instead of change in incidence of distinct motor patterns."[31,111-113] Abo-Yaqoub et al. showed in their study that the difference between the two groups were in isolated head anteflexion (**Figs. 3A to C**), isolated eye blinking, facial expressions, mouth movements (**Figs. 4A to C**), finger movements (**Figs. 5A to C**), isolated hand movements, hand-to-face movements (**Figs. 6A to D**), and general movements (**Figs. 7A to D**). For isolated leg movements (**Figs. 8A to D**) and cranial sutures, the difference was not significant.[114]

Athanasiadis et al. in 2013 applied KANET test to assess and compare fetal behavior and neurodevelopment in 152 pregnant women, classified as low-risk (n = 78) and high-risk (n = 74) pregnancies in the second and third trimester.[42] The neurodevelopmental score was statistically significantly higher in the low-risk group compared to the high-risk group.[42] Though the score was higher in diabetes subgroup compared to the IUGR and the pre-eclampsia subgroup.[114]

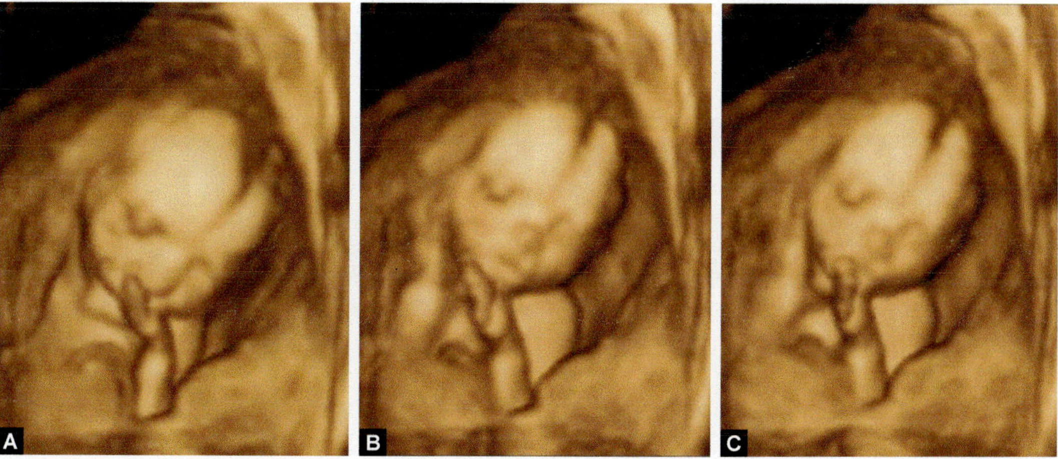

Figs. 3A to C: Anteflexion of the fetal head seen in (A), reverted back to the neutral position in (B) and (C) again shows a slight anteflexion.

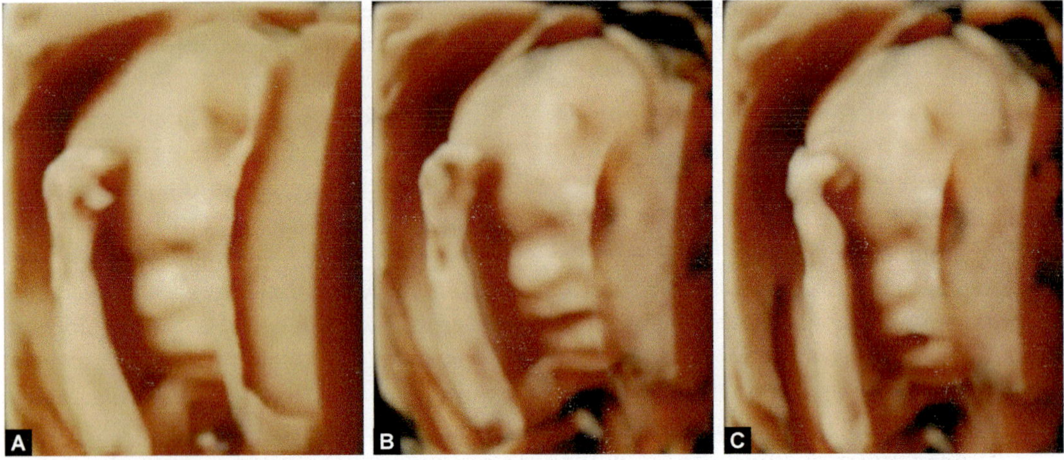

Figs. 4A to C: The series of images from (A) to (C) shows opening of the fetal mouth.

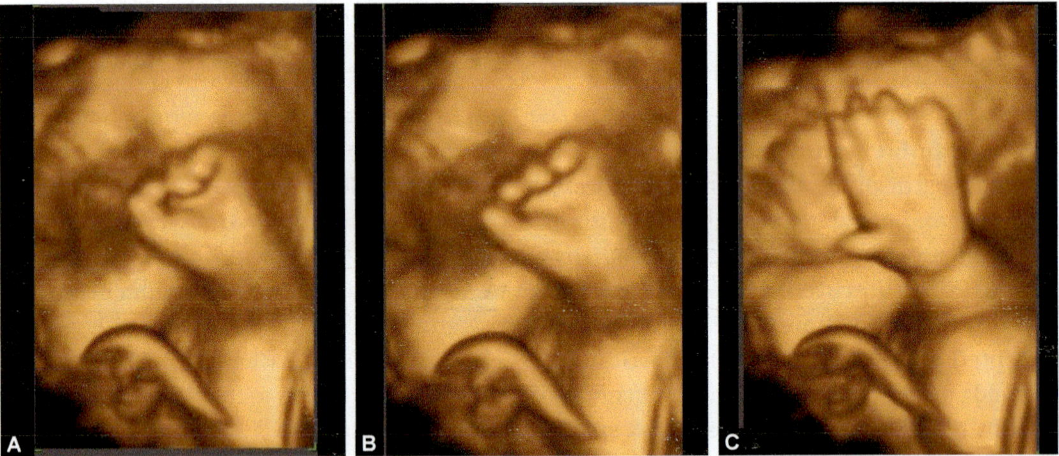

Figs. 5A to C: Movement of thumb noted as thumb fixed to fingers and flexed in (A), thumb close to fingers but extended in (B), and thumb separate from fingers in (C).

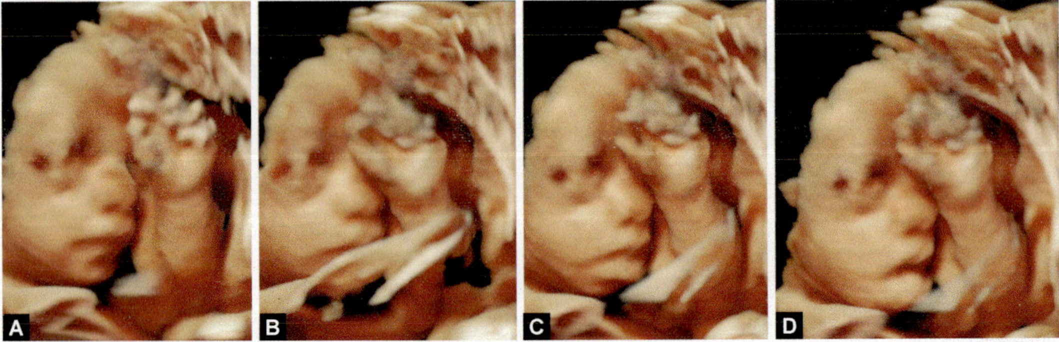

Figs. 6A to D: (A) The image of the fetal face with eye open and hand close to the chin; (B) The hand raised to fetal eye and eye is hidden by the hand; (C) Supination of the hand and abduction of thumb and extension of fingers; (D) Supination of the hand and abduction of thumb and extension of fingers; and open mouth.

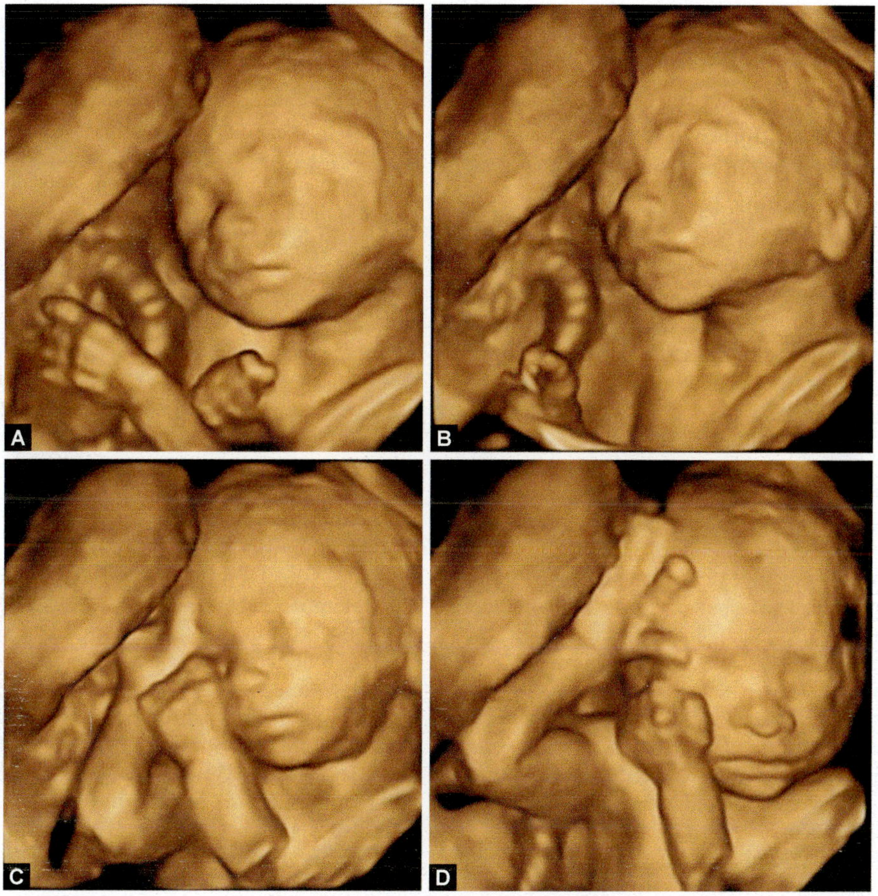

Figs. 7A to D: Fetal head rotation and anteflexion movement with movement of the hand seen from (A) to (D), as a part of general movement.

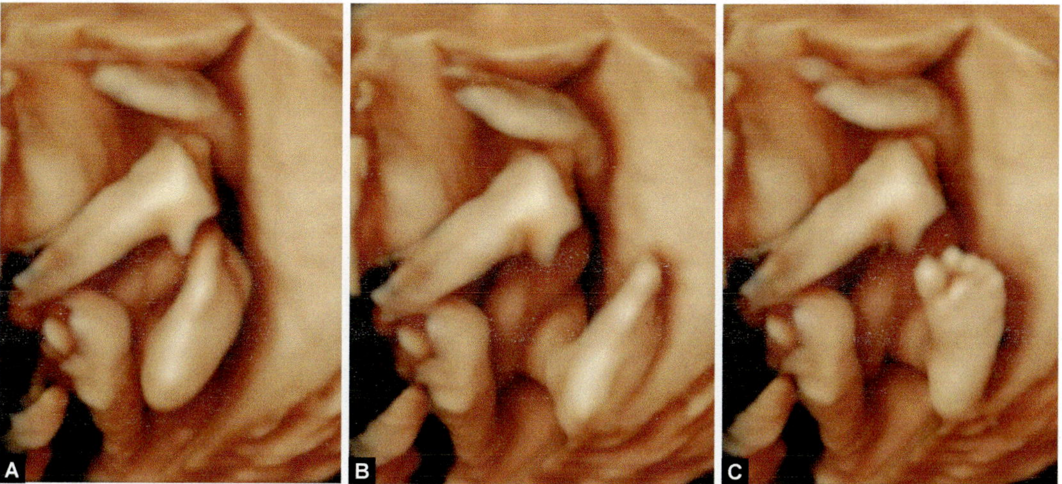

Figs. 8A to C: Partially flexed leg is seen in (A) and extension of the same is seen in (B and C).

CONCLUSION

Inadequate glycemic control and vascular pathologies are the chief causes of neurological developmental inadequacies in fetuses of diabetic mothers. These can be assessed and predicted antenatally by KANET test.

REFERENCES

1. Roodenburg PJ, Wlasimiroff JW, van Es A, Prechtl HH. Classification and quantitative aspects of fetal movements during the second half of normal pregnancy. Early Hum Dev. 1991;25(1):19-35.
2. de Vries JI, Fong BF. Normal fetal motility: An overview. Ultrasound Obstet Gynecol. 2006;27:701-11.
3. Prechtl HFR. Qualitative changesof spontaneous movements in fetus and preterm infant are amarker of neurological dysfunction. Early Hum Dev. 1990;23:151-8.
4. DiPietro JA. Neurobehavioral assessment before birth. Mental Retar Dev Disabil Res Rev. 2005;11:4-13
5. Kurjak A, Predojevic M, Stanojevic M, Salihagic-Kadic A, Miskovic B, Badreldeen A, et al. Intrauterine growth restriction and cerebral palsy. Acta Inform Med. 2010;18(2):64-82.
6. Einspieler C, Prechtl HF, Ferrari F, Cioni G, Bos AF. The qualitative assessment of general movements in preterm, term and young infants review of the methodology. Early Hum Dev. 1997;50(1):47-60.
7. Moster D, Wilcox AJ, Vollset SE, Markestad T, Lie RT. Cerebral palsy among term and post-term births. JAMA. 2010;304(9):976-82.
8. Yigiter AB, Kavak ZN. Normal standards of fetal behavior assessed by four-dimensional sonography. J Matern Fetal Neonatal Med. 2006;19(11):707-21.
9. Rees S, Harding R. Brain development during fetal life: influences of the intrauterine environment. Neurosci Lett. 2004;361(1-3):111-4.
10. Kurjak A, Carrera JM, Stanojevic M, Andonotopo W, Azumendi G, Scazzocchio E, et al. The role of 4D sonography in the neurological assessment of early human development. Ultrasound Rev Obstet Gynecol. 2004;4(3):148-59.
11. Araki M, Nishitani S, Ushimaru K, Masuzaki H, Oishi K, Shinohara K. Fetal response to induced maternal emotions. J Physiol Sci. 2010;60:213-20.
12. Salihagic-Kadic A, Medic M, Kurjak A, Andonotopo W, Azumendi G, Hafner T, et al. Four-dimensional sonography in the assessment of fetal functional neuro-development and behavioural patterns. Ultrasound Rev Obstet Gynecol. 2005;5:154-68.
13. Andonotopo W, Kurjak A, Azumendi G. Ultrasound studies on early pregnancy. In: Kurjak A, Carrera JM (Eds). Atlas of Clinical Applications of Ultrasound in Obstetrics and Gynecology. New Delhi: Jaypee Brothers Medical Publishers; 2005.
14. Azumendi G, Arenas JB, Andonotopo W, Kurjak A. Three dimensional sonoembryology. In: Kurjak A, Arenas JB (Eds). Textbook of Transvaginal Sonography. London: Taylor and Francis; 2005. p. 407.
15. Kurjak A, Predojvic M, Stanojevic M, Talic A, Honemeyer U, Kadic AS. The use of 4D imaging in the behavioural assessment of high risk fetuses. Imaging Med. 2011;3(5):557-69.
16. Kurjak A, Carrera JM, Medic M, Azumendi G, Andonotopo W, Stanojevic M. The antenatal development of fetal behavioural patterns assessed by four dimensional sonography. J Matern Fetal Neonatal Med. 2005;17(6):401-16.
17. Andonotopo W, Medic M, Sahilagic-Kadic A, Milenkovic D, Maiz N, Scazzocchio E. The assessment of fetal behavior in early pregnancy: Compariosion between 2D and 4D songraphic scanning. J Perinat Med. 2005;33(5):406-14.
18. de Vries JIP, Visser GHA, Prechtl HFR. The emergence of fetal behavior I. Qualitative aspects. Early Hum Dev. 1982;7(4):301-22.
19. D'Elia A, Pighetti M, Moccia G, Santangelo N. Spontaneous motor activity in the normal fetus. Early Hum Dev. 2001;65(2):139-44.
20. Kurjak A, Stanojevic M, Andonotopo W, Salihagic-Kadic A, Carrera JM, Azumendi G. Behavioral pattern continuity from prenatal to postnatal life: A study by four-dimensional (4D) ultrasonography. J Perinat Med. 2004;32: 346-53.
21. Robertson SS, Dierker LJ. Fetal cyclic motor activity in diabeteic pregnancies: Sensitivity to maternal blood glucose. [Online] Available from www.interscience.wiley.com [Last accessed Sep., 2021].
22. Yan F, Dai SY, Akther Nm Kuno A, Yanagihara T, Hata T. Four dimensional sonographic assessment of fetal epression in early third trimester. J Gynecol Obstet. 2006;94(2):108-13.
23. Einspieler C, Prechtl HFR, Bos AF, Ferrari F, Cioni G. Prechtl's method on the qualitative assessment of general movements in preterm, term and young infants. Cambridge: Mac Keith Press; 2004.
24. Robertson SS. Mechanism and function of cyclicity in spontaneous movement. In: Smotherman WP, Robinson SR (Eds). Behavior

of the Fetus. Caldwell, NJ: Telford Press; 1988. pp. 77-94.

25. Nijhuis JG (Ed). Fetal Behaviour: Developmental and Perinatal Aspects. Oxford: Oxford University Press; 1992.
26. Kurjak A, Luetic AT. Fetal neurobehavior assessed by three-dimensional/four dimentional sonography. Zdrav Vestn. 2010;79:790-9.
27. Ameil-Tison C, Gosselin J, Kurjak A. Neurosonography in the second half of fetal life: A neonatologist's point of view. J Perinat Med. 2006;34:437-46.
28. Kurjak A, Azumendi G, Vecek N, Kupesic S, Solak M, Varga D, et al. Fetal hand movements and facial expression in normal pregnancy studied by four-dimensional sonography. J Perinat Med. 2003;31(6):496-508.
29. Ten Hof J, Nijhuis JM, Mulder EJH, Nijhuis JG, Narayan H, Taylor DJ, et al. Longitudinal study of fetal body movements: Nomograms, Intrafetal consistency and relationships with Episodes of heart rate patterns A and B. Pediatric Res. 2002:52(4);568-75.
30. Kurjak A, Andonotopo W, Stanojevic M, Milenkovic D, Azumendi G, Hafner T, et al. Longitudinal study of fetal behaviour by four dimensional sonography. Ultrasound Rev Obstet Gynecol. 2005;5(4):259-74.
31. Kostovic I, Rakic P. Development of prestriate visual projections in the monkey and human fetal cerebrum revealed by transient cholinesterase staining. J Neurosci. 1984;4(1):25-42.
32. Joseph R. Fetal brain and cognitive development. Dev Rev. 2000;20(1):81-98.
33. Prechtl HF, Einspieler C. Is neurological assessment of the fetus possible? Eur J Obstet Gynecol. 1997;75(1):81-4.
34. Hadders-Algra M, Klip-Van den Nieuwendijk A, Martijn A, van Eyken L A. Assessment of general movements: towards a better understanding of a sensitive method to evaluate brain function in young infants. Dev Med Child Neurol. 1997;39(2):89-99.
35. Salihagic-Kadic A, Medic M, Kurjak A. Neurophysiology of fetal behavior. Ultrasound Rev Obstet Gynecol. 2004;1-12:2-11.
36. Kurjak A, Carrera JM, Andonotopo W, Azumendi G, Medic MA, Salihagic-Kadic A. Behavioural perinatology assessed by four dimensional sonography. Textbook Perinatal Med. 2003;42:582-88.
37. Einspieler C, Prechtl HFR, Bos AF, Ferrari F, Cioni G. Prechtl's method on the qualitative assessment of general movements in preterm, term and young infants. Cambridge: Mac Keith Press; 2004.
38. DeBoer T, Wewerka S, Bauer PJ, Georgieff MK, Nelson CA. Explicit memory performance in infants of diabetic mothers at one year of age. Dev Med Child Neurol. 2005;47(8):525-31.
39. Cioni G, Prechtl HFR, Ferrari F, Paolicelli PB, Einspieler C, Roversi MF. Which better predicts later outcome in full term infants: quality of general movements or neurological examination? Early Hum Dev. 1997;50(1): 71-85.
40. Widness JA, Susa JB, Garcia JF, Singer OB, Sehgal P, Oh W, et al. Increased erythropoiesis and elevated erythropoietin in infants born to diabetic mothers and in hyperinsulinemic rhesus fetuses. J Clin Invest. 1981;67:637-42.
41. Petry CD, Eaton MA, Wobken JD, Mills MM, Johnson DE, Georgieff MK. Iron deficiency of liver, heart, and brain in newborn infants of diabetic mothers. J Pediatr. 1992;121:109-14.
42. Barks JD, Sun R, Malinak C, Silverstein FS. gp120, an HIV-1 protein, increases susceptibility to hypoglycemic and ischemic brain injury in perinatal rats. Exp Neurol. 1995;132:123-33.
43. Mills JL. Malformations in infants of diabetic mothers. Birth Defects Res A Clin Mol Teratol. 2010;88(10):769-78.
44. de Ungria M, Rao R, Wobken JD, Luciana M, Nelson CA, Georgieff MK. Perinatal iron deficiency decreases cytochrome c oxidase (CytOx) activity in selective regions of neonatal rat brain. Pediatr Res. 2000;48:169-76.
45. Churchill JA, Berendes HW, Nemore J. Neuropsychological deficits in children of diabetic mothers: A report from the collaborative study of cerebral palsy. Am J Obstet Gynecol. 1969;105:257-68.
46. Stehbens JA, Baker GL, Kitchell M. Outcome at ages 1, 3, and 5 years of children born to diabetic women. Am J Obstet Gynecol. 1977;127:408-413.
47. Felig P, Marliss E, Ohman JL, Cahill GF. Plasmo amino acid levels in diabetic ketoacidosis. Diabetes. 1970;19:727-8.
48. Jovanovic L, Peterson CM, Saxena BB, Dawood YM, Saudek CD. Feasibility of maintaining normal glucose profiles in insulin-dependent pregnant diabetic women. Am J Med. 1980;68:105-12.
49. Morokuma S, Fukushima K, Yumoto Y, Uchimura M, Fujiwara A, Matsumoto M, et al. Simplified ultrasound screening for fetal brain function based on behavioral pattern. Early Hum Dev. 1982;6(2):177-95.
50. Horimoto N, Koyanagi T, Maeda H, Satoh S, Takashima T, Minami T, et al. Can brain impairment be detected by in utero behavioural patterns? Arch Dis Child. 1993;69(1 Spec No): 3-8.

51. Nijhuis JG, Prechtl HF, Martin CB, Bots RS. Are there behavioral states in the human fetus? Early Hum Dev. 1982;6(2):177-95.
52. Kurjak A, Andonotopo W, Hafner T, Salihagic-Kadic A, Stanojevic M, Azumendi G, et al. Normal standards for fetal neurobehavioral development—longitudinal quantification by four-dimensional sonography. J Perinat Med. 2006;34(1):56-65.
53. Stanojevic M, Antsaklis P, Kadic AS, Predojevic M, Vladareanu R, Vladareanu S, et al. Is Kurjak antenatal neurodevelopmental test ready for routine clinical application? Bucharest Consensus Statement. Donald Sch J Ultrasound Obstet Gynecol. 2015: 9(3):260-5.
54. Rosier-van Dunne FM, van Wezel-Meijler G, Bakker MP, Odendaaal HJ, de Vries JI. Fetal general movements and brain sonography in a population at risk for preterm birth. Early Hum Dev. 2010;86:107-11.
55. Kurjak A, Stanojevic M, Andonotopo W, Scazzocchio-Duenas E, Azumendi G, Carrera JM. Fetal behavior assessed in all three trimesters of normal pregnancy by four-dimensional ultrasonography. Croat Med J. 2005;46(5):772-80.
56. Stanojevic M, Talic A, Miskovic B, Vasilj O, Naim Shaddad A, Ahmed B, et al. An attempt to standardize Kurjak's antenatal neurodevelopmental test: Osaka consensus statement. Donald Sch J Ultrasound Obstet Gynecol. 2011;5(4):317-29.
57. Ahmed B, Azumendi G, Vasilj O, AndonotopoW, Turudic T, Salihagic-Kadic A. New scoring system for fetal neurobehavior assessed by three-and fourdimensional sonography. J Perinat Med. 2008;36:73-81.
58. Low JA, Galbraith RS, Muir DW, Killen HL, Pater EA, Karchmar EJ. Factors associated with motor and cognitive deficits in children after intrapartum fetal hypoxia. Am J Obstet Gynecol. 1984;148:533-9.
59. Nelson C, Silverstein FS. Acute disruption of cytochrome oxidase activity in brain in a perinatal rat stroke model. Pediatr Res. 1994;36:12-9.
60. Visser GH, Mulder EJ, Tessa Ververs FF. Fetal behavioural teratology. J Matern Fetal Neonatal Med. 2010;23(Suppl 3):14-6.
61. Visser GH, Bekedam DJ, Mulder EJ, van Ballegooie E. Delayed emergence of fetal behavior in type-1 diabetic women. Early Hum Dev. 1985;12(2):167-72.
62. Aladjem S, Feria A, Rest J, Gull K, O'Connor M. Effect of maternal glucose load on fetal activity. Am J Obstet Gynecol. 1979;134:276-80.
63. Eller DP, Stramm SL, Newman RB. The effect of maternal intravenous glucose administration on fetal activity. Am J Obstet Gynecol. 1992;167:1071-4.
64. Gelman SR, Spellacy WN, Wood S, Birk SA, Buhi WC. Fetal movements and ultrasound: Effect of maternal intravenous glucose administration. Am J Obstet Gynecol. 1980;137:459-61.
65. Goodman JD. The effect of intravenous glucose on human fetal breathing measured by Doppler ultrasound. Br J Obstet Gynaecol. 1980;87:1080-3.
66. Miller FC, Skiba H, Klapholz H. The effect of maternal blood sugar levels on fetal activity. Obstet. Gynecol. 1978;52:662-5.
67. Richardson B, Briggs ML, Toomey C, Burry KJ, O'Grady JP. The effect of maternal glucose administration on the specificity of the nonstress test. Am J Obstet Gynecol. 1983;145:141-6.
68. Allen CL, Kisilevsky BS. Fetal behavior in diabetic and nondiabetic pregnant women: An exploratory study. Dev Psychobiol. 1999;35:69-80.
69. Edelberg SC, Dierker L, Kalhan S, Rosen MG. Decreased fetal movements with sustained maternal hyper-glycemia using the glucose clamp technique. Am J Obstet Gynecol. 1987;156:1101-5.
70. Holden KP, Jovanovic L, Druzin ML, Peterson CM. Increased fetal activity with low maternal blood glucose levels in pregnancies complicated by diabetes. Am J Perinatol. 1984;1:161-4.
71. Bocking AD. Observations of biophysical activities in the normal fetus. Clin Perinatol. 1989;16:583-94.
72. Bocking A, Adamson L, Carmichael L, Patrick J, Probert C. Effect of intravenous glucose injection on human maternal and fetal heart rate at term. Am J Obstet Gynecol. 1984;148:414-20.
73. Bocking A, Adamson L, Cousin A, Campbell K, Carmichael L, Natale R, et al. Effects of intravenous glucose injections on human fetal breathing movements and gross fetal body movements at 38 to 40 weeks' gestational age. Am J Obstet Gynecol. 1982;142:606-11.
74. Reece EA, Hagay Z, Roberts AB, DeGennaro N, Homko CJ, Connolly-Diamond M, et al. Fetal Doppler and behavioral responses during hypoglycemia induced with the insulin clamp technique in pregnant diabetic women. Am J Obstet Gynecol. 1995;172:151-5.
75. Patrick J, Campbell K, Carmichael L, Natale R, Richardson B. Patterns of gross fetal body movements over 24-hour observation intervals during the last 10 weeks of pregnancy. Am J Obstet Gynecol. 1982;42:363-71.
76. Ornoy A, Ratzon N, Greenbaum C, Peretz E, Soriano D, Dulitzky M. Neurobehaviour of school

age children born to diabetic mothers. Arch Dis Child Fetal Neonatal Ed. 1998;79(2):F94-9.

77. Wolf A. Developmental evaluation on early school age chil-dren born to gestational diabetic mothers. MSc thesis. Jerusalem, Israel: Hebrew University: 1997.
78. Mulder EJ, Leiblum DM, Visser GH. Fetal breathing movements in late diabetic pregnancy: relationship to fetal heart rate patterns and Braxton Hicks' contractions. Early Hum Dev. 1995;43(3):225-32.
79. Edelberg SC, Dierker L, Kalhan S, Rosen MG. Decreased fetal movements with sustained maternal hyperglycemia using the glucose clamp technique. Am J Obstet Gynecol. 1987;156:1101-5.
80. Schulte FJ, Lasson U, Parl U, Nolte R, Jurgens U. Brain and behavioral maturation in newborn infants of diabetic mothers. II. Sleep cycles. Neuropadiatrie. 1969;1(1):36-43.
81. Robertson SS, Dierker LJ. Fetal cyclic motor activity in diabetic pregnancies: Sensitivity to maternal blood glucose. Dev Psychobiol. 2003;42:9-16.
82. Devoe LD, Youssef AA, Castillo RA, Croom CS. Fetal biophysical activities in third-trimester pregnancies complicated by diabetes mellitus. Am J Obstet Gynecol. 1994;171:298-303.
83. Dierker LJ Jr., Pillay S, Sorokin Y, Rosen MG. The change in fetal activity periods in diabetic and nondiabetic pregnancies. Am J Obstet Gynecol. 1982;143:181-5.
84. Doherty NN, Hepper PG. Habituation in fetuses of diabetic mothers. Early Hum Dev. 2000;59:85-93.
85. Kainer F, Prechtl HF, Engele H, Einspieler C. Assessment of the quality of general movements in fetuses and infants of women with Type I diabetes mellitus. Early Hum Dev. 1997;50:13-25.
86. Mulder EJ, O'Brien MJ, Lems YL, Visser GH, Prechtl HF. Body and breathing movements in near-term fetuses and newborn infants of type I diabetic women. Early Hum Dev. 1990;24:131-52.
87. Mulder EJ, Visser GH. Growth and motor development in fetuses of women with Type I diabetes: I. Early growth patterns. Early Hum Dev. 1991a;25:91-106.
88. Mulder EJ, Visser GH. Growth and motor development in fetuses of women with Type I diabetes: II. Emergence of specific movement patterns. Early Hum Dev. 1991b;25:107-15.
89. Mulder EJ, Visser GH. Impact of early growth delay on subsequent fetal growth and functional development: A study on diabetic pregnancy. Early Hum Dev. 1992;31:91-5.
90. Mulder EJ, Visser GH, Bekedam DJ, Prechtl HF. Emergence of behavioural states in fetuses of Type I diabetic women. Early Hum Dev. 1987;15;231-51.
91. Mulder EJ, Visser GH, Morssink LP, de Vries JI. Growth and motor development in fetuses of women with Type I diabetes: III. First trimester quantity of fetal movement patterns. Early Hum Dev. 1991;25:117-33.
92. Aberg A, Westbom L, Kallen B. Congenital malformations among infants whose mothers had gestational diabetes or preexisting diabetes. Early Hum Dev. 2001;61:85-95.
93. deRegnier RA, Nelson CA, Thomas KM, Wewerka S, Georgieff MK. Neurophysiologic evaluation of auditory recognition memory in healthy newborn infants and infants of diabetic mothers. J Pediat. 2000;137:777-84.
94. Nelson CA, Wewerka S, Thomas KM, Tribby-Walbridge S, deRegnier R, Georgieff M. Neurocognitive sequelae of infants of diabetic mothers. Behavioral Neurosci. 2000;114:950-6.
95. Reece EA, Homko CJ Infant of the diabetic mother. Sem Perinatol. 1994;18:459-69.
96. Reece EA, Homko CJ. Why do diabetic women deliver malformed infants? Clin Obstet Gynaecol. 2000;43: 32-45.
97. Rizzo T, Metzger BE, Burns WJ, Burns K. Correlations between antepartum maternal metabolism and child intelligence. New Eng J Med. 1991;325:911-6.
98. Rizzo TA, Metzger BE, Dooley SL, Cho NH. Early malnutrition and child neurobehavioral development: Insights from the study of children of diabetic mothers. Child Dev. 1997;68:26-38.
99. Schwartz R, Teramo KA. Effects of diabetic pregnancy on the fetus and newborn. Sem Perinatol. 2000;24:120-35.
100. Vaarasmaki MS, Hartikainen A, Anttila M, Pramila S, Koivisto M. Factors predicting peri- and neonatal outcome in diabetic pregnancy. Early Hum Dev. 2000;59:61-70.
101. Robertson SS. Fetal cyclic motor activity in diabeties pregnancies: Sensitivity to maternal blood glucose. Dev Psychobiol. 2003;42(1):9-16.
102. Ornoy A, Ratzon N, Greenbaum C, Peretz E, Soriano D, Dulitzky M. Neurobehaviour of school age children born to diabetic mothers. Arch Dis Child Fetal Neonatal Ed. 1998;79:F94-F99.
103. Acardo PJ, Blondis TA, Whitman BY. Disorders of attention and activity level in a referral population. Pediatrics. 1990;85:426-31.
104. Ornoy A, Ariel L, Tennenbaum A. Inattention, hyperactivity and speech delay at 2-4 years of age as a predictor for ADD-ADHD syndrome. Israel J Psychiatry. 1993;30:155-63.
105. Smith TR. Impaired motor skill (clumsiness) in otherwise normal children: A review. Child Care Health Dev. 1992;18:283-99.

106. Petersen MB, Pedersen SA, Greisen G, Pedersen JF, Mølsted-Pedersen L. Early growth delay in diabetic pregnancy: Relation to psychomotor development at age 4. Br Med J. (Clin Res Ed). 1988;296:598-600.
107. Sells CJ, Robinson NM, Brown Z, Knopp RH. Long-term developmental follow-up of infants of diabetic mothers. J Pediatr. 1994;125:S9-17.
108. Vladareanu R, Lebit D, Constantinescu S. Ultrasound assessment of fetal neurobehaviour in high-risk pregnancies. Donald Sch J Ultrasound Obstet Gynecol. 2012;6(2):132-47.
109. Talic A, Kurjak A, Ahmed B, Stanojevic M, Predojevic M, Kadic AS, et al. The potential of 4D sonography in the assessment of fetal behavior in high-risk pregnancies. J Matern Fetal Neonatal Med. 2011;24(7):948-54.
110. Bekedam DJ, Visser GHA, de Vries JJ, Prechtl HFR. Motor behaviour in the growth retarded fetus. Early Hum Dev. 1985;12(2):155-65.
111. Cioni G, Prechtl HF. Preterm and early post term motor behaviour in low-risk premature infants. Early Hum Dev. 1990;23(3):159-91.
112. Seme-Ciglenečki P. Predictive value of assessment of general movements for neurological development of high-risk preterm infants: comparative study. Croat Med J. 2003;44(6):721-7.
113. Abo-Yaqoub S, Kurjak A, Mohammed AB, Shadad A, Abdel-Maaboud M. The role of 4-D ultrasonography in prenatal assessment of fetal neurobehaviour and prediction of neurological outcome. J Matern Fetal Neonatal Med. 2012;25(3):231-6.
114. Athanasiadis AP, Mikos T, Tambakoudis GP, Theodoridis TD, Papastergiou M, Assimakopoulos E, et al. Neurodevelopmental fetal assessment using kanet scoring system in low and high-risk pregnancies. J Matern Fetal Neonatal Med. 2013;26(4):363-8.

19 CHAPTER

Common Ultrasound-guided Invasive Diagnostic Procedures

Sonal Panchal, Chaitanya Nagori

INTRODUCTION

With the advancing ultrasound technology, it is now possible to diagnose not just major fetal abnormalities but also subtle anatomical variations in the fetuses that can be markers to chromosomal anomalies. Along with this in the last few years, there has been a fast advancement in genetics also. Both these together has made it possible to diagnose chromosomal abnormalities and genetic diseases antenatally. Common indications for these procedures are:

- Advanced maternal age
- Structural abnormalities seen in the fetus on ultrasound
- Siblings with chromosomal abnormalities
- Family history of chromosomal or genetic abnormalities
- High-risk calculation on other screening tests
- History of abortions
- Familial metabolic disorders

The commonly used procedures for the purpose are:

- Chorionic villus biopsy
- Amniocentesis

CHORIONIC VILLUS BIOPSY

Indications of chorionic villus sampling (CVS) are given in **Box 1**.[1]

BOX 1: Common indications for chorionic villus sampling.

- Chromosomal abnormalities
  - Advanced maternal age
  - High risk after prenatal screening of first or second trimester
  - Previous pregnancy with chromosomal abnormality
  - Family history of chromosomal rearrangement
  - Ultrasound marker for chromosomal abnormalities
- Monogenic disorders
  - Thalassemia
  - Duchenne/Becker muscular dystrophy
  - Hemophilia A and B
  - Cystic fibrosis
  - Congenital adrenal hyperplasia
  - Other monogenic diseases
  - Paternity testing
- Metabolic disorders
  - Mucopolysaccharidoses
  - Lipidoses
  - Amino acid disorders
  - Carbohydrate metabolism disorders

Contraindications

- In women with hepatitis B and C, the procedure is better avoided. There is some literature evidence to suggest that in females with high level of antigen E, there is a risk of transmission.[2] Risk of vertical transmission was also reported in women with human immunodeficiency virus (HIV) before antiretroviral treatment.[3]
- Active vaginal bleeding
- Active cervicovaginal infections
- *Rh incompatibility*: Isoimmunization may worsen. In these cases, amniocentesis or cordocentesis is a better option.[4,5] Anti-D immunoglobulin is to be given in all cases with Rh incompatibility in case the procedure is done.

Method

This procedure can be performed transcervically or transabdominally. It was first published in 1968 and then transcervical route was used and the chorionic material was retrieved through a hysteroscope.[6] In 1983, Brambati in Milan introduced a 1.5-mm polythene tube with a soft stainless still malleable obturator in a 1-mm diameter internal barrel.[7] In 1984, transabdominal route was selected for a fine needle approach.

Transcervical CVS is done by a 1.55-mm diameter, 26 cm long polythene catheter, or a biopsy forceps **(Fig. 1A)**. The catheter or forceps is advanced transcervically under full antisepsis with patient in lithotomy position. If required to straighten the uterocervical curvature, a tenaculum may be used. The procedure is done under guidance of transabdominal ultrasound to guide the catheter to chorion frondosum. The catheter is attached to a 10-mL syringe filled with 3–4 mL of normal saline. Once the position of the needle tip is confirmed on ultrasound, suction is applied with the syringe as the catheter is gradually pulled out. The negative pressure sucks the chorionic tissue in the syringe. The aspirated fluid is emptied into the petri dish. Chorionic villi are seen as tiny tissue bands with branching; 5–40 mg of tissue specimen is considered as sufficient **(Fig. 1B)**.

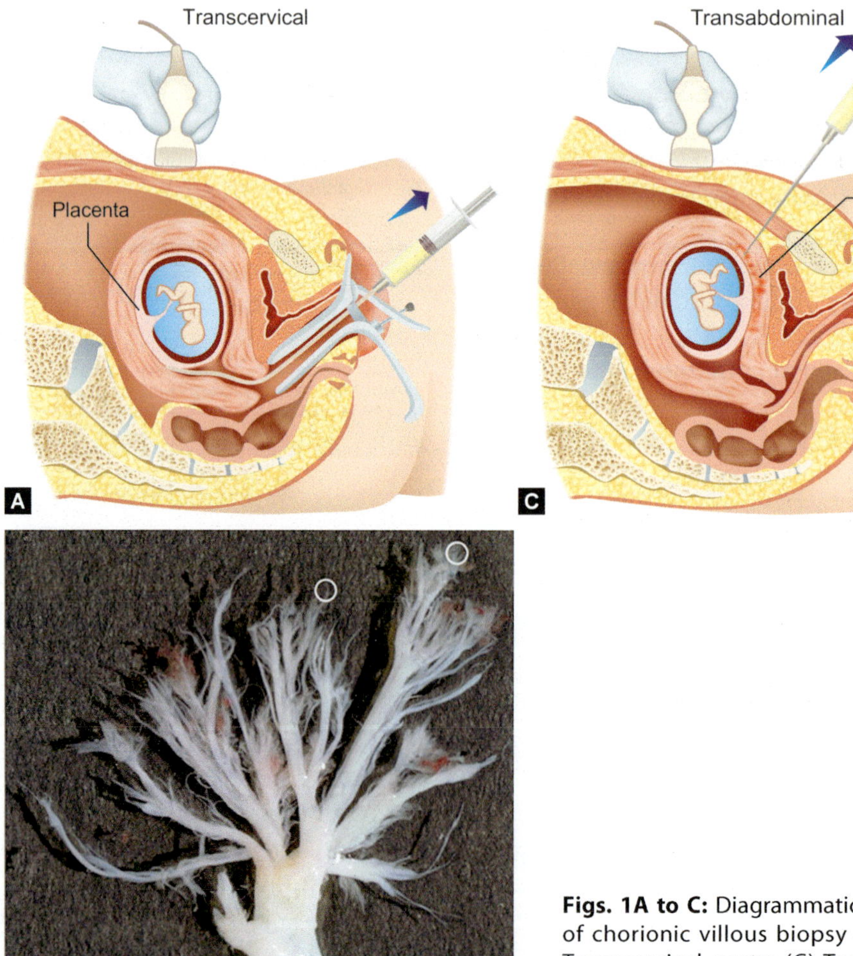

Figs. 1A to C: Diagrammatic presentation of chorionic villous biopsy on: (A and B) Transcervical route; (C) Transabdominal route.

Transabdominal CVS uses an aspiration needle with transabdominal ultrasound guidance using a biopsy guide or by a freehand technique **(Fig. 1C)**. A 20-gauge, 9–12 cm long needle is inserted percutaneously targeting the placenta. Another method is two-needle technique. An 18-gauge, 15 cm long biopsy needle guide is advanced until the placental limit followed by 20–22 gauge, 20 cm long aspiration needle through it. This approach is not feasible in cases with posterior placenta, bowel adhesions, retroverted, retroflexed uterus, etc.

Comparing the two techniques, Cochrane review as a result of a meta-analysis has shown that transabdominal route is safer in terms of total pregnancy loss and spontaneous miscarriage rate (9% vs. 7.4% and 7.9% vs. 4.5%).[8]

But studies have shown variable reports about which method is safer. This is because of the operator's experience. Transcervical CVS appears to be clinically more demanding requiring multiple insertions (11.2% vs. 4.1%) and causing more vaginal bleeding (10% vs. 1.6%).[9]

The material can be used for direct preparations from syncytiotrophoblast layer or from tissue culture of chorionic villus mesenchymal core. Fluorescent in situ hybridization (FISH) can diagnose trisomy 21, 13, or 18 in 24 hours. Polymerase chain reaction (PCR) is used for diagnosis of monogenic disorders.

Procedure can be used for multiple pregnancies also. In these cases, continuous observation of the needle tip is required. Workers have also used both the approaches together in multiple pregnancies.[10]

Timing

The procedure is best done between 11 and 13 weeks. Studies have shown that CVS done at or after 10 weeks of gestation does not increase the background population risk of fetal limb reduction defects. This was claimed to be common in a study when this procedure was done at 7–8 weeks.[11] No statistically significant increase in procedure-related pregnancy loss rate has been documented,[12] though the risk does vary from operator to operator depending on the experience. Some studies have mentioned marginally increased pregnancy loss rate as compared to amniocentesis.[13] Pregnancy loss rate was found to be higher in mothers older than 35 years and gestational age of <8 weeks.[14] Potential risk of vaginal bleeding and post-CVS infections is there, but bleeding is mostly self-limiting.

Efficiency and Reliability of Procedure

Chorionic villi samples can be successfully obtained in 99% of cases.[14,15] Multiple insertions may be required in 5.5% of cases and when more than three insertions are required, fetal loss rate is as high as 10%.[16,17] In 1.1–3%, a second invasive procedure is required. The reason for the failure of the procedure and need for the repeat procedure are maternal contamination, confined placental mosaicism, and culture failures.

Contamination with maternal decidual tissue is more likely when the sample size is small. Biopsies with >10 mg are considered as accurate for analysis.[1] Contamination is found in only 0.9% of cases.[15] Placental mosaicism is because of discrepancy between the chromosomal constitution of fetus and placenta.[18] Mosaicism develops due to: (i) meiotic error in one of the two gametes leading to trisomic conceptus[19] or (ii) mitotic postzygotic errors that produce mosaic morula and percent of aneuploid cells that depend on the timing of nondysjunction.[20] It has been proved that pregnancies with placental mosaicism have higher risk of fetal growth restriction and perinatal death.

Risk of Fetal Loss

A systematic review that analyzed fetal loss rates after amniocentesis and CVS showed only marginally increased pregnancy loss with

CVS as compared to amniocentesis (2.0% vs. 1.9%) when CVS was done abdominally and between 10 and 14 weeks.[16]

AMNIOCENTESIS (FIG. 2)

Amniocentesis is transabdominal aspiration of amniotic fluid. It was first done in 19th century to treat polyhydramnios.[21] In 1950, it was used for the first time for diagnostic purpose in Rhesus isoimmunization and also for fetal sex determination.[22] In late 1960s, amniotic fluid was used for prenatal invasive for congenital fetal chromosomal abnormalities and metabolic and enzymatic diseases.[23,24]

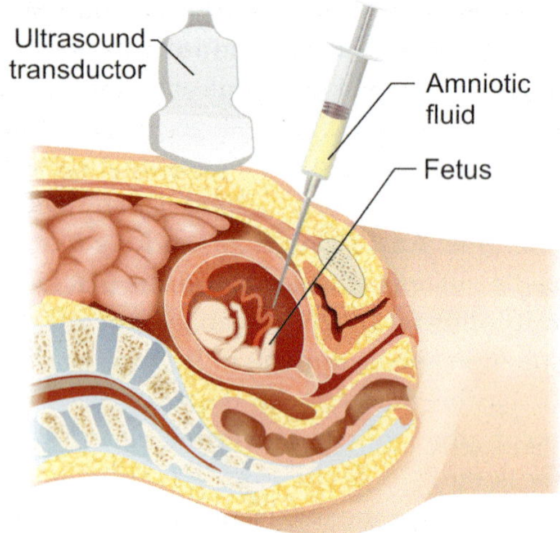

Fig. 2: Diagrammatic presentation of amniocentesis procedure.

Indications of Amniocentesis

- Chromosome and deoxyribonucleic acid (DNA) analysis—fetal karyotyping for chromosomal abnormalities, FISH for DNA study by direct probing for gene diseases like hemophilia, beta-thalassemia, cystic fibrosis, etc.
- Fetal infections by PCR, diagnosis toxoplasmosis, cytomegalovirus (CMV), etc.
- Lung maturity by quantitative and qualitative analysis of amniotic fluid. Lung maturity can be assessed by lecithin-sphingomyelin ratio and also by concentration of phosphatidylglycerol in amniotic fluid.
- In cases of premature rupture of membranes for diagnosis of chorioamnionitis.
- For diagnosis of fetal metabolic diseases and other conditions such as cystic fibrosis, congenital adrenal hyperplasia, etc.
- For treatment of oligohydramnios or polyhydramnios.

Timing

It is usually done between 15 and 18 weeks, when done for diagnosis of chromosomal or genetic abnormalities. But, it may be later if done for other indications such as chorioamnionitis or lung maturity. Early amniocentesis between 11 and 14 weeks can lead to fetal abnormalities such as clubfeet.

A detailed ultrasound assessment of the fetus is required before amniocentesis is done. Plan the entry site and the path of the needle based on the position of placenta, fluid quantity, and fetal position. The path selected should be away from the fetal face. Avoid placenta in the path and especially umbilical cord. Antiseptics are used to clean the entry site of the needle and the surrounding area. Disposable 22 gauge spinal needle is used. It is carefully slided into the amniotic fluid under continuous ultrasound monitoring. When needle is in position, the stellate is removed, 10 cc syringe is attached to the needle, and suction is applied to aspirate amniotic fluid. Needle may be repositioned after replacing the stellate, if fluid cannot be aspirated. It is most commonly due to membrane getting entangled in the needle tip. First 1–2 cc of amniotic fluid that is aspirated is discarded. Though the possibility is less, it may contain maternal cells. Approximately, 20 cc of fluid is aspirated. Place in the stellate after the aspiration is complete, pull out the needle, press the puncture site for about 2 minutes, and seal it with aseptic dressing. Check with ultrasound that there is no active bleeding. Advise to rest and avoid intercourse for at least 3–4 days preferably a week. Uterine cramps are common after the procedure. We prefer to give progesterone to support the pregnancy and pacify the uterus. Antibiotic cover is given to avoid postprocedural infection. Leaking and bleeding are a rare complication in expert hands and must be reported to the operator.

Complications

Maternal Complications

- Uterine contractions
- Blood group sensitization
- Infection

The rest of the complications are rarest of the rare and include damage to intra-abdominal organs and bleeding.[25]

Fetal Complications

- Fetal loss
- Needle puncture injuries
- Placental abruption
- Preterm labor
- Rupture of membranes
- Amniotic infections
- *Fetal loss*: The National Institute of Child Health and Human Development (NICHD) in its study concluded that the fetal loss rate in control group was 3.2% as compared to 3.5% in the amniocentesis group.[25] This risk was unrelated to previous miscarriage, volume of aspirated fluid, or number of attempts. The Canadian Collaborative Study also assessed the fetal loss rate to be approximately the same, but showed higher fetal loss rates with large bore (>19 gauge) needle and multiple punctures.[26] A randomized controlled trial from Denmark in 1986 used 20 gauge needle and did procedure at 16–18 weeks that showed 1.7% fetal loss rate in procedure group as compared to 0.7% in control group.[27] Systematic review of 29 controlled and uncontrolled trials has concluded 0.6% excess procedure-related pregnancy loss.[28] Fetal loss rate raises significantly and reaches 33%, if amniotic fluid contains blood.[29] Bloody or discolored amniotic fluid is also accompanied by high alpha-fetoproteins and prenatal results are not good. But, more commonly discolored amniotic fluid is because of blood that is derived from the mother and does not affect the development or multiplication of the cells and, therefore, does not affect the results.
- *Preterm delivery*: Increased incidence of preterm delivery before 37 weeks of gestation is observed in patients undergoing second trimester amniocentesis after taking into account other risk factors and confounding variables [odds ratio: 1:59; 95% confidence interval (95% CI): 1.31–1.92].[30]
- *Fetal trauma due to needle*: Its attribution is generally by association only. There is no direct evidence. Ultrasound guidance helps prevent it.[31]
- *Alloimmunization*: Fetomaternal hemorrhage during the procedure occurs in about 50% of cases and carries 1% greater risk than the background risk of 1.5% for alloimmunization.[32] Therefore, rhesus-negative mothers must be given 300 g anti-D immunoglobulin G (IgG) immediately after the procedure, if indirect Coombs test is negative.[33] Respiratory distress and orthopedic abnormalities such as talipes equinovarus, congenital dislocation, and subluxation of hip may occur as a result of chronic oligohydramnios that follows amniocentesis.
- Transmission of viral diseases is likely and, therefore, amniocentesis is not done in HIV-positive mothers.
- *Uterine contractions, leakage of the amniotic fluid, and vaginal bleeding*: These are quite common (2–3%), but are transient and self-limiting. Fluid leakage occurs in about 1% of women, the amount is little, and prognosis is good.[34,35]

Amniocentesis in Multiple Gestations

This needs expertise and is preferred to be done by expert fetal medicine specialist. It can be done in three different ways:[36]

1. Each gestational sac is separately and sequentially punctures and in this case, methylene blue or other marker dye is used to identify the sac that is already punctured
2. Single needle is used to puncture both the sacs. First puncture is done close to the septum and the second sac punctures through the septum
3. Two different needles are used to puncture two sacs simultaneously under ultrasound visualization.

The risk of fetal loss after amniocentesis in multiple gestations is higher than in singleton pregnancies, but this is related to multiple gestations and not due to the procedure.[37] The risk does not increase, if amniocentesis is done after multifetal pregnancy reduction.[38]

SUMMARY

Chorionic villus sampling and amniocentesis are prenatal invasive procedures for diagnosis of genetic, chromosomal, and metabolic disorders. These are simple to do, though have a learning curve and are very safe in experienced hands.

REFERENCES

1. Grigoriadis T, Mesogitis S, Anstaklis AJ. Chorionic villus sampling. In: Anstaklis A, Troyano JM (Eds). Donald School Textbook of Interventional Ultrasound. New Delhi: Jaypee Brothers Medical (P) Pvt. Ltd.; 2008. pp. 142-55.
2. Davis G, Wilson RD, Desilets V, Reid GJ, Shaw D, Summers A, et al. Amniocentesis and women with hepatitis B, hepatitis C or human immunodeficiency virus. J Obstet Gynecol Cam. 2003;25:145-52.
3. Tess BH, Rodrigues LC, Newell ML, Dunn DT, Lago TD. Breastfeeding, genetic, obstetric and other risk factors associated with mother-to child transmission of HIV-1 in Sao Paulo State, Brazil. Sao Paulo Collaborative Study for Vertical Transmission of HIV-1. AIDS. 1998;12: 513-20.
4. Moise KJ, Carpenter RJ. Increased severity of fetal hemolytic disease with known rhesus alloimmunization after first trimester transcervical chorionic villus biopsy. Fetal Diagn Ther. 1990;5:76.
5. Mohr J. Fetal genetic diagnosis: development of techniques for early sampling of fetal cells. Acta Pathol Microbiol Scand. 1968:73:73-7.
6. Kazy Z, Rozovsky SI, Bakharev AV. Chorion biopsy in early pregnancy: a method of early prenatal diagnosis for inherited disorders. Prenat Diagn. 1982;2:39-45.
7. Brambati B, Oldrini A, Aladerum SA. Transcervical specimen of chorionic villi in the 1st trimester of pregnancy. Hum Genet. 1983;63:349-57.
8. Alfirevic Z, Mujezinovic F, Sundberg K. Amniocentesis and chorionic villus sampling for prenatal diagnosis. Cochrane Database Syst Rev. 2003;3:CD003252.
9. Smidt-Jensen S, Permin M, Philip J, Lundsteen C, Zachary JM, Fowler SE, et al. Randomised comparison of amniocentesis and transabdominal and transcervical chorionic villus sampling. Lancet. 1992;340:1237-44.
10. Brambati B, Tului L, Lanzani A, Simoni G, Travi M. First-trimester genetic diagnosis in multiple pregnancy: principles and potential pitfalls. Prenat Diagn. 1991;11:767-74.
11. Christiaens GC, Van Baarlen J, Huber J, Leschot NJ. Fetal limb constriction: a possible complication of CVS. Prenat Diagn. 1989;9:67-71.
12. Multicentre randomized clinical trial of chorion villus sampling and amniocentesis. First report. Canadian Collaborative CVS-Amniocentesis Clinical Trial Group. Lancet. 1989;1:1-6.
13. Medical Research Council European trial of chorion villus sampling. MRC working party on the evaluation of chorion villus sampling. Lancet. 1991;337:1491-9.
14. Brambati B, Tului L, Cislaghi C, Alberti E. First 10,000 chorionic villus samplings performed on singleton pregnancies by a single operator. Prenat Diagn. 1998;18:255-66.
15. Brun JL, Mangione R, Gangbo F, Guyton F, Taine L, Roux D, et al. Feasibility, accuracy and safety of chorionic villous sampling: a report of 10,741 cases. Prenat Diagn. 2003;23:295-301.
16. Mujezinovic F, Alfirevic Z. Procedure-related complications of amniocentesis and chorionic villus sampling: a systematic review. Obstet Gynecol. 2007;110:687-94.
17. Jackson LJ, Wapner RJ. Risks of chorionic villus sampling. Clin Obstet Gynecol. 1987;1:513.
18. Crane JP, Cheung SW. An embryogenic model to explain cytogenetic inconsistences observed in

chorionic villus versus fetus tissue. Prenat Diagn. 1988;8:119-29.
19. Wolstenholme J. Confined placental mosaicism for trisomies 2, 3, 7, 8, 9, 16 and 22 and their incidence, likely origins and mechanisms for cell lineage compartmentalization. Prenat Diagn. 1996;16:511-24.
20. Wapner RJ. Invasive prenatal diagnostic techniques. Semin Perinatol. 2005;29:401-4.
21. Schatz F. Eine besondere art von einseitiger polyhydramnie mit anderseitiger oligohydramnie bie eineligen zwillingen. Arch Gynecol. 1882;19:329.
22. Bevis DCA. The composition of liquor amnii in heamolytic disease of the newborn. J Obstet Gynaecol Br Emp. 1953;60:244-51.
23. Jacobson CB, Barter RH. Intrauterine diagnosis and management of genetic defects. Am J Obstet Gynecol. 1967;99(6):796-807.
24. Nadler HL, Gerbie AB. Role of amniocentesis in the intrauterine detection of genetic disorders. N Engl J Med. 1970;282:596-9.
25. Midtrimester amniocentesis for prenatal diagnosis. Safety and accuracy. JAMA. 1976;236: 1471-6.
26. Simpson NE, Dallaire L, Miller JR, Siminovich L, Hamerton JL, Miller J, et al. Prenatal diagnosis of genetic diseases in Canada: report of a collaborative study. Can Med Assoc J. 1976;115:739-48.
27. Tabor A, Philip J, Madsen M, Bang J, Obel EB, Norgaard-Pedersen B. Randomised controlled trial of genetic amniocentesis in 4,606 low-risk women. Lancet. 1986;1:1287-93.
28. Seeds JW. Diagnostic midtrimester amniocentesis: How safe: Am J Obstet Gynecol. 2004;191: 608-16.
29. Karpa E, Schiller HA. Meconium staining of amniotic fluid of midtrimester amniocentesis. Obstet Gynecol. 1977;50:475.
30. Medda E, Donati S, Spinelli A, Di Renzo GC, EUROPOP Group Czech Republic, EUROPOP Group Finland, et al. Genetic amniocentesis: a risk factor for preterm delivery? Eur J Obstet Gynecol Reprod Biol. 2003;110:153-8.
31. Raymond GV. Rare neurologic injury from amniocentesis. Birth Defects Res Clin Mol Teratol. 2003;67:205-6.
32. Tabor A, Bang J, Norgaard-Pedersem B. Fetomaternal hemorrhage associated with genetic amniocentesis: results of a randomized trial. Br J Obstet Gynecol. 1987;94:528-35.
33. American College of Obstetricians and Gynecologists. Prevention of D isoimmunization related to amniocentesis. Am J Med Genet. 1983;16:527-34.
34. Borgida AF, Mills AA, Feldman DM, Rodis JF, Ergan JF. Outcome of pregnancies complicated with rupture of membranes after genetic amniocentesis. Am J Obstet Gynecol. 2000;183:937-9.
35. Bahado-Singh R, Schmitt R, Hobbins JC. New technique for genetic amniocentesis in twins. Obstet Gynecol. 1992;79:304.
36. Elias S, Gerbie ABM, Simpson JL. Genetic amniocentesis in twin gestations. Am J Obstet Gynecol. 1998;138:169.
37. Weisz B, Rodeck CH. Invasive diagnostic procedures in twin pregnancies (review). Prenat Diagn. 2005;25:751-8.
38. Anstaklis A, Daslalakis G, Papantoniou N, Mesogitis S, Michalas S. Genetic amniocentesis in multifetal pregnancies reduced to twins compared with nonreduced twin gestations. Fertil Steril. 2000;74:1051-2.

20 CHAPTER

Three-dimensional and Four-dimensional Ultrasound for Fetal Anomalies

Sonal Panchal, Chaitanya Nagori

INTRODUCTION

Invention of three-dimensional (3D) and four-dimensional (4D) ultrasound has made a dramatic improvement in fetal imaging. 3D ultrasound helps see the fetus in perspective, appreciate depth, and thus allows better demonstration of limb and facial defects of the fetus, that are diagnosed or suspected on two-dimensional (2D) ultrasound but are better demonstrated and confirmed on volume ultrasound. 4D ultrasound is a real-time 3D, where 3D reconstruction is so fast, 16–32 frames/minute, that it appears real time. 4D ultrasound allows not only to demonstrate structural abnormalities but also allows to study abnormalities of movements that may be because of abnormalities of the limbs such as flexion or extension deformities or even because of major neurological abnormalities. Apart from this because of better spatial resolution, abnormalities of fetal internal organs are also better demonstrated.

TIPS FOR VOLUME ULTRASOUND FOR SECOND- AND THIRD-TRIMESTER FETUS

- Use convex volume probe.
- Use volume angle large enough to include the whole structure of interest.
- Acquisition can be done with multiplanar or render mode, though it is better to acquire with optimally selected render mode preset.
- Rendering for internal structures is done with surface texture, in combination with maximum or minimum transparent mode.
- Rendering for limbs and facial defects is best done with surface smooth and gradient modes in combination or by high-definition (HD) live mode. Changing light direction does help in better demonstration of subtle abnormalities. Silhouette mode may be added as and when required, especially for anechoic structures and bones.
- Inversion mode rendering or sonography-based automated volume count (sonoAVC) general may be used for assessment of fluid-filled structures/lesions (hydrocephalus, hydronephrosis, duodenal atresia, etc.).
- Though for better understanding of related anatomy, tomographic ultrasound imaging (TUI) with or without volume contrast imaging (VCI) is used.
- For better understanding of anatomy, align the sectional planes in anatomical identifiable orthogonal planes before interpretation.
- Generally "updown" render direction is used but for spatial temporal image correlation (STIC) volumes and 3D power Doppler "frontback" render direction is used. Though render direction may be changed as per requirement.
- Using curved render line is often required for fetal volume imaging.
- Virtual organ computer-aided analysis (VOCAL) may be used for volume calculation of fetal organs or lesions (e.g., lung volume in diaphragmatic hernia, renal volume in dysplastic kidneys, etc.).
- Angiomode or glass body mode is especially useful when vascular abnormalities are suspected.

- STIC is an excellent tool for assessment of the fetal heart.
- Omniview is widely used for assessment of fetal spine, limbs, corpus callosum, etc.

APPLICATIONS FOR DETECTION OF CONGENITAL DEFECTS IN THE FETUSES

We shall now discuss the applicability of volume ultrasound for diagnosis of congenital defects, system by system. Since the role of volume ultrasound in first trimester has already been discussed in the previous chapter, we shall start discussion here from the time of nuchal scan.

Facial Abnormalities

Volume ultrasound is the only modality that actually allows to study the fetal face. Surface smooth in a combination with gradient light is the rendering mode to be used to demonstrate the fetal face. HD live is a better render mode (**Figs. 1A and B**).

Scanning the face profile and using updown viewing direction is the most common way of demonstrating the fetal face. Though fetus being actively moving in the second trimester, 4D instead of 3D is better used. Best time is between 23 and 30 weeks, but proper fetal position is essential. To get a proper position, pressing mother's abdomen repeatedly, turning mother to one or another side or reexamining after a few minutes would help when fetus is not in a favorable position to see the face. The absolute essential is fluid interface. In 90% of cases, correct and reproducible face images can be produced in the second trimester. Though this reduces to only 30% after 34 weeks due to the obligatory position that the fetus has to attain with its growing size. Fetal limbs overlap on fetal face to accommodate its growing size in relatively small intrauterine space. It is true that when volume of the face is acquired and rendered to demonstrate facial abnormalities suspected on 2D ultrasound, front of the face is required and in that case, on 2D ultrasound, a profile view of the fetus is required (**Fig. 2**). But when fetal face is to be rendered for photographic purpose only, whatever may be the position of the fetus seen on 2D ultrasound, face can be rendered, the only requirement is that there should be an adequate fluid interface (**Figs. 3A and B**).

Three-dimensional ultrasound has an important role in the diagnosis of facial

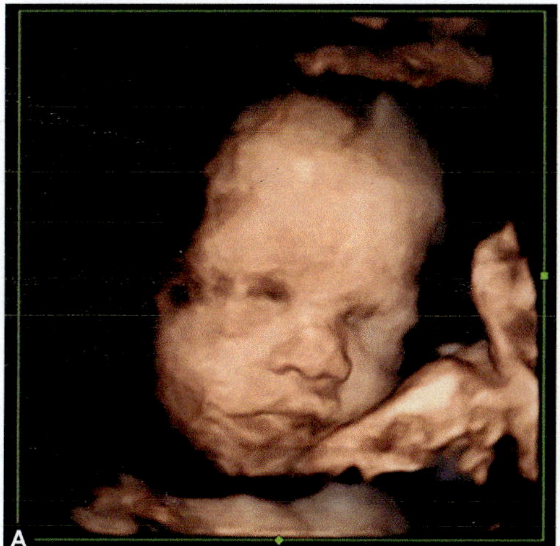

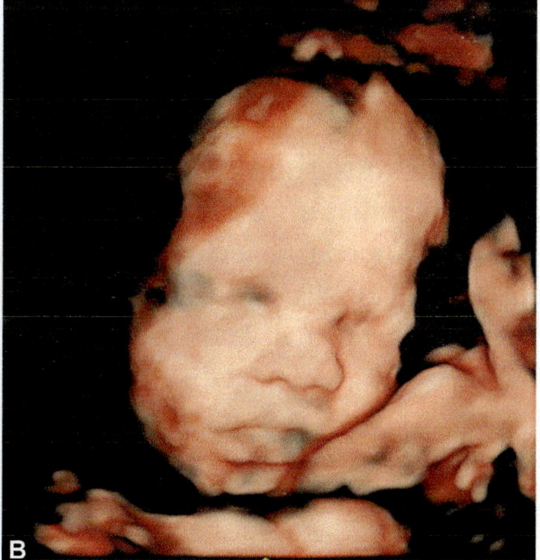

Figs. 1A and B: (A) Fetal face rendered in surface mode; (B) The same face as in Figure 1A is rendered in high-definition (HD) live mode.

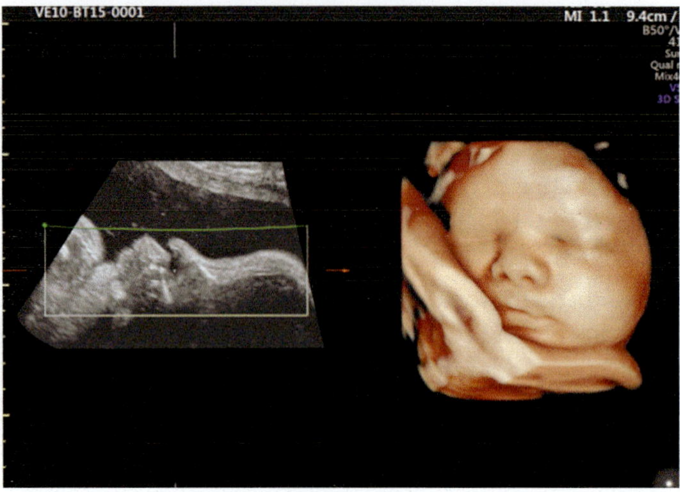

Fig. 2: Fetal front face on render is seen when the acquisition plane shows fetal face profile, when updown render mode is selected.

cleft, micrognathia, nasal abnormalities, ear abnormalities, including low set ears and eye abnormalities (**Figs. 4A and B**). Merz et al. have reported well-defined facial images as early as 9th week of pregnancy.[1] Defects of the orbits such as hypertelorism, hypotelorism, single orbit, and microphthalmia (**Fig. 5**), commonly a part of genetic syndromes, may be suspected by 2D ultrasound, but the confirmation and demonstration are not possible without the use of volume ultrasound.

Cleft lip is suspected on 2D ultrasound as a cut in the upper lip (**Figs. 6A and B**). It may be central, unilateral, or bilateral. Surface rendering and HD live are the best modes to demonstrate the defect. Rotten and Levaillant have proved that 3D and 4D ultrasound are superior to 2D ultrasound for diagnosis of facial clefts.[2] Rendering for the palate can also be done with flipped face technique[3] (**Fig. 7**). 3D ultrasound can also pick up isolated soft palate defects as shown in studies by Pilu et al.[4] Another technique to detect the cleft palate is the 3D "reverse face" view[5] (**Figs. 8A and B**). After acquiring the face volume, the viewing direction is changed to back instead of front, to see the facial bones from inside the skull. Maxilla and palate can be reliably studied as early as 11 weeks.

Though cleft lip is very well demonstrated on surface rendering (**Fig. 9**), cleft palate needs studying the multiplanar planes. Cleft palate can be diagnosed by TUI in axial plane, just caudal to the orbital plane[6] (**Fig. 10**). TUI in coronal plane is also useful for demonstration of the connecting passage between the oral and nasal cavity in cleft palate (**Fig. 11**). Diagnosis of cleft lip and palate is almost 100%, including the cleft of soft palate also.[2,4,7] Omniview with VCI is suggested by Benacerraf et al.[8] Omniview is used with three polylines (**Fig. 12**).

Early diagnosis of median cleft syndrome is possible in which the frontal bones and nasal bones are largely separated with hypertelorism, flat nasal bridge, rudimentary nostrils, and other facial abnormalities.[9] A rare condition where the cleft of the lip extends up to the medial angle of the eye (**Fig. 13**) can be diagnosed by volume ultrasound only as it is not easy to document the facial extension on 2D ultrasound. Generalized information of the facial bony defects available on 3D multiplanar mode or TUI helps decide the surgical approach. Cleft lip with volume ultrasound is best diagnosed between 20 and 24 weeks.

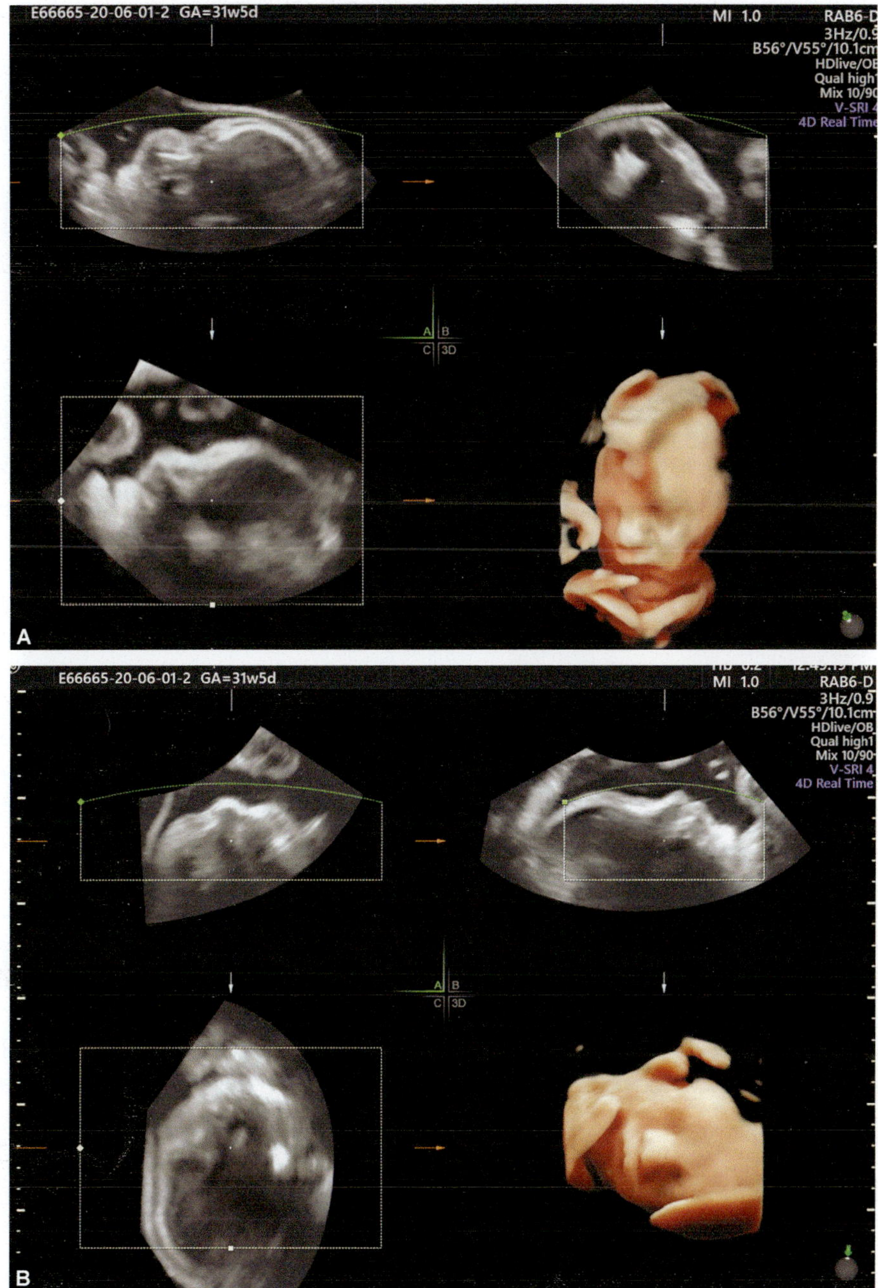

Figs. 3A and B: Fetal face in any position can still be rendered and show the face of the fetus on rendered image, though not the front of the face.

Micrognathia

Three-dimensional ultrasound shows the precise alignment of orthogonal planes in which accurate measurements can be made and allow creation of rendered casts of the mandibular bone. Micrognathia is diagnosed subjectively by rendered 3D image of fetal face (**Fig. 14**) or objectively by measurement of inferior facial angle[10] and jaw index: Anteroposterior (AP) diameter of

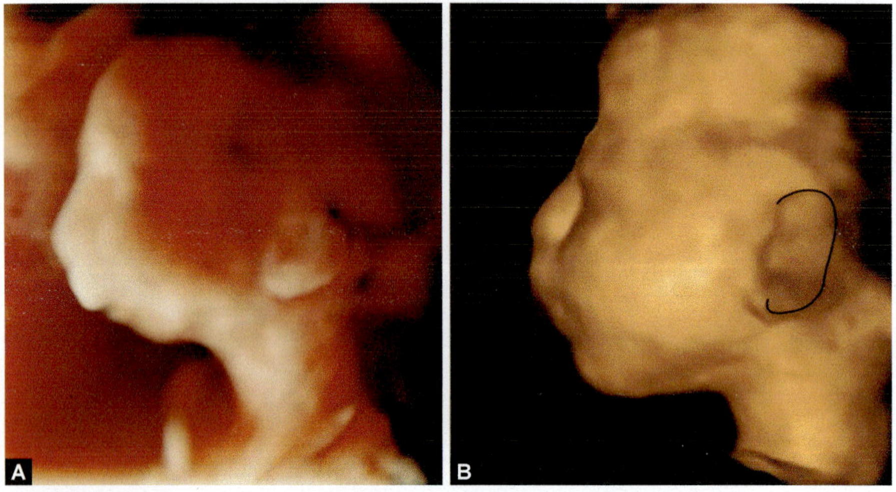

Figs. 4A and B: (A) Rendered image of fetal profile showing flat nasal bridge and micrognathia; (B) Rendered image of fetal profile showing micrognathia and low set ears.

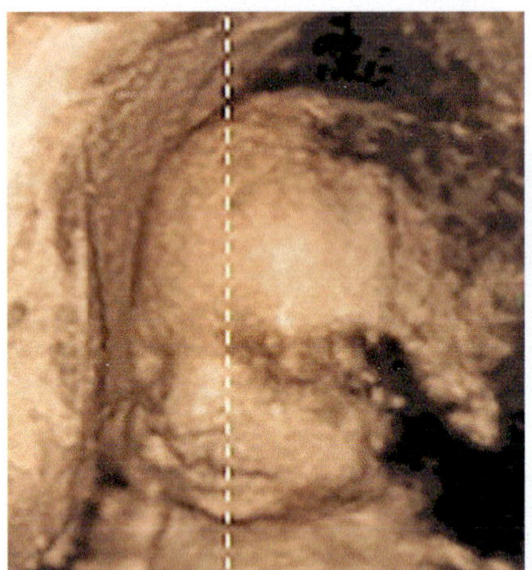

Fig. 5: Hypertelorism and cleft lip seen on 3D rendered image of fetal face.

mandible/biparietal diameter (BPD) (<0.23 is micrognathia)[11,12] (**Figs. 15A and B**).

Ear Abnormalities

Size, morphology, and placement of the ear are important for the diagnosis of chromosomal abnormalities. 70% of trisomy 21 babies have helix-lobe lengths of more than two standard deviations from mean. Detection of ear appendices may be a marker of renal malformation. Size and shape of the ear may sometimes be assessed on 2D ultrasound, but position of the ear can only be assessed by volume ultrasound (**Figs. 16A and B**). Therefore low-placed ears, an

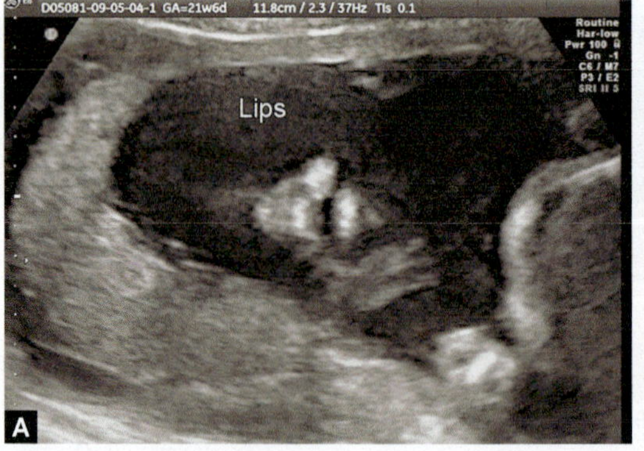

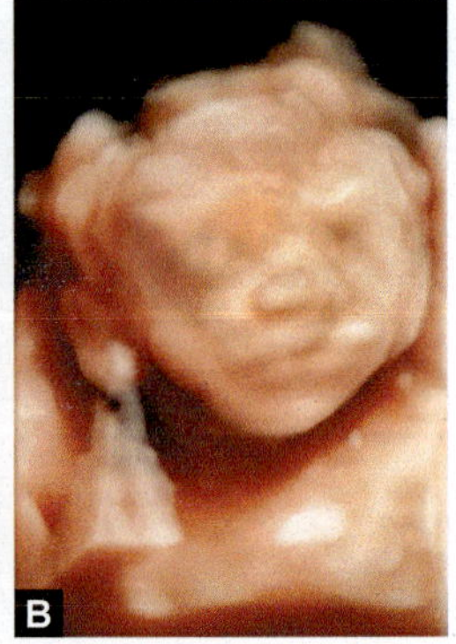

Figs. 6A and B: (A) B-mode ultrasound image of fetal lips in coronal plane with break in the upper lip shadow-cleft lip; (B) Three-dimensional (3D) ultrasound high-definition (HD) live rendered image of fetal face with cleft lip.

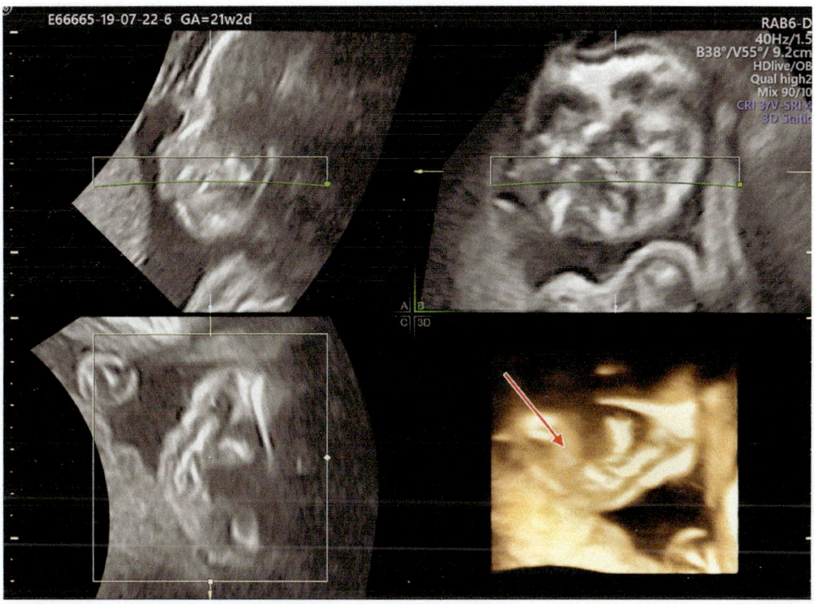

Fig. 7: Cleft palate shown on flipped face rendering.

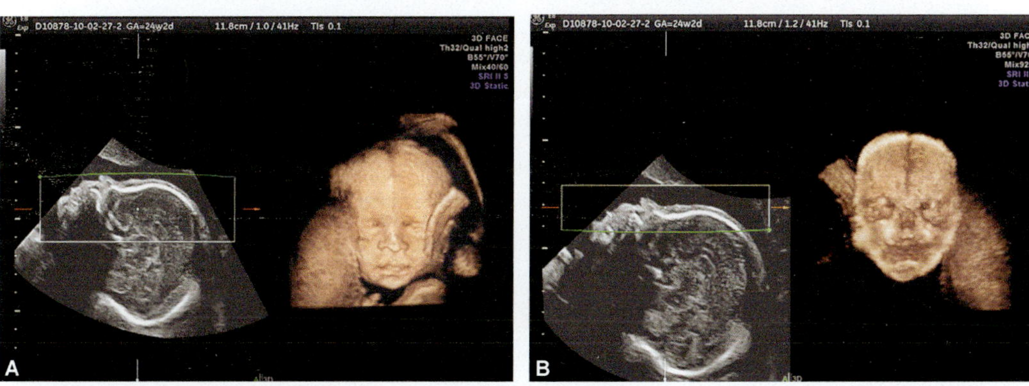

Figs. 8A and B: Profile of the face on B-mode, which was rendered in "updown" direction, shows the face and when render direction was reversed, it shows the bony face for the assessment of the cleft palate—reverse face view.

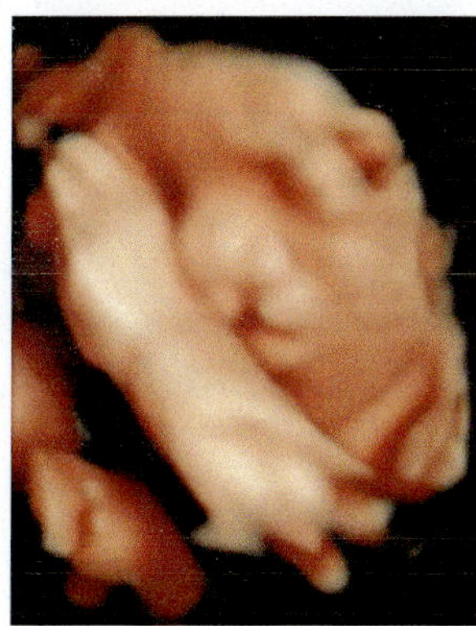

Fig. 9: High-definition (HD) live rendered image of fetal face showing cleft lip.

important marker for trisomy 21, can only be demonstrated by volume ultrasound.

Abnormal profiles such as frontal bossing can also be better demonstrated on volume ultrasound.

Nasal bone is usually seen on the midsagittal plane. But coronal plane-retronasal triangle view is also used to confirm both the nasal bones. Using 3D ultrasound with maximum mode rendering has been proved to be more reliable between 18 and 33 weeks of gestational age for the diagnosis of absence or hypoplasia of the nasal bones[13] (**Fig. 17**). If the gap

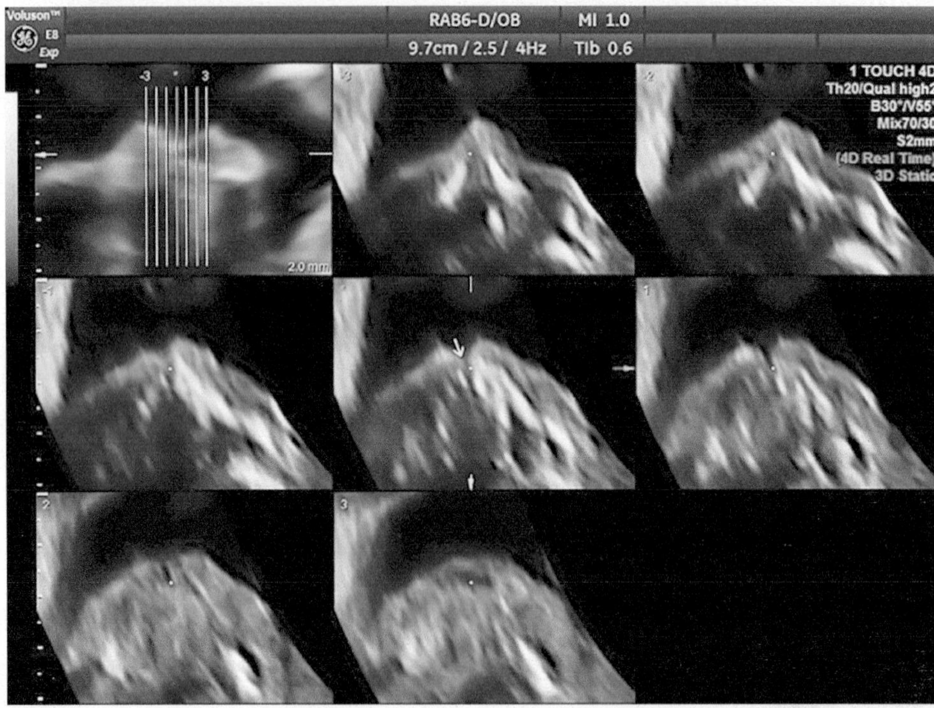

Fig. 10: The same fetus as in **Figure 9**, on axial plane tomographic ultrasound imaging (TUI) shows the cleft in the palate.

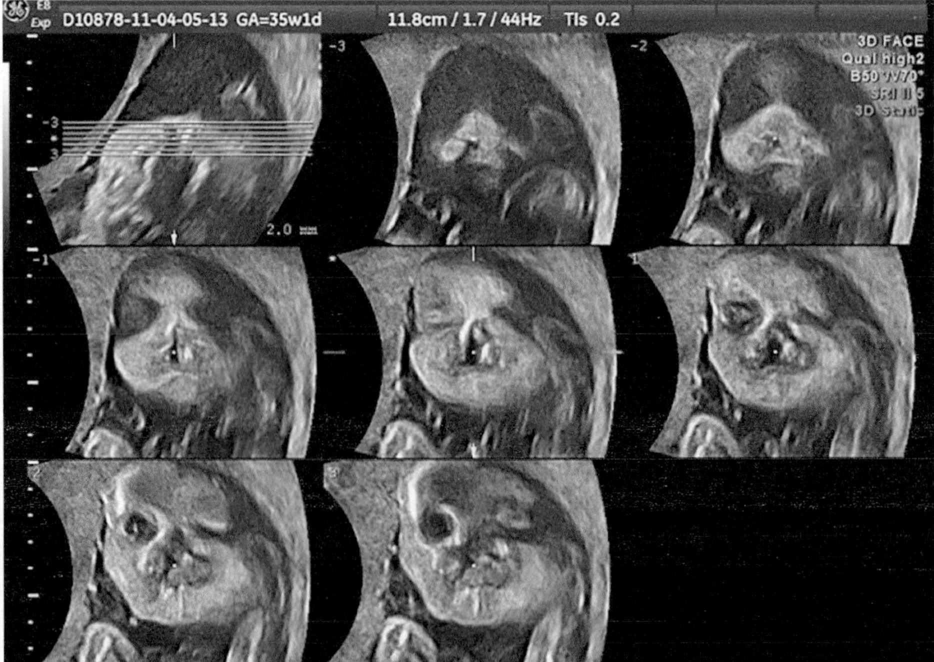

Fig. 11: The same fetus as in **Figure 9**, on coronal plane tomographic ultrasound imaging (TUI) shows the gap in the maxilla, the gap extending toward the nasal cavity.

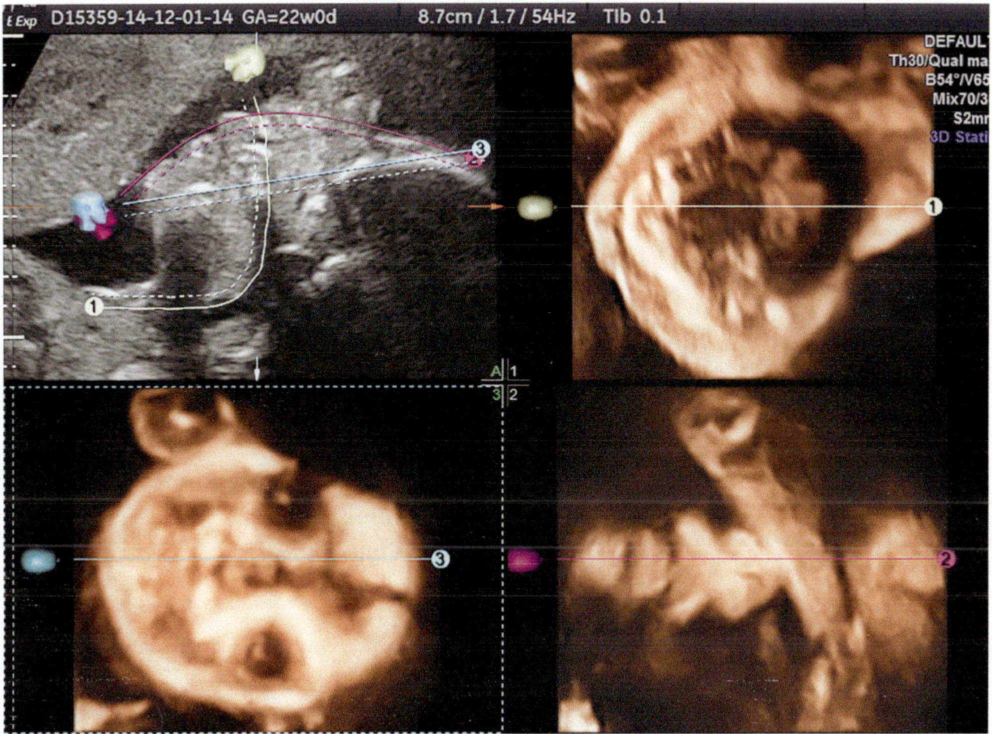

Fig. 12: Demonstration of the palate with omniview on omniview 1 and omniview 3. Omniview 2 shows coronal plane of lips.

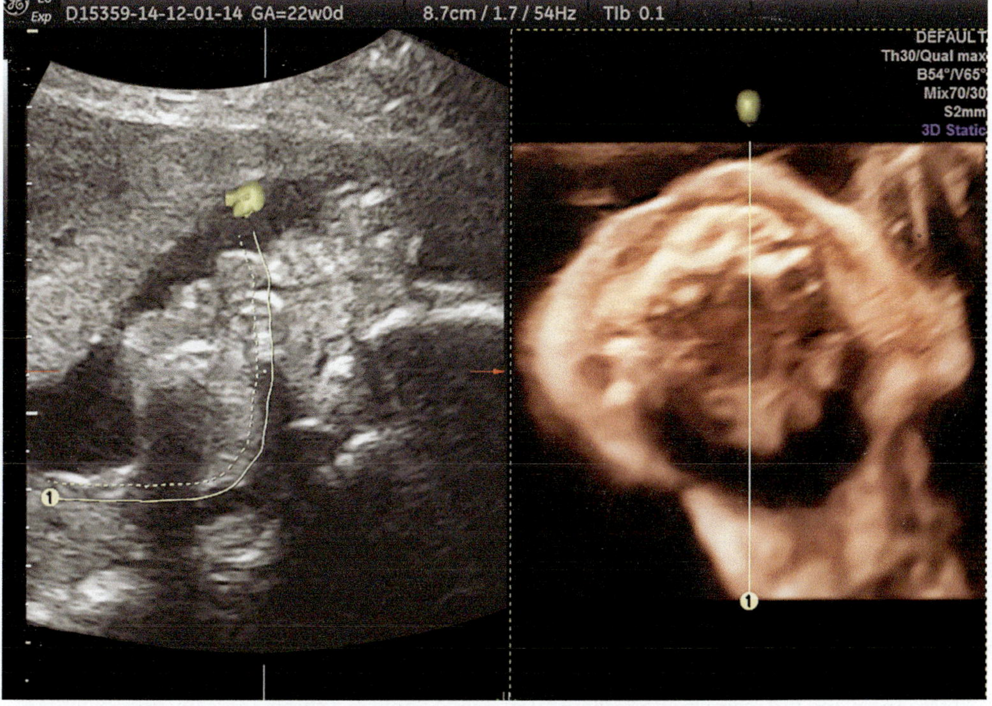

Fig. 13: Omniview shows the entire palate.

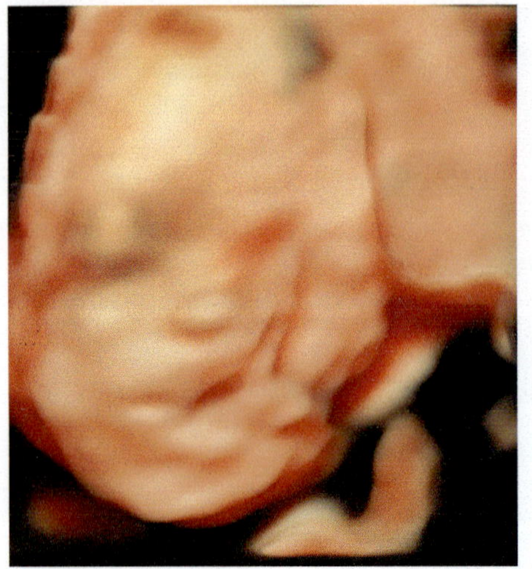

Fig. 14: High-definition (HD) live rendered image of fetal face with facial cleft extending to medial angle of the eye.

between the two nasal bones is >0.6 mm, it indicates absent nasal bone at 12 weeks scan.

Flat nasal bridge is an important sign for aneuploidy, though can be diagnosed on B-mode ultrasound, it may be more easily understandable for the nonscan person by 3D ultrasound (**Fig. 18**).

Orbital Abnormalities

Sepulwada et al. have documented the diagnosis of congenital dacryocystocele by 3D ultrasound as reliable as with magnetic resonance imaging (MRI).[14] 3D ultrasound also has a role in the diagnosis of rare fetal tumors including palatal teratoma, epulis, hemangiomas of face and neck, epignathus, etc. It helps in the assessment of the extension of the tumor and if at all involvement of the airway.

Apart from the defects or anatomical variations, only volume ultrasound can show the fetal expressions that represent the fetal behavior and neurological development of the fetus.

The *expressions* recorded so far are as follows:

- Yawning (**Fig. 19**)
- Smiling (**Fig. 20**)
- Swallowing
- Sucking
- Blinking (**Figs. 21A and B**)
- Grimacing (**Fig. 22**)
- Mouthing (**Fig. 23**)
- Tongue expulsion.

Lot more about this is discussed in Chapter 18 of this book.

Cranial Abnormalities

Skull bones and sutures can be visualized by 3D ultrasound[15] (**Fig. 24**), which is difficult with

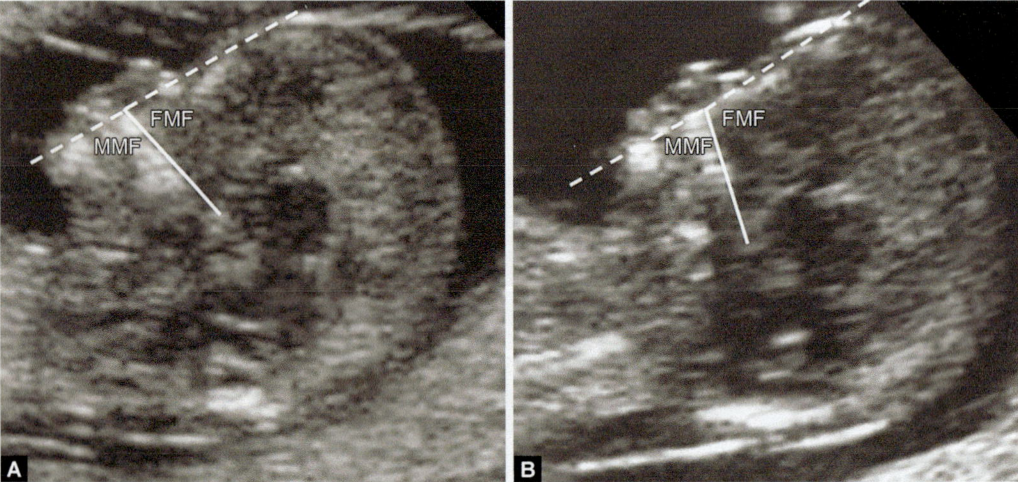

Figs. 15A and B: Mid-sagittal view of the fetal face demonstrating the measurement of the frontomaxillary facial (FMF) angle and the mandibulomaxillary facial (MMF) angle in a chromosomally normal fetus (A) and a fetus with trisomy 18 (B).

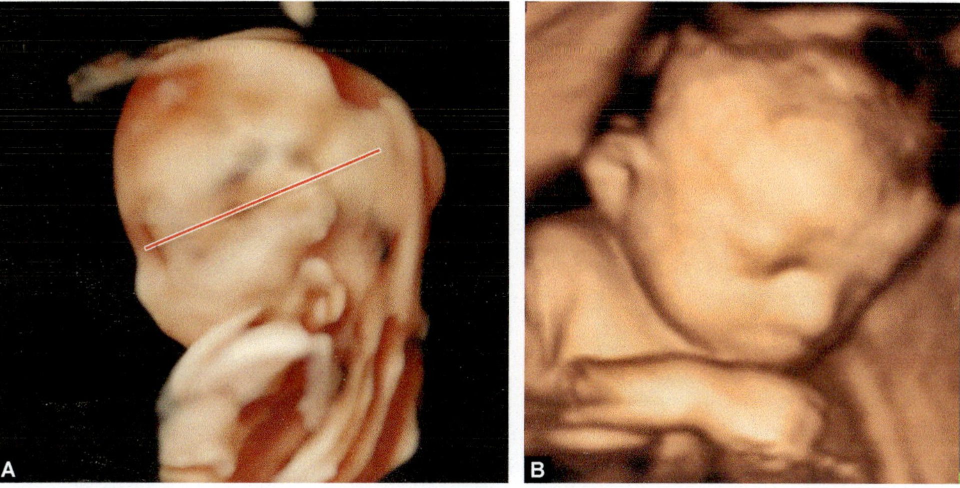

Figs. 16A and B: (A) Normal position of the ear on rendered image of fetal head; (B) Low placed ear on rendered image of fetal head.

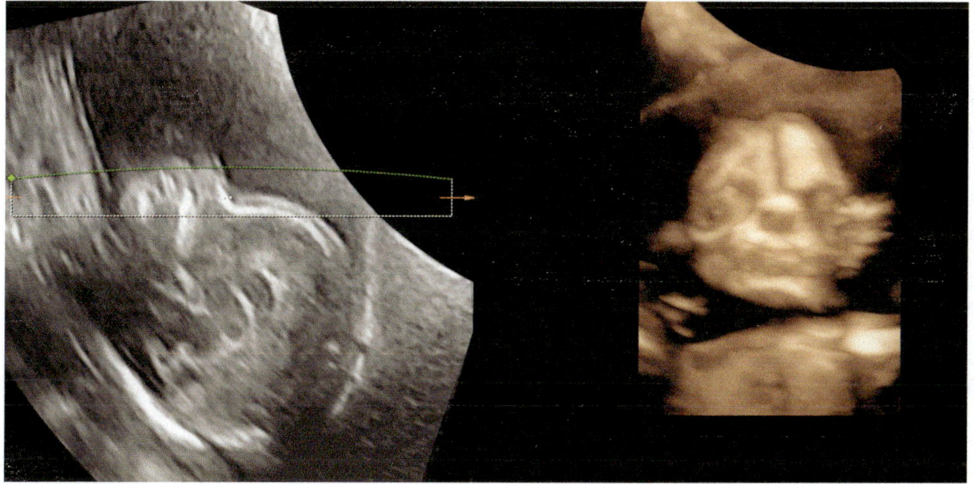

Fig. 17: Maximum mode of fetal face to show maxillary triangle and nasal bones.

2D ultrasound due to natural curve of the skull. Maximum transparency mode is used for this. Excessive diastases of the sutures can be seen in cranium bifidum occultum and premature closure can diagnose craniostenosis and microcephaly early.[16]

Volume ultrasound shows fontanelle very clearly (**Fig. 25**). Paladini et al. have documented that the size of anterior fontanelle increases as gestational age increases, but in relation to the fetal head volume its size decreases with advancing gestational age. The anterior fontanelle is larger in trisomy 21.[17] Features of fetal head dysmorphism such as flattening or prominence of occipital bones or frontal bones, and altered facial angles—superior or inferior can be diagnosed by volume ultrasound only. Small meningoceles that are easily overlooked by 2D ultrasound would be clearly demonstrated by volume ultrasound (**Fig. 26**).

Central Nervous System

In late second and third trimesters, if the fetus is in cephalic presentation, transvaginal approach can be a better approach to study the

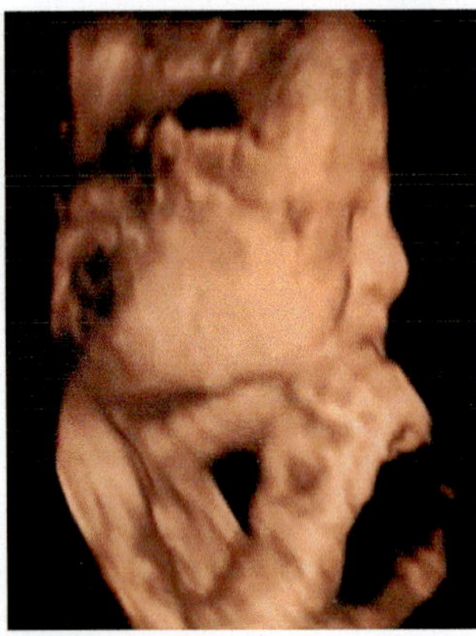

Fig. 18: Surface rendered three-dimensional (3D) ultrasound image of fetal face in profile shows flat nasal bridge and retrognathia.

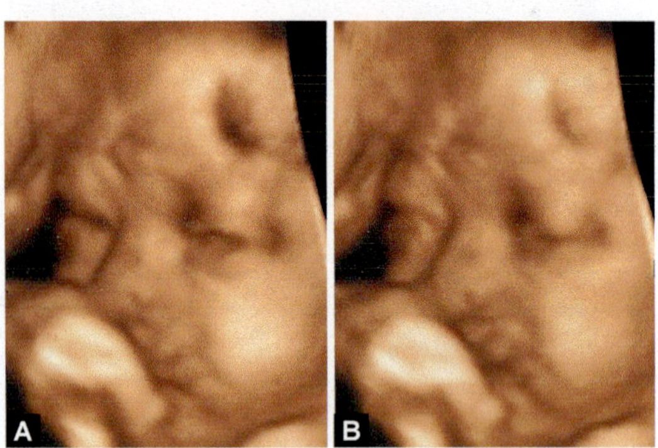

Figs. 21A and B: Opening and closing of eyes of the fetus.

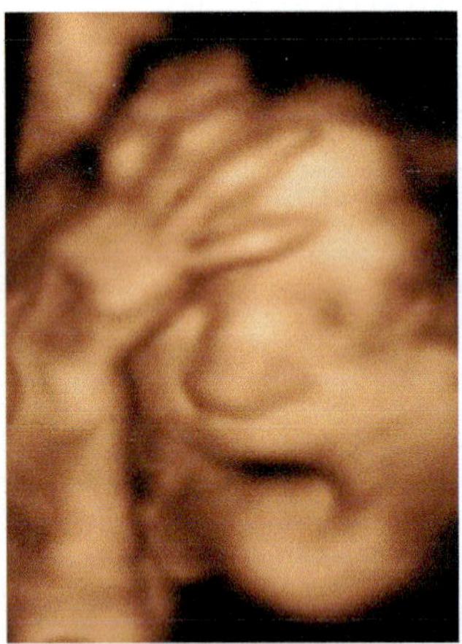

Fig. 19: Yawning fetus.

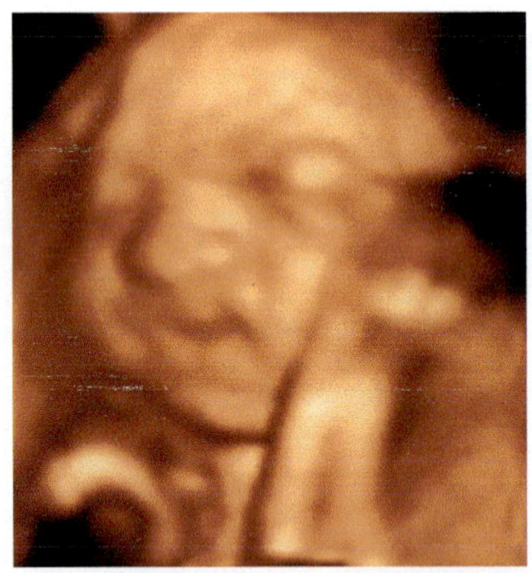

Fig. 22: Grimacing fetus.

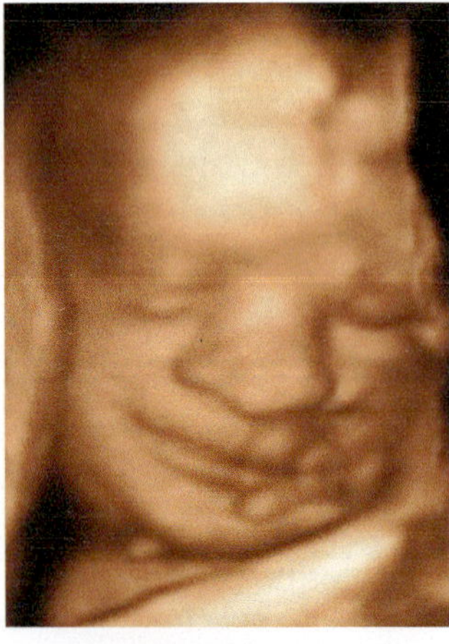

Fig. 20: Smiling fetus.

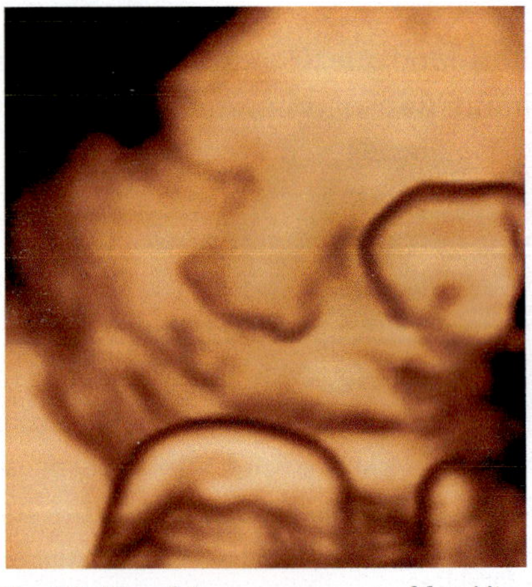

Fig. 23: Mouthing movement of fetal lips.

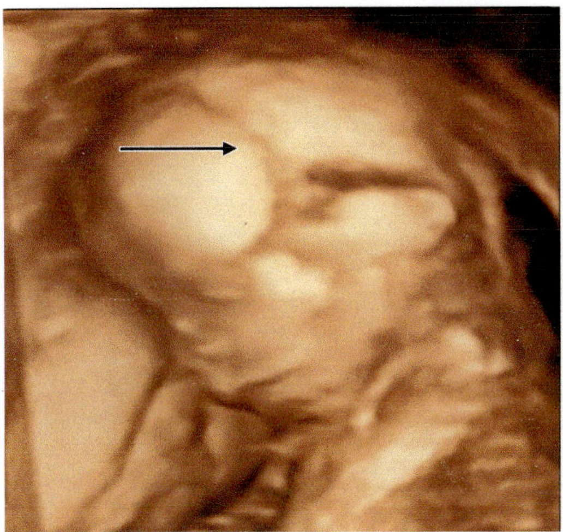

Fig. 24: Cranial sutures (arrow) seen on surface rendered three-dimensional (3D) ultrasound image of the fetal head.

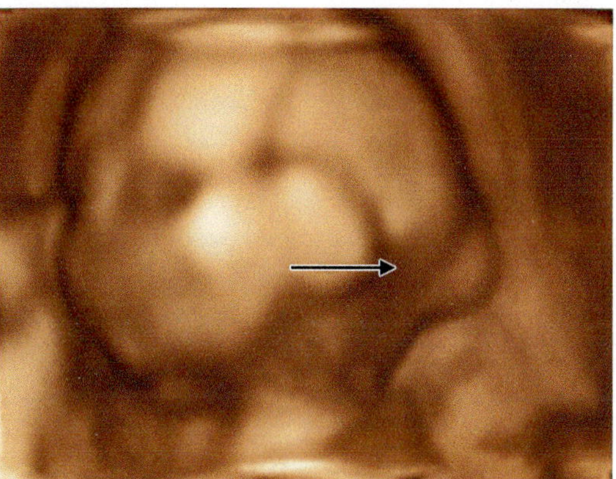

Fig. 26: Small occipital meningocele (arrow) seen on surface rendered three-dimensional (3D) ultrasound image of the fetal head.

fetal brain. Placenta and thick skull bones may be obstructing the vision on transabdominal approach. Gentle pressure on the fetal head with a steady hand while acquiring the volume of the head can avoid bone shadowing and help better visualization of the brain. When transvaginal route is used, the fontanelle which is open is used as an acoustic window (**Fig. 27**). Once the fetal brain volume is acquired, it is then possible to navigate in the stored volume. By multiplanar display, the brain anatomy can be studied in detail. Development of brain in the second trimester has three developmental landmarks which are as follows:

- Development of lateral ventricle into frontal, occipital, and temporal horns
- Development of corpus callosum
- Development of cerebellum and its vermis.

Whenever any abnormality of the fetal brain is suspected on B-mode ultrasound due to simple signs such as mild ventriculomegaly to major abnormalities such as hydrocephalus or midline shift, a detailed neurosonogram is required. Using TUI in all the three orthogonal planes, all the coronal, sagittal, and axial sections required for a detailed neurosonogram can be achieved by one single sweep of the fetal head. This consists of the following (**Figs. 28A to C**):

- Three axial planes:
  - Transventricular
  - Transthalamic
  - Transcerebellar
- Four coronal planes:
  - Transfrontal plane (frontal two planes)
  - Transcaudate plane (midcoronal one plane)
  - Transthalamic plane (midcoronal two planes)

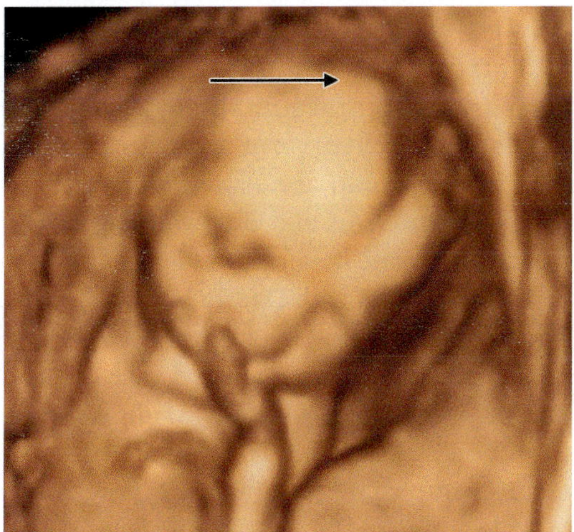

Fig. 25: Anterior fontanelle (arrow) seen on surface rendered three-dimensional (3D) ultrasound image of the fetal head.

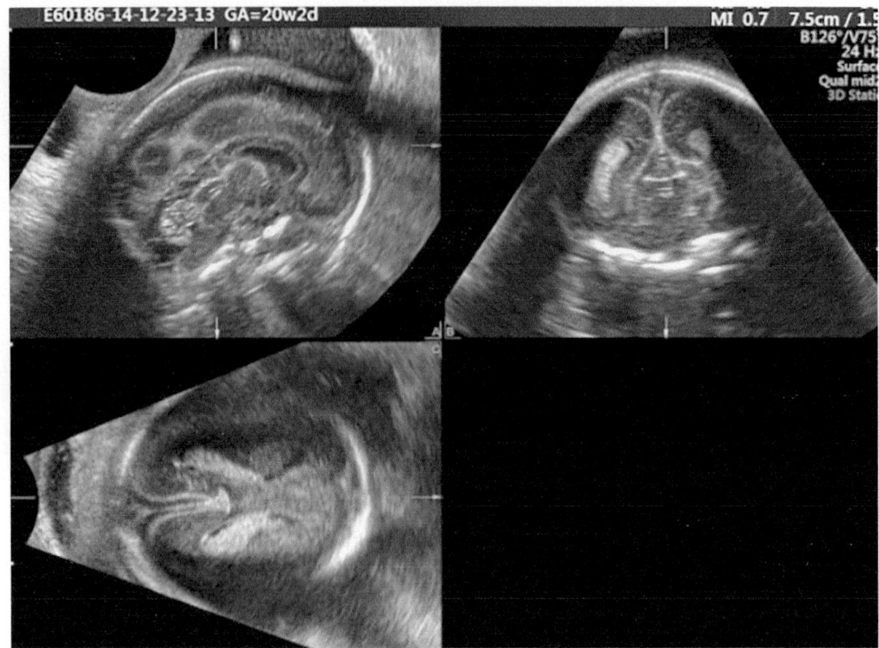

Fig. 27: Three-dimensional (3D) ultrasound acquired volume of fetal brain, through transvaginal route displayed as multiplanar images.

    - Transcerebellar plane (occipital one and two planes)
- Three sagittal planes:
    - Midsagittal
    - Two parasagittal sections.

Virtual organ computer-aided analysis (VOCAL) may be used for volume calculation of dilated ventricles and intracranial lesions. VCI in coronal plane depicts the midline structures such as corpus callosum, brainstem, cerebellar vermis, and optic chiasma.

Agenesis of corpus callosum and cerebellar vermian hypoplasias—Dandy walker syndrome can be demonstrated using VCI C in axial or coronal plane (**Figs. 29A and B**). Transvaginal transfontanelle 3D ultrasound has been preferred for confirmation of corpus callosum in some studies.[18] Volume acquisition if it is done from sagittal plane, corpus callosum appears echolucent, whereas if acquisition is done in axial plane, corpus callosum appears echogenic.[19] Normal corpus callosum and cerebellar vermis with ventriculomegaly is most likely due to aqueduct stenosis. In case of mild ventriculomegaly, it is essential to confirm the status of corpus callosum and cerebellar vermis. Ventriculomegaly can be quantitatively evaluated and clearly delineated using inversion mode for rendering and also by sonoAVC general (**Figs. 30A and B**).

Paladini and Volpe[20] have suggested measuring tentorovermian angle, tentoro-clivus angle, clivo-vermian angle, etc., to diagnose vermian abnormalities (**Fig. 31**). Both tentoro-clivus and clivo-vermian angles can demonstrate the upward displacement of vermis in fetuses with Dandy-Walker variant. The normal tentoro-clivus angle is 4 ± 4.2 and normal clivo-vermian angle is 47.8 ± 7.3 (**Fig. 32**). This study concludes that 3D ultrasound is the modality of choice to demonstrate the key features important for diagnosis of posterior fossa lesions like the upward displacement of the tentorium, the counterclockwise rotation, and the significant hypoplasia of the cerebellar vermis.[20]

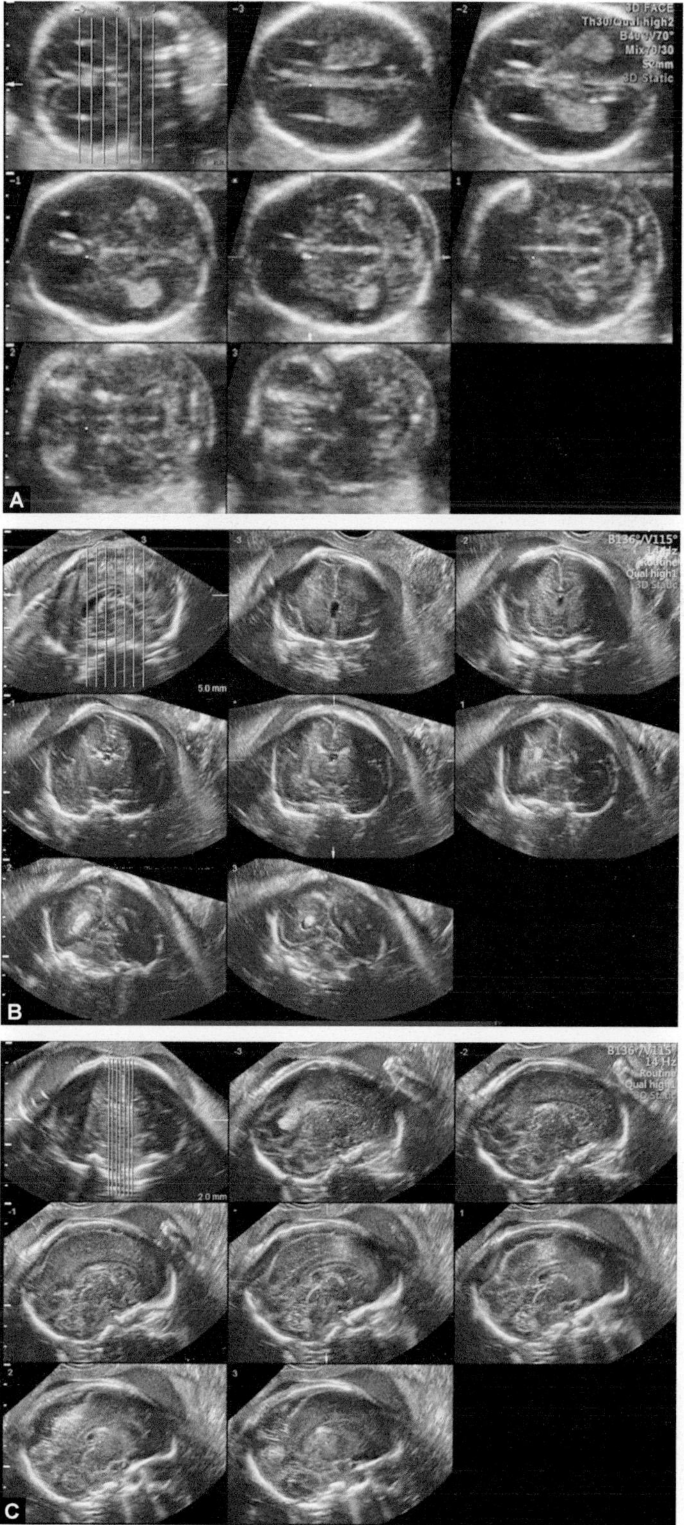

Figs. 28A to C: Tomographic ultrasound imaging (TUI) of the fetal head in axial, coronal and sagittal sections. Ultrasound of sections of detailed neurosonogram.

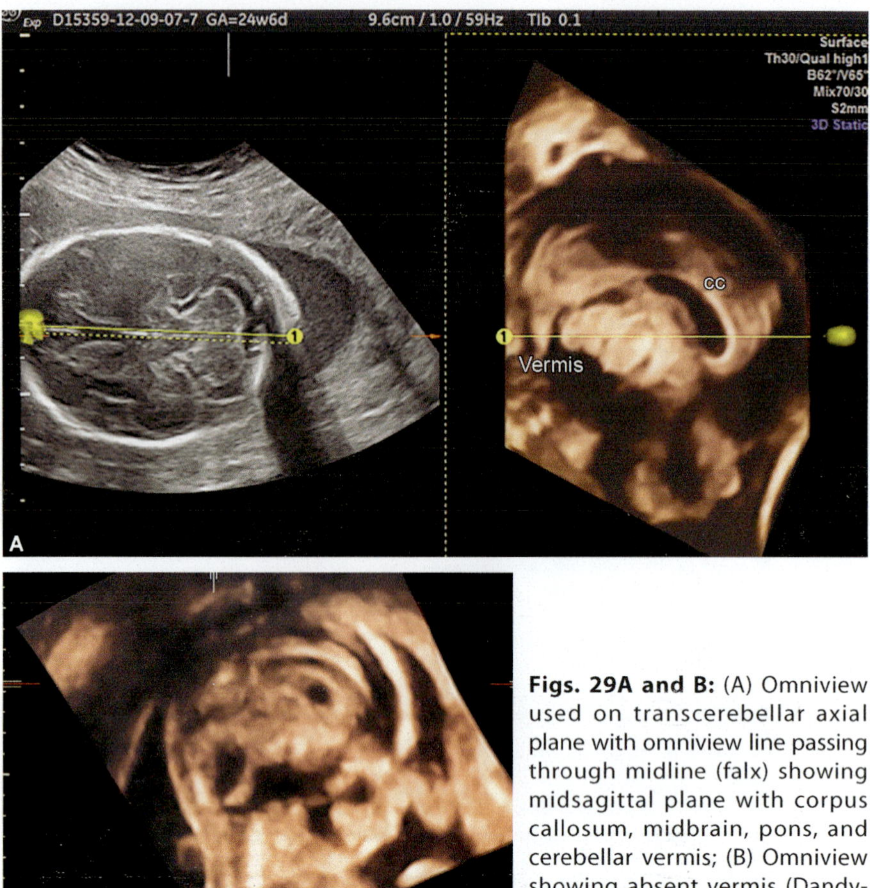

Figs. 29A and B: (A) Omniview used on transcerebellar axial plane with omniview line passing through midline (falx) showing midsagittal plane with corpus callosum, midbrain, pons, and cerebellar vermis; (B) Omniview showing absent vermis (Dandy-Walker syndrome).

Skull base development can be assessed by measurement of anterior skull base length and posterior cranial fossa length and skull base angle.[21] Brain growth leads to higher increment in posterior cranial fossa length leading to 6° flexion in the skull base angle.[21] Craniofacial variability index (CVI) can assist in fetal facial anatomy to study craniofacial development.[22] Sections of the skull required for all these measurements can be all achieved and

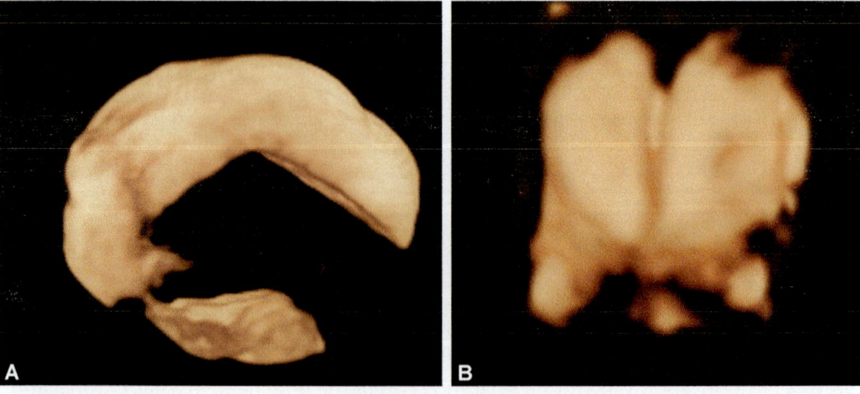

Figs. 30A and B: Inversion mode showing dilated lateral ventricles in sagittal plane and coronal plane.

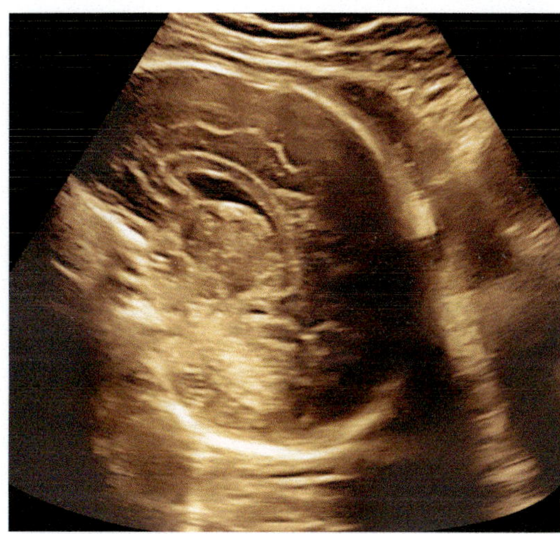

Fig. 31: Mid-sagittal plane of the fetal head.

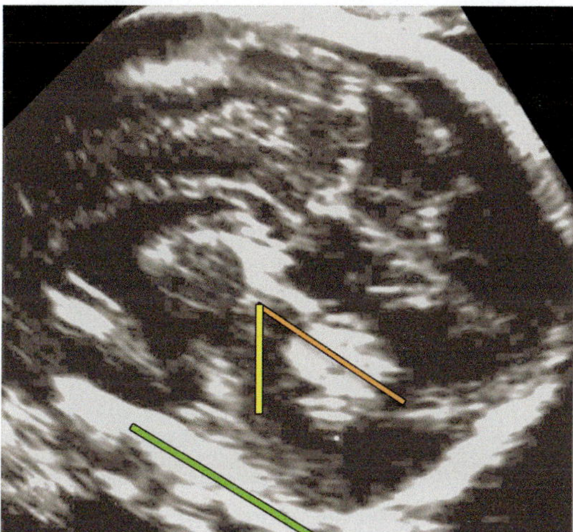

Fig. 32: Mid-sagittal plane of the fetal head showing measurement of tentoro-clivus and clivo-vermian angles.

measured by TUI and multiplanar mode. This technique has proved to be almost as sensitive as computed tomography (CT) scan or MRI for study of the brain lesions. 3D ultrasound may be applied to every central nervous system (CNS) abnormality diagnosed with traditional 2D technique and may offer further information useful for correct diagnosis. It can delineate the exact nature and anatomic level of anomaly.

Three-dimensional power Doppler also delineates the cerebral vasculature and its abnormalities (**Fig. 33**). Several workers have proved the role of 3D power Doppler for demonstration of vein of Galen aneurysm and have also claimed the technique to be comparable with MRI.[23] Though power Doppler does show the vascular architecture in detail, especially with transvaginal approach. 3D power Doppler may be added to the information.

Study of *fetal motor and behavioral pattern* is essential for complete evaluation or functional integrity of fetal CNS. Only 4D ultrasound allows the evaluation of fetal motor and behavioral patterns. With 4D ultrasound, it is possible to better define the degree of normality and pathology of fetal neurological functions in utero and to find out which fetuses are at risk of bad neurological outcome. Kurjak et al. have described patterns of neurodevelopmental behavior during the three trimesters of pregnancy using 4D ultrasound.[24] The changes in the motor pattern express the evolution of the maturative process of CNS during intrauterine life. These fetal behavior and movements can help diagnosis of abnormal motor development (**Figs. 34A to C**). Delayed motor development is seen in fetuses of diabetic mothers. Infolding of the thumb in the fist of the fetus is typically described as neurological thumb being a sign (**Fig. 35**) of some neurological deficit. Fetuses with arthrogryposis show early disturbances

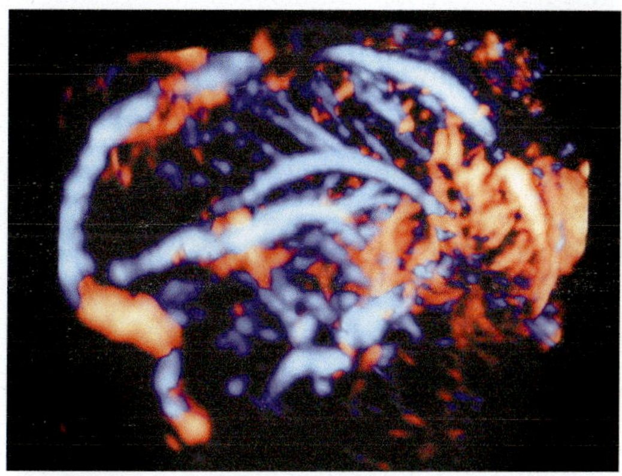

Fig. 33: Cerebral vasculature seen on three-dimensional (3D) power Doppler angiomode.

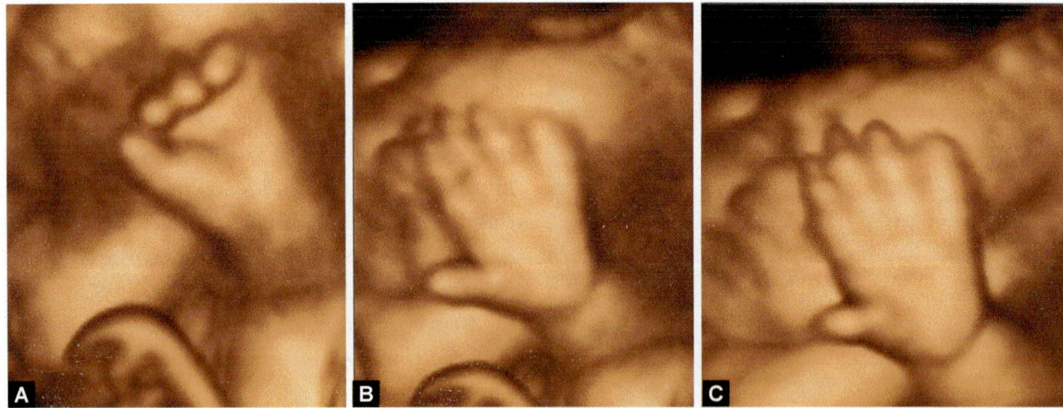

Figs. 34A to C: Movements of hand documented by series of images.

in motor development with absent limb movement and joint contractures (**Figs. 36A and B**). Fetal functional neurology has been discussed in detail in Chapter 8 of this book.

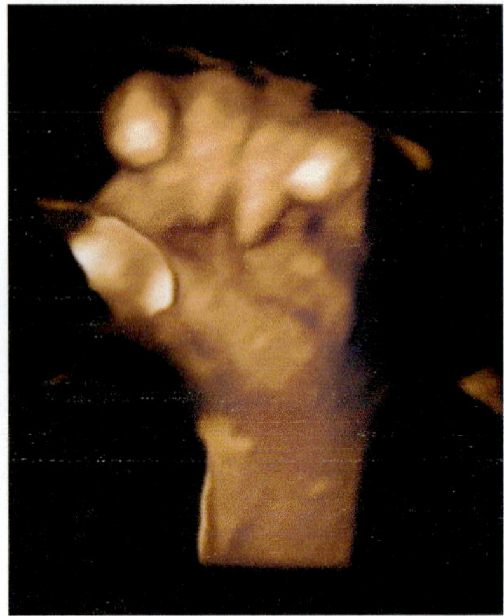

Fig. 35: Neurological thumb (thumb folded inside the fist).

Neck Abnormalities

Chiefly cystic hygroma and thyroid goiter are the two most common lesions seen in the fetal neck. Though these can be diagnosed on B-mode ultrasound, 3D ultrasound can be used for better demonstration of the same.[25,26]

Apart from these various studies have shown 3D ultrasound has been used for diagnosis of trisomy 18, and rare abnormalities of the face such as Treacher Collins syndrome, cebocephaly, and otocephaly (**Figs. 37A and B**).

Spinal Abnormalities

Evaluation of the CNS cannot be called complete without evaluation of the spine. Evaluation of the spine in sagittal, coronal, and axial all three planes is essential to diagnose spinal abnormalities correctly. All the three views cannot be achieved in one fetal position on 2D ultrasound. 3D ultrasound saves examination time and clearly can show all the three views at a time on multiplanar mode along with the overlying skin surface by using maximum mode transparent rendering

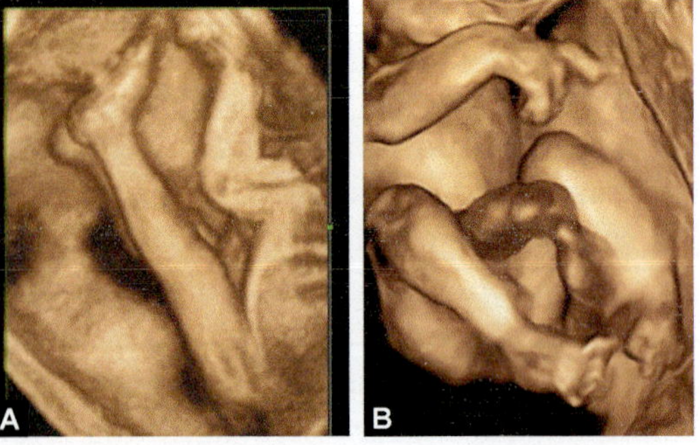

Figs. 36A and B: (A) Persistent extension deformity of lower limbs seen on three-dimensional (3D) ultrasound surface rendered image; (B) Multiple joint abnormalities of upper and lower limbs seen on 3D ultrasound surface rendered image.

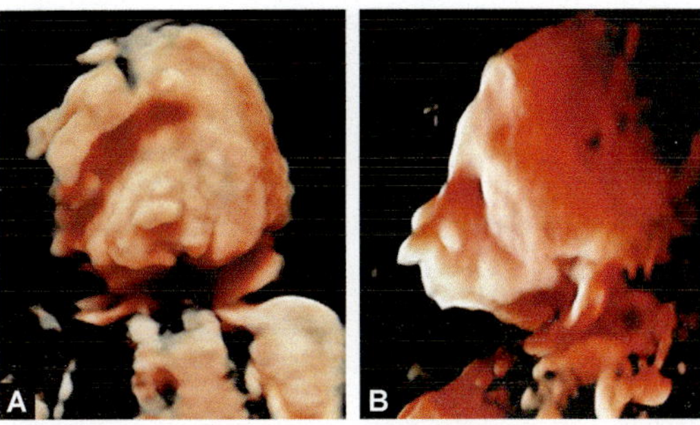

Figs. 37A and B: Coronal and sagittal plane high-definition (HD) live rendered images of major fetal facial abnormality.

and surface rendering (**Fig. 38A**). Using 4D VCI C can also show coronal view even when on 2D ultrasound only axial section is seen (**Figs. 38B and C**). Spinal column abnormalities such as spinal canal defects, hemivertebrae, and diastematomyelia can all be well demonstrated by 3D ultrasound (**Figs. 39A to D**).

Using MagiCut and 3D rotation, it is also possible to see each vertebrae separately on transverse section (**Fig. 40A**) and to define the extent of lesion, especially in cases of open spinal canal defects. In case of lesions such as teratomas or spinal canal defects and meningomyeloceles (**Figs. 40B and C**), 3D ultrasound allows to exactly define the number of involved vertebrae. Volume ultrasound has almost 100% sensitivity and very high specificity for diagnosis of spinal abnormalities. Longitudinal scan of the fetus is used with maximum mode to evaluate the thoracic cage, clavicle, and scapulae (**Fig. 41**). HD live is an even better mode to evaluate the spine. The settings for this are important. To render the bones on HD live,

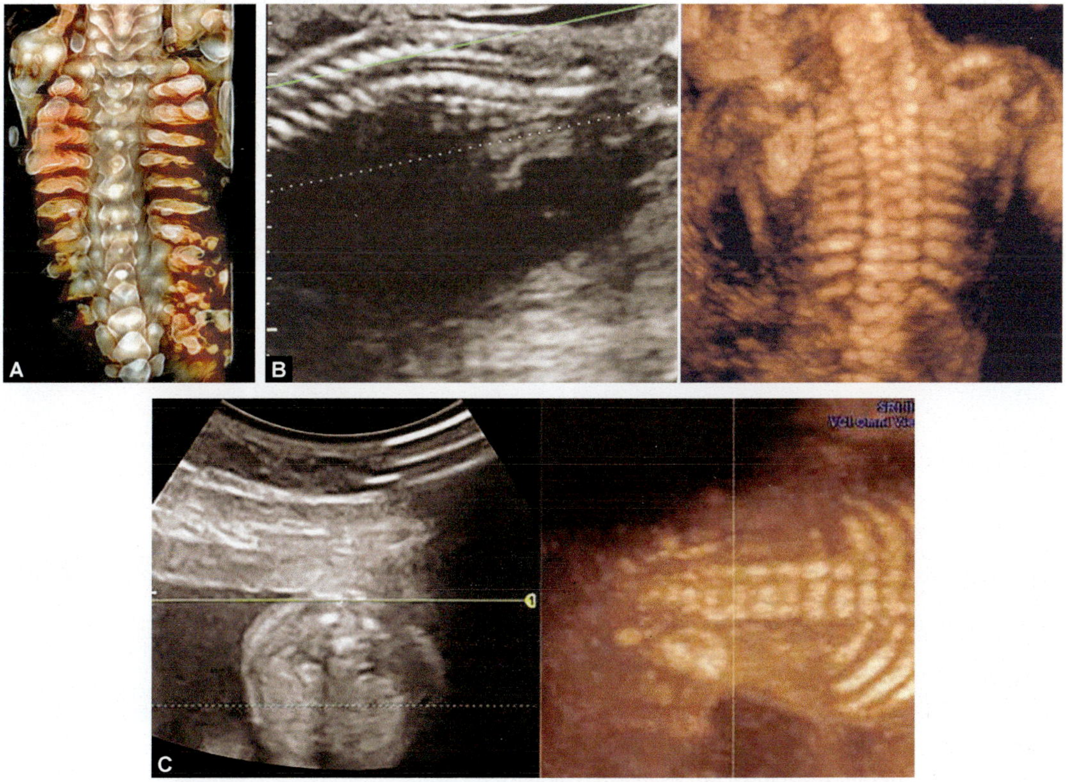

Figs. 38A to C: (A) Three-dimensional (3D) ultrasound high-definition (HD) live silhouette rendered image of normal spine; (B) Normal spine: Volume contrast imaging (VCI); (C) Omniview is used on axial section of trunk to image the spine in coronal plane.

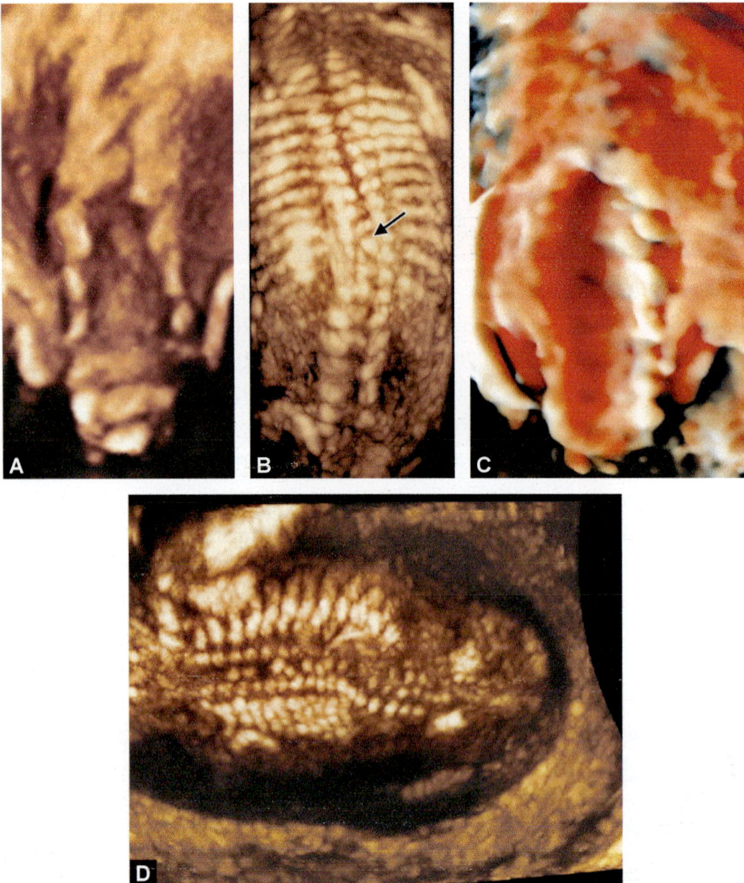

Figs. 39A to D: (A) Large open spinal canal defect of the lumbar spine rendered by three-dimensional (3D) ultrasound with combination of surface and maximum mode; (B) Hemivertebrae in lower thoracic spine rendered by 3D ultrasound with combination of surface and maximum mode; (C) Large open spinal canal defect with a large myelomeningocele rendered on high-definition (HD) live; (D) Multiple vertebral abnormalities rendered on maximum mode.

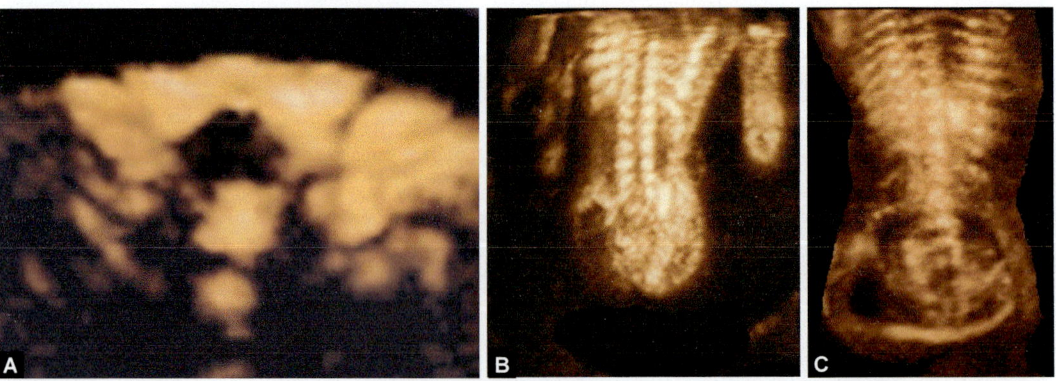

Figs. 40A to C: (A) Single vertebra rendered in transverse section using rendering the spine in coronal plane, selecting the vertebra, scooping it out by MagiCut and then x rotation; (B) Coronal plane of spine rendered in maximum mode showing absence of the sacral spine with soft tissue mass lesion—sacrococcygeal teratoma; (C) Coronal plane of the spine rendered in maximum mode showing widening of the sacral spine with a round echolucent lesion— sacral meningocele.

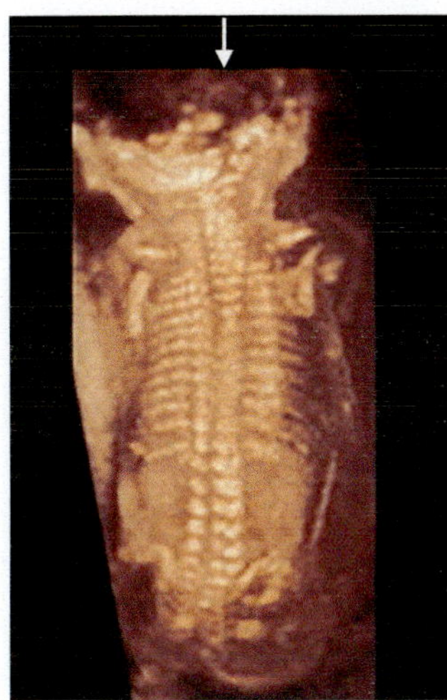

Fig. 41: Longitudinal scan of the fetus is used with maximum mode to evaluate the thoracic cage, clavicle, and scapulae.

usually zero threshold and high silhouette is used.

Chest

Multiplanar mode and TUI allow to study the spatial relationship between lungs, heart, esophagus, and diaphragm[27] (**Figs. 42A to C**). Trachea and esophagus morphology can be studied (**Fig. 43**), thus helping to diagnose tracheoesophageal fistulae early and to decide the type in utero. It is important to mention here that tracheoesophageal fistula is searched for on 2D ultrasound only in high risk cases or in those fetuses in whom stomach is persistently small or not seen. Randomly seeing for the esophagus and trachea for every scan is not done. Moreover, it is also important to note here that not all patients with tracheoesophageal fistula will show small or absent stomach shadow.

Diaphragmatic hernia can be easily diagnosed by 2D ultrasound. 3D ultrasound with VOCAL and 3D-4D multiplanar mode is useful for assessment of fetal lung volume, which is the prognosis deciding parameter in cases of diaphragmatic hernia and pulmonary hypoplasia also.

Studies have evaluated the potential of 3D power Doppler to predict neonatal outcome and pulmonary arterial hypertension in fetuses with congenital diaphragmatic hernia and have found that severity of pulmonary arterial hypertension was associated with progressive reduction in prenatal vascular indices.[28,29] Pulmonary hypoplasia may also be due to oligohydramnios due to any cause, premature rupture of membranes, chylothorax, etc., and it may be the deciding factor for prognosis. Lung volume assessment as mentioned earlier can help predict the prognosis in these cases too. To calculate the lung volume, 3D volume of the thorax is acquired in axial plane including the entire thorax, volume angle about 50–60° depending on the gestational age. Lung volume assessment is also helpful in cases with congenital cyst adenomatoid malformation of the lung (**Fig. 43**). Select either lung, one after the other, and use VOCAL to calculate the volume. Though sequestration of the lung and

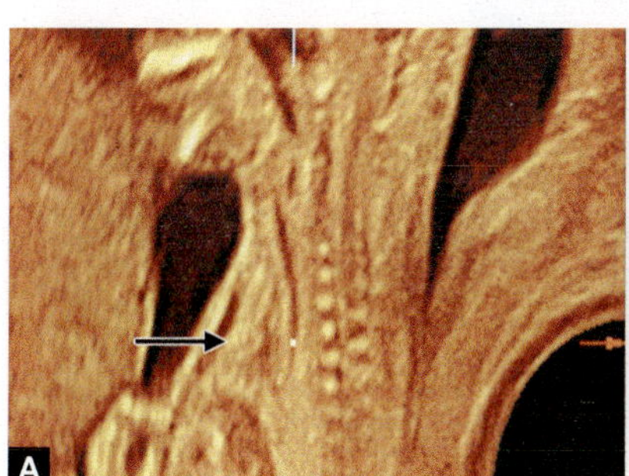

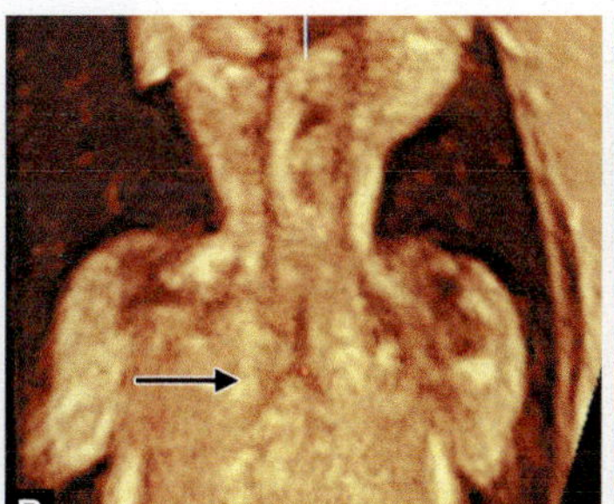

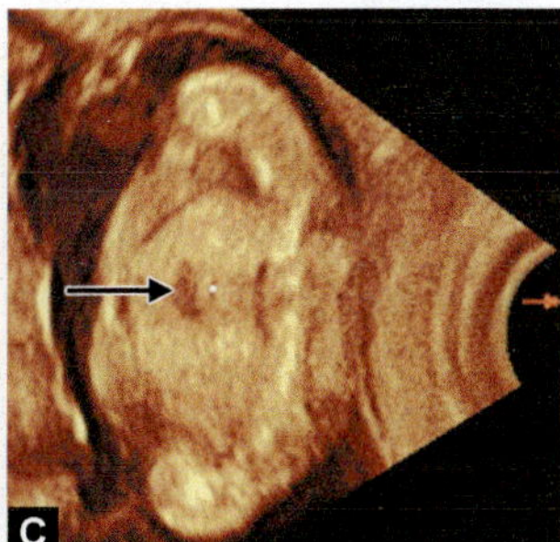

Figs. 42A to C: Multiplanar images of the fetal thorax, explaining the spatial relation of thoracic anatomy. Arrow showing tracheal bifurcation at the reference dot.

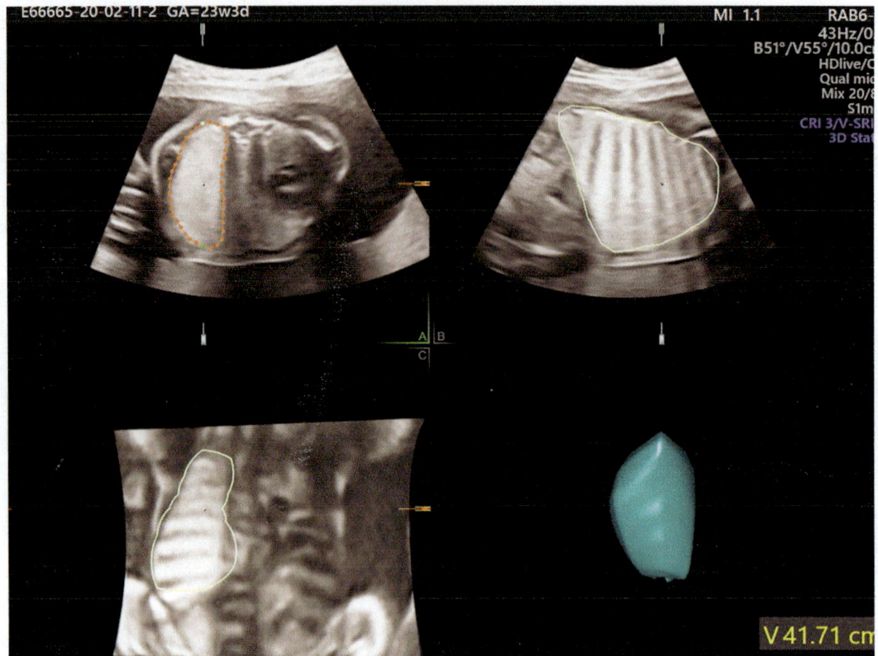

Fig. 43: VOCAL calculated lung volume from the multiplanar image of thorax.

cystic adenomatoid malformation of the lung is diagnosed on B-mode ultrasound, 3D power Doppler may give more confident diagnosis by identification of the vessels (**Fig. 44**).

Abdomen

Using transparent mode and multiplanar mode, the abdominal organs can be very well identified with definition of all tissue planes. 3D ultrasound is an effective tool for the diagnosis of gastrointestinal malformations and gives additional information over 2D ultrasound for pediatric surgeons for surgical planning and for counseling with parents. Inversion mode helps to define cystic lesions and can be best used to confirm the diagnosis of pyloric stenosis, duodenal atresia, posterior urethral valves, obstructive uropathy, etc. (**Figs. 45A to C**). All abdominal masses may be better evaluated by multiplanar mode for their origin and extension.

Hydronephrosis, hydroureter, and even the bladder abnormalities including posterior urethral valve can be well demonstrated by 3D ultrasound (**Fig. 45D**). Congenital renal tumors, nephroblastoma, its extent can be assessed by 3D ultrasound TUI and 3D power Doppler also helps to assess the extent of the lesion. VOCAL may be used to calculate the tumor volume, volume of dilated pelvicalyceal

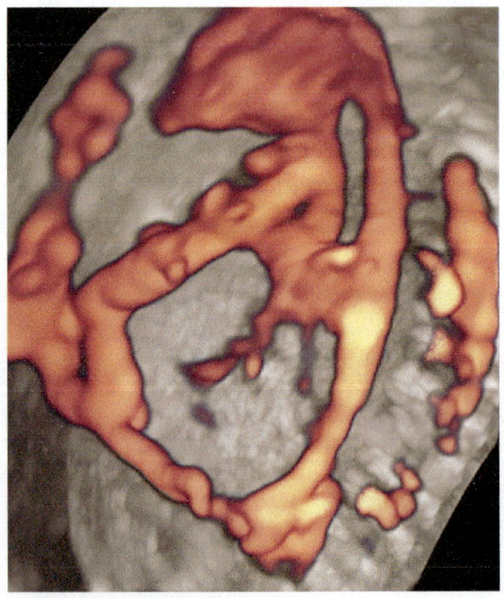

Fig. 44: Three-dimensional (3D) power Doppler image showing fetal trunk vasculature.

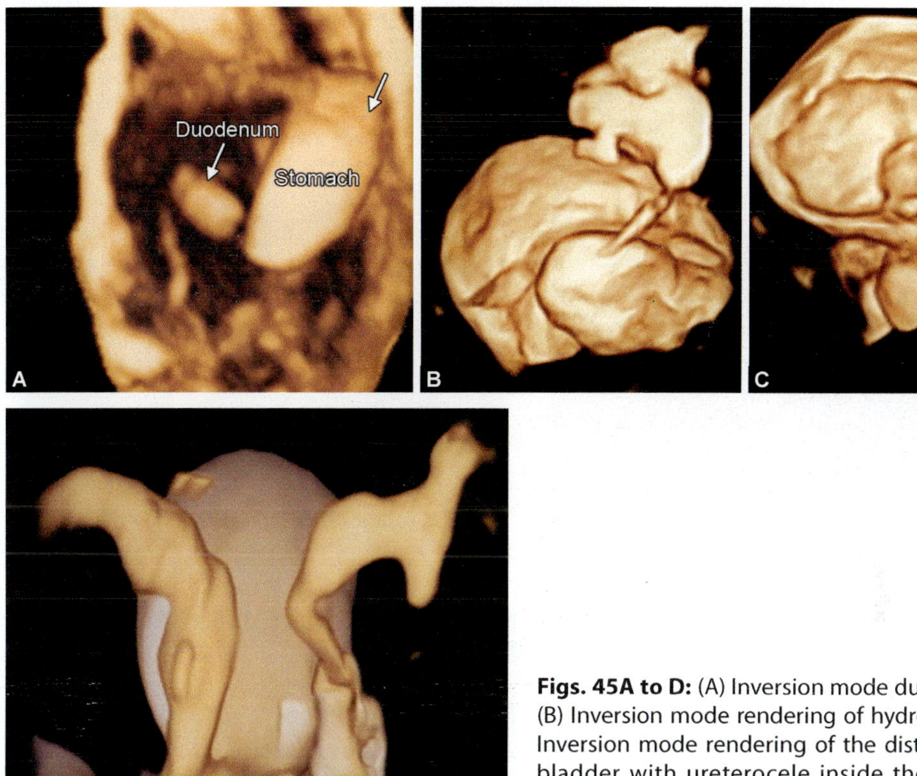

Figs. 45A to D: (A) Inversion mode duodenal atresia; (B) Inversion mode rendering of hydronephrosis; (C) Inversion mode rendering of the distended urinary bladder with ureterocele inside the bladder; (D) Bilateral hydronephrosis and hydroureter shown on inversion mode rendering.

system, distended bladder, and these can be of help for comparison for follow-up of these lesions and to prognosticate them. Surface rendering allows clear visualization of genitals and thus can be a helpful tool to demonstrate the abnormalities of the genitals that may be of major importance for the family. Hypospadias is seen as "Tulip sign"[22] and clitoral hypertrophy can be diagnosed in the third trimester.

Anterior abdominal wall defects are usually diagnosed on 2D ultrasound but are well demonstrated on volume ultrasound. 3D ultrasound with power Doppler is very useful to differentiate the bowel-containing from the liver-containing omphalocele. Use of 3D multiplanar display is more accurate than the use of 2D ultrasound for measuring the size of omphalocele. Omphalocele and gastroschisis can be confidently differentiated by 3D ultrasound.

Three-dimensional ultrasound with VOCAL can be used to calculate the liver volume as for the lungs. Liver volume has been considered as a parameter that correlates with fetal growth retardation.[30] Study of the abdominal vasculature is facilitated by 3D power Doppler.

Limb Abnormalities

Though limb abnormalities are fairly well demonstrated on 2D ultrasound, 3D ultrasound produces a more understandable picture for patient explanation. Accurate analysis of majority of bony structures can be done by using maximum mode rendering of 3D ultrasound or omniview, though in general limb abnormalities can also be

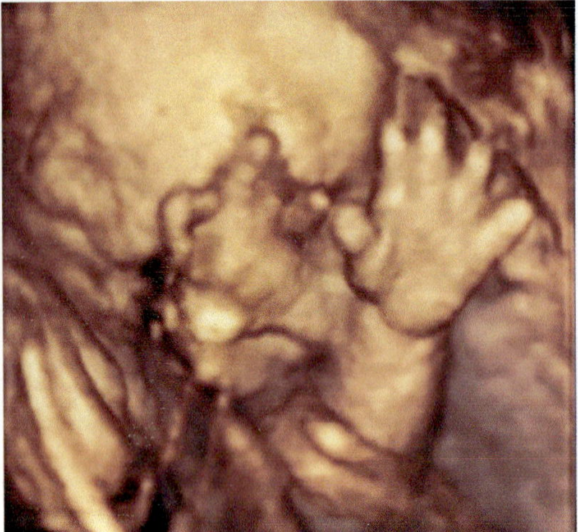

Fig. 46: Surface rendered image of fetal hand.

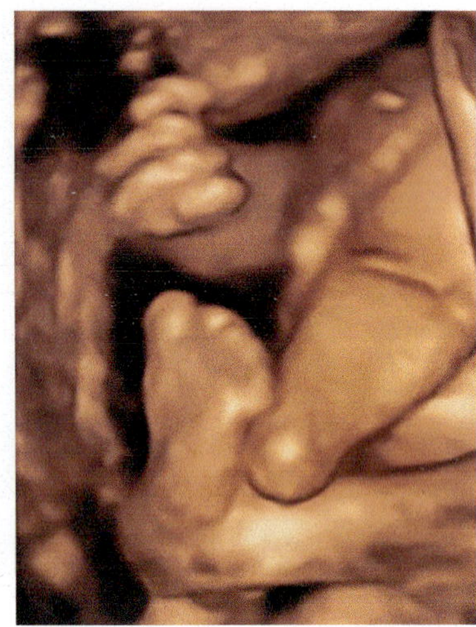

Fig. 47: Surface rendered image of fetal hand and foot.

demonstrated well by surface mode (**Figs. 46 and 47**). 3D–4D ultrasound enables detailed examination of fingers and toes with almost 100% certainty of detecting agenesis and extra digits (**Figs. 48A to C**). Motor abnormalities and abnormal attitude of fingers, toes, or hands and legs such as club feet (**Figs. 49A and B**), overriding of fingers, flexion/extension deformities the joints as in (arthrogryposis), or thumb in the fist may be manifestations of chromosomal or neurological abnormality. Club feet can also be well ruled out or demonstrated with omniview when rendering is difficult due to fetal position or reduced amniotic fluid amount.

Placenta

It is known that pregnancy-induced hypertension occurs only after at least 70% of the placental vasculature is obliterated. 3D power Doppler with angiomode of the placental vasculature may show obliteration of the placental vessels and pruning effect and help to predict pregnancy-induced hypertension much earlier (**Figs. 50A and B**). Morbidly adherent placenta, though is diagnosed by B-mode ultrasound, 3D

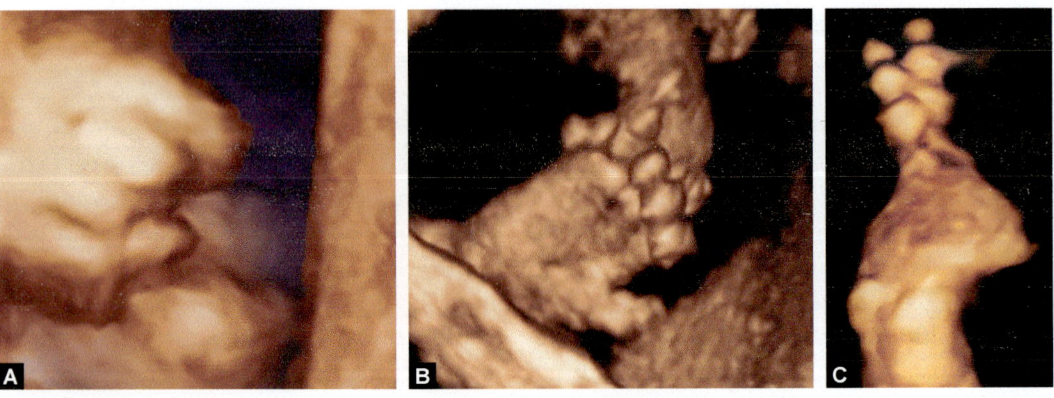

Figs. 48A to C: Surface rendered image of: (A) Overriding of fingers; (B) Polydactyly; (C) Radial aplasia.

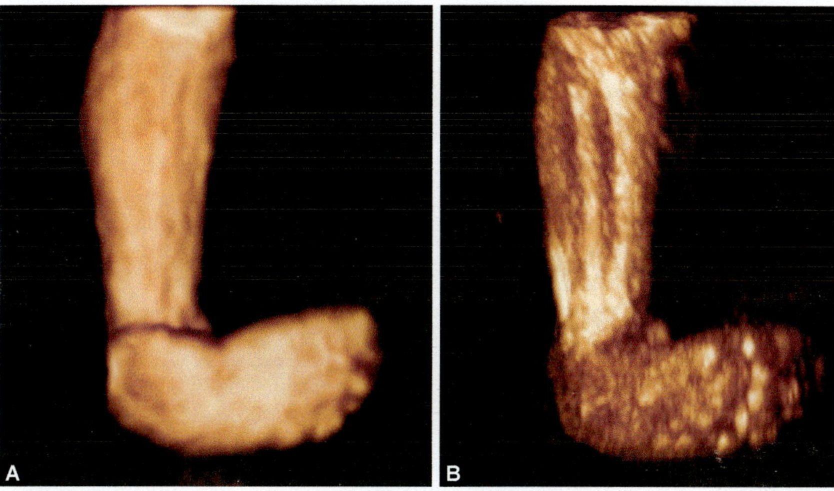

Figs. 49A and B: Clubfoot rendered on: (A) Surface mode; (B) Maximum mode after MagiCut.

power Doppler helps to assess the extent of vascularity and thus confirms the penetration of the placenta (**Figs. 50C and D**).

Normal cord vessels can be visualized on color Doppler and 3D ultrasound added to this gives more real-life and clear image (**Fig. 51A**).

Cord abnormalities such as hypercoiling (**Fig. 51B**) and abnormal cord insertion also can be confirmed with 3D Doppler. Cord round the neck, true knot in cord can be more confidently diagnosed by 3D Doppler (**Figs. 52A and B**).

Benacerraff et al.[31] has described a novel use of 3D ultrasound in offline fetal evaluation. According to her study, five volume sweeps should be taken of every fetus, and they are examined offline. This method has proved to be successful in detailed evaluation of fetal anatomy and very sensitive for diagnosing fetal anomalies. These sweeps are axial section of fetal head, axial section of fetal thorax, axial section of fetal abdomen, longitudinal sweep of lower limbs, and longitudinal section of head.

THREE-DIMENSIONAL AND FOUR-DIMENSIONAL FETAL ECHOCARDIOGRAPHY

Cardiac evaluations have been made less time-consuming and much easier with advancing technology. New 4D ultrasound technology with STIC can be used for offline 4D cardiac evaluation. It is one of the best teaching and learning tools, especially in cases with cardiac abnormalities. After optimizing the 2D image, a single sweep is taken from the upper abdomen to the upper chest in 7.5–15 seconds. Hundreds of images of the heart during different phases of cardiac cycle are captured and stored. The computer depending on its calculated heart rate divides these images into systolic and diastolic phase and synchronizes one after the other in correct sequence of events and then plays the entire clip of the cardiac cycle continuously as a volume. This can be seen in all three planes like any other volume imaging, X, Y, and Z (sagittal, axial, and coronal) (**Fig. 53**) and can be run as a continuous cardiac cycle. This acquisition and display can also be done with color or power Doppler (**Fig. 54**). Volume of the heart can be acquired in with the heart on 2D seen as four chamber heart view. Before acquisition, it must be confirmed that you have selected the fetal cardiac preset that has more bright gray map and high contrast. If the volume is to be acquired with color Doppler, the color settings in the cardiac preset has high pulse repetition frequency (PRF) and high wall motion filter. The color gains should be

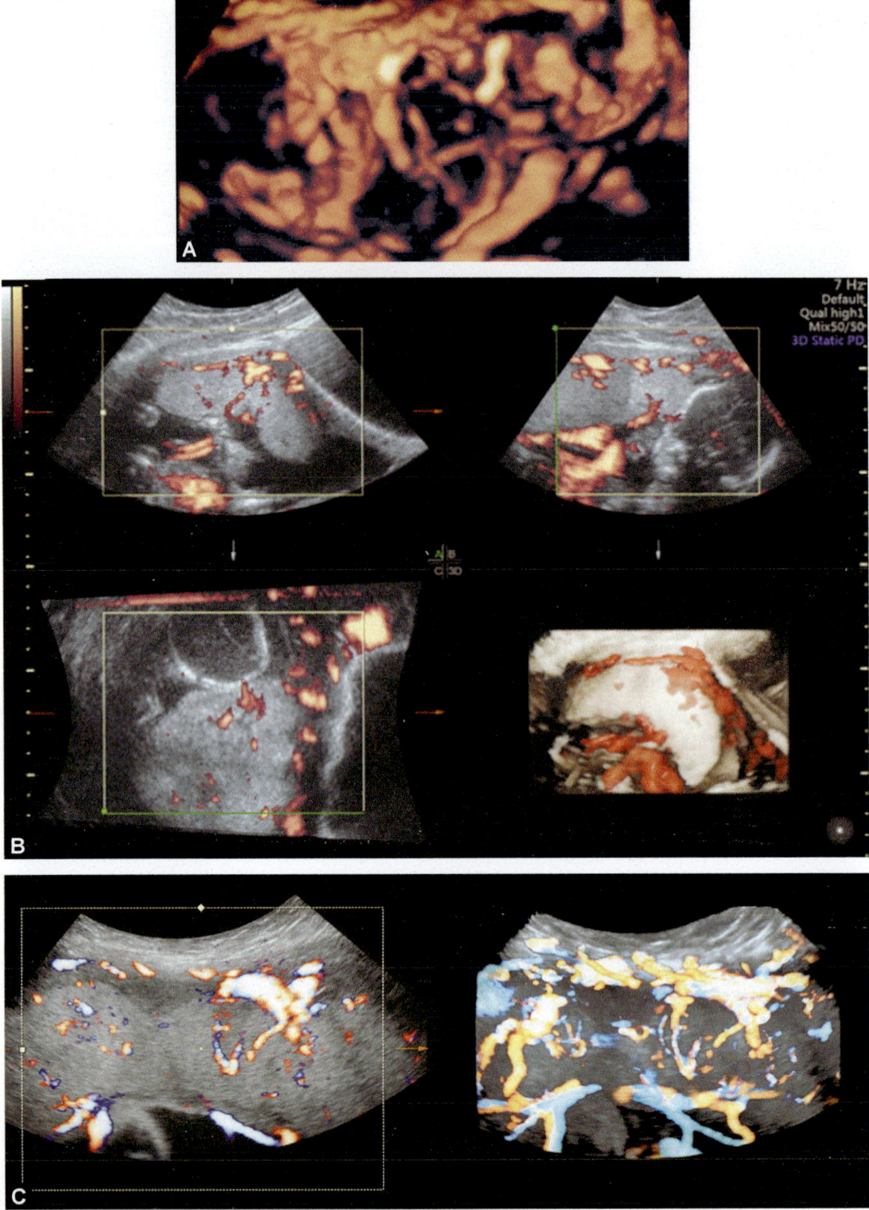

Figs. 50A to C: (A) Normal placental vasculature on three-dimensional (3D) power Doppler; (B) 3D power Doppler multiplanar and rendered image showing scanty placental vascularity with pruning of vessels; (C) 3D high-definition (HD) flow showing normal placental vasculature.

set such that it fills up the cardiac chambers completely and does not spill out. The best possible volume quality is selected according to the fetal movements. Though it is best to wait for the fetus to calm down before STIC volume is acquired. Fetal movements can lead to significant distortions in the image. The volume angle selected is between 20 and 35° depending on the gestational age so that the volume contains upper thorax to upper abdomen. Stomach should be seen in the lower most section and it should extend just

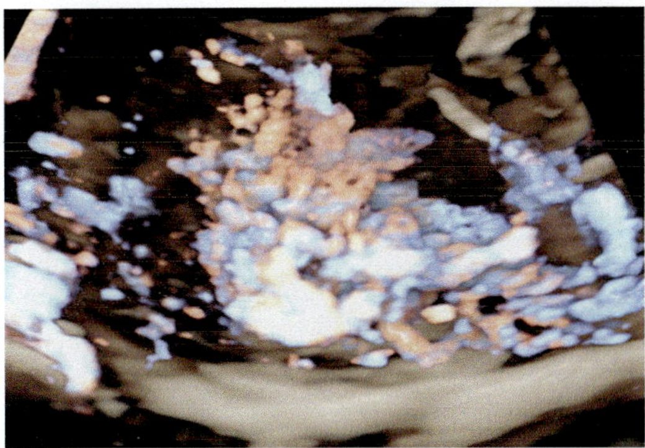

Figs. 50D: Placental increta with placental vasculature extending till uterine serosa.

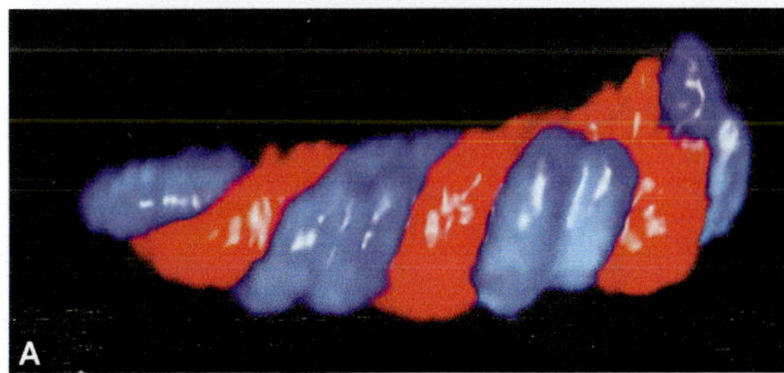

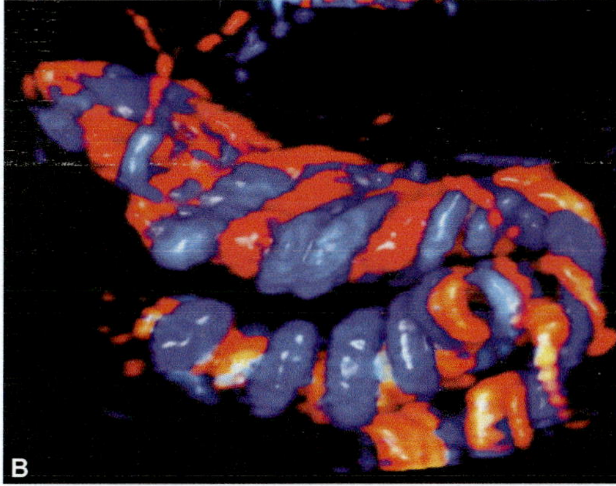

Figs. 51A and B: (A) Normal cord on three-dimensional (3D) power Doppler with MagiCut; (B) Hypercoiling of cord.

beyond the three vessel trachea view. Once the volume is acquired, usually z rotation is used to achieve an apical four chamber view. The x and y rotations may be used to correct any errors in the four chamber section. Once that image is perfect, then the analysis is started. Analysis is started with the reference point on the crux of the heart. Rendering is usually done in front back or back front

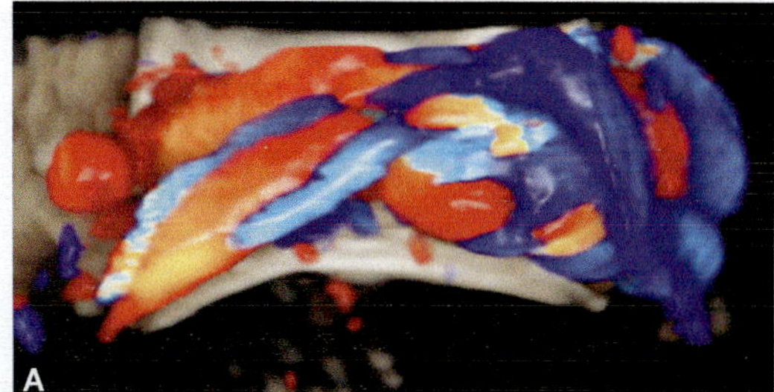

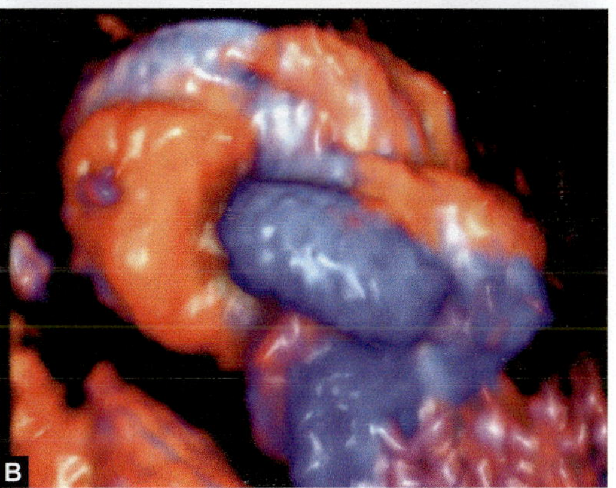

Figs. 52A and B: (A) Two loops of cord round the neck; (B) True knot in the cord. Both images are rendered in three-dimensional (3D) power Doppler with MagiCut.

direction. The render box size and position is adjusted according to what structure is to be rendered. Though usually front back render direction is selected.

Walking through these sections give all the planes required for complete cardiac evaluation, like four chamber view, left ventricular outflow tract view, right ventricular outflow tract view, three vessel view, short axis view, aortic arch view, ductus arch view, etc. These views can be seen simultaneously by using TUI with 3D or 4D (**Fig. 55**). The image can also be seen as live 3D by various rendering modes.

Inversion mode of rendering can be a useful tool to demonstrate small septal defects difficult to image otherwise and also for demonstration of outflow tracts and great vessels (**Fig. 56**). HD live and glass body mode is used for valvular defects, outflow tract defects, and septal defects. Angiomode is

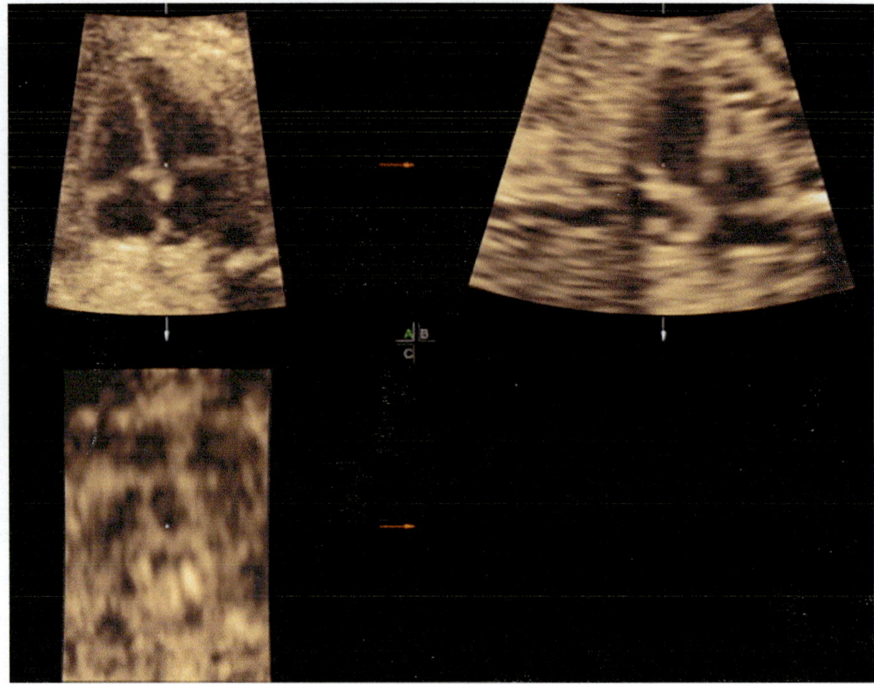

Fig. 53: Multiplanar display of the spatial temporal image correlation (STIC) acquired volume of the fetal heart.

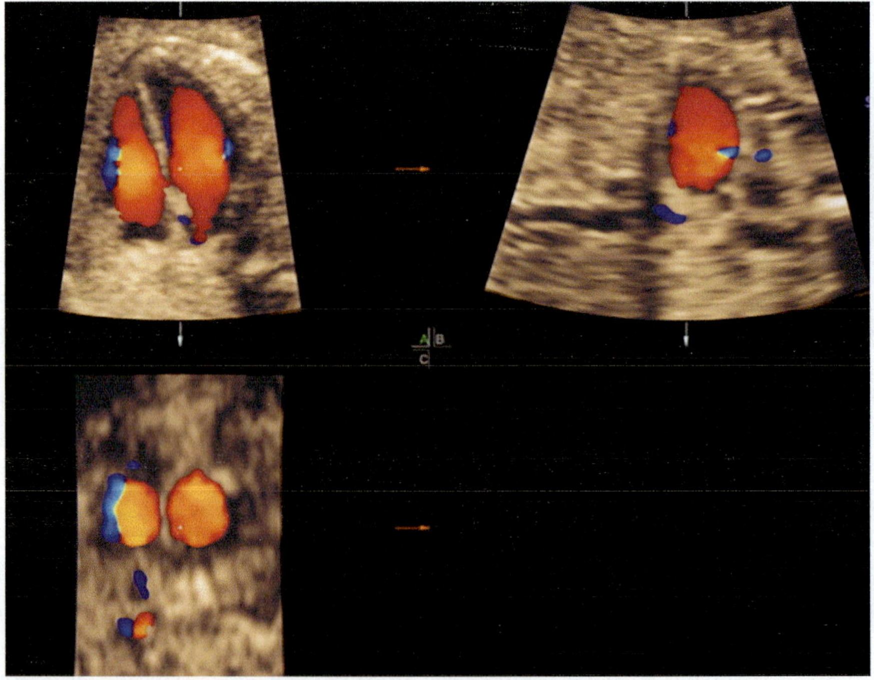

Fig. 54: Multiplanar display of the spatial temporal image correlation (STIC) acquired volume of the fetal heart with color Doppler.

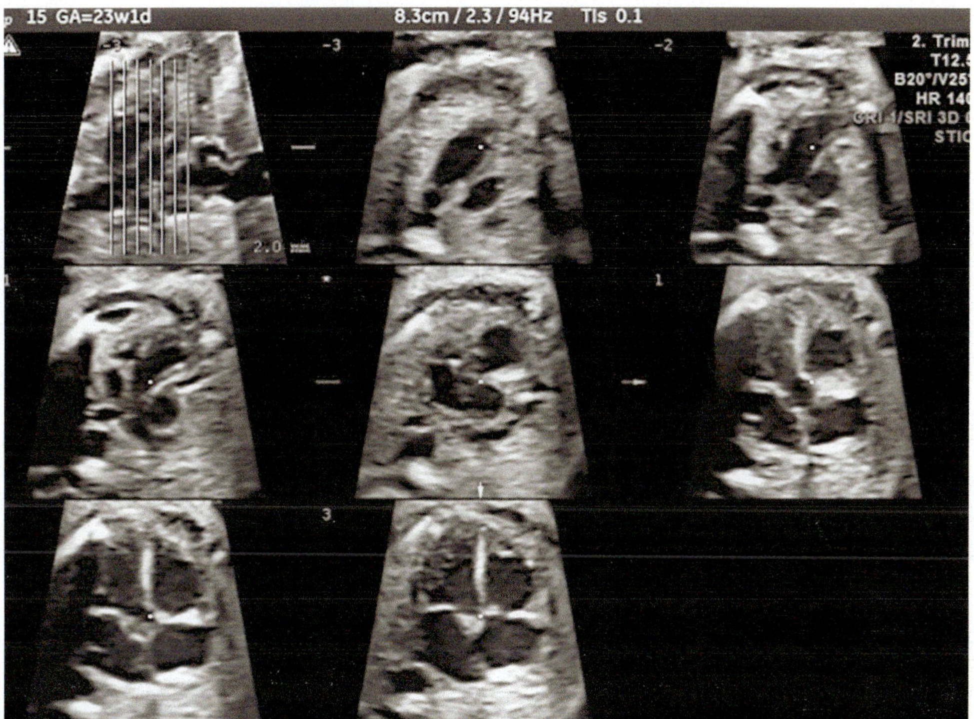

Fig. 55: Tomographic ultrasound imaging (TUI) of the spatial temporal image correlation (STIC) acquired volume of the fetal heart.

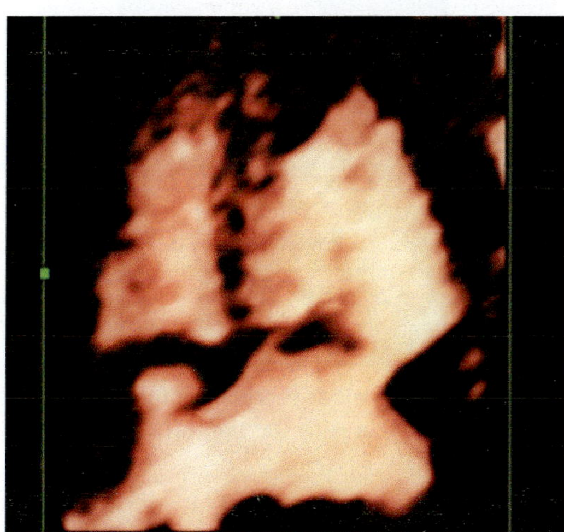

Fig. 56: Inversion mode rendering of the heart.

especially useful for the study of the arch views and relationship of great vessels and study of their branches or vascular abnormalities. Rendering from different directions can give all those views of the heart that were never possible by any other modality, e.g., basic view or surgical view of the heart, which shows relationship of all the four valves, that is very informative for outflow tract relationship, inflow tract abnormalities, and important for surgeons. For this view, the render direction selected is updown. Individual valves can be studied by omniview or rendering.

VCAD can be more useful for beginners. When working with this, the essential views of the heart are only a button touch away. No manual rotations or walking through are necessary. Volume of the heart is acquired as usual. The A plane is manipulated (rotation and zoom-unzoom) to match the predrawn four chamber heart diagram of the heart (**Fig. 57**). The predrawn diagram is placed on A image that is showing four chamber view of the heart and then various sections required are automatically achieved by only a button touch. This makes cardiac evaluation much quicker

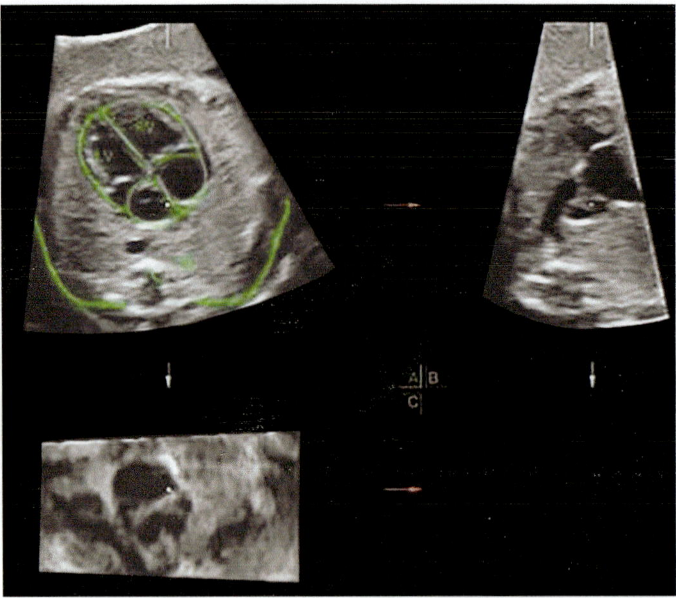

Fig. 57: VCAD used on spatial temporal image correlation (STIC) acquired volume of the heart.

both online and offline. Using rendering, the heart is reconstructed in four chamber view and then is cut by a line from apex to base, closely placed near the septum and then rotating it shows the interventricular septum enface. This view is excellent for demonstration of location and extent of ventricular septal defect (VSD). In cases of cardiac tumors or also for study of the chordae tendinae, the viewing line is placed parallel to interventricular septum in the ventricle of interest. Relationship of the two arches can be best studied when the volume is acquired in sagittal plane of the fetus and the viewing line is placed cephalic to the arches, either on inversion mode or on angiomode (**Fig. 58**). These are just a few narrated here for the reader's interest but there can be lot of innovations in this.

Omniview also can be used to save time and also for some difficult to get image planes. It is chiefly used on outflow tracts or three vessel or three vessel trachea view. To establish the identity of a particular vessel especially in cases of suspected abnormalities, omniview may be used to see the long axis of the vessel or its relationship to surrounding structures.

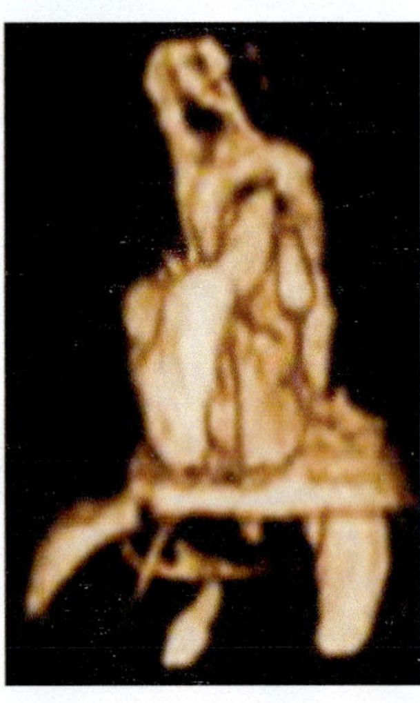

Fig. 58: Inversion mode rendering of the fetal heart and outflow tracts with the two arches in coronal plane.

Conjoined Twins

In conjoined twins, practicability and the consequent morbidity of the fetuses after separation depend on the degree of codivision of organs and vascular structures. Therefore, detailed and accurate anatomic and vascular map is fundamental for evaluation of joined organs in conjoined fetuses and is of

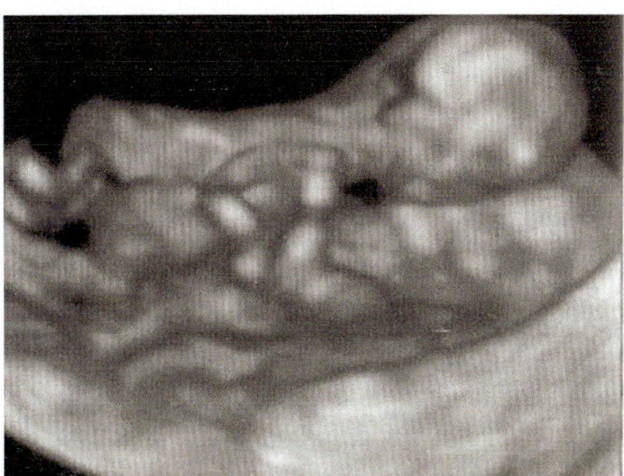

Fig. 59: Surface rendered image of thoracopagus conjoined twins.

fundamental importance to decide the line of treatment. Moreover defects such as orofacial cleft, diaphragmatic hernia, imperforate anus, and neural tube defects are also common. Bega et al. have reported that combining multiplanar display and surface rendering can assess these fetuses fairly reliably, as early as 10 weeks.[32] 3D ultrasound can be of great help in classifying more accurately the type of conjoined twins and color Doppler may be of further help (**Fig. 59**).

LIMITATIONS OF THREE-DIMENSIONAL AND FOUR-DIMENSIONAL ULTRASOUND

As for 2D ultrasound, maternal obesity, maternal scar, maternal movements, excessive fetal movements, and air, calcifications or bones that come in way of sound propagation are obstacles for 3D ultrasound also. Oligohydramnios does not permit sufficient fluid interface that is an absolute essential for surface rendering and so is not a favorable factor for reconstruction and surface rendering.

CONCLUSION

Volume ultrasound is a very valuable tool for diagnosis and demonstration of fetal abnormalities in spite of these limitations. Volume ultrasound gives better accuracy with a shorter examination time. 3D orientation and multiplanar imaging give unlimited tomograms, with only limited probe manipulation and minimize the fetal exposure to ultrasound.

REFERENCES

1. Merz E, Weber G, Bahlmann F, Miric-Tesanic D. Application of transvaginal and abdominal three dimensional ultrasound for detection or exclusion of fetal malformations of fetal face. Ultrasound Obstet Gynecol. 1997;9(4):237-43.
2. Rotten D, Levaillant JM. Two and three dimensional sonographic assessment of fetal face.2. Analysis of cleft lip. Alveolus and palate. Ultrasound Obstet Gynecol. 2004;24(4):402-11.
3. Platt LD, DeVore GR, Pretorius DH. Improving cleft palate/cleft lip antenatal diagnosis by three dimensional sonography the 'flipped face' view. J Ultrasound Med. 2006;25(11):1423-30.
4. Pilu G, Segata M. A novel technique for visualization of the normal and cleft fetal secondary palate: angled insonation and three dimensional ultrasound. Ultrasound Obstet Gynecol. 2007;29(2):166-9.
5. Campbell S, Lees C, Moscoso G, Hall P. Ultrasound antenatal diagnosis of cleft palate by a new technique: the 3D "reverse face" view. Ultrasound Obstet Gynecol. 2005;25(1):12-8.
6. McGahan MC, Ramos GA, Landry C, Wolfson T, Spwell BB, D'Agostini D, et al. Multislice display of the fetal face using three dimensional ultrasonography. J Ultrasound Med. 2008;27(11):1573-81.
7. Kurjak A, Azumendi G, Andonotopo W, Salihagic-Kadic A. Three and four dimensional ultrasonography for the structural and functional evaluation of the fetal face. Am J Obstet Gynecol. 2007;196(1):16-28.
8. Benacerraf BR, Sadow PM, Barnewolt CE, Estroff JA, Benson C. Cleft of secondary palate without cleft lip diagnosed with three-dimensional ultrasound and magnetic resonance imaging in fetus with Fryn's syndrome. Ultrasound Obstet Gynecol. 2006;27(5):566-70.
9. Sleurs E, Goncalves LF, Jhonson A, Espinoza J, Devers P, Chaiworapongsa T, et al. First trimester ultrasonic findings in a fetus with frontonasal malformation. J Matern Fetal Neonatal Med. 2004;16(3):187-97.
10. Rotten D, Levaillant JM, Martinez H, Ducou H, Le Pointe D, Vicaut E. The fetal mandible: a 2D and 3D sonographic approach to the diagnosis of retrognathia and micrognathia. Ultrasound Obstet Gynecol. 2002;19(2):122-30.

11. Paladini D, Morra T, Teodoro A, Lamberti A, Tremolaterra F, Martinelli P. Objective diagnosis of micrognathia in the fetus: The Jaw Index. Obstet Gynecol. 1999;93(3):382-6.
12. Borenstein M, Perisco N, Strobl I, Sonek J, Nicolaides KH. Frontomaxillary and mandibulomaxillary facial angles at 11 + 0 to 13 + 6 weeks in fetuses with trisomy 18. Ultrasound Obstet Gynecol. 2007;30(7):928-33.
13. Benoitt B, Chaoui R. Three dimensional ultrasound with maximal mode rendering: a novel technique for diagnosis of bilateral or unilateral absence or hypoplasia of nasal bones in second trimester screening for Down's syndrome. Ultrasound Obstet Gynecol. 2005;25(1):19-24.
14. Sepulwada W, Wojakowski AB, Elias D, Otano L, Gutierrez J. Congenital dacrocystocoele prenatal 2 and 3 dimensional sonographic findings. J Ultrasound Med. 2005;24(2):225-30.
15. Krakow D, Santulli T, Platt LD. Use of three dimensional ultrasonography in differentiating craniosynostosis from severe fetal molding. J Ultrasound Med. 2001;20(4):427-31.
16. Dikkeboom CM, Roelfsema NM, Van Adrichem LN, Wladimiroff JW. The role of three dimensional ultrasound in visualizing the fetal cranial sutures and fontanels during the second half of pregnancy. Ultrasound Obstet Gynecol. 2004;24(4):412-6.
17. Paladini D, Vassallo M, Sglavo G, Pastore G, Lapa dula C, Nappi C. Normal and abnormal development of the fetal anterior fontanelle: a three dimensional ultrasound study. Ultrasound Obstet Gynecol. 2008;32(6):755-61.
18. Timor-Tristch IE, Monteagudo A, Mayberry P. Three dimensional ultrasound evaluation of fetal brain: the three horn view. Ultrasound Obstet Gynecol. 2000;16(4):302-6.
19. Plasencia W, Dagklis T, Borenstein M, Csapo B, Nicolaides KH. Assessment of corpus callosum at 20-24 weeks gestation by three dimensional ultrasound examination. Ultrasound Obstet Gynecol. 2007;30(2):169-72.
20. Paladini D, Volpe P. Posterior fossa and vermian morphometry in the characterization of fetal cerebellar abnormalities: a perspective three dimensional ultrasound study. Ultrasound Obstet Gynecol. 2006;27(5):482-9.
21. Roelfsema NM, Grijseels EW, Hop WC, Wladimiroff JW. Three dimensional sonography of prenatal skull base development. Ultrasound Obstet Gynecol. 2007;29(4):372-7.
22. Roelf NM, Hop WC, van Adrichem LN, Wladimiroff JW. Craniofacial variability index in utero: a three dimensional ultrasound study. Ultrasound Obstet Gynecol. 2007;29(3):258-64.
23. Ruano R, Benachi A, Aubry MC, Brunelle F, Dumez Y, Dommergues M. Perinatal three dimensional color power Doppler ultrasonography of vein of Galen aneurysms. J Ultrasound Med. 2004;22(12):1357-62.
24. Kurjak A, Pooh RK, Merce LT, Carrera JM, Slihagic-Kadic A, Andonotopo W. Structural and functional early human development assessed by three dimensional and four dimensional sonography. Fertil Steril. 2005;84(5): 1285-99.
25. Bonilla Musoles F, Raga F, Villalobos A, Blanes J, Osborne NG. First trimester neck abnormalities: three dimensional evaluation. J Ultrasound Med. 1998;17(7):419-25.
26. Nath CA, Oyelese Y, Yeo L, Chavez M, Kontopoulos EV, Giannaina G, et al. Three dimensional sonography in the evaluation and management of fetal goiter. Ultrasound Obstet Gynecol. 2005;25(3):312-4.
27. Gerards FA, Twisk JW, Bakker M, Barkhof F, van Vugt JM. Fetal lung volume: three dimensional ultrasonography compared with magnetic resonance imaging. Ultrasound Obstet Gynecol. 2007;29(5):533-6.
28. Spaggiari E, Strinneman JJ, Sonigo P, Khen-DuNlop N, De Saint Blanquat L, Ville Y. Prenatal prediction of pulmonary arterial hypertension in congenital diaphragmatic hernia. Ultrasound Obstet Gynecol. 2015;45(5):572-7.
29. Harting MT. Congenital diaphragmatic hernia associated pulmonary hypertension. Semin Peadiatr Surg. 2017;26(3):147-53.
30. Kuno A, Hayashi Y, Akiyama M, Yamashiro C, Tanaka H, Yanagihara T, et al. Three dimensional sonographic measurement of liver volume in small for gestational age fetus. J Ultrasound Med. 2002;21(4):361-6.
31. Benacerraf BR, Bromley B, Shipp TS, Can 3D volume sets alone be used to detect fetal malformations? ISUOG. 2006;28(4):359-9.
32. Bega G, Wapner R, Toaff-Lev A, Kuhlman K. Diagnosis of conjoined twins at 10 weeks using three dimensional ultrasound: a case report. UOG; 2000;16(4):388-90.

21

CHAPTER

Sonography-based Volume Computer-aided Display in Labor

Sonal Panchal, Chaitanya Nagori

INTRODUCTION

Delivery of the fetus is a complex process that includes several adaptations in maternal pelvis and fetal adjustments that can help fetal passage through barely accommodating pelvic outlet and vagina. This process can be successfully completed only by a perfect materno-fetal coordination. In approximately 5% of cases, this process does not succeed and leads to obstructed labor, which leads to fetal distress, need for cesarean section, postpartum hemorrhage and several complications, and also sometimes fetal loss. It is one of the major causes of materno-fetal morbidity and mortality. These can be prevented by either prelabor evaluation of the patient to anticipate the problem or take relevant actions beforehand. Even if it was not anticipated, its diagnosis in early stage can guard against a lot of these complications. For a long era, this entire complex process was monitored by bimanual clinical examination and it was only a subjective assessment, which grossly depended on the clinician's feel and experience-based intuition.

B-mode ultrasound was then used for several years to follow the position of the fetal head in relation to pubic symphysis using a translabial scan route. This did help in the decision-making, but the precise assessment was not possible and so till three-dimensional (3D) ultrasound became available, the labor/delivery of the fetus was monitored chiefly by clinical judgment.

It was a combination of 3D ultrasound with the artificial intelligence, which made a huge difference in the way the process of labor can be monitored. Several patients of normal delivery were closely observed with 3D ultrasound during the entire labor process. All the data of the changes in the capacity of the pelvic outlet, its shape, and the changes in the fetal position accordingly was fed into the computer memory for it to understand that anything deviating from the fed data could be abnormal. Based on this, a new software was developed—sonography-based volume computer-aided display (SonoVCAD) labor.

PROCESS OF SECOND-STAGE LABOR

It consists of following major events related to the fetal head.

- Descent of the head
- Rotation of the head
- Anterior angulation of the head
- Finally again rotation of the fetus after fetal head is expelled out for the shoulder to deliver. This means the fetal head is already outside the maternal body and can be seen during this phase of delivery.

But, the previous three movements of the head cannot be seen in vivo. These are judged by per vaginal examination, the correct perception of which requires a lot of tactile training and it is subjective.[1] In spite of that, vaginal manual assessment may fail to define the position of the head in 30–60% of cases.[2] Two-dimensional (2D) ultrasound is, otherwise, also used during labor to assess fetal viability and presentation.[3] 2D ultrasound allowed to observe the descent of the fetal head, though not accurately. 3D ultrasound has proved itself to be a very accurate and helpful modality for monitoring of second

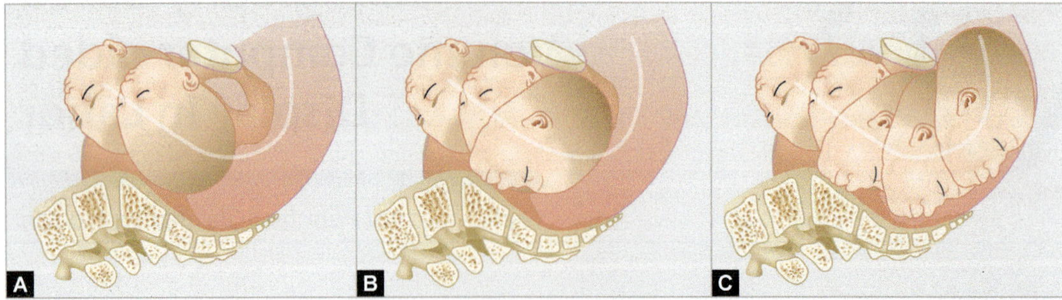

Figs. 1A to C: Diagrammatic representation of progress of fetal head during second stage of labor.

stage of labor. It is used along with the routine digital assessment to assess advancement of the labor.

Understanding the Path of the Fetal Head during Labor (Figs. 1A to C)

This is a curvilinear path. In sagittal plane, the head first progresses toward the posterior aspect of the mother, then horizontally, and then anteriorly or upward[4] (this is associated with internal rotation).

Method

Patient is in semi-recumbent position with knees flexed. Scan is done with 4–8 MHz or 2–5 MHz convex volume probe with a wide insonation angle. The scan depth is adjusted to about 15 cm. The scan is performed with the margin of the probe resting on the pubic symphysis. The probe lies below the symphysis pubis on the labia majora in the midsagittal plane. Probe is covered with a sterile glove with jelly between the probe and the glove. Before acquiring the volume, confirm that pubic symphysis and fetal skull contour are clearly seen **(Fig. 2)**. A large volume sweep is taken. Since this is a dynamic phase of labor and the patient is in quite severe pain and may move, so low quality volume is acquired as the acquisition will be faster. Looking at the multiplanar image and identifying the anatomy.

A second volume is acquired after asking the patient to push. This will help the assessment of head progression. This scan is repeated at regular intervals and may or may not be associated with digital assessment. It is always better to use VCI for better contrast and perfect delineation of edges.

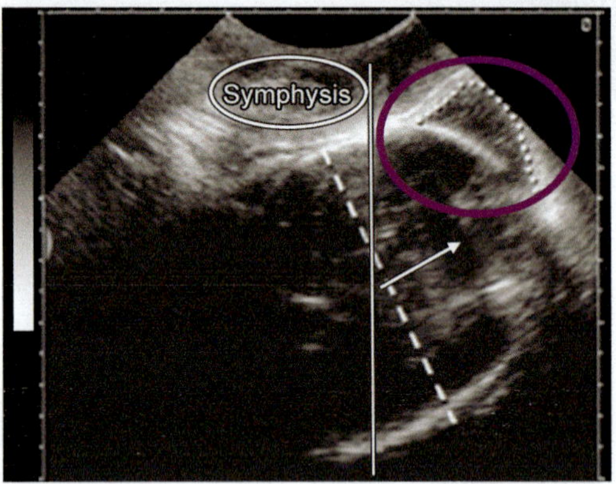

Fig. 2: B-mode ultrasound image on sagittal plane showing symphysis pubis, fetal head, and caput. White bold line indicates lower margin of pubic symphysis and bold arrow indicates the direction of progression.

Analysis and Calculations

This is done on multiplanar mode. Pubic bone is used as a landmark. When calculations are clicked on a "T"-shaped diagram, it appears on the image. This is to be placed on the caudal margin of the pubic bone both in A (sagittal) and B (transverse section of pelvis) image **(Figs. 3A and B)**.

Draw the outline of the fetal head in image A **(Fig. 4)**. This gives the relationship of the pubic bone to head position. The time of acquisition is automatically noted. It is essential to mark the volume with identification of the patient, so that the data of the subsequent assessments done during the labor are all stored in the same

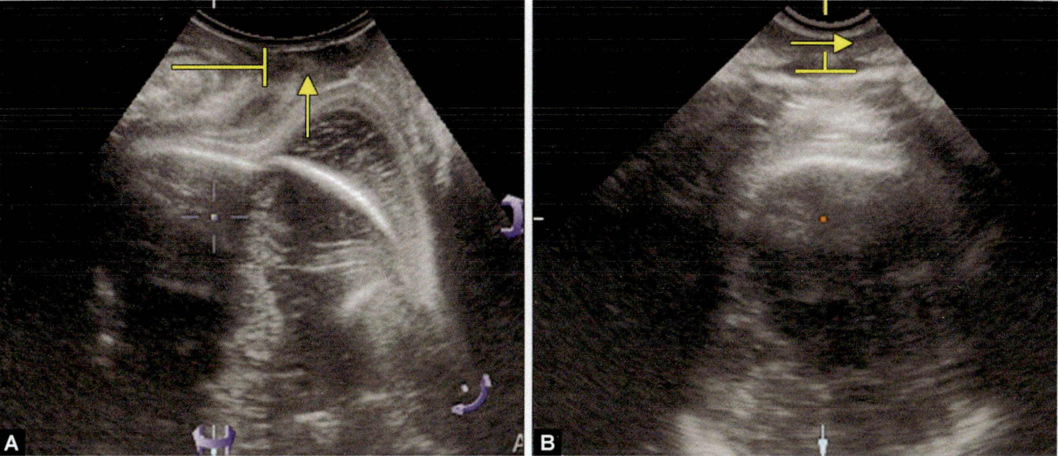

Figs. 3A and B: "T" placed on the causal margin of the pubic bone in A (sagittal) and B (transverse section of pelvis) image (yellow arrows).

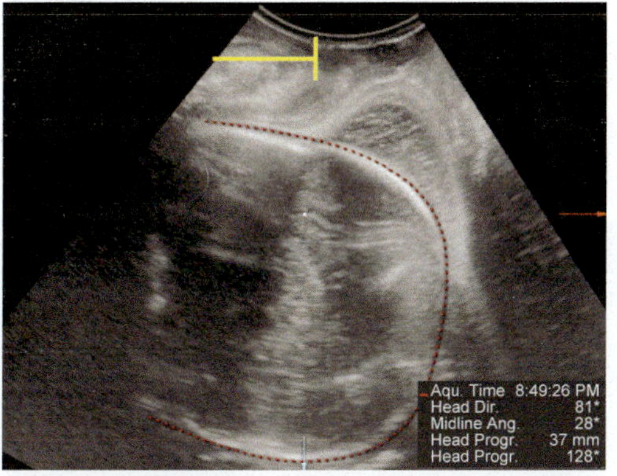

Fig. 4: Red dotted line marking fetal head outline.

name and volume. These can be overlapped and the progression of the labor is normal or otherwise can be judged objectively.

The calculations measure the head direction in relation to the pubic bone as angle. Midline angle is the amount of rotation of the head **(Fig. 5)** again measured as angle. Head progression is measured as descent in millimeters and also as angle because the initial descent is associated with angulation of the head to adapt to the curve of the vaginal canal (measured as angle in head progression) initially downward and posteriorly and then downward and anteriorly. This is followed by rotation of the head (measured as midline angle) to bring the occiput anteriorly, then extension for expulsion of head, and finally rotation again for delivery of the shoulder.

After drawing the head contour on image A, maximum anteroposterior diameter of the head is measured as a straight line. A perpendicular is drawn on this line to the farthest point on the fetal head curvature as shown in **Figures 6A and B**. The direction of this line tells the direction of the head progression. It has been shown that when head to perineal distance on transperineal ultrasound is measured as ≤4 cm, the chances of vaginal delivery were as high as 93% as compared to when it was ≥5 cm (18%).[5] On the B plane, pubic symphysis is seen anteriorly and the head in axial section is seen as a complete circle. On this plane, an occipito-frontal line is drawn. This line becomes vertical as the labor progresses.

Angle of progression is measured on the A plane as a line drawn from the lower margin of symphysis pubis as marked by the "T" sign to touching the head tangentially on its leading surface **(Fig. 7)**.

Angle of progression is the radial measurement of the fetal head progression in birth canal. This has been proved to be an objective, accurate, and reproducible means of assessing the head descent. When this angle was 120°

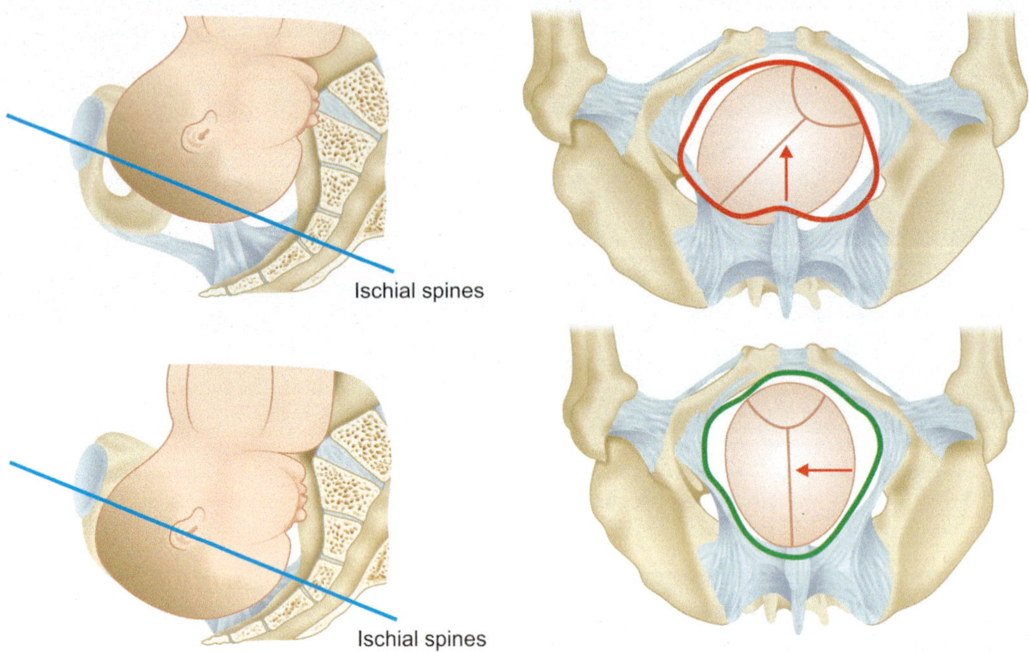

Fig. 5: Diagrammatic presentation of fetal head rotation during second stage of labor.

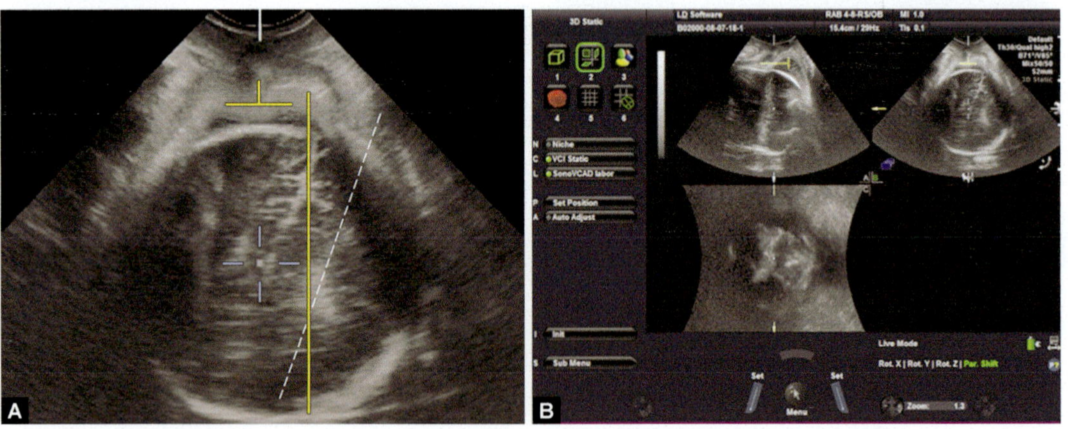

Figs. 6A and B: Measuring head rotation during second stage of labor.

or more, probability of spontaneous vaginal delivery was high.[6,7] If the angle of progression was ≥110°, than the chance of vaginal delivery was as high as 88% as compared to only 38% when it was <100° **(Fig. 8)**.

All the measurements are displayed at a time and when another volume is taken, the results overlap and give comprehensive report.

When *SonoVCAD labor is used* along with 3D acquisition, line passing through the inner part of the symphysis pubis is automatically traced on the sagittal plane (plane A) once the cranial and caudal edge of the pubic bone are identified. When the lateral edges of the bone are marked on B plane (axial image), the inferior margin of the symphysis pubis is automatically traced. Confirm on

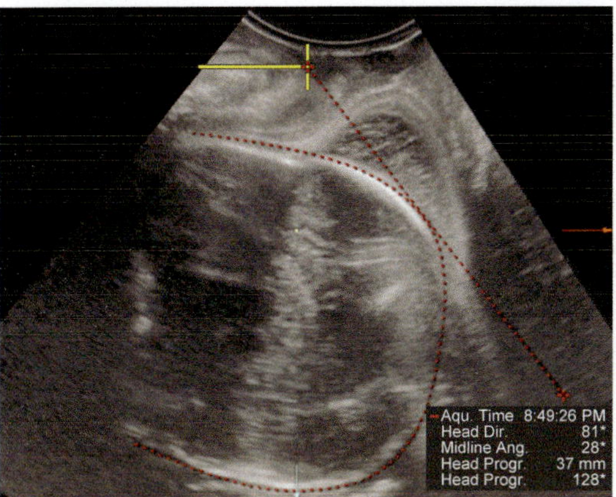

Fig. 7: Measurement of angle of progression on the sonography-based volume computer-aided display (SonoVCAD) image.

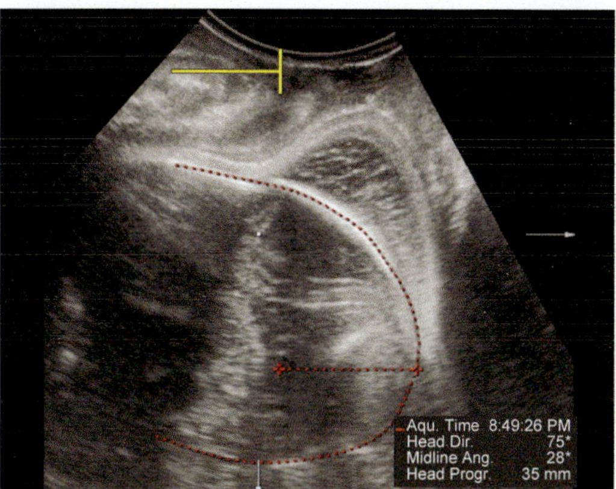

Fig. 9: Measurement of head progression.

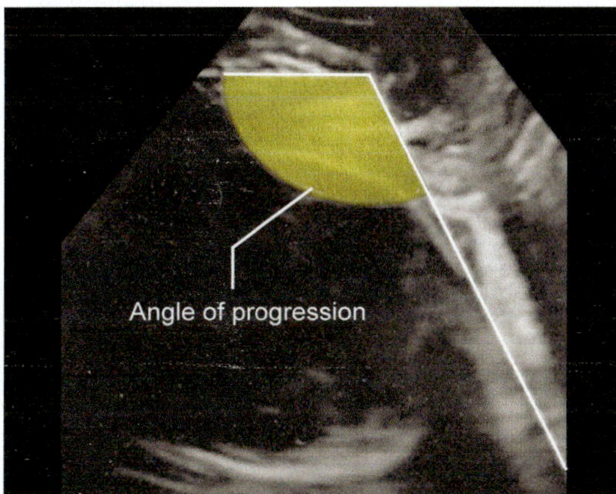

Fig. 8: Measurement of angle of progression.

coronal plane (C plane) that the orientation of the image is correct. Once this is done, the software allows the marking of occiput position and fetal head station.

Head progression is the distance (in cm) between infrapubic line and lowest part of fetal skull (excluding the caput)[8] **(Fig. 9)**. Head direction is the angle between the infrapubic line and automatically drawn perpendicular to biparietal diameter, major longitudinal axis of fetal head.[4]

Angle of progression is measured by line automatically drawn between long axis of pubic bone and a line from inferior margin of pubic bone to lowest convexity of fetal skull. On axial plane, "midline angle" is calculated. This is the angle between the anteroposterior axis of pelvis and midline of head. The occiput and the frontal margin are to be marked by the operator.

The volumes acquired during the later stages of labor are also all aligned in the same anatomical position and the results are superimposed on the previous ones, each one showed dashed lines of different colors **(Figs. 10A and B)**.

Advantages of Ultrasound

Determination of head position is more accurately assessed by ultrasound than by digital examination.[9] There has been a significant correlation between the fetal head direction and the clinically established station of the fetal head. A strong correlation was also found between midline angle below 45° and a station ≥3 cm, particularly in cases of anterior occiput.[10]

Quantification of head engagement is highly reproducible by translabial ultrasound and correlates with findings of clinical assessment.[8] Advantage of the 3D ultrasound is that it allows more accurate alignment of anatomical landmarks of both fetus and mother and allows comparison of serial measurements, this helps to assess the progression of labor more objectively **(Fig. 11)**.

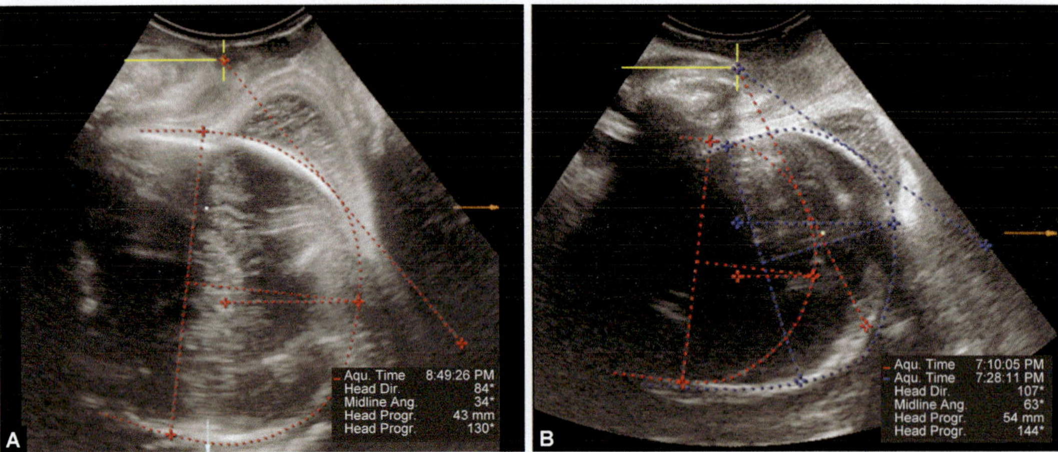

Figs. 10A and B: Sonography-based volume computer-aided display (SonoVCAD) labor showing angle of progression and progression distance in the image on left side and the image on right side shows similar measurements in two colors indicating measurements taken at two different times and compares the progression of labor over the time.

Spontaneous vaginal delivery was associated with lower head-perineum distance (33.2 mm ± 7.8 mm vs. 40.1 mm ± 9.5 mm, P = 0.001) and head-symphysis distance (13.1 mm ± 4.6 mm vs. 19.5 mm ± 8.4 mm, P < 0.001), narrower midline angle (29.6° ± 15.3° vs. 54.2° ± 23.6°, P < 0.001), and wider angle of progression at pushing effort (153.3° ± 19.8° vs. 141.8° ± 25.7°, P = 0.02) and delta angle of progression (17.3° ± 12.9° vs. 12.5° ± 11.0°, P = 0.04). On logistic regression analysis, the midline angle and the head-symphysis distance proved to be independent predictors of spontaneous vaginal delivery.[11]

Sonography-based volume computer-aided display has been proved to be a very useful tool to follow and closely observe the second stage of labor. It gives an objective

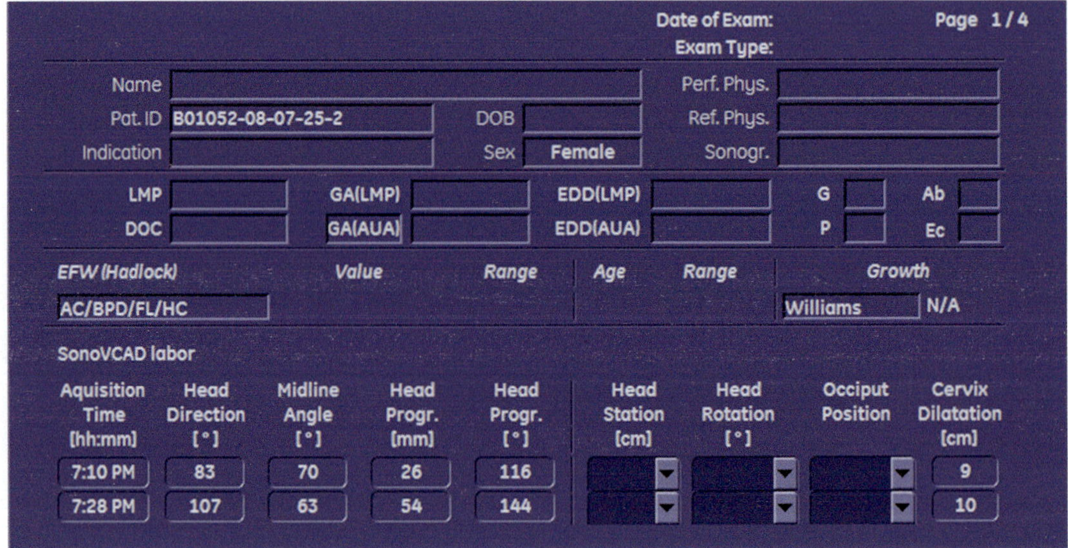

Date of Exam: Page 1/4
Exam Type:

Name | Perf. Phys.
Pat. ID B01052-08-07-25-2 | DOB | Ref. Phys.
Indication | Sex Female | Sonogr.

LMP | GA(LMP) | EDD(LMP) | G | Ab
DOC | GA(AUA) | EDD(AUA) | P | Ec

EFW (Hadlock) | Value | Range | Age | Range | Growth
AC/BPD/FL/HC | Williams N/A

SonoVCAD labor

Aquisition Time [hh:mm]	Head Direction [°]	Midline Angle [°]	Head Progr. [mm]	Head Progr. [°]	Head Station [cm]	Head Rotation [°]	Occiput Position	Cervix Dilatation [cm]
7:10 PM	83	70	26	116				9
7:28 PM	107	63	54	144				10

Fig. 11: Result sheet for sonography-based volume computer-aided display (SonoVCAD) labor.

evidence of obstructed labor and helps timely decision on the mode of delivery and prevents fetal morbidity.

REFERENCES

1. Phelps JY, Higby K, Smyth MH, Ward JA, Arredendo F, Mayer AR, et al. Accuracy and intraobserver variability of stimulated cervical dilatation measurements. Am J Obstet Gynecol. 1995;173(3):942-5.
2. Sherer DM, Miodavnik M, Bradley KS, Langer O. Intrapartum fetal head position I: comparison between transvaginal digital examination and transabdominal ultrasound assessment during the active stage of labor. Ultrasound Obstet Gynecol. 2002;19(3):258-63.
3. Heazell A, Raouf S, Bhatti NR, Smewing S. P03.11: A prospective study of the use of ultrasound scanning on the delivery suite. Ultrasound Obstet Gynecol. 2004;24(3):285.
4. Henrich W, Dudenhausen J, Fuchs I, Kamena A, Tutschek B. Intrapartum translabial ultrasound (ITU) sonographic landmarks and correlation with successful vacuum extraction. Ultrasound Obstet Gynecol. 2006;28(6):753-60.
5. Eggebø TM, Hassan WA, Salvesen KÅ, Lindtjørn E, Lees CC. Sonographic prediction of vaginal delivery in prolonged labor: a two-center study. Ultrasound Obstet Gynecol. 2014;43(2):195-201.
6. Barbera AF, Pombar X, Perugino G, Lezotte DC, Hobbins JC. A new method to assess fetal head decent in labor with transperineal ultrasound. Ultrasound Obstet Gynecol. 2009;33(4):313-9.
7. Kalache K, Dueckelmann AM, Michaelis SAM, Lange J, Cichon G, Dudenhausen JW. Transperineal ultrasound imaging in prolonged second stage of labor with occipitoanterior presenting fetuses: how well does the 'angle of progression' predict the mode of delivery. Ultrasound Obstet Gynecol. 2009;33(3):326-30.
8. Deitz HP, Lanzarone V. Measuring engagement of the fetal head: validity and reproducibility of a new ultrasound technique. Ultrasound Obstet Gynecol. 2005;25(2):165-8.
9. Rozenberg P, Porcher R, Salomon HJ, Boirot F, Morin C, Ville Y. Comparison of learning curves of digital examination and transabdominal sonography for the determination of fetal head position during labor. Ultrasound Obstet Gynecol. 2008;31(3):332-7.
10. Ghi T, Farina A, Pedrazzi A, Rizzo N, Pelusi G, Pilu G. Diagnosis of station and rotation of the fetal head in the second stage of labor with intrapartum translabial ultrasound. Ultrasound Obstet Gynecol. 2009;33(3):331-6.
11. Dall'Asta A, Angeli L, Masturzo B, Volpe N, Schera GBL, Pasquo ED, et al. Prediction of spontaneous vaginal delivery in nulliparous women with a prolonged second stage of labor: the value of intrapartum ultrasound. Am J Obstet Gynecol. 2019;221(6):642.e1-13.

22

CHAPTER

Basics of Transvaginal Scan

Sonal Panchal, Chaitanya Nagori

INTRODUCTION

Detailed evaluation of the female genital tract is essential for any gynecological disease and basis of success of any assisted reproductive technology (ART). Ultrasound (US) is the most convenient and reliable modality for evaluation of uterus, fallopian tubes, and ovaries. Though these pelvic organs can be assessed by transabdominal, transrectal, and transvaginal US, transvaginal route gives best visibility and accuracy of diagnosis.

This is so because:

- Transvaginal probe can be placed close to these organs—uterus, tubes, and ovaries.
- Transvaginal probe is a high-frequency probe and therefore has better resolution.
- The additional advantage is that the patient does not have to tolerate the inconvenience of full bladder.

But transvaginal route cannot be used in virgins or in patients with local vaginal problems, and in these patients, transabdominal or transrectal route should be preferred. Transabdominal route has a disadvantage of poor resolution because of more distance of the pelvic organs from the probe, maternal fat, maternal bowel loops, and the low-frequency (3–5 MHz) probe that has inherently lower resolution than the high resolution, high-frequency transvaginal probe. Approximately 42% of ovarian details are missed by transabdominal scan.[1] Though a transabdominal scan is recommended before transvaginal scan is done for the first time in any patient.

Transrectal sonography in such cases is preferable and informative as compared to transabdominal approach. The probe used is transvaginal, dedicated transrectal, or endocavitary probe (**Figs. 1A and B**), a high frequency probe, so resolution is very similar to that of a transvaginal examination. But the disadvantage is that rectal placement is much more painful than transvaginal placement and needs bowel preparation. Moreover, the orientation of pelvic organs that appear on the image created by transrectal scan is different from that of a transvaginal scan (TVS), and so interpretation may be a little difficult.

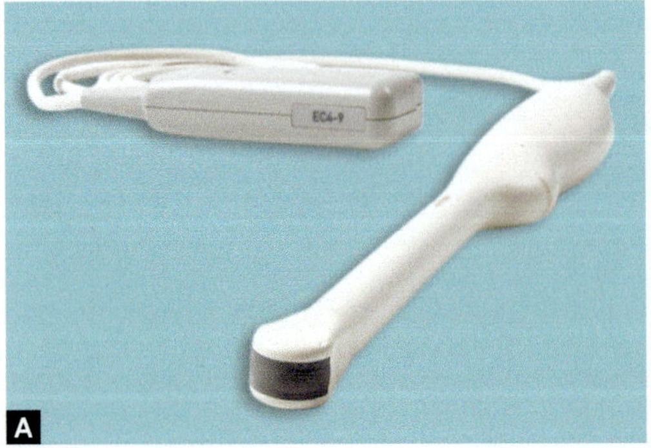

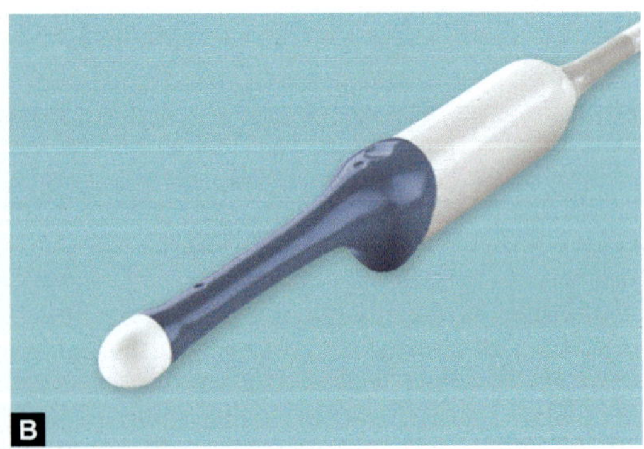

Figs. 1A and B: (A) Endocavitary (transvaginal) probe; (B) Endocavitary (transvaginal) volume probe.

Though commonly gynecologists use transvaginal endocavitary probe for transrectal assessment also, it is better to use dedicated transrectal probe. The basic difference between the two probes is that transvaginal probe is end-firing probe whereas transrectal probe is side-firing probe. It is more convenient to use side-firing probe for transrectal approach as less manipulation of the probe will be required and will cause less discomfort.

Though we shall discuss here in detail the scanning methods by transabdominal and transvaginal route, we shall discuss TVS first as this is the most commonly used one.

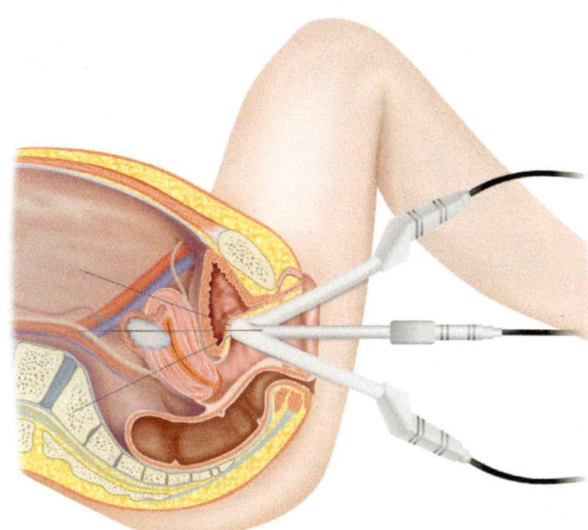

Fig. 3: To allow up and down movement of the probe as shown in the diagram, the gap of the gynecology couch is convenient.

TRANSVAGINAL SCAN

Method

At least a verbal consent of the patient is essential. Patient is asked to empty the bladder. Patient is undressed, placed in lithotomy-like position (**Fig. 2**) on the gynecology couch in the same way as for per speculum or per vaginal examination and is adequately covered with a clean sheet, so that she does not feel uncomfortable. Maintaining privacy and dignity of the patient is of utmost importance. Gynecology couch, as it has a gap in the center, allows easy probe movements (**Fig. 3**). A pillow under the patient's buttocks may help to raise the buttocks if the scan is done on flat bed. But with this position also, the probe movement is restricted, and the comfort of the examination is not sufficient. US jelly is put on the head of the transvaginal probe, and then the probe is covered with the condom, not leaving any air between the probe and the condom. A small amount of jelly is then placed over the condom on the probe head, and the probe is gently slided into the patient's vagina (**Fig. 4**). Counseling the patient before examination and explaining the whole procedure helps eliminate the anxiety and resistance.

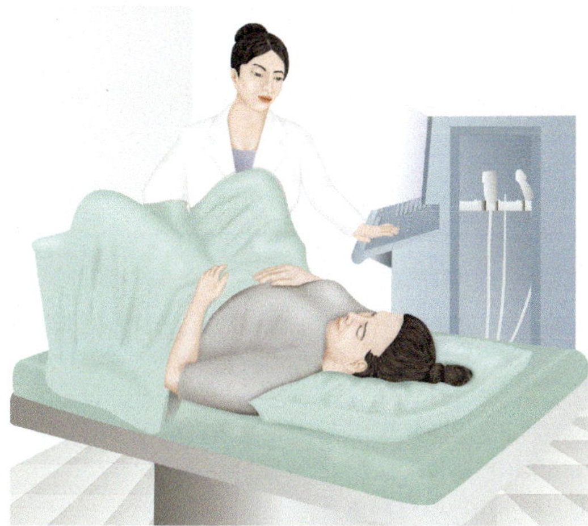

Fig. 2: Diagrammatic presentation of the patient position and preparation for transvaginal scan.

Prescan protocol for transvaginal scan

- Ask the patient to empty the bladder immediately before the scan.
- Patient is placed in lithotomy/lithotomy-like position.
- Examination is preferably done on gynecology couch.
- Cover the patient adequately.
- Counsel the patient about the procedure.
- Privacy is essential to avoid patient's anxiety.

Tips for Probe Insertion

In the case of difficulty in introduction of the probe or patient's resistance to introduction of the probe, she is advised to take deep long breaths with open mouth, that is, deep

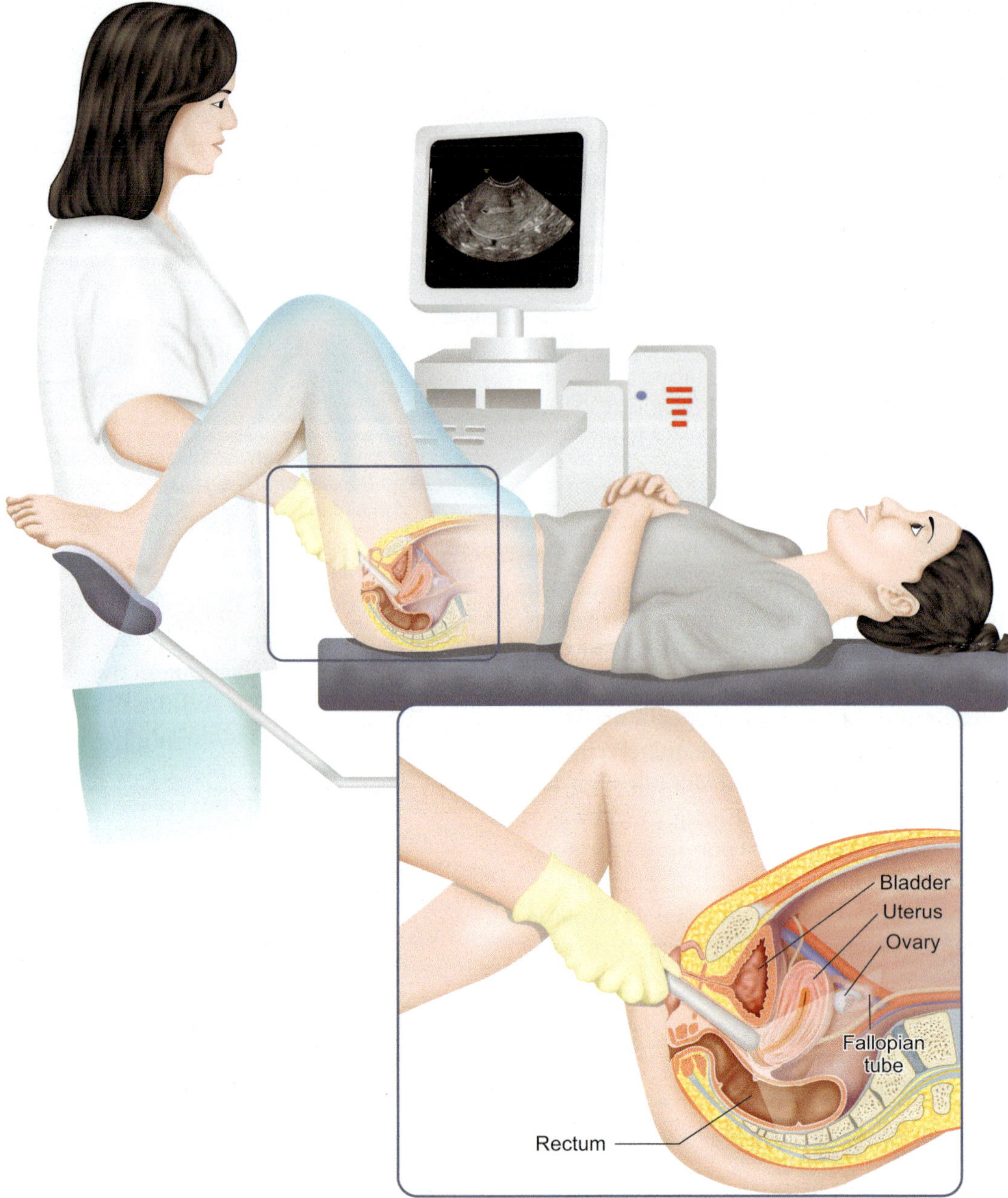

Fig. 4: Position of the probe in the vagina.

inspirations and long complete expirations, which allows relaxation of the introitus. In spite of that, if introduction of probe is difficult, the pressure should be exerted posteriorly toward the rectum which will make introduction of the probe into the vagina easier.

Basic Probe Movements

There are basic four types of probe movements used for TVS:

1. In and out (**Fig. 5**)
2. Side-to-side or spanning movement (**Fig. 6**)

3. Rotation movement or screwing movement (**Fig. 7**)
4. Up and down or anteroposterior movement (in relation to the patient) (**Fig. 8**).

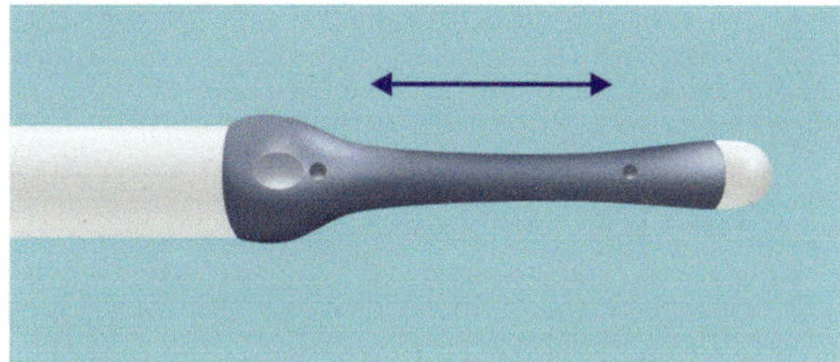

Fig. 5: Arrow showing in and out movement direction of the probe.

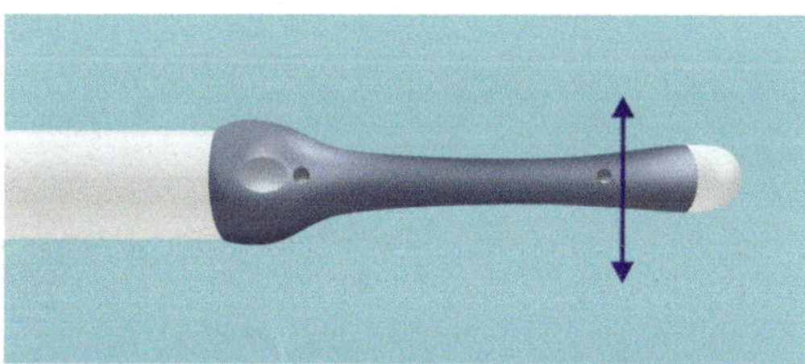

Fig. 6: Arrow showing side-to-side movement (spanning movement) of the probe.

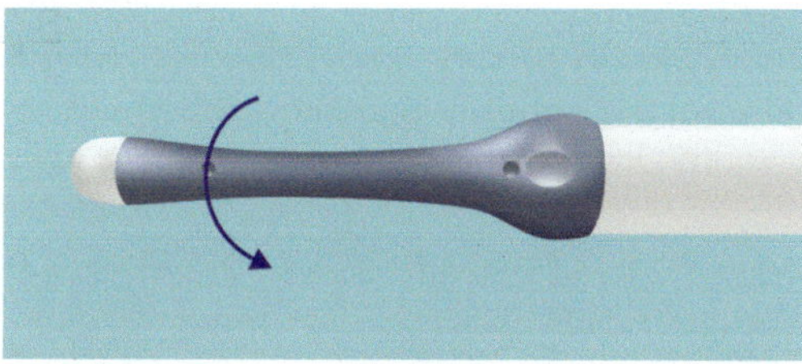

Fig. 7: Arrow showing rotation movement of the probe.

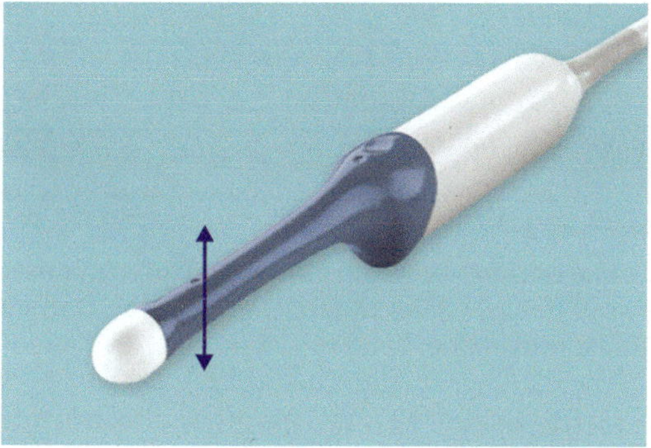

Fig. 8: Arrow showing up and down movement of the probe.

In and Out Movement

It is used for the probe entry and exit from the vagina. This movement helps to slide the tissue planes over one another. It is used to diagnose adhesions between uterus and ovaries, ovaries or uterus with bowel loops, or anterior and posterior vaginal walls with bladder wall or rectal wall.

Side-to-side Movement or Spanning Movement

This is moving the probe from right side of the patient to the left side of the patient or vice versa, without rotation. But spanning may be done with the probe rotated in any direction. It is used for the survey of anatomy of entire pelvis or any pelvic organ individually.

Rotation Movement or Screwing Movement

Rotation movement of the probe does not include movement of the probe position. It is only clockwise or anticlockwise rotation of the probe. This movement is used to visualize a particular organ or lesion in different axis. Rotation of the probe can be done in clockwise or anticlockwise direction.

Up and Down Movement

This is only angulating the probe toward roof or floor, that is, toward patient's anterior or posterior aspect. Moving the handle up directs the probe head down (posterior aspect of patient), and moving the handle down directs the probe head up (toward patient's anterior aspect). This movement along with the spanning movement is used for survey of the anatomy and to find out the position of structure or an organ in the pelvis.

Equipment Settings and Optimizing the Image

Usually, there are presets on all US equipments for different probes and different scans, and there is one for gynecological scan also. The advantage of using a good and proper preset is that one has to manipulate the equipment settings minimally and still get good quality images with majority of the scans. A good quality B-mode image is a primary requirement for good quality color Doppler, volume US images and, over and above all, for correct diagnosis. Though most of the times the presets work well, several parameters need to be adjusted when scanning each patient, due to variations in physique, habitus, and anatomy. Even if the physics part of it is omitted, it is essential to know about the knobs, what they do, and when to use them. This has been discussed in **Chapter 3** of this book.

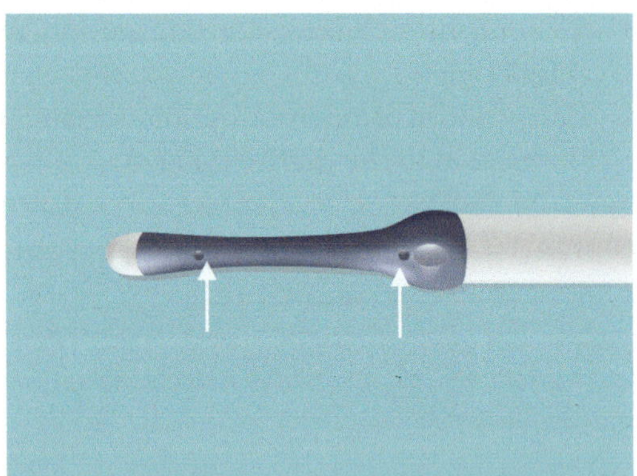

Fig. 9: Transvaginal volume ultrasound probe showing pits for fixation of biopsy guide, shown by arrow, which act as indicators to define the position of the probe, which is indicated on ultrasound image.

Systematic Scan

Probe is introduced in the longitudinal position. That is the position in which the indicators (arrow) on the probe remain up, facing the roof of the room that is on anterior aspect of the patient (**Fig. 9**). These indicators on the probe match the indicator [logo of the company-circle on the screen (**Fig. 10**) on the screen. This means that if the indicator on the screen is on the right side of the screen, the structures anteriorly placed are on the right side of the screen and vice versa. Uterus is normally seen in the midline with this probe position. If uterus is not seen in the center, the probe is spanned from one side in the pelvis to the other side to search for the uterus. Once the uterus is located with the probe in the same position (without rotation), it is spanned from right to left side of the patient, scanning the uterus in long axis from one side to other.

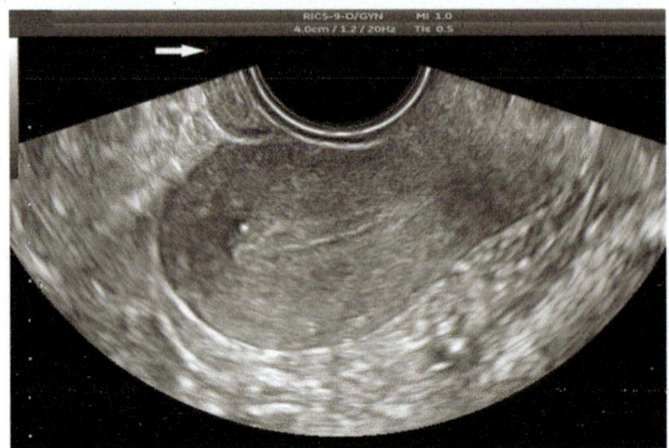

Fig. 10: The company logo (shown by arrow) on this longitudinal section of the uterus.

Now rotate the probe 90° anticlockwise. This maneuver will give transverse view of the uterus (**Fig. 11**) with the right side of the patient on right side of the screen. In this transverse position also, the whole uterus is evaluated from the fundus to the cervix by moving the probe up and down in the vagina. Now span the probe toward right side, in transverse position only at the level of uterine cornu, gradually look at the adnexa, and follow it to the ovary. Extend the movement up to the lateral pelvic wall if ovary is not located. Locate and assess the ovary in a true transverse

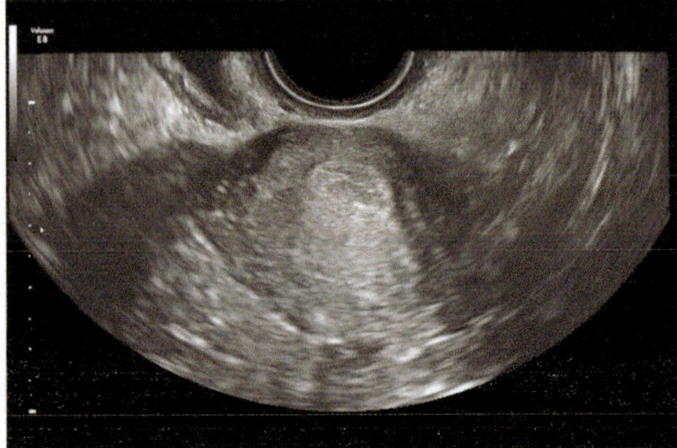

Fig. 11: Anticlockwise 90° rotation of the probe from a position in which long axis of uterus is seen shows transverse section of the uterus on B-mode ultrasound image.

section and then rotate it 90° to get a true long axis of the ovary, the largest longitudinal diameter can be achieved by spanning the probe across the ovary, after the ovarian long axis is seen. Ovaries are located medial to external iliac vessels and anterior to internal iliac vessels. Therefore, on transverse section, external iliac vessels are seen posterior to the ovary, and on longitudinal section, internal iliac vessels are seen posterior to the ovary. Assess the ovaries for any pathology. Then span the probe, come back to the midline, and follow the same procedure for the opposite adnexa. In and out movement of the probe with the ovary in view or pressing on the abdomen when probe is looking at the ovary and checking the sliding of the organs against each other confirms mobility of the ovaries and rules out adhesions. This is also known as Timor-Tritsch sign or a sliding organ sign.

Come back to the midline and angulate the probe head posteriorly and look for fluid in pouch of Douglas. While removing the probe gently, have a close look at the cervical canal. Finally slide the probe against the anterior vaginal wall and posterior vaginal wall and check for mobility of tissue planes by eliciting sliding sign on in and out movement of the probe. This completes the two-dimensional or B-mode routine TVS.

Color, pulse, or power Doppler can be added as and when required.

Systematic transvaginal scan

- US jelly is put on the head of the transvaginal probe.
- Probe is covered with the condom, not to allow any air between the probe and the condom.
- Small amount of jelly is placed over the condom on the probe head.
- Probe is gently introduced into the patient's vagina.
- Mobility of tissue planes between urethra and vagina and vagina and rectum is checked as probe advances in the vaginal canal.
- Uterus is seen in the midline normally.
- Uterus is screened from one side to the other in long axis along with cervix, and then probe is rotated 90° and uterus is screened in transverse plane.
- With the probe in the same direction, the probe is spanned toward lateral pelvic wall to find the ovaries.
- Ovary is screened in longitudinal and transverse plane.
- Both ovaries and uterus are checked for mobility by probe movement in and out or by pressure on abdomen when probe is in place.
- Check for fluid in pouch of Douglas.

Which Vessels to Interrogate and How to Trace them?

For color Doppler of the uterine artery, the probe is brought back in the midline in longitudinal plane and then again moving laterally, serpiginous tubular structure is seen at the level of internal os, which is the uterine artery (**Fig. 12**). It can also be traced in transverse axis of the uterus, moving the probe to the level of internal os, when vessels will be seen on both the sides [**Fig. 13 (arrow)**]. On abdominal scan, moving from midline laterally at the level of symphysis pubis shows iliac vessels, which are large prominent vessels running mediolaterally, superoinferiorly. After tracing these vessels, the probe, if angled slightly medially, shows a vessel perpendicularly crossing these vessels, this is uterine artery. Color Doppler is also

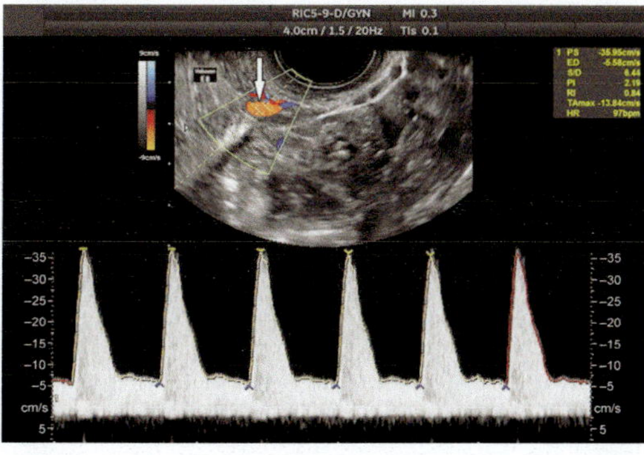

Fig. 12: Color Doppler and spectral Doppler image of uterine artery (arrow), seen on the long section of the uterus, seen on the lateral-most aspect of the uterus.

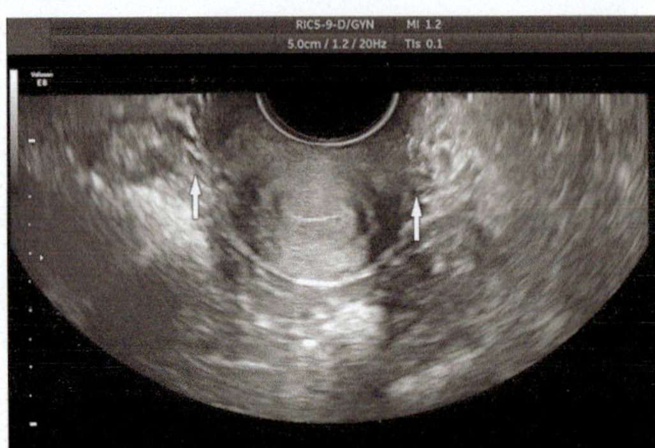

Fig. 13: Transverse section of the uterus at the level of internal os showing lucent serpiginous vascular structures on both sides (arrows)—uterine arteries.

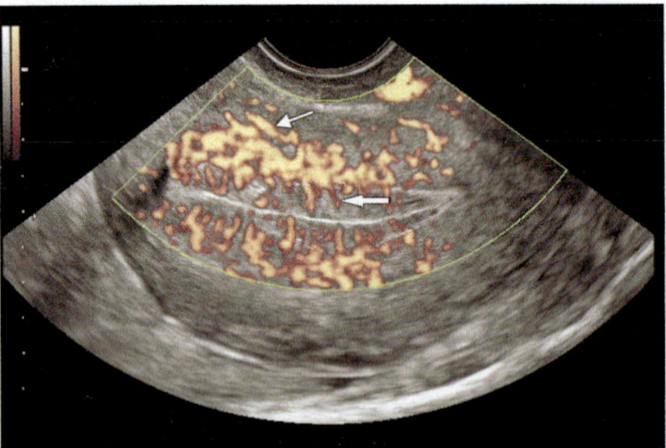

Fig. 14: Power Doppler showing uterine vasculature with arcuate arteries parallel to the endometrium (thin arrow) and spiral arteries perpendicular to the endometrium, penetrating the endometrium (thick arrow).

used to evaluate the endometrial flow. The blood vessels entering the endometrium are branches of spiral artery and are seen as vessels perpendicular to the endometrium (**Fig. 14**).

Moving laterally from the transverse section of uterus toward adnexa will show another vascular structure heading toward the ovary; this is the ovarian vessel. Ovarian artery blood flow is not usually assessed. It is the ovarian stromal blood flow or perifollicular flow that is considered to be relevant during cycle assessment. The ovarian stromal vessels are studied for baseline scan. These are the vessels that are lying in the ovarian stroma (and not close to the follicles. Once ovary is located, Doppler is switched on with the color box covering almost the entire ovary. As the blood vessels are located, pick up the brightest ones and keeping the vessel in view, rotate the probe to confirm that this vessel is not a continuity of the mail ovarian vessel. If so span the probe on either side or pick up another brightest vessel. Preovulatory scan shows follicles in the ovary with perifollicular flow. Perifollicular vessels are those that overlap on the follicular wall. If vessels are seen around the follicle but follicle wall is also seen, these are not perifollicular vessels. Color or power Doppler or even HD flow may be used to document the perifollicular flow and then after assessing for the brightest color spots, pulse wave Doppler sample volume is placed over that color spot to assess the flow quantitatively.

The settings of the color and the power Doppler must be standardized for follicular and endometrial monitoring. Pulse repetition frequency is set at 0.3 and wall motion filter at the lowest. Whereas for gynecological lesions, the pulse repetition frequency can be set from 0.3 to 0.6.

3D Volume US and 3D Power Doppler Techniques in Gynecology and Infertility

It is out of the scope of this book to explain the basics of 3D US and all the applications of volume US as such. We shall therefore discuss only the relevant applications of volume US here. Volume US combined with TVS has revolutionized the gynecological imaging. Multiple planes and sections available on the tissue blocks of volume US have made the understanding of the complex anatomy easy. The availability of coronal section is of prime importance. Volume of US has also made volume calculations more accurate.

This is of importance for gynecological masses as well as for infertility assessment. New software of volume calculation like SonoAVC has great application in infertility for follicular assessment as well as for other fluid-filled masses of fallopian tubes or ovaries and also for volumetric assessment of early pregnancy. New rendering mode—HD live is very helpful for assessment of uterus, for hystero-contrast-salpingography—HyCoSy and for assessment of fetal development.

Acquiring the Volume

The area of interest is first selected on the B-mode scan. This area should ideally be placed in the center of the monitor screen. The B-mode image should be optimized. The volume box is switched on and is placed over the area of interest. The volume box should be large enough to include the area of interest with at least 5–10 mm of margin on all sides. To select the volume angle, probe is manually angulated up and down or side to side depending on orientation of the image to assess the depth the organ of interest. Quality of the volume is selected depending on whether the structure or organ of interest is steady and stable or has movements. Higher quality takes longer time to acquire as it contains more B-mode frames in the volume block, whereas lower quality volume takes shorter time to acquire. Having adjusted the region/area of interest, angle of acquisition, and quality, acquisition is started. The transducer head takes an automatic sweep, and the acquired volume is displayed on the screen as three images of three orthogonal planes—*x*, *y*, *z* axes.

Multiplanar Imaging

Walking through each image would take through the complete anatomical details included in the volume box in individual plane. This is multiplanar imaging. This is the study of sectional planes and makes the understanding of anatomical relationship of various structures clear. A dot is seen in each image, and this is the point at which the orthogonal planes intersect. This point is known as the reference point as it represents the same anatomical landmark in all three sections. Coronal section is the most important, as this is the plane which is inaccessible on B-mode US imaging (**Fig. 15**).

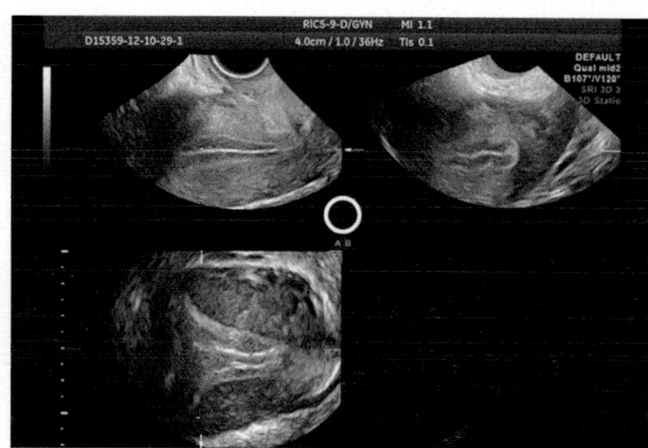

Fig. 15: Multiplanar image acquired by 3D ultrasound. The sections are longitudinal, transverse, and coronal sections of the uterus in clockwise manner starting from upper left corner and as seen in the symbol in the center of the image marked by the circle, these are known as sections A, B, and C, respectively.

Rendering

Viewing the whole tissue block as a whole from any one side is known as rendering (**Fig. 16**). When the image rendering is selected, a box appears on each image. In two of the three images, the box is drawn by three yellow lines and one green line, and in the third image, the box has all yellow lines. The resulting rendered image will be similar to the image in this latter box. The green line on the box is the viewing line. This line can be curved and is aligned with the curve of the organ of interest. For gynecological scans and infertility scans almost always up-down rendering direction is used. Rendering can be done in various modes and even combination of various rendering modes can be used, viz., surface modes, transparent modes, inversion, angiomode, etc. (**Figs. 17A to D**). For tissue rendering that is required for uterus and ovaries, commonly a combination of surface texture or smooth with transparent or gradient light mode is used. Though rendering can be done for straight as well as curved

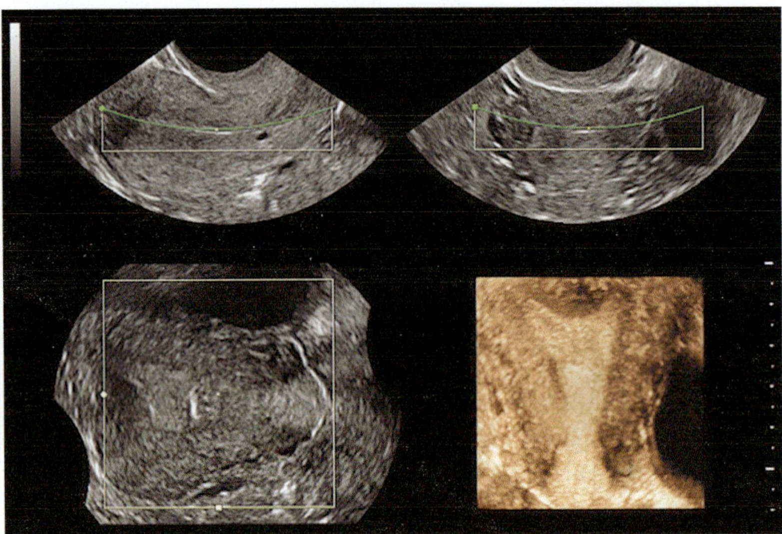

Fig. 16: 3D ultrasound-acquired image of the uterus showing three sectional planes in black and white and a sepia-colored image representing the rendered volume. The sectional images show the box; this is known as rendering box. It selects the part of the acquired volume to be seen on the rendered image. Two out of three boxes show a green line. This line is the viewing line, it can be straight or curved. It acts as a window through which the rendered volume is seen. The green line can be changed to make any side of the box on any of the three sectional planes and that decides the rendering direction. In this, it is up–down rendering direction, which is almost always used for all gynecological rendering.

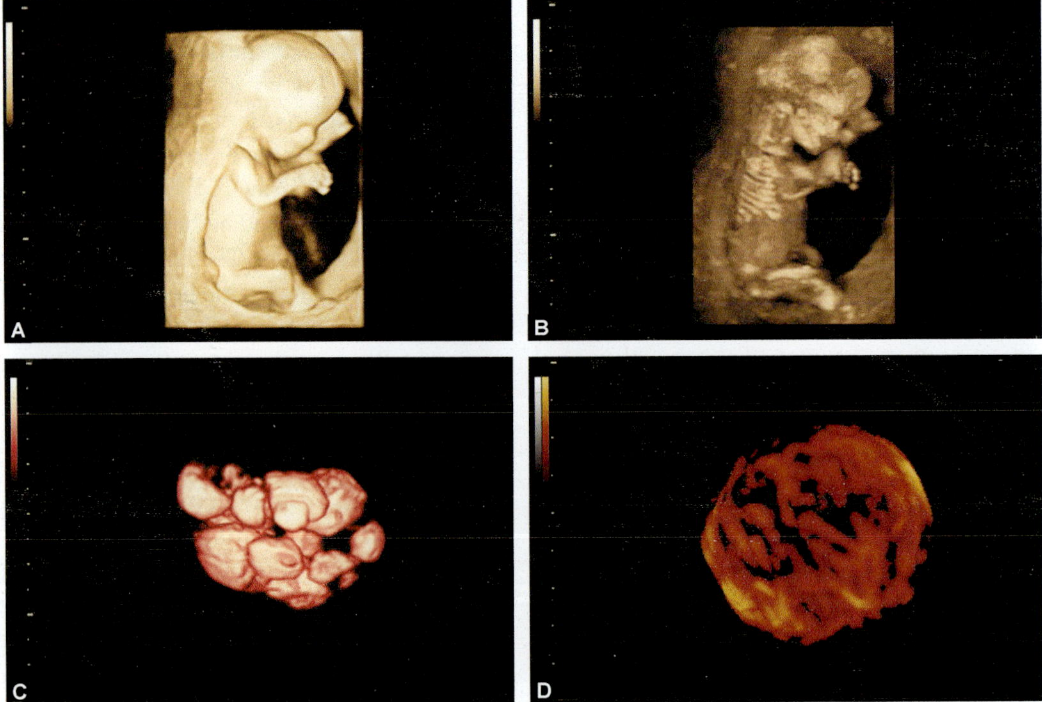

Figs. 17A to D: The volume acquired by 3D/4D ultrasound can be rendered in various modes or combination of any two modes, for example—a few are: (A) Surface mode to see the surfaces; (B) Transparent (maximum) mode to see the internal anatomy, viz., bones; (C) Inversion mode fluid filled structures appear echogenic and solid looking; (D) Angiomode shows only blood vessels as in angiography.

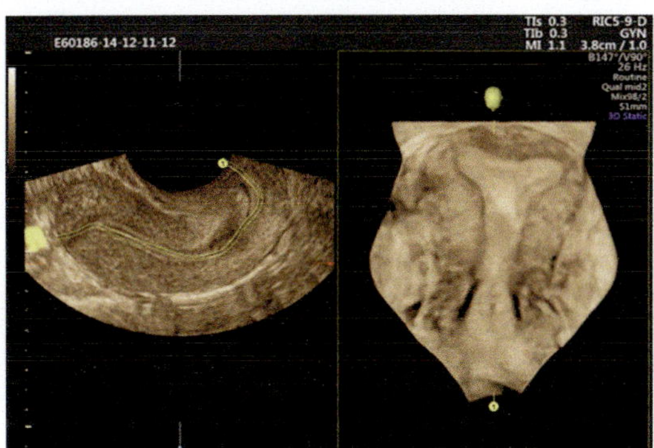

Fig. 18: Volume ultrasound of uterus with omniview. This software allows to see the coronal section of the said structure in the plane of the line drawn. This can be used on 3D acquired volume as well as on live 4D volume.

surfaces, it is difficult to render the uterus or any other surfaces with acute curves. It is in these cases that Omniview is used (**Fig. 18**) and has been described later in this chapter. For 3D power Doppler angiographies, the acquisition is done with power Doppler, and rendering is done in glass body or angiomode (**Figs. 19A and B**) to see the soft tissue details and vascular anatomy together or only blood vessels, respectively. Using volume histogram with the volume that is acquired with power Doppler allows quantitative assessment of the global vascular indices.

On omniview, if a line is drawn on the sectional plane on a static 3D or a live 3D (4D) image, the orthogonal plane of the imaging plane can be immediately reconstructed. Omniview when used with thick slices, improves the contrast markedly, and this is known as volume-contrast imaging (VCI) (**Figs. 20A and B**). VCI can be used in any plane on static 3D US and on scanning plane (VCI A) and coronal plane on 4D US. VCI A is very useful for visualization of subtle lesions like small polyps, small submucosal fibroids, etc.

Volume calculations have become very accurate on 3D US using VOCAL software. After volume acquisition, any one section is selected and that is rotated 180° in all. This total rotation is done step by step. This angle can be selected from 6°, 12°, 15°, or 30° steps. At each step, the margins of the organ or lesion of interest are outlined, and when 180° rotation is complete, volume of the organ is displayed on the monitor screen (**Fig. 21**).

Another software that is of great help in infertility practice is SonoAVC. It calculates the volume of all fluid-filled structures and color codes these (**Fig. 22**). It is therefore of great help for calculation of antral follicles or for calculation of follicular diameter or volume of multiple pretrigger follicles of controlled ovarian hyperstimulation (**Fig. 23**). SonoAVC can also be used for volume calculation of hydrosalpinx, cystic adnexal lesions, or early gestational sac, etc., and any fluid-filled structures (**Figs. 24A and B**).

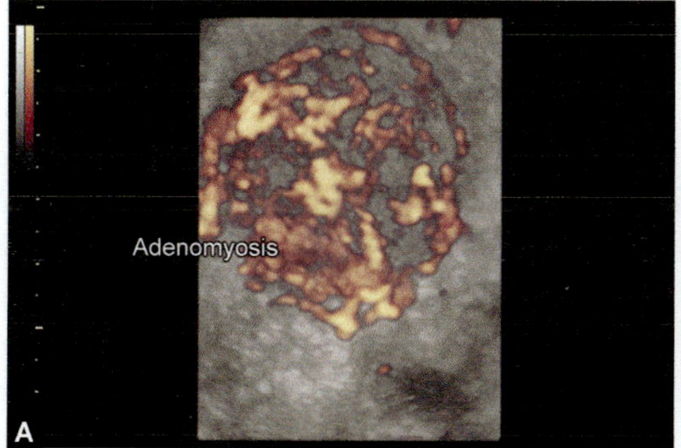

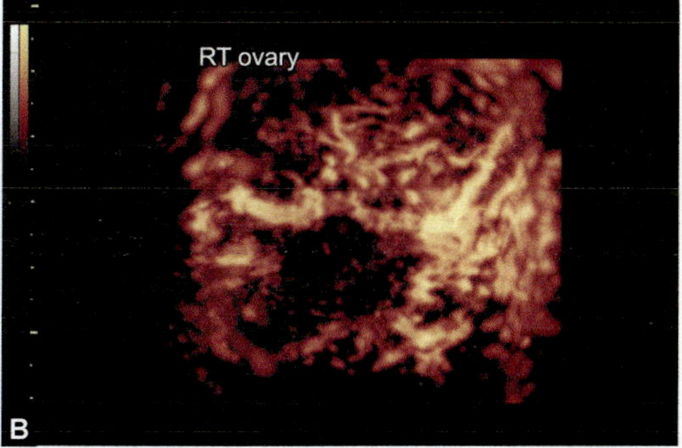

Figs. 19A and B: 3D power Doppler volume rendered in glass body mode: (A) which shows the soft tissue details and also the vascular details; (B) angiomode which shows the vascular details only as in angiography.

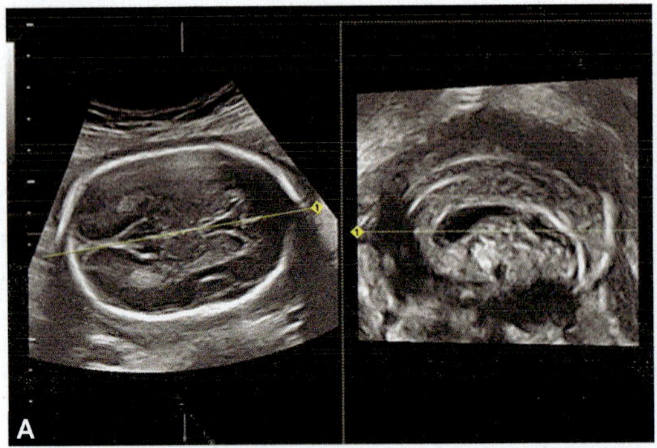

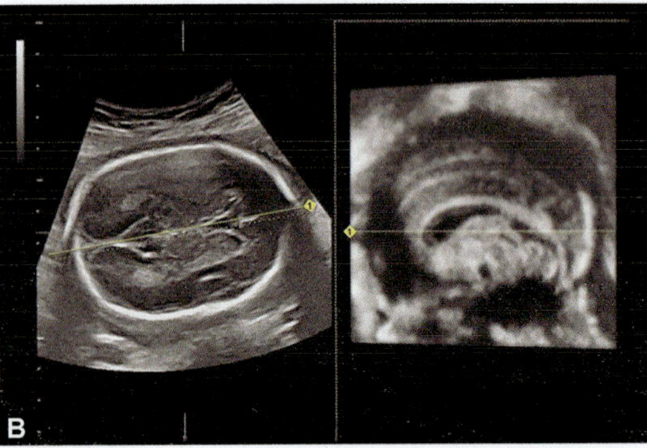

Figs. 20A and B: 3D ultrasound of the head with omniview: (A) Midsagittal view of the head when line for omniview is drawn across the cavum septum pellucidum on the transthalamic axial plane of the head; (B) Same image when coupled with VCI shows better contrast and better delineation of corpus callosum and midline structures.
(VCI: volume contrast imaging)

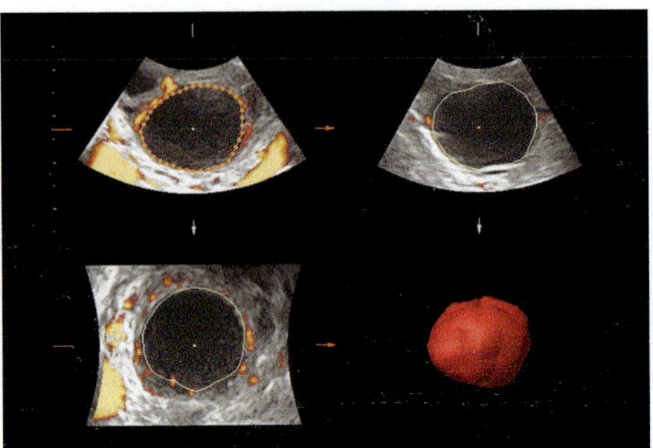

Fig. 21: 3D ultrasound of the follicle with VOCAL software used to define and calculate the volume of the follicle as seen on the fourth image.

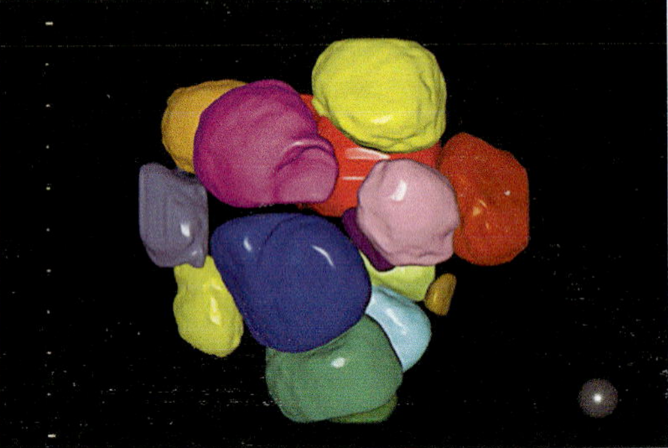

Fig. 23: SonoAVC is also used for counting and measurement of the pre-hCG follicles, especially when there is multifollicular development.

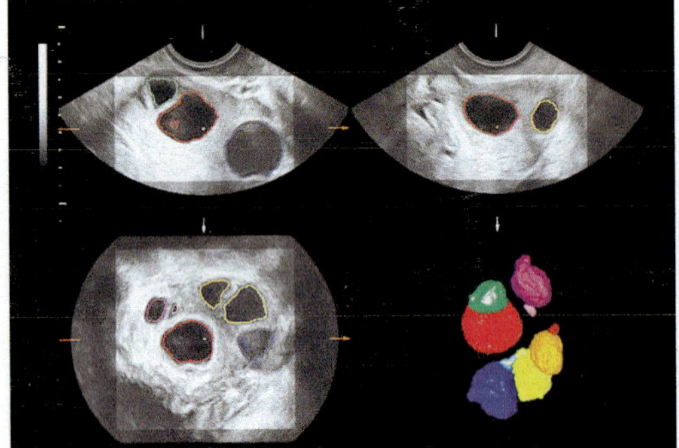

Fig. 22: 3D volume of the ovary rendered by SonoAVC, which shows individual follicle identified by a different color, also calculates volume of each follicle.

TRANSRECTAL SCAN

This route for pelvic scan requires bowel preparation ideally but is not mandatory. The patient position generally for transrectal scan is left lateral with the right lower limb of the patient fully flexed and pressed over the abdomen. But with this position, the image orientation is markedly different from that on the TVS and therefore difficult to understand and interpret. I prefer to do a transrectal scan with the patient in lithotomy-like position. This helps to get the same orientation as with the TVS and therefore easy to interpret (**Fig. 25**).

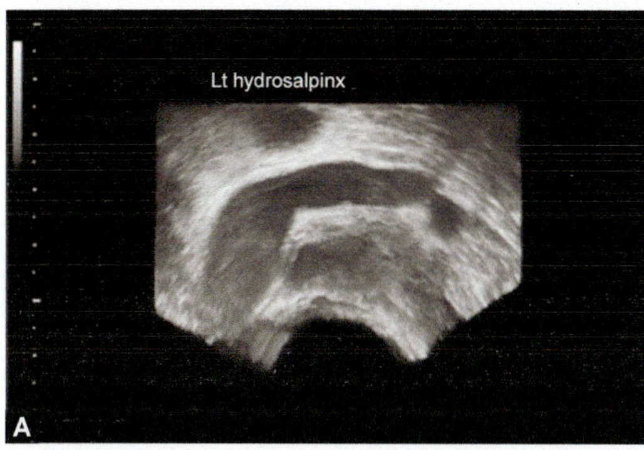

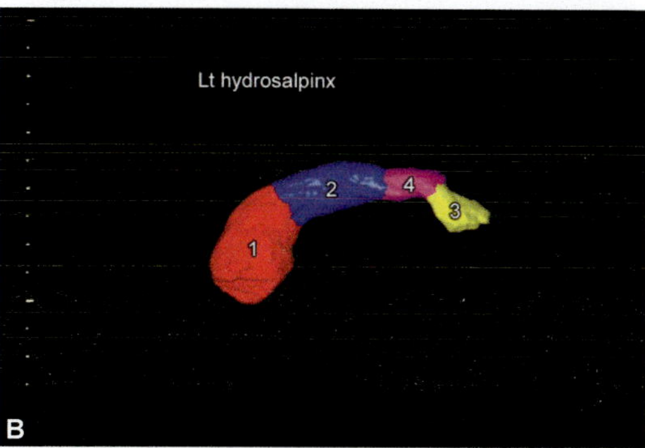

Figs. 24A and B: SonoAVC is based on inversion mode principle and therefore can be used for assessment of the volume of any cystic structures or lesions. Hydrosalpinx is shown on B-mode in part (A) and shown on sonoAVC with volume calculation in the lower right corner in part (B).

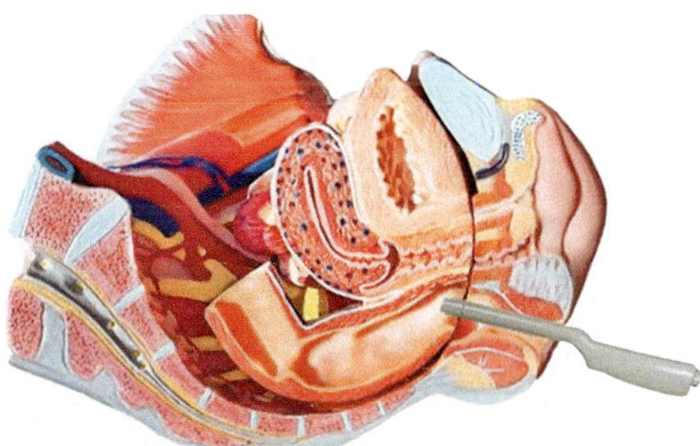

Fig. 25: Diagrammatic demonstration of probe position in a transrectal scan.

TRANSABDOMINAL SCAN

These scans need to be done with a full bladder for evaluation of the uterus and the ovaries and all other pelvic structures. The marker on the probe for the longitudinal scan should always be toward the head end of the female, and therefore on the image, the logo indicates the cephalic end of the patient (**Fig. 26A**). For the transverse section, the probe is always rotated anticlockwise so that the right side of the patient is seen on the right side of the image (**Fig. 26B**). The ovaries can be located by rocking the probe on either side from the longitudinal midsagittal plane of the uterus.

TO SUMMARIZE

- Optimize B-mode images: Adjust angle, focal zones, focal depth, contrast (dynamic range), gains, zoom probe power, and probe frequency.

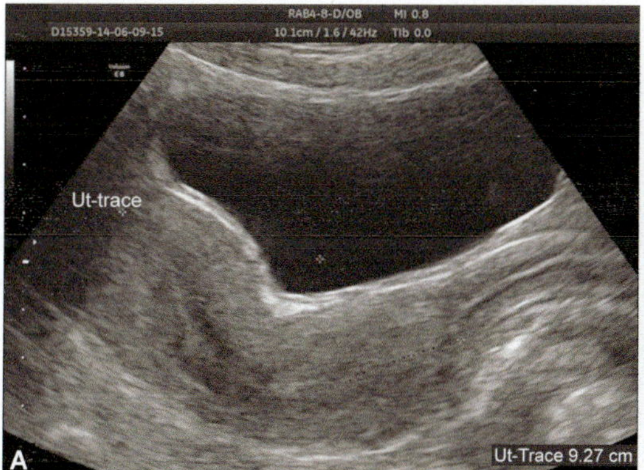

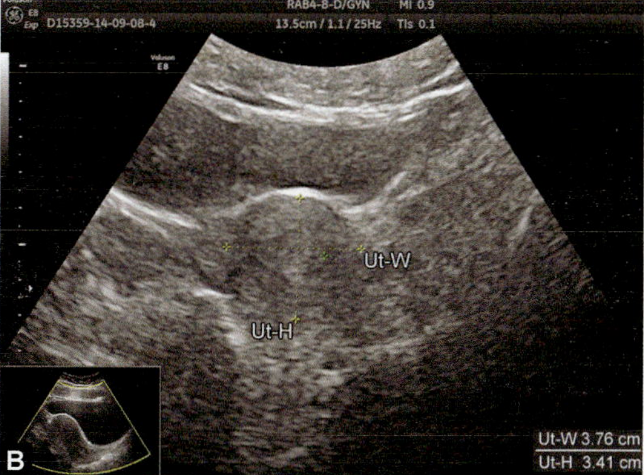

Figs. 26A and B: B mode ultrasound image of the transabdominal scan of the pelvis, showing the uterus in long axis (A), and in transverse section (B).

- Doppler is optimized by: Size of color box or sample volume, gains, pulse repetition frequency (PRF), wall filter, probe power, Doppler angle.
- 3D is a value-adding modality with: Multiplanar imaging, omniview, VCI, tomographic ultrasound imaging (TUI), rendering, VOCAL, and SonoAVC.

REFERENCE

1. Hull MGR. Polycystic ovarian disease: clinical aspects and prevalence. Res Clin Forums. 1989;11:21-34.

23 CHAPTER

Normal Uterus

Sonal Panchal, Chaitanya Nagori

INTRODUCTION

Uterus is a major pelvic organ, not only for its size, but also because it forms the main midline anatomical landmark. Change in its position or orientation may be a clue to uterine or any other pelvic pathology. But, it must be remembered that uterus is a mobile organ and can be seen in different positions even when normal. Moreover, study of uterine morphology also will lead to diagnosis of uterine pathology.

Uterus is best assessed by transvaginal route. The pelvic anatomy as it appears on transvaginal scan is a sagittal section **(Fig. 1)** and transverse section **(Fig. 2)** anatomy. The pelvic anatomy as it is studied and explained in anatomy literature is in coronal plane **(Fig. 3)**. Therefore, pelvic anatomy as it appears on transvaginal scan must be correctly understood to make correct diagnosis (figures of pelvic anatomy in sagittal, transverse, and coronal planes).

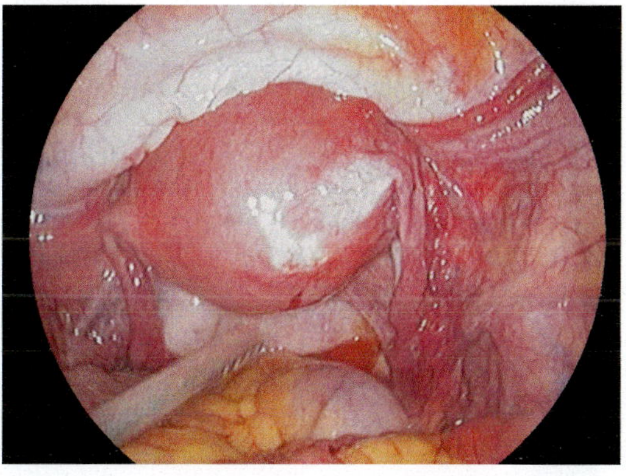

Fig. 2: Female reproductive organs in transverse plane.

But, it is usually preferred to do trans-abdominal scan of the pelvis before trans-vaginal scan. This helps a more generalized idea about the pelvic anatomy. This scan is done on full bladder **(Figs. 4A and B)**.

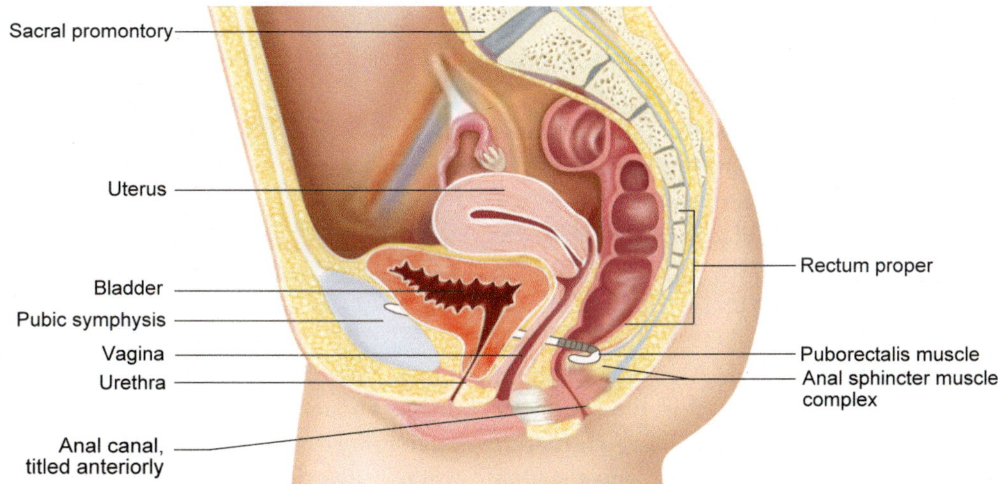

Fig. 1: Female reproductive organs in sagittal plane.

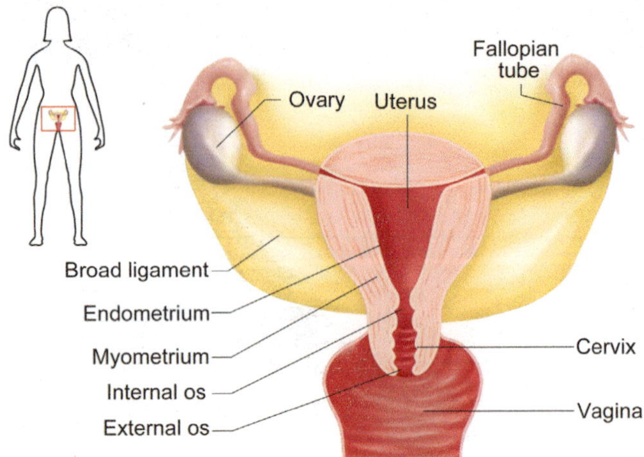

Fig. 3: Female reproductive organs in coronal plane.

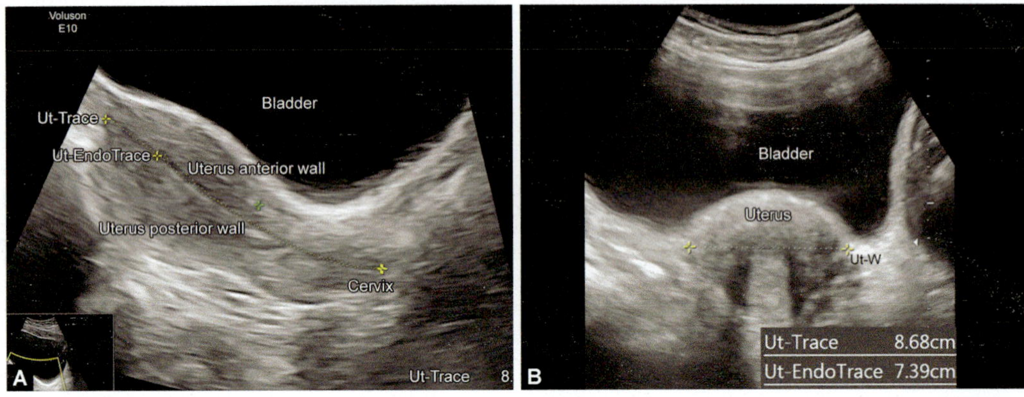

Figs. 4A and B: Uterus on transabdominal ultrasound in: (A) Long section; (B) Transverse section.

SCANNING AND ORIENTATION OF IMAGE

It has been universally accepted that transvaginal is the route of choice for ultrasound assessment of the pelvis organs. The endocavitary (transvaginal) probe is introduced through the introitus in such a way that the markers **(Fig. 5)**, as shown on the probe, face the roof of the room and anterior aspect of the patient. On the resultant image, the logo of the manufacturer corresponds to these indicators **(Fig. 6)**. This image on the screen can be oriented in four different ways **(Figs. 7A to D)** by using right-left reverse switch and up-down reverse switch of machine **(Fig. 8)**. No one orientation of the image is better than the other. One can use the orientation that is convenient to one's self. We will use the orientation shown in **Figure 8** for all our descriptions and discussions.

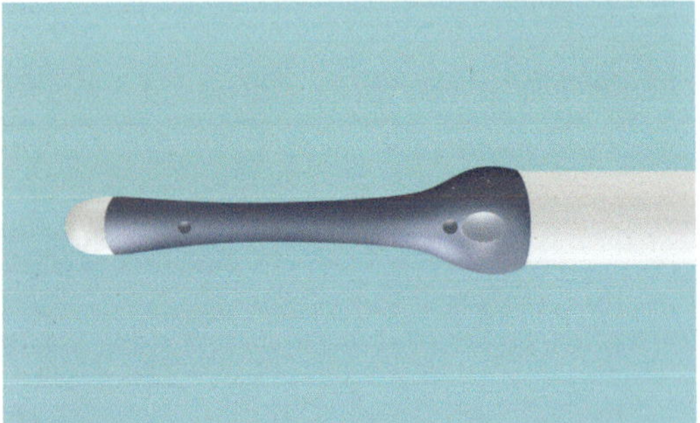

Fig. 5: Volume transvaginal probe, markers on the probe are displayed.

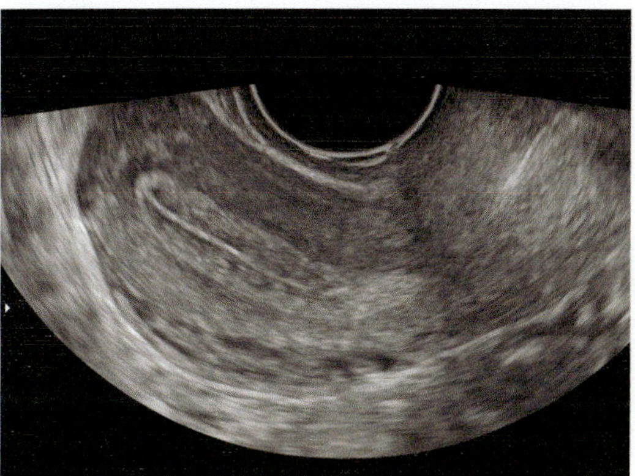

Fig. 6: B mode ultrasound image of the midsagittal plane of the anteverted anteflexed uterus.

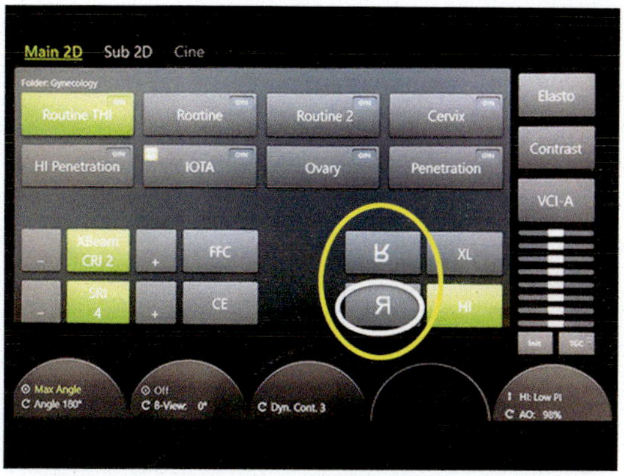

Fig. 8: Touch screen of the scanner with the reverse switches shown by yellow circle.

ORIENTATION AND POSITION OF THE UTERUS

As the probe slides in the vaginal canal, this probe position, with markers toward the roof, normally shows the long axis of the uterus. Uterus may be anteverted or retroverted and anteflexed or retroflexed. Version indicates the direction of cervix from external os to internal os, whereas flexion indicates the direction of fundus of the uterus **(Figs. 9A and B)**. Some authors also describe the angle and version as angle between vagina and cervix and angle

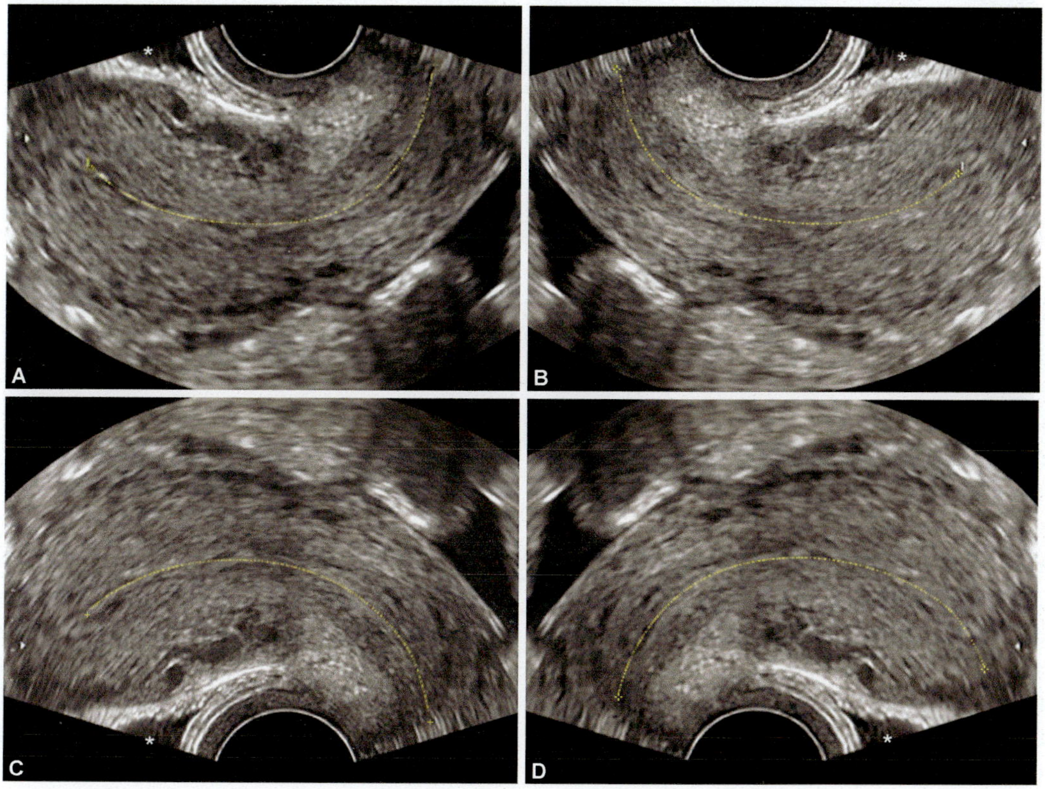

Figs. 7A to D: Four different image orientations: (A) Logo above left; (B) Logo above right; (C) Logo below left; (D) Logo below right.

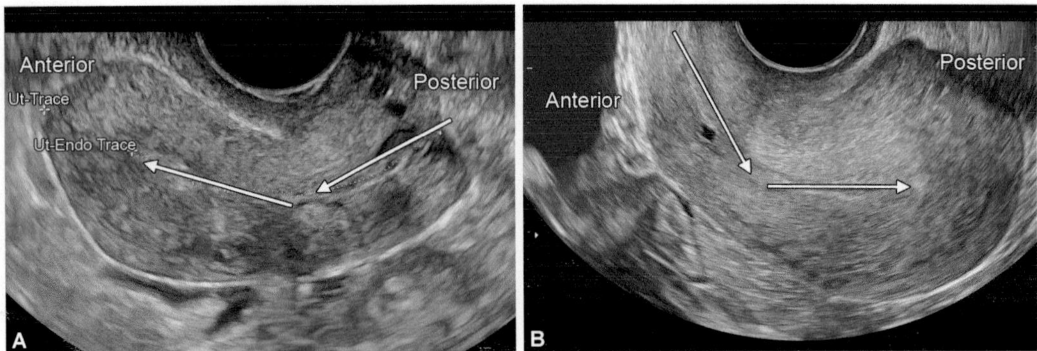

Figs. 9A and B: B mode ultrasound image of sagittal section of uterus, with arrows indicating the direction of cervix and the direction of the uterus in relation to cervix. (A) Anteverted anteflexed uterus; (B) Retroverted retroflexed uterus.

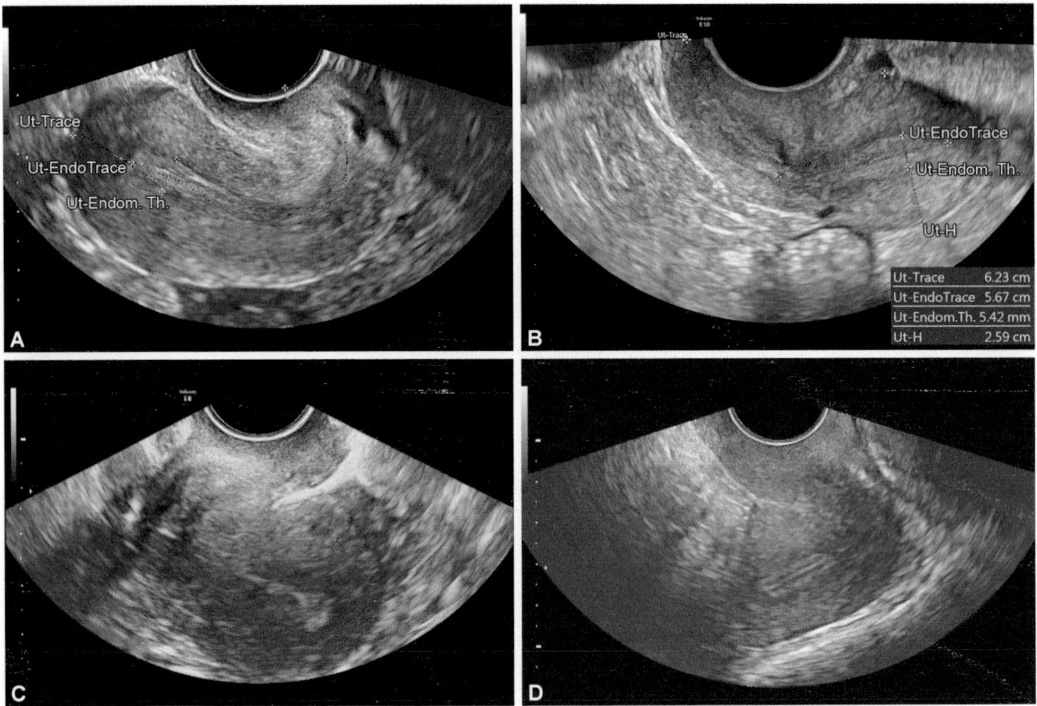

Figs. 10A to D: (A) Anteverted anteflexed uterus; (B) Retroverted retroflexed uterus; (C) Anteverted retroflexed uterus; (D) Retroverted anteflexed.

between cervix and uterus, respectively. Anteversion is when the cervix from external os to internal os is directed from posterior to anterior and retroversion is when the cervix from external os to internal os traverses from front to back. When anteflexed, the uterine fundus will be directed toward the indicator on the screen and urinary bladder is also seen on the same side of the screen; when retroflexed, the uterine fundus will be on the opposite side of the indicator and the urinary bladder **(Figs. 10A to D)**. In other words, if cervix forms an obtuse angle with vagina, it is anteverted and if it forms acute angle with vagina, it is retroverted. If uterus forms obtuse angle with anteverted cervix, it is anteflexed and if it forms acute angle with anteverted cervix, it is retroflexed. If uterus forms an acute angle

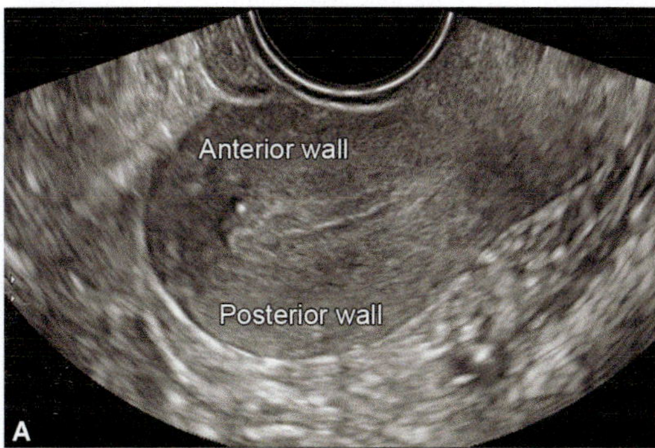

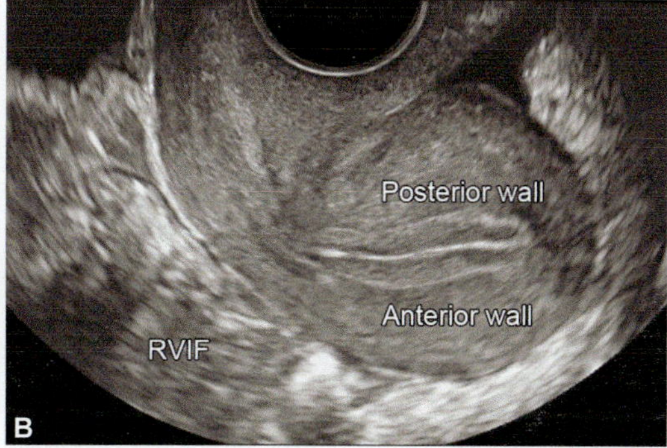

Figs. 11A and B: Anterior and posterior myometrial walls demarcated in: (A) Anteverted uterus; (B) Retroverted uterus.

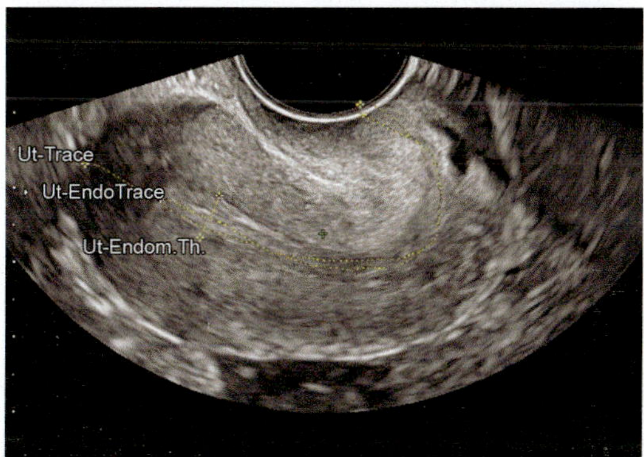

Fig. 12: Midsagittal plane of the uterus as seen on transvaginal probe introduction when uterus is normally positioned.

with retroverted cervix, it is anteflexed and if it forms an obtuse angle with retroverted cervix, it is retroflexed. Though these may change if there is acute anteflexion or retroflexion. If in doubt, one can correlate the position of the uterine fundus in relation to urinary bladder for confirmation. It is important to mention here that in an anteverted uterus, the myometrial wall close to the probe is anterior myometrium, whereas with retroverted uterus, the myometrial wall close to the probe is the posterior myometrial wall **(Figs. 11A and B)**.

The uterus that is normally positioned, whether anteverted or retroverted, is seen in its midsagittal plane with the probe in the midline **(Fig. 12)**. A uterus that is not normal in position will not be seen in midsagittal plane in this probe position or will be partially seen. If uterus is deviated to right or left, it will be seen in true long axis only when the probe is spanned on right or left side, respectively. If one can see the true long axis of the uterus when the probe head faces left side, the uterus is deviated to left side and if it is seen in its true long axis when probe head faces right side, it is deviated to right side. If the uterus is not seen in long axis only on spanning movement, it means that it is not only deviated but is also twisted. Deviation or twisting of the uterus is usually a sign of extrauterine pelvic pathology.

ENDOMETRIUM: POINTS TO OBSERVE AND REPORT

- Symmetry of the endometrial shape (pear shaped)
- Central endometrial line
- Endometrial-myometrial junction
- Intraendometrial lesions such as polyps and adhesions
- Morphology corresponding to the phase of the cycle.

Endometrium has smooth margins, is pear shaped, broadest just caudal to the fundal end, and narrows down smoothly toward cervix **(Fig. 13)**. The central line that demonstrates the endometrial cavity is always seen as a smoothly curved line. Any irregularities in this line indicate an intraendometrial lesion **(Fig. 14)**. In all the phases of the menstrual cycle, there is a thin hypoechoic zone

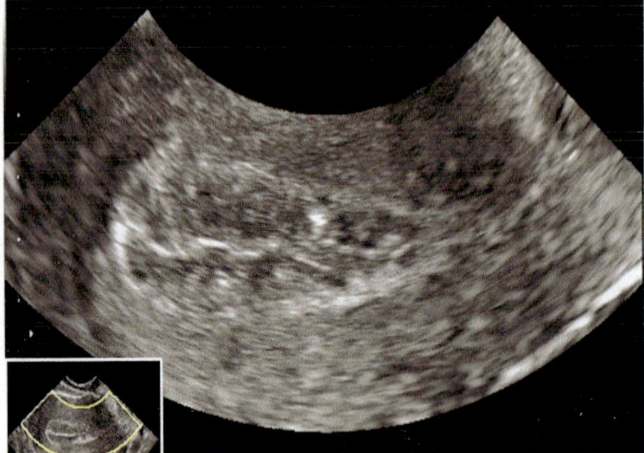

Fig. 13: Normal endometrium.

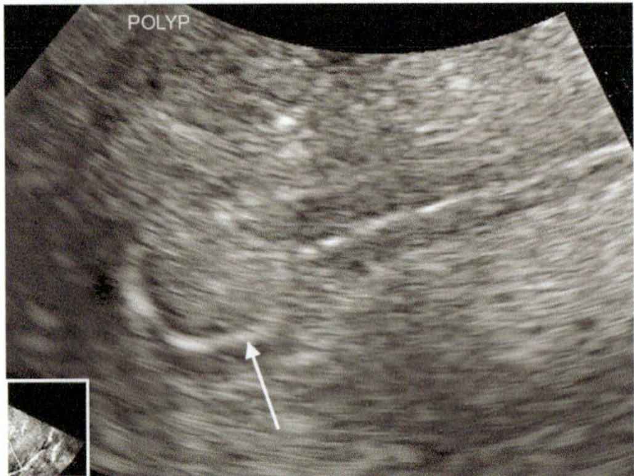

Fig. 14: Deviation of the central endometrial line is seen in the fundal endometrium due to polyp.

seen surrounding the echogenic outline of endometrium. This is known as endometrial-myometrial junction or junctional zone **(Fig. 15)**. It is actually the innermost layer of the myometrium. It is composed of longitudinally and circularly oriented, closely packed smooth muscle fibers parallel to the endometrium.

The junctional zone normally increases in thickness with age to reach its peak at 41–50 years[1] and the junctional zone slightly increases in thickness throughout the menstrual cycle.[2] It shows cyclical changes. It is thickest in the early proliferative phase, thinnest in the preovulatory phase, and again increases in thickness in the secretory phase in conception cycles, but decreases further in nonconception cycles. Endometrial-myometrial junction can be always seen on B-mode scan, but is much better appreciated on three-dimensional (3D) ultrasound in coronal plane **(Fig. 16)**. Breach or irregularity of this zone is suggestive of pathology that involves endometrium and/or myometrium. The pathologies that commonly alter the junctional zone are adenomyosis, endometritis and malignancies **(Figs. 17A to C)**.

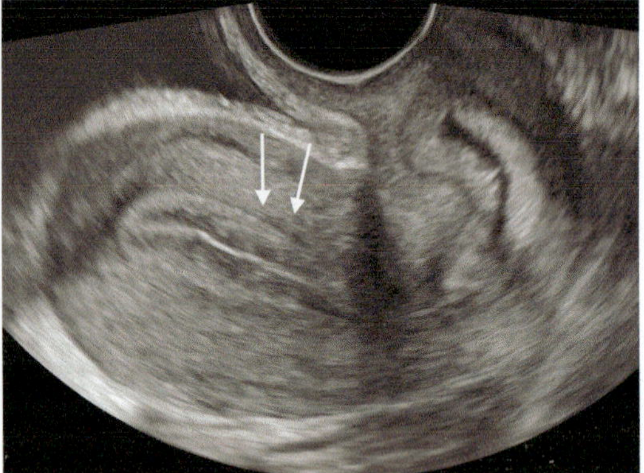

Fig. 15: Midsagittal plane of the uterus, with arrows showing hypoechoic endometrio-myometrial junction outlining the endometrium.

Looking at the endometrium: Any echogenic solid lesion in between the lines of endometrium is suggestive of pathologies such as polyps and synechiae **(Figs. 18A and B)**. There may also be fluid with or without echogenicities, in the endometrium, normally

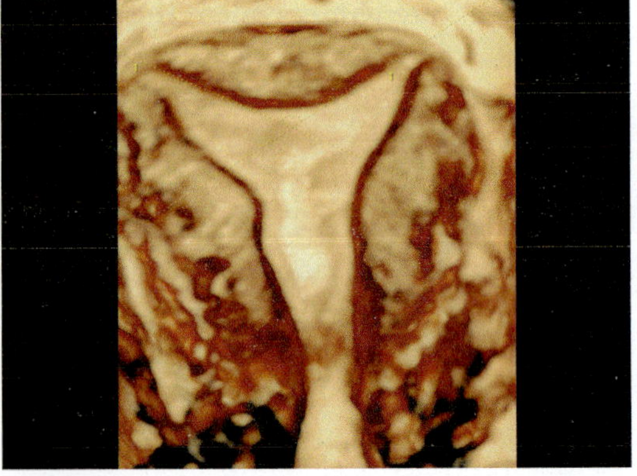

Fig. 16: Coronal plane of the uterus on 3D rendered image showing endometrio-myometrial junction as hypoechoic zone surrounding the endometrium.

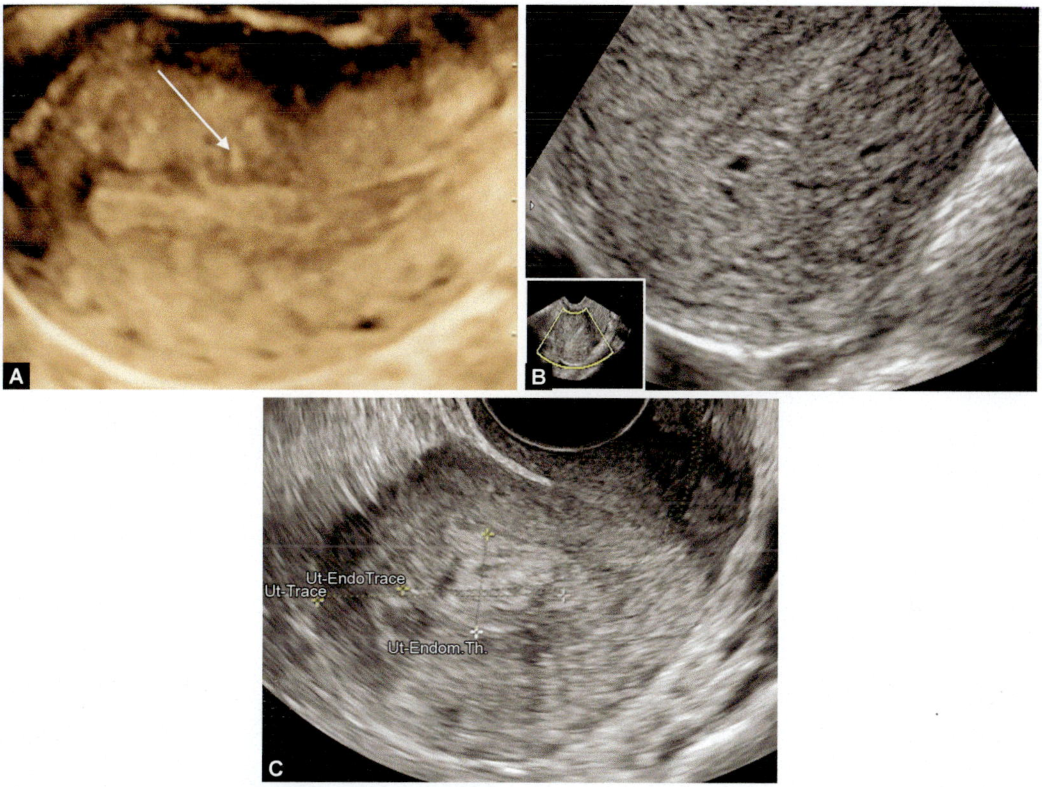

Figs. 17A to C: (A) Irregular and interrupted endometrio-myometirlal junction with thin endometirum and heterogenous myometrium due to adenomyosis; (B) Thick endometrium with inaccessible junctional zone in early proliferative phase due to acute endometritis; (C) Thick heterogenous endometrium with obliterated junctional zone, possibly die to malignancy of the endometrium.

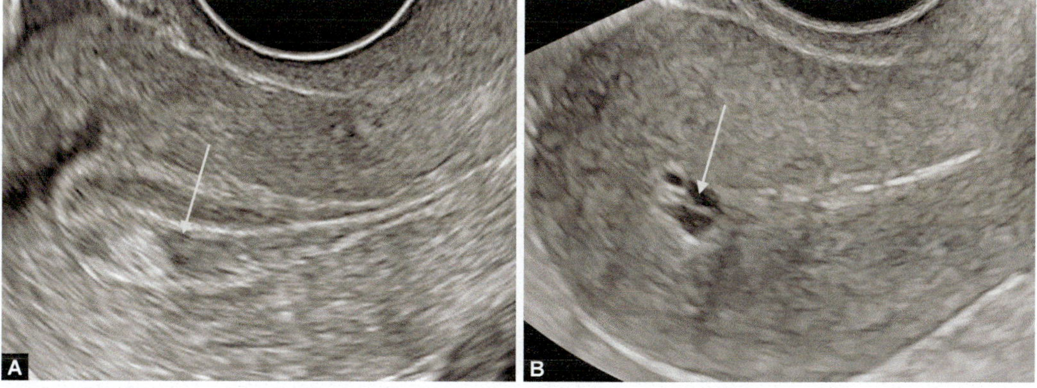

Figs. 18A and B: (A) Endometrial polyp as shown by the arrow—round/oval echogenic solid lesion in endometrium; (B) Endometrial synechiea as shown by the arrow—linear echogenic strand in the endometrial cavity across the two lips of endometrium.

during the menstrual phase or pathologically due to endometritis (acute or chronic) **(Figs. 19A and B)**. Though minimal fluid temporarily (for a few hours) may be seen normally in the endometrium in the preovulatory period. Depending on the phase of the cycle,

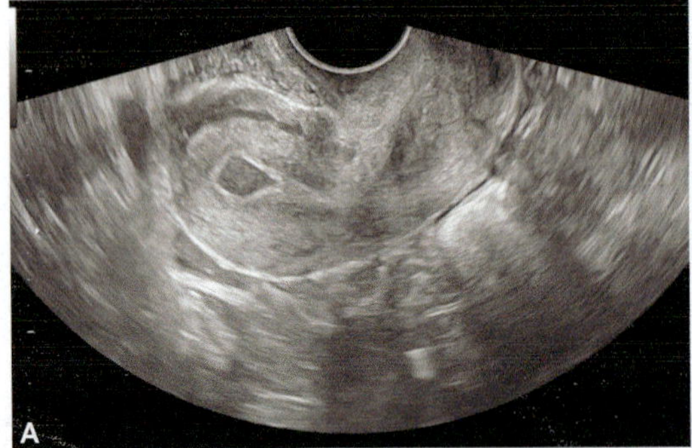

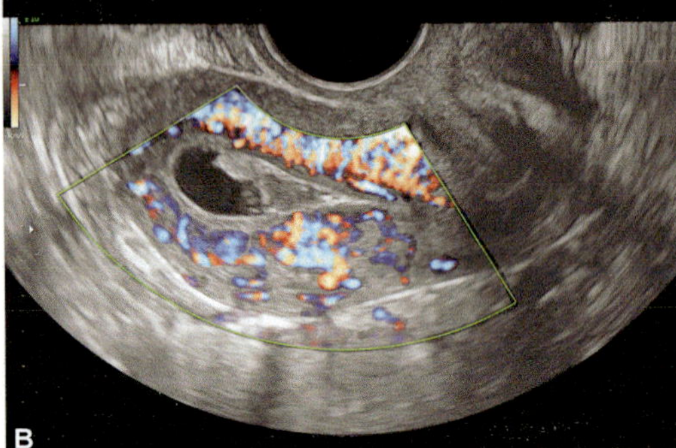

Figs. 19A and B: (A) Fluid in the endometrial cavity with ground glass echogenecity—most likely blood, often seen in the menstrual phase of the cycle; (B) Heterogenous contents in the endometrial caivty with marked blood flow in the subendometrium, possibly due to acute endometritis.

endometrium is expected to be thin linear in early follicular phase, triple line in preovulatory phase, and thick and echogenic in secretory phase **(Figs. 20A to C)**. 3D ultrasound is also the most efficient modality for assessment of endometrial and subendometrial pathologies.

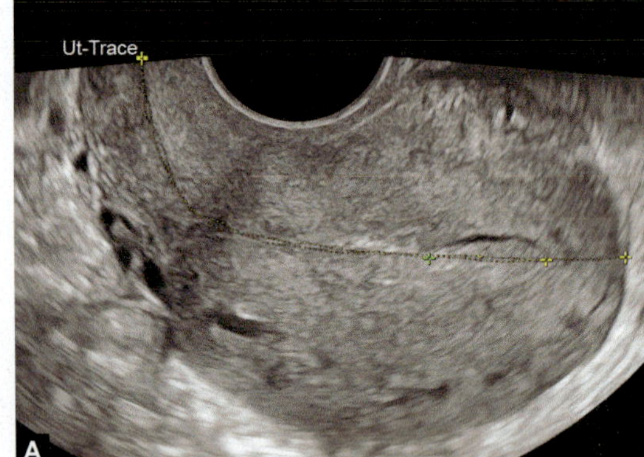

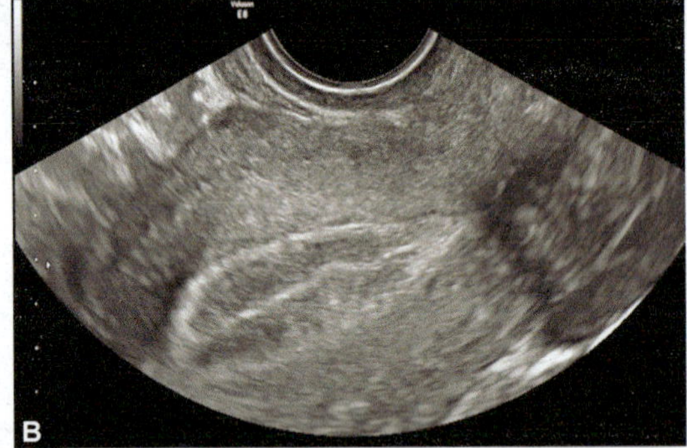

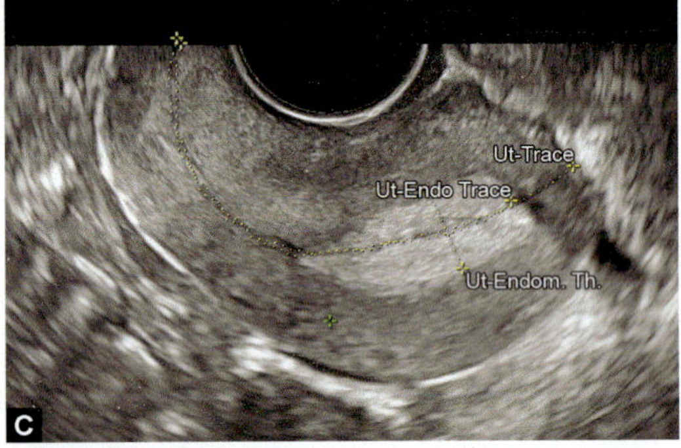

Figs. 20A to C: (A) Thin linear endometrium of early proliferative phase; (B) Multilayered endometrium of preovulatory phase; (C) Hyperechoic endometrium of secretory phase.

MYOMETRIUM: POINTS TO OBSERVE AND REPORT

- Thickness of the myometrium
- Homogenicity of the myometrium
- If heterogeneous, cause of heterogenicity—mass lesions, adenomyosis, scar tissues, etc. **(Figs. 21A and B)**
- Thickness of the myometrium, if asymmetrical anterior and posterior wall or localized, needs a mention.
- Myometrium is homogeneously echogenic normally and both anterior and posterior myometrial walls are almost equal in thickness **(Fig. 22)**. Any generalized heterogenicity or localized hypo-/hyperechogenicity is suggestive of a pathology

SEROSA: POINTS TO OBSERVE AND REPORT

- Smoothness of contour
- Continuity
- Maintenance of tissue interface
- Mobility of the uterus.

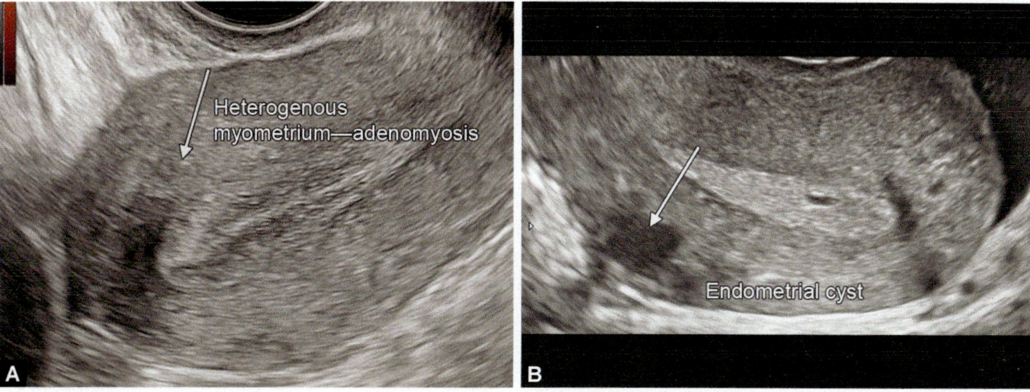

Figs. 21A and B: (A) Generalized heterogenous myometrium with hyperechoic tiny dots and lines (marked by arrow) due to adenomyosis; (B) Arrow showing well-defined hypoechoic roundish lesion—fibroid. Fundal myometrium is also heterogenous with hyperechoic dots and lines and anechoic areas due to adenomyosis.

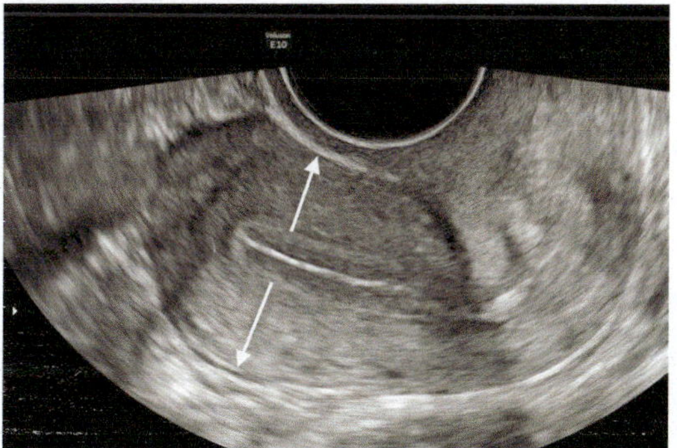

Fig. 22: Midsagittal plane of the uterus showing measurement of myometrial wall thickness.

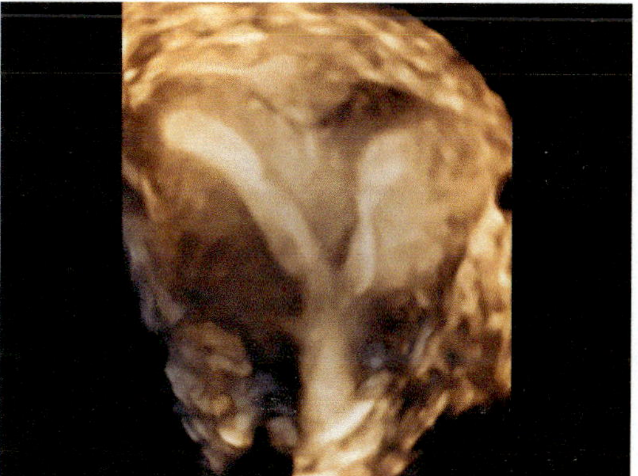

Fig. 23: Coronal plane of the uterus as seen on the 3D rendered image of the uterus, with division of the endometrial cavity and fundal serosal notch suggesting duplication abnormality.

Outer layer of uterus is covered by peritoneum and is the serosal layer. It defines the margins of uterus and, therefore, its integrity is essential to confirm that the uterus is normal. Any mass lesion in the uterus changes the contour of the uterus and, therefore, the smooth pear shape is distorted. In and out movement of the probe confirms the mobility of the uterus and rules out adhesions as bowel loops or sometimes ovary can be seen sliding over the surface of the uterus.

It is the fundal contour and the endometrial cavity contour that diagnose the Müllerian duct abnormalities. These are diagnosed with highest accuracy on 3D ultrasound **(Fig. 23)**. This is so because 3D ultrasound allows the assessment of the uterus in coronal plane and also allows to see the fundal and the endometrial contour together.

CERVIX: POINTS TO OBSERVE AND REPORT

- *Length and mucus*: The cervical length is assessed by identifying the internal os and the external os. Internal os can be identified by two landmarks: (1) The entry of uterine vessels on transverse section **(Fig. 24)** and (2) Cervical glands surrounding the cervical mucosa on longitudinal section **(Fig. 25)**. Thickness of endometrial-myometrial junction is narrowest at the internal os and beyond

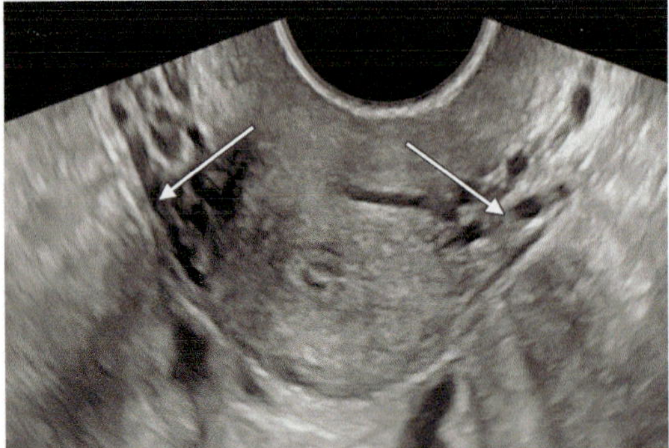

Fig. 24: Transverse section of the uterus at the level of internal os showing uterine vessels on both the sides as multiple anechoic areas.

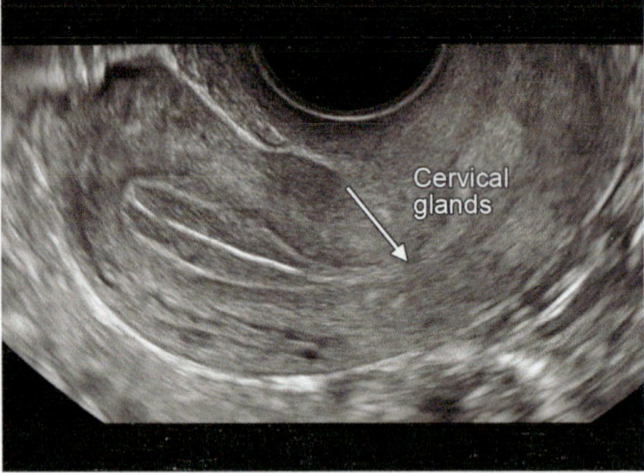

Fig. 25: Points arrow showing internal os in midsagittal plane.

that toward cervix is markedly thickened hypoechoic zone because of these cervical glands making a triangle. It is important to note here that the cervical gland layer appears hypoechoic generally except in periovulatory phase when it appear hyperechoic. The apex of this triangle is internal os. Presence of fluid (mucus) in the cervical canal may also define the cervical canal.

- Cervical lesions such as polyps, fibroids, and nabothian cysts **(Figs. 26A to D)**.

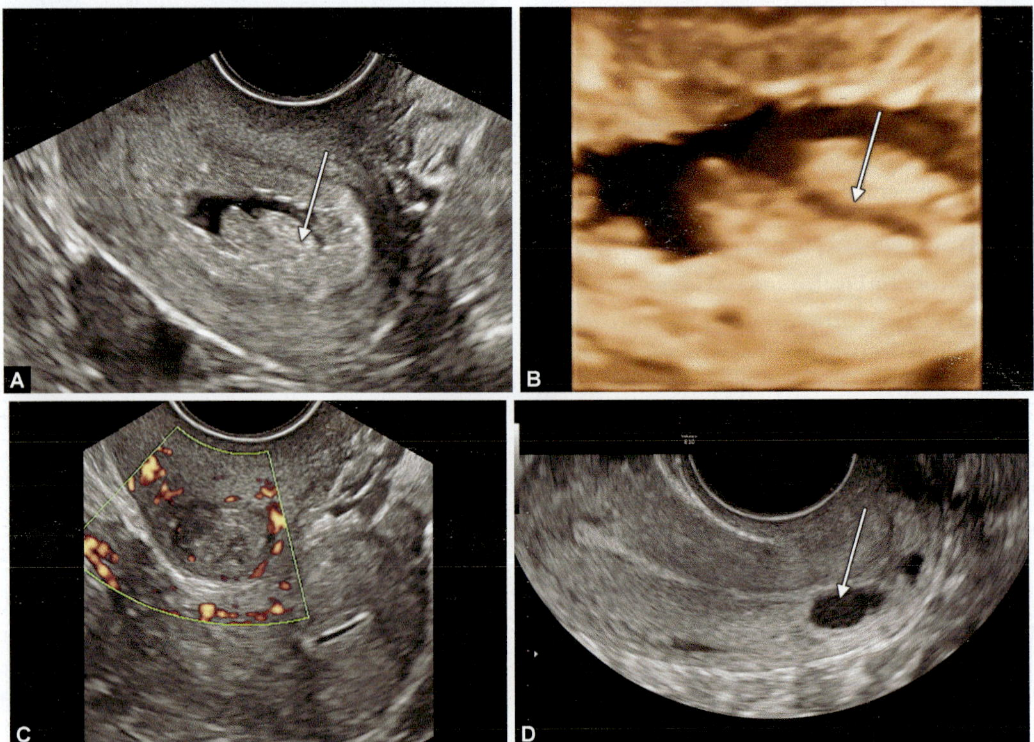

Figs. 26A to D: (A and B) Cervical polyps seen on 2D ultrasound image and on 3D rendered image (arrows); (C) Round hypoechoic lesion with peripheral vascularity is seen in the cervix—cervical fibroid; (D) Arrow showing anechoic well-defined oval lesion, adjacent to cervical lumen—nabothian cyst.

- Serosal integrity as for the body of the uterus is also essential for the cervix.

MEASUREMENTS

Uterocervical length is measured as a complete length from the fundal serosa to the external os. It should ideally be measured by a line trace **(Fig. 27)**. It can be best measured as a continuous tracing from the fundal serosal tip to the external os or it can be a summation of two measurements: (1) fundus to internal os and (2) internal os to external os, but this may lead to errors and, therefore, should not be used. Physiological uterocervical length is also measured in this view **(Fig. 27)**. This physiological uterocervical length or endometrial length must be used for intrauterine insemination (IUI) and embryo transfer. The line is drawn from the fundal tip of the endometrium to the external os. This length is always better measured as a trace rather than separately measuring the uterine length and cervical length by straight lines. The endometrial thickness is measured from anterior outer margin to posterior outer margin of peripheral hyperechoic lines of endometrium and at the thickest part of the endometrium. This is usually about 1–2 cm caudal to the fundal end of the endometrium. The thickness of the endometrium is always measured perpendicular to the central line of the endometrium. If there is fluid in the endometrium, the thickness of two lips is measured separately and then added for correct assessment of the endometrial thickness **(Figs. 28A and B)**.

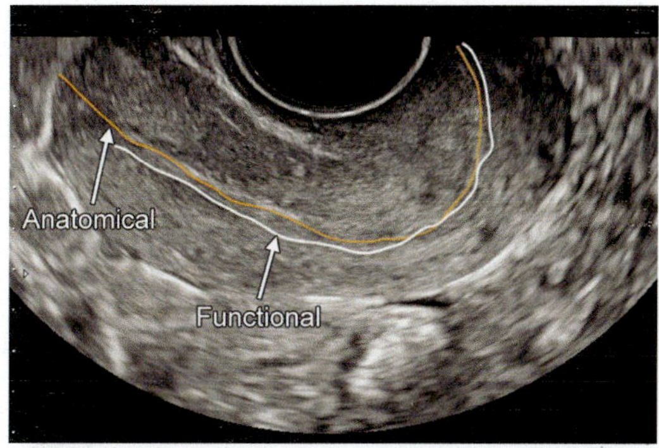

Fig. 27: Midsagittal plane of uterus showing anatomical and functional uterocervical length.

Visual assessment of symmetry of thickness of anterior and posterior myometrium is done and if in doubt, actual measurements may be taken. Myometrium is measured from outer margin of outer hyperechoic line of endometrium to the serosa perpendicular to the central line of the endometrium **(Figs. 29A and B)**. On transverse section, measure the transverse diameter of the uterus.

CYCLICAL CHANGES

Endometrium and uterus are receptor organs to the reproductive steroids—estrogen, progesterone, and androgen. Receptivity of endometrium to embryo is affected by

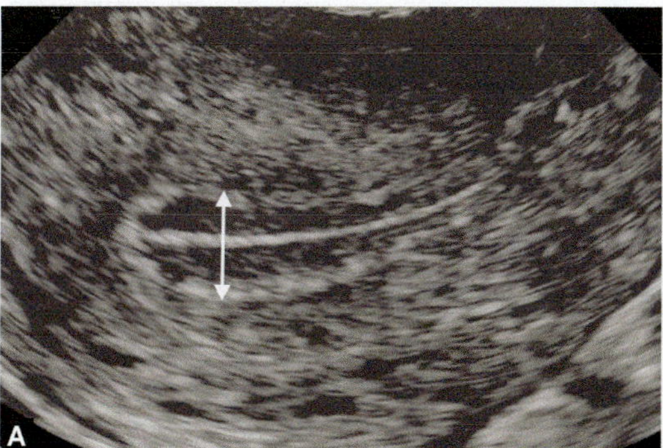

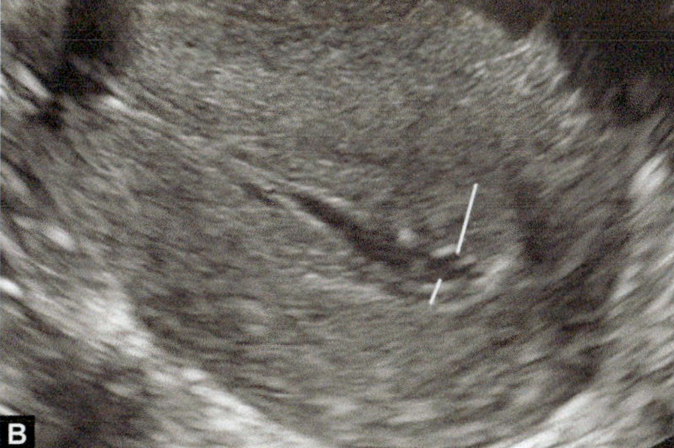

Figs. 28A and B: (A) Endometrial thickness measurement; (B) Endometrial thickness measurement in case of fluid in endometrial cavity.

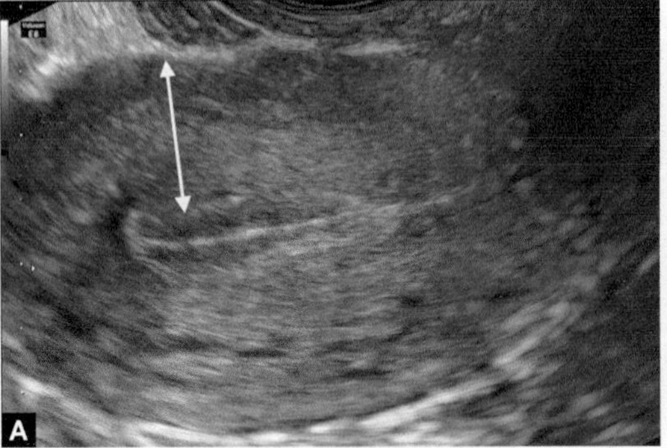

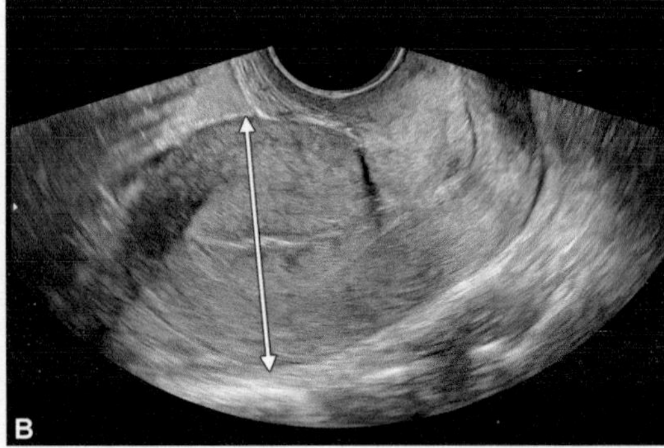

Fig. 29A and B: (A) Myometrial thickness measurement on midsagittal plane; (B) Midsagittal plane of the uterus showing AP diameter measurement.

the delicate equilibrium of these steroids. The changes in these hormones reflect as morphological and vascular changes in the endometrium. These can be studied by ultrasound and Doppler. Therefore, monitoring of continuous changes occurring in the uterus and endometrium is as important as monitoring of the follicle. This not only helps to understand the physiology, but also helps to understand the endometrial behavior in response to drugs and chemicals used to treat subfertile patients. At the start of the menstrual cycle when the whole endometrium has shed off, the endometrium appears thin and linear. Endometrial thickness is <5 mm in early follicular phase and slightly more echogenic than the myometrium. At this stage, estrogen and progesterone levels are at the baseline levels and, therefore, endometrium at this stage also does not show any blood flow normally. During menstruation, at times, blood may be seen in the endometrial cavity **(Figs. 30A and B)**. This is usually seen as heterogeneous echoes with echogenic and anechoic areas due to clotted blood and serum. Fresh blood appears hyperechoic and may often be mistaken for thick endometrium on B-mode alone.

But, Doppler is of help to differentiate between the two. Even a single vessel entering into the depth of the endometrium confirms the thick endometrium, blood never shows any blood vessels inside. It grows at a rate of 1–2 mm/day in early follicular phase after the menstruation starts. Endometrium starts becoming triple line **(Fig. 31A)** from 6 days before luteinizing hormone (LH) surge.

Endometrial thickness can be correlated with the rise in estradiol.[3] Multilayered

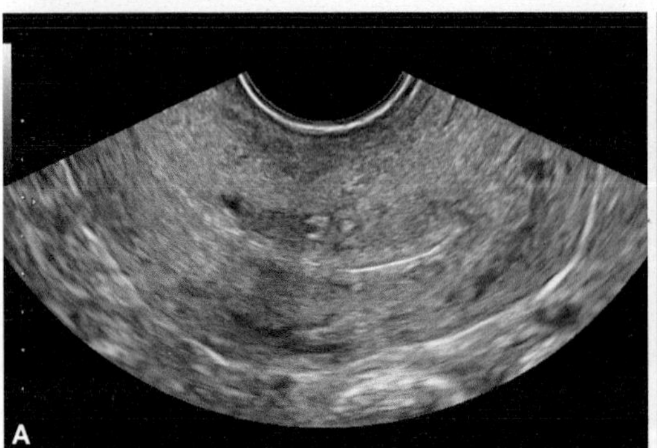

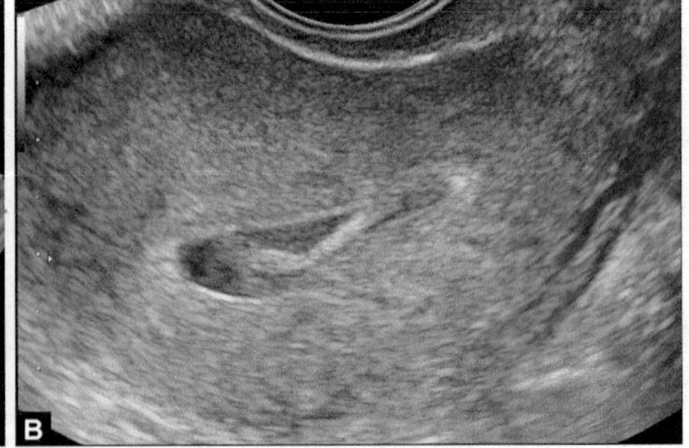

Figs. 30A and B: (A) Single line endometrium of early proliferative phase; (B) Heterogenous content in the endometrial cavity in early proliferative phase due to blood.

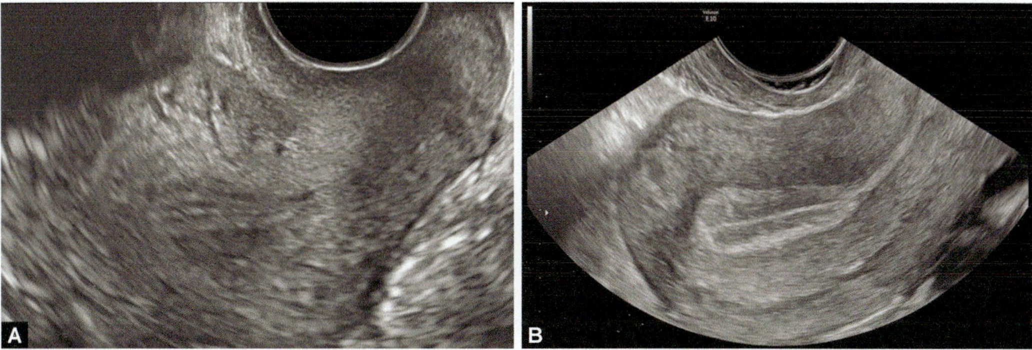

Figs. 31A and B: (A) Multilayered endometrium in mid-proliferative phase; (B) Preovulatory multilayered endometrium.

endometrium grows to a thickness of 10–12 mm at ovulation **(Fig. 31B)**,[4] though relationship of endometrial thickness to histological dating is controversial. Endometrial wave-like activity can be seen on ultrasound throughout the menstrual cycle and is highest in the periovulatory period and in 30–40% of spontaneous cycles, its rate is 3–4/min.[5] This peristalsis initiates in the endometrial-myometrial junctional zone, the innermost layer of the myometrium. At 24–36 hours before ovulation, cervix shows mucus as anechoic strip in the cervical canal **(Fig. 32)**. At times, minimal endometrial fluid is also seen as a result of estrogen rise **(Fig. 33)**. Endometrial and subendometrial vascular flow increases to its maximum 3 days prior to ovulation **(Fig. 34)** and then decreases until fifth postovulatory day (due to probably vasodilatation of subepithelial capillary plexus leading to stromal edema) and then again increases for the rest of the luteal phase.[6] The proliferative phase flow is thought to be due to vasodilatory effect of estrogen and the secretory phase vascularity can be attributed

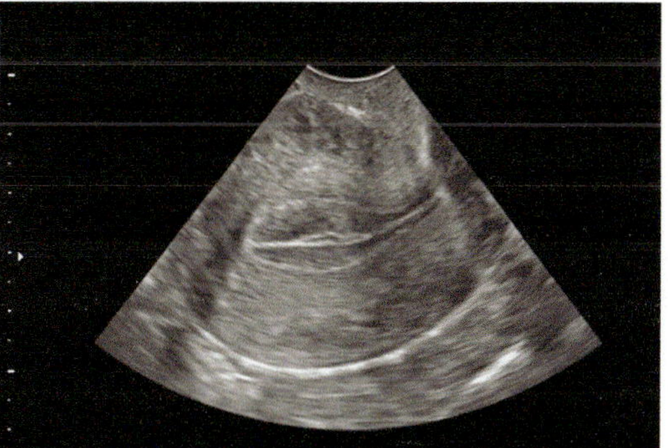

Fig. 33: Preovulatory endometrium with fluid slit in the cavity.

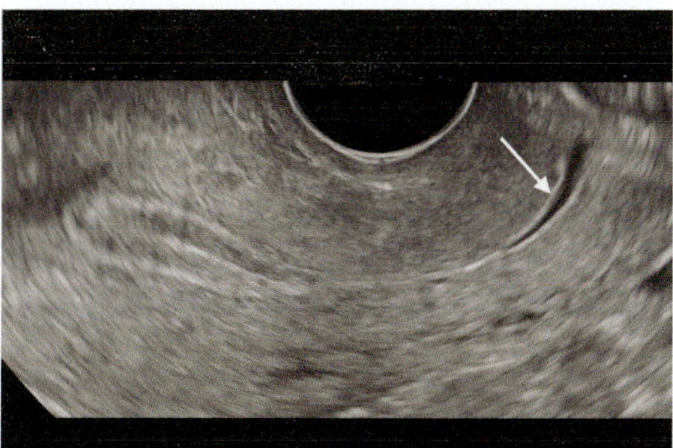

Fig. 32: Preovulatory multilayered endometrium with fluid in cervical canal (arrow): preovulatory cervical mucus.

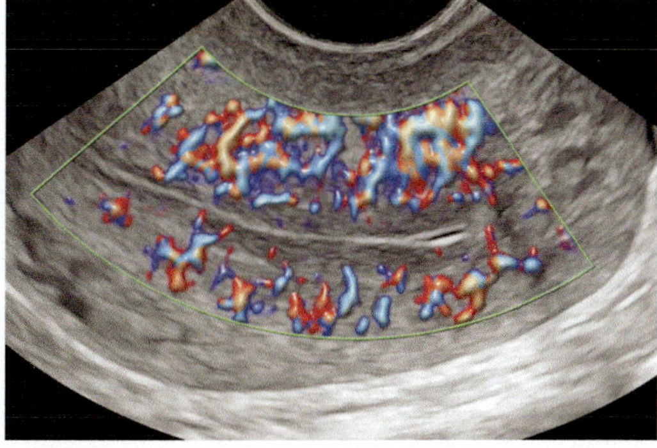

Fig. 34: Preovulatory multilayered endometrium with fluid slit in endometrial cavity and blood flow seen in the endometrium on HD flow.

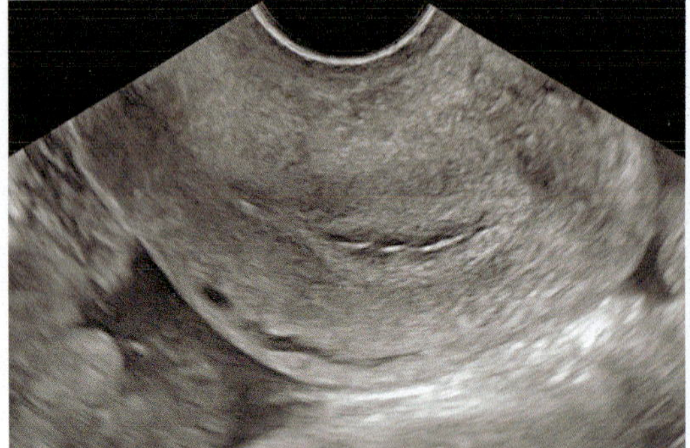

Fig. 35: Fluffy outer margin of multilayered endometrium due to early progesterone exposure.

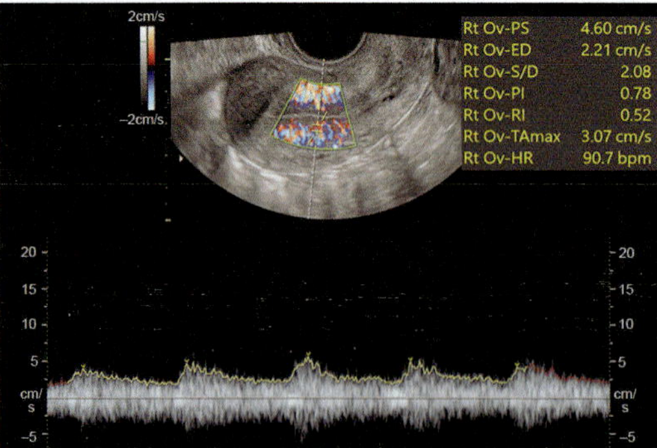

Fig. 36: Pulsed wave Doppler of preovulatory endometrium.

to serum progesterone levels. Blood flow in the uterine vascular bed can be correlated to the estrogen/progesterone ratio.[7] With the start of the LH surge, the outer hyperechoic line of the endometrium starts getting blurred and fluffy, even before ovulation **(Fig. 35)**. At start of the LH surge, the spiral vessels that supply the endometrium show resistance index (RI) of <0.6 **(Fig. 36)**.

During the secretory phase, the endometrium starts becoming echogenic from the periphery and proceeds toward the central line and is described as "endometrial ring sign" **(Fig. 37)**.[8] Its thickness decreases by 0.5 mm on the day of LH surge and then increases by 2 mm in the luteal phase.[9] At about midluteal phase, the whole endometrium appears thickened and hyperechoic.

The endometrial blood flow resistance remains low till the midluteal phase.

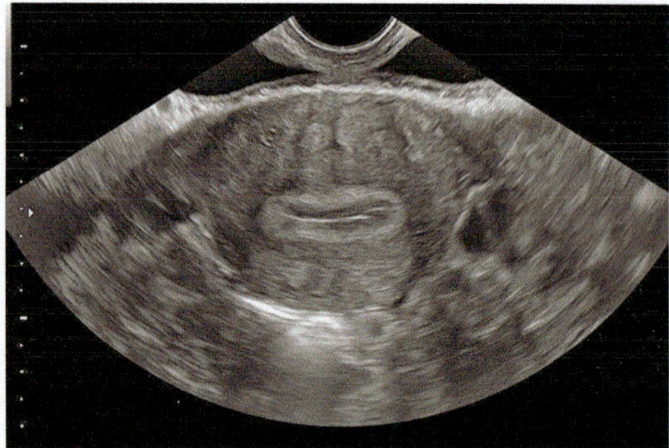

Fig. 37: Endometrial ring sign of early secretory phase.

Uterine artery usually shows a moderate-to-high resistance flow and variations in resistance according to phase of the cycle and is also affected by age. At the time of LH surge, the uterine artery resistance also falls to pulsatility index (PI) < 3.2. The RI of the uterine artery flow is 0.88 ± 0.04 till day 13 of the 28-day menstrual cycle.[10] It is due to postovulatory drop in serum estradiol concentration that leads to increased resistance in uterine artery 3 days after LH peak with highest resistance on day 16.[11,12] The uterine artery resistance then falls and reaches its lowest during the peak luteal function in the midluteal phase. Persistently low resistance in the uterine artery is maintained till the midluteal phase. In conception cycles, this resistance remains low or keeps on falling further, whereas in nonconception cycles, the resistance of the uterine artery increases beyond the midluteal phase with decreasing progesterone levels.

Though, in anovulatory cycles, this fall is not seen and there is persistent rise in the uterine artery RI.[10] Blood flow to the endometrium, which is by spiral arteries, follows a similar pattern as the uterine arteries but shows a lower resistance and lower velocity than the uterine arteries.[13]

POSTMENOPAUSAL UTERUS

As the menopause set, in the body of the uterus significantly decreases in size and the uterocervical ratio from 2:1 reduces

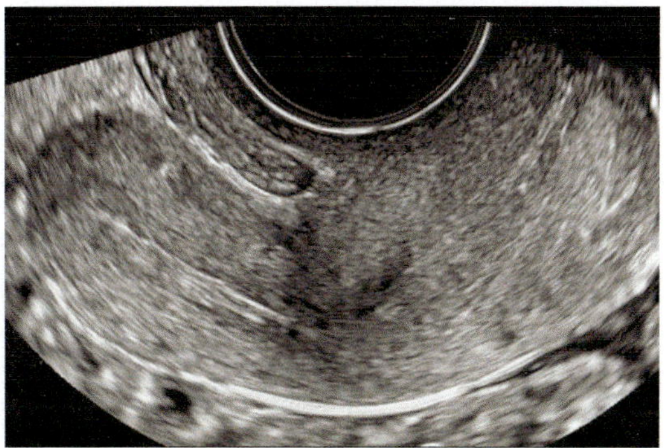

Fig. 38: Postmenopausal uterus with altered uterocervical ratio.

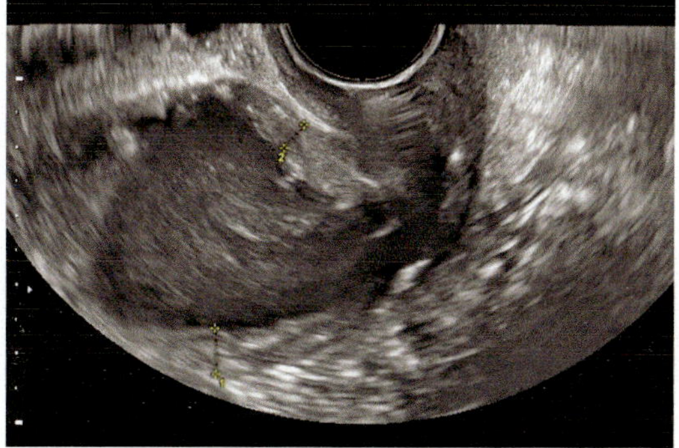

Fig. 39: Blood in endometrial cavity with thin myometrium and irregular inner margins suggestive of endometrial malignancy with possible extension into myometrium.

and reaches 1:1, but in some cases and several years after menopause also reaches 1:2 **(Fig. 38)**. Average uterine size in the postmenopausal age group is 4.5 × 1.5 × 2.5 cm.[14] Myometrium of the uterus gradually decreases in thickness over the years of menopause and appears less echogenic than during the reproductive years. The junctional zone is not distinguishable unless the patient is on hormone replacement therapy.[15] Though if junctional zone is visible, it must be clearly seen as an area of low homogeneous echogenicity with regular thickness. Break in the junctional zone thickness indicates a strong possibility of malignancy in postmenopausal years, especially when associated with thickened heterogeneous endometrium.[16] Endometrium appears thin, single line, and is similar to what it appears in early follicular phase.[17] Endometrial thickness of 4–5 mm is considered as normal in different literature evidences, though hormone replacement therapy increases the thickness of the endometrium. It has been documented to be higher in estrogen with progesterone replacement as compared to only estrogen or only progesterone replacement. The maximum thickness accepted is 8 mm. It is found to be thinnest after progesterone withdrawal.[18] Postmenopausal women on antihypertensive therapy show a thicker endometrium (up to 6.2 mm) as compared to untreated hypertensive women (4.3 mm).[19] Occasionally, some amount of fluid may be seen in the endometrium in postmenopausal women.[17] The most common cause speculated for the same a senile cervical stenosis leading to pooling of minimal endometrial secretions. But, it is essential to exclude the possibility of cervical malignancy and endometrial malignancy also in all these cases. Endometrial malignancy typically shows absolutely irregular margins and can be well appreciated due to fluid in the endometrial cavity **(Fig. 39)**. Tubal malignancy is also a rare possibility.

During the postmenopausal years, Doppler studies show very high resistance flow in the uterine artery. Normal uterine artery RI during reproductive years is 0.84 ± 0.6. There is a significant increase in resistance in the flow of the uterine artery and, in turn, there is high resistance flow in its branches also. It is not uncommon to see almost total absence of Doppler signals in the myometrium and subendometrium in postmenopausal uterus. Radial and arcuate vessels also show calcifications in menopausal uterus. This is more common in diabetic patients.

SUMMARY

Uterus is the receptor organ for ovarian steroids and its anatomy keeps on changing throughout the menstrual cycle. Being hormone dependent, its anatomy also changes during the life cycle. The assessment of the normalcy or otherwise of the uterus, thus, needs to be diagnosed in the light of these physiological changes. It is, therefore, essential to understand the changing ultrasound anatomy of the uterus with different phases of life cycle and menstrual cycle.

REFERENCES

1. Hauth EA, Jaeger HJ, Libera H, Lange S, Forsting M. MR imaging of the uterus and cervix in healthy women: determination of normal values. Eur Radiol. 2007;17:734-42.
2. Wiczyk HP, Janus CL, Richards CJ, Graf MJ, Gendal ES, Rabinowitz JG, et al. Comparison of magnetic resonance imaging and ultrasound in evaluating follicular and endometrial development throughout the normal cycle. Fertil Steril. 1988;49:969-72.
3. Bakos O, Lundkvist O, Bergh T. Transvaginal sonographic evaluation of endometrial growth and texture in spontaneous ovulatory cycles—a descriptive study. Hum Reprod. 1993;8:799-806.
4. Kupesic S. The first three weeks assessed by transvaginal color Doppler. J Perinat Med. 1996;24:301-17.
5. Ijland MM, Evers JLH, Dunselman GAJ, Katwijk CV, Lo CR, Hoogland HJ. Endometrial wavelike movements during menstrual cycle. Fertil Steril. 1996;65:746-9.
6. Rainne-Fenning NJ, Campbell BK, Kendall NR, Clewes JS, Johnson IR. Quantifying the changes in endometrial vascularity throughout the normal menstrual cycle with three-dimensional power Doppler angiography. Hum Reprod. 2004;19:330-8.
7. Killam AP, Rosenfeld C, Battaglia FC, Makowski EL, Meschia G. Effect of estrogens on the uterine blood flow in oophorectomized ewes. Am J Obstet Gynecol. 1973:115;1045-50.
8. Bald R, Hackeloer BJ. Ultraschall-darstellung verschiedener endometriumformen. In: Otto R, Jan FX (Eds). Ultra-schalldiagnostik 1982. Stuttgart: Thieme Medical Publishers; 1983. p. 187.
9. Randall JM, Fisk MM, McTavish A, Templeton AA. Transvaginal ultrasonic assessment of endometrial growth in spontaneous and hyperstimulated menstrual cycles. Br J Obstet Gynecol. 1989;96:954-9.
10. Kurjak A, Kupesic-Urek S, Schulman H, Zalud I. Transvaginal color Doppler in the assessment of ovarian and uterine blood flow in infertile women. Fertil Steril. 1991;56:870-3.
11. Goswamy RK, Steptoe PC. Doppler ultrasound studies of the uterine artery in spontaneous ovarian cycles. Hum Reprod. 1988;3:721-5.
12. Sholtes MCW, Wladimiroff JW, van Rijen HJM, Hop WCJ. Uterine and ovarian flow velocity waveforms in the normal menstrual cycle: a transvaginal study. Fertil Steril. 1989;52:981-5.
13. Andreotti RF, Thompson GH, Janowitz W. Endovaginal and transabdominal sonography of ovarian follicle. J Ultrasound Med. 1989;8:555-60.
14. Kulenkampff D, Puchta J, Osmers R. Sonographic appearance of the myometrium. In: Osmers R, Kurjak A (Eds). Ultrasound and the Uterus. Carnforth, New York: Parthenon Publishing; 1995. pp. 53-9.
15. Rempen A. Normal sonographic features of the uterus. In: Osmers R, Kurjak A (Eds). Ultrasound and the Uterus. Carnforth, New York: Parthenon Publishing; 1995. pp. 1-12.
16. Kurjak A, Shalan H, Sosic A, Benic S, Zudenigo D, Kupesic S, et al. Endometrial carcinoma in postmenopausal women: evaluation by transvaginal color Doppler ultrasonography. Am J Obstet Gynecol. 1993;169:1597-603.
17. Osmers R, Puchta J, Suren A. Pathological findings of the postmenopausal endometrium. In: Osmers R, Kurjak A (Eds). Ultrasound and the Uterus. Carnforth, New York: Parthenon Publishing; 1995. pp. 31-44.
18. Affinito P, Palomba S, Sammartino A, Bonifacio M, Nappi C. Ultrasonographic endometrial monitoring during continuous-sequential hormonal replacement therapy regimen in postmenopausal women. Maturitas. 2001;39:239-44.
19. Alcazar JL. Endometrial sonographic findings in asymptomatic, hypertensive postmenopausal women. J Clin Ultrasound. 2000;28:175-8.

24 CHAPTER

Normal Ovaries

Sonal Panchal, Chaitanya Nagori

SELECTION OF GONADS

The gonads differentiate into ovary or testis at 6–9 weeks of gestation. If there is absence of sex-determining region on the Y chromosome (SRY), then the gonad differentiates into ovary. It is also controlled by dosage-sensitive sex reversal, adrenal hypoplasia congenita, critical region on the X chromosome, gene 1 (DAX-1) or Wnt family member 4/R-spondin-1 (WNT4/RSPO1). The later antagonizes testis formation and promotes testis formation.

DEVELOPMENT OF THE OVARY

In the dorsal wall endoderm of yolk sac near the allantois, the primordial germ cells (PGCs) first appear as a cluster of about 100 cells at 3–4 weeks of gestation.[1] Then, these cells migrate to the hindgut and dorsal mesentery by 4–5th weeks of gestation. Germ cells colonize as gonadal tissue that is essential for formation of ovary and germ cells migrate to the gonadal ridge. If this does not occur, the gonads may not develop and just remain as cord-like structures.[2] Colonized germ cells then further develop into a full fledge ovary.

STRUCTURE OF THE OVARY

The ovary consists of stroma and follicles and/or corpus luteum. The ovary has outer cortex and central medulla. The cortex is an outermost part of connective tissue (stroma) with inside follicles and corpora lutea at several development stages. The medulla is the inner region that contains loose connective tissue, highly vascularized, and originating from ovarian arteries. The vessels of medulla form plexus that give rise to small branches destined to stroma and to follicles and the corpus luteum. The branches of smaller diameter that enter the cortex of the ovary tend to spiralize. Small arteries, leading to the periphery of the follicle, subdivide forming a basket-like network around the follicle. The medullary stroma consists of loose connective tissue and considerable vascularity as compared to cortex that is tough and less vascular. There is no clear delineation between the cortex and the medulla.

Follicles are present in different stages of development and can be classified as preantral (primordial, primary, and secondary) and antral (tertiary and preovulatory) follicles.[3] These are surrounded by somatic cells (granulosa and theca cells). The primordial follicles are very small in size with single layer of squamous, flattened granulosa cells. As the granulosa cells proliferate, they form multiple layers and this stage is secondary antral follicle. Development of the follicle occurs as addition in the granulosa cell layers and this can be divided into different classes. The development classification is—class 1 and 2 (early preantral follicle, less than four granulosa layers) and class 3 (five to seven granulosa cell layers).[4]

This is followed by initiation of zona pellucida assembly and fluid accumulation between the granulosa cells. The fluid accumulated between the granulosa cells accumulates to make the antrum and the follicles are then named as tertiary follicles. The theca layer develops that separates the stroma from the granulosa cell layer. The theca layer then divides into theca externa and theca interna.[4] It is because of this fluid pocket that these are called antral follicles. The antral fluid is rich in hormones, growth factors, and cytokines and supplies nutrition to the oocyte. Antral follicles with lowest androgen/estrogen ratio in the fluid host a healthy oocyte.[5] Formation of follicular antrum can be considered as an end to the oocyte growth at that stage. These are 2–5 mm in diameter and are considered as markers of ovarian reserve. Beyond this stage of growth, the granulosa cells differentiate into mural granulosa cells and cumulus cells. Mural granulosa cells line the walls of the follicle and are responsible for steroid secretion. These cells penetrate through the zona pellucida by transzonal cytoplasmic projections with gap junctions at their tips and make cumulus-oocyte complex. Cumulus cells are in close proximity of the oocyte.

DEVELOPMENT OF THE OVUM (OOGENESIS)

The germ cells in the gonadal ridge proliferate fast by mitosis and from 100 cells at 3–4 weeks of gestation become about 10,000 cells at 6 weeks, 6 lacs cells at 8 weeks, and 6 million cells at 20 weeks of gestation. Maximum number of oocytes is reached to a total of 6–7 millions in both ovaries.[6] The primordial germ cells when reach gonads are called oogonia. Mitosis stops by 28 weeks of gestation. Along with mitosis, oogonial atresia also starts around 8 weeks of gestation and is maximum around 20 weeks of gestation. As a result of mitosis and atresia happening simultaneously, about 1 million germ cells are left in an ovary at birth and only 3–4 lacs germ cells are left at puberty.[7] Oogonia are bound together forming clusters of cells called syncytium. Meiosis starts in all the cells in the syncytium simultaneously. As the meiosis starts, these are called primary oocytes. Meiosis starts at around 8-13 weeks of gestation. Primary oocytes get arrested at the prophase stage of first meiotic division by a protracted resting phase called dictyate, which follows the diplotene stage and preceeds diakinesis. At this stage, chromatin is encapsulated by a nuclear structure called germinal vesicle (GV). The meiosis then resumes just prior to ovulation. Primary oocyte surrounded by flat pregranulosa cells is a primary follicle, starts forming at about 15 weeks of gestation, and ends by about 6 months of postnatal life. This follicle is barely 30–60 μm in diameter. Flat pregranulosa cells develop into cuboidal granulosa cells and the primary oocyte gets a protective cover of zona pellucida by the combined stimulatory and inhibitory effect of certain growth factors and extracellular matrix components with autocrine and paracrine effect, as the primordial follicle progresses to become a primary follicle.[8-10]

DEVELOPMENT OF THE FOLLICLE

Oogonium, as it develops, is contained in densely packed shell of somatic cells and the two together make follicles. Follicle supports oocyte growth. Around fourth month of gestation, the ovarian cortex shows initiation of vascularization. This is beginning of folliculogenesis. The follicular growth can be divided into four distinct stages: (1) Activation of primordial follicles and transition, (2) From primary to preantral follicles, (3) From preantral to tertiary/antral follicles, and (4) From dominant follicles to ovulation.[11,12]

The initial follicular growth is slow and is controlled by the proliferation of granulosa cells. Follicle-stimulating hormone (FSH) enhances the expression of growth factor receptors and exerts indirect mitogenic effect on the granulosa cells. This is considered as the first phase of follicular development. Beyond this, the follicle grows fast as the antrum enlarges with fluid and is also associated with steroidogenesis. It is in this phase that the follicular cells also start differentiating. This phase also is gonadotropin dependent.[11,12]

Folliculogenesis can be divided into primordial follicle, primary follicle, secondary/preantral follicle, antral follicle, dominant follicle, and Graafian or mature follicle. The process of maturity from primordial follicle to primary follicle is hormone independent and is a long process and the estimation of this time is difficult, though that from primary follicle to secondary follicle takes about 120 days. Primordial follicle consists of a nongrowing oocyte, the growth of which is arrested in the diplotene stage of meiotic prophase. It is surrounded by single layer of spindle-shaped granulosa cells (**Fig. 1**).[13,14]

It promotes the primordial to primary transition, preantral follicular growth, and recruitment of theca cells.[14,15]

This is followed by proliferation of granulosa cells and also increase in the size of the follicle. As a final stage of preantral follicular development, the vascular endothelial growth factor (VEGF) expression is stabilized at high levels and follicular walls show widespread capillary network near the basal membrane. These blood vessels are still immature and get stabilized in the course of development in presence of high levels of angiogenic factors.[16] Cell proliferation precedes angiogenesis. In the late secondary and tertiary phases of follicular development, 25–30% of proliferating cells in the inner thecal layer are of endothelial cell origin.[17]

The negative influence primarily on the granulosa layer is due to incompatible vascular network and finally resulting into apoptosis.[18,19]

After the secondary or the preantral follicle is formed, selection of a dominant follicle and growing into maturity take about 85 days. The most active phase of this entire follicular development is the phase from dominance selected to Graafian follicle and that usually takes only about 14 days.[20]

Recruitment and atresia of the follicles maintain a pool of antral follicles and decide the final ovarian reserve. Recruitment of the follicles is initial and cyclical. This process

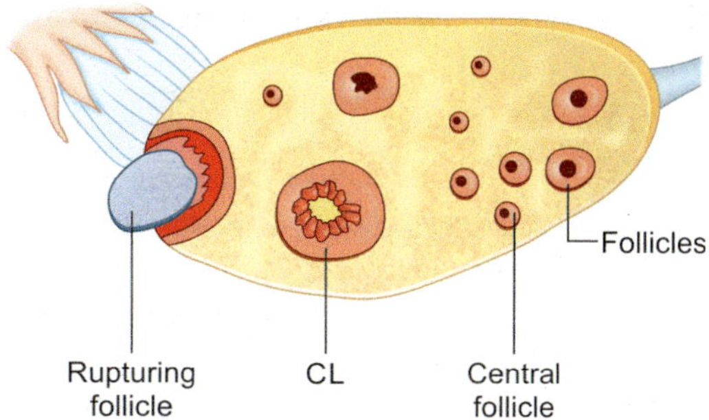

Fig. 1: Diagrammatic presentation of follicles at different stages of development.

starts immediately after the follicle formation and continues till life. After this recruitment, the follicle grows but the oocyte inside is still resting in prophase of meiosis I. Atresia of the oocytes is sort of a continuous process and starts as early as 8 weeks of gestation. Oocytes that are not surrounded by granulosa cells, that mean the ones that are not in the follicle, undergo apoptosis. Those follicles, which enter the initial recruitment, progress till antral stage and undergo atresia. Atresia of the follicles is a continuous process and is in proportion to the total number of follicles present. This means that the rate of atresia is maximum before birth and significantly high before puberty. Out of total 6–7 million of total oocytes developed up to 6–8 weeks of gestation, the total number left before birth is only 2 million and that number decreases to only 300,000 at puberty and only about 400 ovulate during the reproductive lifespan of a female.[6] But, once the puberty starts, few antral follicles enter the cyclical recruitment and escape atresia. These may progress to dominance, maturity, and ovulation. In all, only about 1% of total ova reach ovulatory stage.

As the follicle grows, layers of granulosa cells increase. The granulosa cell layer is surrounded by basal lamina and surrounding that are two layers of theca cells—(1) theca interna and (2) theca externa. The secondary/preantral follicle hosts primary oocyte that is protected in zona pellucida. Between the two theca layers is the intricate capillary network.

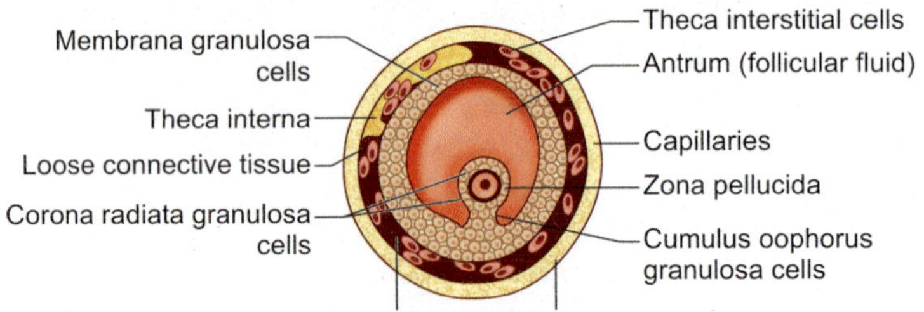

Fig. 2: Diagram of Graafian follicle.

The entire secondary follicle measures 120–150 μm in diameter. These follicles have FSH receptors. Cyclical recruitment is FSH dependent and starts after puberty as FSH increases in circulation. FSH rescues the cohort of small antral follicles from atresia that contain the primary oocytes capable of resuming meiosis and grow further. Of these, the dominant follicle is later on selected.

This is actually a preovulatory phase and the follicles may also be named as tertiary Graafian follicle **(Fig. 2)**. The ovum is secured in the granulosa cells. The granulosa cells are now segregated into those around the oocyte–cumulus oophorus and the mural granulosa cells lining the follicle. Outside this is the basal laminar layer. Outside this layer is the theca cell layer. Theca interna is vascular and theca externa is a connective tissue layer, less vascular, and it is the layer which is the one in relation to the stroma.

After the reinitiation of meiosis I, there is maturation of oocyte but the nuclei break down and chromosome condenses. This is the GV stage. Then, the chromosomes are arranged in metaphase I (MI), anaphase I, telophase I, and finally meiosis I is completed. The oocyte when finishes its first meiotic division contains 2N haploid and becomes secondary oocyte. A haploid secondary oocyte and first polar body are formed. This oocyte is located eccentrically in the follicle and is surrounded by zona pellucida, corona radiata, cumulus oophorus, large antral cavity, granulosa cells, basal lamina, and two layers of theca. Soon after its formation, secondary oocyte goes into meiosis II and gets arrested at the metaphase stage. This stage is also known as metaphase II (MII) oocytes.[21]

Just before ovulation at the luteinizing hormone (LH) peak, the oocyte-cumulus complex becomes free floating in the follicular fluid as the dispersion of the cumulus cells as an effect of FSH surge and preovulatory progesterone rise. At ovulation, corona radiata is expelled into the peritoneal cavity and the secondary oocyte is still arrested in meiosis II till fertilization occurs.[22,23]

After the LH peak in 10–12 hours, ovulation occurs. This is about 24–36 hours after estradiol peak.[24,25]

After rupture, change in the morphological and biochemical configuration of the theca interna and granulosa cells leads to formation of the corpus luteum. The chief changes essential for normal luteal function of corpus luteum are luteinization of the steroidogenic cells and angiogenesis. Corpus luteum is formed of luteal cells, epithelial cells, leukocytes and fibroblasts, pericytes, smooth muscle cells, fibrocytes, and immune cells.[26]

OVARIES AND ULTRASOUND

Anatomical location of ovaries and fallopian tubes is not amenable to any direct inspection. Modality of choice for assessment of these pelvic organs is transvaginal ultrasound. It is the primary examination after clinical assessment, as it gives more information than any other single test and is noninvasive. Ultrasound can be done by transabdominal, transvaginal **(Figs. 3A and B)**, or transrectal route.

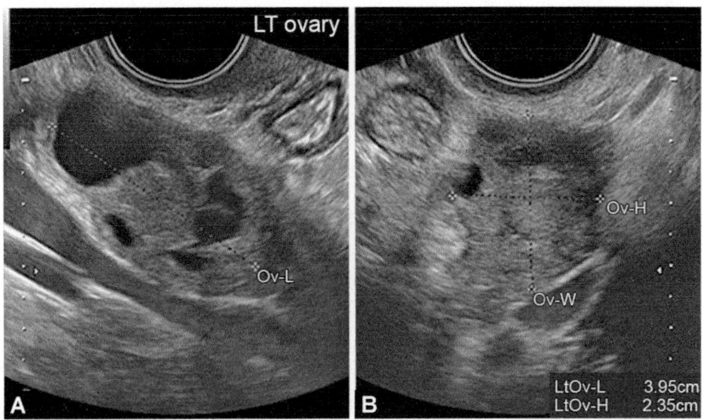

Figs. 3A and B: B-mode ultrasound showing ovary on transvaginal scan.

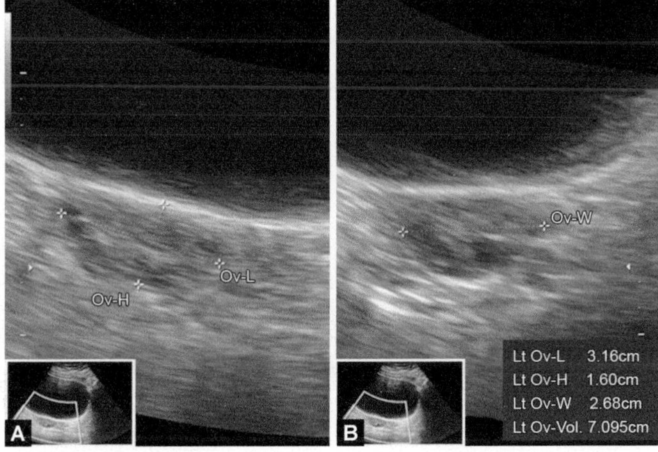

Figs. 4A and B: Ovaries as seen on transabdominal scan.

Advantages of Transvaginal Route

- Probe closest to pelvic organs
- High resolution due to high frequency probe
- No bowel preparation
- No bladder distension

Transabdominal or transrectal routes may be required in:

- When patient is virgin
- When patient is noncooperative
- When there is severe vaginismus or vaginal disease
- Rarely when vagina is absent

Disadvantages of Transabdominal Scan

- It gives little details about the anatomy of the ovaries due to low resolution of the low frequency probe. This is also because the transabdominal probe is placed far from the reproductive organs **(Figs. 4A and B)**.
- Full bladder is required, which causes lot of discomfort to the patient.

Transrectal scan has disadvantages of discomfort, but still gives resolution comparable with the transvaginal scan as it uses a high frequency endocavitary probe.

Ultrasound Modalities Used for Assessment of Ovaries

B-mode ultrasound and Doppler are satisfactorily sufficient for assessment of ovarian pathologies and three-dimensional (3D) power Doppler is of help to differentiate between benign and malignant lesions and also to understand the related anatomy.

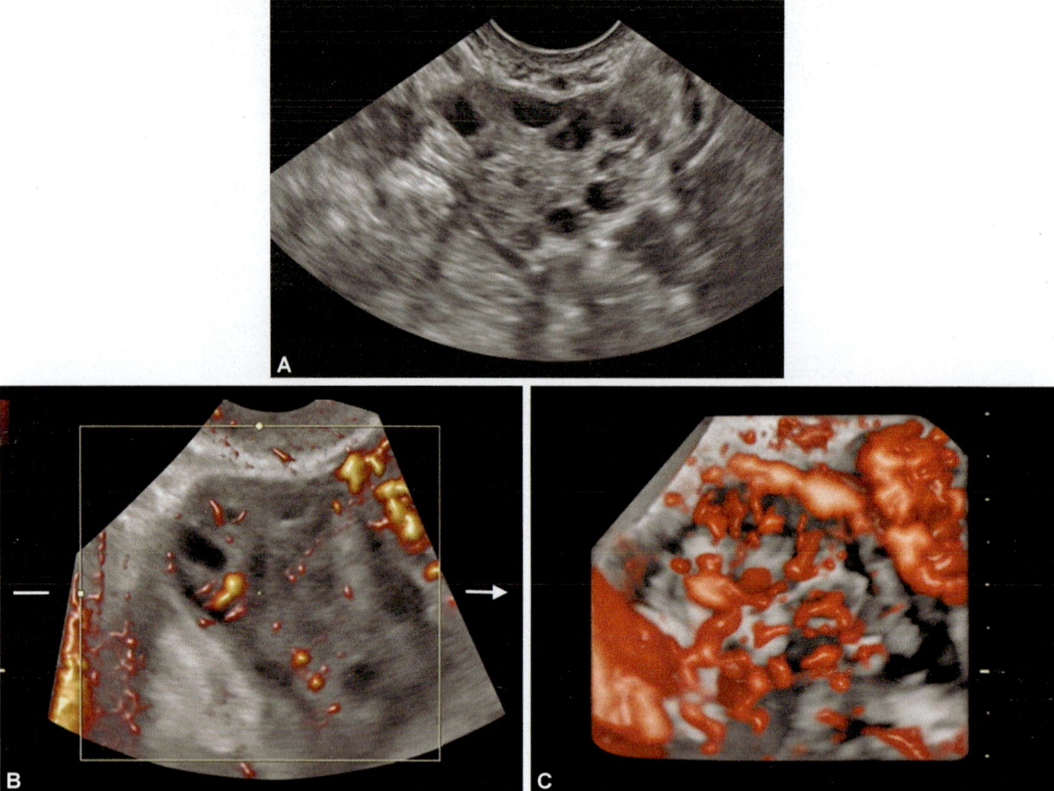

Figs. 5A to C: B-mode power Doppler and three-dimensional (3D) power Doppler images of ovary.

Three-dimensional power Doppler further helps in more precise volume calculations that may be of help for planning of radio or chemotherapy and for the follow-up of treatment too **(Figs. 5A to C)**.

The same modalities also help to understand the physiology better. Assessment of global vascularity helps to interpret the hormonal status. 3D power Doppler helps in better assessment of ovarian volume and assessment for follicle number by sonography-based automated volume calculation (SonoAVC) **(Figs. 6A and B)**.

LOCATION OF OVARIES

Ovaries are situated on both sides of cervix close to lateral pelvic walls in Waldeyer's fossa. Ovaries are mobile and may also be seen in cul-de-sac or in front of or above the uterus. On transvaginal scan, these are located just anteromedial to internal iliac vessels. This is the area between the internal iliac and external iliac vessels almost perpendicular to each other **(Fig. 7)**.

OVARIAN VASCULATURE

Ovarian arteries arise from abdominal aorta below the origin of renal arteries.

These vessels run downward and laterally and through infundibulopelvic ligament enters the pelvis to reach the ovary via mesovarium after crossing the external iliac vessels from lateral to medially to enter ovary from lateral aspect. After entering the ovary, it branches into several spiral branches **(Fig. 8)**. Ovarian branch of uterine artery is the second source.

OVARIAN MORPHOLOGY

Ovaries are ellipsoid, 3 × 2 × 2 cm in size, and 6–10 cc in volume. Maximum volume of the

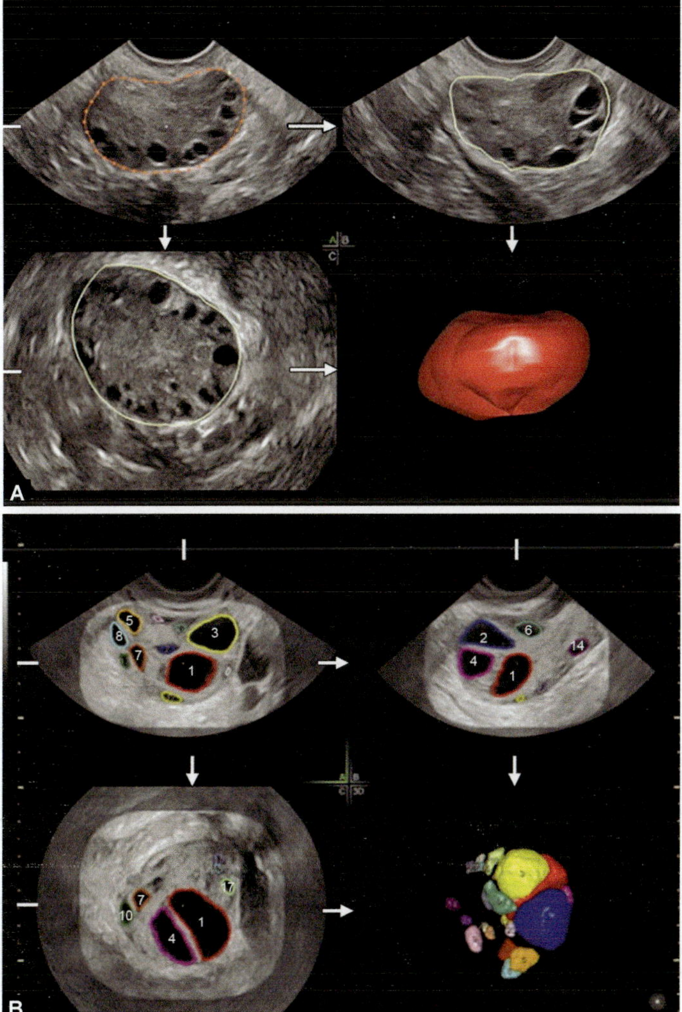

Figs. 6A and B: 3D ultrasound acquired volume of the ovary with: (A) VOCAL calculated ovarian volume; (B) SonoAVC for follicular assessment.
(3D: three-dimensional; VOCAL: virtual organ computer-aided analysis; SonoAVC: sonography-based automated volume calculation)

ovary mentioned in literature is 14–16 cc.[27] Severe polycystic ovaries may be even larger. But, the size and morphology both vary with the age and hormonal status.

Ovarian morphology is ever-changing in response to ever dynamic endocrinological system. Therefore, to understand the normal and abnormal ovarian morphology, it is essential to understand and correlate the hormonal changes to ovarian morphology.

Ovaries have:
- Homogeneous hypoechoic stroma
- Anechoic follicles varying from 2 to 25 mm in size

In utero:
- At 20 weeks of gestation, a female fetus has 7 million follicles.[28] These are primordial follicles, which grow into primordial, primary, and secondary follicles, which are all microscopic in size and, therefore, not seen on scan.

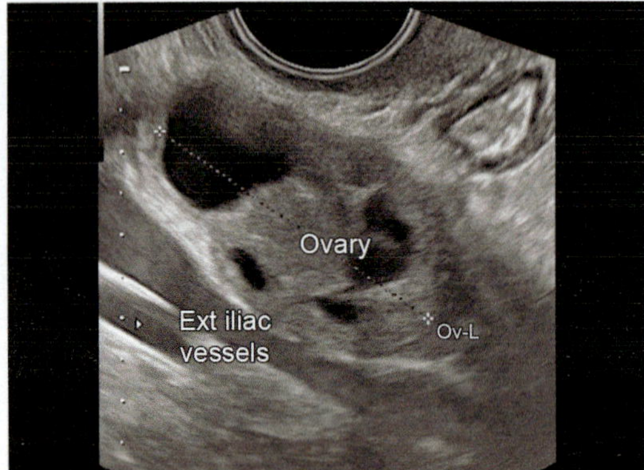

Fig. 7: B-mode image of the ovary and its relation to external iliac vessels.

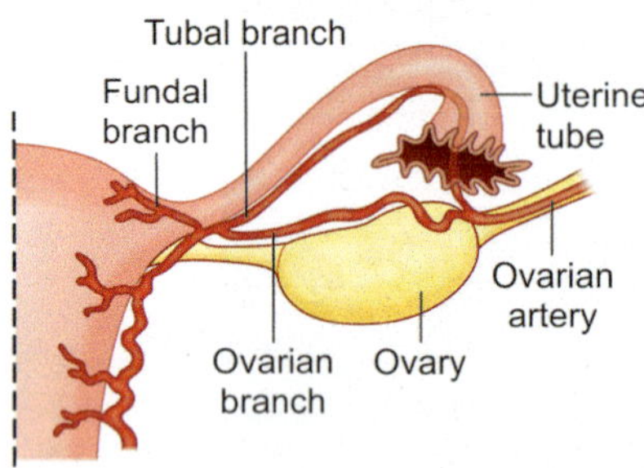

Fig. 8: Ovarian vascular supply.

In newborn (because of withdrawal from maternal pregnancy hormones):

- At birth and till 3 months of age, the size is 1.2 cc
- Decreases to 1.1 cc from 4 to 12 months
- Reduces up to 0.7 cc from 1 to 2 years of age[29]

In childhood:

- The size may further reduce till the age of 3 years to 0.5 cc
- Then, it starts growing to reach an average size of 2.8 cc at 18 years.[30] The growth is faster around 8 years because of adrenarche and gradual rising FSH levels and also before and during puberty

In adolescence:

- At menarche, the ovaries have 250,000–300,000 oocytes
- With hormonal stimulation during adolescence, these follicles grow into preantral and antral follicles when these become visible due to fluid collection
- In absence of or when the hormonal environment is unfavorable, these follicles undergo atresia
- With each ovulatory cycle, when one follicle matures, there is atresia of several other follicles
- The number of small antral follicles (2–6 mm) is significantly related to age and also, independent of age, to all endocrine ORTs tested, suggesting the number of small antral follicles represents the functional ovarian reserve[31]
- Dominant follicle, if does not grow to mature and ovulate, as in adolescence, it may lead to long cycles
- This may lead to multifollicular appearance in adolescence

Multicystic ovary:

- Normally seen at puberty
- Different sized follicles distributed throughout the ovary because of incomplete pulsatile gonadotropin stimulation
- No excess of stroma

OVARIAN FOLLICLE TRACKING

Follicular tracking is serial ultrasonographic study of the ovary during the follicular phase of the menstrual cycle. The aim is to estimate follicular maturity, so that the time of ovulation can be predicted. During follicular tracking, the mean diameter of each of the follicles is measured and their growth followed. US is often used in conjunction with serum measures of estradiol, LH, and progesterone to improve accuracy.

Continuous and complex hormonal changes occurring during the menstrual cycle reflect as morphological and vascular changes in ovaries and uterus. Therefore, tracking these changes by ultrasound (US) and Doppler can explain the physiology. Transvaginal US is the modality of choice to study these changes. The accuracy of diagnosis and monitoring

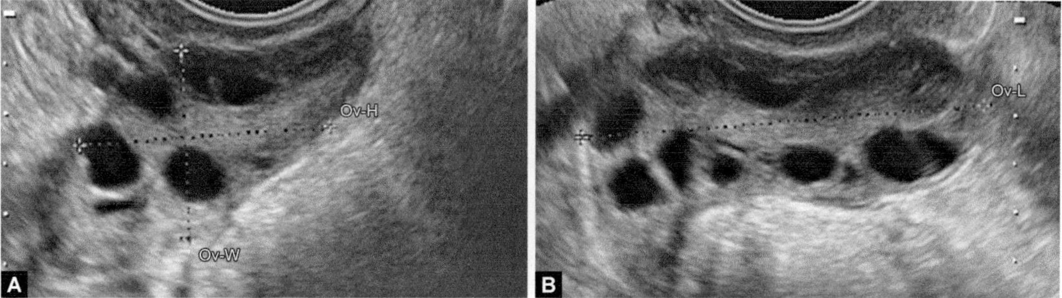

Figs. 9A and B: B-mode ultrasound of baseline ovary showing antral follicles.

of infertility treatments such as ovulation induction have greatly increased because of the availability of sophisticated US technology and equipment.[32]

Population of the antral follicles drastically decreases during the luteal phase of the previous cycle. A new cohort of small antral follicles develops during the menstruation phase. During the course of sequential cellular proliferation and differentiation, primordial follicles develop into intermediate, primary, and, eventually, secondary preantral follicles. This is a phase of slow follicular growth and takes about 150 days. Secondary antral follicles are the first follicular structures to be visualized and beyond this is a phase of accelerated follicular growth. Monitoring of a menstrual cycle should start in early proliferative phase, preferably day 2–3 of the cycle. At this time, estrogen, progesterone, FSH, and LH are at baseline levels. Early antral follicles (1–2 mm) are the first follicular structures that may be visualized on US **(Figs. 9A and B)**. A cohort of small antral follicles develops during the luteal phase of previous menstrual cycles independently of gonadotropin stimulation. Follicles up to 2 mm in diameter grow independent of gonadotropins (FSH).[33]

Further development of the follicle is only possible in the presence of appropriate levels of gonadotropin; subsequently, the most mature follicle is selected and the others become atretic. Before day 5 of the cycle, selection of the dominant follicle occurs. Between days 5 and 7, dominance of the follicle becomes apparent. Follicle that is 10–12 mm in size is known as a dominant follicle and it is this follicle that is most likely to grow to become a mature follicle. It is interesting to know that often first largest follicle on baseline scan is not the dominant follicle. A normal growth rate of a healthy follicle is approximately 2 mm/day and reaches a size of 18–24 mm by the time of ovulation[34] **(Figs. 10A to C)**.

In response to LH surge, resulting preovulatory changes in follicle are seen as appearance of a sonolucent halo surrounding the follicle and appearance of cumulus (a small solid projection from the follicle wall) within 24 hours before ovulation. Ovulation is characterized by a blurring of the follicular borders, the appearance of intrafollicular echoes **(Fig. 11)**, and the appearance of free fluid in the pouch of Douglas. But absence of free fluid does not indicate absence of ovulation. Ovulation results in collapse of the follicle with irregular contour followed by filling of its cavity with echogenic fluid, now called as corpus luteum. Corpus luteum typically has variable appearances with ground-glass echogenicity in lumen or lace-like echogenicities **(Figs. 12A and B)** and has circumferential blood flow referred to as a "ring of fire" **(Fig. 12C)**. Secretory changes are seen in the endometrium in the form of echogenicity of the endometrium, which starts from outside and proceeding to the central

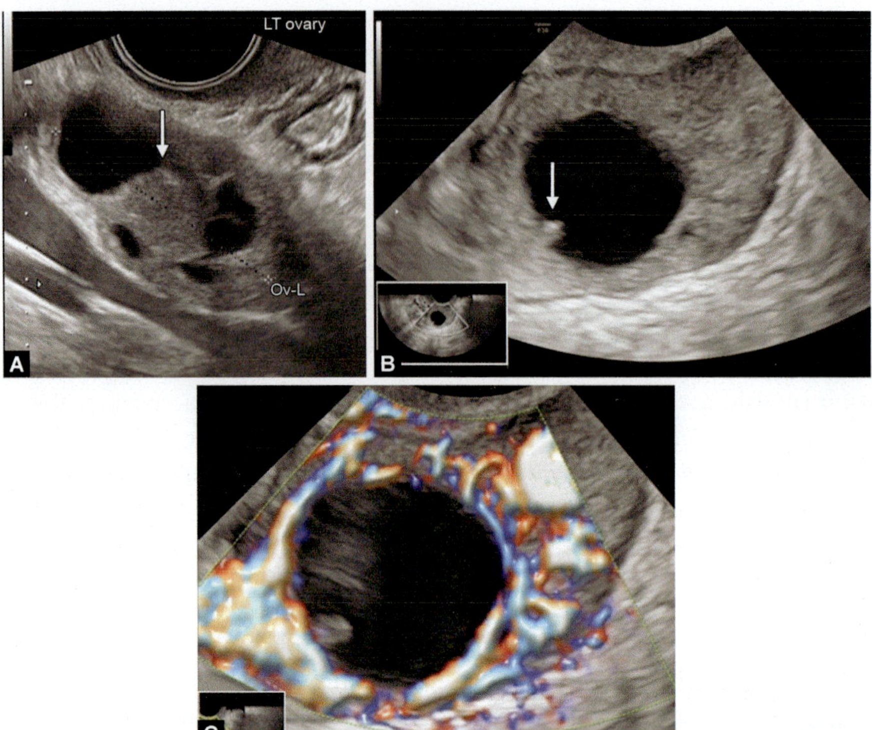

Figs. 10A to C: (A) B-mode image of ovary showing dominant follicle (white arrow); (B) Mature follicle on B-mode and also showing cumulus (white arrow); (C) Doppler showing perifollicular flow in a mature follicle.

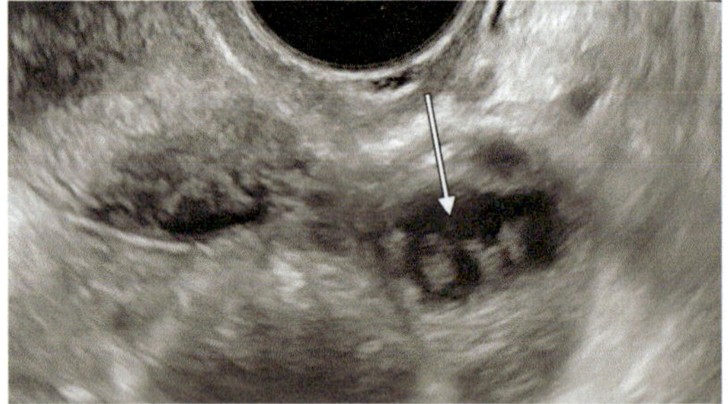

Fig. 11: Freshly rupture follicles seen on B-mode ultrasound (white arrow).

line making a ring sign of the endometrium[35] **(Fig. 13)**.

The corpus luteum has a limited life expectancy and resolves if pregnancy does not occur at the end of the luteal phase. Rarely, ovulation fails to occur leading to a luteinized unruptured follicle (LUF) in which, despite the absence of follicular rupture and release of the oocyte, the unruptured follicle undergoes luteinization under the action of LH. US, but not the midluteal progesterone levels (aids in diagnosing this condition), as there is normal production of progesterone. LUF is diagnosed on ultrasound by low-level echoes in lumen and hyperechoic walls and high resistance peripheral flow **(Fig. 14)**.

Blood flows close to the follicle can be seen by Doppler when follicle reaches 10 mm in diameter and this may be used as a hemodynamic parameter of its growth, maturation, and ovulation. Resistance index (RI) of these vessels is reported as 0.54 ± 0.04. RI starts falling 2 days prior to ovulation and reaches its nadir of 0.44 ± 0.04 at ovulation.[36] Just prior to rupture, the vascularity surrounding the follicle increases along with the increase in its flow velocity.[37] The mean changes in peak systolic velocity (PSV) follow the mean rise in LH by approximately 12 hours. PSV increases 29 hours before the time of follicular rupture and continues for at least 72 hours after corpus

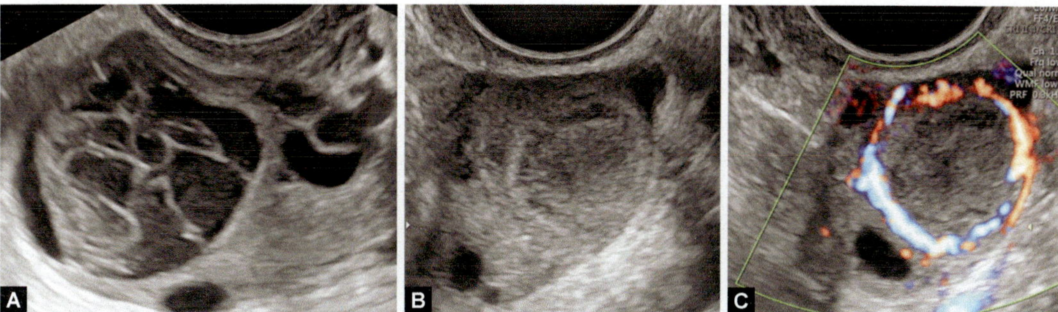

Figs. 12A to C: (A) B-mode image of corpus luteum showing fishnet (hemorrhagic) appearance; (B) B-mode image of corpus luteum with ground-glass echogenicity; (C) Doppler showing tight of vascularity around corpus luteum.

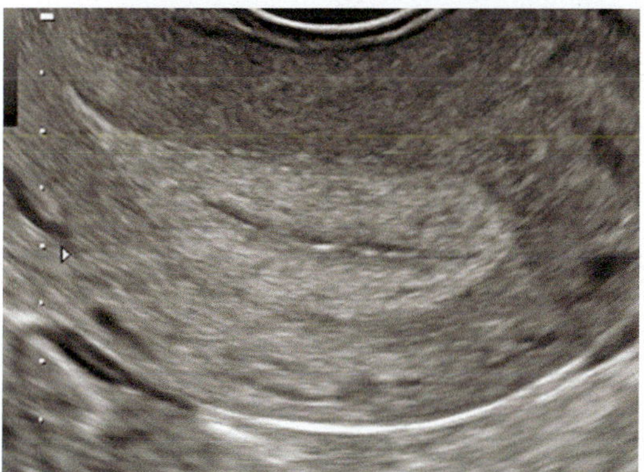

Fig. 13: Secretory endometrium on B-mode ultrasound.

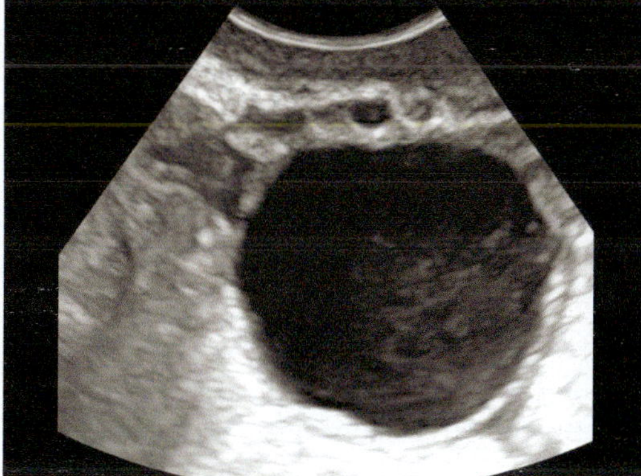

Fig. 14: B-mode image of luteinized unruptured follicle (LUF).

luteum is formed.[38] Three to seven times increase in the blood flow are noted in the dominant ovary (ovary from which ovulation occurs) during the luteal phase.[39] The flow is highest in the midluteal phase, which declines till menstruation in the absence of conception.

Resistance index of the corpus luteum has been suggested as an adjunct to plasma progesterone assay as an index of luteal function.[40] A healthy corpus luteum will show a vascular ring surrounding itself on color Doppler and on power Doppler, these vessels show RI 0.35–0.50, pulsatility index (PI) 0.70–0.80, and PSV 10–15 cm/s[41,42] **(Fig. 15)**.

This resistance starts increasing on day 23 of the cycle in a nonconception cycle to RI 0.5–0.55. Based on these values, abnormal parameters indicate luteal phase problems such as LUF **(Figs. 5A to C)** or luteal phase defect.[41]

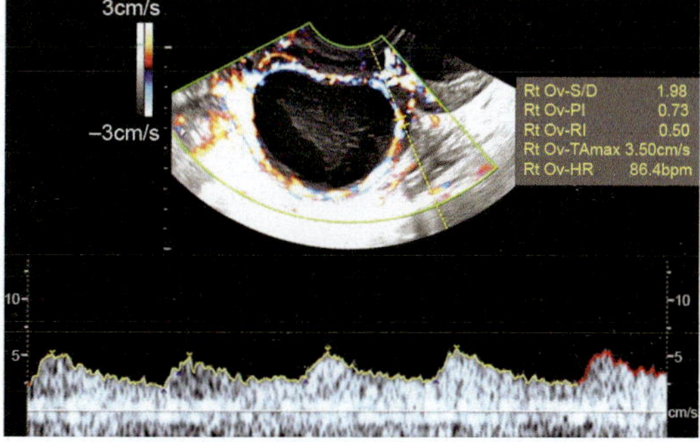

Fig. 15: Spectral Doppler image of corpus luteum showing low resistance flow.

PERIMENOPAUSAL OVARY

It is a state of:

- Follicle depletion (at menopause, 100–1,000 follicles are left)
- Decreased recruitment of antral follicles
- Low inhibin

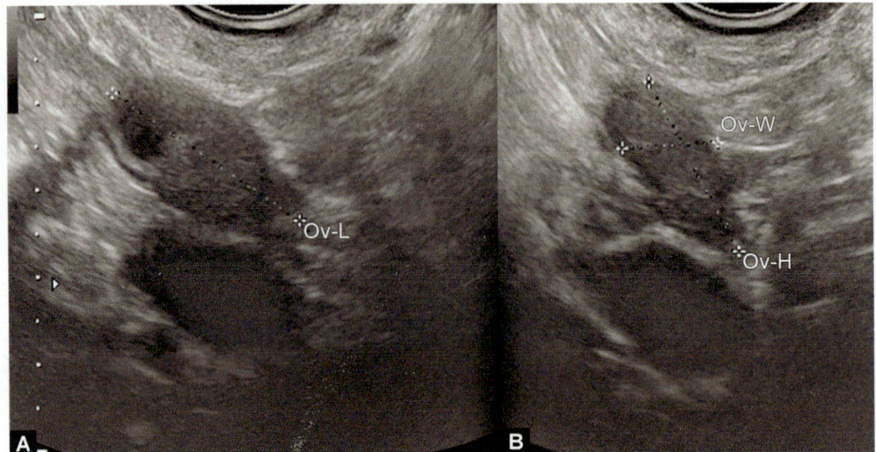

Figs. 16A and B: Postmenopausal solid-looking ovary on B-mode ultrasound.

- High FSH (early follicular development and short cycles)
- On ultrasound, it shows ovary with usually one to three antral follicles with ovarian volume of usually 2–3 cc. Doppler shows scanty flow in the stroma with higher resistance than in the ovaries of reproductive age **(Figs. 16A and B)**.

MENOPAUSE

- Climacteric is a period of prolonged estrogen withdrawal, decreased frequency of ovulation, and gradual disappearance of secondary sex characters
- Insufficient follicle maturity—insufficient estrogen—no menstruation—menopause
- Low estrogen and inhibin and high FSH
- Small homogeneous ovaries with follicle depletion (1–2 cc) **(Figs. 16A and B)**
- Though in multiparous women, the ovaries are a little larger comparatively
- Scanty and high resistance (RI > 0.65) vascularity

CONCLUSION

- Ovaries have a dynamic anatomy whether considered from birth till menopause or in individual menstrual cycle
- Correct understanding of reproductive physiology is, therefore, required to understand normal and abnormal changes in these organs.

REFERENCES

1. McKay DG, Hertig AT, Adams EC, Danziger S. Histochemical observations on the germ cells of human embryos. Anat Rec. 1953;117:201-19.
2. Merchant-Larios H, Centeno B. Morphogenesis of the ovary from the sterile W/v mouse. Prog Clin Biol Res. 1981;59:383-92.
3. Hulshof SCJ, Figueiredo JR, Bekers JF, Bevers MM, Van Den Hurk R. Isolation and characterization of preantral follicles from fetal bovine ovaries. Vet Q. 1994;2:78-80.
4. Martelli A, Russo V, Mauro A, Di Giacinto O, Nardinocchi D, Mattioli M, et al. Insights into Ovarian Follicle Angiogenesis: Morphological and Chronological Vascular Remodeling from Primordial to Ovulating Follicles. Vasc Med. 2017;2:1009.
5. Anderson CY. Characteristics of human follicular fluid associated with successful conception after in vitro fertilization. J Clin Endocrinol Metab. 1993;77:1227-34.
6. Baker TG. A quantitative and cytological study of germ cells in human ovaries. Proc R Soc Lond B Biol Sci. 1963;158:417-33.
7. Oktem O, Oktay K. The ovary: anatomy and function throughout human life. Ann N Y Acad Sci. 2008;1127:1-9.
8. Oktay K, Briggs D, Gosden BG. Ontogeny of follicle-stimulating hormone receptor gene expression in isolated human ovarian follicles. J Clin Endocrinol Metab. 1997;11:3748-51.
9. Eppig JJ. Oocyte control of ovarian follicular development and function in mammals. Reproduction. 2001;6:829-38.

10. Skinner MK. Regulation of primary follicle assembly and development. Hum Reprod Update. 2005;5:461-71.
11. Cao G, Fehrenbach ML, Williams JT, Finkelstein JM, Zhu JX, Delisser HM. Angiogenesis in platelet endothelial cell adhesion molecule-1-null mice. Am J Pathol. 2009;175:903-15.
12. Rutkowski JM, Ihm JE, Lee ST, Kilarski WW, Greenwood VI, Pasquier MC, et al. VEGFR-3 neutralization inhibits ovarian lymphangiogenesis, follicle maturation, and murine pregnancy. Am J Pathol. 2013;183:1596-607.
13. van Wezell L, Umapathysivam K, Tilley WD, Rodgers RJ. Immunohistochemical localization of basic fibroblast growth factor in bovine ovarian follicles. Mol Cell Endocrinol. 1995;11:133-40.
14. Nilsson EE, Detzel C, Skinner MK. Platelet-derived growth factor modulates the primordial to primary follicle transition. Reproduction. 2006;13:1007-15.
15. Matos MH, den Hurk RT, Lima-Verdei B, Luque MCA, Santos KDB, Martins FS, et al. Effects of fibroblast growth factor-2 on the in vitro culture of caprine preantral follicles. Cells Tissues Organs. 2007;18:112-20.
16. Robinson RS, Woad KJ, Hammond AJ, Laird M, Hunter MG, Mann GE. Angiogenesis and vascular function in the ovary. Reproduction. 2009;138:869-8.
17. Wulff C, Wiegand SJ, Saunders PTK, Scobie GA, Fraser HM. Angiogenesis during follicular development in the primate and its inhibition by treatment with truncated Flt-1Fc (vascular endothelial growth factor trapA40). Endocrinology. 2001;142:3244-54.
18. Martelli A, Berardinelli P, Russo V, Mauro A, Bernabò N, Gioia L, et al. Spatiotemporal analysis of vascular endothelial growth factor expression and blood vessel remodeling in pig ovarian follicles during the periovulatory period. J Mol Endocrinol. 2006;36:107-19.
19. Mauro A, Martelli A, Berardinelli P, Russo V, Bernabò N, Di Giacinto O, et al. Effect of antiprogesterone RU486 on VEGF expression and blood vessel remodeling on ovarian follicles before ovulation. PLoS One. 2014;9:1-13.
20. Gougeon A. Regulation of ovarian follicular development in primates: facts and hypothesis. Endocr Rev. 1996;17:121-55.
21. Trounson A, Anderiesz C, Jones G. Maturation of human oocytes in vitro and their developmental competence. Reproduction. 2001;121:51-75.
22. Fritz MA, McLachlan RJ, Cohen NL, Dahl KD, Bremmer WJ, Soules MR. Onset and characteristics of the midcycle surge in bioactive and immunoactive luteinizing hormone secretion in normal women: influence of physiological variations in preovulatory ovarian steroid hormone secretion. J Clin Endocrinol Metab. 1992;75:489-93.
23. Temporal relationships between ovulation and defined changes in the concentration of plasma oestradiol-17 beta, luteinizing hormone, follicle-stimulating hormone, and progesterone. I. Probit analysis. World Health Organization, Task Force on Methods for the Determination of the Fertile Period, Special Programme of Research, Development and Research Training in Human Reproduction. Am J Obstet Gynecol. 1980;138:383-90.
24. Xie Q, Cheng Z, Chen X, Lobe CG, Liu J, Robinson RS, et al. The role of Notch signaling in ovarian angiogenesis. J Ovarian Res. 2017;10:13.
25. Torres-Ortiz MC, Gutiérrez-Ospina G, Gómez-Chavarín M, Murcia C, Alonso-Morales RA, Perera-Marín G. The presence of VEGF and Notch2 during preantral-antral follicular transition in infantile rats: anatomical evidence and its implications. Gen Comp Endocrinol. 2017;249:82-92.
26. Retamales I, Carrasco I, Troncoso JL, Heras JL, Devoto L, Vega M. Morpho-functional study of human luteal cell subpopulations. Hum Reprod. 1994;9:591-6.
27. Higgins RV, van Nagell JR, Woods CH, Thompson EA, Kryscio RJ. Interobserver variation in ovarian measurements using transvaginal ultrasound. Gynecol Oncol. 1990;39(1):69-71.
28. Faddy MJ, Gosden RG, Gougeon A, Richardson SJ, Nelson JF. Accelerated disappearance of ovarian follicles in mid-life: implications for forecasting menopause. Hum Reprod. 1992;7:1342-6.
29. Cohen HL, Shapiro MA, Mandel FS, Shapiro ML. Normal ovaries in neonates and infants: a sonographic study of 77 patients 1 day to 24 months old. Am J Roentgenol. 1993;160:583-6.
30. Bridges NA, Hindmarsh PC, Cooke A, Brook CGD, Healy MJR. Standards of ovarian volume in childhood and puberty. Fertil Steril. 1993;60:456-60.
31. Haadsmaet ML, Bukman A, Groen H, Roeloffzen EM, Groenewoud ER, Heineman MJ. The number of small antral follicles (2-6 mm) determines the outcome of endocrine ovarian reserve tests in a subfertile population. Hum Reprod. 2007;22:1925-31.
32. Kyei-Mensah A, Zaidi J, Pittrof R, Shaker A, Campbell S, Tan SL. Transvaginal three-dimensional ultrasound: accuracy of follicular volume measurements. Fertil Steril. 1996;65:371-6.
33. Hackeloer BJ, Sallam HN. Ultrasound scanning of ovarian follicles. Clin Obstet Gynecol. 1983;10:603-20.

34. Hackelöer BJ, Fleming R, Robinson HP, Adam AH, Coutts JR. Correlation of ultrasonic and endocrinologic assessment of human follicular development. Am J Obstet Gynecol. 1979;135:122-8.
35. Bald R, Hackeloer BJ. Ultraschall-darstellung verschiendener endometrium formen. In: Otto R, Jan FX (Eds). Ultraschall diagnostik 1982. Stuttgart: Thieme Medical Publishers; 1983. p. 187.
36. Kurjak A, Kupesic-Urek S. Infertility. In: Kurjak A (Ed). Transvaginal Color Doppler. Carnforth, UK: Parthenon Publishing; 1991. pp. 33-8.
37. Bourne T, Jurkovic D, Waterstone J, Campbell S, Collins WP. Intrafollicular blood flow during human ovulation. Ultrasound Obstet Gynecol. 1991;1:53-9.
38. Bourne TH, Athanasiou S, Bauer B. Ovulation and the periovulatory follicle. In: Bourne TH, Jauniaux E, Jurkovic D (Eds). Transvaginal Color Doppler. Berlin: Springer-Verlag; 1995. pp. 119-30.
39. Niswender GD, Moore RT, Akbar AM, Nett TM, Diekman MA. Flow of blood to the ovaries of ewes throughout the estrous cycle. Biol Reprod. 1975;13:381-8.
40. Glock JL, Brumsted JR. Color flow pulsed Doppler ultrasound in diagnosing luteal phase defect. Fertil Steril. 1995;64:500-4.
41. Kupesic S, Kurjak A. The assessment of normal and abnormal luteal function by transvaginal color Doppler sonography. Eur J Obstet Gynecol. 1997;72:83-7.
42. Salim A, Kurjak A, Zalud I. Ovarian luteal flow in normal and abnormal early pregnancies. J Matern Fetal Invest. 1992;2:119.

25

CHAPTER

Uterine Müllerian Abnormalities

Sonal Panchal, Chaitanya Nagori

INTRODUCTION

Uterine abnormality is the cause of majority of the gynecological complaints and ultrasound is now considered as a first-line investigation for its assessment. Uterus can be visualized on ultrasound by transabdominal route as well as transvaginal route. Though the assessment by transvaginal ultrasound [transvaginal sonography (TVS)] is the best choice, transabdominal scan is usually preferred before the transvaginal scan, if the patient is being assessed for a particular complaint for the first time. Transabdominal scan gives a better idea about the gross anatomy, but has a disadvantage of having lower resolution than the transvaginal route due to lower frequency probe used for transabdominal scan and also due to more distance of the uterus from the probe. Therefore, for the detailed study of the intrauterine anatomy, transvaginal route is preferred. In cases, when this is not possible or permissible, transrectal route may be used. Doppler is very essential for differential diagnosis of various uterine pathologies. Volume ultrasound [three-dimensional-four-dimensional (3D-4D) ultrasound] can significantly increase to the details available and is considered essential for the diagnosis of Müllerian abnormalities and endometrial pathologies of the uterus. Sensitivity of the volume ultrasound (US) for the detection of congenital uterine abnormalities is almost 98% and, therefore, it is also known as "virtual hysteroscopy".[1] Saline infusion sonohysterography is also a useful modality for evaluation of the endometrial pathologies.

MÜLLERIAN DUCT ABNORMALITIES

Uterus is formed by the fusion of the two paramesonephric (Müllerian) ducts at 10 weeks of gestation followed by resorption of fused midline tissues occurring by 20th week by apoptosis **(Fig. 1)**. Arrest of these processes at different stages may result into various Müllerian duct abnormalities.

- Failure of one or more Müllerian duct to develop
- Failure of the Müllerian ducts to canalize
- Failure to fuse or abnormal fusion of Müllerian ducts
- Failure of resorption of midline uterine septum.

Incidence of Müllerian duct abnormalities is 0.1–3.8% in normal fertile females, but reaches 6.7% in infertile patients.[2] For the ease of differentiating and diagnosing, these abnormalities are classified into groups. In 2003, the American Fertility Society (AFS) published a classification system[3] **(Fig. 2)**.

But, in 2013, the European Society of Human Reproduction and Embryology (ESHRE) and the European Society for Gynecological Endoscopy (ESGE) joined together and devised a new classification system named ESHRE-ESGE classification for Müllerian abnormalities[4,5] **(Fig. 3 and Table 1)**. This is claimed to be more suitable classification system for the accurate and clear diagnosis and is correlated with clinical management with simple categorization of female genital tract anomalies. The system is based on anatomy and cervical and vaginal anomalies are classified independently

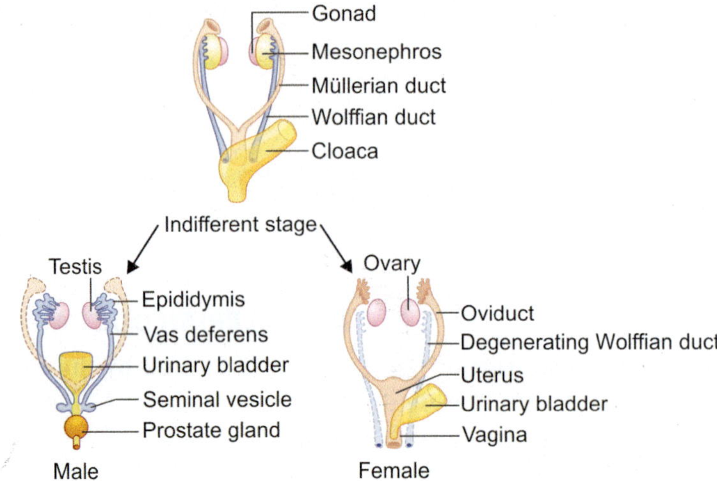

Fig. 1: Diagrammatic explanation of development of reproductive tract in male and female.

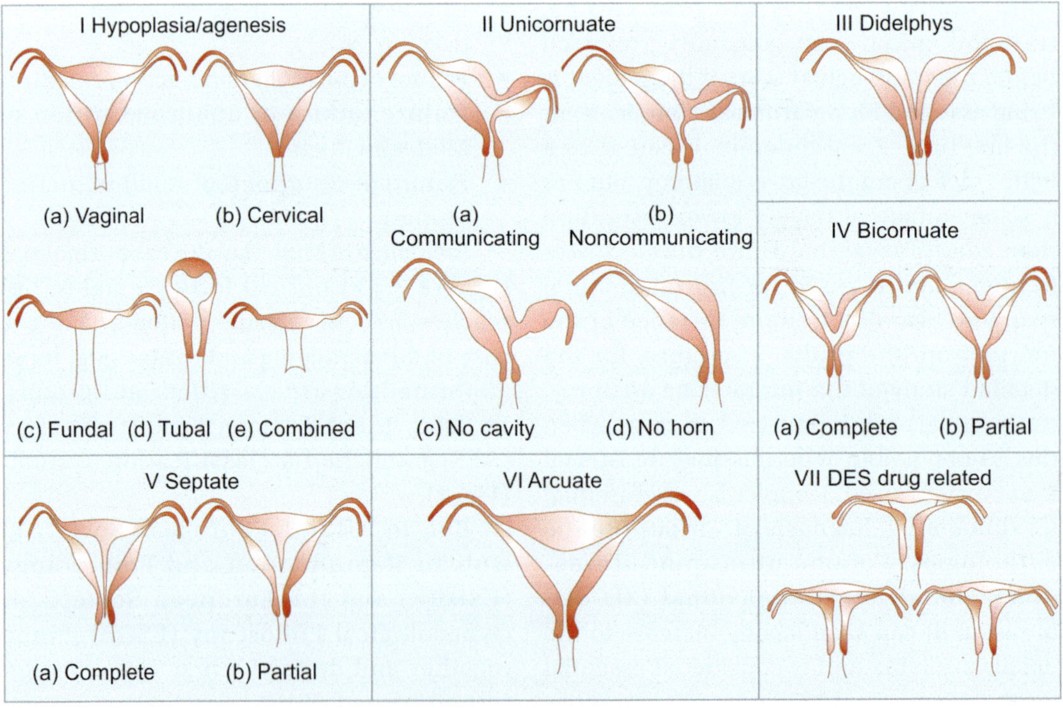

Fig. 2: Uterine abnormalities: The American Fertility Society classification. (DES: diethylstilbestrol)

from uterine abnormalities into subclasses having clinical significance. It is thought to be more practical also because according to this system, the uterus's own myometrial wall thickness measurement is used as a standard to evaluate the abnormalities of the shape, unlike the AFS classification, that uses absolute measurements for differentiation between different subgroups such as bicornuate, septate, and arcuate. This system has been

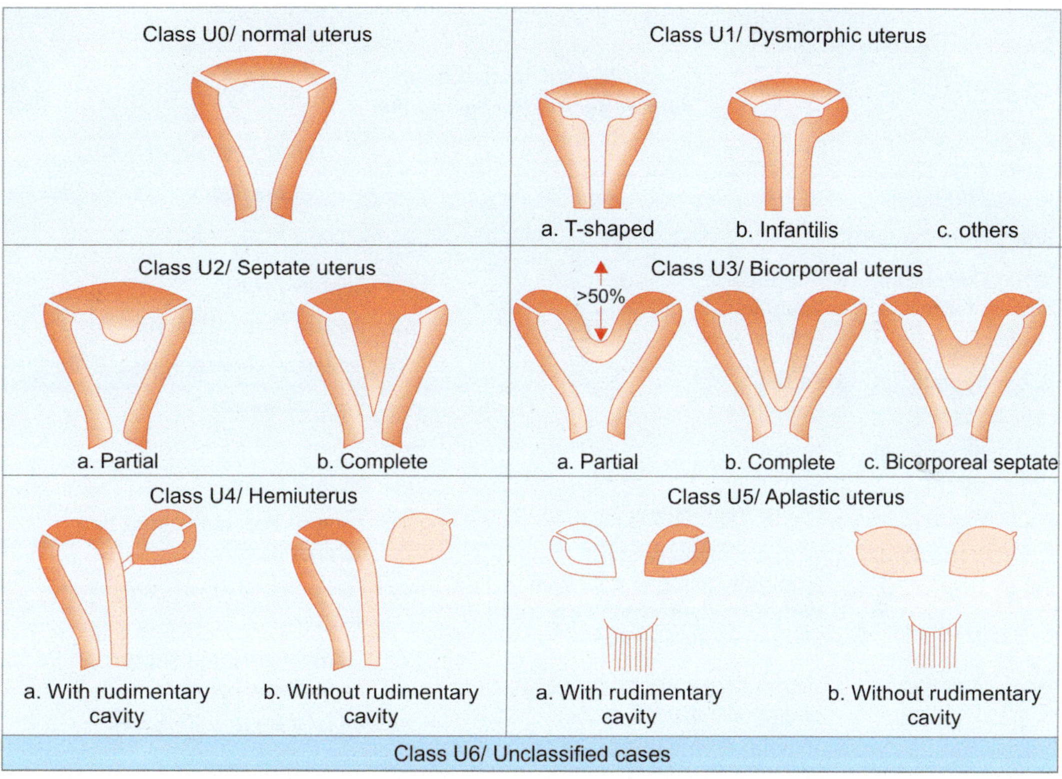

Fig. 3: Classification of female genital tract anomalies.[6]

developed by common working group under the name CONgenital UTerine Anomalies (CONUTA).[6]

This classification system can be explained as follows.

Class U0—Normal Uterus

Class U0 is a normal uterus. It shows a straight or convex contour of the uterine fundus and that of the endometrium also. But, even when the endometrial contour is concave, if the depth of the indentation at the fundal midline does not exceed 50% of the uterine wall thickness, it is still considered a normal uterus **(Fig. 4)**. This means that when the uterus is seen in the midcoronal plane, the vertical distance between the highest point on the endometrium to the intercornual line is defined as myometrial wall thickness and this distance is the standard of measurement for evaluation of any Müllerian abnormality.

This later condition was named as arcuate uterus. On 3D US, endometrial cavity is concave at fundus **(Fig. 5A)**. External fundal contour is flat or convex **(Fig. 5A)**. These features are common in the AFS and the ESHRE-ESGE classification. But according to the AFS classification, distance between line touching the tips of endometrial cavities and the deepest point between the endometrial cavities is <10 mm **(Fig. 5B)** and angle between the cavities is >105° **(Fig. 5C)**.

Class U1—Dysmorphic Uterus

Usually, dysmorphic uteri are smaller in size. Normal uterine is fundal shape, but with an abnormal shape of the endometrial cavity excluding septa.

Class U1a—T-shaped Uterus

Narrow uterine cavity is due to thickened lateral walls with normal uterocervical ratio (2:1).

TABLE 1: ESHRE/ESGE classification of female genital tract anomalies.[6]

ESHRE/ESGE classification Female genital tract anomalies 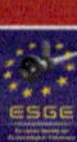				
Uterine anomaly			***Cervical/Vaginal anomaly***	
	Main class	***Subclass***	***Coexistent class***	
U0	Normal uterus		C0	*Normal cervix*
U1	Dysmorphic uterus	a. T-shaped b. Infantilis c. Others	C1	Septate cervix
			C2	Double "normal" cervix
U2	Septate uterus	a. Partial b. Complete	C3	Unilateral cervical aplasia
			C4	Cervical aplasia
U3	Bicorporeal uterus	a. Partial b. Complete c. Bicorporeal septate	V0	Normal vagina
			V1	Longitudinal nonobstructing vaginal septum
U4	Hemiuterus	a. With rudimentary cavity (communicating or not horn) b. Without rudimentary cavity (horn without cavity/no horn)	V2	Longitudinal obstructing vaginal septum
			V3	Transverse vaginal septum and/or imperforate hymen
U5	Aplastlc	a. With rudimentary cavity (bi- or unilateral horn) b. Without rudimentary cavity (bi- or unilateral uterine remnants/Aplasla)	V4	Vaginal aplasia
U6	Unclassified malformations			
U			C	V

(ESGE: European Society for Gynecological Endoscopy; ESHRE: European Society of Human Reproduction and Embryology)

Lateral wall thickness of the uterus is confirmed by as follows: measure the myometrial wall thickness. Draw a line from cornu to the internal os. Draw a perpendicular on that line from the deepest point on the lateral endometrial cavity. The part of that perpendicular, lateral to the line connecting os to cornu, if it measures 1.4 times or more of the myometrial wall thickness, is T-shaped uterus **(Fig. 6A)**. T-shaped uterus was fairly a confusion when AFS classification is used. Any narrow cavity was considered to be T-shaped uterus. According to a still one more classification system called CUME classification (congenital uterine abnormalities by experts),[7] T shaped uterus is a uterus with narrow cavity, in which the lateral inner angle of the endometrial cavity is <40 degree, the angle on the lateral endometrial wall—outer

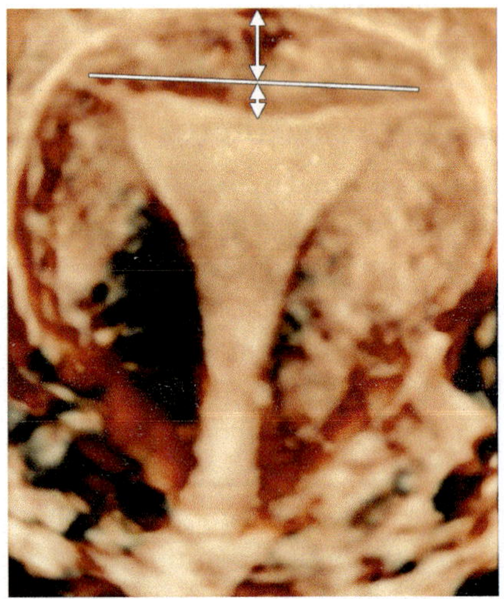

Fig. 4: Three-dimensional (3D) ultrasound image of the normal uterus showing interostial line (black) and the two white arrow lines, the longer one indicating uterine wall thickness.

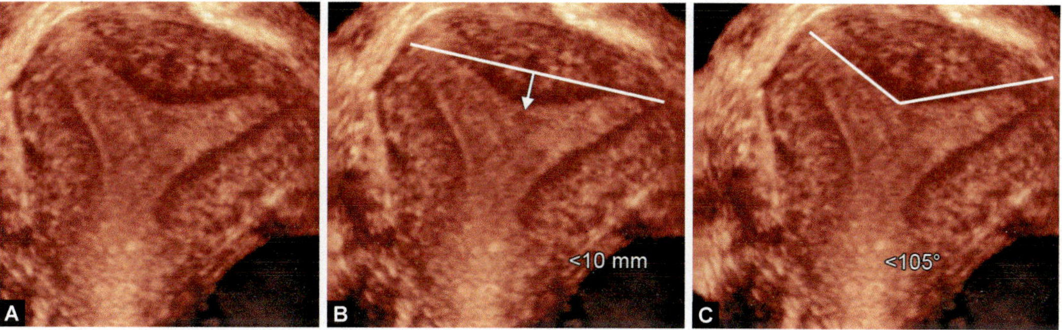

Figs. 5A to C: Three-dimensional (3D) US arcuate uterus.

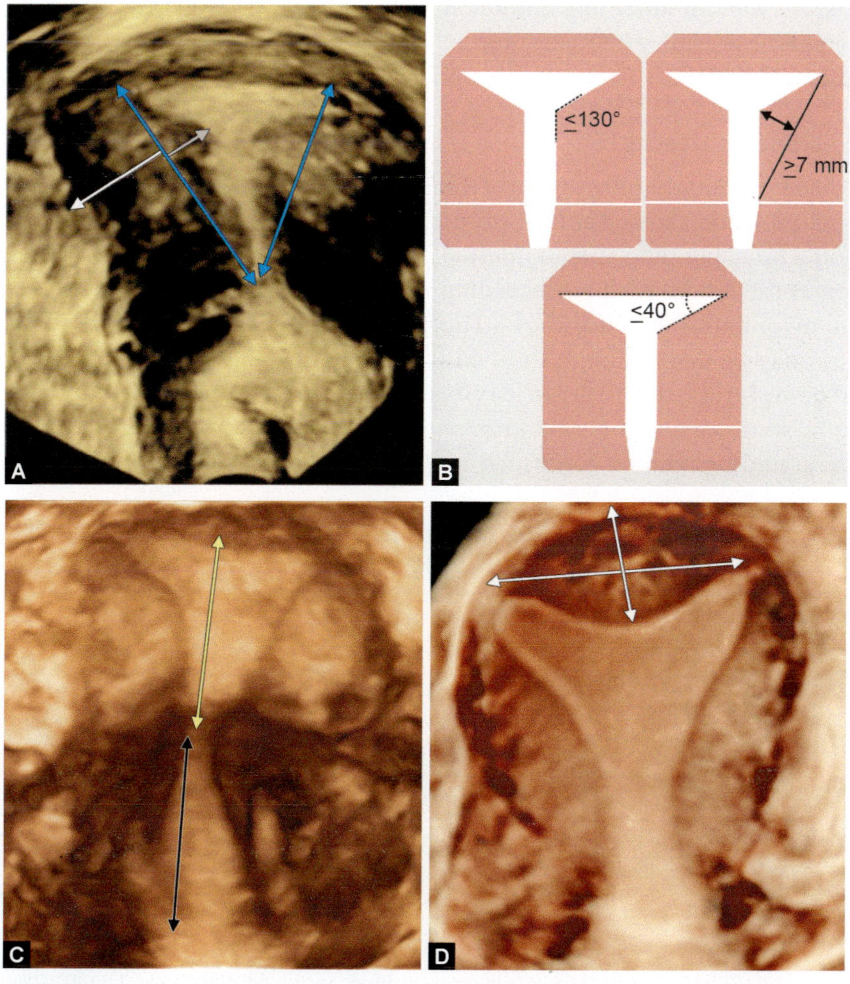

Figs. 6A to D: (A) Class U1a: T-shaped uterus; (B) Diagrammatic presentation of T-shaped uterus according to CUME classification; (C) Class U1b: Hypoplastic uterus; (D) Class U1c: Dysmorphic uterus.

angle is >130 degree and the distance between the line drawn from endometrial cornu to internal os and the deepest point on the lateral endometrial wall is >7 mm is a T-shaped uterus (**Fig. 6B**).

Class U1b—Uterus Infantilis

Narrow uterine cavity is without lateral wall thickening and an inverse uterocervical ratio (**Fig. 6C**). Uterus infantilis according to the AFS classification is hypoplastic uterus.

Class U1c—Others

Minor deformities of the uterine cavity including those with an inner indentation at the fundal midline level of <50% of the uterine wall thickness (**Fig. 6D**).

Class U2—Septate Uterus

Normal fusion but abnormal absorption of the midline septum is the cause. Septate uterus shows normal fundal outline and an internal indentation at the fundal midline exceeding 50% of the myometrial wall thickness. The indentation may be deep enough to divide partly or completely the uterine cavity including in some cases of cervix and/or vagina. These findings can be confirmed on 3D ultrasound. B-mode ultrasound may only raise the doubt of duplication abnormality.

Class U2a—Partial Septum

Septum partially dividing the uterine cavity short of the internal cervical os (**Fig. 7A**).

Class U2b—Complete Septum

Septum fully dividing the uterine cavity up to the level of the internal cervical os (may or may not have cervical and vaginal septum) (**Fig. 7B**).

Preovulatory or secretory phase is the best phase to diagnose congenital uterine abnormalities on 3D US. Septate uterus on the AFS classification also is defined by flat or convex fundus and division of the endometrial cavity. But, unlike considering the indentation of endometrial cavity of >50% of myometrial wall thickness, septate uterus on the AFS classification is diagnosed by no/minimal indentation on the fundus (**Fig. 8A**), angle between cavities is <75° (**Fig. 8A**), at least 5 mm of uterine wall can be seen above the line joining tips of two endometrial cavities (**Fig. 8B**), and distance between this line and deepest point between endometrial cavities are >10 mm (**Fig. 8B**). It has also been observed

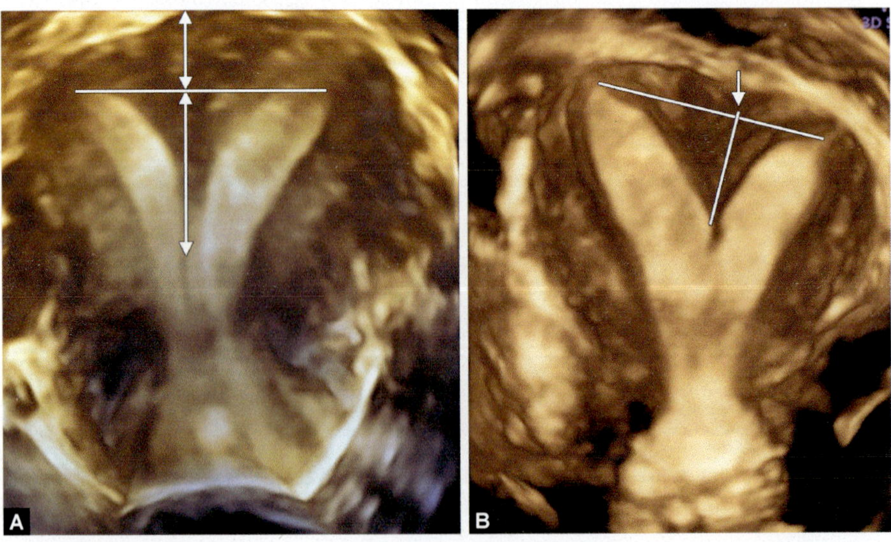

Figs. 7A and B: (A) Class U2a: Complete septum septum; (B) U2b: Partial septum.

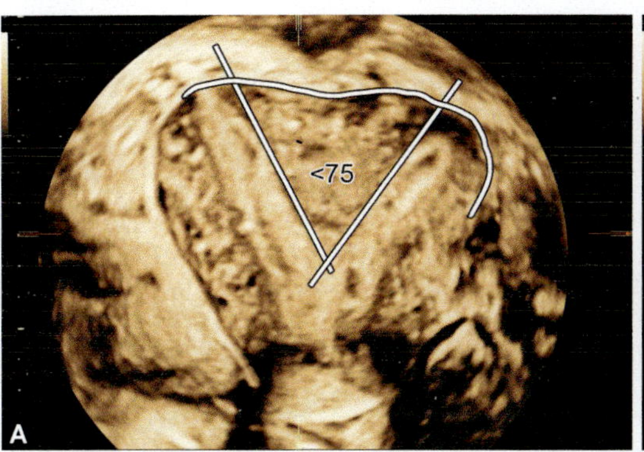

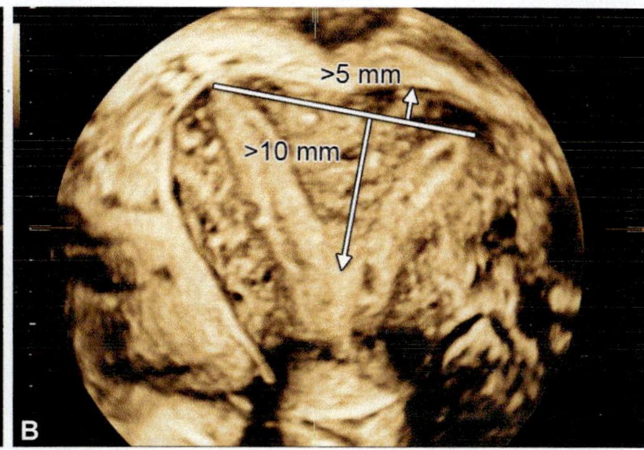

Figs. 8A and B: 3D ultrasound images of uterus showing AFS classification criteria of septate uterus.

that medial margins of the endometrial cavities are more commonly straight in septate uterus **(Fig. 8A)**.

It has been described in several studies that septae are avascular. But, there are controversies regarding this. Vascularity may be seen in 71.22% of septae with resistance index (RI) between 0.68 and 1.00 (0.84) **(Fig. 9)**.[8]

Septate uterus has maximum implications on fertility and pregnancy outcome among all Müllerian duct abnormalities:[9-11]

- Infertility
- Frequency of ectopic 27.34% as compared to 13.3% otherwise
- *First trimester abortions*: 28–45%
- *Second trimester abortions*: 5%
- Premature deliveries
- Dystocia

Different theories have been developed to rationalize these complications.

- It has been confirmed by histological studies that septae have less connective tissue and more muscle tissue and interlacing of these muscle fibers. There are vessels within these myometrial fibers also. Because of the interlacing arrangement of myometrial fibers when uterus contracts, the contractions in the septal region are incoordinated. This causes abortions or do not allow the embryo to implant.[12] More the muscular tissue in the septum, more the vascularity and more incoordinated contractions, therefore, more vascularized septae—more complications.

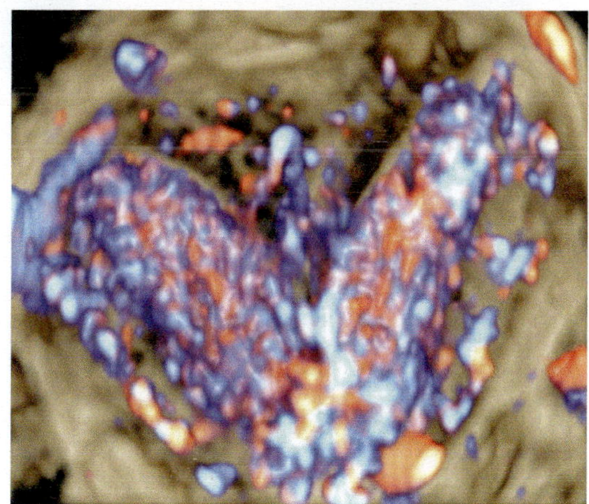

Fig. 9: Vascularity in septum seen on three-dimensional (3D) power Doppler.

- Less connective tissue leads to poor decidualization and so low implantation rate.[13]
- There is decrease in sensitivity of endometrium to estrogens on endometrium overlying the septum, due to less and irregularly distributed glandular ostia and incomplete ciliogenesis, is thought to be a cause of infertility.[14]

Size of septum and implications: It was thought that if the septum divides at least two-thirds of the uterine cavity **(Figs. 10A and B)**, it was more likely to cause complications but studies have shown that there is no correlation between the septal height and thickness and the incidence of abortions.[8] But, still there are other studies that show that whether septate or arcuate uterus, the length of remaining uterine cavity was significantly shorter and distortion

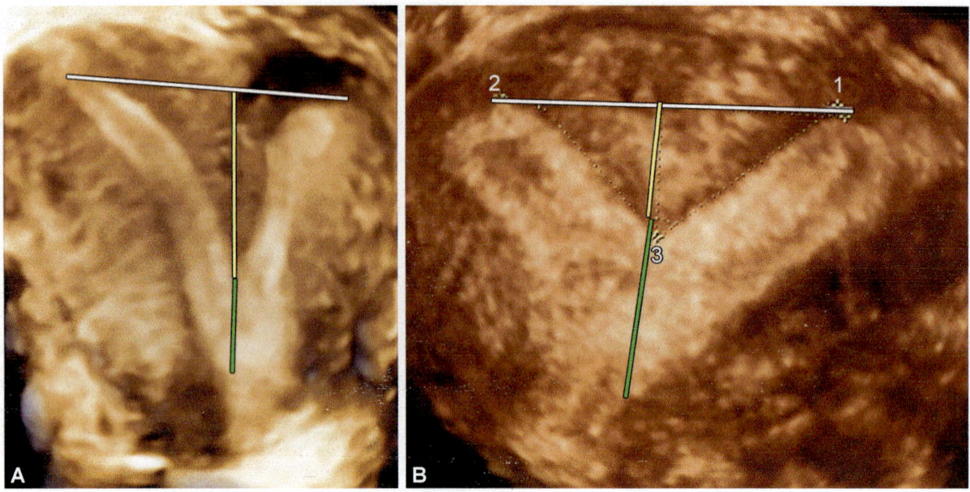

Figs. 10A and B: 3D ultrasound image of septate uterus showing measurement of the septum (yellow line) and the residual endometrial cavity (green line).

ratio was significantly higher in patients with recurrent miscarriage.[15]

Pitfalls in ultrasound-based differential diagnosis: The reliability of color and pulse Doppler for diagnosis of septum is reduced, if there is another intracavitary lesion such as polyp, submucous leiomyoma, or fundal fibroid. Small uterine cavity due to adhesions, shadowing due to fibroids, may affect 3D US diagnosis. With this marked confusion in the diagnosis of septate uterus, CUME (congenital uterine abnormalities by experts) classification has made the diagnosis comparatively simpler. According to this the fundal notch of <1 cm and the endometrial notch of >1 cm, are diagnostic of septate uterus.

Class U3—Bicorporeal Uterus

External indentation at the fundal midline exceeding 50% of the uterine wall thickness and the inner indentation at the midline level that divides the cavity as happens also in case of septate uterus.

Class U3a—partial bicorporeal uterus, where the external fundal indentation is partly dividing the uterine corpus above the level of the cervix **(Fig. 11A)**.

Class U3b—complete bicorporeal uterus, with external fundal indentation completely dividing the uterine corpus up to the level of internal os **(Fig. 11B)**.

Class U3c—bicorporeal septate uterus, which is an absorption defect in addition to the main fusion defect. The width of the midline fundal indentation exceeds by 150% to the uterine wall **(Fig. 11C)**.

In the AFS system, this duplication abnormality was known as bicornuate uterus or uterus didelphys. Though, with this classification, the cervical shape was of importance to differentiate between bicornuate and uterus didelphys. Uterus didelphys has two separate uteri and cervix **(Figs. 12A and B)**. Two separate vagina may be seen on per speculum examination. It has best prognosis of all malformations—fetal survival of up to 64%. Premature deliveries are common.

On ultrasound, uteri may be closely placed in the center of pelvic cavity and show division of the endometrial cavity or may be placed far lateral on the lateral pelvic walls and look like unicornuate uterus one on each side. Two horns may show symmetrical or asymmetrical development. Always look for the ovaries in vicinity of the uterus. This

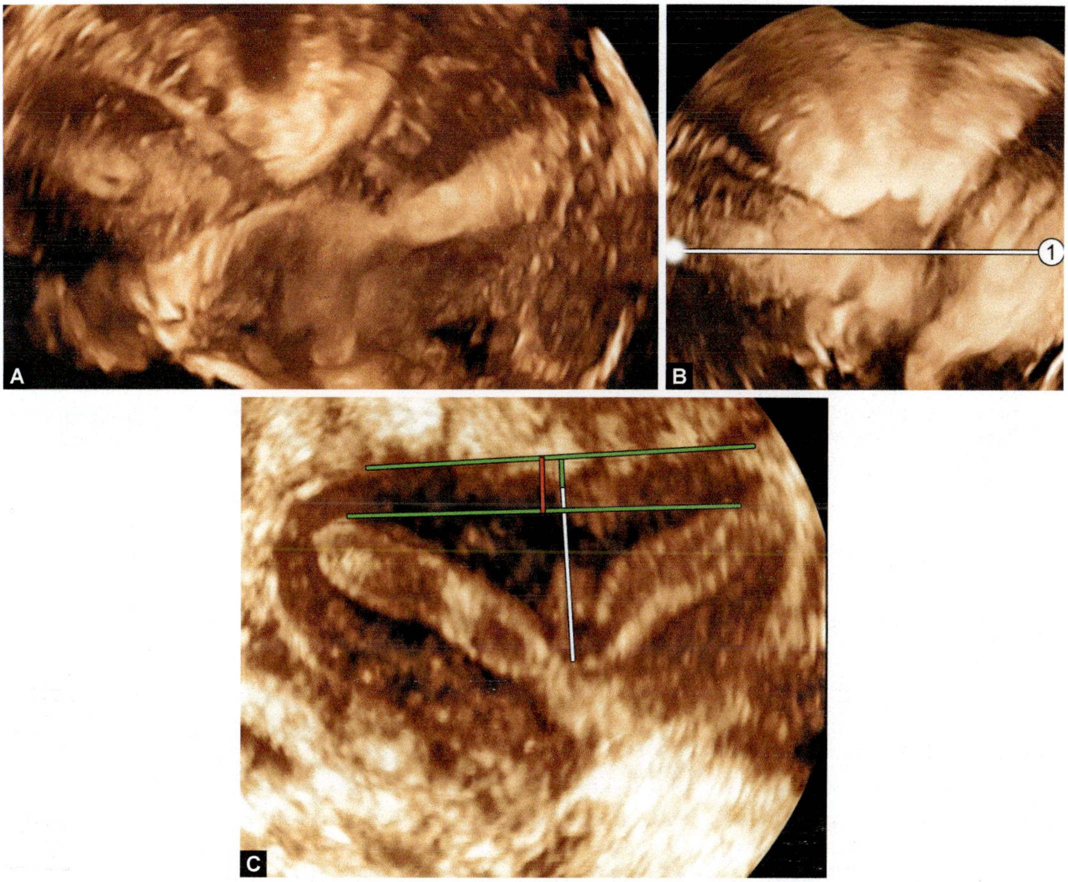

Figs. 11A to C: (A) Class U3a: Partial bicorporeal uterus; (B) Class U3b: Complete bicorporeal uterus; (C) Class U3c: Bicorporeal septate uterus.

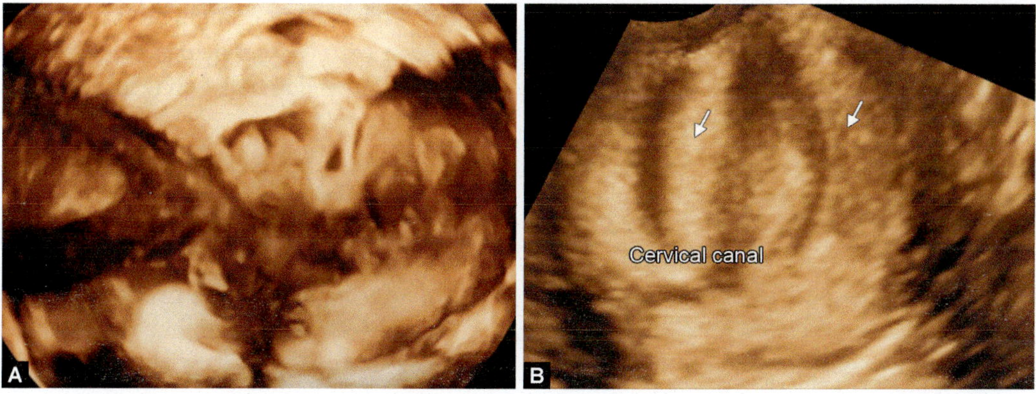

Figs. 12A and B: (A) 3D ultrasound image of two separate corpora of didelphys uterus; (B) Two separate cervices on 3D rendered image.

abnormality is commonly associated with tubal and renal abnormalities.

On B mode on transverse section tracing the uterus from the cervix to the fundus, it will show widening and division of the endometrial cavity toward fundus with indentation on the endometrial fundus looking like a figure of eight **(Fig. 13A)**.

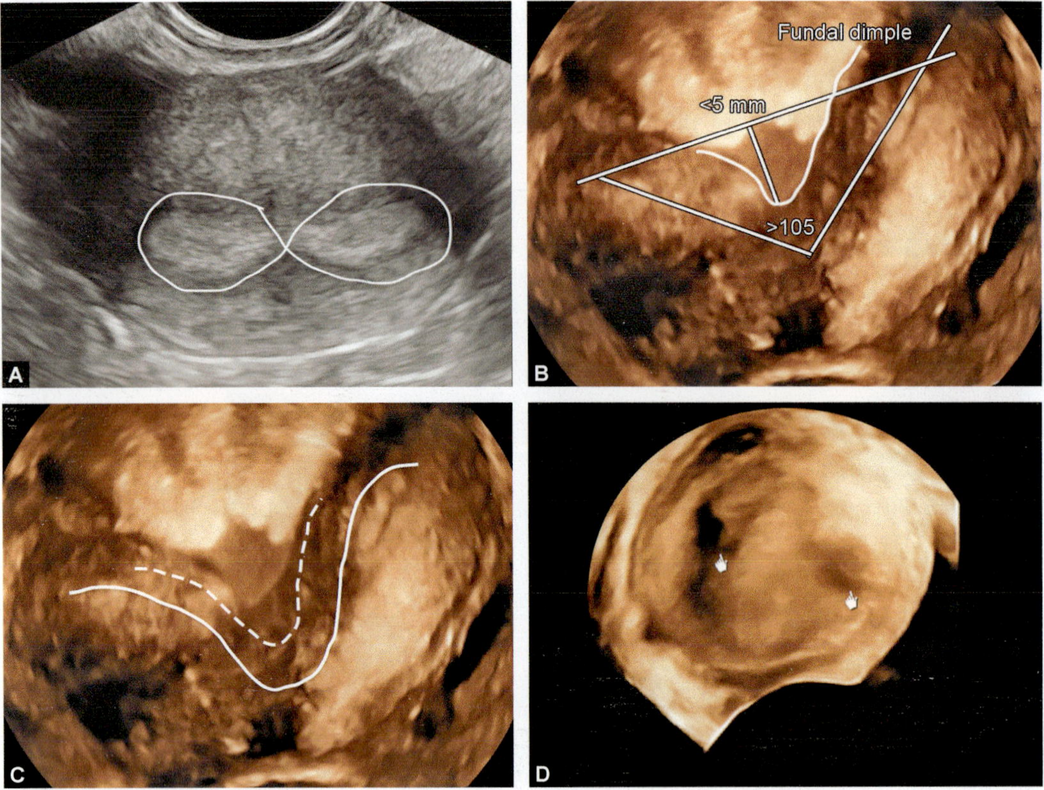

Figs. 13A to D: (A) B mode image showing transverse section of the uterus with 'figure of 8' endometrium; (B) 3D ultrasound image of the uterus showing criteria of bicornuate uterus according to AFS classification; (C) D ultrasound image of the uterus showing criteria of bicorporeal uterus according to ESHRE ESGE classification; (D) 3D ultrasound image of the axial section of the cervix showing single muscular complex with two cervical canals separated by thick muscular wall.

Volume US has a very important role to play in the diagnosis of bicornuate uterus as it shows uterus in coronal view.

- Fundus of the uterus shows a dimple **(Fig. 13B)**.
- If a straight line is drawn joining the top of the endometrial cavities, the fundus dimple is <5 mm above this line **(Fig. 13B)**.

Two signs seen on hysterosalpingogram (HSG) are also appreciated on 3D US.

- Angle between the two cavities is >105° **(Fig. 13B)**.
- Endometrial cavities appear convex medially meaning they are leaf shaped[3] (**Fig. 13C**—bold line).
- One more feature seen on 3D US is that myometrial layers can be seen dipping in between the endometrial cavities (**Fig. 13C**—dashed line). Single cervical complex is seen with two cervical canals and thick muscular wall in between **(Fig. 13D)**.

On color Doppler:

- Blood vessels are seen in between the two endometrial cavities with same resistance index as myometrium between 0.58 and 0.84.
- The uterine arteries on two sides may or may not show a difference in resistance indices depending on the amount of unification.
- The vessels in between the two endometrial cavities form a V or a Y **(Fig. 14)**.

Class U4—Hemiuterus

Class U4—hemiuterus is a formation defect. It is unilateral uterine development. The

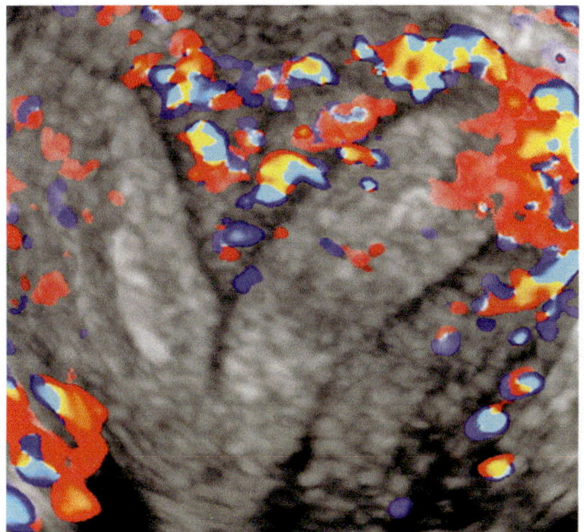

Fig. 14: Dipping of myometrial layers in bicornuate uterus.

contralateral part could be either incompletely formed or absent. This group is further divided into two subclasses depending on the presence or absence of a functional rudimentary cavity.

Class U4a or hemiuterus with a rudimentary (functional) cavity, which may be communicating or noncommunicating with hemiuterus **(Figs. 15A and B)**.

Class U4b or hemiuterus is without rudimentary (functional) cavity with nonfunctional contralateral uterine horn or by aplasia of the contralateral part **(Fig. 15C)**.

On TVS, in most of the cases, uterus is not seen in midline. Normal looking uterine contour in its long axis is seen on one side in pelvis. No uterine shadow or a rudimentary horn is seen on other side. Ovary is seen near the respective horn. On transverse scan at the level of uterine fundus, a beak-like projection from the endometrial shadow, cornu, is seen only on one side. 3D ultrasound is ultimate and clearly shows a banana-shaped

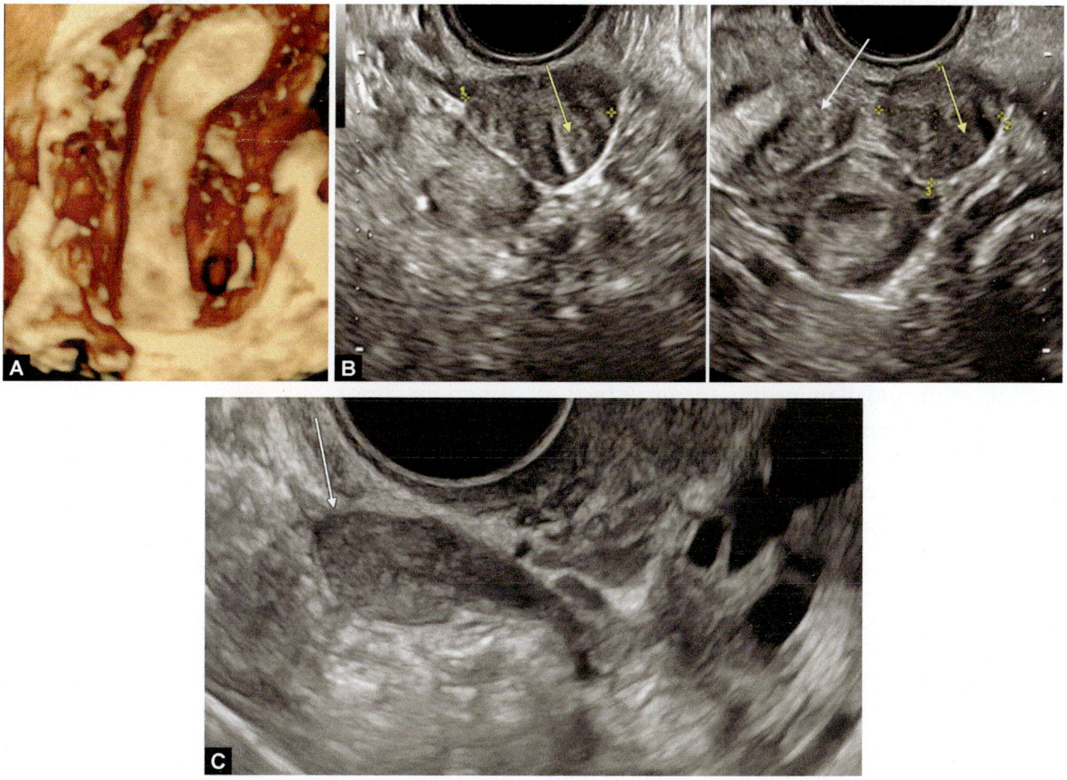

Figs. 15A to C: (A) Class U4: Hemiuterus on three-dimensional (3D) ultrasound; (B) Class U4a: Hemiuterus (white arrow) with functional rudimentary horn (yellow arrow) on B mode; (C) B-mode image of the rudimentary horn of uterus.

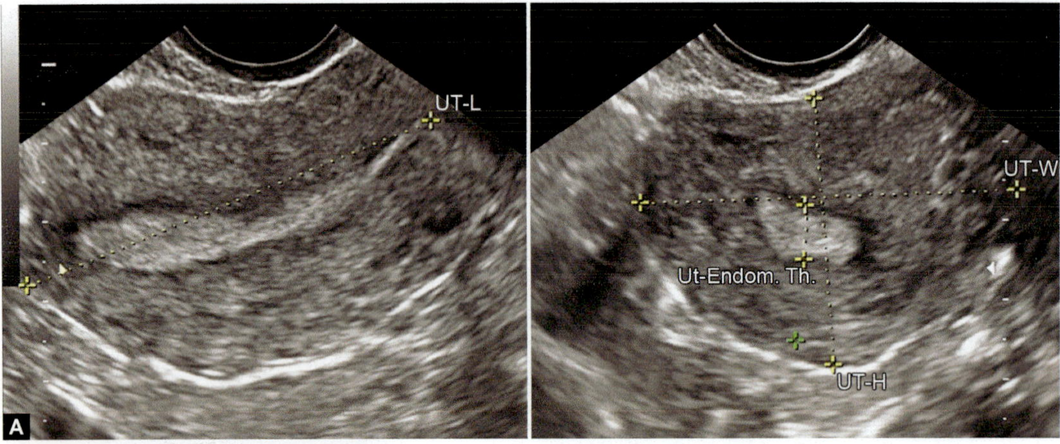

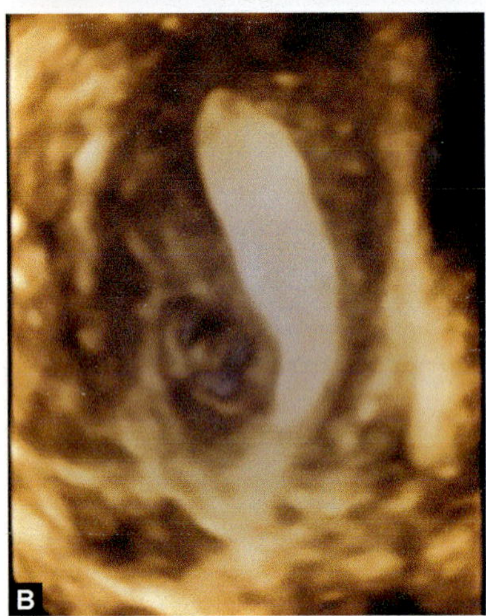

Figs. 16A and B: (A) B mode image of the uterus in long and transverse section, with only one cornu seen on the transverse section; (B) 3D ultrasound image of the unicornuate uterus.

uterine cavity **(Figs. 16A and B)**. Ultrasound recognition of hemiuterus by the ESHRE-ESGE classification and of unicornuate uterus by the AFS classification is the same.

Class U5—Aplastic Uterus (Uterus Aplasia)

It refers to absence of any fully or unilaterally developed uterine cavity. Unilateral or bilateral rudimentary horns with cavity may be seen in some, while in others, there could be uterine remnants without cavity. Coexistent defects (e.g., vaginal aplasia/Mayer-Rokitansky-Küster-Hauser syndrome) are common with this group of abnormalities.

Class U5a—aplastic uterus with rudimentary (functional) bilateral or unilateral functional horn.

Class U5b is aplastic uterus without rudimentary (functional) cavity.

It is suspected in patients with primary amenorrhea. Transabdominal scan with full bladder shows convex base with no dimple **(Fig. 17)**. This indicates complete absence of uterus and karyotyping is essential in these patients. If rudimentary horns or uterus is seen anywhere in pelvis, it is not uterine aplasia, but it is hypoplastic uterus. It is identified by pear-shaped isoechoic structures with or without thin echogenic line in the

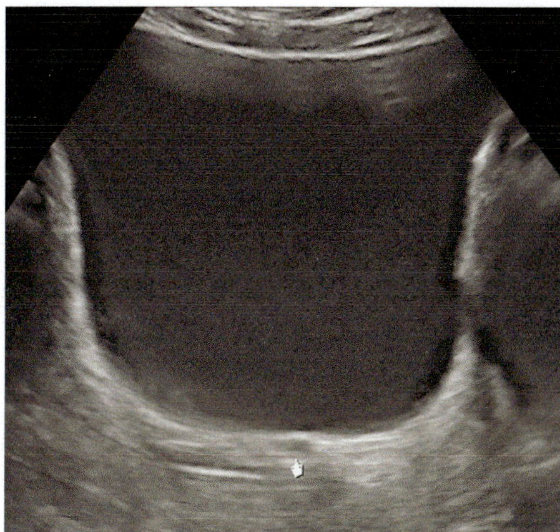

Fig. 17: B mode ultrasound image of the trans-abdominal scan, with full bladder showing a tiny dimple at the bladder base.

center. Ovaries may be seen in close vicinity to these horns. This on the AFS classification is agenesis of the uterus.

Class U6-Unclassified Cases

These are infrequent anomalies and subtle changes or combined pathologies could not be allocated correctly to one of the six groups.

The classification of cervical canal anomalies and vaginal anomalies is also an additional advantage.

C0—normal cervix **(Fig. 18A)**, C1—septate cervix **(Fig. 18B)**, and C2—double normal cervix can be confidently diagnosed by 3D ultrasound **(Fig. 18C)**. Unilateral cervical aplasia, which constitutes C3 class, cannot be easily diagnosed on ultrasound. Cervical aplasia is rare.

TABLE 2: Sensitivity and specificity of various ultrasound methods.

Ultrasound	*Sensitivity*	*Specificity*
TVS	95.21%	92.21%
TVCD PD	99.29%	97.23%
Volume USG	98.38%	100%
Sonohysterography	98.18%	100%

(PD: power Doppler; TVCD: transvaginal color Doppler; TVS: transvaginal sonography)

Sensitivity and specificity of various ultrasound methods for the diagnosis of congenital uterine abnormalities are given in **Table 2.**[13]

Congenital uterine abnormalities are commonly associated with congenital renal abnormalities such as ectopic kidney or unilateral absent kidney. Therefore, an abdominal scan is essential in all patients with congenital uterine malformations.

CONCLUSION

Müllerian duct abnormalities are more commonly found in patients presenting for infertility or recurrent abortions. 3D ultrasound is the modality of choice for diagnosis of these

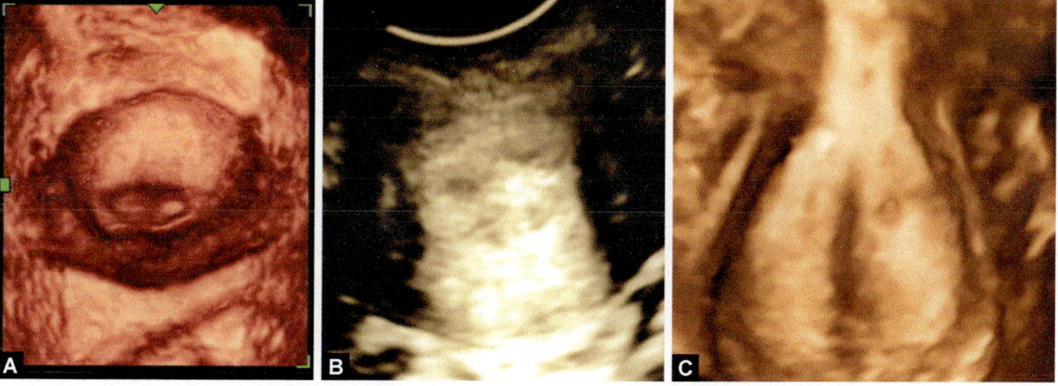

Figs. 18A to C: (A) Single normal cervix—C0; (B) Cervix with septum in transverse section—C1; (C) Normal double cervix in long section—C2.

abnormalities. For differential diagnosis of these abnormalities, the ESHRE-ESGE classification (2013) and the AFS classification are the two popular systems. Though the ESHRE-ESGE system is claimed to be more practical and accurate, in borderline or confusing cases of duplication abnormalities, features of the AFS system such as angle between the endometrial cavities may be taken into consideration as an additional sign.

REFERENCES

1. Richman TS, Viscomi GN, deCherney A, Polan ML, Alcebo LO. Fallopian tube patency assessed by ultrasound following fluid injection. Work in Progress. Radiology. 1984;152:507-10.
2. Raga F, Bonilla-Mosules F, Blanes J. Congenital Müllerian anomalies: diagnostic accuracy of three-dimensional ultrasound. Fertil Steril. 1996;65:523-8.
3. The American Fertility Society classification of adnexal adhesions, distal tubal occlusion, tubal occlusion secondary to tubal ligation, tubal pregnancies, Müllerian anomalies and intrauterine adhesions. Fertil Steril. 1998;49:944-55.
4. Rock JA, Roberts CP, Jones HW. Congenital anomalies of the uterine cervix: lessons from 30 cases managed clinically by a common protocol. Fertil Steril. 2010;94:1858-63.
5. Grimbizis GF, Tsalikis T, Mikos T, Papadopoulos N, Tarlatzis BC, Bontis JN. Successful end-to-end cervico-cervical anastomosis in a patient with congenital cervical fragmentation: case report. Hum Reprod. 2004;19:1204-10.
6. Grimbizis GF, Gordts S, Sardo ADS, Brucker S, Angelis CD, Gergolet M, et al. The ESHRE/ESGE consensus on the classification of female genital tract congenital anomalies. Hum Reprod. 2013;28:2032-44.
7. Ludwin A, Martins WP, Nastri CO, Ludwin I, Coelho Neto MA, Leitao VM, et al. Congenital uterine malformations by experts (CUME): better criteria for distinguishing between normal/arcuate and septate uterus? Ultrasound Obstet Gynecol. 2018;51(2):282.
8. Kupesic S, Kurjak A. Septate uterus: detection and prediction of obstetrical complications by different forms of ultrasonography. J Ultrasound Med. 1998;17:631-6.
9. Gaucherand P, Awada A, Rudigoz RC, Dargent D. Obstetrical prognosis of septate uterus: a plan for treatment of the septum. Eur J Obstet Gynecol Reprod Biol. 1994;54:109-12.
10. Fedele L, Arcaini L, Parazzini F, Vercillini P, Nola GD. Metroplastic hysteroscopy and fertility. Fertil Steril. 1993;59:768-70.
11. Heinonen PK, Saarikoski S, Pystynen P. Reproductive performance of women with uterine anomalies: an evaluation of 182 cases. Acta Obstet Gynecol Scand. 1982;61:157-62.
12. Dabirashrafi H, Bahadori M, Mohammad K, Alavi M, Moghadami-Tabrizi N, Zandinejad K, et al. Septate uterus: new idea on the histologic features of this abnormal uterus. Am J Ob Gyn. 1995;172(1Pt 1):105-7.
13. Salle BL, Sergeant P, Galcherand P, Guimont I, Hilaire PDS, Rudigoz RC. Transvaginal hysterosonographic evaluation of septate uteri: a preliminary report. Hum Reprod. 1996;11:1004-7.
14. Fedele L, Bianchi S, Marchini M, Franchi D, Tozzi L, Dorta M. Ultrastructural aspects of endometrium in infertile women with septate uterus. Fertil Steril. 1996;65:750-2.
15. Salim R, Woelfer B, Backost M. Reproducibility of three-dimensional ultrasound diagnosis of congenital uterine anomalies. Ultrasound Obstet Gynecol. 2003;21:578-82.

26

CHAPTER

Myometrial Pathologies of Uterus

Sonal Panchal, Chaitanya Nagori

INTRODUCTION

Uterus, a central landmark organ in the pelvis, is also a pivotal organ of female reproductive system. Myometrium—the muscle layer of the uterus forms the major bulk of the uterus mass. It protects the endometrial cavity and is surrounded by the serosa. It defines the margins of uterus and therefore its integrity confirms that the uterus is normal. The inner most layer of the myometrium is known as endometrial-myometrial junctional zone (JZ). This layer is structurally and functionally different form the rest of the myometrium. Myometrium is normally homogeneously hypoechoic, and serosal surface is smooth and regular. Any mass lesion in the uterus changes the contour of the uterus and therefore the smooth pear shape is distorted.

Distortion of the shape or change in echogenicity suggests myometrial lesion.

SCAN ROUTES AND MODALITIES

Myometrial evaluation on ultrasound can be done by transabdominal route or by transvaginal route. Actually both are supplementary to each other. Transabdominal scan is of use to define the extent and margins of the myometrium. It is especially required in cases with large uterus or in cases in which due to space occupying lesions like fibroid, the uterus is pushed upwards and its superior margin cannot be accessed by transvaginal scan. Whereas the detailed morphology of the myometrium can be better studied by transvaginal scan due to proximity of probe to the uterus and better resolution due to high frequency probe. Uterus is evaluated in sagittal and transverse planes on B-mode ultrasound. Coronal plane of the uterus may be best evaluated by 3D ultrasound. For assessment of the vascular changes, Doppler is the modality of choice. Uterus is evaluated in a systematic manner on transvaginal scan.

METHOD OF ASSESSMENT OF THE UTERUS

Patient is first asked to empty the bladder and is placed in lithotomy position on the gynec couch in the same way as for per speculum or per vaginal examination. Ultrasound jelly is put on the head of the transvaginal probe and then the probe is covered with the condom, not to allow any air between the probe and the condom. A small amount of jelly is then placed over the condom on the probe head and the probe is gently slided into the patient's vagina. In case of difficulty in introduction or patient's resistance to introduction, she is advised to take deep long breaths with open mouth, i.e., deep inspirations and long complete expirations. Counseling the patient before examination and explaining the whole procedure and adequate privacy helps eliminate the anxiety and resistance. Probe is introduced in the longitudinal position with indicator on the probe facing the patient's anterior aspect (**Fig. 1**).

This indicator of the probe also matches the logo on the screen. This means that if the indicator on the screen is on the right side of the screen, the structures anteriorly placed are on the right side of the screen (**Fig. 2**). This

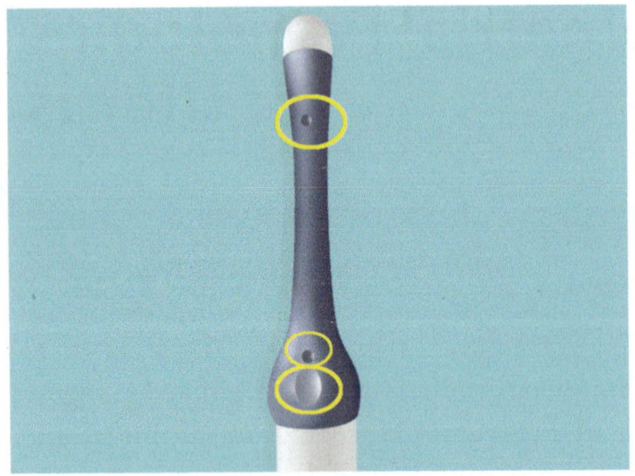
Fig. 1: Image of the transvaginal volume probe sowing the markers.

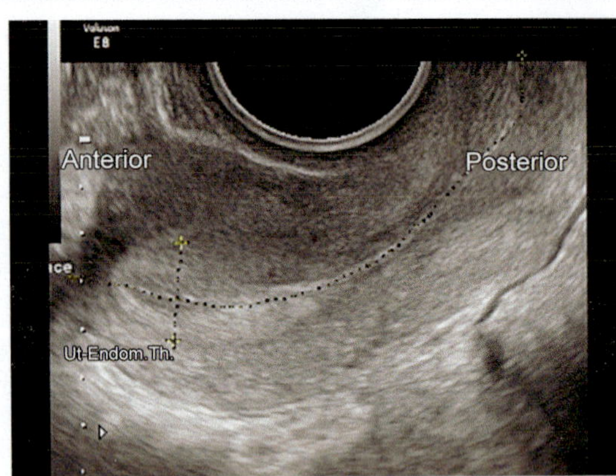

Fig. 2: Midsagittal section of the uterus on B-mode on transvaginal scan indicating anterior and posterior aspect of the patient.

shows long axis of the patient and longitudinal axis of the patient normally corresponds to the long axis of the uterus. That means the uterus must be seen in the sagittal plane on this view. It may be anteverted or retroverted. When anteverted the uterine fundus will be directed toward the indicator on the screen and urinary bladder is also seen on the same side of the screen, when retroverted fundus will be on the opposite side of the indicator and the urinary bladder (**Figs. 3A and B**). If the uterus is not seen in this view, it means that the uterus is deviated toward one side. When it is deviated, it would indicate that either it is pulled on the side of the pathology like adhesions or is pushed away by the pathology which is on the opposite side, say a mass.

Once the midsagittal plane of the uterus is seen, span the probe from one side to another, without rotating it, for the anatomical survey of the uterus in longitudinal axis. The spanning should extend from one side of the uterus across the midsagittal plane to the other side, till the uterus goes out of vision. Then the probe is realigned in the midsagittal plane of the uterus and then rotate the probe 90° anticlockwise. This maneuver will give transverse view of the uterus with the right side of the patient on right side of the screen (**Fig. 4**). In this transverse position also the

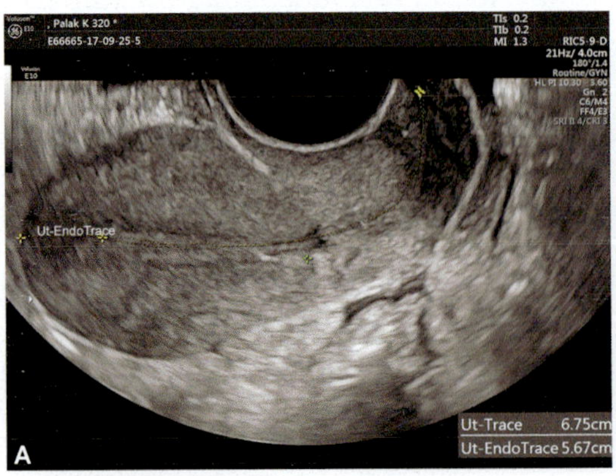

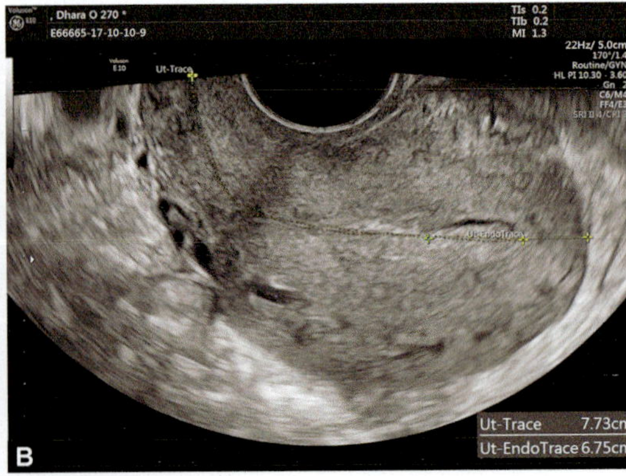

Figs. 3A and B: (A) Midsagittal section of the uterus showing anteverted anteflexed uterus; (B) Midsagittal section of the uterus showing retroverted retroflexed uterus.

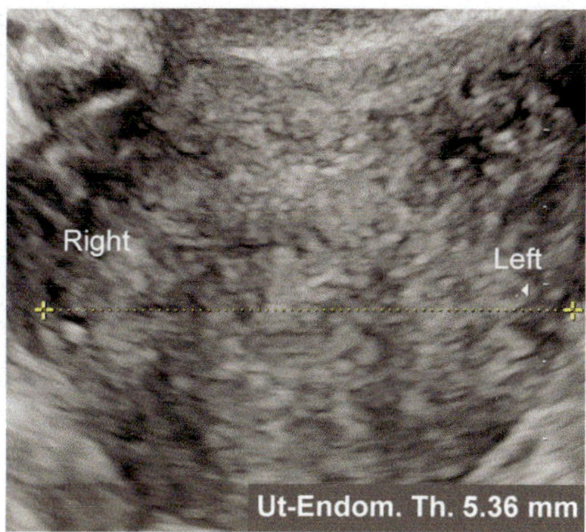

Fig. 4: Transverse section of the uterus with right and left side of the patient marked on the image.

whole uterus is evaluated from the fundus to the cervix by moving the probe up and down in the vagina. This survey should give a complete idea about the anatomy of the uterus and the exact location of any fibroids, etc. Any localized lesion if seen in the uterus, its location in all three planes (sagittal, axial, and coronal) must be confirmed. This understanding of the orientation of the image and the uterus and the probe movement is essential to correctly diagnose the location of the lesions in the myometrium.

Myometrial lesions like fibroids and adenomyosis are among the most common uterine pathologies and still these are the ones that bring most surprises on surgery as these are most inaccurately reported. The inaccuracy is because of random terms used for the description of ultrasound image and nonspecific terms used for localization. It is for this that a consensus was formed to describe the myometrial appearance or lesions and was termed as morphological uterus sonographic assessment (MUSA).

Morphological uterus sonographic assessment:[1] It accurately describes the measurement techniques, specifies on the terms used for various ultrasound pictures, clearly defines the reporting formats and also helps to identify reliable characters of benignity.

MEASUREMENTS

The length of the uterus is measured as length of the three different segments. *Fundal length* is the distance from the fundal serosa to the fundal end of the endometrial cavity, in the line that is in continuity with the endometrial cavity. The second segment is the *length of the endometrial cavity* measured as a trace from fundal tip of the endometrium to the internal os. The third segment is the *cervical length*, length from the internal os to external os, measured as a trace (**Fig. 5**).

The *antero-posterior diameter* is measured in this same midsagittal plane as the longest diameter on the uterus body, perpendicular to the endometrial cavity (**Fig. 6**). The probe is then rotated for the transverse section (90° anticlockwise) to achieve the transverse section of the uterus. The broadest distance on this section, side to side is the *transverse diameter*

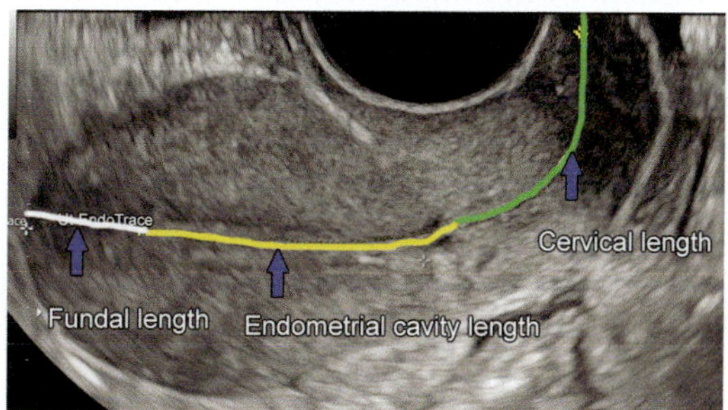

Fig. 5: Longitudinal measurements of the uterus on midsagittal section of the uterus, measured according to MUSA.

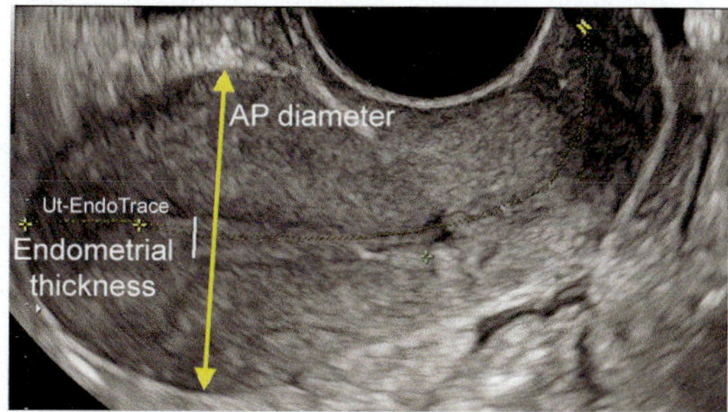

Fig. 6: AP diameter and endometrial thickness of the uterus on midsagittal section of the uterus, measured according to MUSA.

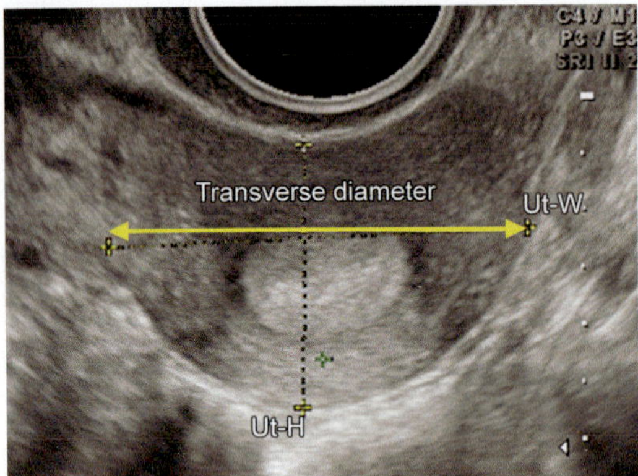

Fig. 7: Transverse diameter of the uterus on transverse section of the uterus, measured according to MUSA.

(**Fig. 7**). The uterine volume is calculated as total length × width × AP diameter × 0.523. The thickness of the *anterior and posterior myometrial walls* may be measured separately in cases where these appear unequal or asymmetrical. This is measured as the longest distance from outer margin of endometrium to the serosa, perpendicular to the central line of the endometrium, both anteriorly and posteriorly (**Fig. 8**). The *endometrial thickness* is also measured on this same plane, at the level where the endometrium is the thickest and the is measured from outer margin of the endometrium to outer margin of the endometrium (anterior and posterior), perpendicular to the central line of the endometrium (**Fig. 6**). *JZ thickness* is the measurement of the thickness of the hypoechoic zone in the most proximity of the outer hyperechoic margin of the endometrium, perpendicular to the endometrial outer margin and if regular it is measured as shown in **Figure 9**. JZ is best assessed on 3D ultrasound with VCI (volume contrast imaging) (**Fig. 10**). If it is irregular the maximum and the minimum thickness of the JZ is measured and is also important to mention the location and extent of the irregularity.

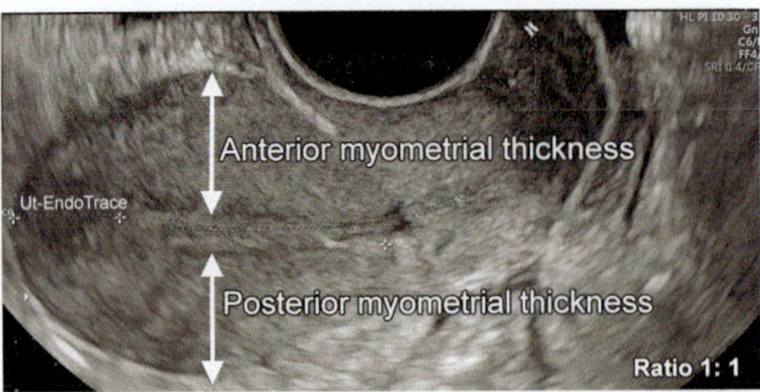

Fig. 8: Anterior and posterior myometrial diameter measured on midsagittal section of the uterus, measured according to MUSA.

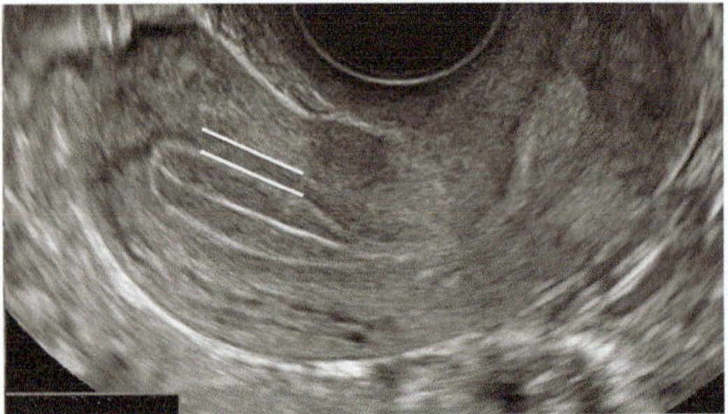

Fig. 9: Junctional zone measurement of the uterus on midsagittal section of the uterus, measured according to MUSA.

DESCRIPTION

Terminology used according to morphological uterus sonographic assessment: Junctional zone qualitatively is described as regular, irregular (**Fig. 11**), interrupted (**Fig. 12**) or inaccessible (**Fig. 13**). The interruption of the JZ may be because of cystic areas, hyperechogenic-dots, buds, or hyperechoic lines (**Figs. 14A and B**). JZ may be interrupted due to focal lesions/contractions. When the entire JZ cannot be identified, it is nonaccessible. But it may also be mentioned as inaccessible when it may not be clearly seen due to poor visibility, in obese patients or when uterus is deep.

If it is irregular, its thickness is measured at the thickest area of the JZ (**Fig. 15**). When JZ is interrupted or irregular, severity of irregularity is documented as a ratio of thickness of the thickest part of the JZ and thickness of the entire myometrial thickness, measured at the same level, in the same image, in the same plane (**Fig. 16**). Magnitude of a JZ irregularity is expressed as the difference between the

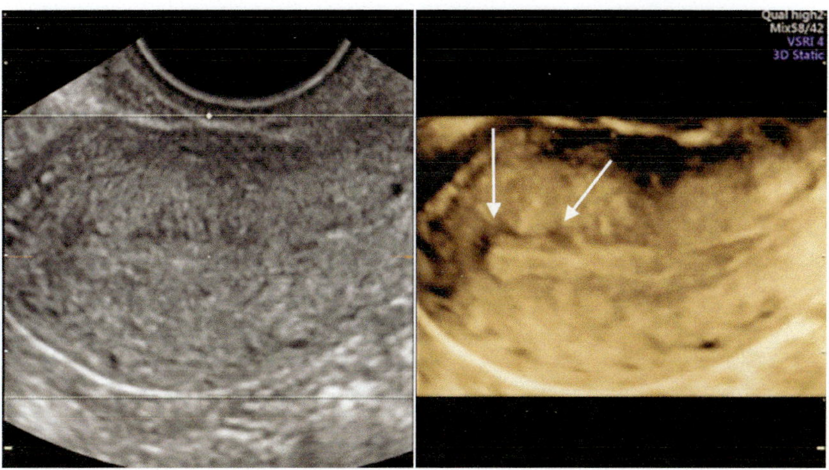

Fig. 10: B-mode and volume contrast imaging in the A plane (VCI-A) of the midsagittal section of the uterus, demonstrating clear delineation of the junctional zone on VCI-A.

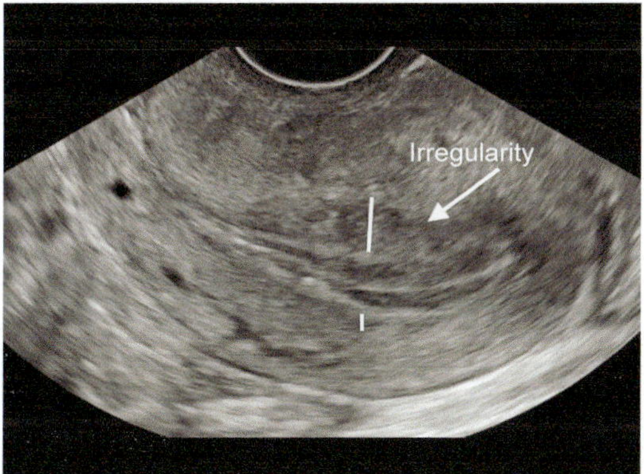

Fig. 11: Transvaginal ultrasound B-mode showing retroverted retroflexed uterus, midsagittal section of the uterus with irregular endometrial–myometrial junction on the posterior aspect.

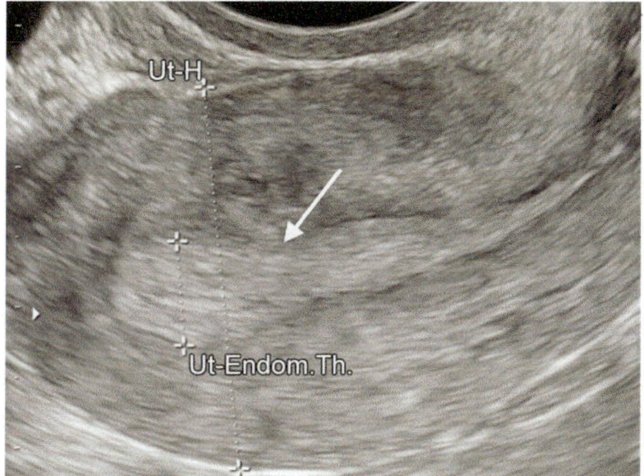

Fig. 12: Transvaginal ultrasound B-mode showing anteverted anteflexed uterus, midsagittal section of the uterus with interrupted endometrial–myometrial junction on the anterior aspect.

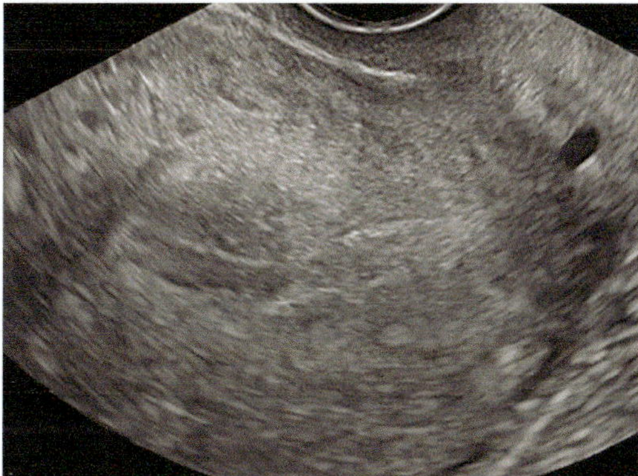

Fig. 13: Transvaginal ultrasound B-mode showing anteverted anteflexed uterus, midsagittal section of the uterus with inaccessible endometrial–myometrial junction on the anterior aspect.

maximum and minimum JZ thickness: (JZdif) = JZmax - JZmin (**Fig. 15**).

It is essential to mention that the irregularity/interruption involves anterior wall, posterior wall, right lateral wall, left lateral walls, or fundus. Extent of the irregularity can be subjectively described as <50% or >50%, for the uterus as a whole or for each location.

MYOMETRIAL DESCRIPTION (FLOWCHART 1)

Myometrium is described as homogeneous or heterogeneous in echotexture/echogenicity (**Fig. 17**). Heterogenicity may be due to cystic

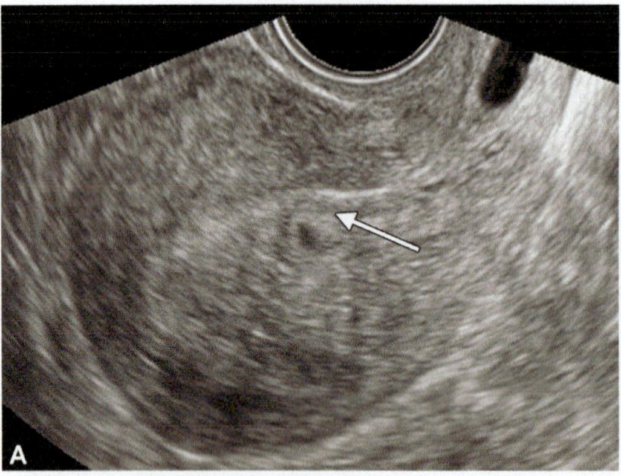

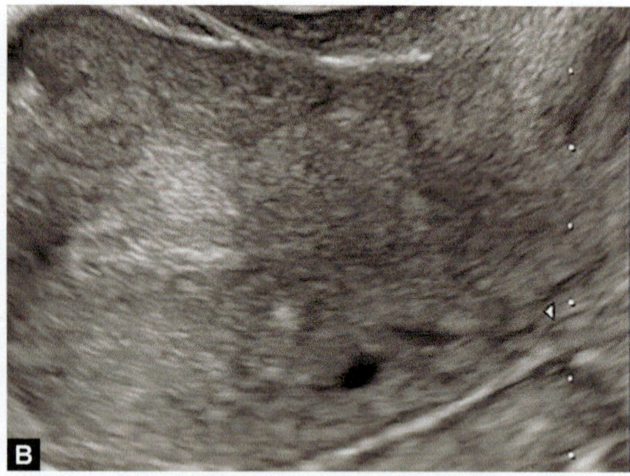

Figs. 14A and B: (A) Transvaginal ultrasound B-mode showing anteverted anteflexed uterus with interruption of the junctional zone because of cystic areas; (B) Transvaginal ultrasound B-mode showing anteverted anteflexed uterus with interruption of the junctional zone because of hyperechoic islands.

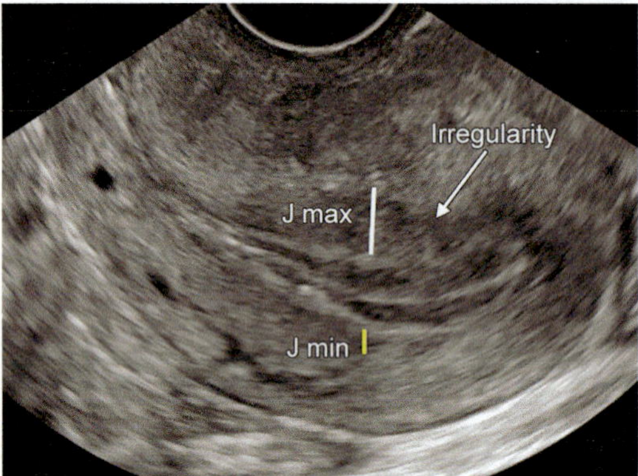

Fig. 15: Transvaginal ultrasound B-mode showing retroverted retroflexed uterus with irregularity of the junctional zone. The white line shows maximum thickness and yellow line shows minimum thickness of the junctional zone.

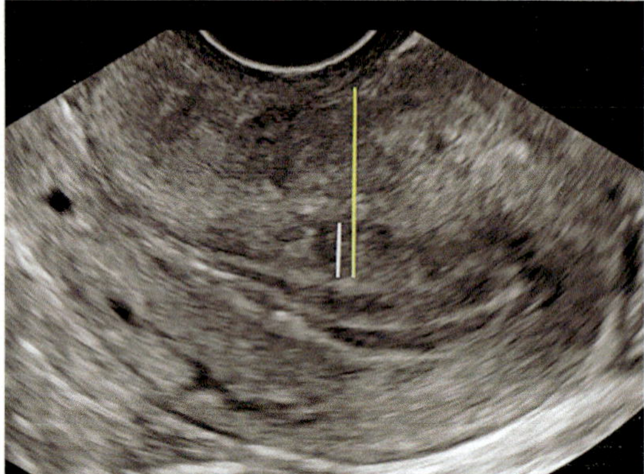

Fig. 16: Transvaginal ultrasound B-mode showing retroverted retroflexed uterus with irregularity of the junctional zone. The white line shows maximum thickness of the junctional zone, and yellow line shows thickness of the posterior myometrium.

Flowchart 1: Assessment for myometrium.

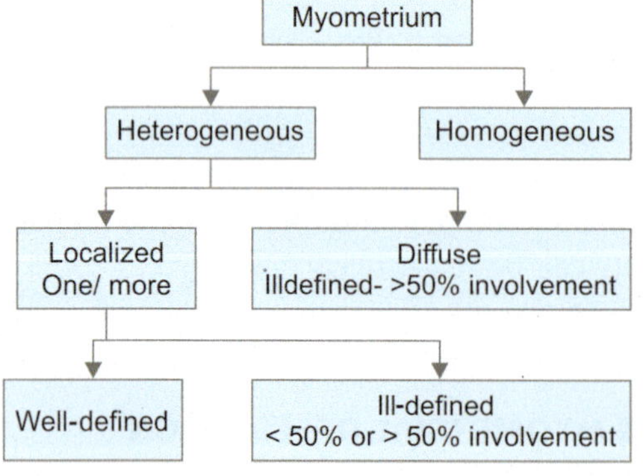

areas, hyperechogenicities, or shadowing (**Figs. 18A and B**). Heterogenicity may be localized (one/more areas) (**Fig. 19A**) or diffuse (**Fig. 19B**).

When the lesion is a localized one, it is essential to mention whether it is well defined (**Fig. 20**) or ill defined (**Fig. 19A**). Its location is described as anterior, posterior, fundal, right lateral, or left lateral and it involves upper, mid, or lower body, or cervix. If the lesion is diffuse, it is described as a global heterogenicity/global involvement of the uterus by the lesion. The size of the lesion is measured as three orthogonal diameters. The longest is measured in the longest plane, the anteroposterior (AP) diameter is the longest diameter perpendicular to this and on a

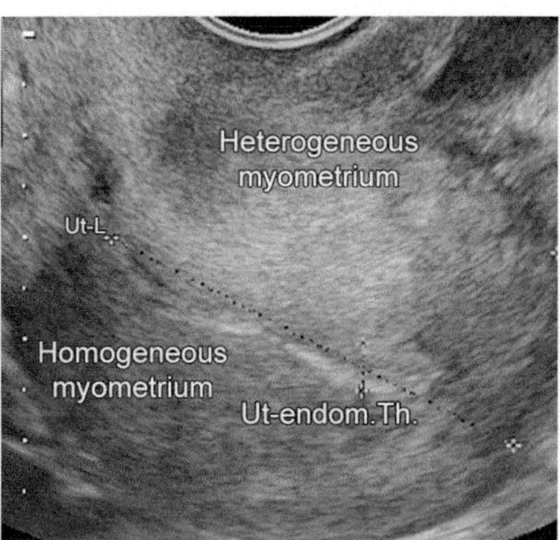

Fig. 17: Retroverted retroflexed uterus on B-mode, transvaginal ultrasound showing heterogeneous and thick posterior myometrium and homogeneous normal anterior myometrium.

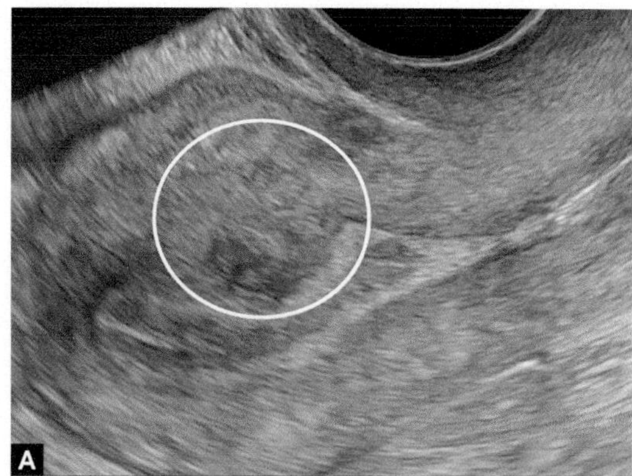

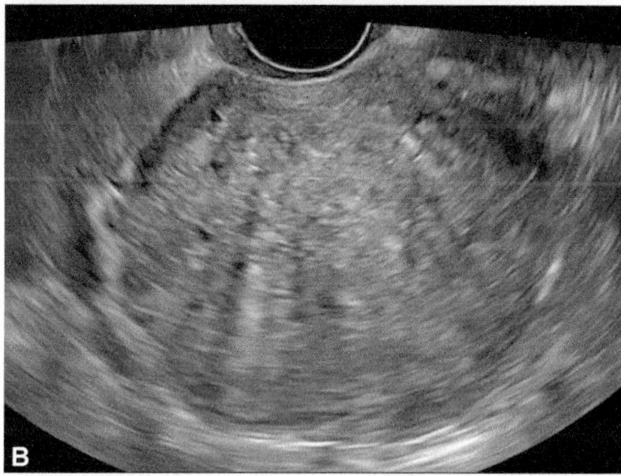

Figs. 19A and B: (A) Anteverted anteflexed uterus on B-mode on transvaginal scan with localized area of heterogeneous myometrium as marked by the circle, though the margins are ill defined; (B) Generalized heterogenicity of the myometrium.

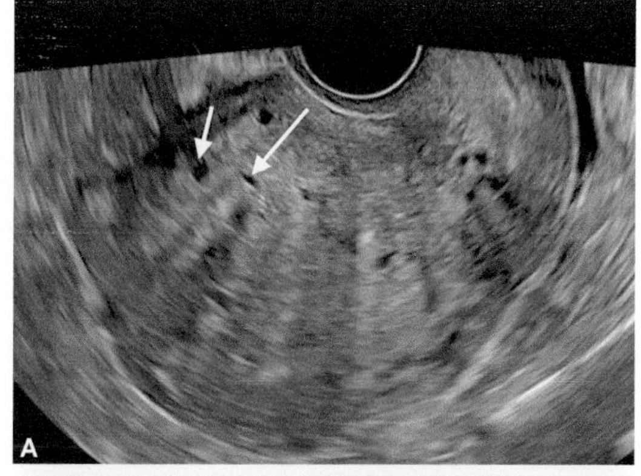

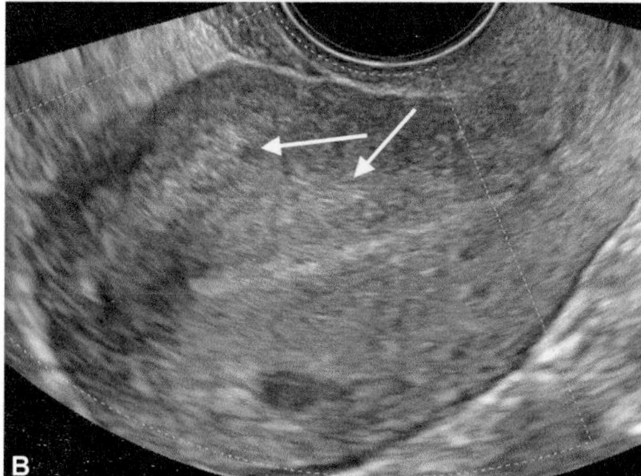

Figs. 18A and B: (A) B-mode ultrasound image of the uterus showing anechoic cystic areas of myometrial cysts marked by arrows; (B) Hyperechoic lines marked by arrows.

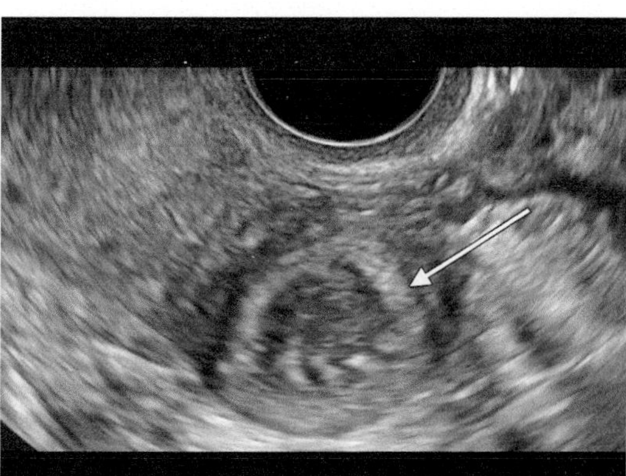

Fig. 20: A well-defined localized lesion is seen in the posterior wall of the uterus as marked by the arrow.

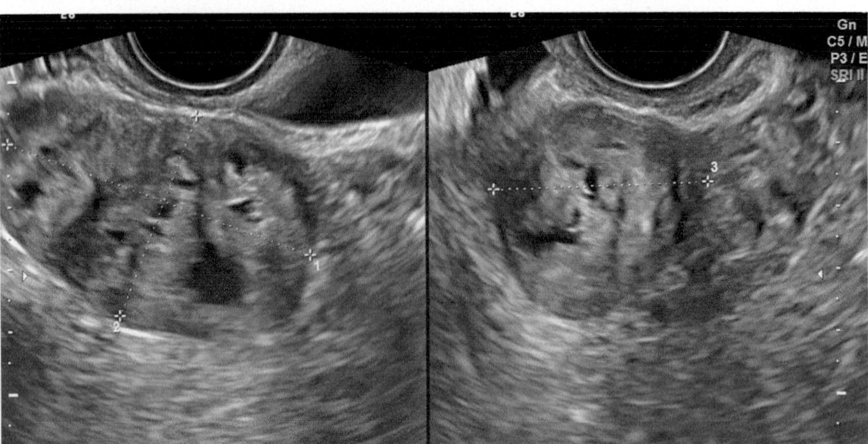

Fig. 21: Measurements of the localized myometrial lesion (fibroid), the long and the AP diameter measured on long section and transverse diameter on transverse section of the lesion.

transverse plane, that is achieved by only 90° rotation of the probe (**Fig. 21**). The site of the lesion is described as anterior, posterior, right or left lateral or fundal and then whether it is involving upper, middle, or lower part of the corpus or cervix is mentioned. Since myometrium is a thick layer of the uterus, most lesions will not involve its entire thickness. Therefore, it is essential to mention, how much thickness of the myometrium is affected by the lesion and also whether it is peripheral layer of the myometrium or central layer of the myometrium that is involved. These lesions are therefore classified according to palm-coein classification.[2] For the exact localization of the lesion and also to get the guidance about the route of surgery, minimum distance of the lesion from endometrium (inner lesion-free margin) or minimum distance from serosa (outer lesion-free margin) must also be mentioned (**Fig. 22**).

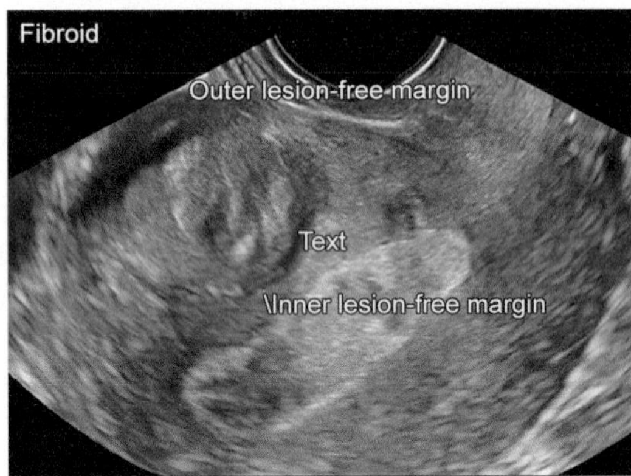

Fig. 22: Transvaginal ultrasound B-mode showing anteverted anteflexed uterus with anterior intramural fibroid showing outer and inner lesion-free margins.

Description of the lesion includes its shape (round, oval, lobulated, irregular), rim/margins (ill-defined, hypoechoic, hyperechoic), and its echogenicity (homogeneous/heterogeneous). Most lesions in the myometrium cast an acoustic shadow and that must also be mentioned. These may be fan shaped (alternate hyper and hypoechoic bands) (**Fig. 23A**) with or without edge shadows (**Fig. 23B**). Amount of shadowing is described as slight, moderate, or strong. The hyper/hypoechogenicity of the lesion is described as follows:

Level of echogenicity: It is compared to that of normal myometrium

- Very hypoechogenic (–)
- Hypoechogenic (–)
- Isoechogenic
- Hyperechogenic (+)
- Very hypogenic (++)
- Detailed description on the echogenicity is required.

When the lesion is diffuse, penetration of the diffuse lesions are described as a ratio between the maximum thickness of the lesion to the total uterine wall thickness and extent

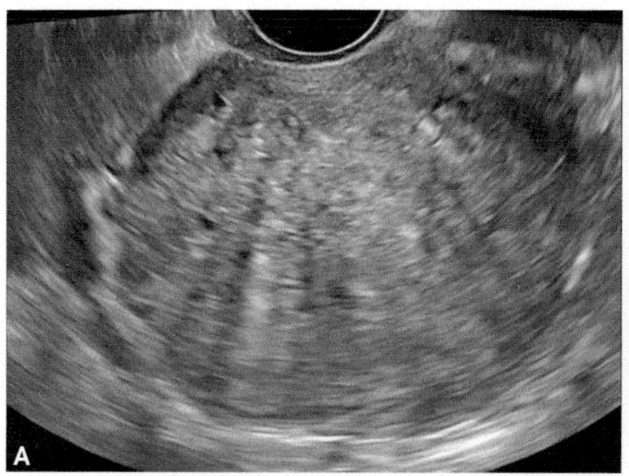

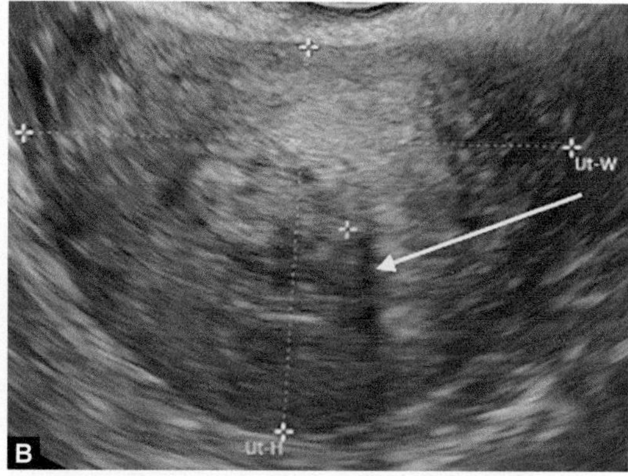

Figs. 23A and B: (A) Fan-shaped acoustic shadowing; (B) Edge shadows as indicated by the arrow.

as >/<50% of the total uterus body length. Ant/ post/lateral/ fundal wall involvement is to be mentioned like localized lesion.

Myometrial heterogenicities: Myometrial echogenicity is called to be heterogeneous either in presence of localized lesion or in presence of myometrial cysts (**Fig. 18A**), hyperechoic islands (**Fig. 24**), hyperechogenic lines (**Fig. 18B**)/dots. These are most often found in the adenomyosis, but may be seen in certain chronic inflammations, postsurgical, vascular abnormalities, etc.

Myometrial cysts: These are anechoic well defined, mostly rounded lesions. The contents may be anechoic, may have low level echogenicities, ground glass echogenicities, or mixed echogenicities. One must mention the number of cysts, locations, and largest diameters of the largest cyst. When these are distributed widely, walls that are involved and the upper, middle, or lower third of the body and whether it is involving >/<50% of the myometrium. If multiple small cysts aggregate, it makes an anechoic lacuna, that may be irregular in shape.

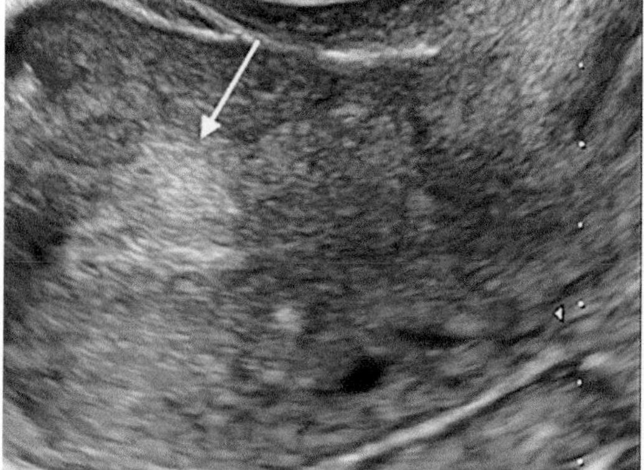

Fig. 24: Transvaginal ultrasound B-mode showing anteverted anteflexed uterus with hyperechoic localized area—hyperechoic island as marked by the arrow.

Hyperechoic islands: These are regular, irregular, or ill-defined hyperechoic areas. Same as for cysts, it is essential to mention the number of hyperechoic islands, size of the largest cyst, and location of each cyst. These are most commonly due to endometrial growth in the myometrium in patients with adenomyosis.

Hyperechoic lines and buds: Hyperechoic lines and buds are seen leading to irregularity or interruption of the JZ. These hyper echoic lines and buds are different from hyperechoic spots. These lines and buds are in continuity with the endometrium and are perpendicular to endometrium or not, needs a mention. These lines and buds affect anterior, posterior, right or left lateral or fundal JZ and what is the extent of the irregular or interrupted endometrium needs to be mentioned. If these are countable, their number needs to be mentioned.

The vascularity study gives more information on these lesions, but it is very essential to evaluate the myometrium on B-mode and adequately analyze it before vascularity studies are done.

DOPPLER STUDIES

The distribution of the vascularity is described as uniform if the entire lesion has uniformly distributed vascularity or nonuniform if it shows heterogeneous distribution of blood vessels in the lesion (**Figs. 25A and B**).

According to MUSA, the vascularity of the myometrial lesions can be scored as score 1—no color, 2—minimal vascularity, 3—moderate vascularity, and 4—abundant vascularity (**Figs. 26A to D**). Scoring is done, taking into consideration, the most vascular area of a

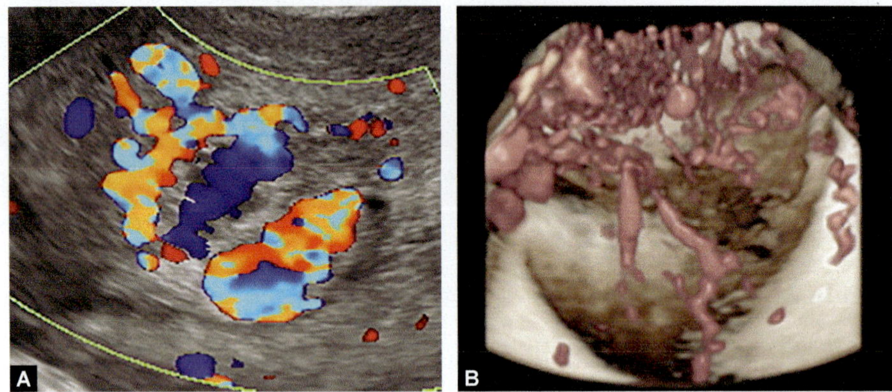

Figs. 25A and B: (A) Homogeneous distribution of the blood vessels in the myometrial lesion on color Doppler; (B) heterogeneous distribution of the blood vessels in the lesion on 3D power Doppler.

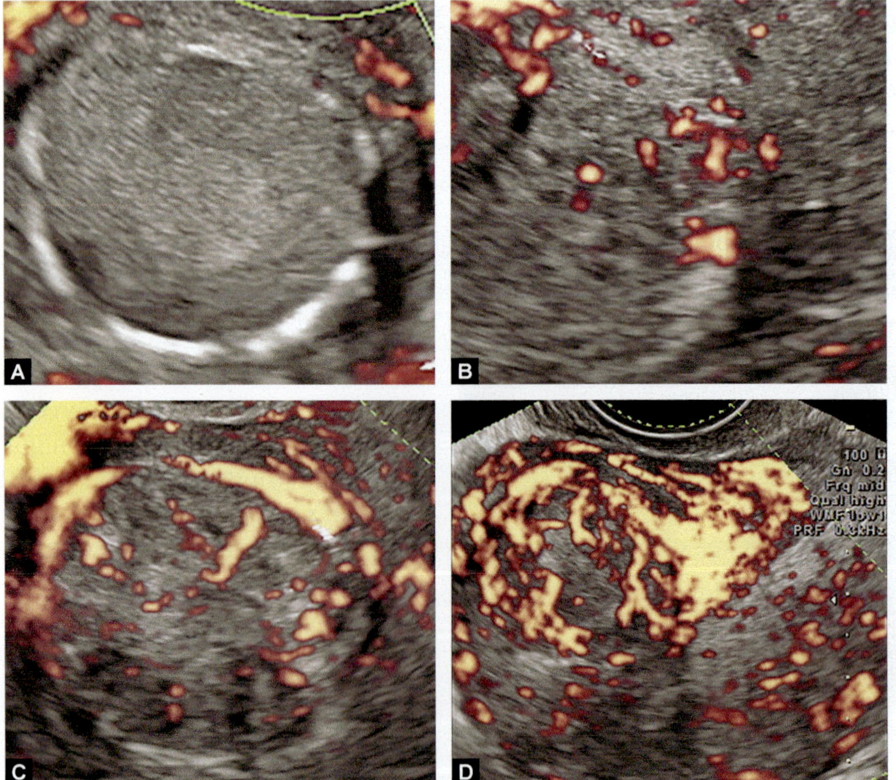

Figs. 26A to D: Vascular score of 1–4, as: (A) Score 1—no color; (B) Score 2—minimal vascularity; (C) Score 3—moderate vascularity; (D) Score 4—abundant vascularity.

lesion. In lesions that show heterogeneous vascular distribution, do mention what percentage of the solid component is vascular. Commonly found myometrial lesions may show circumferential (**Fig. 27A**), intralesional, both (**Fig. 27B**) or translesional (**Fig. 27C**) vascularity. Circumferential is a peripheral vascularity of a lesion (like seen in a fibroid). The vessels that are seen in the lesion are intralesional vessels. Lesions like degenerated fibroids may show both circumferential and intralesional vascularity. Lesions like adenomyosis will show vessels traversing perpendicular to the uterine cavity/serosa crossing the lesion. These are described as translesional vessels.

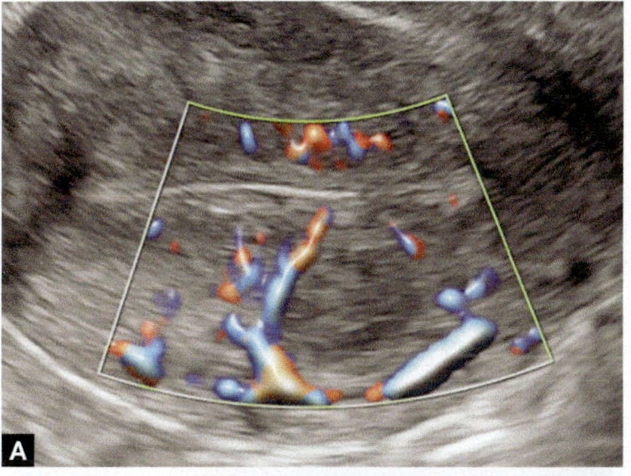

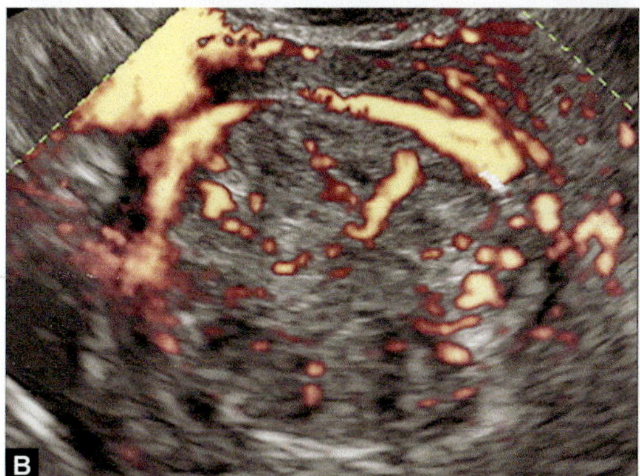

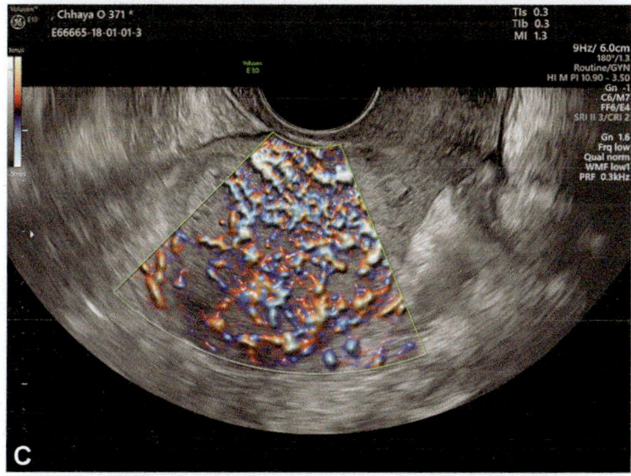

Figs. 27A to C: (A) Circumferential vascularity in a fibroid as seen on high-definition (HD) flow; (B) Circumferential and intralesional vascularity in a fibroid as seen on power Doppler; (C) Translesional vascularity in adenomyosis as seen on HD flow.

Further description about the vessels that can be studied by Doppler is the number of vessels (single/multiple), diameter of vessels as compared to normal myometrial vessels (large/ small), whether all vessels in the lesion have an equal diameter (**Fig. 28A**) or they vary in diameter. It is essential to specifically mention whether the variability in diameter is seen in individual vessels also or is seen in different vessels. This may be reported as abnormal tortuous vessels, irregular caliber, when individual vessel shows variability in caliber (**Fig. 28B**).

The branching pattern of the vessels is especially different in benign and malignant lesions and so documenting the regular/ irregular branching pattern is important. Branching pattern of vessels in malignant lesions are typically described as lack of hierarchy in branching, varying branching angles, and chaotic vessel pattern.

The reporting should include:

- Size
- Symmetry of myometrial walls
- Echogenecity
- Junctional zone—regular, irregular, ill-defined
- Extent and magnitude of irregularity
- *Lesion*: Well defined/ill defined, number, location, size, maximum diameter, echogenecity of the lesion (cysts, hyperechoic islands, buds, lines, spots, shadowing)
- *Mapping* of lesions
- *Vascularity*—Pattern, score, branching pattern, number of vessels, diameter

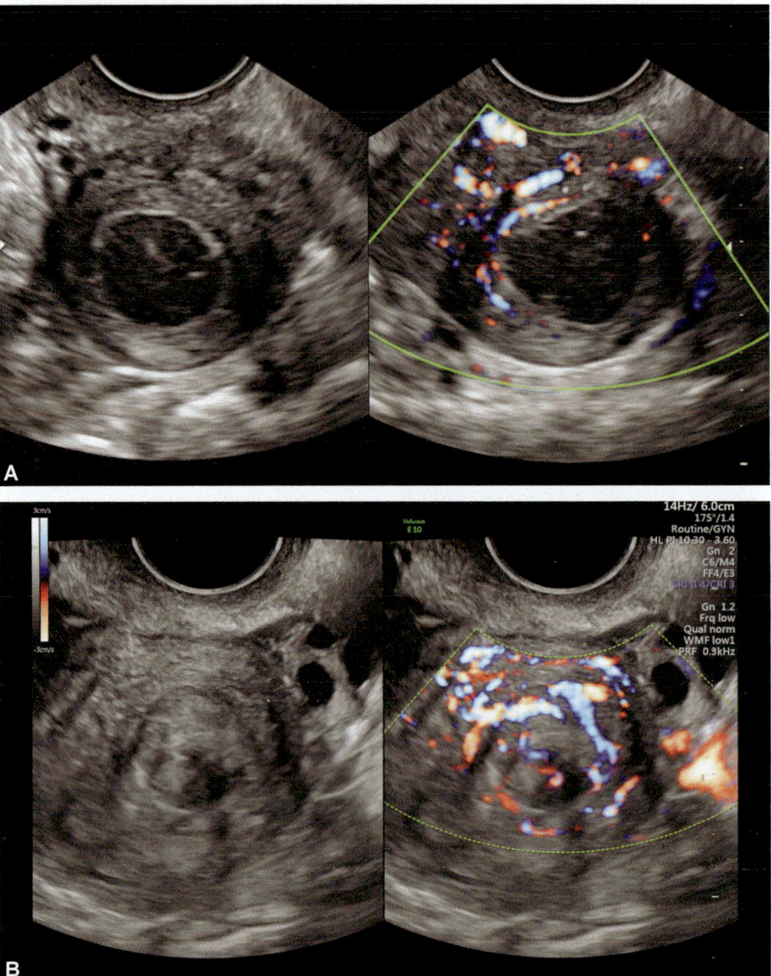

Figs. 28A and B: (A) All vessels in the lesion showing almost equal diameter on HD flow; (B) Abnormal tortuous vessels, irregular caliber, when individual vessel shows variability in caliber as seen on power Doppler.

- *If the lesion is present, is it relevant to the symptoms.*

Keeping into consideration the descriptive terms discussed, let us now look into the ultrasound presentation of common myometrial lesions, with special consideration on their Doppler findings.

Myometrial lesions commonly seen are fibroids, adenomyosis, adenomyomas, and leiomyosarcomas. Fibroids and adenomyosis are among the most common pathologies found in patients presenting with various gynecological complaints and also with infertility.

ADENOMYOSIS

Adenomyosis is an ectopic growth of endometrium into the myometrium, and is common in multiparous women. But it is seen in women with a history of any obstetric event or any surgical procedure disturbing the endometrium. Pathologically, adenomyosis is defined as endometrial glands and stroma in the myometrium of half of one low-power field beneath the endomyometrial junction. Adenomyosis is often an incidental finding on ultrasound. But these patients may present with menorrhagia, metrorrhagia, pelvic pain, dysmenorrhea, and dyspareunia. Patients with adenomyosis often present with infertility and one of the major causes for this is inadequate endometrial receptivity. This may be due to physical compression effect and thickened endometrium, but may also be due to inadequate development of estrogen receptors due to altered vascularity. Pathologies such as leiomyomas (6–28%) and endometrial hyperplasia may coexist with adenomyosis. On clinical examination, the uterus feels bulky and is tender on palpation.

On ultrasound: Depending on the severity of the adenomyosis, the uterus may or may not appear bulky. It may cause symmetrical or asymmetrical thickening of myometrium. Adenomyosis may be diffuse and focal.[3]

The affected myometrium shows a coarse heterogeneous echogenicity. Heterogeneous echogenicity has a sensitivity of 88% for diagnosis of adenomyosis[3] (**Fig. 29**).

The endometrial tissue that proliferates inside the myometrium tends to bleed on progesterone withdrawal during menstrual cycle. This gives the uterus a typically speckled appearance resembling "salt and pepper" (hyperechoic areas and hypoechoic areas)[4] (**Fig. 30**). Adenomyosis presents with alternate hyper and hypoechoic zones, typically described as "rain in forest" or a "vanishing blind" appearance of the myometrium (**Fig. 31**).

Anechoic irregular cystic spaces of 5–7 mm in diameter will disrupt the homogeneous echo pattern of the myometrium (**Fig. 32**). These are myometrial cysts. Myometrial cysts have 98% specificity and 78% accuracy for diagnosis of adenomyosis. The myometrial cysts typically have hyperechoic margins. This probably is the active endometrial tissue. These echogenic flecks seen at the endometrial-myometrial junction are collapsed myometrial cysts. Hyperechoic areas in myometrium may be due to fresh bleed or collapsed endometrial cavities. In some cases, hyperechoic spots or areas are also seen in the subendometrial myometrium and these may be islands of

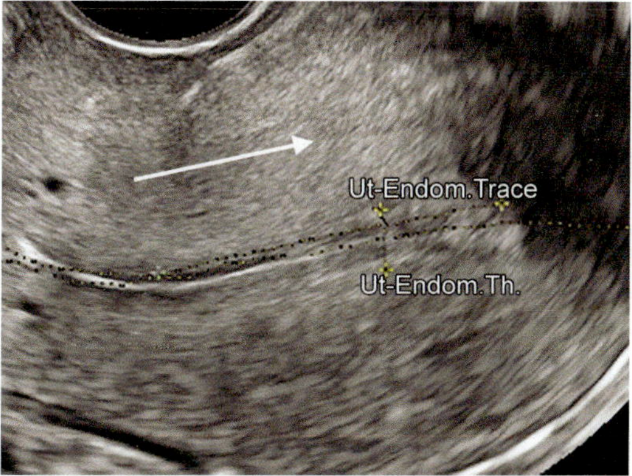

Fig. 30: "Salt and pepper" appearance of adenomyosis as seen on transvaginal B-mode ultrasound of the uterus, marked by arrow.

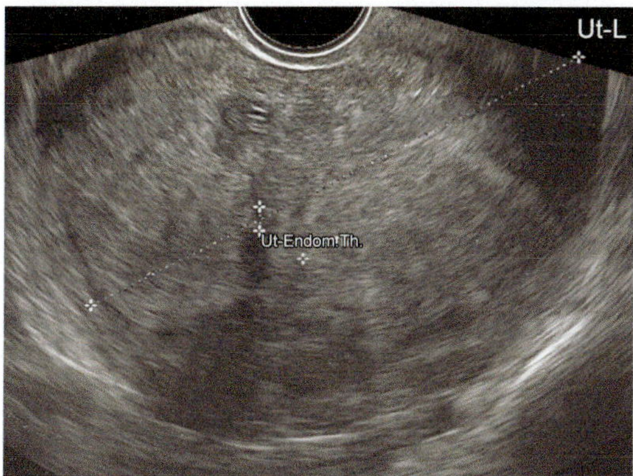

Fig. 29: Heterogeneous myometrial echogenicity of adenomyosis as seen on B-mode transvaginal ultrasound.

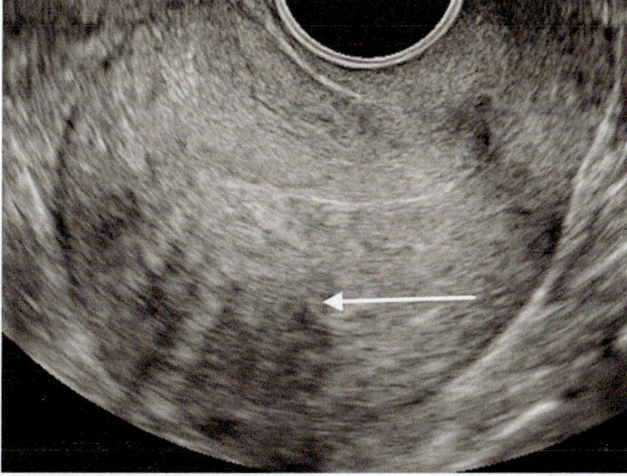

Fig. 31: "Rain in forest" or "vanishing blind" appearance of adenomyosis as seen on transvaginal B-mode ultrasound of the uterus, marked by arrow.

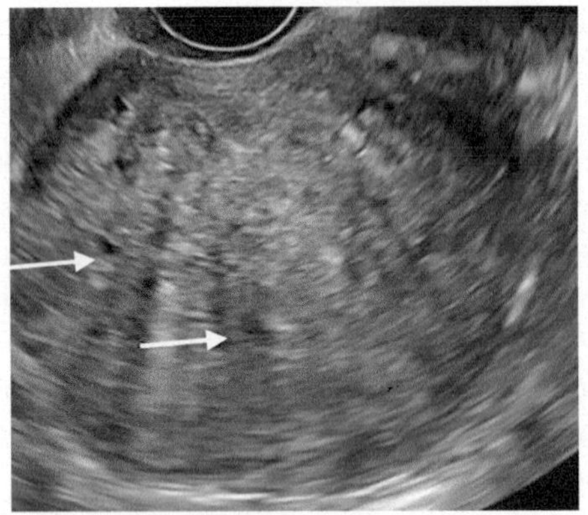

Fig. 32: Myometrial cysts (as marked by arrows) are seen in the heterogeneous adenomyotic myometrium.

active endometrial tissue. These may be named as endometrial buds. Fan-shaped acoustic shadowing is typical of adenomyosis (**Fig. 33**).

Typically the myometrium shows alteration in the echogenicity depending on the phase of the menstrual cycle. Adenomyosis being an invasive lesion has indistinct margins.

Junctional zone is irregular or interrupted and in severe cases may also be inaccessible. High-resolution ultrasound now can show the endometrial strands extending into the myometrium, interrupting the JZ (**Fig. 34A to C**).

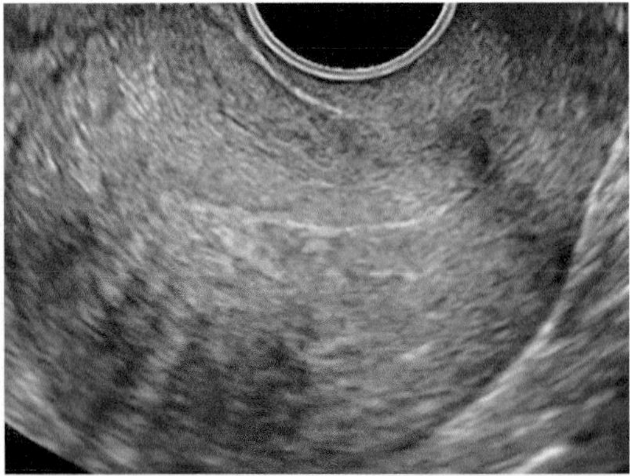

Fig. 33: "Fan-shaped acoustic shadowing of adenomyosis as seen on transvaginal B-mode ultrasound of the uterus.

Adenomyotic uteri may commonly show an abnormal curvature of the fundal endometrial cavity, in a direction opposite to the normal direction of the fundus (**Fig. 35**). This is described as question mark sign of the uterus.[5]

The more difficult situation is the adenomyoma. This is a localized adenomyosis, with heterogeneous echogenicity and less defined margins, and so is difficult to differentiate from degenerated fibroid as this also has heterogeneous echogenicity. But the main differentiating points between the adenomyoma and the fibroid are capsular vascularity seen in the fibroid with intralesional vascularity, that is never seen in adenomyoma (**Fig. 36**), edge shadows along with fan-shaped shadows, displacement of but intact JZ, whereas adenomyoma shows translesional vascularity, no edge shadows, and irregularity or disruption of JZ.

On color Doppler: Affected myometrium shows markedly increased vascularity with vascular dilatation (**Fig. 37**). These vessels have resistance index (RI) of 0.56 ± 0.12. Diameter of these vessels is larger than those of normal myometrium.[6]

Vascularity in adenomyosis is a penetrating type—translesional in distribution as described earlier. Decreased uterine artery resistance and increased velocity is also noted.

Though *sonohysterography* is not a routine investigation for adenomyosis, if done by chance, it shows contrast (negative or positive), percolating into the myometrium.

Endometrial strands extending into myometrium are also seen on *3D US*. When seen on *3D power Doppler* also a vascular fibroid shows circumferentially arranged blood vessels, while in adenomyoma the vascular arrangement is radial or penetrating (**Figs. 38A and B**). It is the JZ assessment that was not adequately possible with B-mode ultrasound always. For these reasons MRI (magnetic resonance imaging) was considered

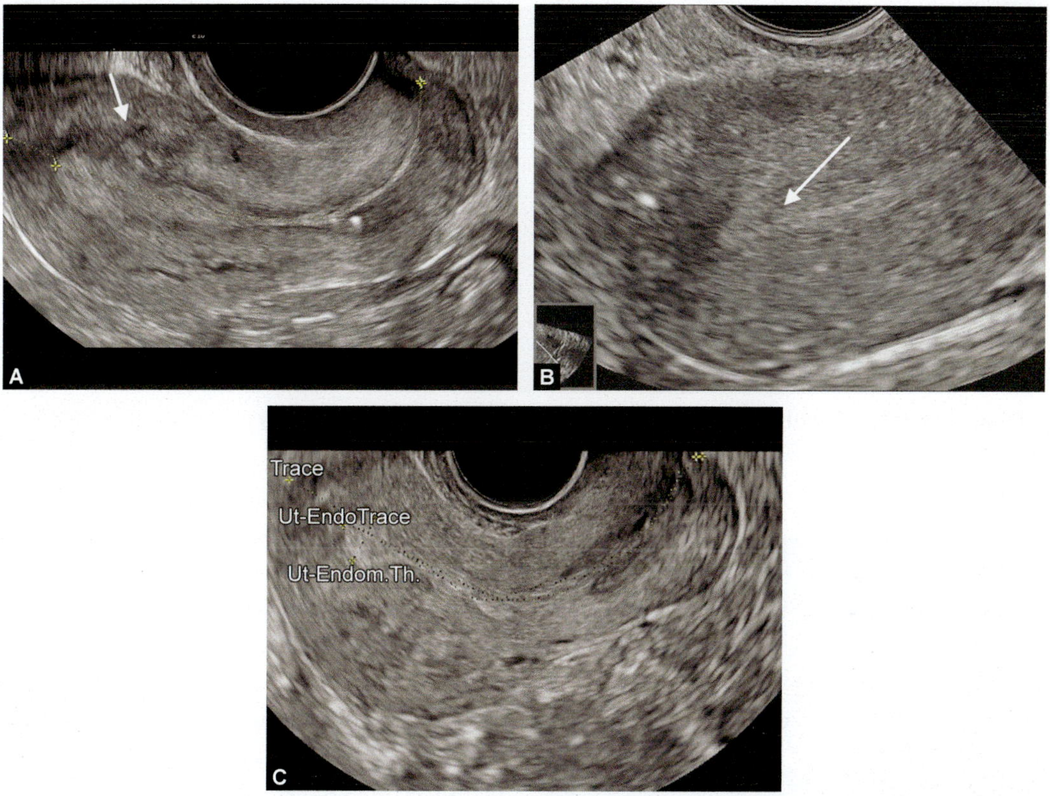

Figs. 34A to C: Transvaginal ultrasound B-mode showing anteverted anteflexed uterus, midsagittal section of the uterus with irregular endometrial–myometrial junction on the anterior aspect (arrow); (B) Transvaginal ultrasound B-mode showing anteverted anteflexed uterus, midsagittal section of the uterus with interrupted endometrial–myometrial junction on the anterior aspect due to endometrial strands extending into myometrium (arrow); (C) Transvaginal ultrasound B-mode showing anteverted anteflexed uterus, midsagittal section of the uterus with inaccessible endometrial–myometrial junction.

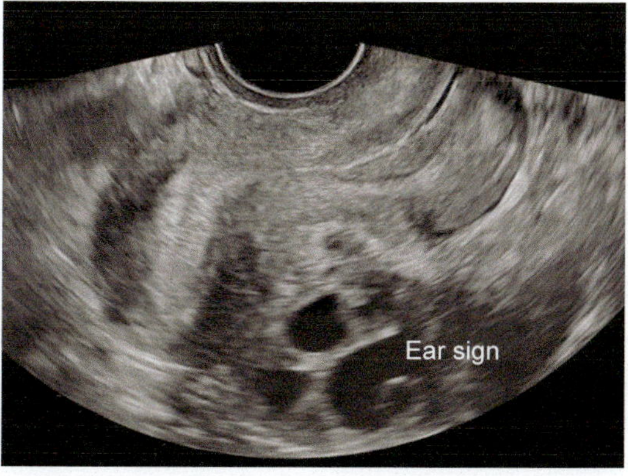

Fig. 35: Transvaginal ultrasound B-mode showing anteverted anteflexed uterus, midsagittal section of the uterus with question mark sign.

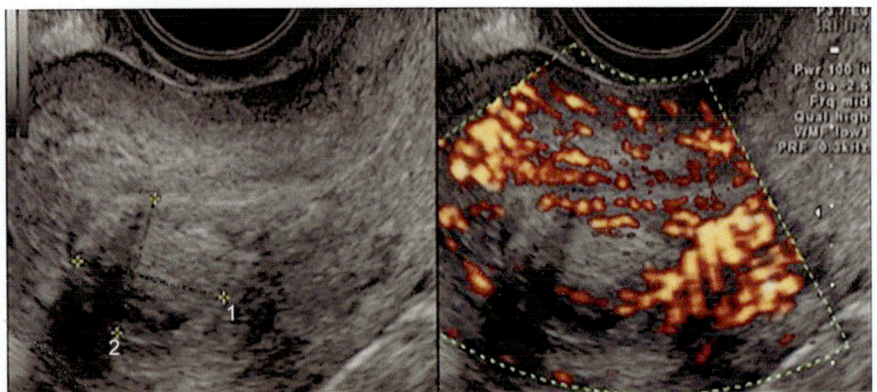

Fig. 36: Absence of circumferential vascularity and only intralesional vascularity in adenomyoma seen as a localized ill-defined lesion on B-mode.

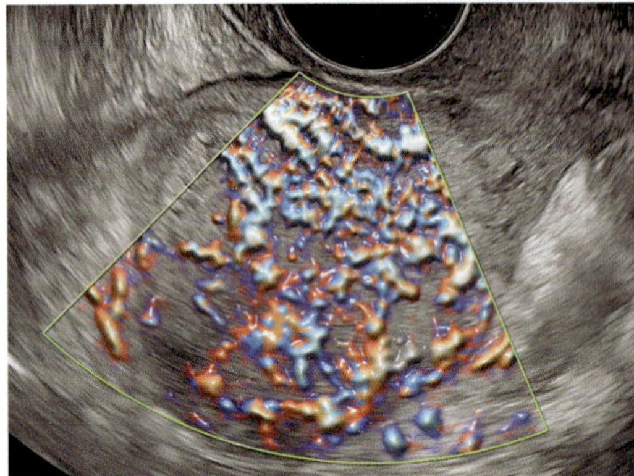

Fig. 37: HD flow showing translesional vascularity with nonparallel arrangement and increased diameter of the blood vessels (than the normal spiral vessels) in adenomyosis.

as an imaging modality for adenomyosis. Difference in the JZ thickness at two different places around the endometrium of >4 mm or a JZ thickness of 12 mm has 88% sensitivity and 85% accuracy for the diagnosis of adenomyosis.[7] Three-dimensional TVS markers:[7,8] JZ (JZ) difference >4 mm and JZ infiltration and distortion have been proved as highly sensitive markers for the diagnosis of adenomyosis (**Fig. 39**).

Elastography is a modality of ultrasound that measures tissue strain. This is useful for differentiating myometrial lesions, though it is more commonly used for differentiating benign from malignant lesions in breast, liver, and other organs. Elastography may be qualitative or quantitative. Qualitative elastography subjectively compares the stiffness/firmness of various tissues, whereas quantitative elastography may measure the firmness objectively.

The tissues with different firmness are seen in different colors of the light spectrum. Blue side of this spectrum demonstrates hard or firm tissues and red side of the spectrum demonstrates soft tissues (**Box 1**). For example, bowel appears red or yellow and myometrium shows uniform blue color. Fibroids are firmer (blue) than the myometrium and adenomyosis is softer (green). Elastography-based diagnosis is in excellent agreement with MRI[9] (**Fig. 40**).

Fibroid: Fibroids are found in 20–40% of women of >30 years of age and are more common in nulliparous. These are mostly an incidental finding, but may sometimes present with dysmenorrhea, menorrhagia, infertility, and pregnancy-related problems.

Fibroids affect fertility because of:

- Distortion of endometrial cavity due to submucous fibroid.
- Pressure of the fibroid and stretching of endometrium overlying it causing

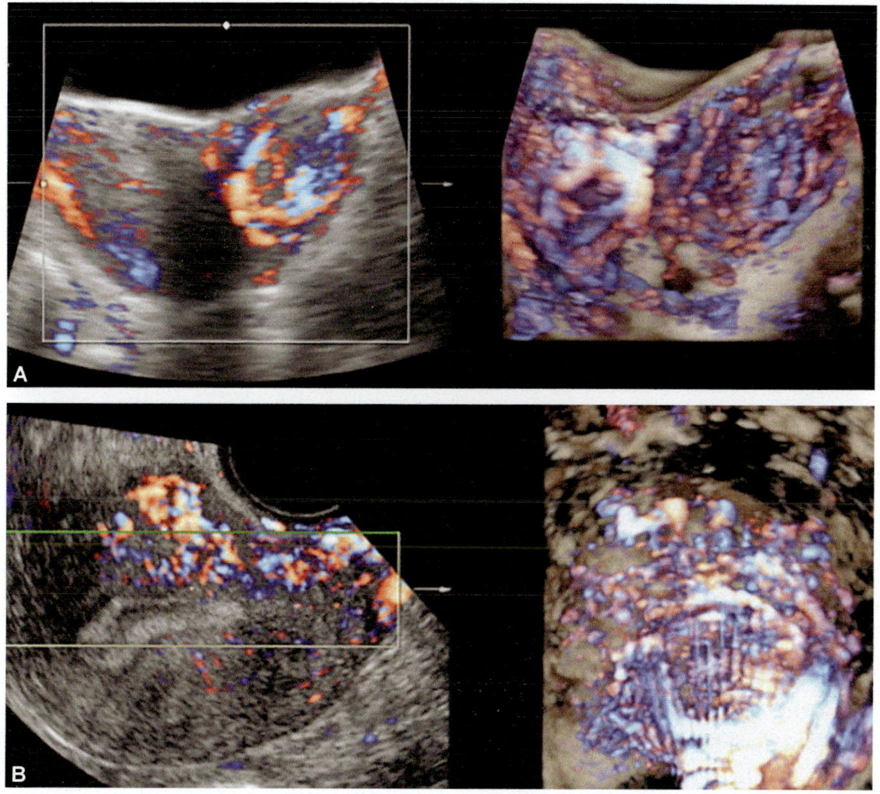

Figs. 38A and B: (A) 3D power Doppler showing vascular fibroid with circumferentially arranged blood vessels; (B) Adenomyoma showing penetrating vascular pattern.

atrophy of endometrial glands and stroma.

Buttram, et al. have shown in their study that fertility is chiefly affected by submucous fibroids due to altered uterine contractility,

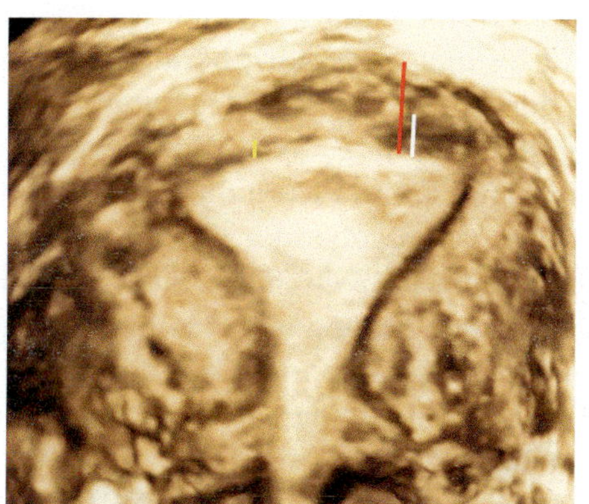

Fig. 39: Irregularity of the junctional zone in adenomyosis as seen on 3D ultrasound with the white line showing J_{max} and yellow line showing J_{min}.

BOX 1: Ultrasound features of adenomyosis.

- Generalized/localized thickening of myometrial wall
- Asymmetrical thickening of anterior and posterior myometrial wall
- Heterogeneous myometrium: Salt and pepper appearance
- "Rain in forest" or "venetian blind" appearance
- Fan-shaped acoustic shadowing
- Irregularity and interruption of endometrial-myometrial junctional zone
- Echogenic flecks, lines, and buds at junctional zone
- Myometrial cysts
- Endometrial strands penetrating into the myometrium
- Question mark sign
- Translesional vascularity
- Vessels with diameter larger than that of normal spiral vessels
- Abnormal orientation of myometrial vessels (chaotic arrangement)

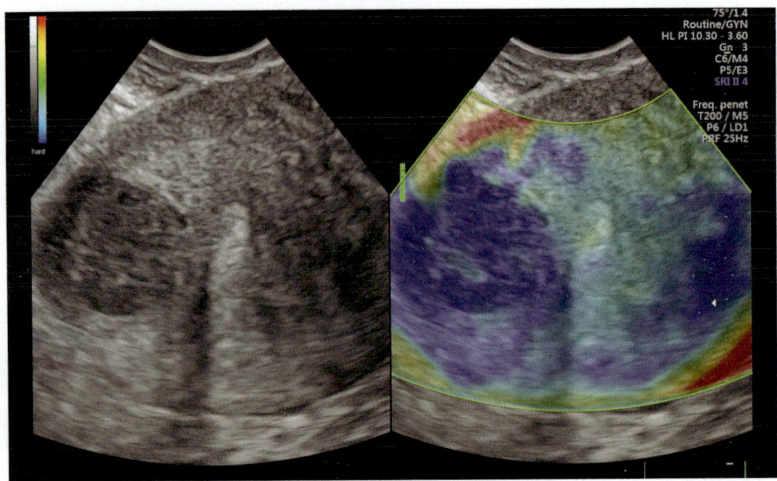

Fig. 40: Elastography showing blue colored fibroid indicating its firm consistency.

deranged cytokine profile, abnormal vascularization, and chronic endometrial inflammation.[10,11] These are benign tumors of myometrial and fibrous tissue origin, arising from the smooth muscle of uterine fundus and corpus. Fibroids are known to have a genetic basis and also have a familial distribution or a hereditary transmission. Loss of tumor suppressor genes may be one of the causes. Estrogen and progesterone appear to promote the growth of fibroids as these have more estrogen and progesterone receptors as compared to normal myometrial tissue. Insulin-like growth factor may also affect the growth of the fibroid.

These may be seen in a variety of locations in the uterus. Depending on their location in relation to myometrium, endometrium, or serosa, these are classified as types subendometrial and subserosal and intramural fibroids.

Subserosal and intramural fibroids were further classified as:

- Type 0: Pedunculated subserosal fibroid
- Type 1: Involvement of <50% of the outer uterine wall
- Type 2: >50% of the myometrial wall
- Type 3: Fibroids extending from mucosa to serosa

Submucosal fibroids were further classified as:[12]
Type 0: If they are pedunculated and 100% in the cavity (**Fig. 41A**).

- Type 1: If the fibroid is >50% in cavity (**Fig. 41B**).
- Type 2: If less than 50% is protruding in the cavity (**Fig. 41C**).

But according to the new FIGO (International Federation of Gynecologists and Obstetricians) classification, that is more commonly used now, fibroids are classified into eight types[2] (**Fig. 42 and Table 1**).

ON ULTRASOUND

On ultrasound fibroid appears as well-defined, hypoechoic, homogeneous, round/oval, solid lesions, with peripheral hypoechoic rim due to displacement of myometrial fibers (**Fig. 43**). When large and especially subserosal or intramural they distort the serosal surface, whereas when subendometrial they distort the endometrial cavity. Fibroids typically show edge shadows along with the linear stripes like fan-shaped acoustic shadowing (**Fig. 44**). Echogenicity increases with increasing amount of fibrous tissue and vascularity.

Degeneration in fibroids leads to heterogenicity of texture and may become hyperechoic (**Fig. 45**). Cystic degeneration

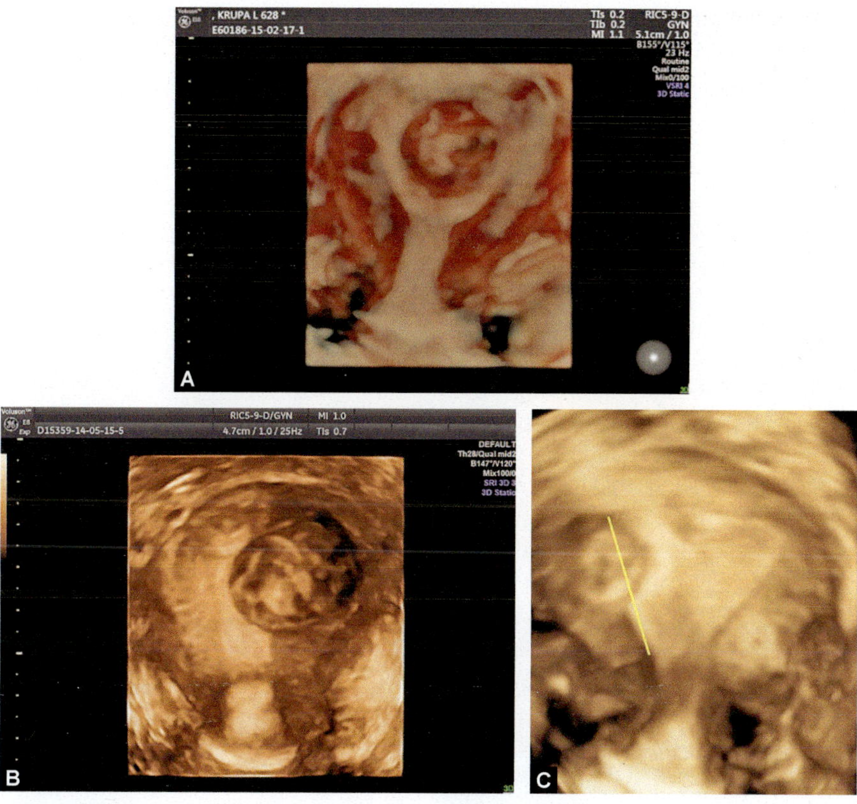

Figs. 41A to C: Submucous fibroids, type 0, 1, and 2 demonstrated on 3D ultrasound on coronal section in (A), (B), and (C), respectively.

leads to anechoic spaces in the fibroid (**Fig. 46**). Red degeneration is the most common form of degeneration in fibroids with pregnancy though red degeneration is not easily diagnosed on ultrasound. When the fibroid undergoes an acute degeneration, patient may present with marked pain, sometimes vomiting and fever and the fibroid shows increase in size. Calcification may be seen in fibroids as hyperechoic (++) areas with posterior shadowing (**Fig. 47**). When uterine artery embolization is done for fibroids, air may be seen in the fibroids as hyperechoic areas with comet shadows.

Fig. 42: Diagrammatic demonstration of types of fibroid according to FIGO classification.

Correct localization of the fibroid on imaging is essential for better planning of the surgery. That is why fibroid mapping is an essential part of reporting a fibroid. This is especially important when there are multiple fibroids. Mapping can be correctly done by survey of the uterus in longitudinal and transverse axis by sweeping across the entire uterus in sagittal and transverse planes on B-mode and also by the use of 3D for assessing the correct location on the coronal plane. In cases with multiple fibroids, when the endometrium is

TABLE 1: Types of fibroid according to FIGO classification.

SM -Submucosal	0	Pedunculated intracavitary
	1	<50% intramural
	2	≥50% intramural
0–Other	3	Contacts endometrium; 100% intramural
	4	Intramural
	5	Subserosal ≥50% intramural
	6	Subserosal <50% intramural
	7	Subserosal pedunculated
	8	Other (secify, e.g., cervical, arasitic)
Hybrid leiomyomas (impact both endometrium and serosa)	Two numbers are listed separated by a hyphen. By convention, the first refers to the relationship with the endometrium while the second refers to the relationship to the serosa. One example is below:	
	2–5	Submucosal and subserosal, each with less than half the diameter in the endometrial and peritoneal cavities, respectively.

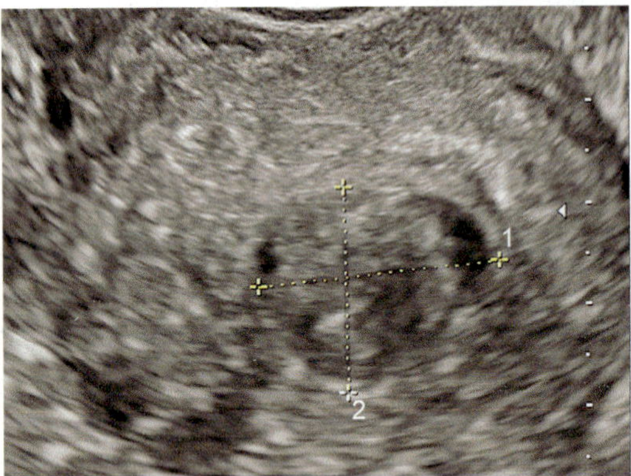

Fig. 43: Round well-defined isoechoic lesion is seen in the myometrium with hypoechoic margins—fibroid, on B-mode transvaginal ultrasound.

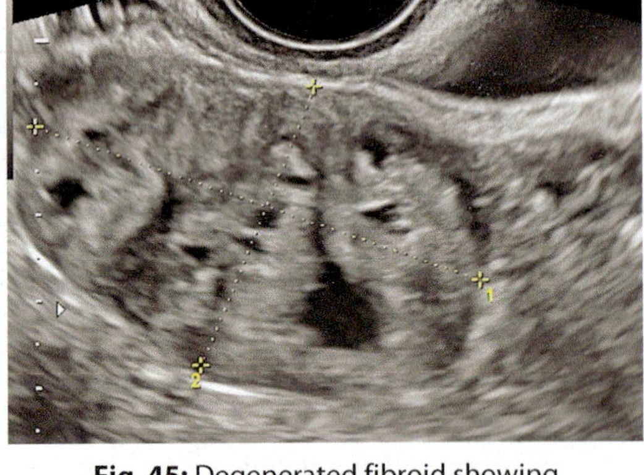

Fig. 45: Degenerated fibroid showing heterogeneous echogenicity.

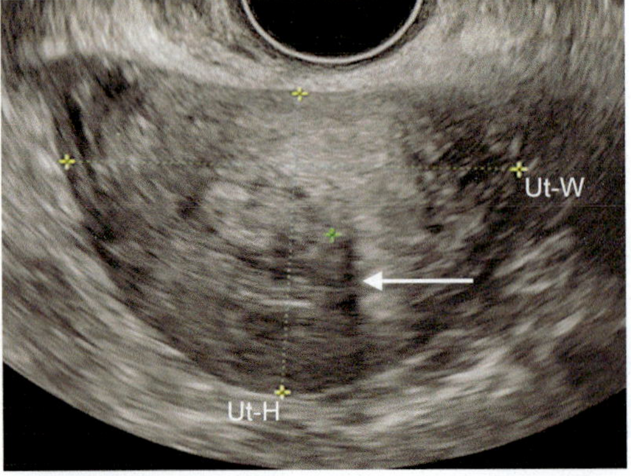

Fig. 44: Arrow showing edge shadow of fibroid on B-mode transvaginal ultrasound.

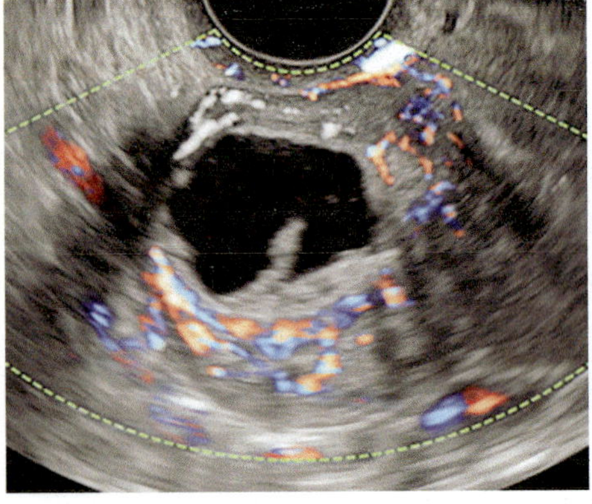

Fig. 46: Cystic degeneration of the fibroid seen as anechoic center with HD flow showing circumferential flow.

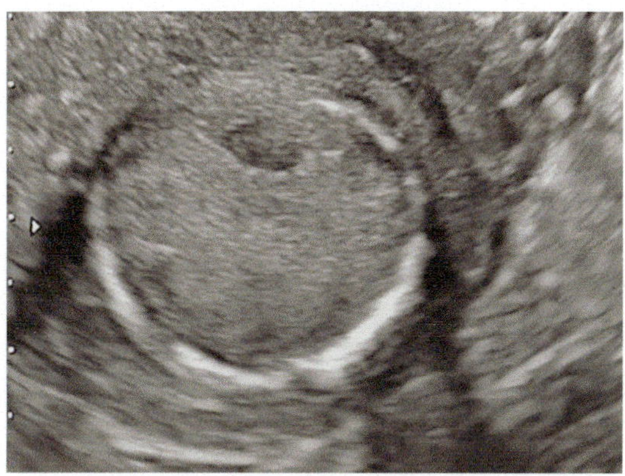

Fig. 47: B-mode transvaginal ultrasound showing fibroid with a calcified rim.

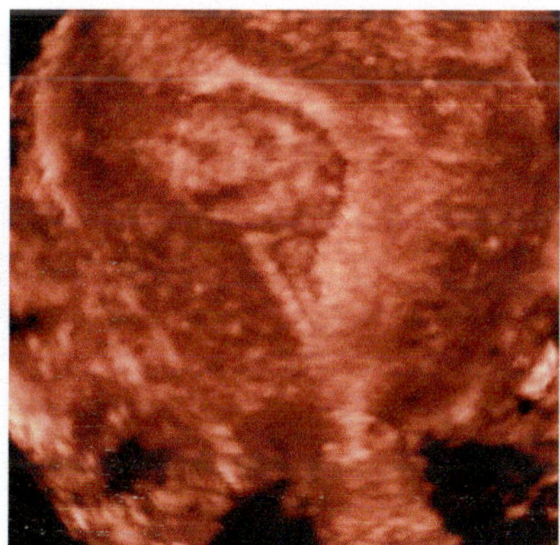

Fig. 48: 3D ultrasound of the uterus showing coronal section of the uterus, with a submucous fibroid showing ill-defined margin on its myometrial surface.

also grossly distorted, establishing the correct location of these fibroids may be difficult and then the endometrial line may be traced from the cervical canal to cephalad. Along with the written report, hand drawn diagram of the uterus with position of fibroids in midsagittal plane, mid coronal plane, and transverse plane is essential (**Fig. 48**).

The correct location of the fibroid can be defined by:

- Its position in the uterus—involving upper, middle, or lower part of the body of the uterus or the cervix
- Involving anterior, posterior, or right/left lateral walls
- Its position/penetration according to the FIGO classification
- Its size—preferably three orthogonal diameters
- Its distance from the endometrium or from the serosa to which ever wall it is closer.

ON DOPPLER

Peripheral vascularity is typical of a fibroid (**Fig. 27A**). These vessels are vessels of displaced muscle fibers and therefore show a resistance index (RI) of 0.54 ± 0.08,[13] similar to that of normal myometrial vessels. Resistance is higher in submucosal fibroids and deep intramural fibroids compared to subserosal fibroids but lower compared to submucosal fibroids. This variability is because of the compression effect of the muscle fibers on the fibroid and therefore on the surrounding vessels. Fibroids with degeneration show intralesional vascularity with low resistance flow and a vascular score of 2–3 (**Fig. 27B**). In addition to the peripheral vascularity, amount of vascularity decides the activity or growth potential of a fibroid. Malignant change leading to leiomyosarcoma shows a resistance as low as 0.37 ± 0.03 RI, with rapid growth in size and disruption of well-defined margins (**Fig. 48**). But resistance indices of vessels cannot be used as only evidence for malignant change, because it is equally low in degenerating fibroid also. In fact even on B-mode ultrasound due to the heterogenicity being a common finding in degenerating as well as malignant fibroid, it is not possible to confidently diagnose a leiomyosarcoma on B-mode or color Doppler. Uteri with fibroids also show higher uterine artery peak velocity and lower RI (mean: 0.74 ± 0.09).[14]

VOLUME ULTRASOUND

Volume ultrasound is especially useful in fibroids to find the relationship of fibroids to the endometrium and assess the distortion or invasion of the endometrium with the fibroid as it can evaluate the lesion in three orthogonal planes. Sonohysterography with saline combined with 3D ultrasound may demonstrate the distortion of the endometrial cavity by submucosal fibroids better.[14,15]

3D power Doppler indices—vascularization index (VI), flow index (FI), and vascularization flow index (VFI) are especially useful for follow-up of fibroids in patients who are on GnRha therapy, menopausal, or pregnant.

Fibroids reporting should include:

- Homogeneous/heterogeneous
- Well defined
- Number
- Location, size, site, penetration
- Mapping
- Vascularity—circumferential, equal diameter homogeneous/heterogeneous distribution
- Red, hyaline, cystic/myxoid or hydropic degeneration
- It is important to have a standard report format for any scan that first describes the ultrasound features of a lesion/organ and then derives the diagnosis.

It is important to have a standard report format for any scan that first describes the ultrasound features of a lesion/organ and then derives the diagnosis.

Diffuse leiomyomatosis is a rare condition in which there is diffuse and uniform involvement of entire myometrium by multiple fibroids (**Fig. 49**).

Fibroids are also seen arising from the cervix and show similar appearances as fibroid in the uterus (**Fig. 50**).

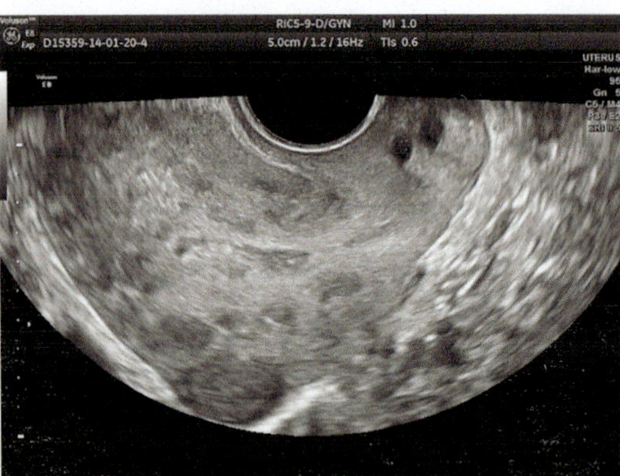

Fig. 49: Multiple fibroids (myomas) spread across the entire uterus leiomyomatosis.

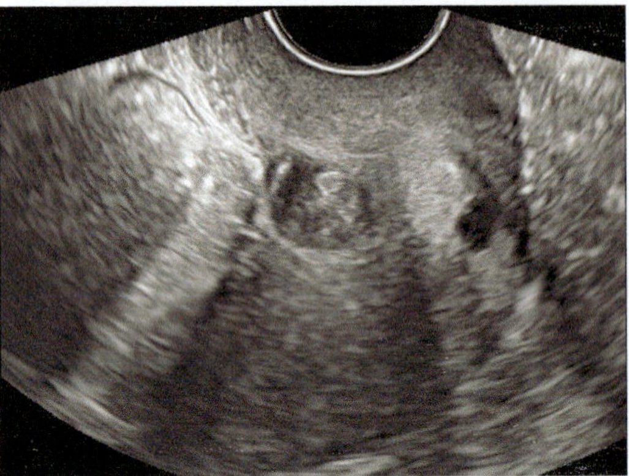

Fig. 50: 2D ultrasound image shows a round hypoechoic lesion in the cervix—cervical fibroid.

DISSEMINATED PERITONEAL LEIOMYOMATOSIS

This is a very rare condition. There are several nodules of smooth muscle seen scattered throughout the peritoneum. It may occur due to seeding during surgeries, especially laparoscopic morcellation. Multiple lesions may distort the pelvic anatomy and therefore lead to symptoms. But may also occur spontaneously at times. It is associated with elevated estrogen levels. According to another hypothesis, it is also thought to be due to metaplasia of subperitoneal mesenchymal cells.[16] Diameter of the lesions may vary from 0.1 to 10 cm. These lesions appear to have estrogen and progesterone receptors and also LH receptors.[17,18]

BENIGN METASTASIZING LEIOMYOMA

In the uterus, it appears like a typical fibroid, but similar lesion may be seen in the lungs and may lead to deterioration of lung function. Oophorectomy may treat the condition. Lung lesions are also seen in another fibroid-like composition called lymphangioleiomyomatosis and this is more serious condition, has a genetic origin.

CONCLUSION

The most common myometrial lesions are adenomyosis and fibroid. Though on B-mode ultrasound, these have certain overlapping features. Doppler is diagnostic for these, due to typical intralesional and peripheral vascularity, respectively.

REFERENCES

1. Van den Bosch T, Dueholm M, Leone FPG, Valentin L, Rasmussen CK, Votino A, et al. Terms, definitions and measurements to describe sonographic features of myometrium and uterine masses: a consensus opinion from the Morphological Uterus Sonographic Assessment (MUSA) group. Ultrasound Obstet Gynecol. 2015;46(5):284-98.
2. Munro MG, Critchley HOD, Broder MS, Frase IS. FIGO classification system (PALM-COEIN) for causes of abnormal uterine bleeding in nongravid women of reproductive age. Int J Gynecol Obstet. 2011;113:3-13.
3. Raine-Fenning N, Jayaprakasan K, Deb S. Three-dimensional ultrasonographic characteristics of endometriomata. Ultrasound Obstet Gynecol. 2008;31:718-24.
4. Aleem F, Pennisi J, Zeitoum K, Predanic M. The role of color Doppler in diagnosis of endometriomas. Ultrasound Obstet Gynecol. 1995;5:51-4.
5. Di Donato N, Bertoldo V, Montanari G, Zannoni L, Caprara G, Seracchioli R. Question mark form of uterus: a simple sonographic sign associated with presence of adenomyosis. Ultrasound Obstet Gynecol. 2015;46(1):126-8.
6. Perrot N, Frey I, Mergui JL, Bazot M, Uzan M, Uzan S. Picture of the month. Adenomyosis: power Doppler findings. Ultrasound Obstet Gynecol. 2001;17(2):177-8.
7. Exacoustos C, Brienza L, Di Giovanni A, Szabolcs B, Romanini ME, Zupi E, et al. Adenomyosis: three-dimensional sonographic findings of the junctional zone and correlation with histology. Ultrasound Obstet Gynecol. 2011;37: 471-9.
8. Kupesic S, Kurjak A, Pasalic L, Benic S, Llijas M. The value of transvaginal colour Doppler in the assessment of pelvic inflammatory disease. Ultrasound Med Biol. 1995;21(6);733-8.
9. Stoelinga B, Hehenkamp WJK, Brolmann, HAM, Huirne JAF. Real-time elastography for assessment of uterine disorders. Ultrasound Obstet Gynecol. 2014;43:218-26.
10. Buttram VC Jr, Reiter R. Uterine lieomyomata: etiology, symptomatology and management. Fertil Steril. 1981:36:433-45.
11. Taylor E, Gomel V. The uterus and fertility. Fertil Steril. 2008;89:1-16.
12. Wamsteker K, de Blok S. Resection of intrauterine fibroids In: Lewis BV, Magos AL (Eds). Endometrial Ablation. Edinburgh, UK: Churchill Livingstone; 1993.
13. Kurjak A, Kupesic S, Miric D. The assessment of benign uterine tumour vascularization by transvaginal colour Doppler. Ultrasound Med Biol. 1992;18:645-9.
14. Balen FG, Allen CM, Gardener JE, Siddle NC, Lees WR. 3-dimensional reconstruction of ultrasound images of the uterine cavity. Br J Radiol. 1993; 66(787):588-91.
15. Weinraub Z, Maymon R, Shulman A, Bukovsky J, Kratochwil A, Lee A, et al. Three dimensional saline contrast hysterosonography and surface rendering of uterine cavity pathology. Ultrasound Obstet Gynecol. 1996;8(4):277-82.
16. Drake A, Dhundee J, Buckley CH, Woolas R. Disseminated leiomyomatosis peritonealis in association with oestrogen secreting ovarian fibrothecoma. BJOG. 2001;108(6):661-4.
17. Akkersdjik GJ, Flu PK, Giard RW, van Lent M, Wallenburg HC. Malignant leiomyomatosis peritonealis disseminata. Am J Obstet Gynecol. 1990;163(2):591-3.
18. Butnor KJ, Burchette JL, Robboy SJ. Progesterone receptor activity in leiomyomatosis peritonealis disseminata. Int J Gynecol Pathol. 1999;18(3): 259-64.

27

CHAPTER

Endometrial Lesions and Doppler

Sonal Panchal, Chaitanya Nagori

INTRODUCTION

Uterus is the central pelvic organ suspended by several ligaments. Endometrium is central in the uterus. It outlines the potential cavity of the uterus. It has cell rich connective tissue composed of superficial functional layer and deeper basal layer **(Fig. 1)**. It is the most dynamic anatomical structure in the uterus. In response to the hormonal changes during the menstrual cycle, the functional layer of the endometrium sheds off completely during the menstruation, then grows gradually during the proliferative phase under the effect of estrogen, gets compacted when exposed to progesterone, and then again under the effect of progesterone and estrogen in luteal phase grows to maximum till midluteal phase and then again starts regressing in a nonconception cycle to breakthrough during menstruation **(Fig. 2)**. Endometrium also has different appearances from neonatal life to menopause. Interestingly, the appearance of the endometrium is almost similar in the neonatal life and at menopause. The endometrium is thin and at times ill-defined and may also at times contain fluid in the cavity.

Endometrium is best evaluated on transvaginal scan during reproductive years, but a prior abdominal scan is recommended for evaluation of the pelvic anatomy.[1] In cases when transvaginal scan is not possible or denied by the patient, transrectal scan is

Fig. 1: Diagrammatic demonstration of the layers of uterine wall.

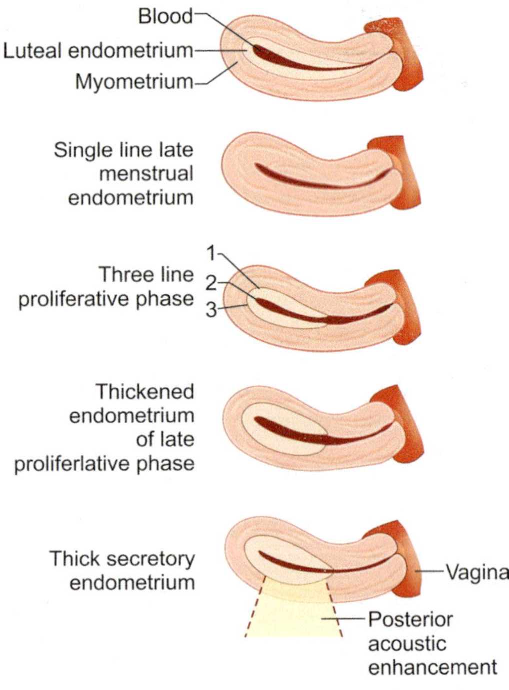

Fig. 2: Diagrammatic demonstration of the changing morphology of the endometrium during the menstrual cycle.

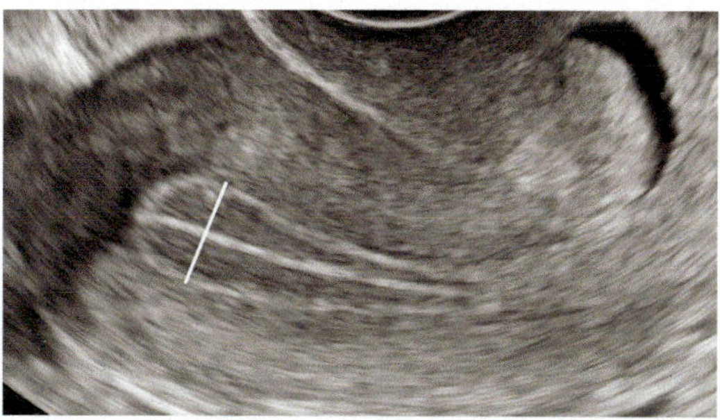

Fig. 3: Midsagittal section of the uterus showing endometrial measurement.

preferred to transabdominal route. Doppler must be used for assessment of the vascularity. Three-dimensional (3D) ultrasound is useful for evaluation of the coronal plane and is a modality with proved ability for assessment of the endometrial-myometrial junction.

Endometrial thickness is measured from outer margin of the hyperechoic line to the outer margin of the hyperechoic line, at the broadest part of the endometrium, perpendicular to the central line of the endometrium **(Fig. 3)**. Normal endometrium appears single line in early proliferative phase, multilayered in late proliferative and periovulatory phase, and hyperechoic in luteal phase.

Endometrial pathologies may be of inflammatory origin, may be due to abnormal response to hormones, or may be benign or malignant neoplasms.

But, before initiating the discussion on the endometrial lesions and their vascular patterns, it is essential to get acquainted with the standard terminology used worldwide. This is described under the International Endometrial Tumor Analysis (IETA) consensus.[2] It can be used to describe the endometrial appearance on B-mode ultrasound, on sonohysterography, and also on Doppler. There are specific terms used for description of each aspect of the endometrium. **Figures 4 to 8** illustrate the appearances with the text mentioned in the figures narrating the terms to be used.

INFLAMMATORY LESIONS

Endometrium is easily susceptible to infections because of its possibly easy access to infections through vagina and cervix. Inflammation of the endometrium may be related to

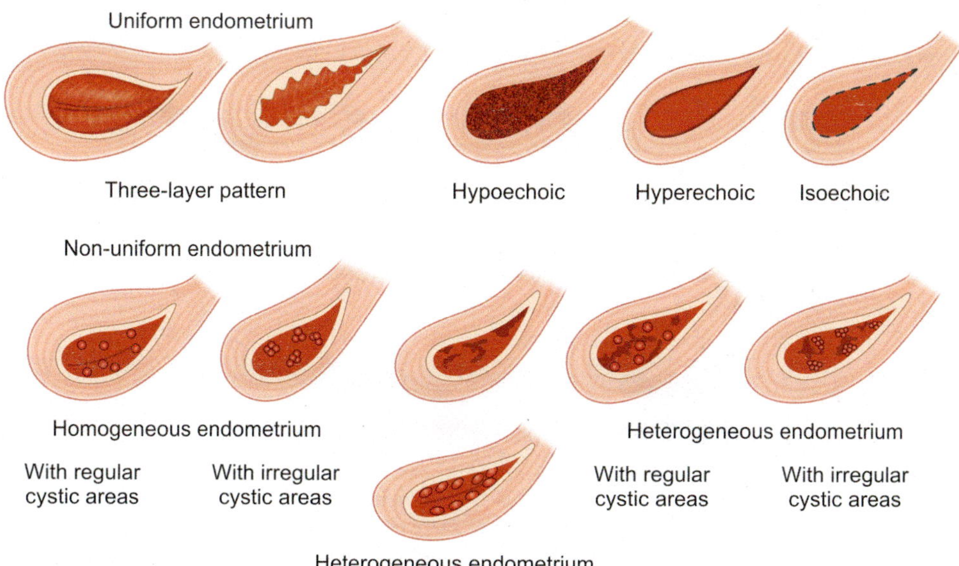

Fig. 4: Diagrammatic demonstration of the uniform and nonuniform endometrium on B mode—International Endometrial Tumor Analysis (IETA) terminology.

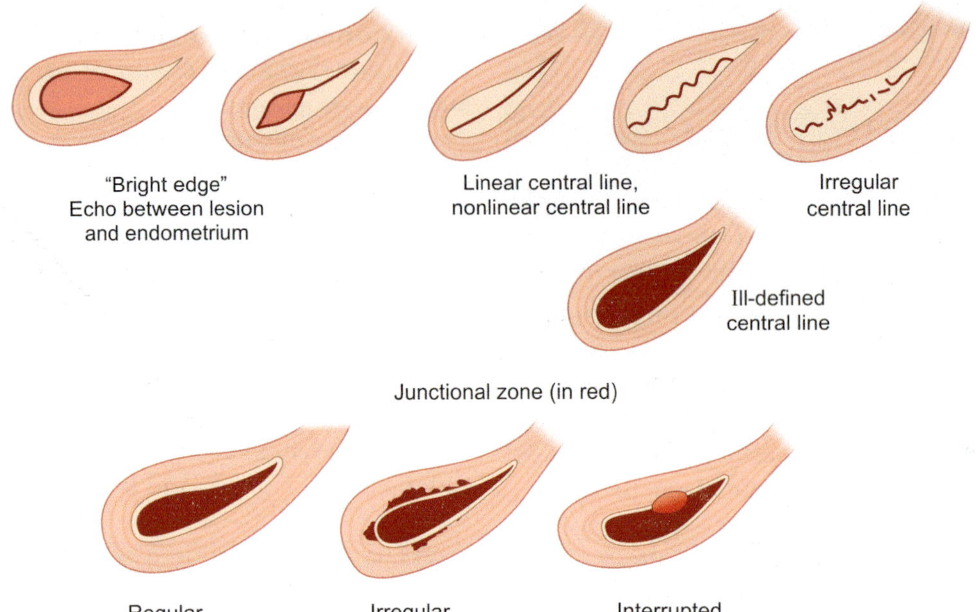

Fig. 5: Diagrammatic demonstration of junctional zone, central line, and edges of the endometrial lesion on B mode—International Endometrial Tumor Analysis (IETA) terminology.

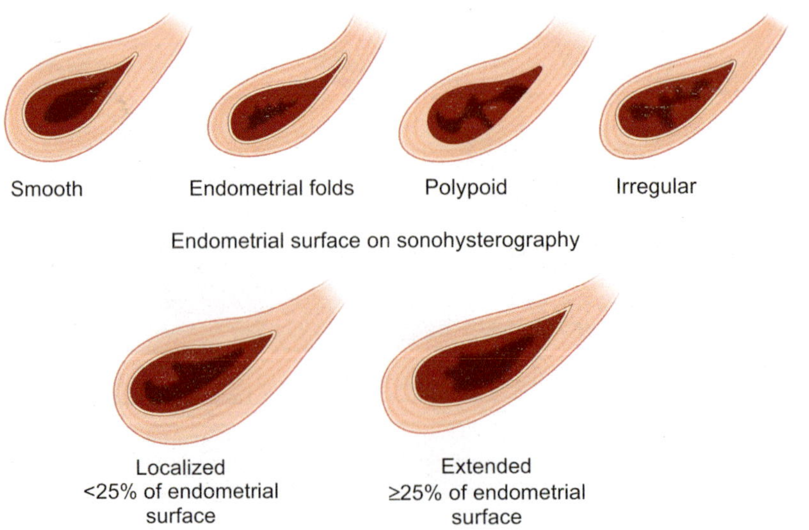

Fig. 6: On sonohysterography, diagrammatic demonstration of endometrial margins and localized lesion on B mode—International Endometrial Tumor Analysis (IETA) terminology.

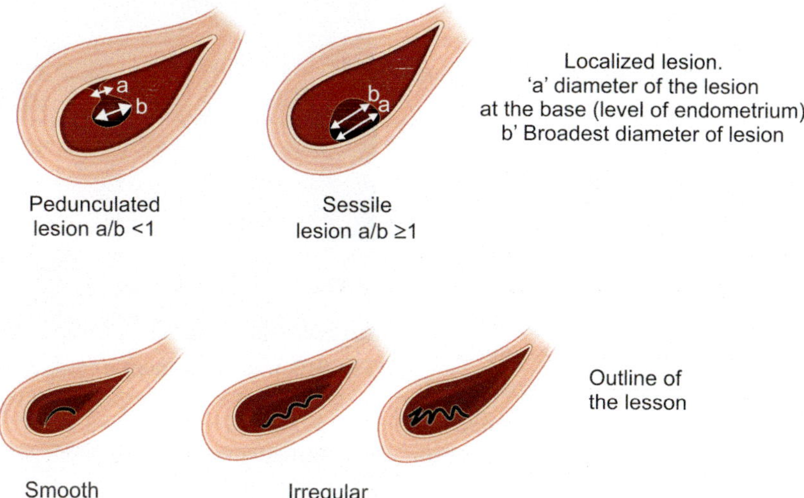

Fig. 7: Diagrammatic demonstration of sonohysterography picture of margins of localized or extended lesion and differentiation between sessile or pedunculated localized lesion on B mode—International Endometrial Tumor Analysis (IETA) terminology.

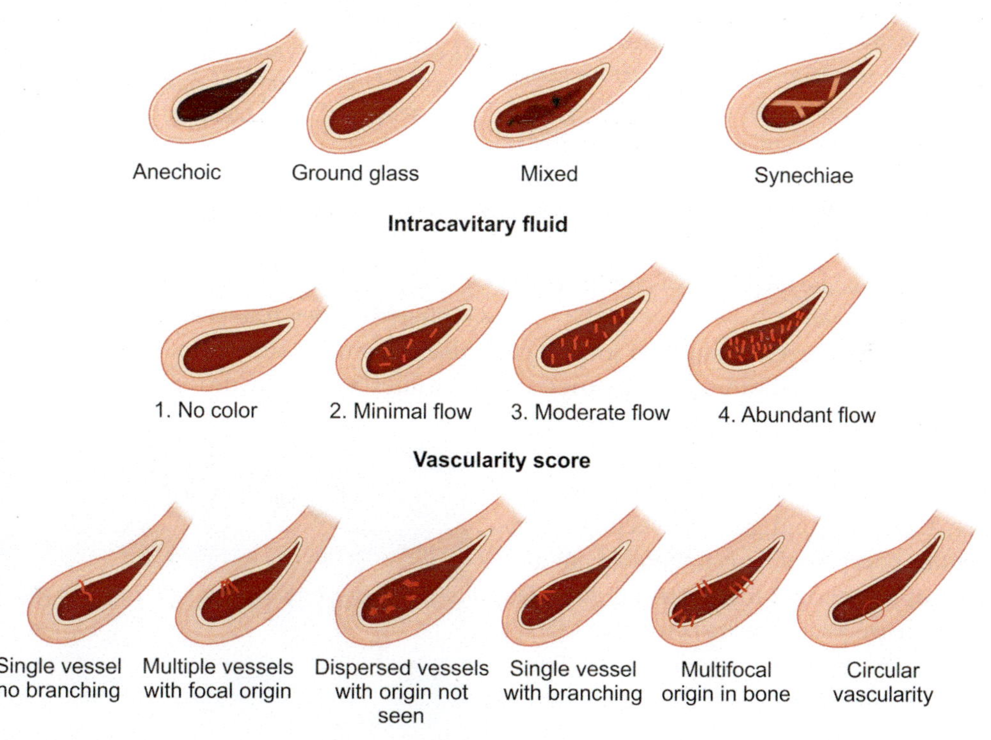

Fig. 8: Diagrammatic demonstration of endometrial contents, vascularity score, and vascular arrangement as by the International Endometrial Tumor Analysis (IETA).

pregnancy or to pelvic inflammatory disease (PID). Inflammation related to pregnancy—postpartum endometritis is more florid and may present with fever, pain, bleeding (secondary hemorrhage), and foul-smelling lochia.

Chronic endometritis may be due to retained products of conception, but also may be due to tuberculosis, intrauterine contraceptive devices, or neoplastic masses such as endometrial carcinoma or a submucus fibroid. This inflammation may be acute or chronic. Patients with acute endometritis may complain of bad odor in the menstrual discharge. At times, it may also present as menorrhagia or metrorrhagia, often associated with acute pelvic pain, whereas patients with chronic endometritis more commonly present with scanty bleeding or amenorrhea.

Acute Endometritis

Acute inflammatory process leads to edema and hyperemia due to neoangiogenesis. Edema involves the endometrium and also the subendometrial tissue due to its close anatomical vicinity. But, the subendometrial layer is also likely to be affected because it is this layer that hosts the dilated spiral vessels, the parent vessels of the endometrial vessels. Extravasation of the fluid from these dilated vessels may also be the cause of edema in the subendometrial layer.

This leads to irregularity and increased thickness of the endometrial-myometrial junctional zone (JZ) **(Fig. 9)**. Endometrial edema may appear as increased thickness of the endometrium with a homogeneous texture. It may have a ground glass-like echogenicity and both because of its echogenicity similar to that of the normal myometrium and also because of irregularity of the JZ may be difficult to distinguish from the myometrium. There may be fluid in the endometrial cavity that is turbid (blood/pus) **(Fig. 10)**.

If it is due to a foreign body such as a gauze or retained products of conception, one may see heterogeneous shadows in the cavity. If it is postpartum, a subinvoluted uterus is seen that appears bulky, heterogeneous, and vascular. In presence of anaerobic infections, air may be seen in the endometrial cavity as bright scattered echoes. If associated with PID, adnexa also will present signs of inflammation such as free fluid (**Fig. 11**), hydrosalpinx, or oophoritis.

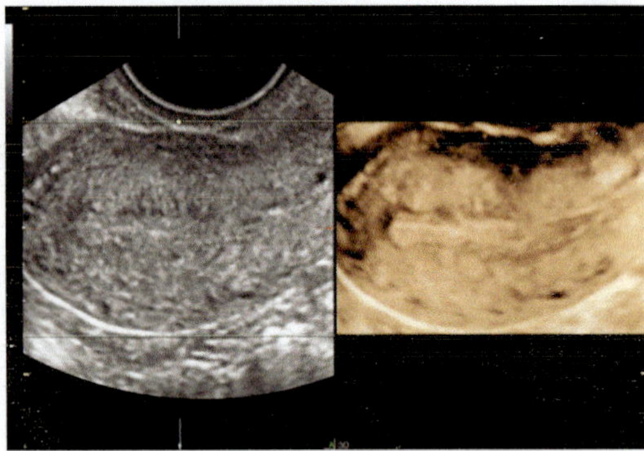

Fig. 9: B mode and volume contrast imaging (VCI) showing irregularity of the junctional zone.

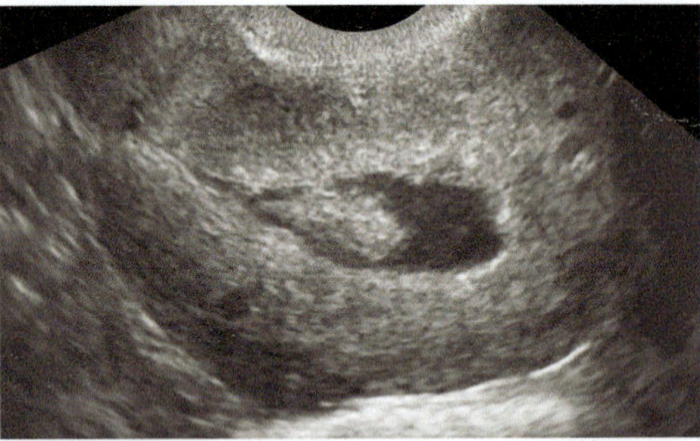

Fig. 10: B-mode ultrasound showing irregular junctional zone endometrial fluid with heterogeneous echogenicity of acute endometritis.

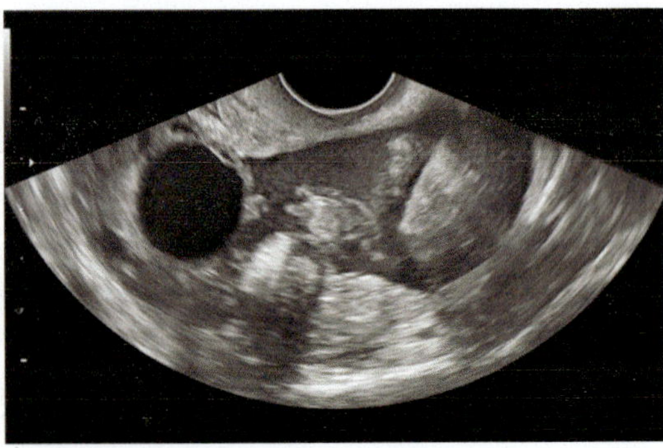

Fig. 11: Acute pelvic infection showing free fluid with low-level internal echogenicities in it.

The neoangiogenesis of inflammation is documented on ultrasound as increased Doppler signals in the endometrium. These vessels typically have larger diameter than the normal spiral vessels and also have low resistance [resistance index (RI) < 0.5] blood flow. As these vessels are newly formed such as other neoangiogenic vessels, these vessels also do not have muscularis layer. The vascular distribution may be heterogeneous due to nonuniform involvement of the endometrium in the inflammatory process.

But, interestingly, the low resistance blood flow in the endometrium cannot always be used as diagnostic criteria for diagnosis of acute inflammatory process. This is so because it is known that normally also during the preovulatory and secretory phase, there is physiological neoangiogenesis in the endometrium and, therefore, normal endometrium appears highly vascular with low resistance blood flow. Therefore, this sign can be used only in a phase of the cycle when normally the endometrium is avascular or has high resistance blood flow. This phase is early proliferative phase.

Thickened endometrium also cannot be used as the diagnostic criteria for acute inflammation in preovulatory and secretory phases for the reasons described earlier, though thickened irregular endometrial-myometrial junction can be used as a strong supportive sign for inflammatory reaction.

Chronic Endometritis

Chronic inflammatory process, instead, results into fibrosis and compromises of the normal endometrial tissue. This does not allow the endometrium to grow in thickness under estrogen or progesterone stimulation. This means that endometrium remains thin even during the preovulatory and the secretory phases when it should, otherwise, grow in thickness. As a result of chronic inflammation, the endometrium also shows scanty high resistance vascularity. Normally, the endometrium shows vascularity reaching the inner layers of the endometrium in the preovulatory and secretory phases with vascular RI of <0.6 and <0.5, respectively. The vascular abundance and resistance may vary according to the severity of the inflammation. It is important to clarify here that the endometrium normally also is thin and avascular or has scanty vascularity in the early proliferative phase. Similar to acute inflammation—acute endometritis, even chronic endometritis shows irregular endometrial-myometrial junction and this may help to suspect chronic endometritis in the early proliferative endometrium (**Fig. 12**).

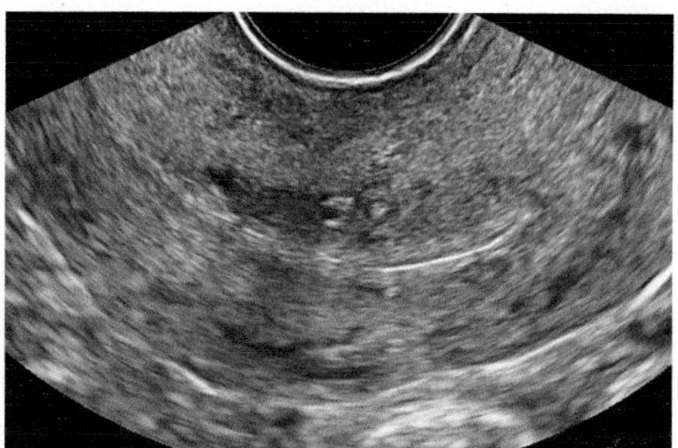

Fig. 12: Irregular endometrial-myometrial junction and thin endometrium of chronic endometritis.

Tuberculous Endometritis (Box 1)

One of the most commonly found, feared of, and difficult to diagnose and treat infection in the developing countries is tuberculosis. In the acute state of the disease, it is not possible to differentiate other infections from tuberculosis. Ultrasound shows irregular endometrial-myometrial junction and

BOX 1: Tuberculous endometritis.

- Persistently thin endometrium
- Irregular junctional zone
- Endometrial, myometrial, and junctional zone calcifications
- Myometrial cysts
- Vertical orientation of interstitial part of tube
- Scarred, contracted endometrial cavity
- Hypo-/avascular endometrium

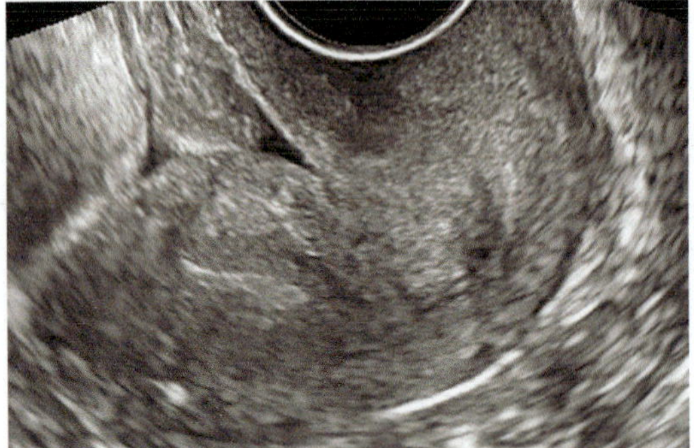

Fig. 13: B-mode ultrasound image showing irregular junctional zone and thin endometrium and hyperechoic flecks in junctional zone.

thickening at times. Sometimes, one may find a fairly normal looking endometrium in patients with tuberculosis.

But, typically, acute tubercular endometritis does not show low resistance blood flow. This may be so because tuberculosis commonly affects end arteries. Chronic tuberculous endometritis, though like other chronic inflammatory endometritis, shows persistently thin endometrium with irregular JZ; it also presents with certain features that are much more commonly seen in tubercular infection as compared to other infections (**Fig. 13**). The most consistent is vertical orientation of the interstitial part of the tube (**Fig. 14**). Fluid collection may be seen in the endometrium, but typically the inner layer of the endometrium appears hyperechoic with irregular endometrial-myometrial junction and no vascularity beyond the JZ (**Fig. 15**). Endometrial, myometrial and endometrial-myometrial JZ calcifications may be seen (**Fig. 16**). Endometrial scarring and synechiae occur due to healing with fibrosis (**Fig. 17**). Fluid may be seen in the endometrial cavity with hyperechoic inner endometrial lining in midproliferative phase. Tuberculous endometritis may also at times present as multiple micropolyps in the endometrium (**Fig. 18**). Tuberculosis may also affect the myometrium and cause myometrial cysts. Though like endometrium, the myometrium also is typically hypovascular.

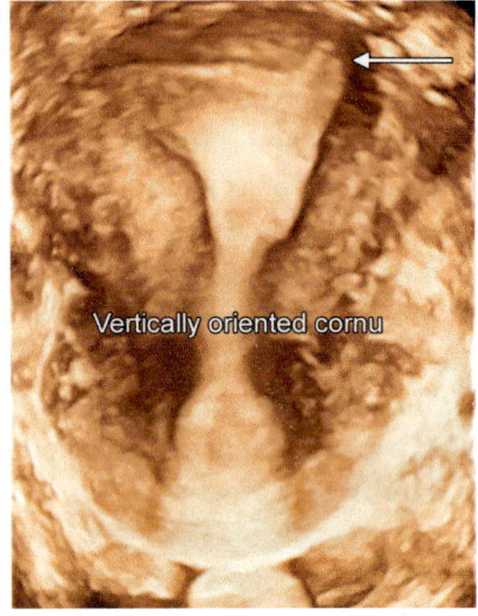

Fig. 14: Three-dimensional (3D) ultrasound of the uterus—coronal plane showing vertical orientation of the cornu (arrow).

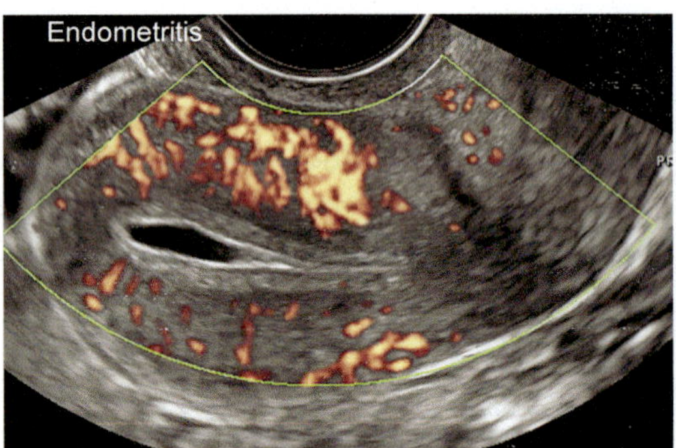

Fig. 15: B-mode ultrasound image of the uterus showing fluid in the endometrial cavity with hyperechoic endometrial margin and absent vascularity in the subendometrial area—chronic endometritis possibly tuberculous.

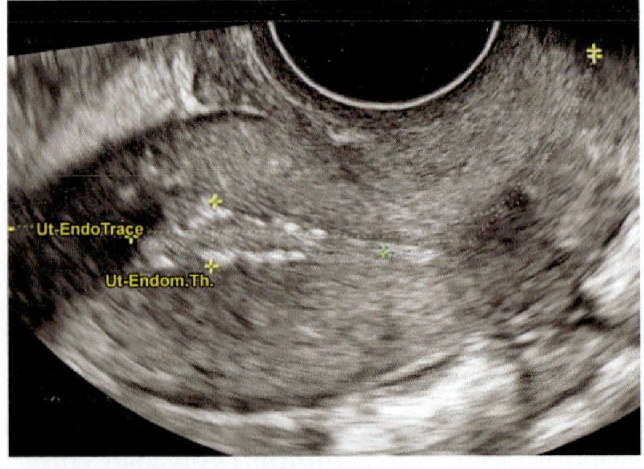

Fig. 16: Endometrial-myometrial junctional calcifications seen on B-mode ultrasound.

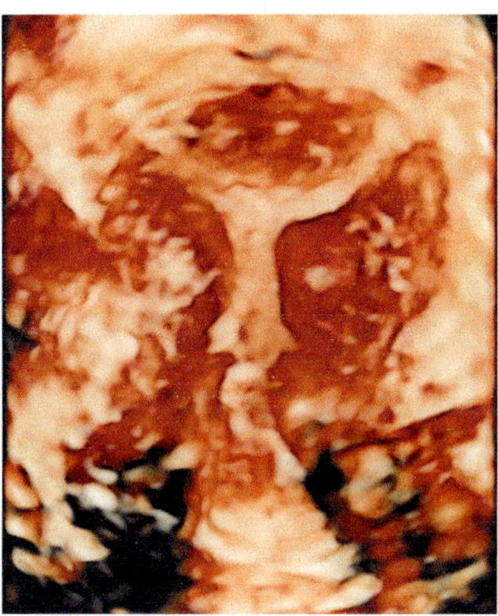

Fig. 17: Three-dimensional (3D) ultrasound image of coronal plane of uterus showing grossly contracted scarred endometrial cavity.

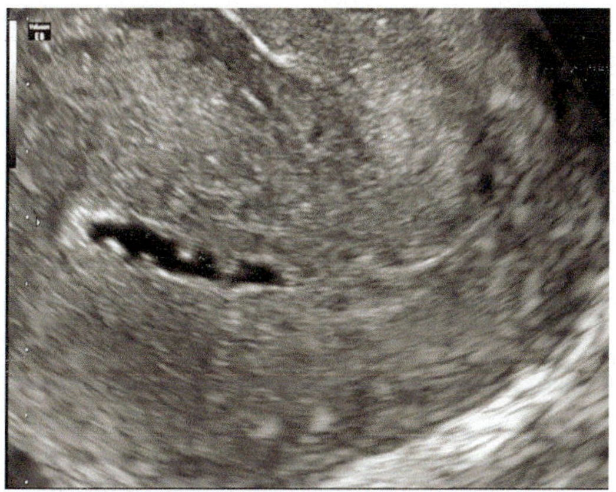

Fig. 18: Micropolyposis seen on sonohysterography on B-mode ultrasound.

ABNORMAL RESPONSE TO HORMONES

It is known that the endometrium has a changing morphology throughout the menstrual cycle. It is the receptor organ for estrogen and progesterone. For the normal menstrual cycle, an alternate predominance of estrogen and progesterone is essential. It is withdrawal of both that leads to breakthrough of the endometrium. Break in this hormonal cycle may lead to abnormalities in the endometrium or even abnormal response of the endometrium to normal hormonal changes may lead to pathologies of the endometrium.

It is due to persistent estrogen exposure that the endometrium keeps on growing to a thickness beyond physiological limits. This is mentioned as 15 mm in literature, but we have observed the endometrium growing to 18 mm thickness in some patients with normal endometrial morphology. Apart from the thickness, endometrium changes its morphology in presence of persistent estrogen exposure. Under the influence of rising estrogen levels, the endometrium grows from single line to multilayered endometrium. With rising estrogen level, the endometrium changes its morphology from multilayered pattern to homogeneous endometrium. This is due to proliferation of endometrial glands.

Persistently high levels of estrogen lead to endometrial hyperplasia due to increased endometrial gland to stroma ratio **(Box 2)**. This, on ultrasound, is seen as mildly hyperechoic endometrium with multiple well-defined round anechoic areas. These anechoic areas are hyperplastic glands. Patients with endometrial hyperplasia present with a period of amenorrhea following by spotting. Endometrium has glandular and stromal components. The abundance of anechoic areas in the thickened endometrium indicates that it is a predominantly *glandular hyperplasia* **(Fig. 19)** and if it has chiefly solid look with only few anechoic areas, it is predominantly *stromal hyperplasia* **(Fig. 20)**. Endometrial hyperplasias may show polypoid endometrium at times. This shows irregular central line on B mode and a polypoid endometrium on sonohysterography.

BOX 2: Endometrial hyperplasia.

- Thick endometrium
- Hyperechoic with cystic areas
- Stromal or glandular predominance
- Intact junctional zone
- Regularly distributed vascularity
- Resistance index (RI) 0.6–0.7

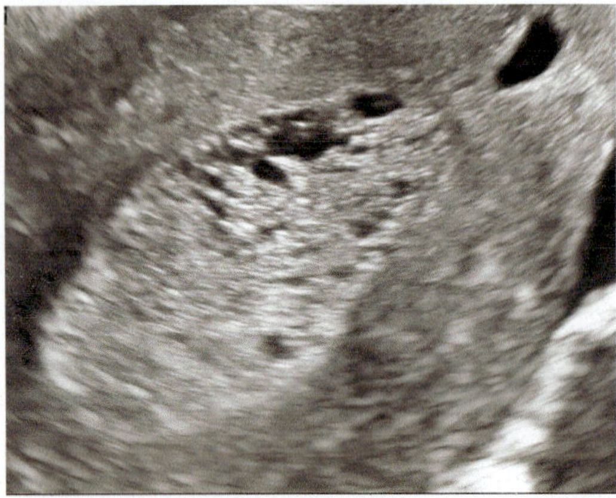

Fig. 19: Cystic endometrial hyperplasia on B-mode ultrasound showing thickened endometrium with hyperechogenicity and multiple anechoic cystic areas.

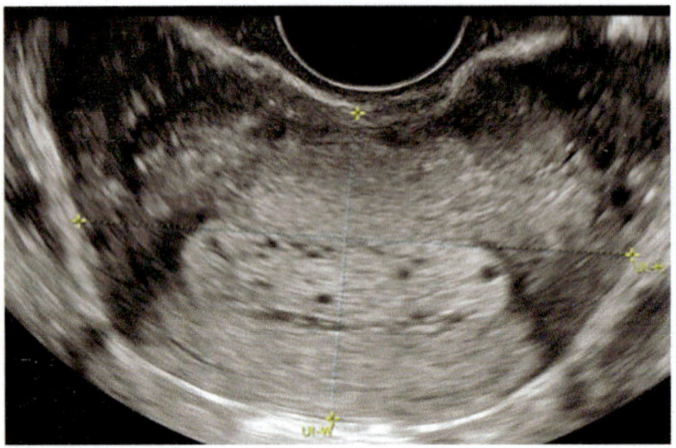

Fig. 20: Hyperechoic endometrium with very few cystic areas—endometrial hyperplasia with stromal predominance.

The endometrial-myometrial junction is typically intact in endometrial hyperplasia. Endometrial hyperplasia on Doppler shows regularly distributed blood vessels throughout the endometrium **(Fig. 21)**. These blood vessels have a moderate resistance flow with RI 0.60–0.70.

Persistent progesterone exposure leads to a compact hyperechoic endometrium with intact endometrial-myometrial JZ. It is the hyperechogenicity that differentiates a hyperestrogenic endometrium from the hyperprogesteronic endometrium. On Doppler, the endometrium that is hyperprogesteronic shows variable vascularity. Actually, the

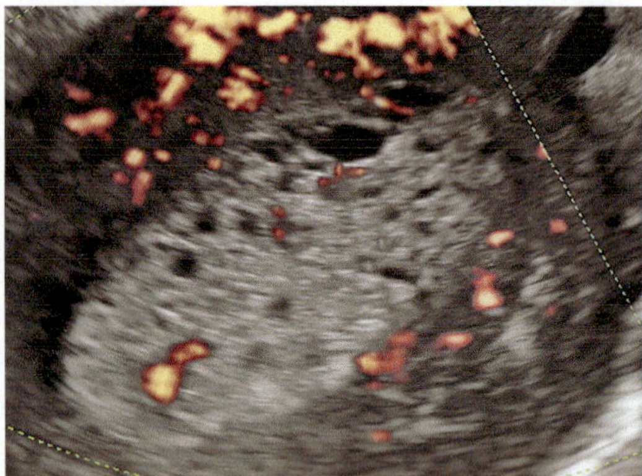

Fig. 21: Cystic glandular hyperplasia on power Doppler showing scanty endometrial vascularity.

vascularity of the progesterone-exposed endometrium depends on the estrogen-progesterone ratio.

Endometrial Metaplasia

Apart from this, endometrial hyperplasia may also be seen as an effect of tamoxifen. Hyperplastic endometrium is seen in the tamoxifen-exposed patients and in endometrial metaplasia. Tamoxifen is widely used for treating breast cancer and has a proestrogenic effect on endometrium. Endometrial metaplasia due to tamoxifen exposure is about progressive changes in the endometrium when the patient is on tamoxifen therapy. On ultrasound, the endometrium shows different pictures at different stages of this progressive change. The changes seen are as follows:

- Echogenic endometrium with good halo and homogeneous echo pattern
- Echogenic endometrium and good boundaries with small echo-free cysts **(Fig. 22)**
- Echogenic nonhomogeneous, small cystic structures, and blurred boundaries
- Echogenic nonhomogeneous endometrium, blurred boundaries, and interrupted halo **(Fig. 23)**
- This last is the nonreversible stage to endometrial malignancy. During this stage, Doppler shows high velocity and low

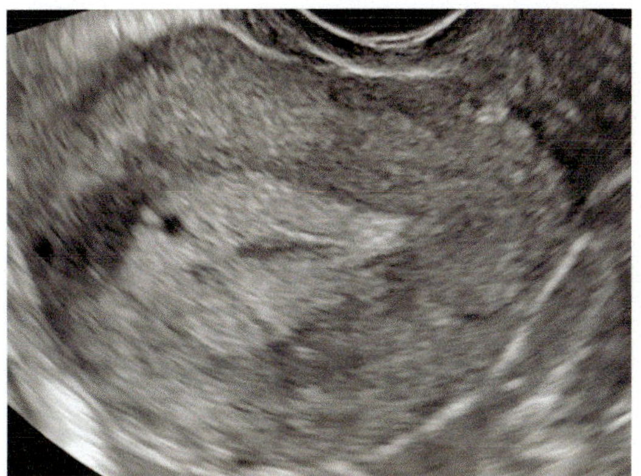

Fig. 22: Endometrium showing well-defined round anechoic lesion—endometrial cyst of endometrial metaplasia.

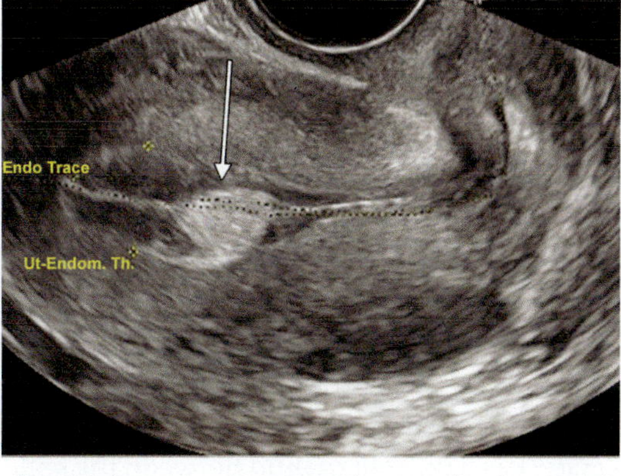

Fig. 24: B-mode ultrasound image of endometrial polyp (arrow).

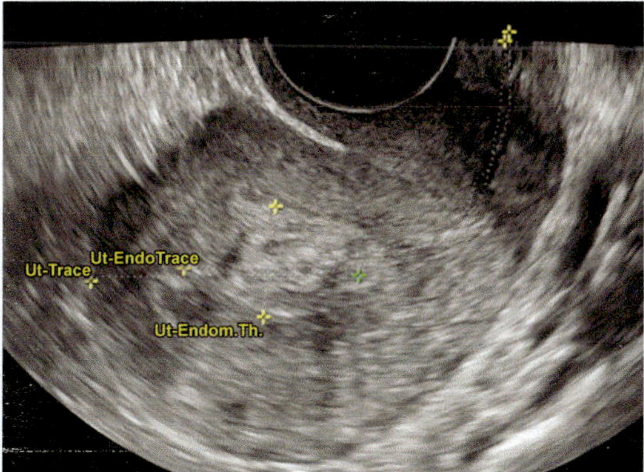

Fig. 23: Echogenic nonhomogeneous endometrium, blurred boundaries, and interrupted halo—tamoxifen effect.

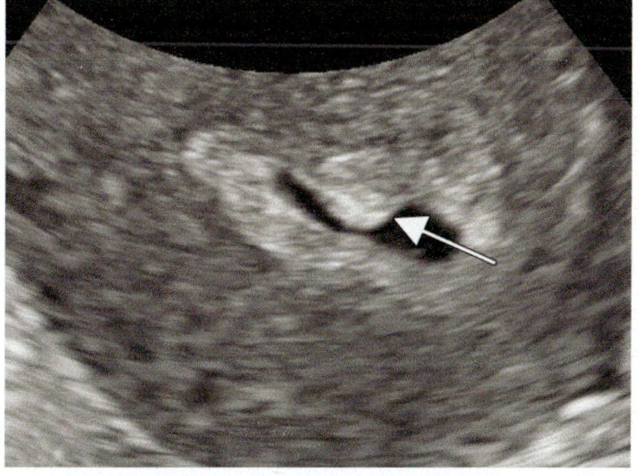

Fig. 25: Endometrial polyp as seen on B-mode ultrasound with saline infusion sonohysterography (arrow).

resistance flow is seen where RI may be as low as 0.39. Lower the resistance, higher is the risk of atypia and malignancy.

Neoplastic Lesions

Polyps

Endometrial polyps are solid projectile lesions of endometrium. These are often diagnosed as an incidental finding. But, some patients may present with intermenstrual spotting and infertility. Sonographically, these are seen as solid echogenic lesions in the endometrial cavity in between the endometrial lines.

Polyps can be diagnosed on B-mode scan and are best visible in the periovulatory phase of the menstrual cycle. The endometrium in this phase is multilayered with the intervening area being hypoechoic. Against this background, these solid soft-tissue lesions standout as homogeneous echogenic round or ovalish lesions with smooth margins **(Fig. 24)**. In the early proliferative phase, before endometrium becomes multilayered, polyp is only seen deshaping the endometrial cavity causing a bulge. Though, at times, if there is fluid in the endometrial cavity, it may help as a negative contrast media and show the polyp as solid soft-tissue projectile lesion in the cavity **(Fig. 25)**. But, I would prefer not to use the menstrual period as a scanning time for endometrial lesions, as there is a strong possibility to misinterpret blood or blood products as endometrial lesions. Pedunculated fibroids also move with peristalsis such as blood clots. Blood clots may appear as solid echogenic structures in the endometrial cavity. In the secretory phase, the endometrium is hyperechoic and obscures the visibility of the polyp, though a good observant will identify the subtle change in echogenicity. Doppler shows a feeding vessel in polyp, unlike the clot, and that is diagnostic. When the endometrial polyp fills up the endometrial cavity, it is a thin slit of fluid between the solid lesion and the endometrial hyperechoic line that indicates the correct diagnosis or one can identify splitting of the two endometrial layers **(Fig. 26)**. Polyps may vary in size from very small ones that may be difficult to visualize on ultrasound to large ones that may mimic thickening of the entire endometrium such as in hyperplasia or malignancy **(Fig. 27)**. Very small polyps may be isoechoic or mildly hyperechoic to the endometrium and sometimes can barely be seen on B-mode ultrasound. The diagnostic clue to such a polyp is an abnormal curve in the central line of the endometrium **(Fig. 28)**. Polyps may be pedunculated or sessile. Sometimes, polyps may show tiny anechoic cystic areas due to dilated endometrial glands. This may be seen in the polyps in patients on tamoxifen therapy also.

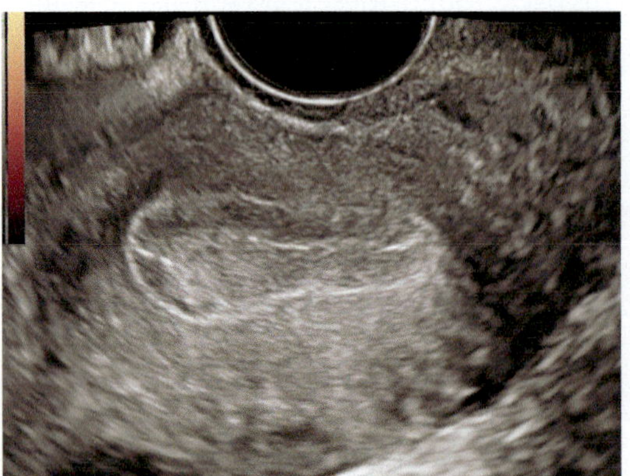

Fig. 26: Large endometrium polyp identified on sonohysterography as the fluid fills up surrounding it on B-mode ultrasound.

Polyps may often be multiple **(Fig. 29)**. In spite of this huge variability in types of polyps and their appearances on ultrasound, its typical vascular supply is diagnostic. Polyp

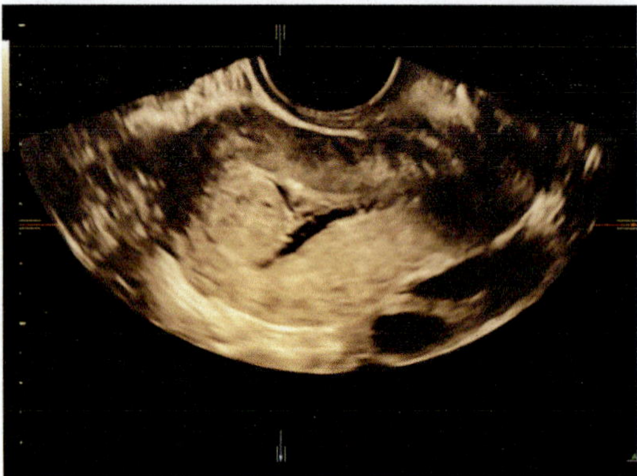

Fig. 27: Large polyp with subtle echogenicity—difficult to differentiate from hyperplasia on B-mode ultrasound.

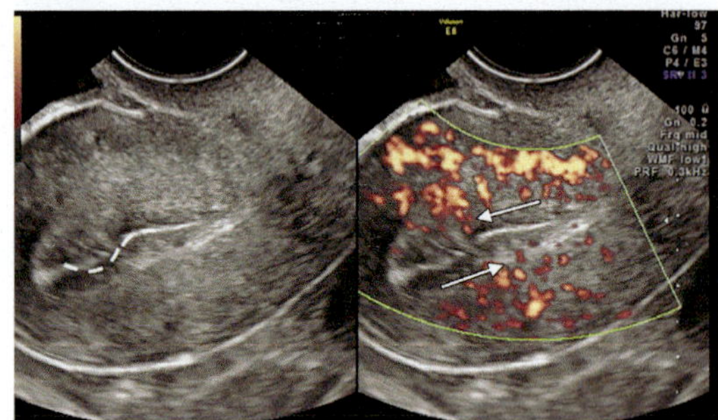

Fig. 28: Polyps with subtle echogenicities can be suspected on B mode by abnormal curvature of the central line and differentiated from hyperplasia by single feeding vessels (arrows).

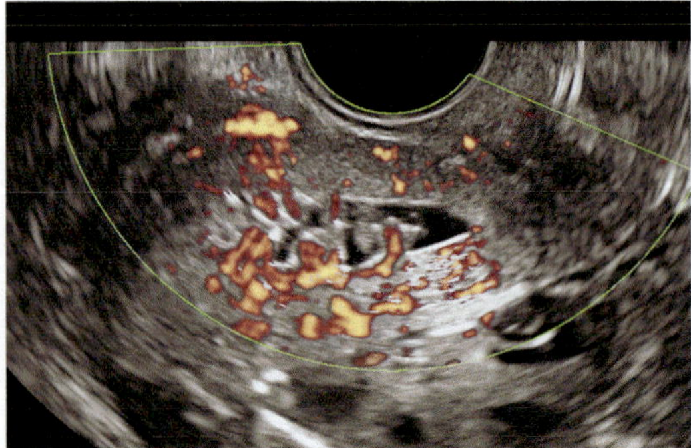

Fig. 29: Sonohysterography with power Doppler showing multiple polyps with single feeding vessel for each.

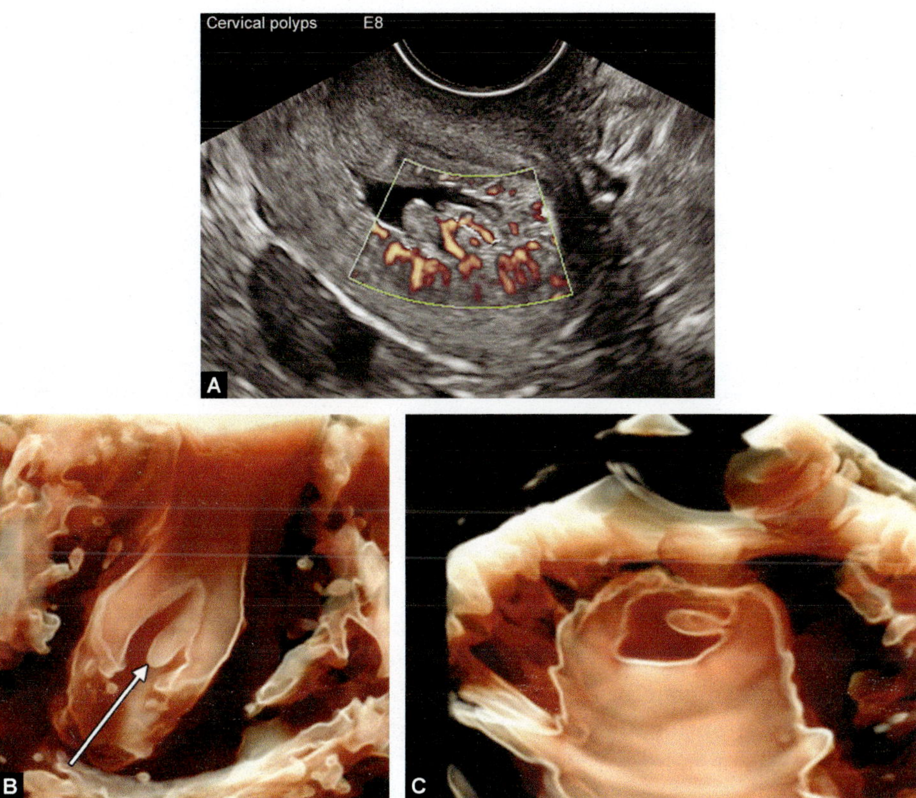

Figs. 30A to C: (A) B mode with power Doppler image of two cervical polyps with feeding vessels; (B and C) 3D ultrasound rendered image of the cervix in longitudinal and transverse planes respectively with cervical polyp.

has a characteristic blood supply by a single feeding vessel or maximum two vessels very closely placed (pedicular vessels especially in sessile polyps). Even when there are multiple polyps, each one has an individual single feeding vessel. Interestingly, when polyps are seen in the cervix, even these show a similar vascular pattern **(Fig. 30A)**. Cervical polyps can be often missed. It is essential to follow the scan during the entry of the probe through the vagina. When there is fluid in the cervix, it is easy to visualize the polyps. Polyps can be well demonstrated by gel vaginosonography **(Figs. 30B and C)**.

Polyps—being benign lesions, these vessels have a high resistance flow (RI about 0.6). But, with RI < 0.45, atypia may be suspected in these polyps.[3] Infection, necrosis, or atypia in the polyp leads to heterogeneous echogenicity on the B mode and Doppler shows abundant branching of the vessels inside the polyp mass **(Figs. 31A and B)**. Adenomyomatous polyp also shows mildly heterogeneous echogenicity and abundant branching of blood vessels **(Fig. 31B)** inside the polyp mass, but the RI of these vessels is almost always >0.5.

Vascular pattern has a high accuracy for differential diagnosis of endometrial lesions. Single vessel pattern for polyp[4] has a sensitivity of 81.2%, specificity of 88.2%, positive predictive value (PPV) of 92.9%, and negative predictive value (NPV) of 71.4% for the diagnosis of polyps. According to another study, the single feeding vessel (pedicle artery) has a sensitivity of 76.4%, specificity of 95.3%, PPV of 81.3%, and NPV of 91.3% for the diagnosis of polyps.[5] Large polyps also have characteristic single feeding vessel, whereas hyperplastic endometrium shows uniformly distributed multiple vessels as discussed

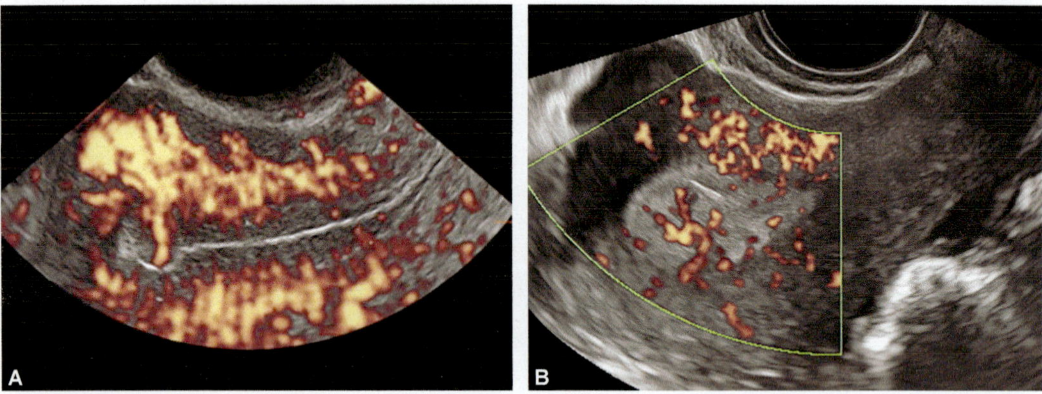

Figs. 31A and B: (A) B-mode image of a polyp with power Doppler showing single feeding vessel with no branching; (B) B-mode image of a polyp with power Doppler showing single feeding vessel with abundant branching.

earlier and malignant endometrial growth shows heterogeneously distributed, increased vascular density **(Fig. 32)**, with vessels of asymmetrical caliber.

Apart from Doppler, sonohysterography is a useful investigation for diagnosis and differential diagnosis of endometrial lesions. It is a simple, painless procedure and does not require any analgesia or anesthesia. It can be used with Doppler or with 3D ultrasound. One can use a dedicated sonohysterography catheter for the procedure, but we prefer to use Foley catheter 6–8 Fr (external diameter 1.6 mm and internal diameter 1.1 mm). The catheter is introduced into the cervix with the balloon fixed in the cervical canal. Balloon is distended with 1.5–2 mL of normal saline or distilled water. After fixing the balloon, 5–7 mL of normal saline is slowly introduced in the endometrial cavity with 10–20 mL syringe. While filling the endometrial cavity with saline, the speculum and anterior retractor, used earlier to visualize the cervix and facilitate the introduction of the probe, are removed from the vagina and the probe is introduced to observe the endometrial cavity as it is being filled up with saline. As the saline fills up and the endometrial cavity distends, the solid lesions of the endometrium can be clearly visualized in the endometrial cavity. It is recommended to fill the catheter with fluid with syringe attached at the time of introduction of the catheter to avoid entry of air bubbles or to keep these to minimum. Air can hamper the visualization of small lesions and may also lead to artifacts.

Once the cavity is distended and the lesion is visualized, either a B-mode sweep in sagittal and axial planes can be taken and stored or a 3D volume of the uterus can be taken. One can also use Doppler after endometrial cavity is filled with saline for differential diagnosis of endometrial lesions.

Fig. 32: B mode with high definition (HD) flow image of the thickened hypervascular endometrium with abundant and heterogeneously distributed vascularity suggestive of malignancy. It is also seen extending into the myometrium suggesting tumor extension into the myometrium.

Endometrial Fibroids

Fibroids are benign neoplasms originating in the myometrium. But, some of these distort the endometrium and some may be pedunculated and grow in the endometrium. Though discussion about the fibroids will be further done in the chapter dedicated on the subject, its discussion here is relevant because these fibroids may mimic polyps and the differential diagnosis may be difficult.

Intraendometrial fibroids also have the same morphology as the other fibroids. This means that these are also hypoechoic to the myometrium, are round/oval and well defined, and have a whorled pattern. In the periovulatory phase, the endometrium is typically hypoechoic to the myometrium and the fibroids may be isoechoic to this and difficult to diagnose, except for abnormal endometrial contour or deviation of the central line. Doppler can be a diagnostic in these cases, as fibroids typically show peripheral vascularity **(Fig. 33)**. Though on B mode also, these fibroids can be better seen in the secretory phase of the menstrual cycle, when endometrium is hyperechoic that acts as a contrast for hypoechoic fibroid **(Fig. 34)**.

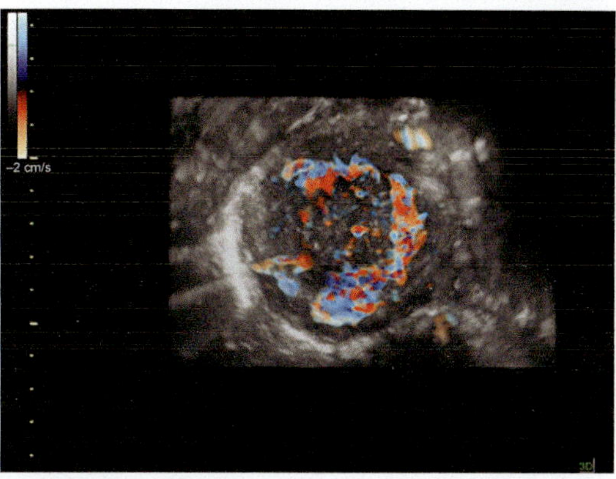

Fig. 34: Subendometrial fundal fibroid on B-mode ultrasound image seen as a round hypoechoic lesion against hyperechoic secretory endometrium.

Fibroid Polyp

This is a confusing and very loosely used term. Large polyps are often termed as fibroid polyps. True fibroid polyps on pathology may have a combination of myometrial and endometrial tissue and may be difficult to correctly diagnose on imaging. A typical fibroid polyp on B mode or on 3D sectional planes may show broad base and a continuity of the myometrial interface may be seen toward the polyp wall **(Fig. 35)**. It has a heterogeneous echogenicity. Doppler, unlike fibroid, typically shows feeding pedicle, but usually this pedicle has multiple vessels. Abundant branching may be seen and this may be mistaken for atypia in the lesion. By tracing these feeding vessels, these show continuity from the myometrial radial vessels rather than from the spiral vessels that are feeders to endometrium **(Fig. 36)**.

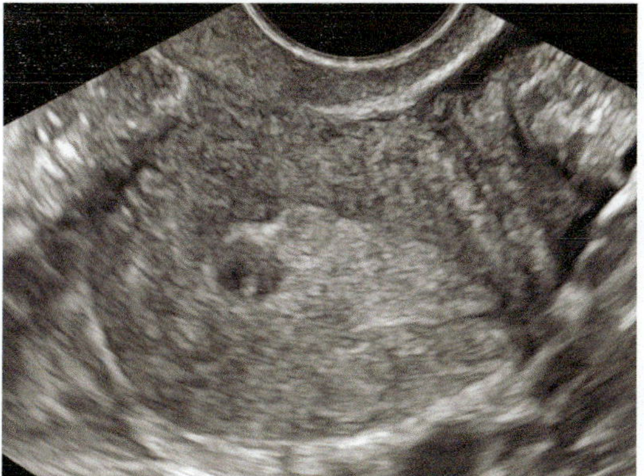

Fig. 33: Subendometrial fibroid on three-dimensional (3D) power Doppler showing peripheral ring of vascularity.

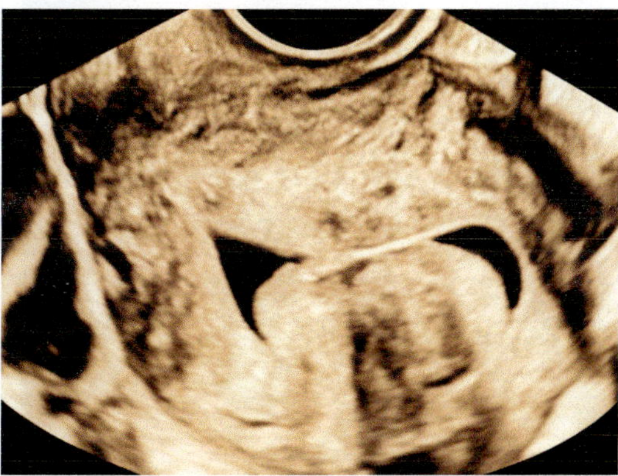

Fig. 35: B-mode ultrasound with sonohysterography showing a large solid sessile lesion protruding in the endometrial cavity possibly fibroid polyp.

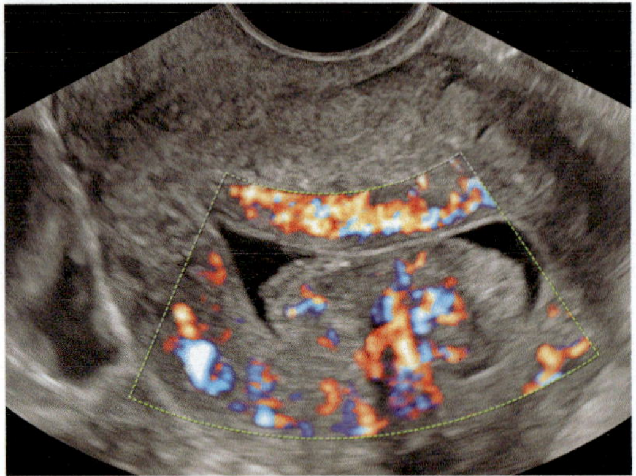

Fig. 36: The same lesion as in Figure 35 with power Doppler showing the feeder extending through myometrium.

Endometrial Synechiae

These are typically avascular lesions of the endometrium. It is known that synechiae occur as a result of surgical insult or inflammation finally leading to fibrosis. Patients present with severe oligomenorrhea or amenorrhea. These appear as soft-tissue strands across the endometrium on B-mode ultrasound, but are often not seen on ultrasound, instead only appear as a thin endometrium. The echogenicity may vary depending on the firmness, thickness, or calcifications of the synechiae **(Fig. 37A)**. Sonohysterography may be a more helpful investigation in these cases **(Fig. 37B)**.

Endometrial Malignancies

Endometrial malignancy is the fourth most common malignancy in United States.[6] Its incidence in Asian countries and New Zealand is 1.5–2.5 times higher than that in European countries.[7] The increased rates of endometrial cancer may be related to obesity, failing fertility, and increased life span.[8] Endometrial malignancy may present with varied menstrual disturbances. Endometrial malignancy on ultrasound may have variable appearance depending on its stage. But, still heterogeneous echogenicity is a consistent finding (**Fig. 38**). Depending on the extent of the disease, there may be focal/diffuse thickening of the endometrium. Endometrial thickness of >15 mm in premenopausal women as mentioned in literature and >5 mm in a postmenopausal patient with bleeding disorders may be suspected of having endometrial malignancy. But, I will like to quote here from our experience that 15 mm is probably a too low cutoff for premenopausal women. We have seen several women with an endometrium of up to 18–19 mm usually in secretory phase or up to 15–16 mm in preovulatory phase. If the echo pattern of the endometrium is normal according to the phase of cycle and JZ is intact, it is very less likely to be malignant. Doppler may help to confirm

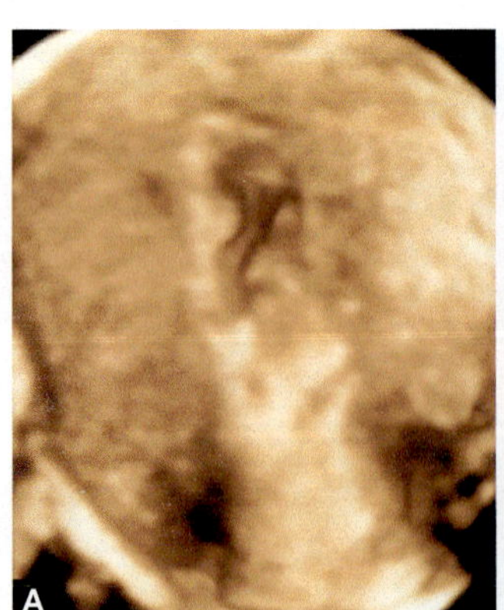

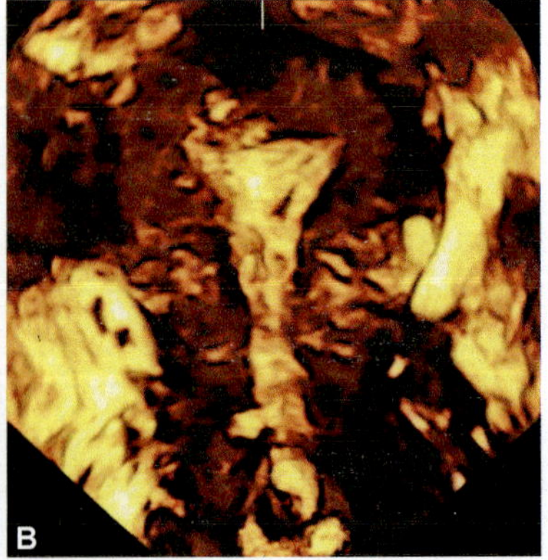

Figs. 37A and B: Three-dimensional (3D) ultrasound image of the coronal plane of the endometrium showing grossly contracted endometrial cavity due to synechiae.

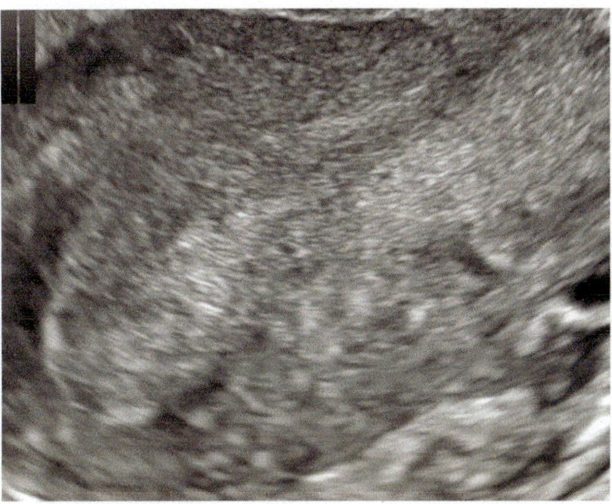

Fig. 38: Thickened endometrium with heterogeneous echogenicity on B-mode ultrasound may lead to suspicion of endometrial malignancy.

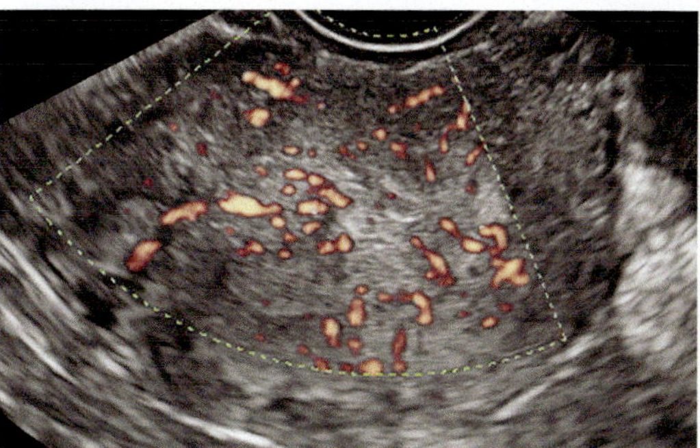

Fig. 39: Thick endometrium with heterogeneous echogenicity and irregular junctional zone with blood vessels of irregular caliber as seen on power Doppler suggest endometrial malignancy.

the regular and symmetrical distribution of blood vessels, thus excluding the doubt of malignancy. Endometrial thickness of <4 mm has a 100% NPV for endometrial cancer.[9]

Interestingly, the endometrial echogenicity varies according to the stage and grade of the disease. Stage 1A cancers are hyperechoic or isoechoic, whereas stage 1B cancers and above have mixed echogenicity or are hypoechoic. Well or moderately differentiated (grade 1–2) tumors are hyperechoic compared to grade 3 and more wide spread lesions that are hypoechoic or heterogeneous.[10] Irregular endometrial surface is another diagnostic criteria for the diagnosis of endometrial malignancy **(Fig. 39)** and this can be best appreciated by sonohysterography. But, if malignancy is suspected either clinically or on ultrasound, sonohysterography is not preferred for the risk of its peritoneal spread and seeding.[11] At times, fluid may be seen in the endometrial cavity. When the endometrial malignancy grows beyond the endometrial margins, it leads to irregularity of the subendometrial halo. Irregular endometrial margin has a positive likelihood of 10 for endometrial malignancy.[12]

On Doppler, it typically shows heterogeneously distributed dense vascularity. Low resistance flow is seen in the premenopausal women with endometrial malignancy, but in early endometrial carcinoma in perimenopausal women, moderate intratumoral resistance may be seen **(Fig. 40A)**. The vascular pattern is of multifocal origin, dispersed vessels, and less commonly single vessel with abundant branching **(Fig. 40B)**. In patients with endometrial malignancy, the uterine artery resistance is also low with uterine artery pulsatility index (PI) < 1.45 and radial artery PI < 1.06.[13]

Typically, the malignant neoangiogenesis shows chaotic vascular branching pattern with microaneurysms, arteriovenous shunts, elongation, and coiling **(Fig. 40B)**. These are appreciated best on the 3D power Doppler (PD) angiography. Combining morphological and 3D PD criteria sensitivity for endometrial carcinoma is 91.67%.[14] 3D ultrasound also plays an important role in diagnosing the extension of the endometrial carcinoma into myometrium **(Fig. 41A)**. Inaccessibility or obliteration of the endometrial-myometrial junction because of myometrial extension of the lesion can be best appreciated on 3D ultrasound. 3D ultrasound can calculate the tumor volume accurately and increasing volume of the endometrium suggests higher grade of endometrial carcinoma and also myometrial invasion.[15] Volume >25 mL has

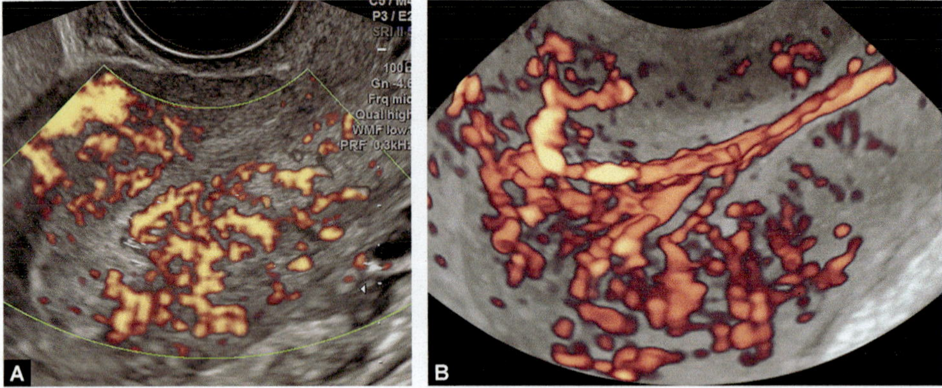

Figs. 40A and B: (A) Heterogeneously distributed dense vascularity with irregular vascular caliber in a heterogeneously thickened endometrium—endometrial malignancy; (B) Three-dimensional (3D) power Doppler showing single vessel with abundant vascular branching in heterogeneously thickened endometrium—endometrial malignancy.

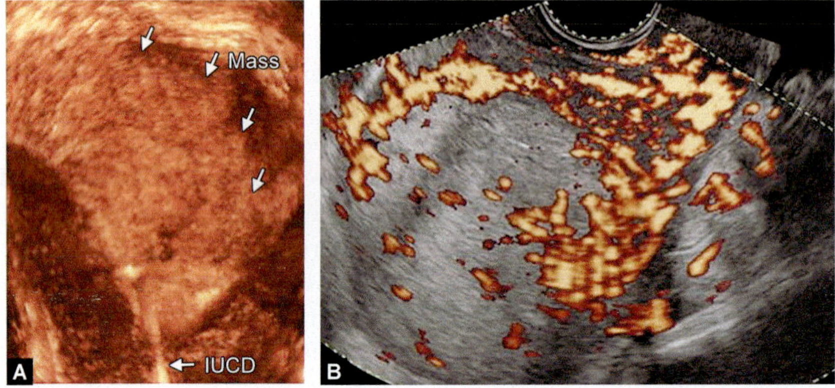

Figs. 41A and B: (A) Three-dimensional (3D) ultrasound image of the uterus in coronal plane with hyperechogenicity extending into the myometrium totally obliterating the junctional zone and has irregular margins of endometrial malignancy with myometrial extension (white arrows); (B) In the same lesion on sagittal plane, the tumoral vascular pattern is seen penetrating into the myometrium.

a high chance of pelvic node involvement at surgery. 3D hysterosonography with transverse plane picture may also show bladder or rectal infiltration. 3D PD is efficient for diagnosis of deep invasion with sensitivity of 100%, specificity of 94.44%, PPV of 83.33%, and NPV of 100%. The tumoral vascular pattern is seen penetrating into the myometrium **(Fig. 41B)**. Higher stages of tumor show lower RI, higher velocity, and higher microvessel density (VI).[16] Though local spread can be well evaluated on ultrasound for final staging of these lesions, modalities such as computed tomography or magnetic resonance imaging are essential.

CONCLUSION

Transvaginal ultrasound is the modality of choice for assessment of the endometrium and diagnosis of endometrial pathologies. Doppler is an essential addition for the differential diagnosis of these pathologies. 3D plays an important role for demonstration of endometrial lesions. 3D PD especially is of importance for diagnosis, assessing the extent, and follow-up of malignant lesions.

REFERENCES

1. Tsuda H, Kawabata M, Kawabata K, Yamamoto K, Hidaka A, Umesaki N. Comparison between transabdominal and transvaginal ultrasonography for identifying endometrial malignancies. Gynecol Obstet Invest. 1995;40:271-3.
2. Leone FPG, Timmerman D, Bourne T, Valentine L, Epstein E, Goldstein SR, et al. Terms, definitions, and measurements to describe the sonographic features of the endometrium and intrauterine lesions: a consensus opinion from the International Endometrial Tumor Analysis (IETA) group. Ultrasound Obstet Gynecol. 2010;35:103-12.
3. Kurjak A, Kupesic S. Transvaginal color Doppler and pelvic tumor vascularity: lessons learned and future challenges. Ultrasound Obstet Gynecol. 1995;6:1-15.
4. Richman TS, Viscomi GN, Cherney AD, Polan A. Fallopian tubal patency assessment by ultrasound following fluid injection. Radiology. 1984;152:507-10.
5. Timmerman D, Verguts J, Konstantinovic ML, Moerman P, van Schoubroeck D, Deprest J, et al. The pedicle artery sign based on sonography with color Doppler imaging can replace second-stage tests in women with abnormal vaginal bleeding. Ultrasound Obstet Gynecol. 2003;22:166-71.
6. Duong LM, Wilson RJ, Ajani UA, Singh SD, Eheman CR. Trends in endometrial cancer incidence rates in the United States, 1999-2006. J Womens Health (Larchmt). 2011;20:1157-63.
7. Blakely T, Shaw C, Atkinson J, Cunningham R, Sarfati D. Social inequalities or inequalities in cancer incidence? Repeated consensus-cancer cohort studies, New Zealand 1981-1986 to 2001-2004. Cancer Causes Control. 2011;22:1307-18.
8. Lambe M, Wigertz A, Garmo H, Walldius G, Jungner I, Hammar N. Impaired glucose metabolism and diabetes and the risk of breast, endometrial, and ovarian cancer. Cancer Causes Control. 2011;22:1163-71.
9. Karlsson B, Granberg S, Wikland M, Ylöstalo P, Torvid K, Marsal K, et al. Transvaginal ultrasonography of the endometrium in women with postmenopausal bleeding—a Nordic multicenter study. Am J Obstet Gynecol. 1995;172:1488-94.
10. Epstein E, Van Holsbeke C, Mascilini F, Måsbäck A, Kannisto P, Ameye L, et al. Gray-scale and color Doppler ultrasound characteristics of endometrial cancer in relation to stage, grade, and tumor size. Ultrasound Obstet Gynecol. 2011;38:586-93.
11. Amant F, Moerman P, Neven P, Timmerman D, Limbergen EV, Vergote I. Endometrial cancer. Lancet. 2005;366:491-505.
12. Epstein E, Valentine L. Gray-scale ultrasound morphology in presence or absence of intrauterine fluid and vascularity as assessed by color Doppler for discrimination between benign and malignant endometrium in women with postmenopausal bleeding. Ultrasound Obstet Gynecol. 2006;28:89-95.
13. Bezircioglu I, Baloglu A, Cetinkaya B, Yigit S, Oziz E. The diagnostic value of Doppler ultrasonography in distinguishing the endometrial malignancies in women with postmenopausal bleeding. Arch Gynecol Obstet. 2012;285:1369-74.
14. Kurjak A, Kupesic S. Three-dimensional ultrasound and power Doppler in assessment of uterine and ovarian angiogenesis: a prospective study. Croat Med J. 1999;40:51-8.
15. Alcazar JL, Jurado M. Three-dimensional ultrasound for assessing women with gynecological cancer: a systematic review. Gynecol Oncol. 2011;20:340-6.
16. Kupesic S, Kurjak A, Zodan T. Staging of endometrial carcinoma by 3D power Doppler. Gynecol Perinatol. 1999;8:1-5.

28 CHAPTER

Ovarian Pathologies and Endometriosis

Sonal Panchal, Chaitanya Nagori

INTRODUCTION

Ultrasound is accepted as the primary imaging modality for evaluation of adnexal masses. Ultrasound is a very useful tool for localizing the origin of pelvic mass and to study the morphological characteristics of the mass. It is based on this morphology that these masses can be categorized as benign, possibly malignant, or malignant. Doppler is an important tool for differential diagnosis of adnexal lesions and pathology of most benign lesions also can be known. Ultrasound-based triage of asymptomatic women diagnosed with a persistent adnexal mass is effective for selecting the surgical approach.[1] Several meta-analyses revealed significant higher performance for combined techniques using morphologic assessment and Doppler ultrasound indices than B-mode evaluation alone.[2] International ovarian tumor analysis (IOTA) is an ultrasound-based very reliable method to differentiate benign from malignant lesions.

Though the protocol that we follow for adnexal lesions is as follows:

- Decide the organ of origin (ovarian or extraovarian)
- Assess the morphology and correlate to physiology
- If physiological correlation of the lesion is excluded, think of physiology-related abnormalities, e.g., hemorrhagic cyst, follicular cyst, etc.
- Think of common pathologies, e.g., simple cyst, endometrioma, dermoids, fibroma, etc.
- Does not fit into any of these, use IOTA to match to simple descriptors first and if does not match to differentiate between benign and malignant pathologies.

OVARIAN LESIONS

Ovaries are physiologically active organs—solid and oval in shape. These are anchored in the pelvis by the mesovarium to the posterior surface of the broad ligament, to the uterus with the utero-ovarian ligament and to the lateral pelvic wall by the suspensory ligament. Continuous change is seen in their morphology throughout the menstrual cycle. This is in the form of follicle recruitment, maturation, rupture, and formation of corpus luteum. Therefore, cystic structures appear and change in morphology from time to time in the ovaries and these are physiological. Apart from these, ovaries also play a host for several other pathological lesions such as endometriomas, dermoid cysts, serous and mucus cystadenomas, endometriomas, fibromas, and ovarian epithelial carcinomas.

To decide the origin of the lesion:

The signs used to confirm the origin of the lesion from the ovary are:

- *Sliding organ sign*: Place a probe in such a way that the lesion and the ovary are seen in the same frame on the screen. Apply pressure with the probe, to separate the two. If probe pressure can displace the two away from each other, or the ovary and the lesion slide over each other, the lesion is not arising from the ovary. If the two cannot be separated or do not slide over

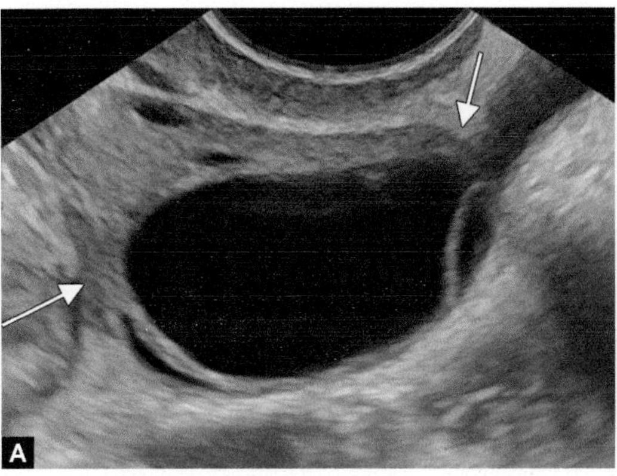

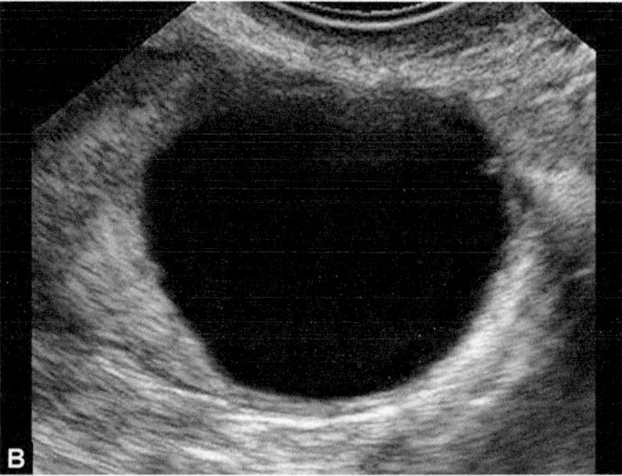

Figs. 1A and B: (A) Anechoic lesion is seen in the ovary. The ovarian tissue forms a beak around the lesion, partially covering the lesion-beak sign. Its anechoic appearance and more brightness of the tissues behind it (posterior enhancement) confirm its cystic nature; (B) Cystic lesion seen in the ovary, covered on all sides by rim of ovarian tissue.

each other, the lesion is either adherent to the ovary or it is arising from the ovary.

- If the lesion is arising from the ovary, the lesion will be completely or partially covered by normal ovarian tissue and is typically described as a "rim sign" or "beak sign," respectively (**Figs. 1A and B**). It is essential that the lesion is well scrolled across to look for rim or beak sign.
- If the sliding sign is negative and beak or rim sign is also absent, it is an extraovarian lesion, adherent to ovary.

Having confirmed the origin of the lesion from the ovary, the differential diagnosis of these lesions can be thought of. We would prefer to do this by dividing these lesions into different categories based on their ultrasound appearance.

ULTRASOUND-BASED CLASSIFICATION OF OVARIAN LESIONS

- Nonseptated clear cysts
- Clear cysts with septa
- Cysts with thick walls and internal echogenicities
- Solid lesions
- Complex lesions with cystic and solid areas

Nonseptated Clear Cysts

These cysts are thin walled, have no internal echogenicities, no septa, or no solid component (**Fig. 2**).

The lesions/structures in this category are:

- Follicular cyst
- Simple cyst of the ovary.

Follicle or Follicular Cyst

It is common to see thin-walled cystic structures with no internal echogenicities in the ovary. These are usually follicles (**Fig. 3**) or follicular (physiological) cysts and have a natural tendency to resolve. Follicle starts growing in early follicular phase. It grows till 18–24 mm in diameter before it ruptures due

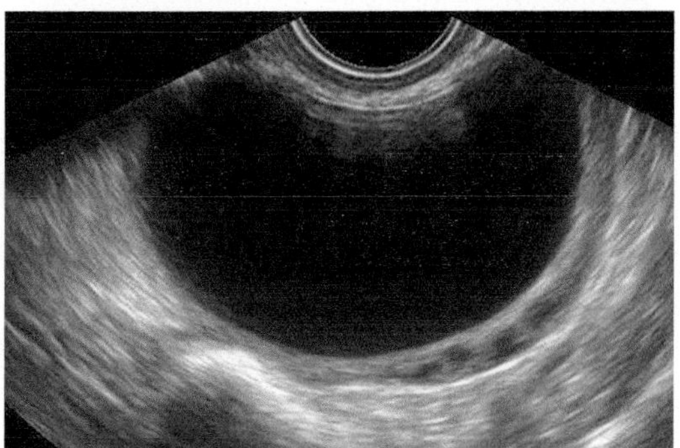

Fig. 2: Typical thin-walled cyst with no internal echogenicities and no septa or solid projections.

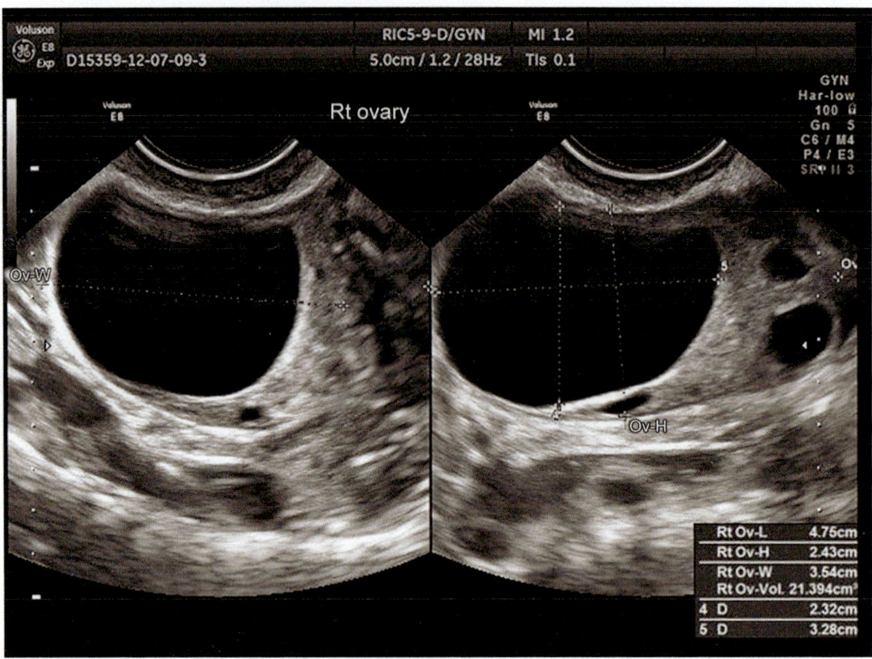

Fig. 3: The most commonly seen anechoic roundish cystic structure in ovary with beak sign follicle—especially when seen in proliferative phase.

to the surge of luteinizing hormone to release the ovum that it contains. If the surge does not occur, the follicle will not rupture and will result in a hormonally inactive/only minimally active structure. This is termed as a follicular cyst when it grows beyond 25 mm and persists in luteal phase of the cycle or even in the subsequent cycle. Contrary to the normal follicle, the follicular cyst shows scanty and high resistance flow (**Fig. 4**). But, it is ultimately a physiological cyst and would resolve on its own over a maximum period of 4–6 weeks. The flow resistance increases, as it regresses or it becomes hormonally inactive. When seen in proliferative phase of the menstrual cycle, the first possibility is thought of the follicle, and follicle when active shows a low-resistance flow on Doppler (**Fig. 5**). If such a lesion is seen in the luteal phase, it is more likely to be a follicular cyst. These cysts do not require any treatment and regress on their own in a period of 4–6 weeks, being physiological in nature. Therefore, before stamping a diagnosis of a simple cyst of the ovary, it is important to reassess such a lesion at least twice at an interval of 2–3 weeks (in two different phases of menstrual cycle) and observe for change in the nature of the lesion or resolution and also Doppler.

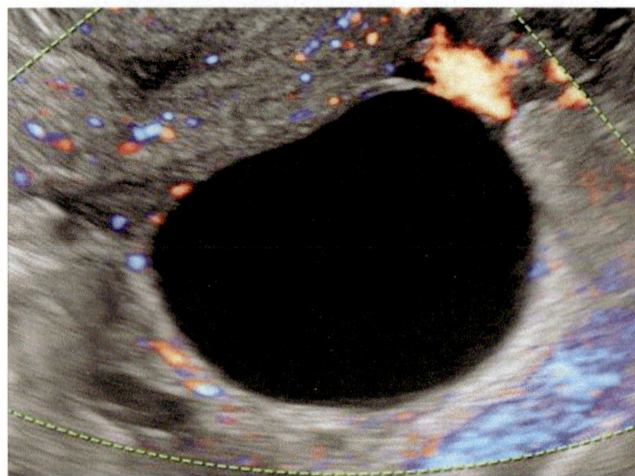

Fig. 4: When a follicle-like structure is seen in secretory phase or very early proliferative phase, it is usually follicular cyst. It is differentiated from a follicle by the Doppler signals, which show scanty flow as seen in the figure.

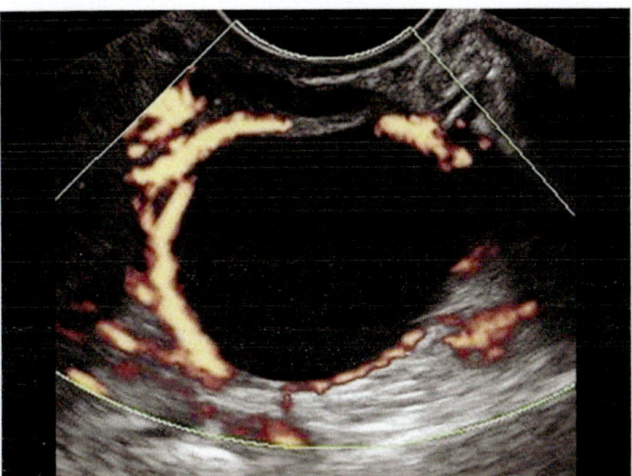

Fig. 5: An active and nearly mature follicle shows Doppler signals covering its circumference—perifollicular vessels. Perifollicular vessels are only those, which obliterate the follicular wall.

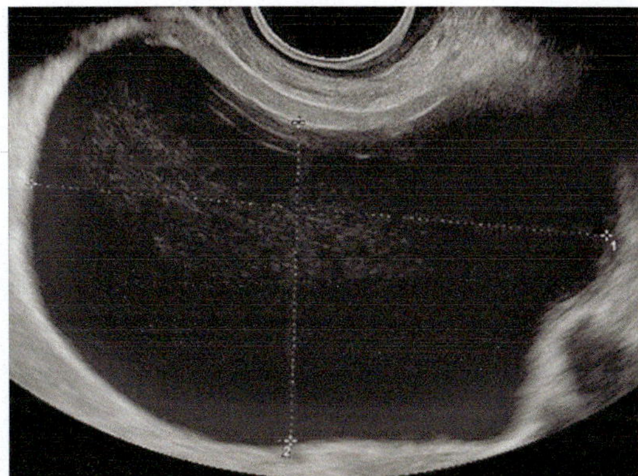

Fig. 6: Thin-walled, anechoic lesion in the ovary with no internal echogenicities, septa, or solid projections, which persists over the menstrual cycles and does not change its character, is a simple cyst of the ovaries.

Simple Cyst of the Ovary

It is a thin-walled intraovarian cystic structure usually >5 cm (**Fig. 6**). Doppler shows no flow. It does not resolve on its own and may require ultrasound-guided aspiration usually. Appearance of echogenicities in this cyst is only due to infection or malignant change (**Fig. 7**).

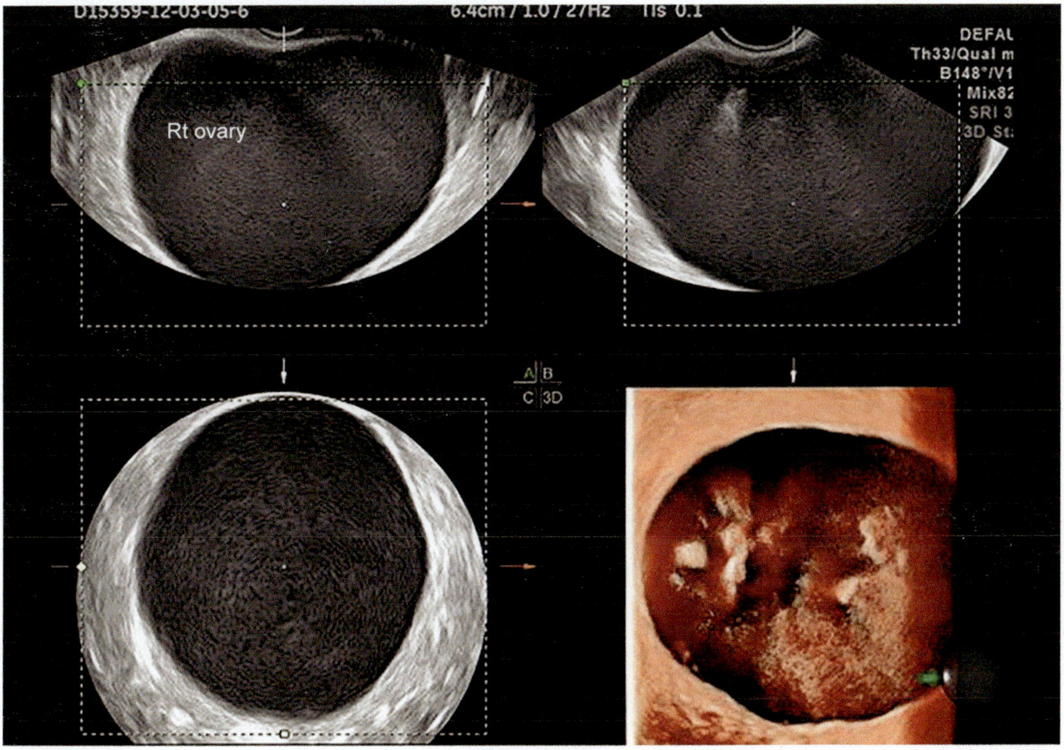

Fig. 7: Appearance of echogenicities in a cyst that appeared anechoic and thin walled earlier indicates either infection or a malignant change in such a cyst.

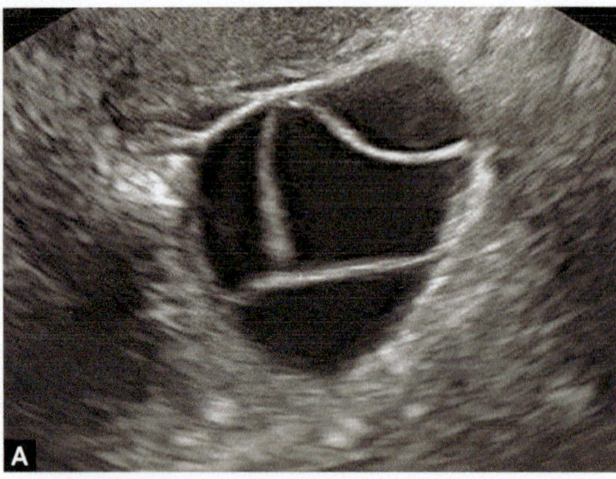

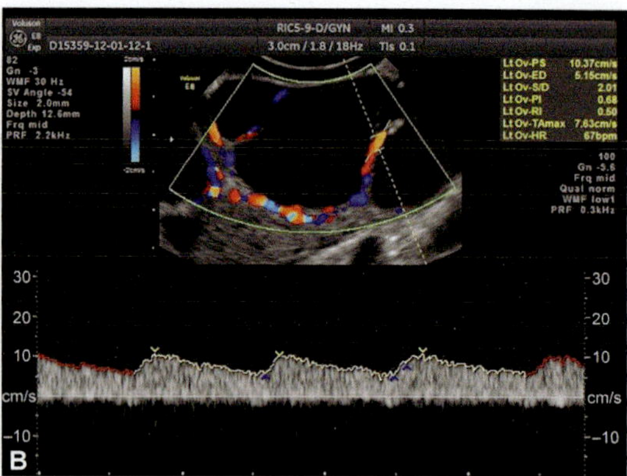

Figs. 8A and B: Thin-walled cystic structure in the ovary with multiple thin septa, but no internal echogenicities. (A) When seen in proliferative phase of the cycle especially in ovulation induction cycles, these are multiple follicles; (B) On Doppler, the septa of such a multiloculated cystic structure, which are actually follicular walls, show abundant low-resistance flow.

Cysts with Septa but no Internal Echogenicities

These cysts show thin walls and thin septa but no internal echogenicities:

- Multiple follicles
- Serous cystadenoma.

Multiple Follicles

Patients on ovulation induction therapy for treatment of subfertility are likely to develop multiple follicles and these often look like multiloculated cyst (**Figs. 8A and B**). Because the fluid inside the follicles is under pressure, the follicle walls are bulging and so the septa often look straight and tight. Because the follicles are vascular, the septa often look vascular.

Serous cystadenoma: It usually has multiple thin, avascular septa and these septa often look loose and curved (**Fig. 9**). The septa are most often avascular. Development of vascularity may be first sign of conversion of this benign lesion to malignant.

Cysts with Internal Echogenicities

The most common lesions in this category are:

- Corpus luteum
- Hemorrhagic cyst
- Luteinized unruptured follicle (LUF)
- Endometrioma.

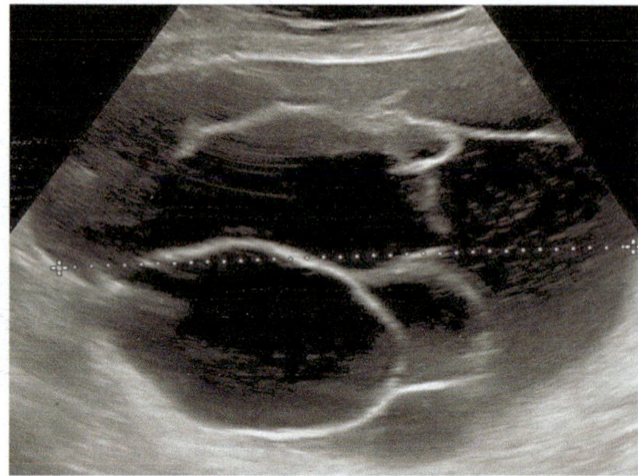

Fig. 9: Thin-walled multiloculated cystic structure with at times loose-looking curved septa, no septal vascularity, persist over the cycles, and may increase in size. The septa of these lesions are usually avascular.

All these structures have thick, shaggy walls with internal echogenicities, but no solid projections or no septa (**Figs. 10A to C**). This means we need to differentiate the internal echogenicities from solid projections. Solid projections arise from the walls of the cyst and, therefore, are attached to the walls, and therefore on eliciting the sliding organ sign, this cannot be separated from the cyst wall or does not slide against the cyst wall. Whereas internal echogenicities are due to debris and

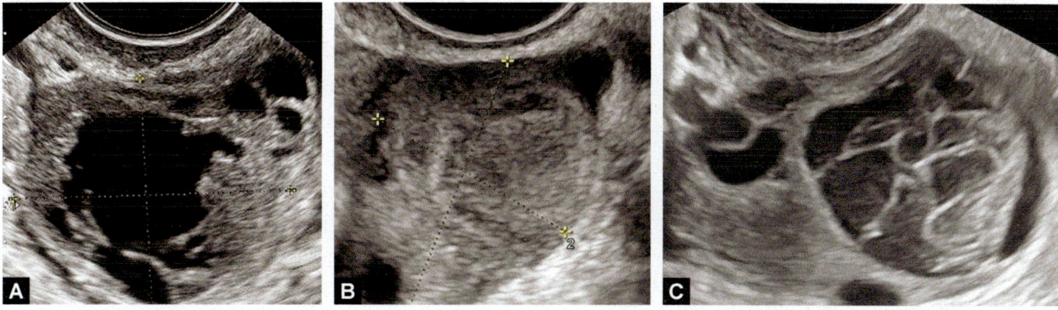

Figs. 10A to C: Intraovarian cystic lesions with thick shaggy walls with different types of internal echogenicity. (A) Ground–glass echogenicity, (B) anechoic contents, and (C) lacelike echogenicity. The most common lesions seen with this appearance are corpus luteum, hemorrhagic cyst, and endometrioma.

debris lies free in the cyst lumen, and therefore on eliciting sliding organ sign, it can be moved and it changes its relative position in the cyst lumen. Moreover, the solid projections usually have a convex surface (**Fig. 11**) in the cyst lumen, whereas debris usually shows flat or concave surface in cyst lumen (**Figs. 12A and B**). This group of lesions does not have actual septa but have linear structures running across the walls (**Fig. 13**). These are fibrin strands. Fibrin strands always show concavity on one of its margins, on rotation or spanning of the probe. This is because fibrin is a result of clot retraction. The appearance of lesions in this group may vary, namely, absolutely isoechoic homogeneous, clear fluid, lacelike or cobweb pattern, or ground–glass appearance. These may be also described as hemorrhagic echogenicities.

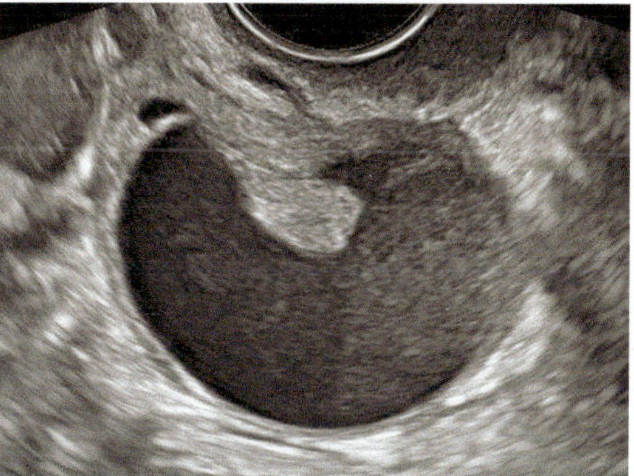

Fig. 11: Cystic lesion with an echogenic solid projection seen arising from the wall of the lesion with its margins convex in the cyst lumen.

Corpus Luteum

Corpus luteum is physiologically active cyst. It appears as a result of rupture of the follicle and ovulation. Its existence usually is till the

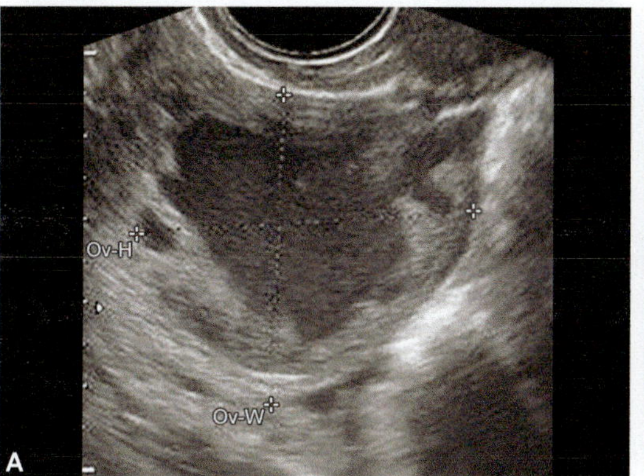

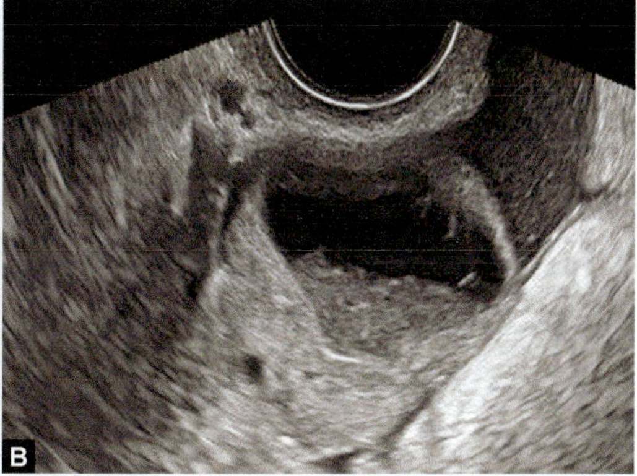

Figs. 12A and B: (A) Cystic lesion showing isoechoic echogenicity overlying on the cyst wall, and parallel to cyst wall suggestive of debris in the cyst; (B) Cystic lesion showing internal echogenicity forming a layer with horizontal upper margin (parallel to the floor)—debris in the cyst.

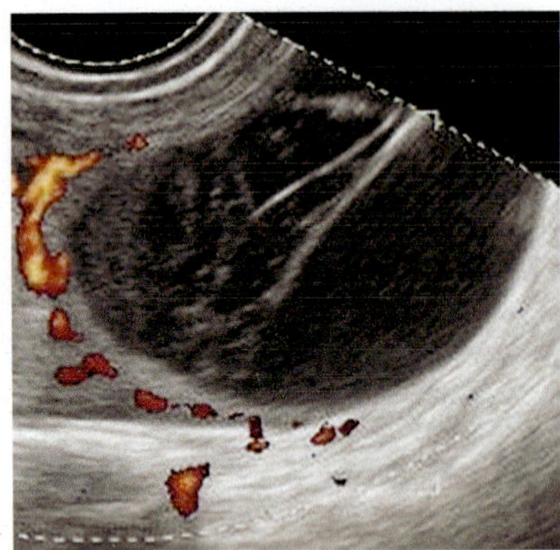

Fig. 13: Cystic lesion with multiple linear echogenicities extending between two walls of the cyst and some of them also crisscrossing. These are fibrin strands and not septa.

end of the luteal phase. But, it may persist till 9–10 weeks in conception cycles. It has thick, crenulated walls. Contents of the cyst show heterogeneous echogenicity with or without septa. The echogenicity and appearance of the contents may vary. It may be a ground-glass echogenicity, cobweb-like or fishnet-like appearance, may show debris-like free-lying echogenicity, and may also sometimes be isoechoic to the ovarian stroma (**Figs. 14A to D**). It is in this later type of corpus luteal morphology that the corpus luteum may only be identified when Doppler is used. Doppler gives almost a complete ring of color with low resistance [RI (resistance index) < 0.5]. That is the most characteristic feature to differentiate it from other lesions with similar appearance on B-mode (**Fig. 15**). More about corpus luteum will be discussed in the relevant chapter.

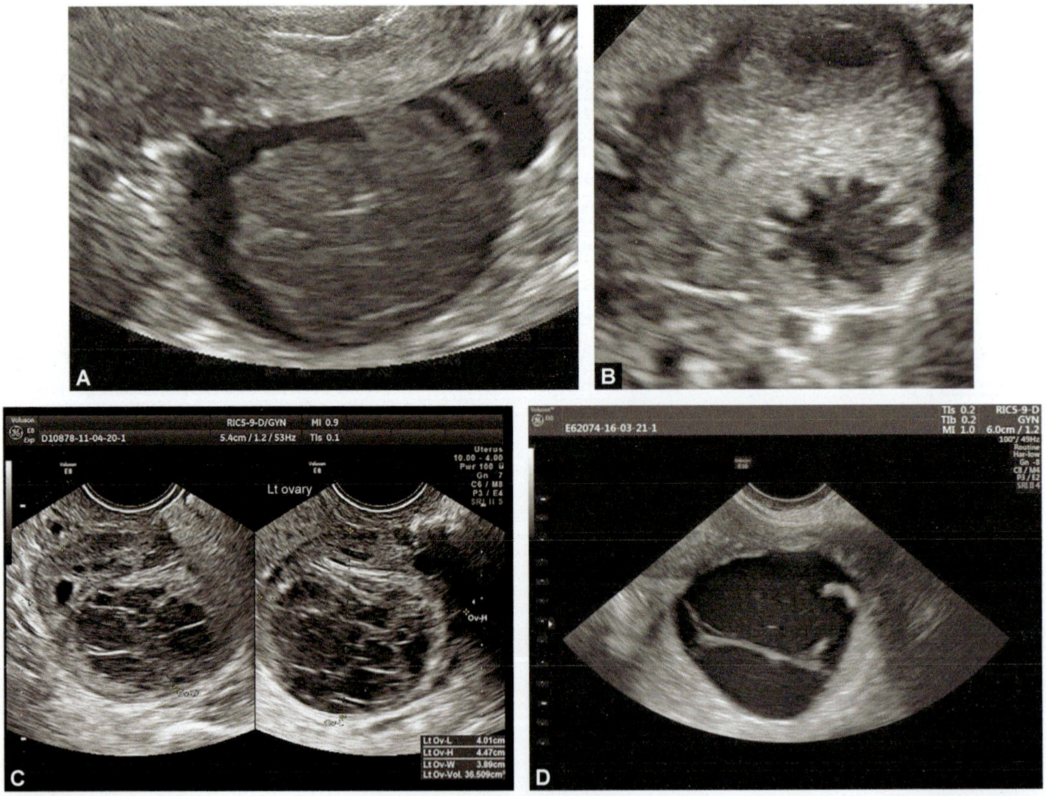

Figs. 14A to D: Corpus luteum is a cystic structure with blood in it, which has appeared as a result of rupture of the follicle. Therefore, it contains clotted blood and fibrin strands and therefore typically presents with thick walls and internal echogenicities such as close-knit net and an echogenicity (A), low-level ground–glass echogenicities (B), fishnet appearance (C), and fibrin strands (D). When such a lesion is seen in the ovary in luteal phase, corpus luteum should be considered as the first probability.

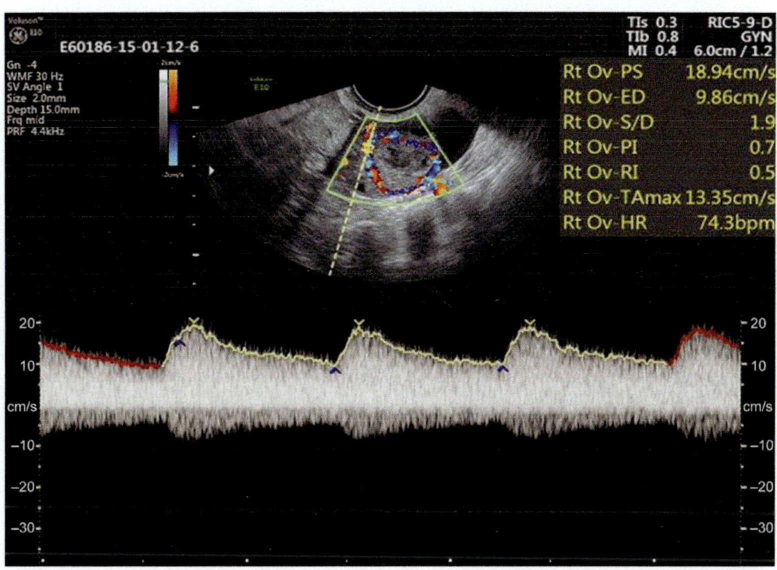

Fig. 15: Corpus luteum shows encircling blood vessels in form of surrounding Doppler signals with low resistance flow seen on spectral Doppler.

Hemorrhagic Cyst

Hemorrhagic cyst is a cyst containing blood in any of its forms. It is most of the times a result of unresolved corpus luteum but is hormonally inactive. It changes echogenicity over time due to fibrinolysis of the clot. The most common appearance is a fishnet appearance, but often fibrin strands are seen (**Figs. 16A to C**). It shows very scanty and high-resistance blood flow. Being physiological in nature, it has a tendency to resolve on its own.

Luteinized Unruptured Follicle

It has thick, hyperechoic, but not shaggy walls, and does not contain blood or blood products. Therefore, it does show low-level internal echogenicity but is less heterogeneous and lacelike or cobweb echogenicity is not likely (**Fig. 17**).

The three above described lesions are physiological ovarian cysts and 53–89% of these show spontaneous regression on follow-up after 4–6 weeks.[3] To avoid confusing these with malignancies, examination must be done in early proliferative phase or two examinations 2–3 weeks apart should be done, so that assessment can be done in two different phases of menstrual cycle and complete or partial resolution of these lesions can be demonstrated, which excludes the possibility of malignancy.

Endometrioma

Endometriosis is detected in 15% of infertile women. It may cause acquired dysmenorrhea, dyspareunia, irregular bleeding, and infertility. One-third to one-half of the ovarian endometriotic cysts are bilateral. Most endometriomas are positioned medially or retrouterine. Features typical of endometriomas are thick shaggy walls with fibrin strands, which may appear like septa, internal echogenicities, ground-glass appearance, fluid–fluid level, linear echogenic flecks in its walls (**Figs. 18A to D**), and pain on pressure with the probe. The fluid–fluid level is an apparent vertical fluid level. But, this is in the longitudinal section of pelvis with patient lying on the examination cot, facing the roof of the room, wherein the left side of the image is anterior (in this orientation of probe and image) (**Fig. 19**), and right

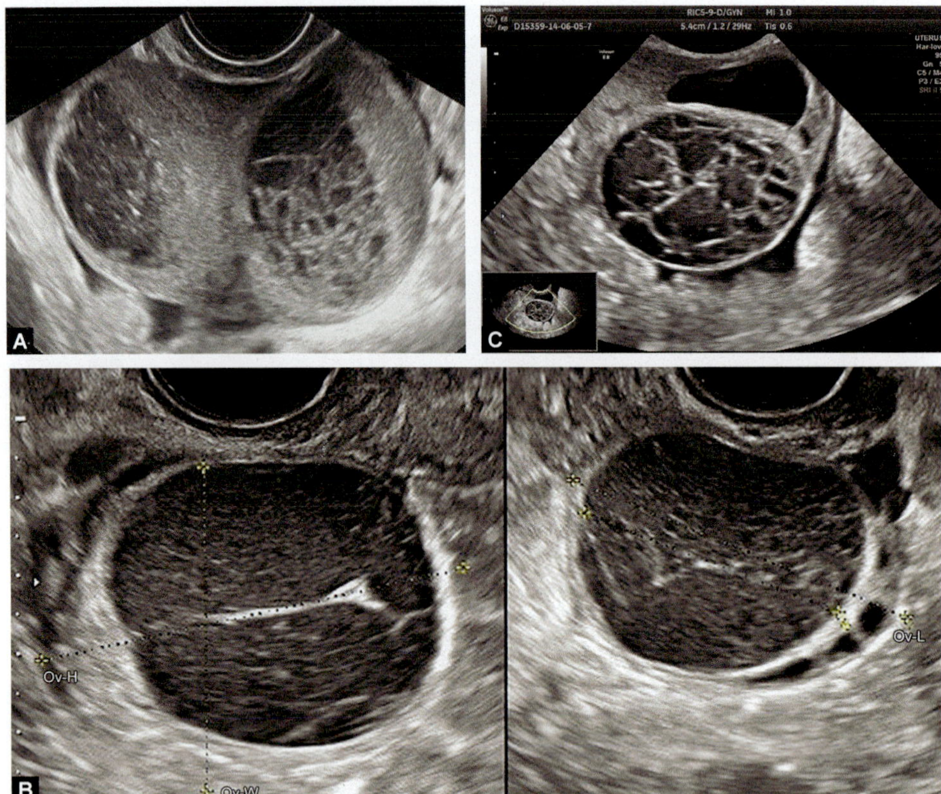

Figs. 16A to C: When a structure with thick shaggy wall and internal echogenicity is seen in the proliferative phase, the diagnosis that should be considered first is hemorrhagic cyst. As the name suggests, it has hemorrhage inside. Close-knit or broad-knit fishnet-like internal echogenicity is characteristic of hemorrhagic cyst. Figures A, B, and C present different B-mode pictures of the hemorrhagic cyst.

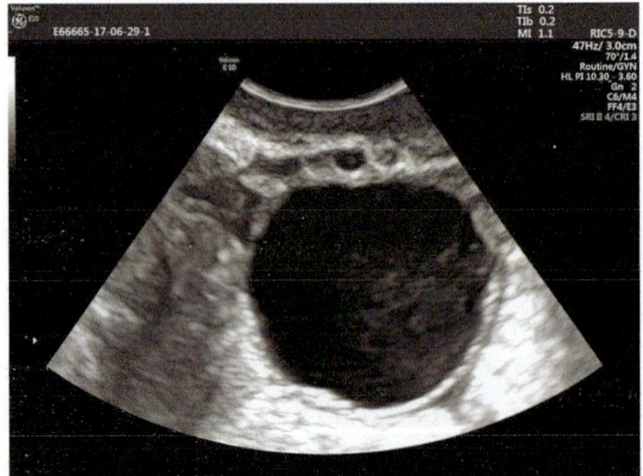

Fig. 17: A thick-walled cystic lesion, with mildly hyperechoic walls and low-level internal echogenicities. Though may be sometimes difficult to differentiate it from corpus luteum, its echogenic walls, absence of fishnet appearance, and high-resistance scanty vascularity are typical. These are because of follicle to luteinizing hormone and no rupture, so no bleeding in the cyst.

side is posterior aspect. The vertical line therefore indicates a transverse plane and therefore it shows anechoic area anteriorly and echogenic area posteriorly. The anechoic area is serum and the echogenic area consists of whole blood due to fresh hemorrhage and debris. The echogenic flecks are believed to be cholesterol or hemosiderin deposits in the cyst walls. These are seen in about one-third of endometriomas. Adhesions are very common in patients with endometriosis. This leads to usually posteriorly placed ovaries. Sometimes, when both ovaries are adherent posterior to the uterus, these are typically known as kissing ovaries (**Fig. 20**). Solid areas may be sometimes seen, these may be blood clots. Streaming sign is often seen in endometriomas. This is slow downward

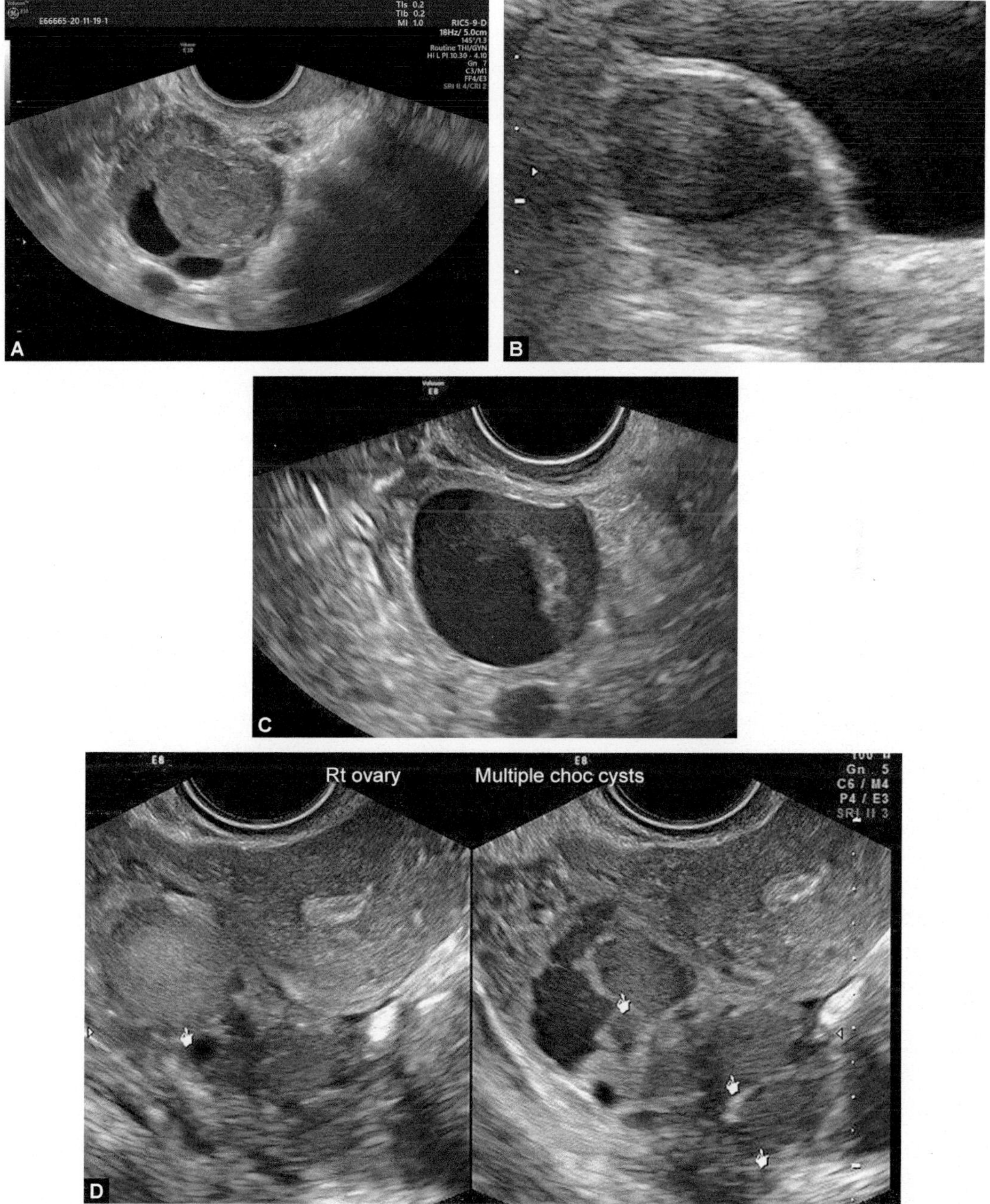

Figs. 18A to D: Endometriomas may present as different ultrasound pictures, though ground–glass appearance is considered to be typical of endometrioma (A), fibrin strands may be seen in the ground–glass cystic lesion, echogenic flecks in the walls are specific of endometrioma (B), it may show lucent areas with echogenicities due to fresh bleed and degenerated blood products (C); endometriomas may be multiple (D).

(toward the gravity) movement of small low-level echogenicities seen in endometrioma typically appreciated on probe movement. This is due to the thick fluid content in these cystic lesions (chocolate cyst). Mean gray value (MGV) of endometrioma is shown to be significantly higher in ovarian endometrioma compared to all other kinds of ovarian cysts.

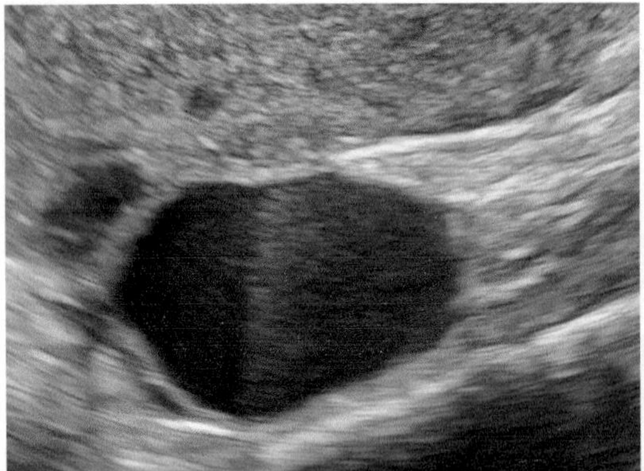

Fig. 19: A vertically oriented fluid–fluid level on an image with longitudinal orientation of probe may be seen in endometrioma. This is because of presence of fluid with two different densities in the cyst (explanation in the text).

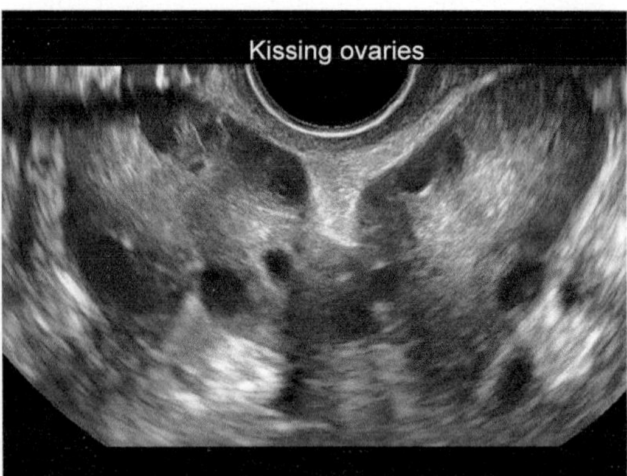

Fig. 20: As adhesions are common with endometriomas and endometriosis, the ovaries get stuck to the uterus and to each other, usually posterior to the uterus and this is known as kissing ovaries.

MGV cut-off >15.560 had a sensitivity of 85% and specificity of 76.5% for diagnosis of endometrioma.[4] Solid components are not a feature of endometrioma. But, when these undergo decidualization, in presence of pregnancy, the walls may grow to produce cauliflower-like solid projections. These may also be vascular and raise a strong suspicion of malignancy. Though actual malignant change in endometrioma also may lead to similar changes in the endometrioma. On Doppler, scattered vascularity at ovarian hilus with moderate vascular impedance has been described in literature. The ovarian hilar RI varies between 0.40 and 0.56. Vascularity may vary between lesions. It is higher during menstruation and in symptomatic patients.[5] Vascularity can be used as a means to decide the mode of therapy for endometriomas. Avascular lesions indicate scarification and are less convenient for delivery of medication and therefore should be considered for surgical therapy.[6]

Kurjak et al. have shown a sensitivity of 83.9%, specificity of 97.1%, positive-predictive value (PPV) 82%, and negative-predictive value (NPV) 97.5% of vaginal sonography for characterization of endometriomas. If CA (cancer antigen) 125 > 35 IU/mL was added as a cut-off to these parameters, the sensitivity and specificity reached 99.04% and 99.64%, and PPV and NPV reached 98.10% and 99.82%.[6] Similar results were also confirmed by several other workers. Apart from the hilar vascularity, endometriomas typically show short-coursed vessels (**Fig. 21**).

The vessels are seen approaching the endometrioma, but do not run along with the wall of the endometrioma. The Doppler picture shows disappearance of these vessels because these vessels take acute turns. 3D power Doppler typically shows multiple short-coursed regularly separated pericystic vessels giving a typical bird's nest appearance (**Fig. 22**).[7] Vascularity is markedly increased and is also low resistance in presence of decidualization or malignant change. Three-dimensional ultrasound allows detection of surface of the endometrioma, visualization of preserved ovarian tissue, and assessment of the ovarian relationship with neighboring pelvic structures in a single image, though 3D ultrasound is not required for the diagnosis of endometrioma (**Fig. 23A**).

Apart from endometriomas, endometriosis is seen in 4–13% of women in reproductive age group and in 25–50% of women with infertility. Endometriosis when extends to >5 mm deep

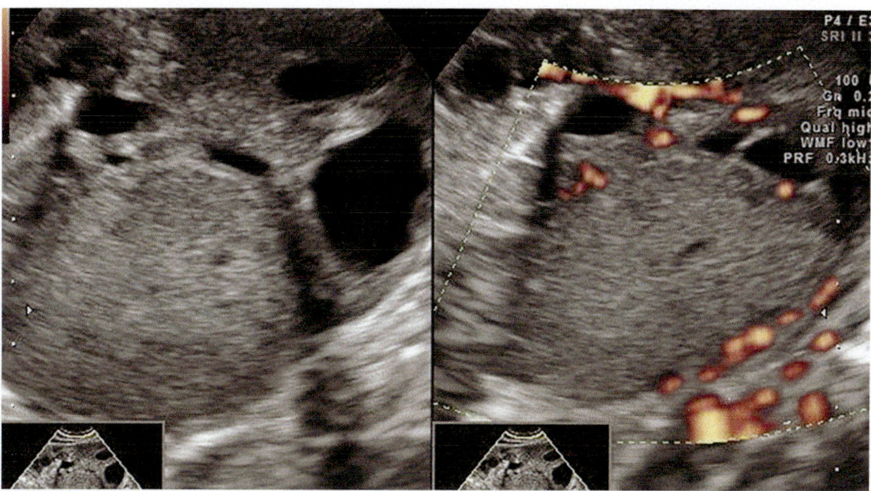

Fig. 21: Endometrioma typically shows multiple vessels coming to the wall of the lesion and then disappear. This is because of acute curves in these vessels. These vessels are described as short-coursed vessels.

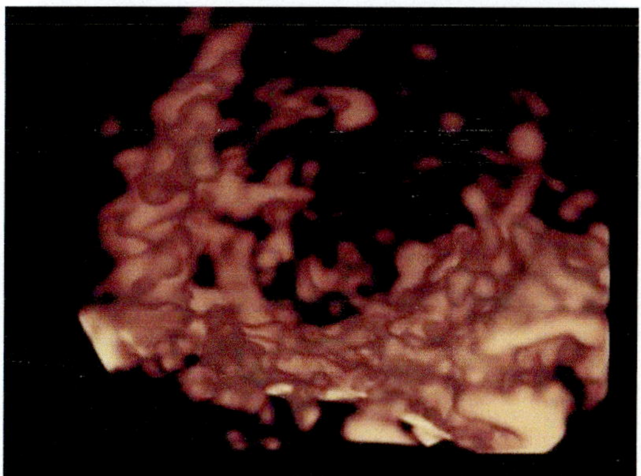

Fig. 22: The short-coursed vessels of endometrioma typically show a bird's nest appearance (crisscrossing weeds) on 3D power Doppler, angio-mode rendering.

from the peritoneal surface, it is termed as deep infiltrating endometriosis, otherwise it is superficial endometriosis.

The latter is difficult to diagnose on ultrasound. It is the deep infiltrating endometriosis (DIE) that leads to dysmenorrhea, dyspareunia, chronic pelvic pain, and often dysuria or pain on defecation, if it involves bladder or bowel, respectively. When in bladder, it may also involve the ureteric insertion and may lead to obstruction and hydronephrosis. The endometriotic patch typically leads to inflammation and fibrosis, leading to distortion of surrounding anatomy.

These generally appear as ill-defined irregular hypoechoic areas with some acoustic shadowing at times. These lesions typically show hyperechoic spots due to hemosiderin and cholesterol deposits. These are tender on probe pressure and are typically hypovascular. Adhesions of involved surfaces are common. Transvaginal scan has shown 81.1% sensitivity and 94.2% specificity for diagnosis of DIE.[8]

Deep infiltrating endometriosis may involve bowel, bladder, uterosacral ligament, vaginorectal septum, most commonly, but may also involve abdominal organs at times.

Rectosigmoid DIE: It usually involves the anterior muscularis of the rectosigmoid part of the large bowel. It is known that the muscularis of the large bowel has inner layer of circular and outer layer of longitudinal muscle fibers. The entire muscularis, which otherwise appears as a hypoechoic linear band, is seen being traversed by an echogenic line that separates these two layers. Discontinuity of this line due to a fusiform or elongated hypoechoic area indicates endometriosis. On transverse section, this typically gives a signet ring appearance. When the submucosa is involved, fibrotic retraction of the lesion in submucosa leads to a typical "red Indian head" appearance (**Fig. 23B**). Negative sliding organ

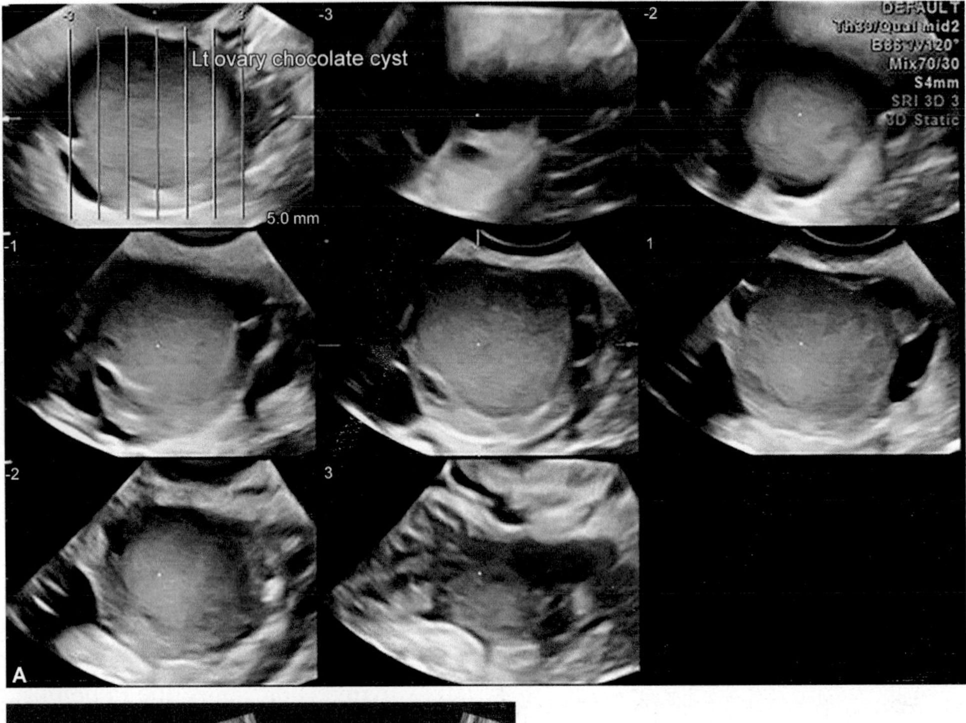

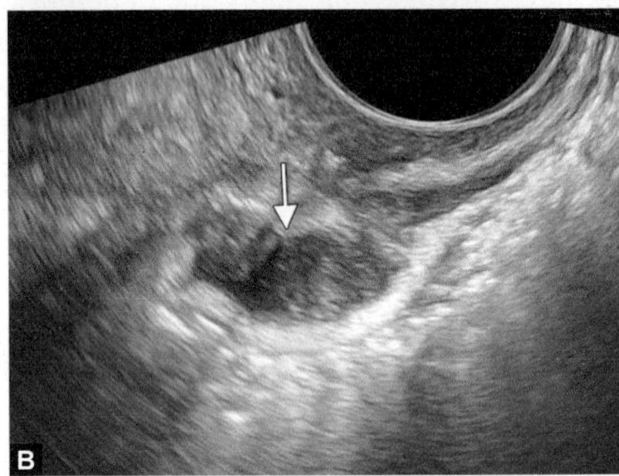

Figs. 23A and B: (A) 3D ultrasound with tomographic ultrasound imaging combined with volume-contrast imaging (thick slice technique for better contrast) showing multiple sections with homogeneously echogenic endometrioma with ovarian parenchyma with follicles surrounding it projections; (B) B-mode ultrasound showing "red Indian head sign".

sign between the uterus and the bowel may be an additional sign. This has a likelihood ratio of 23.6 for rectal DIE.[9] This lesion may extend into the posterior vaginal wall.

Vaginal DIE: It is seen as localized heterogenous thickening of the vaginal wall, though the margins are not well defined. When the lesion extends from the rectum, the rectovaginal septum is typically not continuous. The vaginal wall thickening can be more clearly appreciated, if the scan is done with the probe placed only superficially in the vaginal canal when the vaginal cavity is filled with gel (gel vaginosonography).

Cervical DIE: It is seen as thick firm cervical wall appears as hypoechoic area on ultrasound with ill-defined margins and also at times associated with acoustic shadowing. And like all other endometriotic lesions, even these lesions are tender on probe pressure.

Uterosacral DIE: These are most difficult to image on ultrasound, unless when there is fluid around. If uterosacral ligament is seen as a thick soft tissue mass instead of a string-like structure, it may indicate DIE.

DIE in the bladder: It may appear as localized thickening of bladder wall, hypoechoic, and hypovascular on ultrasound. Trigone is the area most commonly affected. When the lesion extends from the anterior vaginal wall as a penetrating lesion, and may involve the bladder diffusely, it gives a typical hourglass shape to bladder.

Solid Lesions

Lesions that can be included in this group are fibroma, fibrothecoma, thecoma, Brenner tumor, etc. All these, except fibromas, are extremely rare. Fibroma is well-defined round/oval lesion with echogenicity like that of a fibroid-hypoechoic (to myometrium), homogeneous, but sometimes may be heterogeneous and may also show calcifications (**Figs. 24A to C**). When homogeneous fibromas are isoechoic to normal ovarian stroma and may be difficult to identify on B-mode scan. The ovary may then look solid. Therefore, Doppler study of a solid-looking ovary is a must. Doppler typically shows a ring of color-like in uterine fibroid (**Figs. 25A and B**). This peripheral vascularity is well appreciated on 3D power Doppler also (**Figs. 26A and B**). Fibromas need to be differentiated from pedunculated subserosal fibroids and that can be done by tracing the blood supply to this lesion to find out, if it is coming from uterus or ovary. Fibromas are often bilateral and may also be associated with ascites and pleural effusion. This complication is known as Meigs' syndrome.

Solid tumors or tumors with solid components may be Sertoli cell tumor, Leydig cell tumor, and Sertoli–Leydig tumor. Small solid tumors are usually Leydig cell tumor. Sertoli cell tumors are larger solid tumors, whereas Sertoli–Leydig tumors are small or

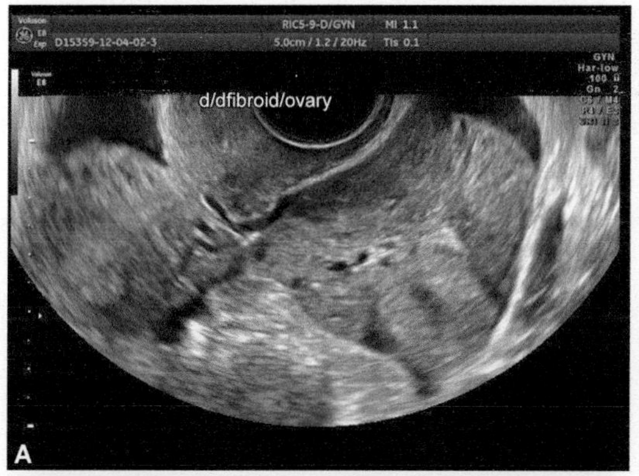

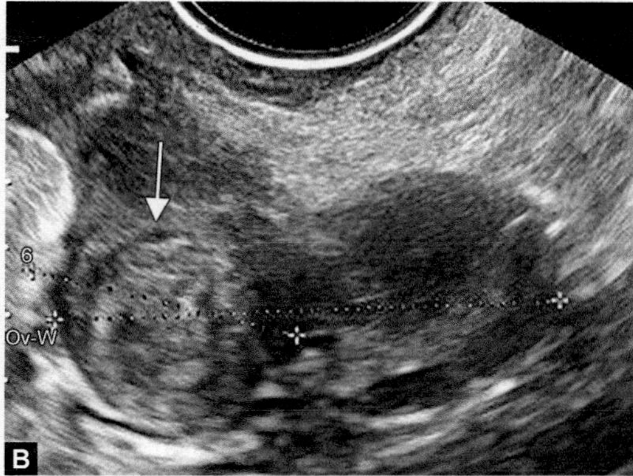

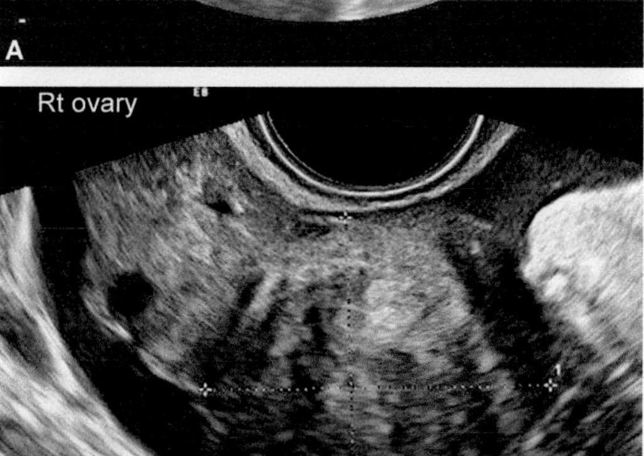

Figs. 24A to C: Solid isoechoic roundish well-defined intraovarian lesion is fibroma (A); fibromas may sometimes show heterogeneous echogenicity (B), and at times may be large and become exophytic (C).

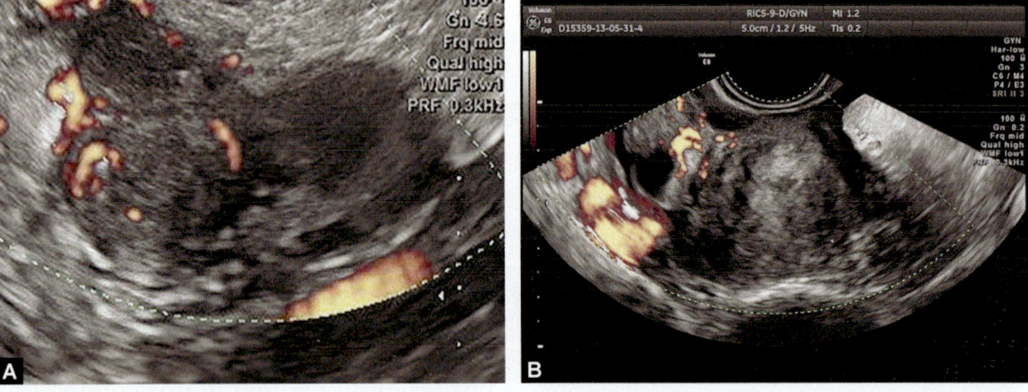

Figs. 25A and B: Ovarian fibroma typically shows peripheral vascularity like fibroids, as seen on power Doppler (A) or color Doppler (B).

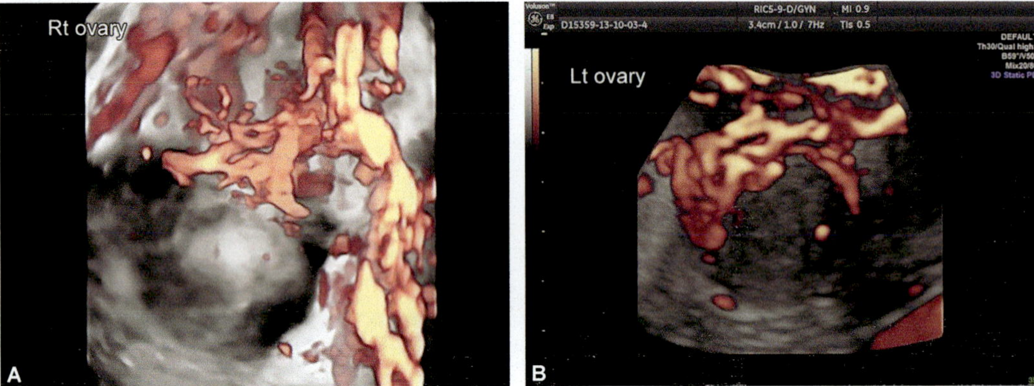

Figs. 26A and B: 3D power Doppler, glass-body rendered image typically shows the peripheral vascularity of ovarian fibroma in both the images.

medium-sized solid tumors or multilocular tumors. On the basis of endocrine symptoms, the woman's age and ultrasound findings may help to suggest a correct diagnosis.[10] Ovarian dysgerminoma also presents as large solid, lobulated highly vascularized adnexal mass with heterogeneous echogenicity in a woman of 20–30 years (**Fig. 27**).

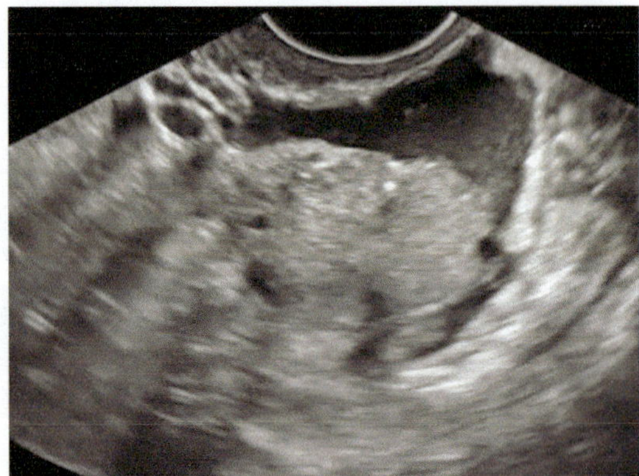

Fig. 27: A solid looking large exophytic ovarian tumor with irregular but well-defined margins is seen with minimal free fluid surrounding the lesion. This lesion possibly may be dysgerminoma.

Solid-looking ovaries may also be seen in ovarian torsion. In ovary with torsion, stroma is hypoechoic with peripherally placed small follicles (**Fig. 28**). Vascularity may or may not be present and that decides the viability of the ovary. On twisting of the pedicle of the ovary, first the venous flow is obliterated as veins have low pressure and thinner walls, and later during the process of torsion, the arteries are also obliterated. The ovaries are considered to be viable as long as the arterial blood flow is seen. It must, therefore, be remembered

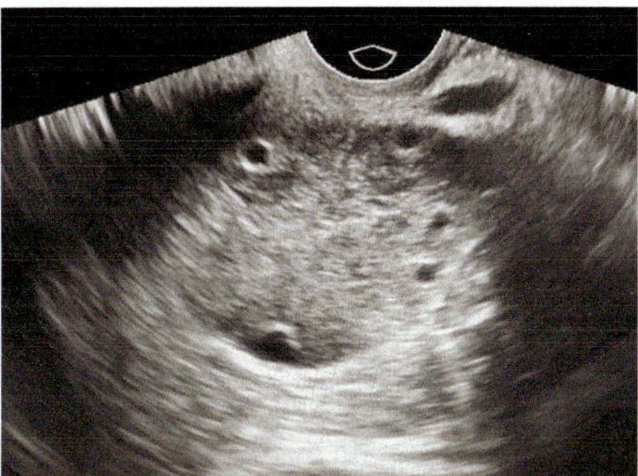

Fig. 28: Ovary showing multiple small follicles in the periphery with hypoechoic stroma, typical of ovarian torsion.

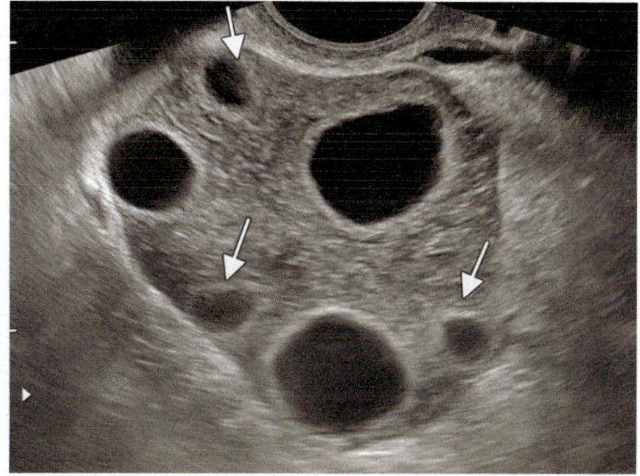

Fig. 30: Small follicles showing complete echogenic rim, which is described as follicular rim sign and is seen in early torsion.
Courtesy: Dr Mala Sibal, Bengaluru, India.

that presence of vascularity does not exclude torsion. Definitive sign of torsion is a whirlpool sign in adnexa (**Fig. 29A**). Because of twisting of vessels in the pedicle, there are multiple circles of vessels, which look like whirlpool.[11] This sign can be seen on B-mode scan as well as on color Doppler (**Fig. 29B**). This whirlpool typically slides with the probe movement in and out as it is not fixed. Follicular ring sign has been described as the earliest sign of ovarian torsion. This is a complete echogenic rim surrounding small follicles (**Fig. 30**).[12] Follicular rings are seen starting early in the course of torsion when venous and lymphatic flow begins to get compromised. They are very distinct at this early stage. As hemorrhage spreads to other areas, the ovarian tissue becomes more echogenic and the follicular rings, though still seen, are less distinct. Follicular ring has also been documented in ovarian tuberculosis but typically the ovaries are hypovascular in these cases.

Complex Lesions with Cystic and Solid Components

Lesions in this group have thick walls, with internal echogenicities and also solid projections arising from the walls. Lesions included in this group are:

- Dermoids
- Epithelial tumors

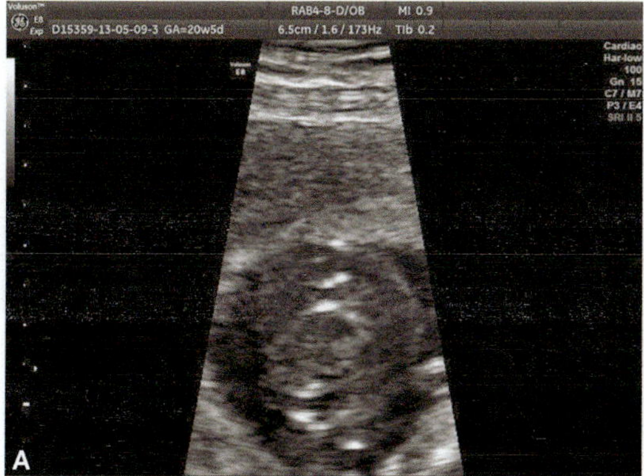

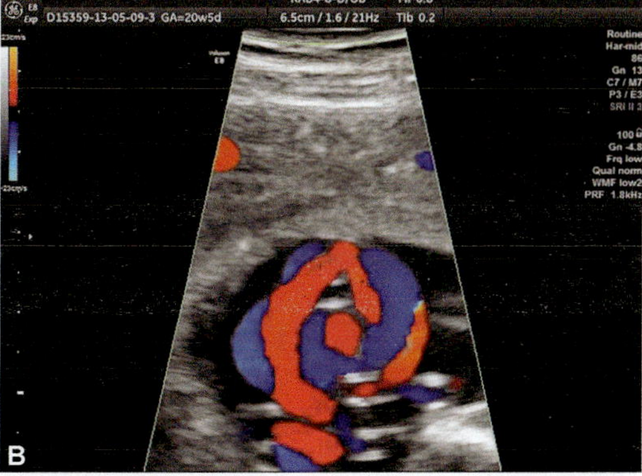

Figs. 29A and B: Whirlpool-like appearance is seen on B-mode image (A) in free fluid due to twisting of the vessels in the pedicle as a result of torsion. This is described as whirlpool sign. Color Doppler (B) shows also the same sign and twisting of blood vessels.

- Endometrioid tumors
- Certain not very commonly seen tumors such as struma ovarii, granulosa cell tumors, or dysgerminomas.

Dermoids

Dermoids or teratomas are often an incidental finding. These are well-defined lesions with thick walls and may show low-level echoes, fluid–fluid level, hyperechoic lines, and dots due to:

Dermoids may present as cystic lesions with low-level echogenicities and dense echogenic areas with posterior shadowing due to bones or teeth, hair, hyperechoic/calcified echoes like teeth or bones with posterior shadowing, regional diffuse bright echoes with or without acoustic shadowing due to hair clumps or fat in Rokitansky protuberance (**Figs. 31A to G**). As compared to the fluid-fluid levels in the endometriomas, dermoids have echogenic fluid anteriorly (on left side) and anechoic fluid posteriorly (on right side). The echogenic layer in dermoid is fat, which is lighter than fluid and therefore floats on the fluid. These features have been assigned definite PPV (positive-predictive value).[13]

- 80% for shadowing echodensity
- 75% for regionally bright echoes
- 50% for hyperechoic lines and dots
- 20% for fluid–fluid level.

Positive-predictive value for dermoid with more than two features is 100%.

Morphologic scoring system for dermoids by Kurjak et al. has sensitivity of 93.1% and specificity of 99.4%. 72% of cystic teratomas are avascular. Vascularity in these teratomas may be an indicator of malignant change. Including color Doppler, sensitivity of 99% and specificity of 99.8% can be achieved.[14]

Dermoids are often an incidental finding and are not an absolute indication for surgery unless these are large (>4 cm), vascular, or interfering with tubo-ovarian relationship in a patient seeking fertility. Dermoids are otherwise avascular but when these undergo malignant change, these develop vascularity. Torsion of the ovary is common when it has a dermoid inside, but in these cases, Doppler may not be of much help in diagnosing torsion as has already been mentioned that dermoids are avascular.

Struma Ovarii

It may be considered a type of dermoid. It is a dermoid-containing thyroid tissue. On ultrasound, this lesion appears as lesion with solid and cystic components. It has pure and impure forms. Struma ovarii typically shows struma pearl. This is a rounded solid ball-like

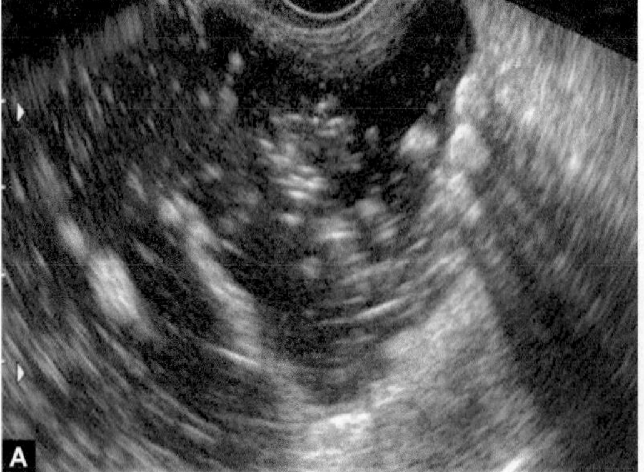

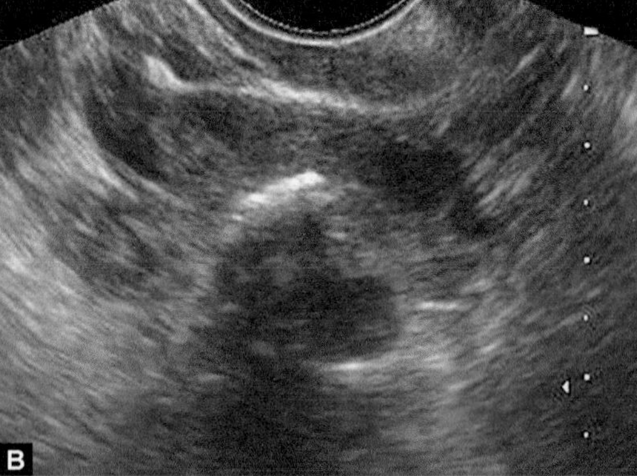

Figs. 31A and B: Dermoids of the ovary may have various appearances and B-mode ultrasound is diagnostic of dermoids. (A) Cystic lesion with echogenic spots and lines seen in the cyst lumen because of hair. Triangular echogenicities with posterior shadowing are due to teeth in the dermoid; (B) Isoechoic mass lesion with hyperechoic blade like lesion with posterior shadowing.

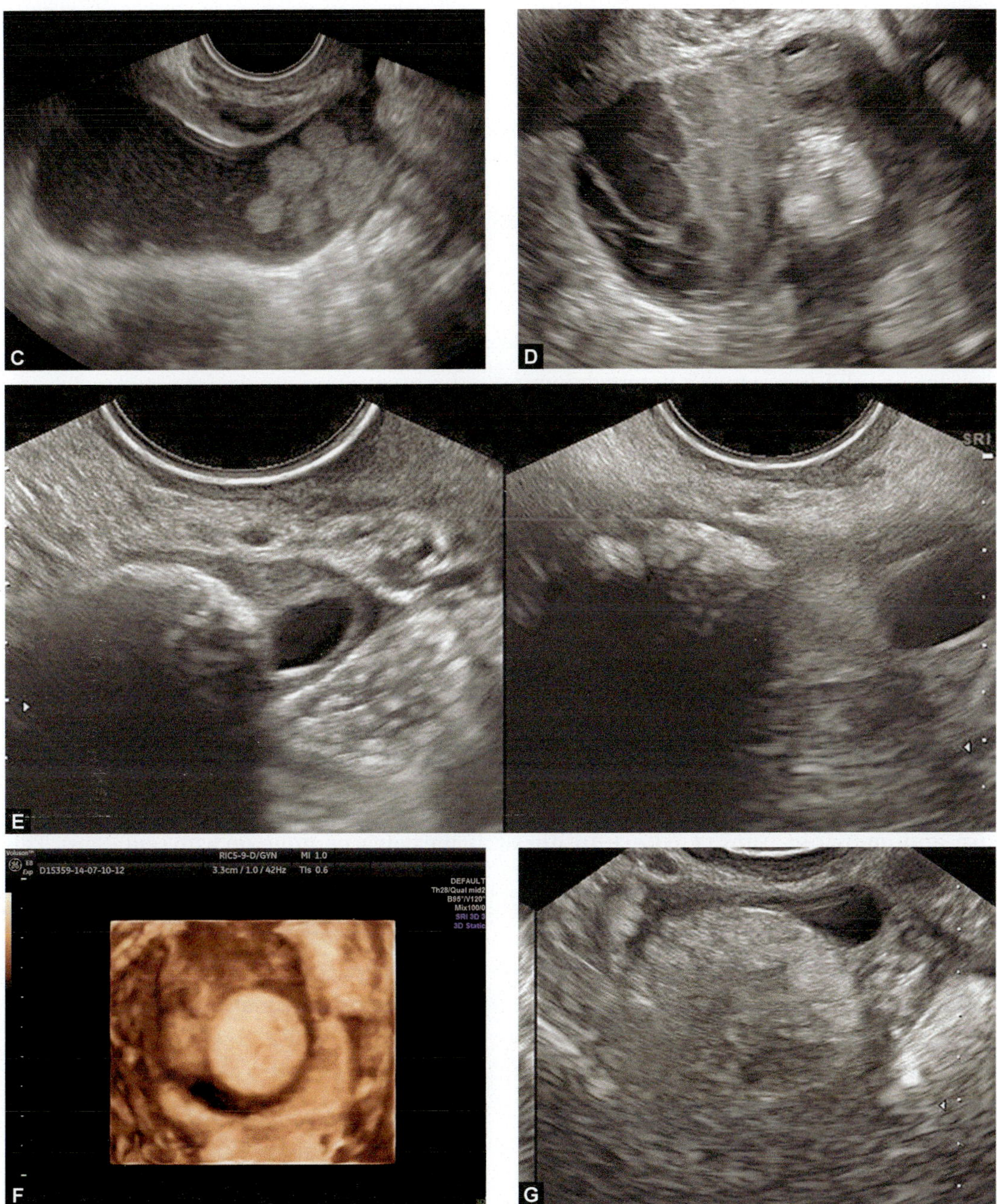

Figs. 31C to G: (C) Cystic lesion with thick shaggy walls, low-level internal echogenicities, and multiple roundish echogenicities, possibly hairballs; (D) Ovary shows a solid echogenic ball-like dermoid; (E) Dermoid is sometimes seen as only an irregular blade of hyperechogenicity with posterior shadowing on B-mode; (F) The same lesion on 3D US shows an echodense ball with not very smooth margins; (G) Dermoid may also present as an intraovarian snowball-like lesion, the posterior margin of which cannot be appreciated.

structures, similar to white balls in dermoid. Struma pearls according to the International Ovarian Tumor Analysis (IOTA) definitions can be called papillary projections. The difference is that the white balls in dermoids are avascular and struma pearls are vascular. Doppler shows flow in the center of lesions in struma ovarii and only at periphery of ovary in dermoids.[15] The solid components are thyroid tissue and cystic components are colloid-rich areas with cystic degeneration.[16] It is because of this colloidal material that the contents of this cystic lesion show low-level echogenicities.

Granulosa Cell Tumor (GCT)

On ultrasound, most GCTs are large multi-locular—solid masses with large number of locules or solid tumors with heterogeneous echogenicity. The septa are thick and show vascularity. These are hypervascular lesions. It may also be associated with endometrial hyperplasia and increased endometrial vascularity due to hyperestrinism, which is due to estrogen secretion from the granulosa cells of the tumor.

Epithelial Tumors

Surface epithelial-stromal tumors account for 60% of ovarian neoplasms and 80–90% of ovarian malignancies. Of all these, 46% are serous, 36.5% are mucinous, and 7.5% are endometrioid tumors. These tumors are chiefly cystic and have septa, internal echogenicities, and projections arising from its walls. Benign and malignant counterparts of these tumors have a similar but overlapping ultrasound appearance.

A benign serous cystadenoma has thin walls, thin septa, no internal echogenicities, no papillarities, no solid projections, and no vascularity in the septa (**Fig. 32**). Whereas serous cystadenocarcinoma has thicker walls, thicker septa (>3 mm), small papillarities, internal echogenicities, and may also show solid areas (**Figs. 33A to C**) and shows significant vascularity (**Figs. 34A and B**). Mucus cystadenoma has thicker walls, thicker septa, shows internal echogenicities, papillarities, and may or may not show solid areas. On ultrasound, therefore, it is not possible to give a histopathological diagnosis. It appears similar to serous cystadenocarcinoma.

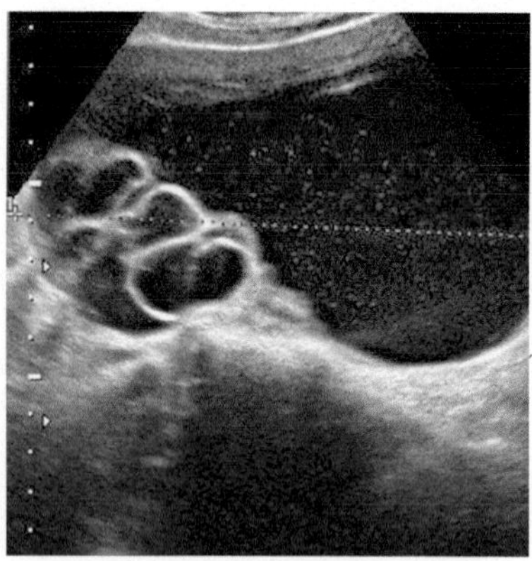

Fig. 32: Serous cystadenoma—thin walled cystic lesion with multiple septa but no internal echogenicity, no papillarities, or solid projections.

Broad ligament fibroid: This is a fibroid arising from broad ligament. On ultrasound, it is a well-circumscribed, usually round, and hypoechoic lesion. It can be separated from both uterus and ovary by probe pressure (sliding organ sign) and shows peripheral vascularity. Tracing the feeding vessel can also help to decide the organ of origin.

Peritoneal inclusion cyst: It is a fluid collection in the pelvic peritoneum with septations. This fluid collection is not under pressure and therefore changes shape on probe pressure. The septa inside move with respiration, pressure, or with pulsations of nearby vessel. These lesions typically do not show any vascularity. Often an ovary may be seen in close vicinity of such a cyst.

Paraovarian cyst: These are remnants of mesonephric ducts. Up to 20% of adnexal masses may be paraovarian cysts. These are benign, avascular lesions with thin walls and anechoic contents. The shape does not change with pressure but can be easily separated from ovary. Adhesions indicate infection and solid projections in it may raise a possibility of malignancy.

Paratubal cysts: These may be mesosalpingeal cysts, fimbrial cysts (hydatid cyst of Morgagni) or those arising from Müllerian duct remnants.

These are connected to fimbria typically and may be multiple.

Depending on ultrasound appearances, these lesions can be divided into benign, possibly malignant, and malignant tumors. Benign tumors have thin walls, clear contents, are usually unilocular, if septate, septa are thin and avascular and show no papillarities and solid projections. Whereas lesions having following features have higher chance of malignancy.[17]

Ovary >20 cm^3 in premenopausal patient, and >10 cm^3 in postmenopausal patient; though this means waiting for too long before diagnosis.

- Cyst wall thickness >3 mm and with papillarities of >3 mm
- Septa thicker >3 mm thickness

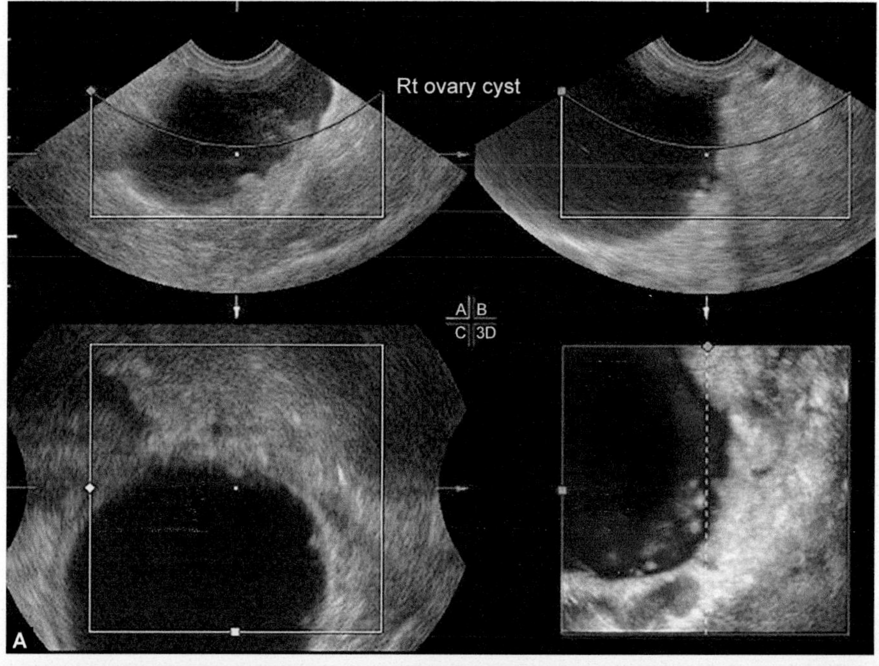

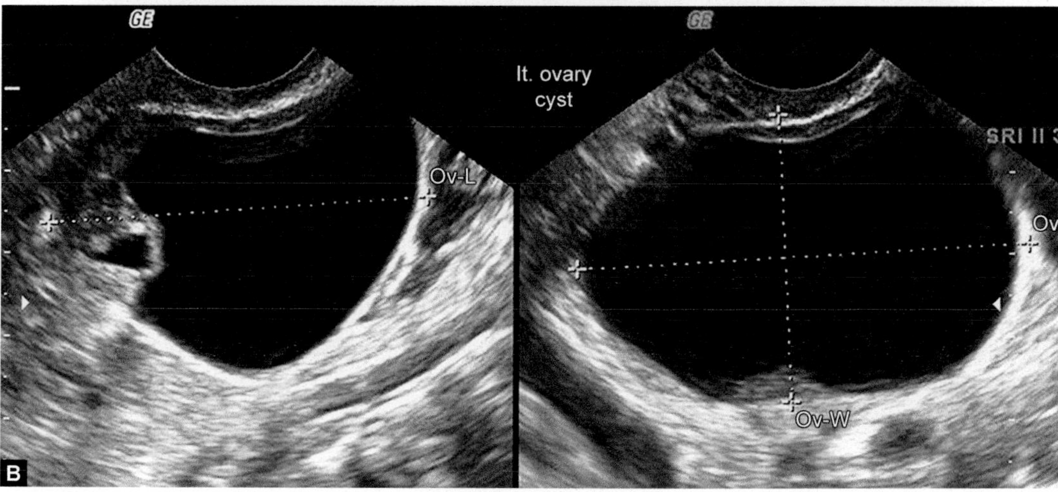

Figs. 33A to C: *Contd...*

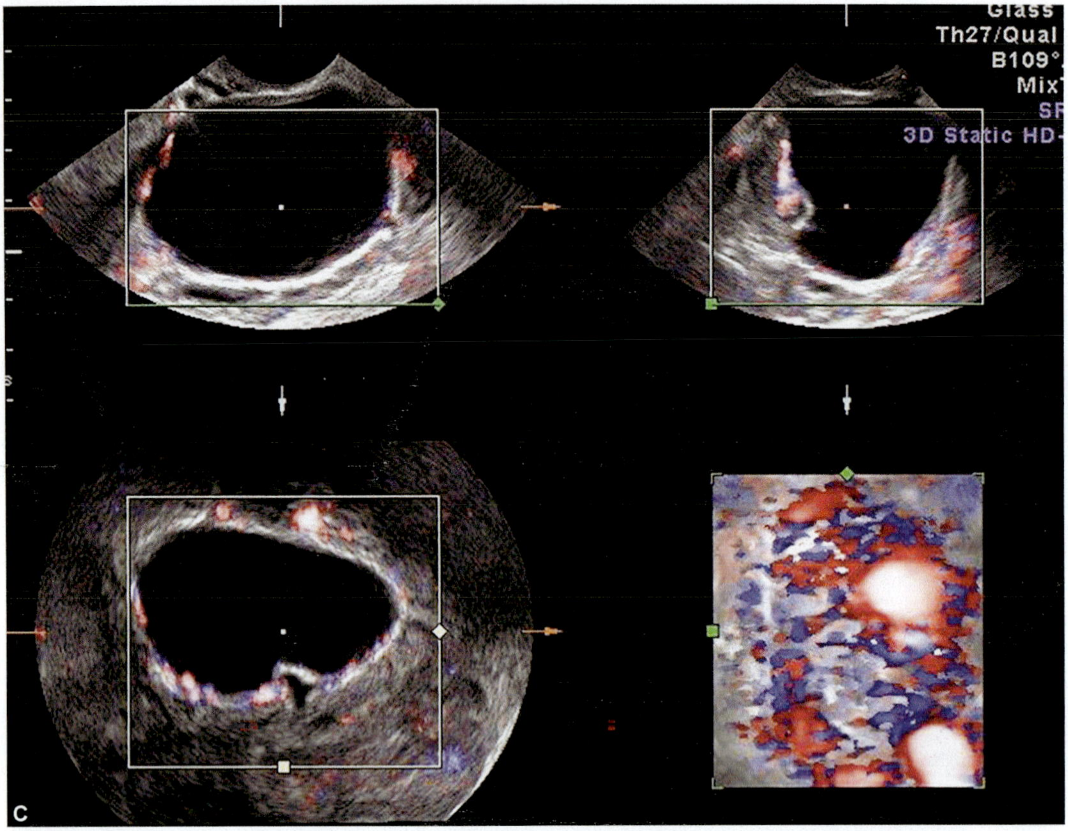

Figs. 33A to C: (A) 3D ultrasound volume of cystic lesion with multiple small papillarities—serous cystadenocarcinoma; (B) B-mode image of a cystic lesion showing only one thick-walled small septum, this was otherwise benign looking, but on 3D power Doppler; (C) It showed abundant vascularity and was proved to be serous cystadenocarcinoma.

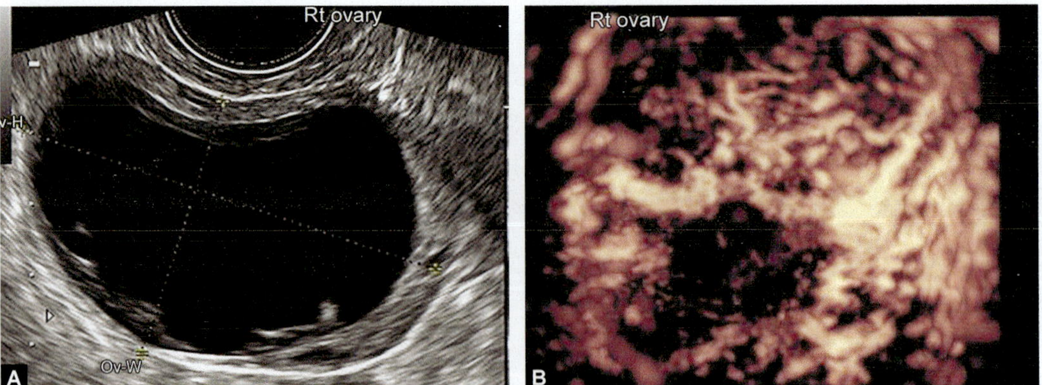

Figs. 34A and B: Nonseptated cystic lesion, with no papillarities or solid projections but shaggy walls seen on B-mode image (A), the same lesion on 3D power Doppler (B) shows abundant vascularity with vessels of variable caliber and branching in various directions, suggestive of a malignant lesion.

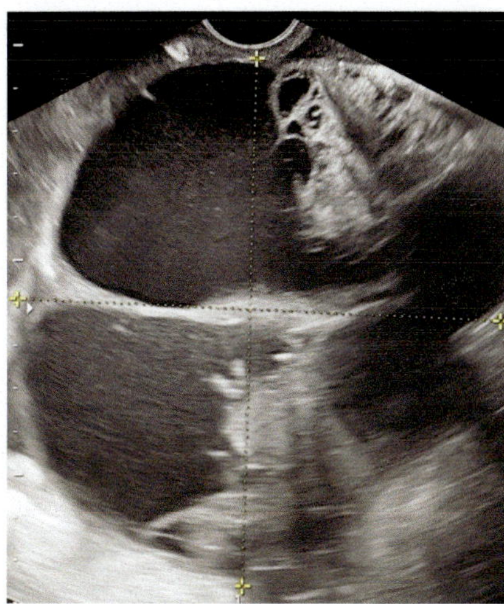

Fig. 35: B-mode image of an ovarian mass lesion showing heterogeneous echogenicity and irregular margins, suggestive of malignancy.

- Solid parts >1 cm Cysts with papillarities, solid projections with irregular margins, and solid projections with vascularity are more likely to recur.[18]
- Mixed or high-level internal echoes
- Irregularity in shape or echogenicity (heterogeneous echogenicity) is the most reliable sign of malignancy. In a study of 309 cases, it has shown a sensitivity of 85%, specificity of 94%, +LR (positive likelihood ratio) of 14, and –LR (negative likelihood ratio) of 0.15 (**Fig. 35**).[19] RI (resistance index) ≤ 0.42 is suggestive of malignancy. RI < 0.41 can be used as a cut-off for the screening of ovarian malignancy and can detect ovarian cancer as early as FIGO (Federation of International Gynecologists and Obstetricians) stage Ia.[20] But, there are pitfalls to this generalization.

Variable caliber of vessels typical of malignant lesion may show variable resistance and velocity. Pre-existing vessels in the lesion may not show low resistance and in postmenopausal patients the resistance may not be as low as described. Therefore, a low resistance has a PPV for malignancy, but high-resistance vessels do not rule out malignancy (**Figs. 36A to D**).

- Bilaterality—ascites
- Adhesions and disturbed relationship with structures around
- *Chaotic vascular architecture*: Dichotomous branching, microaneurysm, and small arteriovenous fistulae are seen on 3D power Doppler.

*Typical vascular criteria seen on 3D PD in malignant tumors (**Fig. 37**)*:[21]

- Loss of tree-like branching pattern of vessels
- Sacculation of arteries and veins
- Focal narrowing of arteries
- Internal shift in velocity within arterial lumen
- "Beach ball" finding of increased and disorganized blood flow
- Increased flow to center of a solid region
- Crowding of vascularity
- Abruptly stopping vessels.

This has improved the predictability of ovarian cancer significantly as seen in several studies. VI (vascularity index) and VFI (vascularity flow index) were significantly higher in advanced-stage tumors and metastatic tumors as compared with early-stage tumors. But 3D PD cannot differentiate between advanced stage tumors and metastatic tumors.[22] 3D PD (3D power Doppler) allows accurate detection of ovarian malignancy at FIGO stage I. *Accuracy for stage I of Ca*:[23]

- 2D US abdominal 69.8%
- TVCD 86%
- 3D US 74.4%
- 3D PD 95.3%
- 3D PD + 3D US 97.7%.

Different scoring systems have been established combining all the above-mentioned features. Using 3D US and 3D power Doppler improves the diagnostic accuracy, as it is superior in evaluating such lesions:[20]

- Papillary projections
- Characteristics of cystic walls, so it is especially helpful in evaluating cystic tumors (surface mode) (**Figs. 38A to D**)

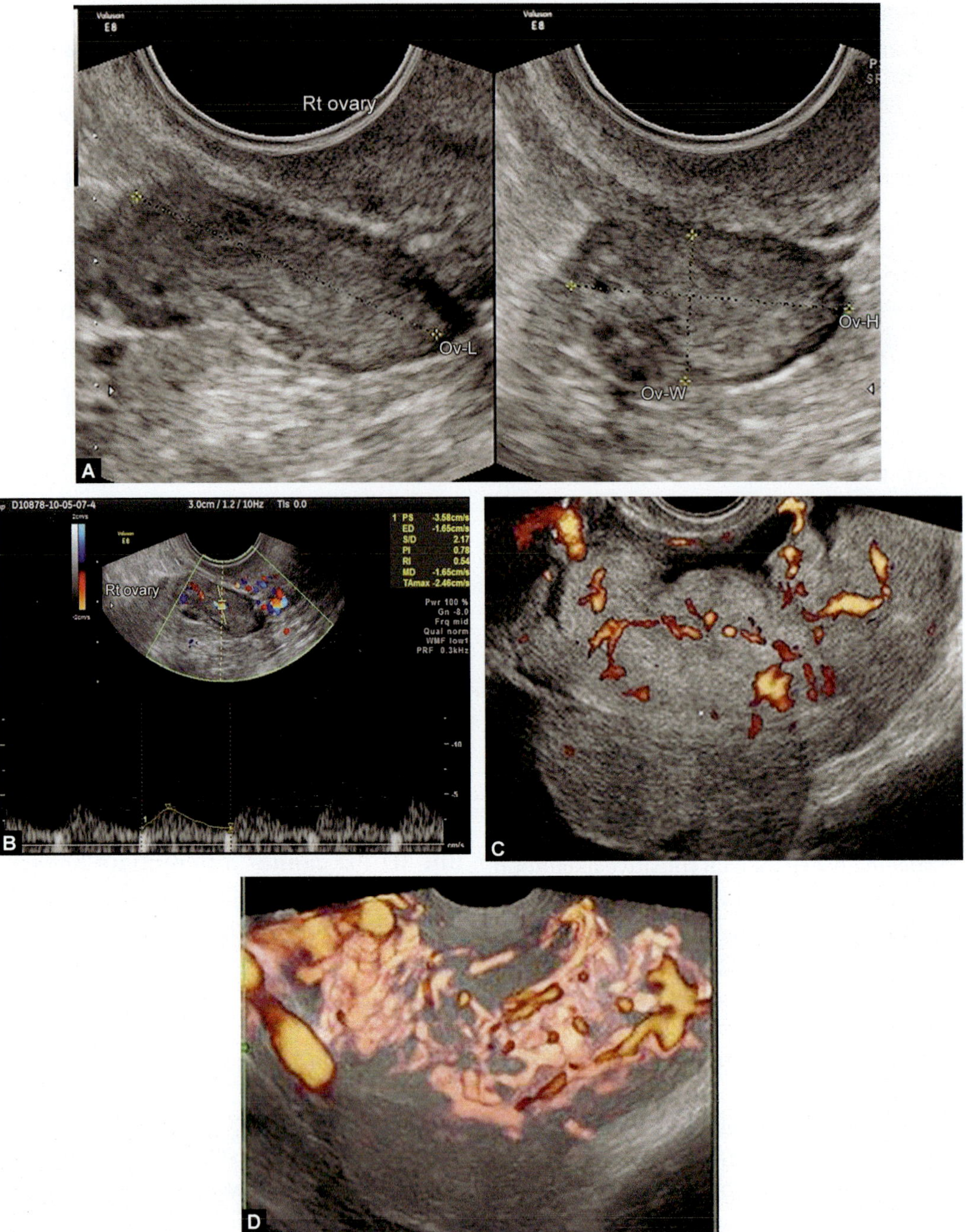

Figs. 36A to D: (A and B) Normal sized but solid-looking ovary in a 58-year-old female, which on Doppler shows a vascularity with moderate resistance. The findings fit into the benign normal-like ovary out of the context of the age, but because this was a postmenopausal ovary, the resistance index is higher in this malignant ovary; (C and D) Isoechoic large lobulated solid lesion on power Doppler shows scanty vascularity, but the blood vessels of variable caliber, raising a suspicion of malignancy. On 3D power Doppler, this lesion shows abundant vascularity, with typical malignant characteristics.

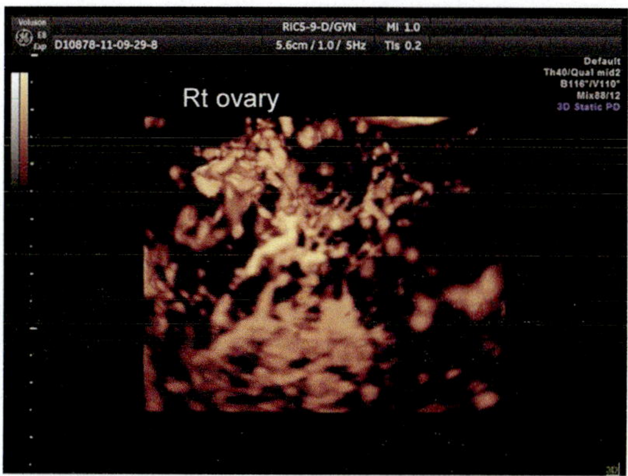

Fig. 37: 3D power Doppler vascular characteristics of malignancy—irregular caliber of vessels, arteriovenous communications, microaneurysms, vascular lakes, and dichotomous branching.

- Calcifications and bone densities (transparent mode)
- Identifying the extent of capsular infiltration of tumors
- Calculating the volume
- 3D PD (power Doppler) has improved specificity (75% as compared to 54%) for ovarian malignancy and staging though the detection rate is 97.7%.[23]

Contrast enhancement on ultrasound further enables the visualization of very small vessels that were not otherwise seen. This improves the definition of small vessels in the tumor and their architecture. Differentiation between benign and malignant lesions by contrast-induced 3D PD shows:[24]

- Sensitivity—100%
- Specificity—93.9%
- PPV—85.7%
- NPV—100%.

The contrasts commonly available are Echovist, Levovist, or SonoVue. These are positive contrast media used for ultrasound. This helps to potentiate the color signals

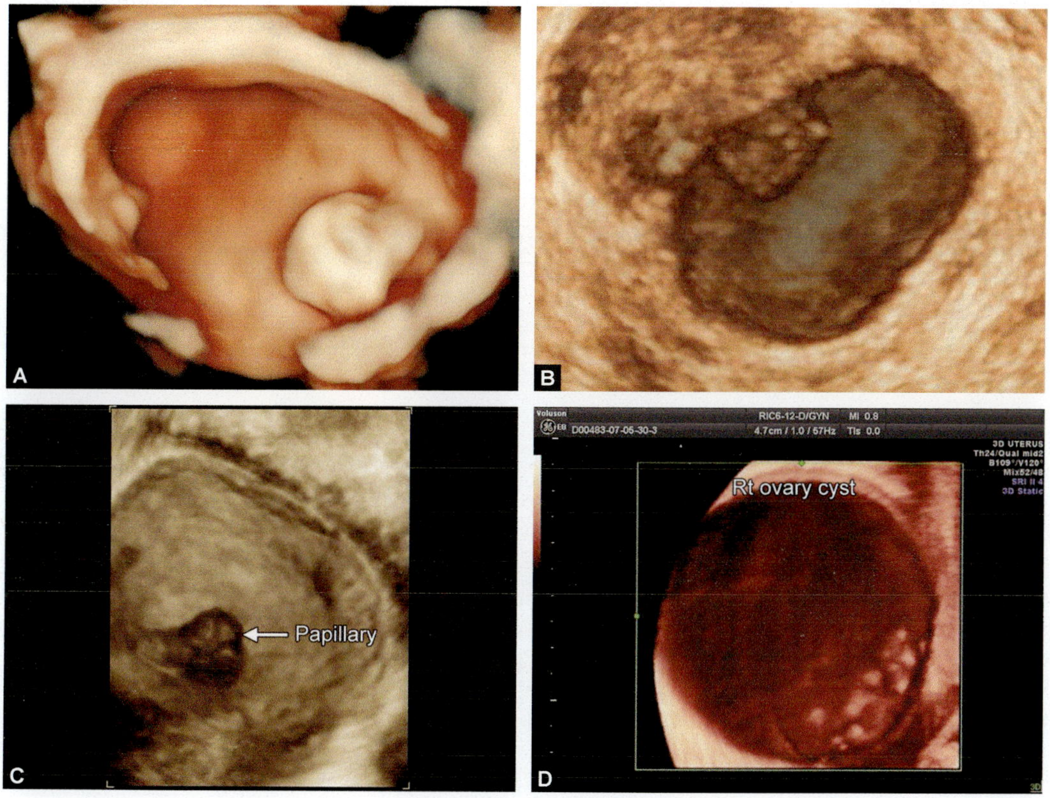

Figs. 38A to D: 3D surface rendering gives better information about irregularity of cyst wall (A), solid projections (B and C), and papillarities (D).

produced due to low velocity flows and thus helps to visualize the vascular details better and thus differentiate between benign and malignant lesions.

Further risk factors such as postmenopausal age and family history of breast or ovarian cancer are also added to it, along with assessment of chemical markers for malignancy such as CA 125. Though it is thought that ovarian malignancies are common in postmenopausal age, there are a few very interesting and noteworthy facts about postmenopausal ovaries. Simple asymptomatic ovarian cyst may be found in 5–17% of menopausal population (**Fig. 39**). Most likely these are inclusion cysts or neoplastic cysts and may resolve spontaneously. Among those which do not resolve, the most common found pathologies are serous cystadenoma, paratubal or paraovarian cysts, endometriotic cyst, mucinous cystadenoma, and hydrosalpinx. Risk of malignancy in unilocular ovarian cystic tumors <10 cm size, in women ≥50 years, is very low.[25] Surgery therefore should be only considered in these cases when there is a positive family history of ovarian, breast, or colon cancer, high CA 125 and sonographic findings suggest malignancy.

According to IOTA simple rules,[26] features of malignant tumors are irregular solid tumor, ascites, at least four papillary projections, irregular multicystic lesion, and very strong blood flow (**Figs. 40A to C**). Whereas features for benign tumor are unilocular tumor, if a solid projection is present, it is <7 mm, acoustic shadow, smooth contour, no blood flow (**Figs. 41A and B**).

Gynecologic imaging report and data system (GIRADS):[27]

- GIRADS reporting system identifies adnexal masses at high risk of malignancy and is useful for clinical decision making
- GIRADS 2: Follow-up scan
- GIRADS 3: Laparoscopic surgery
- GIRADS 4 or 5: Refer to gynecologic-oncologist. This system has:
  - Sensitivity—100%
  - Specificity—93.9%
  - PPV—85.7%
  - NPV—100%.

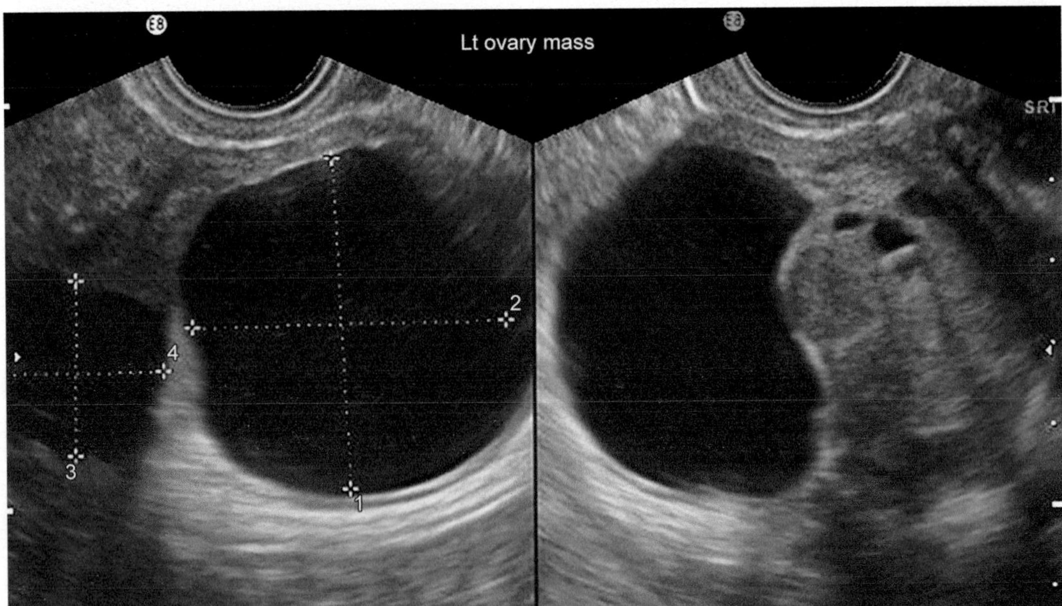

Fig. 39: Simple ovarian cyst in a postmenopausal woman, with thin walls, no internal echogenicities, papillarities, or solid projections.

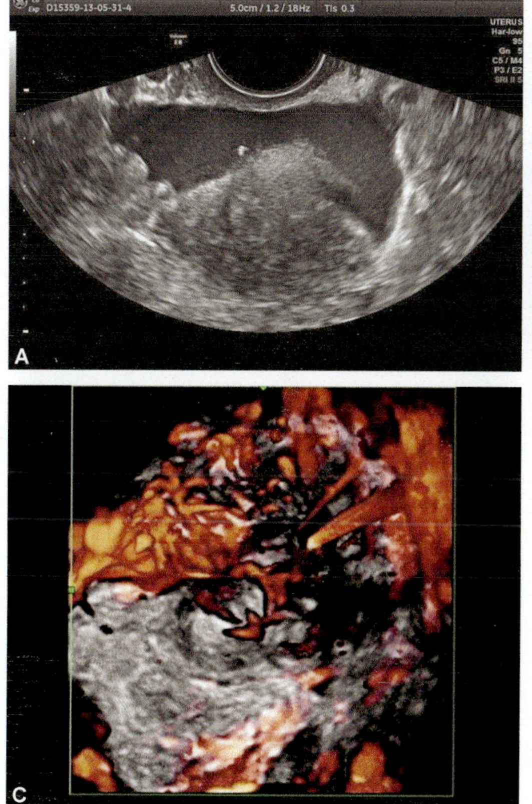

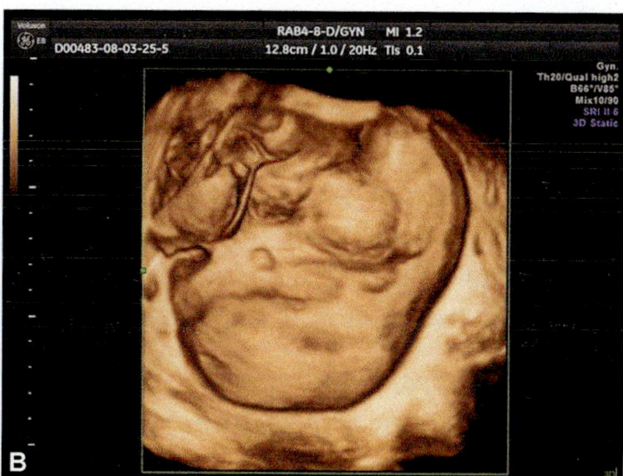

Figs. 40A to C: A solid tumor with irregular margins (A) confirmed by 3D ultrasound (B) and abundant vascular density seen on 3D power Doppler (C), suggestive of the malignant nature of the tumor.

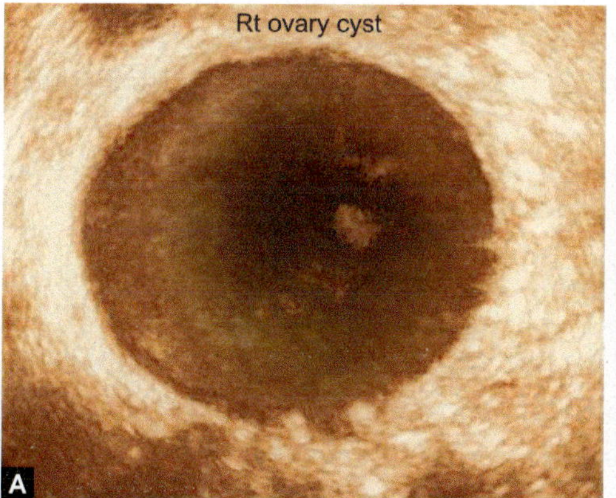

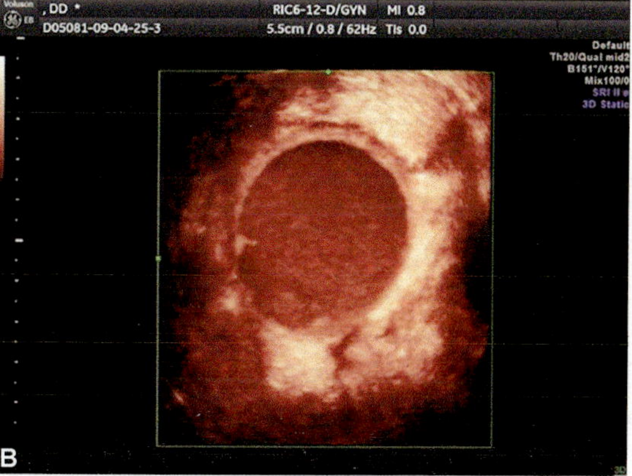

Figs. 41A and B: 3D ultrasound showing a unilocular tumor with single small solid projection of <7 mm (A) and smooth contour (B) suggestive of a benign tumor.

According to the reference mentioned, GIRADS 1 indicates normal ovary, GIRADS 2 is lesion thought to be functional in origin, GIRADS 3 neoplastic adnexal lesions but thought to be benign such as simple cyst, endometrioma, dermoid, paraovarian cyst, hydrosalpinx, peritoneal inclusion cyst, pedunculated myomas, etc., GIRADS 4 is the lesion in which one or two malignant features according to IOTA guidelines are present, and

GIRADS 5 is the one that has >3 malignant features according to IOTA guidelines.

As has been discussed, for differentiation of benign and malignant lesions or assessing the risk of malignancy, it is essential to discuss and understand the basic principles of IOTA and also understand the standard terminology used for the description of ovarian lesions:

International ovarian tumor analysis (IOTA): According to IOTA, adnexal lesion is:

- It is a part of the ovary or an adnexal mass that as judged from ultrasound is inconsistent with normal physiology.
- It may be inside or outside the ovary.
- The size of both the lesion and the ovary are measured separately.
- In some cases, normal ovarian tissue is not seen or it is not indistinguishable from the lesion when measurements of both become the same.

Functional or pathological:

- Information of the phase of the menstrual cycle and any drugs taken is important.
- A thorough knowledge of the classical appearances of the physiological structures—follicle, corpus luteum, etc. is essential.

And lastly:

- Benign or malignant
- Specific diagnosis
- *Prevalence of lesions*:
  - Borderline tumors: 5–6%
  - Metastatic tumors: 7–8%
  - Benign tumors: 50–60%

These questions can be answered by the following strategy (in that order):

- Correct terminology for description
- Easy descriptors—pattern recognition
- Simple rules
- Logistic regression
- Expert opinion.

Descriptions and definitions according to IOTA:
Septum: Thin strand of tissue running across the cystic cavity from one to another internal surface of the cyst. Septa are incomplete when in one or more sections, it appears not extending till the opposite wall. Whether complete/incomplete, it is called thin when <3 mm and thick when >3 mm in thickness.

It is measured at maximum thickness of the septum at any point other than its interface with the cyst wall. Measurement is taken when the septum appears perpendicular/oblique to the sound beam and not parallel.

Solid component: It exhibits high echogenicity suggesting presence of tissue (e.g., myometrium, ovarian stroma, fibroids, etc.). Irregular thick wall, regular septa, or normal ovarian tissue is not considered a solid tissue.

Though in case of doubt, the blood clot or solid component, it is considered a solid component.

Solid papillary projection: Solid projection from the cyst wall into the cavity with ≥3 mm in height. In cases of cystic lesions with small diameter, there may be confusion between incomplete septum and papillary projection. These must be considered as solid papillary projection. This applies for hydrosalpinges also with cog-wheel appearance.[28]

Though these are not solid projections:

- Reflective avascular area in the center of the dermoid[29]
- Sludge on internal walls (these are described as irregular walls).

Papillary projection: If it is <3 mm in height, it is only irregularity.

It is important to understand that papillary projection is a solid component, but solid component is not always a papillary projection. Height of the papillary projection is measured from inner margin of wall to the upper margin of the solid projection/papillary projection. And, the breadth of the base is measured. When papillary projections are present, their number, size, and vascularity of each should be mentioned.

Internal wall of a cystic lesion is described as smooth or irregular. Naturally, a solid projection makes it irregular. But in solid lesion, the same description is applicable for external walls: Regular/smooth wall. Irregular wall may have papillary projection.

Contents of cystic lesion:

- Anechoic
- Low level echoes (like in mucinous tumors or amniotic fluid)
- Ground glass
- Hemorrhagic (with fibrin strands—star shaped, cobweb like, and jelly like)
- Mixed (hypo-hyperechoic).

Mixed cystic lesions:

- Mixed
- Mixed (fat-fluid) level
- Mixed (abscess).

Acoustic shadowing: Loss of acoustic echo behind sound absorbing structure.

Ascites: Fluid outside the pouch of Douglas.

Terminology used is standardized.

Timmerman et al. have divided the tumors as:

- *Unilocular (also includes lesions with incomplete septa)*: Cystic lesion with no septum or solid component. Though incomplete septum may be included in this group.
- *Unilocular solid*: Unilocular cyst with measurable solid component or at least one papillary structure.
- *Multilocular*: Cyst with at least one septum.
- *Multilocular solid*: Multilocular cyst with at least one measurable solid component.
- *Solid*: Tumor with a solid component of 80% or more.
- *Not classifiable*: May be because of poor visualization, due to strong acoustic shadowing, or obesity.

Possibility of malignancy for each type of lesion:

- Unilocular 0.6%
- Unilocular solid 37%
- Multilocular 10%
- Multilocular solid 43%
- Solid 65%
- This means existence of solid component in a lesion increases the risk of malignancy significantly.

Vascularity score:

Color Doppler or Power Doppler (more sensitive) settings are adjusted at PRF 0.3.

Or, Velocity scale 3–6 cm/s, balance 220 and adjust Doppler gain to just below artifact level:

- No flow = 1
- Minimal flow = 2
- Moderate flow = 3
- Strong flow throughout = 4

Several areas in a tumor may be sampled for vascularity. It is a subjective/semiquantitative assessment.

Simple descriptors:

These are based on pattern recognition/subjective evaluation. This has 92% sensitivity and 93% specificity for differentiation of benign from malignant lesions.

- Simple descriptors can diagnose 43% of lesions
- Simple rules can add to accuracy and it reaches 75%
- Logistic regression leads to increased diagnostic performance.

This is a three-stage approach for differentiation of benign from malignant lesions by calculating the risk of malignancy.

Simple descriptors:

- *Endometriotic cyst*: Thick irregular internal walls and ground-glass appearance with echogenic foci (hemosiderin deposits) and amorphous material
- *Dermoid*: Unilocular cyst with mixed echogenicity and posterior shadowing
- *Simple cyst*: Unilocular thin-walled cyst with anechoic contents
- *Cystadenofibroma*:
  - Cystic lesion with anechoic contents
  - Small papillary projection with hyperechogenicity and posterior shadowing, but no vascularity.

If simple descriptors cannot identify the pathology, use simple rules.

For benign lesions:

- Unilocular cyst
- Presence of solid component for largest diameter of <7 mm
- Acoustic shadowing
- Smooth multilocular tumor with largest diameter of <100 mm.
- No blood flow (color score 1).

For malignant lesions:

- Irregular solid tumor
- Presence of ascites
- At least four papillary structures
- Irregular multilocular solid tumor with largest diameter of >100 mm
- Very strong blood flow (color score 4).

How to use these simple rules:

- If one or more features of benign—benign lesion
- One or more features of malignant—malignant lesion
- If one or more features from both—inconclusive—then logistic regression (LR) is applied.

Logistic regression, if these do not help. This is of two types:

LR1 has 12 features and LR2 has 6. LR2 is simpler and is the one that is commonly used. Each feature when present carries a particular value in numbers and multiplying them all, if it is >10 indicates malignancy. But these numbers are not to be remembered and the calculations are not to be done manually.

LR1 includes 12 demographic and ultrasound variables:

1. Personal history of (h/o) ovarian cancer
2. Current hormonal therapy
3. Age
4. Maximum diameter of lesion
5. Pain during examination
6. Ascites
7. Flow in papillary projection
8. Purely solid tumor
9. Maximum diameter of solid component
10. Irregular internal cyst wall
11. Acoustic shadows
12. Color score.

LR2 includes 6 demographic features:

1. Age
2. Ascites
3. Flow in solid papillary projection
4. Maximum diameter of solid component
5. Irregular internal walls
6. Acoustic shadows.

LR1 has sensitivity and specificity of 92% and 87% respectively and LR2 has a sensitivity and specificity of 92% and 96% respectively for estimating the risk of malignancy. According to IOTA, if the estimated probability of malignancy according to LR2 is 25%, it is high risk and if it is <5%, it is low risk. Adding CA125 has not added to this accuracy of diagnosis.

And, if that also does not help, expert opinion is the answer.

CONCLUSION

Ultrasound is a very efficient tool for assessment of adnexal lesions. With advent of new ultrasound technologies such as Doppler, 3D US, 3D power Doppler, and contrast-enhanced ultrasound, this efficacy has further increased. Dynamic assessment by ultrasound and clinical correlation add to the efficiency of ultrasound as a modality for assessment of adnexal lesions. Pelvic US is especially important to decide the site of origin of the lesion, differentiation of pathological and physiological lesions and for differentiation of benign from malignant masses, which will help to decide the line of treatment. Ultrasound is also useful for management of some of these lesions, for example, for cyst aspirations or biopsies under ultrasound guidance.

Points to remember when evaluating the adnexal mass:

- Assess morphology.
- Decide the organ of origin.
- Assess the lesion in two orthogonal planes.
- Assess the lesion at least twice at an interval 2–3 weeks, if there is any doubt for diagnosis.
- Doppler is an important tool for definitive diagnosis.
- Think of more physiological causes.

REFERENCES

1. Alcazar JL, Royo P, Jurado M, Mínguez JA, García-Manero M, Laparte C, et al. Triage for surgical management of ovarian tumours in asymptomatic women: assessment of an ultrasound-based scoring system. Ultrasound Obstet Gynecol. 2008;32:220-5.
2. Kinkel K, Hricak H, Lu Y, Tsuda K, Filly Ra. US characterization of ovarian masses: a meta-analysis. Radiology. 2000;217:803-11.
3. Osmers R. Sonographic evaluation of ovarian masses and its therapeutic implications. Ultrasound Obstet Gynecol. 1996;8:217-22.
4. Alcazar JL, Leon M, Galvan R, Guerriero S. Assessment of cyst content using mean gray value for discriminating endometrioma from other unilocular cysts in premenopausal women. Ultrasound Obstet Gynecol. 2010;35:228-32.
5. Alcazar JL. Transvaginal colour Doppler in patients with ovarian endometriomas and pelvic pain. Hum Reprod. 2001;16:2672-5.
6. Kurjak A, Kupesic S. Scoring system for prediction of ovarian endometriosis based on transvaginal colour and pulsed Doppler sonography. Fertil Steril. 1994;62:81-8.
7. Raine-fenning N, Jayaprakasan K, Deb S. Three-dimensional ultrasonographic characteristics of endometriomata. Ultrasound Obstet Gynecol. 2008;31:718-24.
8. Vimercatti A, Achilarre MT, Scardapane A, Lorusso F, Ceci O, Mangiatordi G, et al. Accuracy of transvaginal sonography and contrast enhanced magnetic resonance colonography for pre-surgical staging of deep infiltrating endometriosis. Ultrasound Obstet Gynecol. 2012;40(5):593-603.
9. Hudelist G, Fritzer N, Staettner S, Tammaa A, Tinelli A, Sparic R, et al. Uterine sliding sign: a simple sonographic predictor for presence of deep infiltrating endometriosis of the rectum. Ultrasound Obstet Gynecol. 2013;41:692-5.
10. Demidov VN, Lipatenkova J, Vikhareva O, Van Holsbeke C, Timmerman D, Valentin L. Imaging of gynecological disease (2): clinical and ultrasound characteristics of Sertoli cell tumours, Sertoli-Leydig cell tumours and Leydig cells tumours. Ultrasound Obstet Gynecol. 2008;31:85-91.
11. Vijayaraghavan SB. Sonographic whirlpool sign in ovarian torsion. J Ultrasound Med 2004;23:1643-9.
12. Sibbal M. Follicular ring sign: a simple sonographic sign for early diagnosis of ovarian torsion. J Ultrasound Med. 2012;31:1803-9.
13. Patel MD, Feldstein VA, Lipson SD, Chen DC, Filly RA. Cystic teratomas of the ovary: diagnostic value of sonography. Am J Roentgenol. 1998;171:1061-5.
14. Kurjak A, Kupesic S, Babic MM, Antsaklis A. Preoperative evaluation of cystic teratoma: what does colour Doppler add? J Clin Ultrasound. 1997;25:309-16.
15. Zalel Y, Seidman DS, Oren M, Achiron R, Gotlieb W, Mashiach S, et al. Sonographic and clinical characteristics of struma ovarii. J Ultrasound Med. 2000;19:857-61.
16. Kim JC, Kim SS, Park JY. MR finding of struma ovarii. Clin Imaging. 2000;14:310-2.
17. Lerner JP, Timor-Tritsch IE, Federman A, Abramovich G. Transvaginal ultrasonographic characterization of ovarian masses with an improved, weighted scoring system. Am J Obstet Gynecol. 1994;51:81-5.
18. Franchi D, Boveri S, Fruscio R, Fischerova D, Guerriero S, Moruzzi MC, et al. Imaging in gynecological disease: ultrasound characteristics of recurrent borderline ovarian tumours. Ultrasound Obstet Gynecol. 2013;41:452-8.
19. Valentin L. Pattern recognition of pelvic masses by gray-scale ultrasound imaging: the contribution of Doppler ultrasound. Ultrasound Obstet Gynecol. 1999;15:338.
20. Kurjak A, Zalud I, Jurkovic D, Alfirevic Z, Miljan M. Transvaginal colour Doppler for the assessment of pelvic circulation. Acta Obstet Gynecol Scand. 1989;68:131-7.
21. Crade M. Tissue block ultrasound and ovarian cancer-a pictorial presentation of findings. Donald School J Ultrasound Obstet Gynecol. 2009;3:41-7.
22. Alcazar JL. Tumor angiogenesis assessed by three-dimensional power Doppler ultrasound in early, advanced and metastatic ovarian cancer:

a preliminary study. Ultrasound Obst Gyn. 2006;28:325-9.

23. Kurjak A, Kupesic S, Sparac V, Prka M, Bekavac I. The detection of stage 1 ovarian cancer by three dimensional sonography and power Doppler. Gynecol Oncol. 2003;90:258-64.
24. Kupesic S, Kurjak A. Contrast enhanced three-dimensional power Doppler sonography for the differentiation of adnexal masses. Obstet Gynecol. 2000;96:452-8.
25. Bailey CL, Ueland FR, Land GL, DePriest PD, Gallion HH, Kryscio RJ, et al. Malignant potential of small cystic ovarian tumours in postmenopausal women. Gynecol Oncol. 1998;69:3-7.
26. Alcazar JL, Pascual MA, Olartecoechea B, Graupera B, Aubá M, Ajossa S, et al. IOTA simple rules for discriminating between benign and malignant adnexal masses: prospective external validation. Ultrasound Obstet Gynecol. 2013;42:467-71.
27. Amor F, Alcazar JL, Vaccaro H, Leon M, Iturra A. GI-RADS reporting system for ultrasound evaluation of adnexal masses in clinical practice: a prospective multicenter study. Ultrasound Obstet Gynecol. 2011;38:450-5.
28. Timor Tritsch IE, Lerner JP, Monteagudo A, Murphy KE, Heller DS. Transvaginal sonographic markers of tubal inflammatory disease. Ultrasound Obstet Gynecol. 1998;12:56-66.
29. Cohen L, Sabbagha R. Echopatterns of benign cystic teratomas by transvaginal ultrasound. Ultrasound Obstet Gynecol. 1993;3:120-3.

29

CHAPTER

Tubal Evaluation by Ultrasound

Sonal Panchal, Chaitanya Nagori

INTRODUCTION

Tubal pathology is a cause of subfertility in 25–35% of subfertile couples. Evaluation of fallopian tubes, therefore, forms an essential part of evaluation of a subfertile female. For correct description of the tubal pathology, it is important to understand the tubal anatomy and to use appropriate terminology for different parts of the tube. The intramyometrial part of the tube is the interstitial part of the tube; this leads to a thick-walled tubal isthmus, followed by thin-walled ampulla, then the broad infundibulum, leading to fimbria. Several investigations have been used since decades to evaluate the tubal patency.

It has been established that when the follicle grows to maturity in the ovary and luteinizing hormone (LH) surge leads to follicle rupture for release of the ovum, the fimbrial end of the tube proceeds to cover the ovulation site. The fimbrial processes cover the ovary like a ball being held in the palm (**Figs. 1A and B**).[1] The ciliary movement in the tubal lumen leads to development of negative pressure that sucks the ovum from the follicle into the tubal lumen. The ovum then advances in the tubal lumen, where the sperms have already reached after a natural intercourse or intrauterine insemination (IUI). Fertilization occurs in the tube and the embryo advances toward uterine cavity for implantation (**Fig. 2**).

Fallopian tubes are not just tubular portals but are motile structures and have peristalsis. This explains that the tubo-ovarian relationship and tubal function in the form of tubal peristalsis and fimbrial function are as

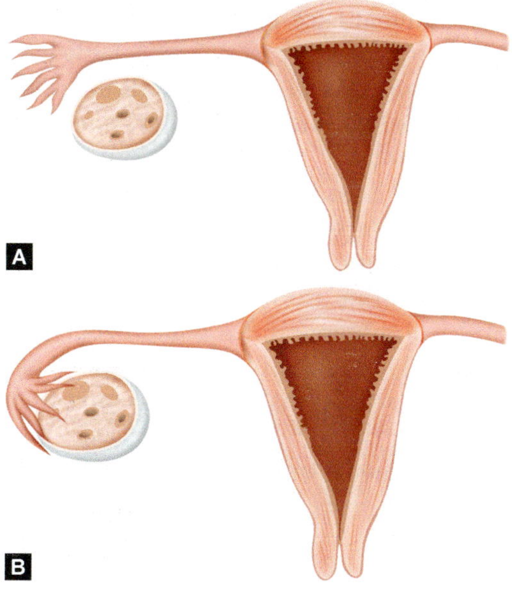

Figs. 1A and B: Diagram of the uterus with fallopian tube of right side showing fimbrial end (A) placed close to the ovary demonstrating normal tubo-ovarian relation and (B) holding the ovary in the first made by fimbrial projections.

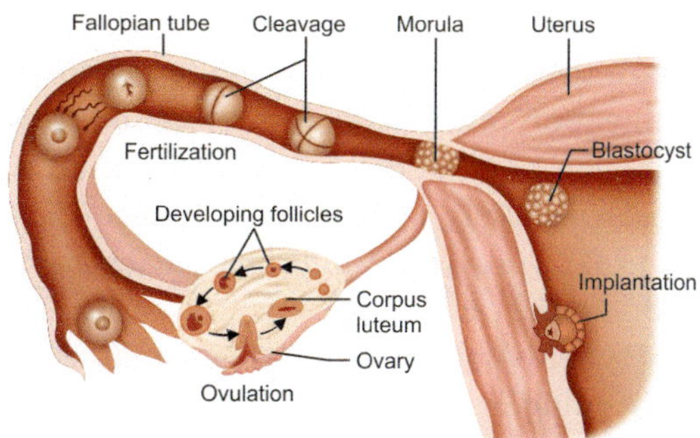

Fig. 2: Diagrammatic presentation of development of the ovum in the ovary and its passage in the fallopian tube, where it fertilizes and progresses toward the endometrial cavity as an embryo.

important as patency of the fallopian tubes for preservation of fertility.

INVESTIGATIONS FOR ASSESSMENT OF TUBAL STATUS

Various nonsurgical and surgical investigative modalities have been employed to assess fallopian tubes. An ideal test should correctly diagnose the tubal disease and should have minimal false-negative test results. It should be accurate, cost-effective, fairly easy to perform, easily available, well tolerated by the patient, and should not have any complications.

Several tests have been tried to assess the tubal status. Hysterosalpingography (HSG) and ultrasound-based techniques such as saline infusion salpingography (SIS) and hystero-contrast-salpingography (HyCoSy) are less invasive and associated with less serious risks. Laparoscopy with chromopertubation is highly invasive but most informative and is considered the gold standard for assessment of tubal patency and pathology.

Hysterosalpingography

Hysterosalpingography is widely used for tubal evaluation in subfertile women. This method is fairly accurate in detecting proximal tubal patency, is safe, not much expensive, and may potentially be associated with increased pregnancy rates.[2] HSG provides optimal delineation of the fallopian tubes, allowing detection of tubal patency, tubal occlusion, tubal irregularity, and peritubal disease (**Figs. 3A to D**). It also gives information about the endometrial cavity.

Hysterosalpingography is generally done in the proliferative phase of the cycle in order to ensure that the woman is not pregnant when the procedure is performed. But, HSG should not be done in patients having any comorbidities such as pelvic inflammatory disease, previous ectopic pregnancies, or endometriosis.

Method

An analgesic or antispasmodic agent is given to the patient, about 1 hour prior to the procedure to reduce lower abdominal discomfort and to avoid tubal spasm. Testing for chlamydia and/or prophylactic antibiotic is recommended to reduce the risk of pelvic infection. Patient is placed in lithotomy position and aseptic precaution is essential. Speculum is used to visualize the cervix. Vagina and cervix are cleaned with antiseptic solution. Anterior cervical lip is grasped with tenaculum; HSG cannula is introduced and stabilized into the cervix. Radio-opaque-contrast solution is introduced through the HSG cannula into uterus. Solution is warmed to body temperature before injection, and very small amount is introduced. Under fluoroscopic guidance, filling of the uterine cavity and passage of the radio-opaque solution into the tubes and its spill from fimbrial end is observed and documented in the form of X-rays.

Hysterosalpingography allows one to study the endometrial cavity and diagnose Müllerian abnormalities and endometrial lesions (**Figs. 4A and B**), in addition to its main use to assess the whole tube, condition of the tubal lumen, and site of block (**Fig. 5**).

In spite of having this important advantage of being able to assess the uterine cavity and fallopian tubes at a time, it has some disadvantages. Radio-opaque contrast used for the procedure contains iodine and therefore has a risk of causing a hypersensitivity reaction and adverse effects. The procedure is to be done in the radiology setup where both the gynecologist and the patient do not feel very comfortable. However, the main disadvantages are exposure to radiation, use of iodinated contrast that has a high adverse reaction rate and its high false-negative rates.

Though HSG has been used for several years for tubal assessment, it has been shown in meta-analysis based on these three studies pooled estimates of sensitivity and specificity for HSG as a test for tubal obstruction of

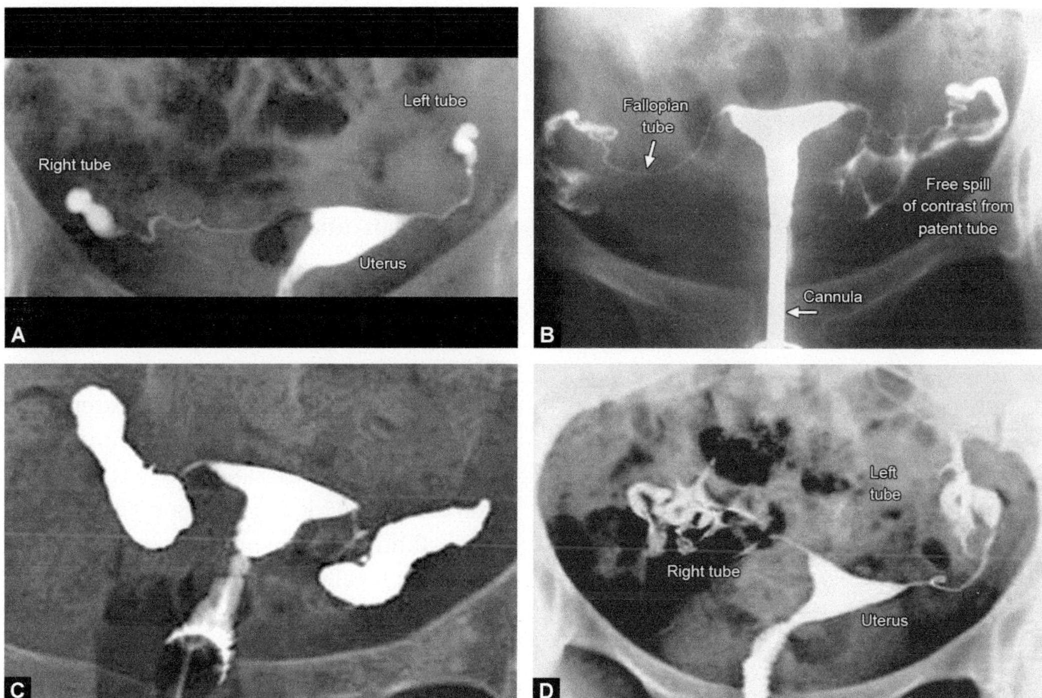

Figs. 3A to D: (A) Hysterosalpingography (HSG) image showing uterus with both the tubes, seen as thin string-like extension from the cornu of the uterus and extending laterally to end in ampulla as slightly dilated contrast-filled tubes; (B) HSG image of contrast-filled uterus and tubes with lateral ends not as distended as in previous picture. Instead, contrast is seen outside the tubal line and its distribution is like it is outlining bowel loops suggesting spill of the contrast in the peritoneum from the lateral end of the tubes; (C) HSG image of contrast-filled uterus and tubes with lateral ends. Contrast is seen outside the tubal line and its distribution is like it is outlining bowel loops suggesting spill of the contrast in the peritoneum from the lateral end of the tubes; (D) HSG image of contrast-filled uterus and tubes with markedly distended lateral ends of both the fallopian tubes. No contrast is seen outside the uterus and tubes, in spite of distended distal ends of tubes suggesting obstruction at lateral (fimbrial) end of the tube—hydrosalpinx.

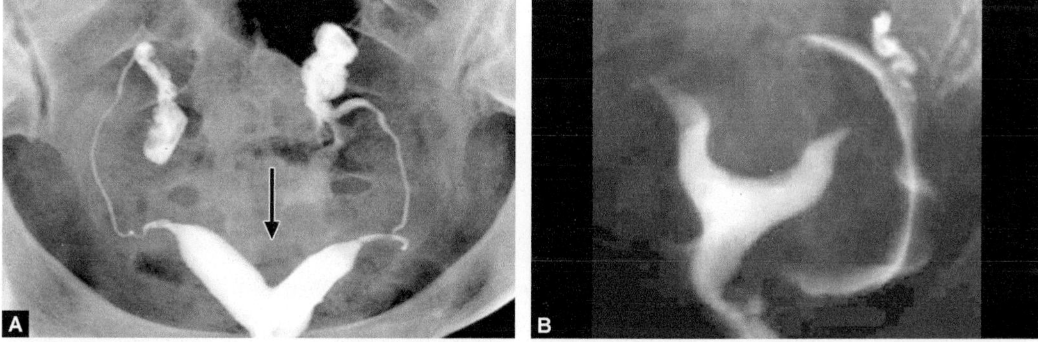

Figs. 4A and B: (A) Hysterosalpingography (HSG) image showing contrast-filled endometrial cavity and tubes. The endometrial cavity is divided into two, with acute angle between two parts of endometrial cavity suggestive of septate uterus. Distal ends of both tubes show mild dilatation, more on left side than right with no spill, suggestive of bilateral fimbrial block of the tubes; (B) HSG image showing a uterine cavity that is divided with the two parts of the endometrial cavity widely split apart suggestive of a wide septum or a bicornuate uterus. The contrast is seen filling only left tube with spill, but right tube is not filled suggestive of right tubal block.

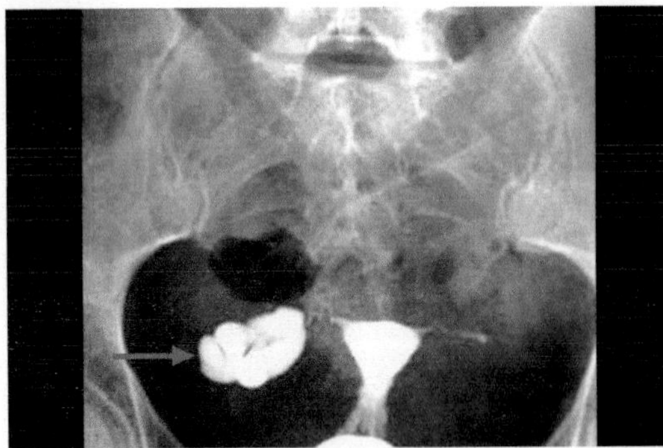

Fig. 5: Hysterosalpingography (HSG) image showing the contrast-filled uterus. Contrast is seen filling the right fallopian tube with grossly distended distal end of the tube and no spill, suggestive of hydrosalpinx. The left tube is filled only up to the mid part, though no dilatation is seen suggestive of mid-tubal block on left side.

0.65 [95% (confidence interval) CI 0.50–0.78] and 0.83 (95% CI 0.77–0.88), respectively. Tubal block seen on HSG will be confirmed by laparoscopy in only 38% of the women.[3] When HSG suggests that the tubes are patent, this will be confirmed at laparoscopy in 94% of the women, and, thus, HSG is a reliable investigation of tubal patency. These findings imply that after abnormal HSG, even in cases of bilateral pathology such as obstruction, it is still worth performing laparoscopy because, in a considerable number of these patients, the laparoscopic diagnosis allows IUI treatment to remain an option.[4]

Use of ultrasound to test tubal patency may potentially avoid the risk of radiation and side effects related to iodine-containing contrast. Moreover, ultrasound is an investigation of choice for assessment of uterus and ovaries and was therefore tried for the assessment of the fallopian tubes also.

Sonohysterosalpingography (Saline Infusion Salpingography—SIS)

While transvaginal ultrasound has now proved its place for assessment of uterus and ovaries, normal fallopian tubes are impossible to visualize on ultrasound without any intervention. This is so because there is no tissue–fluid interface present when the tubes are normal. Fallopian tubes can be identified only when there is fluid in the tubal lumen or outside the tubes. This means that tubes can be identified on ultrasound when either there is hydrosalpinx or free fluid in pelvis (**Figs. 6A and B**) or fluid is introduced in the tubal lumen or in the pelvis. Fluid can be introduced using a catheter through cervix to visualize and assess the fallopian tubes by ultrasound.

Sonographic evaluation of tubes was initially described by various authors, Nanini,[5] Richman,[6] and Randolph,[7] who performed abdominal sonography following intracervical injection of fluid, but was reported first by Richman. For this procedure, 200 mL of saline

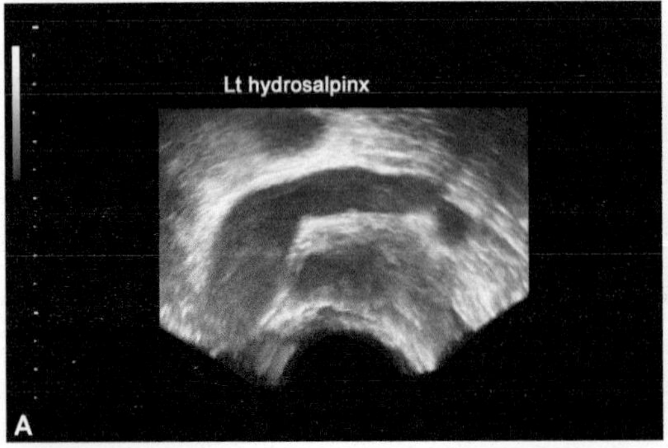

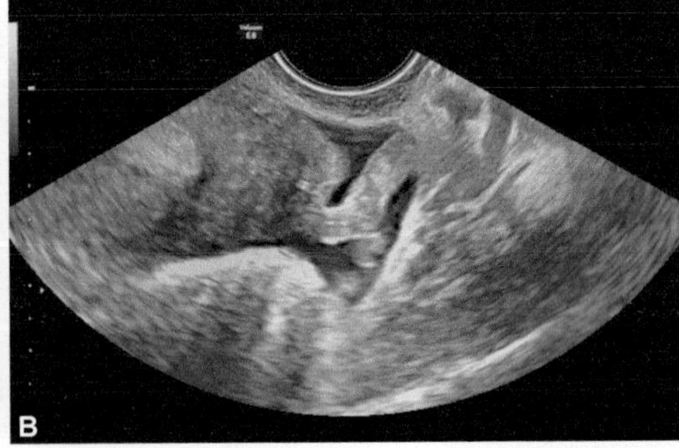

Figs. 6A and B: (A) 3D ultrasound multiplanar image of the distended fallopian tube (fluid-filled tubular structure) is seen with closely placed ovary—hydrosalpinx; (B) B-mode ultrasound image of left adnexal region showing anechoic free fluid with an echogenic tubular structure floating in it, suggestive of fallopian tube, floating in free fluid in pelvis. Uterus in its transverse section with echogenic endometrium is seen in continuity with the tube.

was introduced transvaginally, through the cervix into the uterus. Fluid would fill up the uterine cavity and pass through the tubes into the pelvic cavity. Retrouterine fluid seen on abdominal ultrasound was accepted as a criterion for patency. Tufekci also reported use of isotonic saline but with transvaginal ultrasound for tubal patency in 1992.[8] Deichert was the first to report on transvaginal sonographic evaluation of tubal patency, following transcervical injection of echogenic ultrasonic contrast fluid.[9] This investigation was given different names by various workers—saline infusion salpingography (SIS), saline sonosalpingography (SSG), saline HyCoSy, etc.

Technique

Saline sonosalpingography is ideally done in mid-proliferative phase (days 6–10 of a typical 28-day cycle), after menstruation stops but before ovulation occurs, to reduce the risk of disturbing an early pregnancy. Oral analgesic, ibuprofen 400–600 mg, may be given 1–2 h before the procedure. Preprocedural screenings for infections such as chlamydia and/or prophylactic oral antibiotics are recommended. Strict asepsis is essential. A detailed transvaginal ultrasound scan is done to assess the position of pelvic organs and to rule out any pathologies, which would come in the way of the procedure. Moreover, any free fluid in pelvis is also checked for.

After finishing the primary preprocedure scan, speculum is placed in the vagina to visualize the cervix. Vagina and cervix are cleaned with antiseptic solution. If required, cervix is fixed with tenaculum and manipulated to align it with uterus. An 8F balloon catheter or a cannula, specially devised for saline infusion sonography or hysterosalpingography, is attached to a 10-mL syringe prefilled with saline. The catheter is introduced through cervix into the uterus. Balloon is distended with 1–2 mL of distilled water or normal saline and is placed just beyond the internal os. Alternatives to this catheter are pediatric feeding tubes or small gage Foley catheter. Once the catheter is fixed, tenaculum and speculum are removed and transvaginal probe is introduced into the vagina for further assessment (**Figs. 7A and B**).

Saline is injected through the catheter slowly. Scanning is done to assess the uterine cavity that is distended by saline and also passage of saline (fluid) seen through the tubes. When uterine cavity is filled with saline, any endometrial pathologies can be

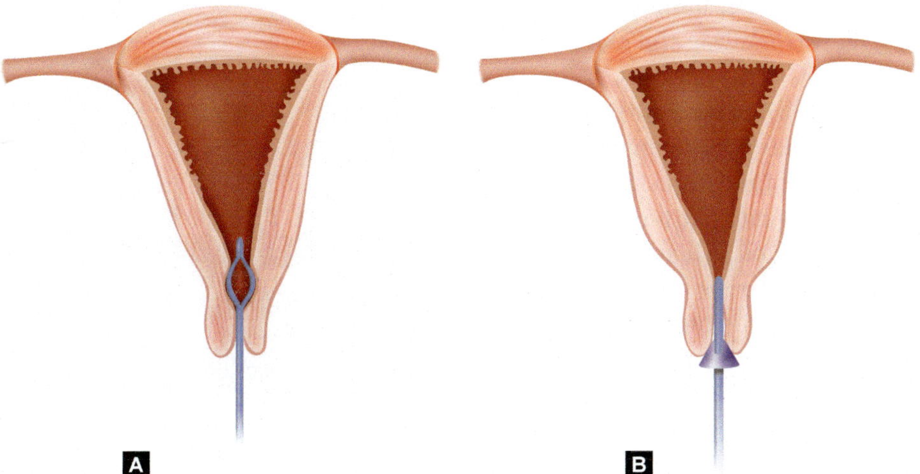

Figs. 7A and B: Diagrammatic representation of the uterus with a balloon catheter in the cervical canal with balloon placed just above the internal os in parts (A) and (B) showing the dedicated sonohysterography cannula in place of catheter with the lock (violet-colored triangle) placed at the external os of cervix.

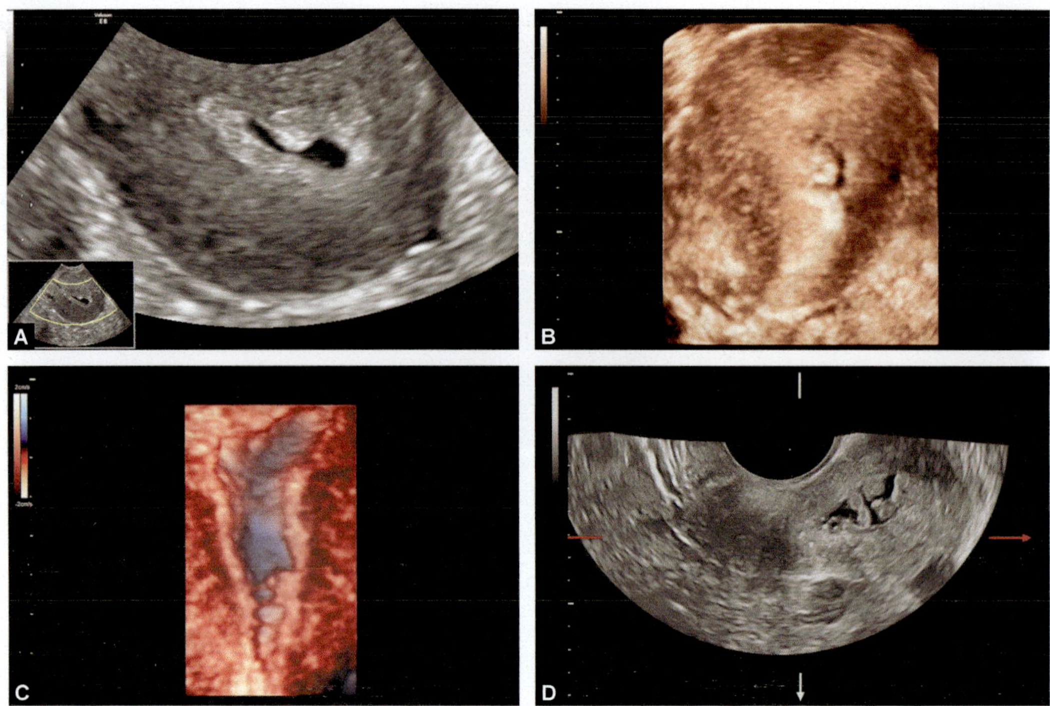

Figs. 8A to D: (A) B-mode ultrasound image of longitudinal section of retroverted uterus with saline infusion sonohysterography showing a solid projection protruding in the endometrial cavity from posterior wall of endometrium, suggestive of a polyp; (B) 3D ultrasound image of uterus in coronal plane with saline infusion sonohysterography, barely showing any endometrial cavity with endometrial calcification. This is suggestive of dense endometrial synechiae with calcifications barely allowing any expansion of endometrial cavity with saline; (C) 3D ultrasound image of uterus in coronal plane with saline infusion sonohysterography, showing multiple synechiae in the lower part of the endometrial cavity, with nearly normal endometrial cavity in fundal area; (D) Sonohysterography with B-mode transvaginal scan showing a retroverted uterus. Multiple solid projections are seen in the endometrial cavity suggestive of multiple endometrial polyps.

demonstrated and diagnosed (**Figs. 8A to D**). Spill of saline from fimbrial end is seen as fluid flow surrounding the ovary and its collection in pelvis on B-mode scanning (**Fig. 9**). Absence of spill may indicate blockage. It is not always possible to document the spill from the fimbrial end of individual tube. In such cases, fluid accumulation in pouch of Douglas confirms patency of at least one fallopian tube (**Fig. 10**). In patients with bilateral block, distension of the uterine cavity causes severe pain and no spill is observed. Once the procedure is completed, the instruments are removed. Patient is informed that she might get some pelvic cramping or spotting, but the symptoms are short termed and she should not worry about it. The accuracy of SIS compared to chromopertubation varies from 81.82[10] to 100%.[11-13]

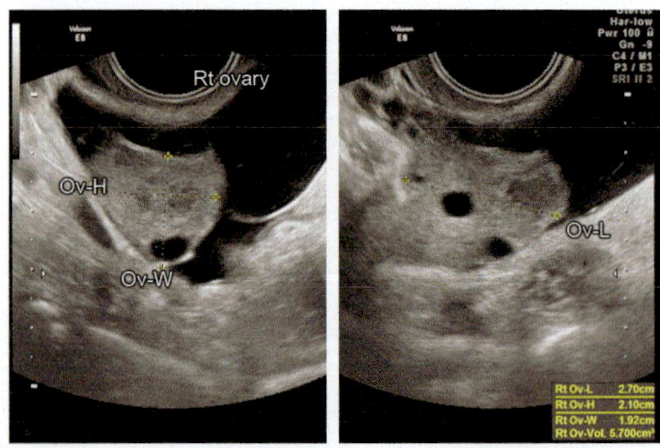

Fig. 9: B-mode transvaginal ultrasound image of adnexal region showing ovary with free fluid in its vicinity. This fluid is collected as a result of spill of saline from the fimbrial end of a patent tube as a result of saline infusion salpingography.

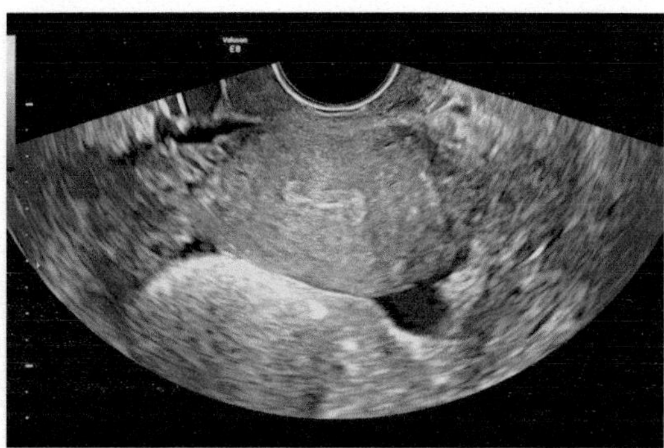

Fig. 10: B-mode image of transvaginal scan pelvis showing free fluid in pelvis. This may be inflammatory or as a result of rupture of the follicle, but in this case, it was because of spill of saline from the fimbrial end of one or both of the fallopian tubes. This is too large an amount to be instilled to assess the patency of the tubes. But when the spill is not evident on either side, in an attempt to establish the patency of the tube, sometimes a large amount of saline may be used for the procedure.

The procedure has no major complication except nausea, vomiting, and mild-to-moderate pain. But, these are rare. The risk of pelvic infection and associated peritonitis is approximately 1%. Vasovagal syncope is rare during or after the procedure. The reported prevalence of complications combined is 8.8%.[14] Failure to perform or complete the procedure was documented in 7% in a meta-analysis of 24 studies and 2,278 procedures.[15]

Reliability of the Procedure

The agreement of transvaginal salpingo-sonography compared with X-ray hystero-salpingography was 94%, the sensitivity 50%, the specificity 97%, the positive predictive value 50%, and the negative predictive value 97%.[16]

Results of SSG correlated positively with laparoscopy in 97% and SSG and HSG showed 93% correlation.[17]

Another study showed sensitivity of SSG as 97.3% for open tubes with specificity of 92%, whereas sensitivity of laparoscopy was 94.6%, and sensitivity of HSG was 94.5%, but with a specificity of only 84%.[18]

Saline infusion salpingography HyCoSy is accurate in determining tubal patency and evaluating the uterine cavity and can supplant HSG as the first-line diagnostic test in an infertility workup.[19]

The shortcoming of the procedure is that even when patency of individual tube can be confirmed, it does not give any information about the site of the block, condition of the lumen, and tubo-ovarian relationship. Some modifications in this technique were tried to overcome this shortcoming.

Modifications

Several modifications have been made to this basic procedure of SIS to improve its diagnostic accuracy as an investigative modality for tubal assessment. The reported modifications are:

- Using pulse Doppler
- Using color Doppler
- Combining air and saline
- 3D saline sonosalpingography.

Using pulse Doppler: If examination during B-mode reveals evidence suggesting tubal occlusion or if a small segment of the tube is not visualized, a pulse Doppler examination can be performed.[20] Doppler gate is placed where the block is suspected. This is exactly the point beyond which the tube is not filled with saline or color flow is not seen on injection of saline when examination is done with color Doppler. The gate is reduced to the width of the tube. Brief injections of fluid/saline lasting for 5s are done while Doppler signals are observed.

Patent tube is indicated by a short-filling phase with rapid, steep increase in Doppler shift followed by slow uniform fall in Doppler shift. Obstruction presents as short, steep Doppler shift with no subsequent noise signals (**Fig. 11**).

Using color Doppler: Color Doppler can be used with saline infusion salpingography. This is more informative when injection of saline is done selectively toward one of the tubes.

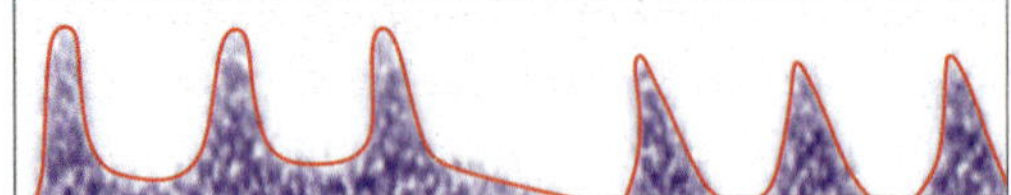

Fig. 11: Diagrammatic representation of the flow pattern in patent and blocked fallopian tube using pulsed Doppler for assessment modality with saline infusion.

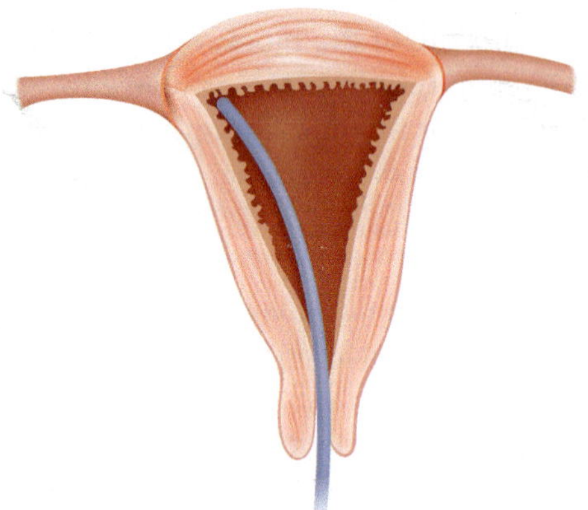

Fig. 12: Diagrammatic representation of the placement of the catheter tip close to the cornu-selective flow of saline into the respective tube. This can make the assessment of tubal patency by saline infusion salpingography more informative.

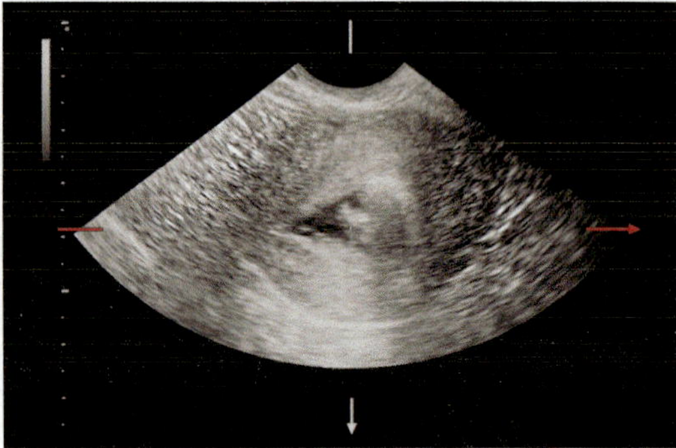

Fig. 13: Transverse section of uterus on B-mode saline infusion hysterosalpingography showing fluid in the endometrial cavity.

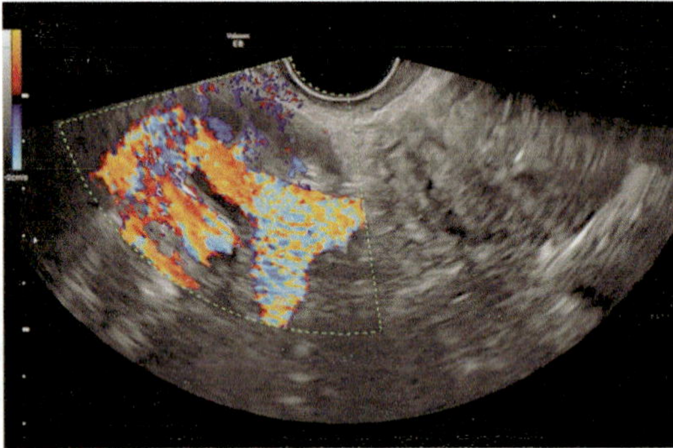

Fig. 14: B-mode transvaginal ultrasound image of pelvis showing uterus and ovary in the transverse section with the color box placed around the ovary, avoiding the myometrium.

Under ultrasound guidance, the tip of the catheter is placed close to either cornu, one by one (**Fig. 12**). First, the probe is placed to see the transverse section of the uterus. Fluid in the uterine cavity confirms the passage of fluid in the uterus, as saline is injected through the cannula in the uterus in short bouts (**Fig. 13**). The field of vision is immediately changed over to ovary and adnexa, by spanning the probe from transverse section of uterus laterally. While injecting saline, color box is placed to visualize the adnexa and ovary (**Fig. 14**). Care must be taken that when the box is placed around the ovary to check the patency by color spill, the box should not include any part of the myometrium. If the box is on the myometrium, false diagnosis is a strong possibility. This is so because, when saline is injected in the uterus, the cavity expands and myometrial fibers also move with expansion and this leads to color signals. Filling up of the box with color signals indicates patency of the tube, and absence of such signals indicates block (**Figs. 15A and B**).[21] The same procedure is repeated on the opposite side. A detailed evaluation for any pathology is important immediately prior to performing the procedure, as hydrosalpinx may create turbulence in the fluid present in the tube and give a false impression of a patent tube.

Adding color Doppler may increase the efficiency and accuracy of SIS for assessment of tubal patency.[22] In a study by Peters and Colum of 129 infertile patients, Doppler SIS showed complete agreement with HSG in 81% cases. When compared with the gold standard test of tubal assessment, chromopertubation, Doppler SIS showed agreement in 86% of cases, while HSG agreed with chromopertubation

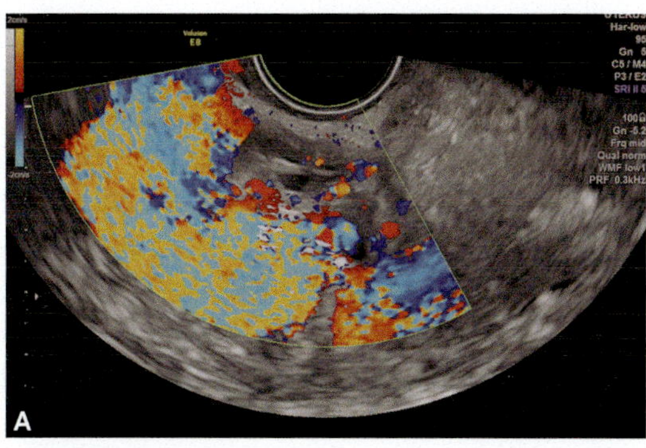

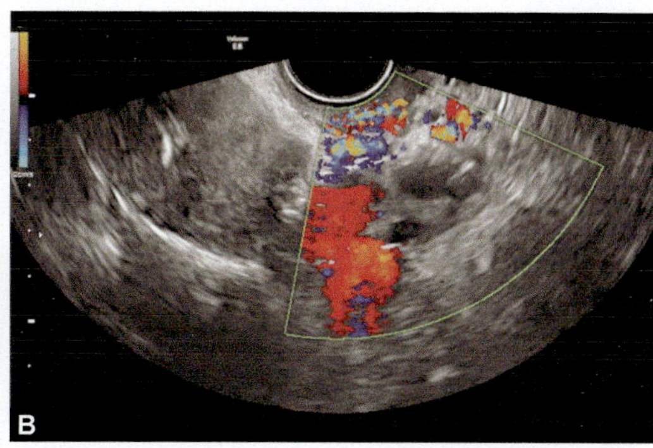

Figs. 15A and B: Color Doppler image of uterus and ovary on transverse section with Doppler box on the ovary showing the color box filled with color on injecting the jet of saline through the catheter placed in the uterus for saline infusion hysterosalpingography (A), this indicates patent tube; Part (B) shows no filling of color box on injection of saline in the uterine cavity indicating a blocked fallopian tube.

only in 75% cases.[21] In a small study by Kupesic et al., 91.5% agreement was seen between color Doppler sonosalpingography and chromopertubation.[11] Correlation of color Doppler sonosalpingography and HSG with chromopertubation was 81% versus 60%, respectively, in one study.[10]

Combining saline with air: When air is mixed with saline, bubbles are formed and that makes saline hyperechoic and this helps better outlining of tubal lumen (**Fig. 16**). This can be performed either by agitating air and saline or by injecting air after saline has been already pushed to fill up the uterine cavity and tubes (**Fig. 17**). The later technique was described by Jeanty et al. and showed 79.4% agreement with results of chromopertubation and showed a sensitivity of 85.7% and specificity of 77.2%.[22]

3D transvaginal three-dimensional saline SHSG (sonohysterosalpingography): Transvaginal three-dimensional saline SHSG provides good visualization of the uterine cavity and myometrial walls in three orthogonal planes. However, it does not diagnose tubal occlusion or depict architecture of the fallopian tube as accurately as X-ray HSG. Although the distal fallopian tube and fimbria were seen with real-time imaging, the proximal tube is not satisfactorily imaged with three-dimensional

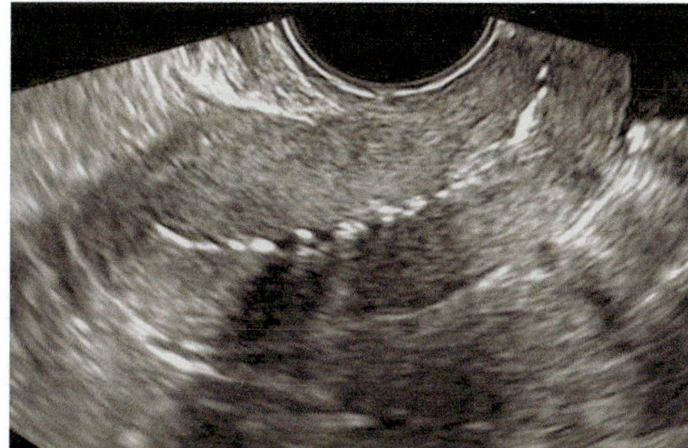

Fig. 16: Longitudinal section of uterus on transvaginal scan when saline mixed with air is being injected into the uterine cavity through a transcervical catheter. The mixture of air and saline is seen as a line of hyperechoic spots unlike saline that would appear hypoechoic.

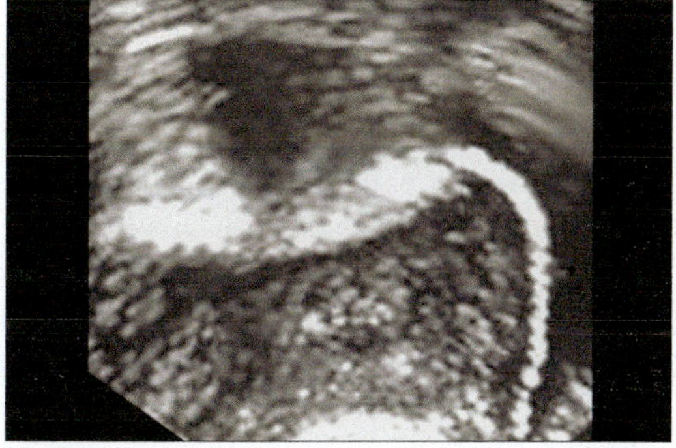

Fig. 17: In the same case as in **Figure 16** when more mixture of air and saline is injected and scanned in transverse section on transvaginal scan shows uterine cavity filled with hyperechogenicity and the same hyperechogenicity is also seen filling the fallopian tube.

power Doppler. This technique may be reserved as an initial screening test to evaluate the uterine cavity and test tubal patency. Patients at high risk for tubal disease by history or with suspected tubal occlusion on three-dimensional saline SHSG should be evaluated by laparoscopy with chromopertubation.[23]

Though Kiyokawa et al., have shown that when 3D was added to saline infusion salpingography, the positive-predictive value, negative-predictive value, sensitivity, and specificity of predicting tubal patency were 100%, 33.3%, 84.4%, and 100%, respectively. Over and above this, this method also has an advantage of assessing the shape of the uterine cavity. The full contour of the uterine cavity was depicted in 96% of cases by 3D HyCoSy and 64% by X-ray HSG.[24] In this study, the contrast used was saline.

Hystero-Contrast-Salpingography

While intracavitary lesions are clearly delineated by anechoic media, very small hollow cavities, such as normal tubes, are not always easily visualized using SIS.[25] Demonstration of the lumen of tubes requires using highly echogenic medium.[26] Hyperechogenic contrast medium enhances echo signals and allows detection of the flow, both by B-mode and Doppler ultrasound.

Experimental and clinical data suggest that insonation of echo-enhancing contrast agents with high acoustic power produces disintegration of microbubbles, resulting in a phenomenon called stimulated acoustic emission (SAE). It is based on this principle that the positive ultrasound contrast media are developed.[27]

While a cheap and cost-effective option is the use of saline mixing with air that produces a high-contrast fluid due to the presence of air bubbles. However, these bubbles stand only for a very short period, and therefore, tubal patency assessment may become practically difficult. Therefore, commercially available contrast media were introduced with microbubbles that can stand for a longer time.

Echovist and Levovist (Schering AG, Berlin) consist of suspension of microbubbles made of special galactose microparticles. These are suspended either in galactose solution, as in Echovist, or in sterile water, as in Levovist. Just before use, these solutions are made by mixing and vigorously shaking the microparticles with the solvent and it can stand for 5–10 minutes. These solutions completely dissolve in the body, within about 30 minutes. These can be used in all patients except those with galactosemia. Nonembryotoxic gel—ExEm-gel (GynaecologIQ BV, Delft, The Netherlands), containing hydroxyethyl cellulose and glycerol, has also been used as an intrauterine-contrast medium for sonohysterography as an alternative to saline. Gel instillation offers a more stable filling of the uterine cavity. This gel and its compounds have been tested extensively and safely used in medicine. When this gel is pushed rigorously through small openings in syringes or tubes, turbulence causes local pressure drops resulting in air dissolving in the solution and yields foam that is stable for several minutes. ExEm-gel (containing 88.25% purified water), however, is rather viscous for passing into the fallopian tubes. Therefore, 10-mL ExEm-gel is diluted with 10-mL purified water (to give a mixture containing 94.12% water) and mixed to create foam. The mixture at this ratio created foam that is sufficiently stable to show echogenicity for ≥5 min and sufficiently fluidy to pass through patent tubes. The viscosity of this foam (270 cP) is comparable with that of Echovist (400 cP).[28]

Hystero-contrast-salpingography is a safe outpatient procedure with a relatively low cost, and its accuracy has been assessed in a meta-analysis, which compared the results of HyCoSy and laparoscopy and dye tests in 428 infertile women. Its sensitivity was 93.3% and specificity was 89.7%.[29]

A meta-analysis of three comparative studies of Echovist-200 [solution of galactose and 1% palmitic acid (Echovist-Schering-AG, Germany)], including 1,007 women, showed that the results of HyCoSy and chromolaparoscopy were identical in 294 of 428 patients (68.7%) or in 688 of 828 individual tubes (83.1%). HyCoSy showed "false" occlusion in 85 tubes (10.3%) and "false" patency in 55 (6.7%). The results of HyCoSy and HSG were identical in 138 of 202 patients (68.3%) or in 320 of 384 individual tubes (83.3%). HyCoSy showed "false" occlusion in 49 tubes (12.8%) and "false" patency in 15 (3.9%). The findings of chromolaparoscopy and HSG agreed in 49 of 77 patients (63.6%) or in 116 of 152 tubes (76.3%). HSG showed "false" occlusion in 19 (12.5%) tubes and "false" patency in 17 (11.2%).[29]

Contrast agent that is more easily available in most countries, including India, is SonoVue (Bracco). This contrast agent consists of sulfur hexafluoride microparticles in normal saline. For assessment of tubal status, 1 mL of SonoVue is further diluted with 4 mL of normal saline and is agitated to create foam for injection into the uterus. This contrast is safe for HyCoSy, as it is for intravascular use also. It is used as an ultrasound contrast agent for vascular studies and for diagnosis of malignancy.

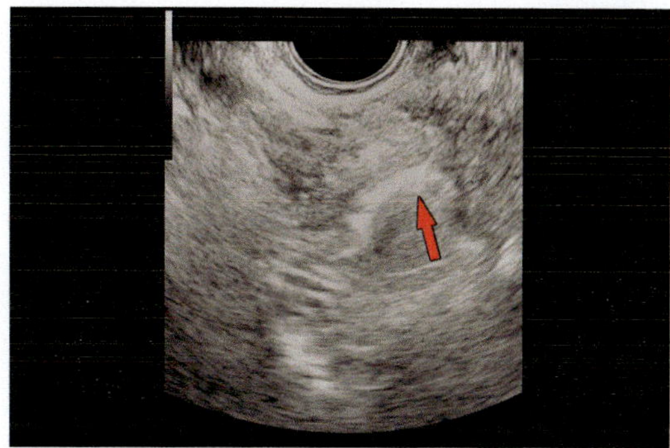

Fig. 18: B-mode transvaginal ultrasound image of the uterus in transverse section with positive contrast (SonoVue—Bracco) showing hyperechoic echoes filling the endometrial cavity and outlining the tube.

This contrast appears white echogenic on ultrasound. The scanning technique is the same as that for saline infusion salpingography. Using positive contrast, it is possible to delineate the whole tube along with the uterine cavity even on B-mode scanning (**Fig. 18**). There is ultrasound equipment with contrast mode (contrast tuned imaging technology based on harmonics) (**Figs. 19A and B**). The advantage is that it enhances the contrast and makes visualization of tubes even better. Using contrast mode with positive contrast actually makes it easier to view the spill from the fimbrial end, if the tube is patent. If the tube is not patent, the contrast column in the tube can identify the site of block.

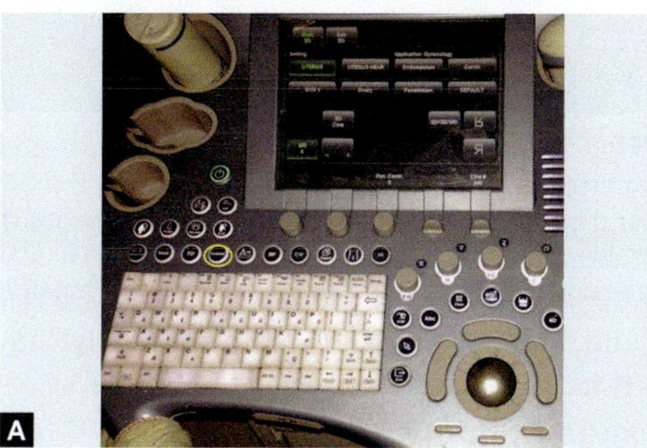

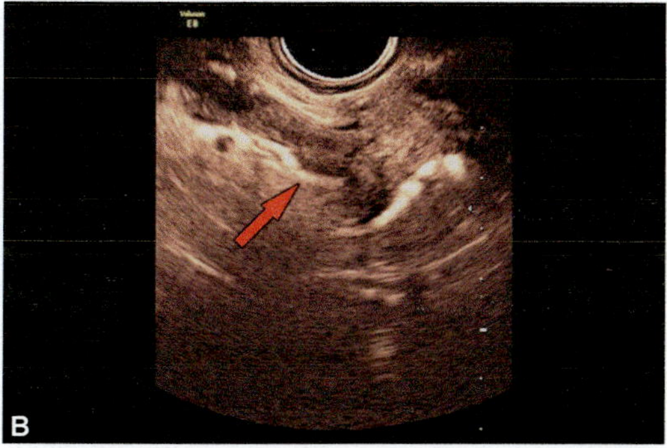

Figs. 19A and B: (A) Keyboard of the ultrasound scanner showing the contrast mode option (highlighted by yellow circle); (B) The same scan as shown in **Figure 18** is here imaged on contrast mode, using harmonics. This makes the passage of contrast much more visible. It shows passage of contrast filling the uterus and tube.

Technique

The technique for HyCoSy is the same as for saline infusion salpingography. As delineation of the tube is better with HyCoSy, total amount of contrast needed is as less as 2–3 mL per tube. For diagnosis of tubal patency, two to three observation phases per tube are needed, with an observation period of continuous flow of about 10 seconds. Visualization of long segments of tube beyond intramural part of the tube usually indicates patency, though whole tube must be observed and spill should be confirmed (**Fig. 20**). Appearance or increase in the fluid in pouch of Douglas may be an indirect sign of tubal patency, the same as for SIS. HyCoSy has several advantages over saline infusion salpingography such as it helps clearer visualization of uterine cavity, better assessment of tubal lumen and fimbriae, clearer visualization of spill, and a more exact localization of site of block (**Figs. 21A and B**).

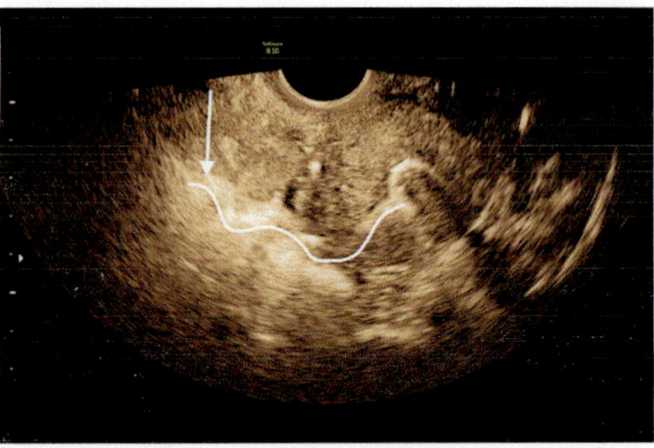

Fig. 20: Contrast-enhanced image of the uterus and right fallopian tube seen highlighted by contrast. Distal end of the tube also shows contrast spill as marked by arrow.

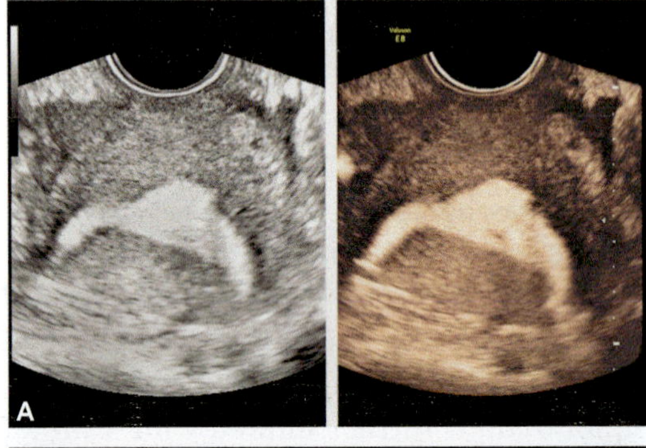

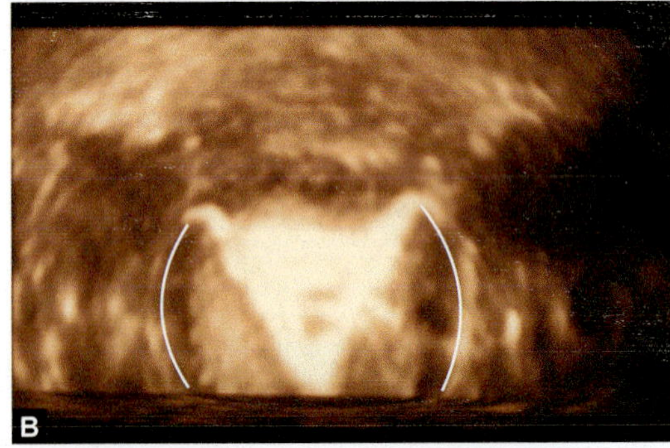

Figs. 21A and B: (A) HyCoSy showing contrast-filled uterus and proximal part of both tubes on B-mode and contrast-enhanced mode; (B) Uterus and both tubes seen on contrast-enhanced mode on HyCoSy.

Compared to conventional HSG, HyCoSy provides a simultaneous ultrasound evaluation of pelvis and a more cost-effective evaluation of tubal pathology and can be successfully used as a first-line noninvasive screening method.[30]

Hystero-contrast-sonosalpingography with contrast is more efficient than with saline solution in determining fallopian tube patency and is as efficient as HSG and can be used instead of HSG for screening infertile patients.[31] In a diagnostic accuracy study of HyCoSy performed with air and saline (hydro-HyCoSy) and with contrast media (SonoVue-HyCoSy) considering hysterosalpingography (HSG) and/or chromopertubation as reference tests, SonoVue-HyCoSy has been found to be more accurate than hydro-HyCoSy for the assessment of fallopian tubes.[32] While the sensitivity, specificity, and positive- and negative-predictive values of hydro-HyCoSy were 91%, 71%, 55%, and 95%, respectively, these were 87%, 84%, 69%, and 94%, respectively for SonoVue-HyCoSy. The diagnostic accuracies of hydro-HyCoSy and of SonoVue-HyCoSy were 77% and 85%, with a Cohen's kappa of 0.52 and 0.66, respectively. In another small study comparing HyCoSy and chromopertubation, there was a high degree of correlation in assessing tubal patency, with sensitivity, specificity, PPV (positive-predictive value), and NPV (negative-predictive value) of 100%, 55.6%, 80%, and 100%, respectively.[30]

Moreover, the amount contrast agent required for adequate examination was also less with positive contrast. Mean volumes of contrast injections required were 35.3 mL of saline, 14.4 mL of Infoson, and 13.8 mL of Iopamiron 370. Infoson-enhanced HyCoSy provided a significantly larger ($p = 0.006$) number of correct diagnoses (20/22 fallopian tubes) than did saline HyCoSy (12/24 fallopian tubes), and the same number as that achieved by hysterosalpingography.

In another comparative study, it has been shown that sensitivity, specificity, and positive- and negative-predictive values of hydro-HyCoSy were 91%, 71%, 55%, and 95%, respectively, while for CnTI (contrast tuned imaging)-SonoVue-HyCoSy, they were 87%, 84%, 69%, and 94%. The diagnostic accuracies of hydro-HyCoSy and of CnTI-SonoVue-HyCoSy were 77% and 85%, with a Cohen's kappa of 0.52 and 0.66, respectively. CnTI-SonoVue-HyCoSy does not require a learning curve period. Yet, another study has shown that HSG and HyCoSy demonstrated a high concordance with laparoscopy (83% and 80%, respectively). The two methods had a high negative-predictive value for tubal disease (HSG, 94%; HyCoSy, 88%), and the positive-predictive values were 47% and 75%, respectively.[33]

The study by Exacoustos et al. has also shown that HSG and HyCoSy had the same high concordance as laparoscopy, 86.7% and 86.7%, respectively.[34]

The study concluded that HyCoSy proved to be superior to conventional HSG in evaluating adjacent myometrial structures, adnexa, and degree of follicular maturation, equal to HSG in visualizing the passage of the contrast medium into the peritoneum but inferior to HSG in imaging the fallopian tubes owing to their tortuosity.[35]

In spite of all advantages, Balen et al. found that both SIS and HyCoSy are insufficiently accurate and inferior to HSG.[36] They quoted a false-positive rate of 9% and false-negative rate of 20% for HyCoSy. This is because fallopian tubes are tortuous and usually not confined to a single plane. Moreover, distal parts of the tube may be obscured by bowel gas.

Modifications of HyCoSy

Additional use of pulsed wave Doppler in HyCoSy can be done as a supplement to gray-scale imaging to improve the diagnostic accuracy in cases of suspected tubal occlusion, and in patients in whom intratubal flow was demonstrated only over a short distance.[12] 3D power Doppler helps to visualize the whole tube and spill.[37] This technique has shown to be superior to conventional HyCoSy with free spill from fallopian tubes demonstrated in 91% of tubes using 3D-power Doppler (PD) as compared to only 46% by conventional HyCoSy, and the contrast agent required was almost half for 3D PD in one study.[37] There are various advantages with 3D HyCoSy techniques, which include simultaneous visualization of the uterine cavity and whole tube, short procedure time and reduced patient discomfort, and requirement of less amount of contrast and storage of the 3D volume, that allows off-line review and reassessment.

Technique of 3D HyCoSy

SonoVue (Bracco) is used as the contrast agent. Patient preparation, catheter placement, and preparation of contrast media were done according to the method described earlier. Scanning is performed using a 3D ultrasound machine (e.g., Voluson E8 Expert BT12; GE Medical Systems). A high-frequency transvaginal volume probe (6–9 MHz) is used for pelvic evaluation. Contrast mode is switched on, on the machine. As the contrast is slowly injected through the balloon catheter into the uterus, transvaginal probe is so oriented that uterine cornu and ovaries are

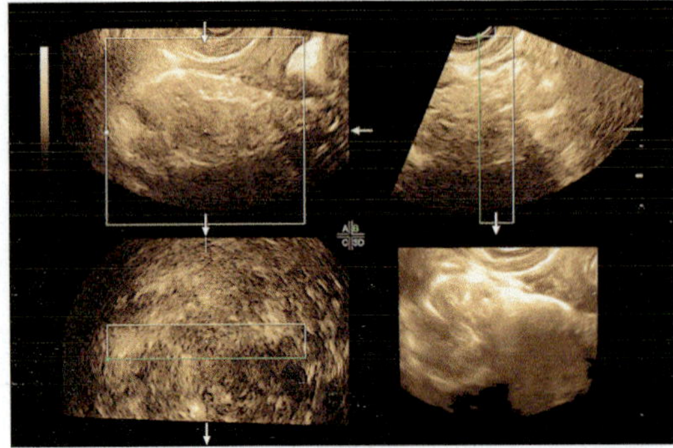

Fig. 22: 3D ultrasound acquired volume of contrast-enhanced sonohysterosalpingography (HyCoSy), showing contrast-filled endometrial cavity and right fallopian tube.

seen on the same plane. Having defined the contrast filling in the tubes, 3D is switched on and volumes are acquired for each side independently (**Fig. 22**).

Rendering is done in front-back viewing direction. Surface-enhanced mode is used. Threshold is set to make the contrast path more obvious. MagiCut (electronic scalpel) is then used to cut all shadows other than the contrast path. Then HD live rendering mode is switched on and direction of the light is adjusted to visualize the fimbriae and spill to its best. After the final picture is ready, both the halves are put together and matched to make a complete picture of uterus and both tubes (**Figs. 23A to D**).

In a series of 65 subfertile women in whom we performed 3D HyCoSy followed by a laparoscopy and dye test to evaluate the diagnostic accuracy of 3D HyCoSy, the results of 3D HyCoSy were consistent with that of laparoscopy except in two women. One of these two patients had unilateral tubal

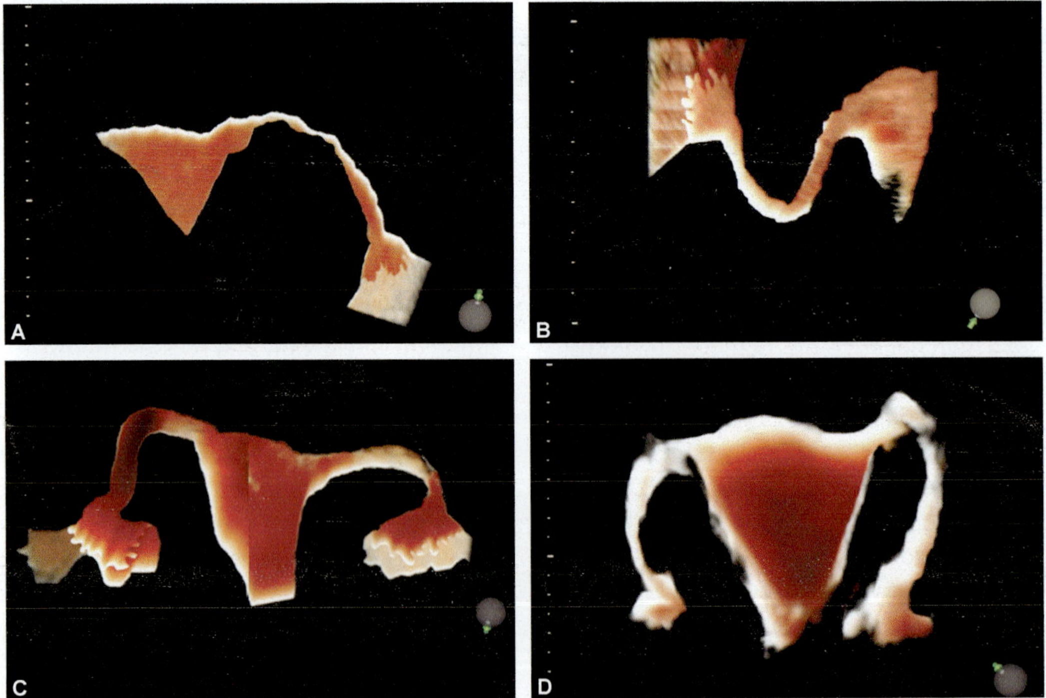

Figs. 23A to D: 3D ultrasound HD live rendered HyCoSy showing endometrial cavity and left and right fallopian tube, respectively, in parts (A) and (B), with clear outlining of fimbria and the contrast spill not only establishing the tubal patency but also showing the entire tubal lumen; Part (C) shows computer-aided unification of both these images resulting in the complete picture of endometrial cavity and both tubes—the entire extent; (D) 3D HyCoSy showing uterus and both tubes with fimbrial ends.

block on HyCoSy, but the tube was patent on laparoscopy with injection of the methylene blue dye with pressure. In the other patient, the fimbrial end of the tube was not clearly visualized on 3D HyCoSy and was thought to be blocked; but on laparoscopy, the distal tubal portion was buried behind the ovary due to endometriosis and the tube was patent. 3D HyCoSy is more informative and reliable than 2D HyCoSy. Whole extent of the tubal lumen and fimbrial condition can be visualized. Relation of fimbrial end of tube to ovary can also be defined (**Figs. 24 and 25**).

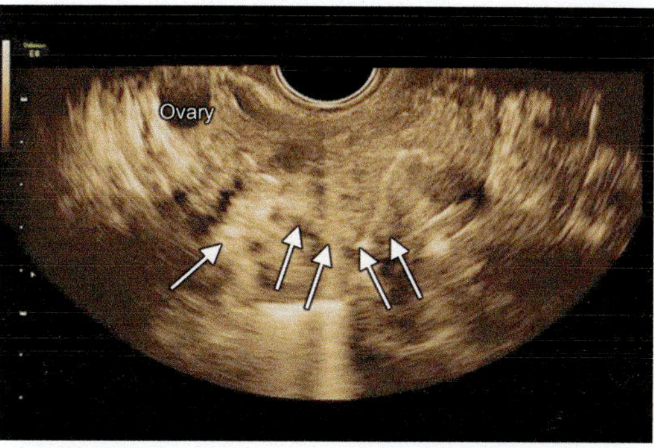

Fig. 24: Contrast-enhanced transvaginal scan transverse section showing the tube and the ovary establishing the tubo-ovarian relationship.

Hystero-contrast-sonosalpingography with automated 3D-CCI (coded contrast imaging) technology retains the advantages of conventional 2D HyCoSy while overcoming the disadvantages. 2D HyCoSy is highly observer dependent and is only accurate in the hands of experienced investigators. By obtaining a volume of the uterus and tubes, automated 3D volume acquisition permits visualization of the tubes in the coronal view and of the tubal course in 3D space and should

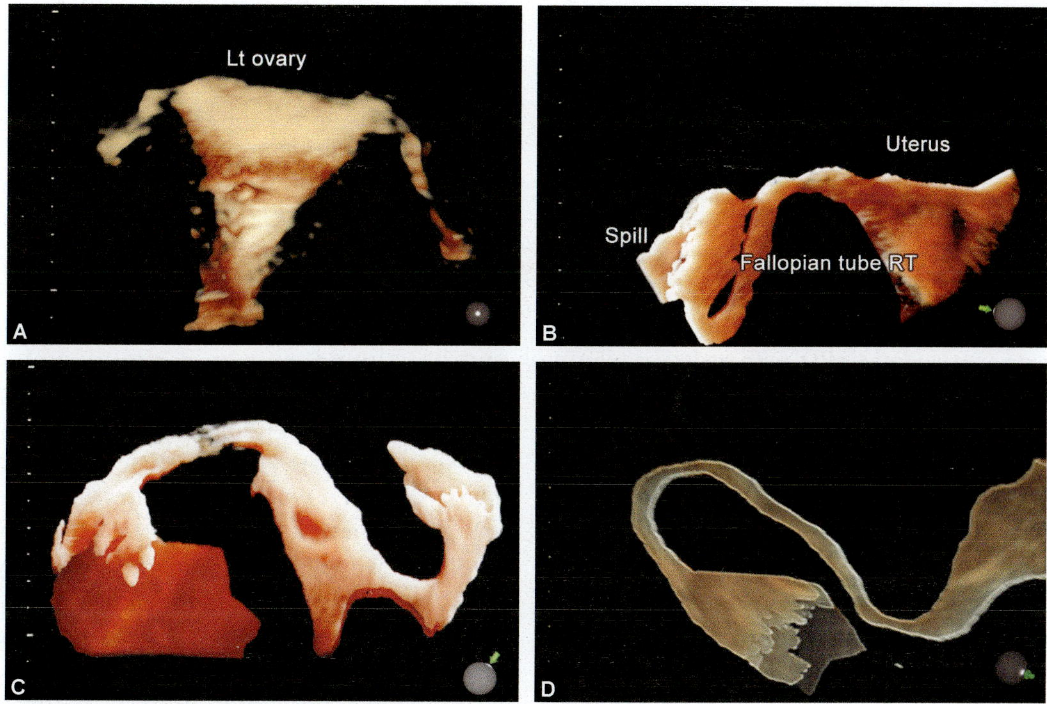

Figs. 25A to D: 3D ultrasound HD live rendered HyCoSy images: (A) normal endometrial cavity with bilateral mid-tubal block; (B) Normal endometrial cavity with left cornual block. Right tube is fully filled with contrast, but the fimbria are pruned and damaged; (C) Deviated uterine cavity with patent tubes. The left tube shows a twisted path as the uterus is deviated and left ovary is also displaced and fixed due to adhesions (D). Normal right tube and normal fimbrial end seen on HD live silhouette mode rendering.

allow less-experienced operators to evaluate tubal patency status relatively easily.[38]

Large studies have reported that 3D HyCoSy is highly accurate with 100% sensitivity, 67% specificity, 89% PPV, and 100% NPV for tubal patency and concordance rate with laparoscopy of 91%.[39] In a study by Kupesic et al., 3D HyCoSy (sensitivity, specificity, PPV, and NPV of 97.9%, 100%, 97.9%, and 100%, respectively) was found to be marginally superior to 2D HyCoSy (sensitivity, specificity, PPV, and NPV of 93.6%, 97.3%, 98.2%, and 97.3%, respectively) for tubal assessment.[40]

It has been shown in another study that for detecting tubal patency among the 150 fallopian tubes assessed, 3D SonoVue-HyCoSy had a sensitivity of 93.5%, specificity of 86.3%, positive- and negative-predictive values of 87.8% and 92.6%, respectively, and diagnostic accuracy of 90%. The test-positive rates of 3D SonoVue-HyCoSy versus lap and dye were not significantly different (82/150 vs. 77/150, $p > 0.05$).[41] Yet another study by Chan et al. has shown that the sensitivity of 3D HyCoSy for detecting tubal patency was 100% with a specificity of 67%. The positive- and negative-predictive values were 89% and 100%, respectively; the concordance rate was 91%. The mean duration (±SD) for the 3D HyCoSy was 13.4 ± 5.5 minutes.

Color-coded 3D PDI with surface rendering allowed visualization of the flow of contrast through the entire tubal length and free spill of contrast was clearly identified in the majority of cases. The 3D-PDI method appeared to have advantages over the conventional HyCoSy technique, especially in terms of visualization of spill from the distal end of the tube, which was achieved twice as often with the 3D technique. The 3D-PDI technique allowed better storage of the information for reanalysis and archiving than conventional HyCoSy. The mean duration of the imaging procedure was less with 3D PDI, but the operator time that included postprocedure analysis of the stored information was similar. A significantly lower volume of contrast medium (5.9 ± 0.6 mL) was used for 3D PDI in comparison with that (11.2 ± 1.9 mL) used for conventional 2D HyCoSy.[37]

CONCLUSION

Tubal evaluation is essential in subfertile patients. HSG has been used for a long time for assessment of tubal patency. Saline infusion salpingography has been proved to be fairly reliable technique for tubal evaluation. Its diagnostic accuracy can be improved by the use of pulse Doppler and color Doppler. Introduction of ultrasound-contrast media and HyCoSy has improved the visibility of the tubal lumen. HyCoSy is accurate in determining tubal patency and evaluating the uterine cavity, suggesting that it could completely supplant HSG as the first-line diagnostic test in an infertility workup.

Evaluative studies of HyCoSy showed good statistical comparability and concordance with HSG and laparoscopy combined with dye.[42] HyCoSy is well tolerated and can be a suitable alternative outpatient procedure.[43] HyCoSy using contrast agent appears to be more efficient than saline solution in detecting tubal obstruction.[44]

These studies confirm that HyCoSy is as efficient as HSG in assessing tubal patency and has the advantage of simultaneous pelvic evaluation for pelvic pathology and ovarian reserve. HyCoSy can, therefore, be considered as first-line investigative tool in low-risk women who are not known to have any reproductive comorbidities. HyCoSy combined with 3D ultrasound has the ability to increase the diagnostic accuracy, but this technique is not widely used because of limited availability of 3D ultrasound. While laparoscopic chromopertubation is the gold standard investigative modality for tubal assessment, its use can be restricted to selective group of women as most women could have less-invasive ultrasound methods to assess tubal patency.

To quote a few other studies that have concluded similar facts are as follows:

- SSG can be used as an initial investigation for infertile patients and laparoscopy can be deferred for 6 months. Meanwhile, endocrinological and immunological causes are ruled out and then, if required, laparoscopy may be done.[17]
- SSG can be used as first ambulatorial evaluation of tubal patency in infertility workup.[45] Royal College of Obstetricians and Gynecologists (RCOG) recommends that where appropriate expertise is available, screening for tubal occlusion using HyCoSy should be considered because it is an effective alternative to HSG for women who are not known to have comorbidities. Women who are thought to have comorbidities should be offered laparoscopy and dye injection, so that tubal and other pelvic pathology can be assessed at the same time.

Because of good degree of statistical comparability and concordance of conventional HyCoSy with HSG and laparoscopy and dye test, the National Institute for Health and Clinical Excellence (NICE) has recommended HyCoSy as a suitable outpatient procedure for tubal patency assessment in women who are not known to have any comorbidities such as pelvic inflammatory disease, previous ectopic pregnancy, or endometriosis.[43] HyCoSy is well tolerated by women and associated risks are minimal with the risk of pelvic infection ≤1%.

REFERENCES

1. Gordts S, Campo R, Rombauts L, Brosens I. Endoscopic visualization of the process of fimbrial ovum retrieval in the human. Hum Reprod. 1998;13(6):1425-8.
2. Mohiyiddeen L, Hardiman A, Fitzgerald C, Hughes E, Mol BW, Johnson N, Watson A. Tubal flushing for subfertility (Cochrane Review). Cochrane Database Syst Rev. 2015;(5):CD003718.
3. Belisle S, Collins JA, Burrows EA, Willan AR. The value of laparoscopy among infertile women with tubal patency. J Soc Obstet Gynaecol Can. 1996;18:326-36.
4. Watrelot A, Dreyfus JM, Andine JP. Evaluation of the performance of fertiloscopy in 160 consecutive infertile patients with no obvious pathology. Hum Reprod. 1999;14:707-11.
5. Nanini R, Chelo E, Branconi F, Tantini C, Scarselli GF. Dynamic echohysteroscopy: a new diagnostic technique in the study of female infertility. Acta Eur Fertil. 1981;12(2):165-71.
6. Richman TS, Visconi GN, deChurney A, Polan ML, Alcebo LO. Fallopian tubal patency assessed by ultrasound fluid injection. Work in progress. Radiology. 1984;152(2):507-10.
7. Randolph JR, Ying YK, Maier DB, Schmidt CL, Riddick DH. Comparison of real time ultrasonography, hysterosalpingography and laparoscopy/ hysteroscopy in the evaluation of uterine abnormalities and tubal patency. Fertil Steril. 1986;46(5):828-32.
8. Tufekci EC, Girit S, Bayirli MD, Durmuşoğlu F, Yalti S. Evaluation of tubal patency by transvaginal sonosalpingography. Fertil Steril. 1992;57(2):336-40.
9. Deichert U, Schlief R, van de Sandt M, Juhnke I. Transvaginal hysterosalpingo-contrast-sonography (Hy-Co-Sy) compared with conventional tubal diagnostics. Hum Reprod. 1989;4:418-24.
10. Stern J, Peters AJ, Coulam CB. Colour Doppler ultrasonography assessment of tubal patency: a comparison study with traditional techniques. Fertil Steril. 1992;58(5):897-900.
11. Kupesic S, Kurjak A. Gynecological vaginal sonographic interventional procedures—what does colour add? Gynecol Perinatol. 1994;3:57-60.
12. Deichert U, Schlief R, van de Sandt M, Daume E. Transvaginal hysterosalpingo-contrast sonography for the assessment of tubal patency with gray-scale imaging and additional use of pulsed wave Doppler. Fertil Steril. 1992;57(1):62-7.
13. Heikkinen H, Tekay A, Volpi E, Martikainen H, Jouppila P. Transvaginal salpingosonography for the assessment of tubal patency in infertile women: methodological and clinical experiences. Fertil Steril. 1995;64(2):293-8.
14. Dessole S, Farina M, Rubattu G, Cosmi E, Ambrosini G, Nardelli GB. Side effects and complications of sonohysterosalpingography. Fertil Steril. 2003;8(3):620-4.
15. de Kroon CD, de Bock GH, Dieben SW, Jansen FW. Saline contrast hysterosonography in abnormal uterine bleeding: a systematic review and meta-analysis. BJOG. 2003;110(10):938-47.

16. Spalding H, Martikainen H, Tekay A, Jouppila P. Transvaginal salpingosonography for assessing tubal patency in women previously treated for pelvic inflammatory disease and benign ovarian tumors. Ultrasound Obstet Gynecol. 1999;14:205-9.
17. Kore S, Hegde A, Nair S. Sonography for assessment of tubal patency: our experience. J Obstet Gynecol India. 2000;50(2):636.
18. Seal SL, Ghosh D, Saha D. Comparative evaluation of sonosalpingography, hysterosalpingography and laparoscopy for determination of tubal patency. J Obstet Gynecol India. 2007;57:158-61.
19. Lucaino DE, Exacoustos C, Johns DA. Transabdominal saline contrast sonohysterography: can it replace hysterosalpingography in low resource countries? Am J Obstet Gynecol. 2011;204:79.
20. Deichert U, van de Sandt M. Transvaginal hysterosalpingo-contrast sonography (Hy-Co-Sy). The assessment of tubal patency and uterine abnormalities by contrast enhanced sonography. Adv Echocontrast. 1993;2:55-8.
21. Peters AJ, Coulam CB. Hysterosalpingography with colour Doppler sonography. Am J Obstet Gynecol. 1991;164(6 Pt 1):1530-2.
22. Jeanty P, Besnard S, Arnold A, Turner C, Crum P. Air-contrast sonohysterography as a first-step assessment of tubal patency. J Ultrasound Med. 2000;19:519-27.
23. Sankpal RS, Confino E, Matzel A, Cohen LS. Investigation of the uterine cavity and fallopian tubes using three-dimensional saline sonohysterosalpingography. Int J Gynaecol Obstet. 2001;73:125-9.
24. Kiyokawa K, Masuda H, Fuyuki T, Koseki M, Uchida N, Fukuda T, et al. Three-dimensional hysterosalpingo-contrast sonography (3D-HyCoSy) as an outpatient procedure to assess infertile women: a pilot study. Ultrasound Obstet Gynecol. 2000;16(7):648-54.
25. Bonilla-Musoles F, Simon C, Sampaio, Sampaio M, Pellicer A. An assessment of Hysterosalpingosonography as a diagnostic tool for uterine cavity defects and tubal patency. J Clin Ultrasound. 1992;20(3):175-81.
26. Emanuel MH, Exalto N. Hysterosalpingo-foam sonography (HyFoSy): a new technique to visualize tubal patency. UOG. 2011;37:498-9.
27. Prefumo F, Serafini G, Martinoli C, Gandolfo N, Gandolfo NG, Derchi LE, et al. The sonographic evaluation of tubal patency with stimu- lated acoustic emission imaging. Ultrasound Obstet Gynecol. 2002;20(4):386-9.
28. Boudghene FP, Bazot M, Robert Y, Perrot N, Rocourt N, Antoine JM, et al. Assessment of fallopian tube patency by HyCoSy: comparison of a positive contrast agent with saline solution. Ultrasound Obstet Gynecol. 2001;18:525-30.
29. Holz K, Becker R, Schürmann R. Ultrasound in the investigation of tubal patency: a meta-analysis of three comparative studies of Echovist-200 including 1007 women. Zentralbl Gynakol. 1997;119:366-73.
30. Korell M, Seehaus D, Strowitzki T, Hepp H. Radiologic versus ultrasound fallopian tube imaging. Painfulness of the examination and diagnostic reliability of hysterosalpingography and hysterosalpingo-contrast-ultrasonography with echovist 200. Ultraschall Med. 1997;18: 3-7.
31. Lanzani C, Savasi V, Leone FP, Ratti M, Ferrazzi E. Two-dimensional HyCoSy with contrast tuned imaging technology and a second-generation contrast media for assessment of tubal patency in an infertility program. Fertil Steril. 2009;92(3):1158-61.
32. Tanawattanachaeron S, Suwajanakorn S, Uerpairojkit B, Boonkasemsamti W, Virutamasen P. Transvaginal hystero-contrast sonography (HyCoSy) compared with chromolaparoscopy. J Obstet Gynecol Res. 2000;26:71-5.
33. Strandell A, Bourne T, Bergh C, Granberg S, Asztely M, Thorburn J. The assessment of endometrial pathology and tubal patency: a comparison between the use of ultrasonography and X-ray hysterosalpingography for the investigation of infertility patients. Ultrasound Obstet Gynecol. 1999;14:200-4.
34. Exacoustos C, Zupi E, Carusotti C, Lanzi G, Marconi D, Arduini D. Hysterosalpingo-contrast sonography compared with hysterosalpingography and laparoscopic dye pertubation to evaluate tubal patency. J Am Assoc Gynecol Laparosc. 2003;10:367-72.
35. Guazzaroni M, Mari A, Politi C, Guazzaroni M, Remedi S, Mallarini G, et al. Ultrasound hysterosalpingography with levovist in the diagnosis of tubaric patency. Radiol Med. 2001;102:62-6.
36. Balen FG, Allen CM, Gardener JE, Siddle NC, Lees WR. 3-Dimensional reconstruction of ultrasound images of the uterine cavity. Br J Radiol. 1993;66(787):588-91.
37. Sladkevicius P, Ojha K, Campbell S, Nargund G. Three-dimensional power Doppler imaging in the assessment of fallopian tube patency. Ultrasound Obstet Gynecol. 2000;16:644-7.
38. Exacoustos C, Di Giovanni A, Szabolcs B, Romeo V, Romanini ME, Luciano D, et al. Automated three-dimensional coded contrast imaging hysterosalpingo-contrast sonography: feasibility in office tubal patency testing. Ultrasound Obstet Gynecol. 2013;41:328-35.

39. Chan CC, Ng EH, Tang OS, Chan KKL, Ho PC. Comparison of three-dimensional hystero-contrast-sonography and diagnostic laparoscopy with chromopertubation in the assessment of tubal patency for the investigation of subfertility. Acta Obstet Gynecol Scand. 2005;84:909-13.
40. Kupesic S, Plavsic BM. 2D and 3D hysterosalpingo-contrast-sonography in the assessment of uter- ine cavity and tubal patency. Eur J Obstet Gynecol Reprod Biol. 2007;133:64-9.
41. Zhou L, Zhang X, Chen X, Liao L, Pan R, Zhou N, et al. Value of three-dimensional hysterosalpingo-contrast sonography with SonoVue in the assessment of tubal patency. Ultrasound Obstet Gynecol. 2012;40:93-8.
42. Tanahatoe S, Hompes PG, Lambalk CB. Accuracy of diagnostic laparoscopy in the infertility work- up before intrauterine insemination. Fertil Steril. 2003;79:361-6.
43. Dijkman AB, Mol BW, van der Veen F, Bossuyt PM, Hogerzeil HV. Can hysterosalpingo-contrast-sonography replace hysterosalpingography in the assessment of tubal subfertility? Eur J Radiol. 2000;35:44-8.
44. Ayida G, Kennedy S, Barlow D, Chamberlain P. A comparison of patient tolerance of hystero-salpingo-contrast sonography (HyCoSy) with Echovist-200 and X-ray hysterosalpingography for outpatient investigation of infertile women. Ultrasound Obstet Gynecol. 1996;7:201-4.
45. Volpi E, De Grandis T, Sismondi P, Giacardi M, Rustichelli S, Patriarca A, et al. Transvaginal salpingo-sonography (TSSG) in the evaluation of tubal patency. Acta Eur Fertil. 1991;22(6):325-8.

30

CHAPTER

Ultrasound Diagnosis of PCOS

Sonal Panchal, Chaitanya Nagori

INTRODUCTION

The polycystic ovary syndrome (PCOS) is a complex endocrine condition in which ovulatory dysfunction and androgen excess are cardinal features.[1] It has metabolic and endocrinal components that are both intricately inter-related. Earliest description of polycystic ovaries appears to date from 1845 as "sclerocystic ovaries".[2] The syndrome was redescribed in 1935 when American gynecologists, Irving F Stein, Sr and Michael L Leventhal, associated the presence of ovarian cysts with anovulation[3] and then was also named Stein-Leventhal syndrome.

Other names suggested were polyfollicular syndrome or ovarian dysmetabolic syndrome. The PCOS is a heterogeneous condition, the pathophysiology of which appears to be both multifactorial and polygenic. There are many extraovarian aspects to the pathophysiology of PCOS, yet ovarian dysfunction is central.[4] PCOS apparently begins in the perimenarcheal period in adolescents and has been characterized as an abnormal and exaggerated transition to puberty involving four key physiological processes—(1) the increase in luteinizing hormone (LH) secretion, (2) the increase in adrenal androgen production, (3) the increase in body mass, and (4) the onset of adult patterns of insulin resistance (IR).[5]

INCIDENCE

Approximately, 20–30% of women in reproductive age have polycystic ovaries and about half of these have signs and symptoms of PCOS. PCOS affects about 10% of women in reproductive age.[6] Though in our experience taking into consideration only the infertile women in the reproductive age group, the incidence of polycystic ovarian syndrome is higher than mentioned in this study.

DIAGNOSIS

Three major ways to diagnosis of PCOS are:

1. Clinical findings
2. Laboratory testing
3. Ultrasound (US) findings.

According to ESHRE/ASRM consensus 2003, the diagnosis of polycystic ovarian syndrome consists of at least two of the three following criteria:[7]

1. Oligo- and/or anovulation
2. *Hyperandrogenism*: Biochemical or clinical
3. *Polycystic ovaries on US*: This means an ovary that is 10 cm^3 in volume and/or has >12 antral follicles. Though certain new amendments and guidelines have been established in ESHRE 2018, still keeping the Rotterdam criteria as a basis.

In 2006, the Androgen Excess PCOS Society suggested a tightening of the diagnostic criteria to all of the following:[1]

- Excess androgen activity
- Oligoovulation/anovulation and/or polycystic ovaries
- Other entities are excluded that would cause excess androgen activity.

According to both these definitions, androgen excess is the key feature for diagnosis of PCOS, and this androgen excess is a result of hyperinsulinemia. Insulin augments Luteinizing hormone (LH)-stimulated androgen production.[8] Androgen excess leads to increased LH and oligoanovulation. Oligoanovulation can be documented on US. Whichever definition is considered, polycystic ovaries on US are one of the key features for diagnosis.

Ultrasound Diagnosis

This assessment is done on baseline US scan. This scan is done on second to 3rd day of menstrual cycle. This scan is done when estrogen and progesterone levels are at baseline, ovaries are silent, and have no active follicle or corpus luteum.

The scan is done using not only B-mode US but also with color Doppler, pulse Doppler, three-dimensional (3D) US, and 3D power Doppler. Using color Doppler in this assessment is mandatory to understand the hormonal dynamics of PCOS, which reflects as vascular and morphological changes in the ovaries and uterus. 3D US is especially useful for volume measurements. Volumes, when calculated by 3D US using VOCAL (volume calculation) software, are much more reliable than volumes calculated by two-dimensional (2D) US. 3D power Doppler assessment has been found to be highly promising, as it gives idea about the global vascularity of ovaries, instead of one or two selected vessels being interrogated on pulse Doppler.

Scanning Technique

B-mode US assessment of the ovaries consists of assessment of ovarian diameters and volume and counting of antral follicles as quantitative assessment and qualitative assessment of stroma. Stromal excess has been described as one of the key features of polycystic ovaries since the earliest documentation of this syndrome.

Once ovary is located, the probe is rotated to find out the long axis of the ovary and then is spanned to find out the longest section of the ovary and is stored as one frame on a dual screen. Then probe is rotated 90° to get a true transverse axis of ovary (**Fig. 1**). Measure the largest longitudinal, transverse, and AP diameter of the ovary in centimeters (cm), and ovarian volume can be calculated by the formula ($x \times y \times z \times 0.523$). The long diameter is measured as the longest diameter on the long section of the ovary. AP diameter is measured as a longest diameter perpendicular to the long diameter in the same section. Transverse diameter is measured as side-to-side diameter on the transverse section.

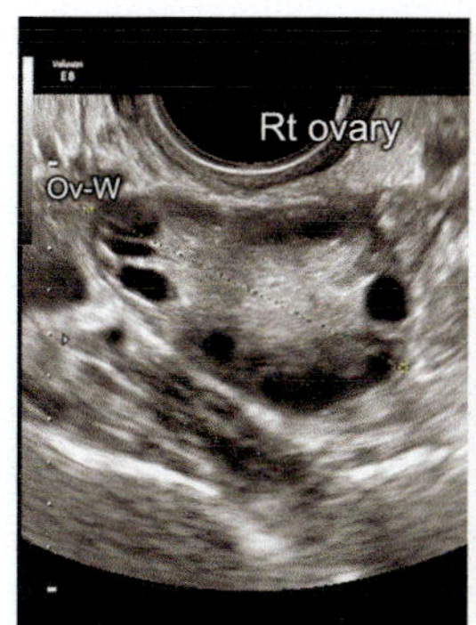

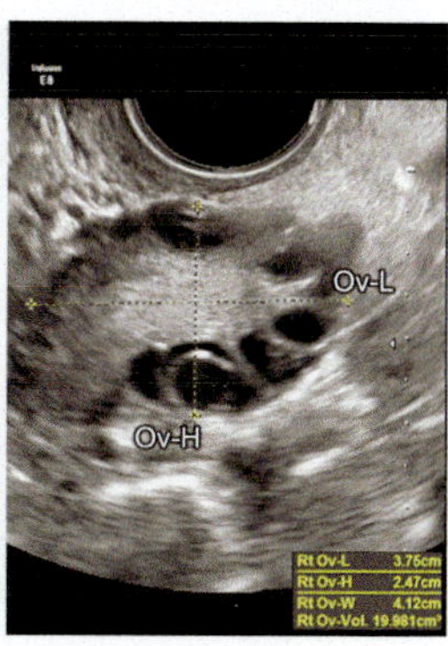

Fig. 1: B-mode US image of ovary in dual frame showing longitudinal and transverse section of the ovary with multiple follicles placed peripherally and central echogenic stroma. The cursors are seen measuring the longitudinal, transverse, and anteroposterior (AP) diameters of the ovary.

Number of antral follicles is counted in the whole ovary by taking a 2D sweep across whole ovary and counting the follicles by eyeballing. As a rule, when counting antral follicles by eyeballing on B-mode US, the probe is only swept from one side of the ovary to other and is never ever rotated. This method is feasible and reliable when number of antral follicles is approximately up to 10–12. But when number of follicles is much more as typically seen in polycystic ovaries, the calculation is likely to be inaccurate. In these cases, 3D US and advanced calculation software are required.

Stromal echogenicity is assessed against echogenicity of myometrium on B-mode US. But, this can be done only if ovary and uterus

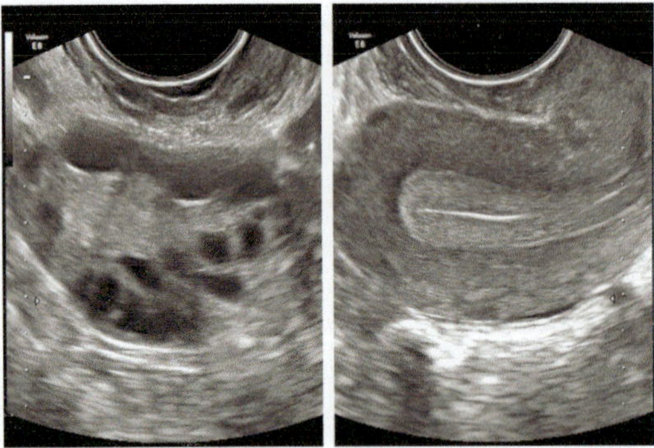

Fig. 2: B-mode ultrasound image in dual frame showing longitudinal section of ovary in the left frame and long section of the uterus in right frame. This image is taken to compare the stromal echogenicity with echogenicity of the myometrium. Stromal echogenicity is more than the echogenicity of the myometrium in polycystic ovaries.

are at almost same depth from the probe (**Fig. 2**). In a normal ovary, ovarian stroma is isoechoic to normal myometrium.

Color or power Doppler box is now placed on the ovary. The color box should be large enough to cover the whole ovary. Doppler is used to see presence of vessels in ovarian stroma. The vessel that is close to any of the follicles is not a stromal vessel (**Fig. 3**). If stromal vascularity is present, spectral Doppler is used for quantitative assessment of the flows—intraovarian resistance index (RI) and peak systolic velocity (PSV) (**Fig. 4**). For color Doppler, pulse repetition frequency

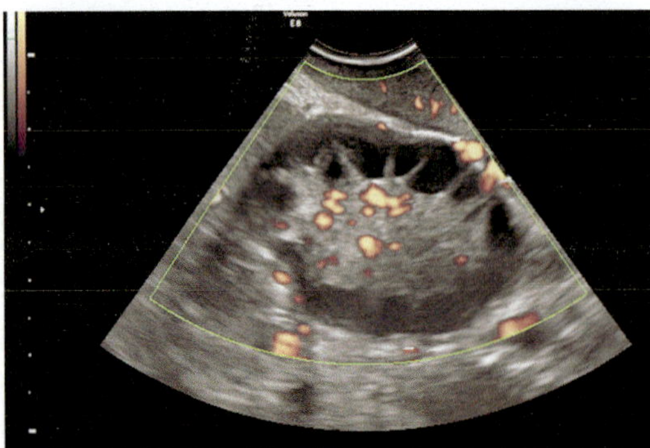

Fig. 3: Power Doppler ultrasound image of ovary showing peripherally distributed follicles and echogenic stroma with color flow in the stroma–ovarian stromal vessels.

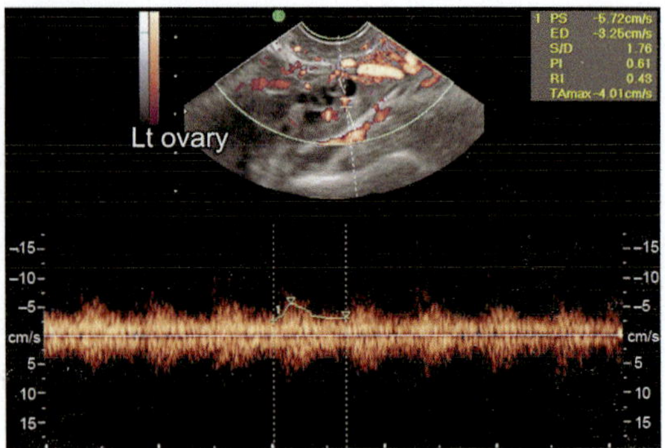

Fig. 4: Spectral Doppler of the ovarian stromal vessels showing low-resistance blood flow.

(PRF) is set at 0.3, wall filters are lowest, with optimum gains and balance settings. For pulse Doppler also PRF around 0.9–1.3 is set, and wall filters are set at 30 Hz as stromal flows on baseline scan are usually low-velocity flows (**Fig. 5**). The vessel selected for interrogation is a vessel that shows brightest color on color Doppler. It is recommended that angle correction is used when assessing the stromal flows.

Having completed the Doppler study, volume studies are initiated. 3D US provides

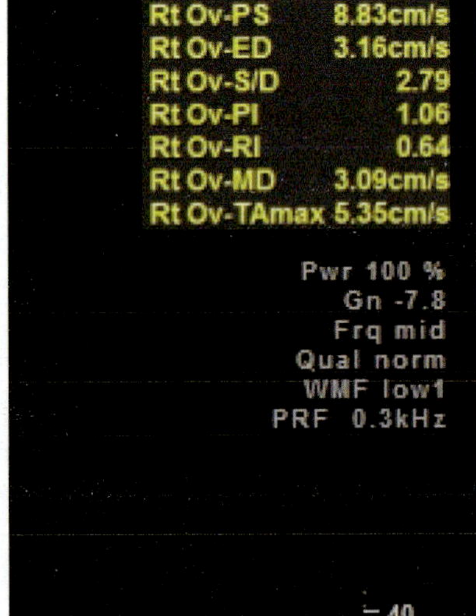

Fig. 5: Cut part of the US scanner screen showing Doppler settings on the machine for assessment of ovarian stromal flows, which are very low velocity flow. The data in white in the last two lines show WMF low and PRF 0.3 (low-pulse repetition frequency). (WMF: wall motion filter)

a new method for objective quantitative assessment of follicle count, ovarian volume, stromal volume, and blood flow in the ovary.[9] Power Doppler box is set to include whole ovary, and then 3D volume of ovary is acquired. Volume and power Doppler box and the volume angle are all set to include the whole ovary in the volume in all three planes. This can be confirmed when the entire ovary is seen in A and B images of the multiplanar image (**Figs. 6A and B**). This volume of ovary is used to calculate ovarian volume, stromal volume, and to count number of antral follicles. Global vascular indices VI (vascularity index), FI (flow index), and VFI (vascularity FI) may be calculated from the same ovarian volume.

Antral follicles are counted by using a software called SonoAVC (automated volume calculation). To use SonoAVC, region of interest (ROI) is selected to include the whole ovary in all three orthogonal planes on acquired ovarian volume. This software is based on inversion mode rendering. Inversion mode (**Fig. 7**) renders fluid-filled structures as solid areas, and this helps to identify very small fluid-filled spaces also clearly. SonoAVC further color codes each follicle (**Fig. 8**) and also measures *x*, *y*, and *z* diameters, mean diameter, and volume of each follicle on report sheet (**Fig. 9**). This is a more precise method than all other methods available at this time to count the number of antral follicles, as there is least chance of follicles being missed or being counted twice. But to avoid undercounting, postprocessing (PP) is required. Actions included in PP are—(1) adding the uncounted follicles, (2) removing the areas that are erroneously counted as follicles, (3) cutting the extra areas that are considered by the software as follicular areas, and (4) merging the two areas that are actually a part of the same follicle but are counted as separate follicles. SonoAVC with PP is a reliable method for measuring total antral follicle count (AFC). Though Jayaprakasan et al. have shown that FNPO (follicle number per ovary) calculated with 2D or 3D have given identical results.[10]

Another study quotes that fewer antral follicles are evident overall when SonoAVC is used to analyze 3D US data. But, it is significantly quicker than 2D US in making measurements.[11]

However, the AFC obtained by SonoAVC-PP is likely to be lower because this method measures and color codes each follicle preventing recounting.

Moreover, intraobserver and interobserver reliabilities of automated AFCs made using 3D US and SonoAVC make it a preferred method.[12] It must still be understood that the inherent intra- and interobserver variation seen in measuring the number of antral follicles can be reduced but not eliminated by the use of 3D US and more recently, automated US.[13]

The cohort of small follicles measuring 1–5 mm does seem to more accurately reflect ovarian reserve and is increased in women with PCOS.[14] Automated 3D measures do provide reliable information on follicle number and size and can be used to individually identify each follicle[11] and appear to be more reflective of ovarian reserve and response, but their accuracy needs to be determined by further work.[15]

A software called virtual organ computer-aided analysis (VOCAL) (volume calculation by computer) is used to calculate ovarian volume. VOCAL calculates volume of any structure by rotating it 180°. A rotating step of 6–30° can be selected (**Figs. 10A to G**). A circumference is drawn around the structure of interest at every rotation step, and at the end of 180°, total volume is calculated. The volume calculated by 3D US and VOCAL is much more accurate than when calculated from three diameters taken in orthogonal planes on B-mode scan. There are two basic methods employed to calculate volume from a 3D data set: the conventional "full planar" method

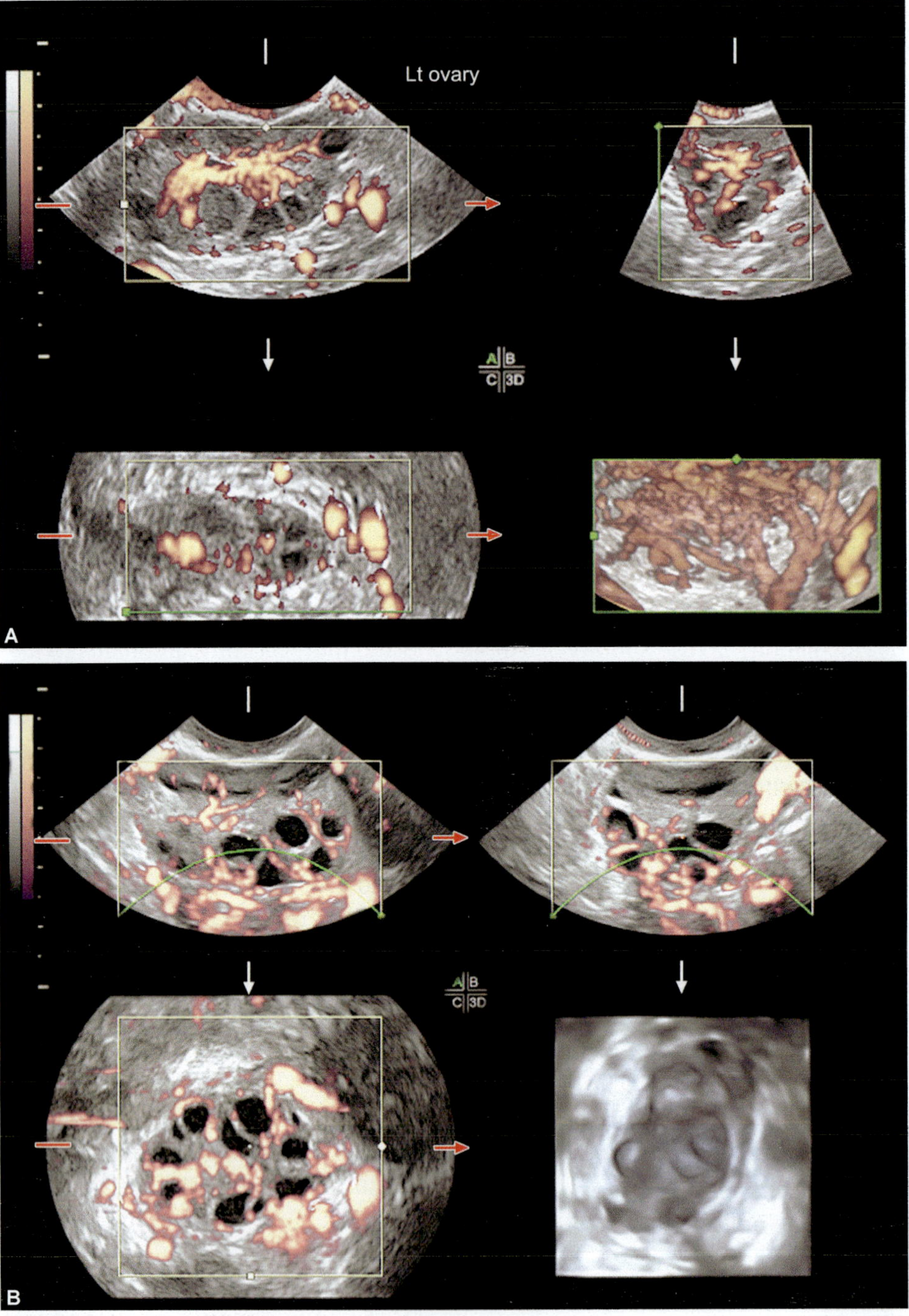

Figs. 6A and B: Both these images are 3D power Doppler acquired images of the ovary. Both images have four images in them. The left upper image is the long axis of the ovary and is known as image A, right upper image is image B (transverse section of ovary here), C is coronal section of ovary, and D is the rendered image. In both images, a sectional image shows whole ovary in long axis. But on B sectional image in part (A), the margins of the ovary are cut from the sides, and therefore, it is an inadequate volume and is not acceptable; In part B, on the b sectional image, the angle is wider and whole ovary is included on this sectional image indicating it has an adequate volume angle and is an acceptable volume.

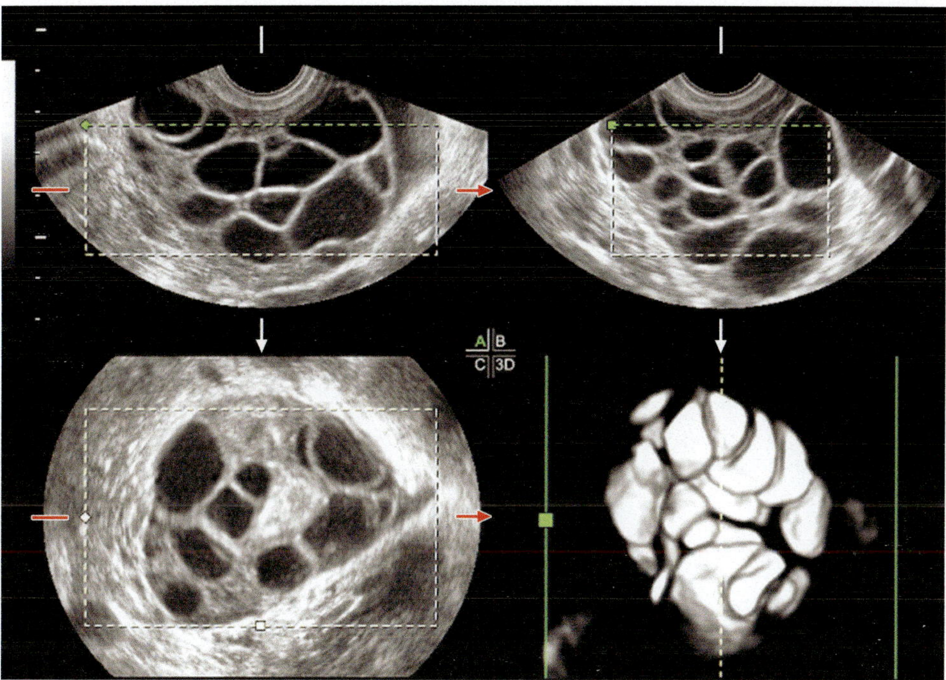

Fig. 7: 3D ultrasound image of a stimulated ovary with multiple follicles rendered on inversion mode.

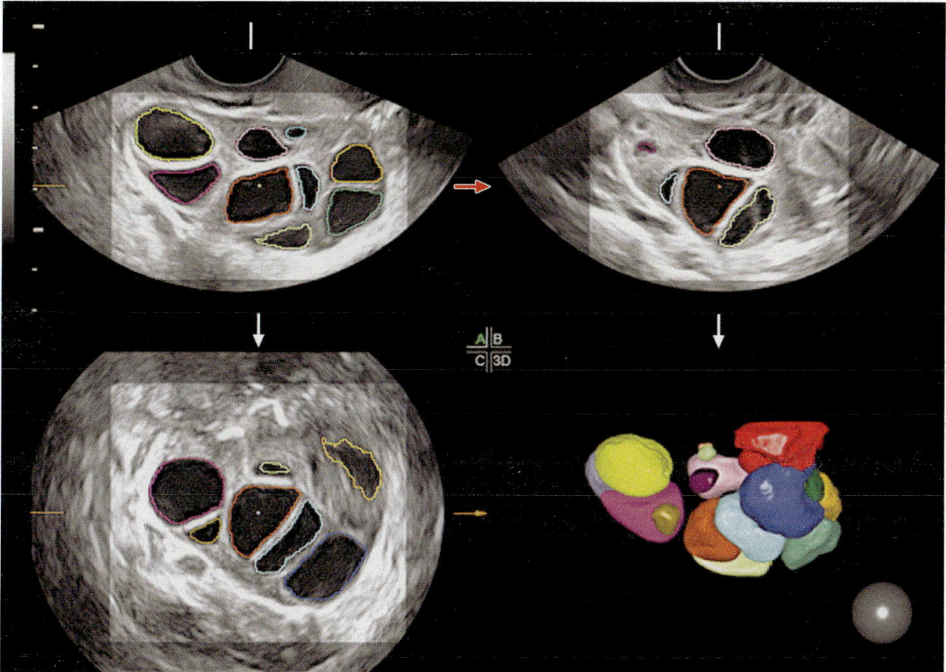

Fig. 8: 3D ultrasound-acquired volume of stimulated ovary showing follicles outlined by different colors on sectional planes and on the rendered image; these follicles are seen like balls of different colors—color coding of follicles rendered in inversion is done by software called SonoAVC.

Name | Pat. ID

Ovary: Left
Total#: 12

Nr.	d(V) mm	dx mm	dy mm	dz mm	mn. d mm	V cm³
1	9.3	17.0	9.6	5.8	10.8	0.42
2	7.6	10.7	8.2	5.2	8.0	0.23
3	7.4	11.0	7.5	5.7	8.1	0.21
4	5.8	6.9	6.4	4.7	6.0	0.10
5	5.7	13.5	7.7	4.2	8.5	0.10
6	5.7	6.6	6.2	4.7	5.8	0.10
7	5.4	6.8	6.6	3.9	5.8	0.08
8	5.0	7.6	5.4	3.7	5.6	0.07
9	4.6	5.6	4.5	4.1	4.7	0.05
10	3.0	5.4	3.0	1.8	3.4	0.01
11	2.2	3.3	2.1	1.6	2.4	<0.01
12	2.1	3.2	2.3	1.7	2.4	<0.01

Ovary: Right
Total#: 10

Nr.	d(V) mm	dx mm	dy mm	dz mm	mn. d mm	V cm³
1	13.1	20.7	15.6	7.9	14.7	1.18
2	9.7	13.6	11.7	6.5	10.6	0.48
3	8.6	10.7	9.0	7.0	8.9	0.33
4	7.2	10.1	7.2	5.5	7.6	0.20
5	7.0	9.6	6.6	5.8	7.3	0.18
6	5.1	7.2	5.7	3.4	5.4	0.07
7	4.7	6.2	5.2	3.4	4.9	0.05
8	4.2	5.7	4.6	3.1	4.4	0.04
9	3.2	3.6	3.4	2.8	3.3	0.02
10	3.1	3.7	3.0	2.7	3.1	0.02

Endo Thickness 4.89 mm

Pelvic Floor

funneling ▪ yes ▪ no

urethral kinking ▪ yes ▪ no

Fig. 9: Report sheet of SonoAVC showing the list of follicles in each ovary with its color coding information *x*, *y*, and *z* diameters and also mean diameter and volume of each follicle.

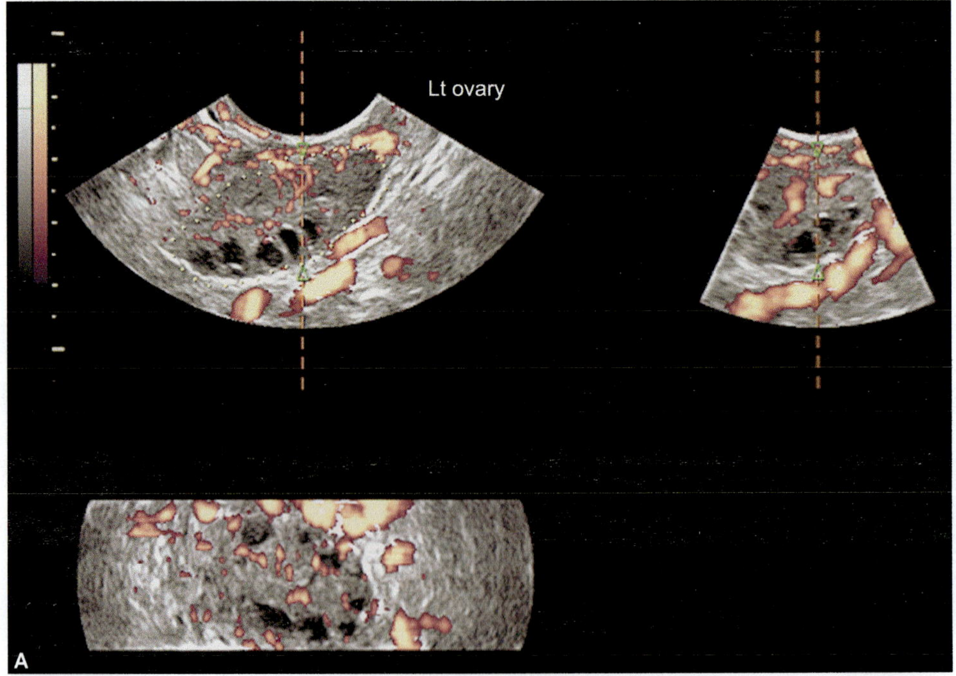

Figs. 10A to G: *Contd...*

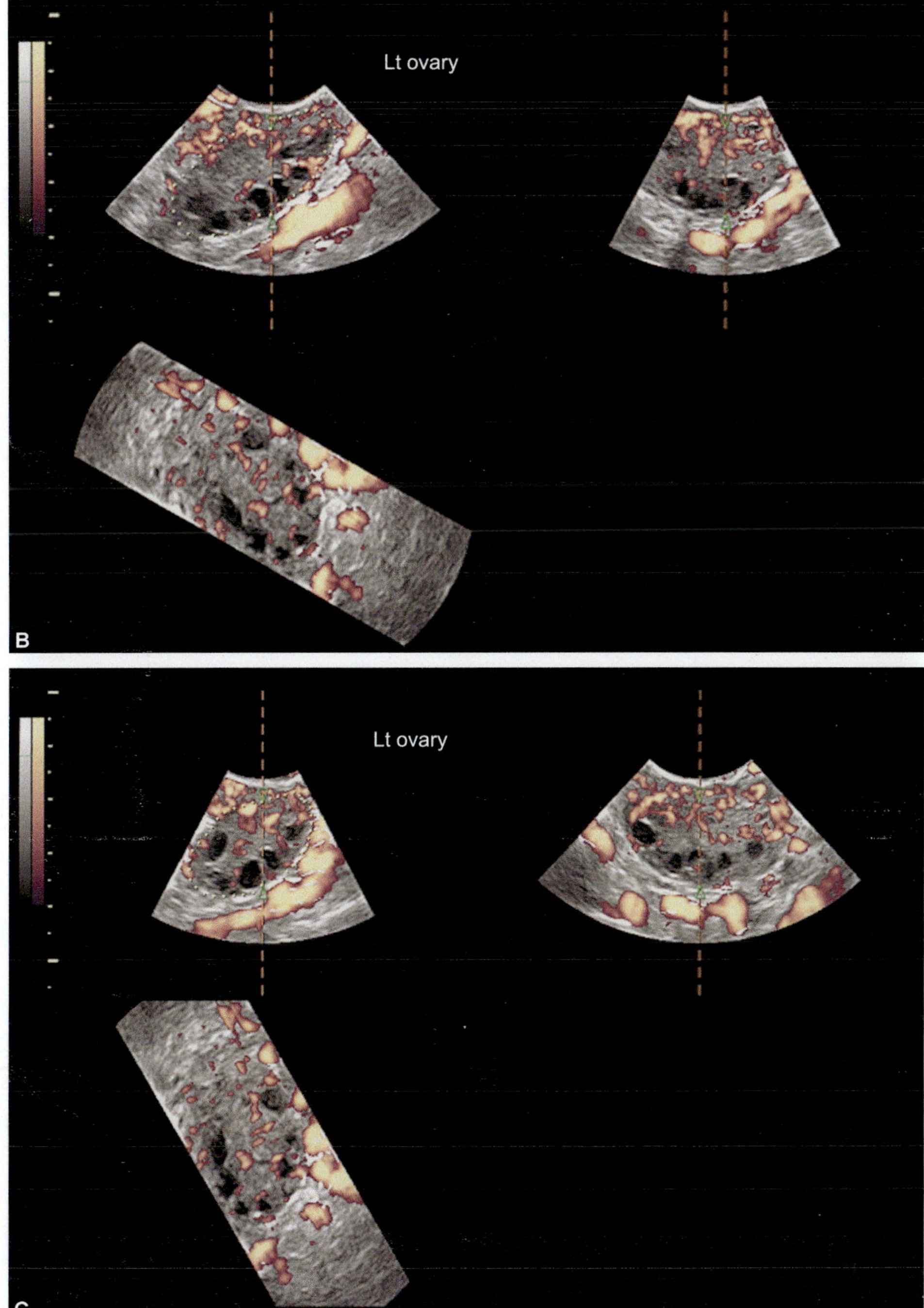

Figs. 10A to G: *Contd...*

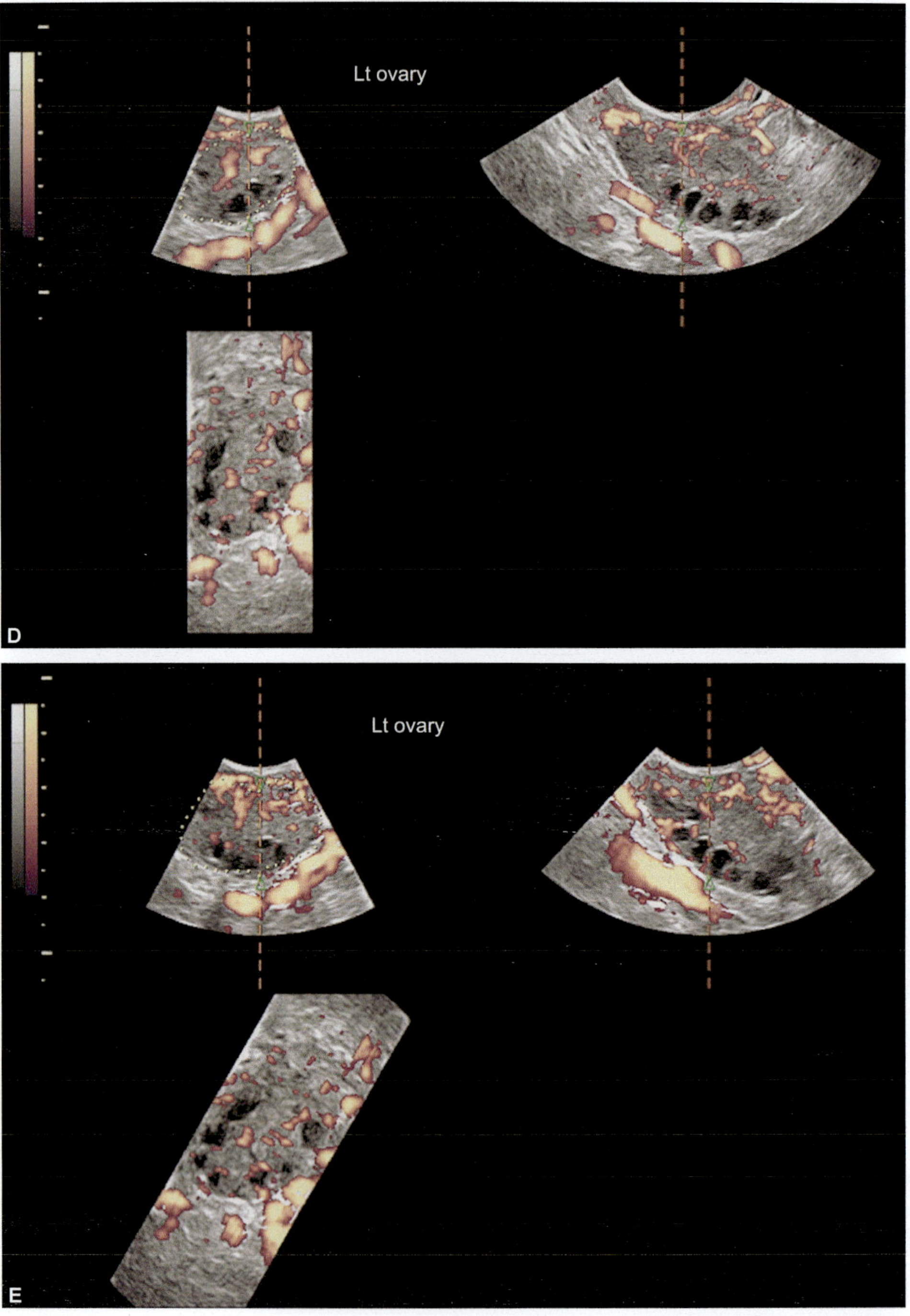

Figs. 10A to G: *Contd...*

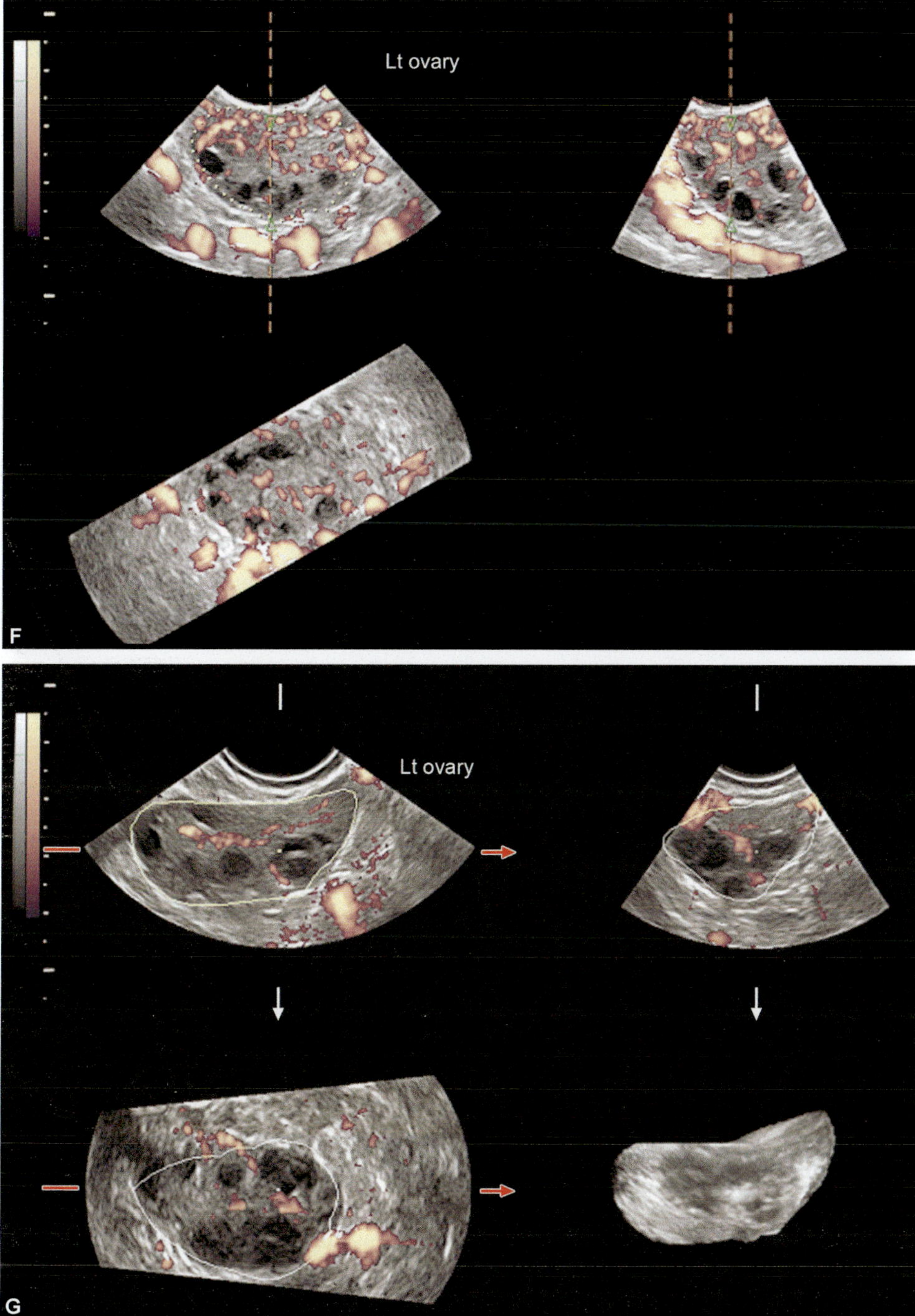

Figs. 10A to G: (A) 3D US-acquired volume of the ovary with power Doppler; (B to F) The rotation of the C images as images A to D rotated for vocal multiple; (G) The calculated ovarian volume by virtual organ computer-aided analysis (VOCA L).

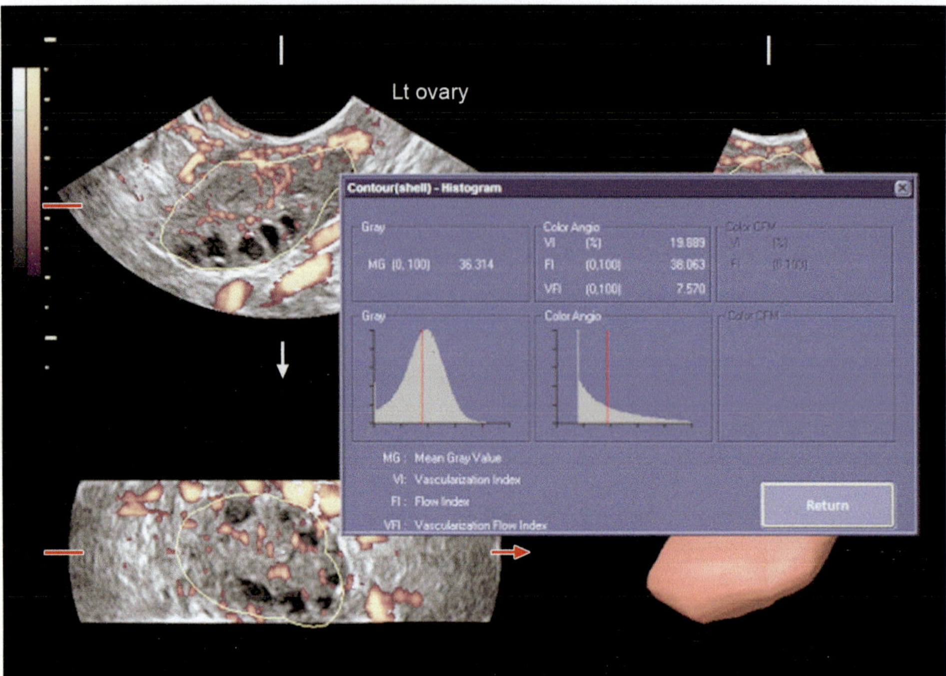

Fig. 11: 3D power Doppler volume with virtual organ computer-aided analysis (VOCAL) with volume histogram showing the 3D power Doppler indices (VI, FI, and VFI) in the blue box. These are global vascular indices giving information about the vascular abundance and intensity in the selected volume.
(VI: vascularity index; FI: flow index; VFI: vascularity flow index)

and the more recently introduced rotational method possible through the virtual organ computer-aided analysis (VOCAL)-imaging program. Volume calculations have proven to be highly reliable and valid both in vitro and in vivo with either method, although the newer rotational method appears statistically superior.[16-19]

On this VOCAL-calculated ovarian volume that is acquired with power Doppler, applying volume histogram gives values of 3D power Doppler indices (**Fig. 11**), VI, FI, and VFI. VI is an index for abundance of flow in the selected volume, FI is an index for average intensity of flow in a selected volume, and VFI is a perfusion index. Applying threshold volume on the same VOCAL-calculated volume will define stromal volume when threshold is set to differentiate follicles from rest of the ovarian tissues (**Fig. 12**).

Ultrasound Findings of Polycystic Ovarian Syndrome

According to Rotterdam criteria, one of the three criteria for diagnosis of polycystic ovarian syndrome is polycystic ovaries on US. And according to the same criteria, the polycystic ovaries on US are ovaries that are >10 cm^3 in volume and/or have >12 antral follicles. This number of 12 follicles has now been changed to 20 per ovary. These ultrasound features need to be confirmed on transvaginal ultrasound with 8 MHz probe. If transabdominal ultrasound is done instead, only volume is to be considered, follicle count is not taken into account.

Ovarian Volume

It has been described by Stein-Leventhal also that patients with polycystic ovarian syndrome have large ovaries. The old descriptions for

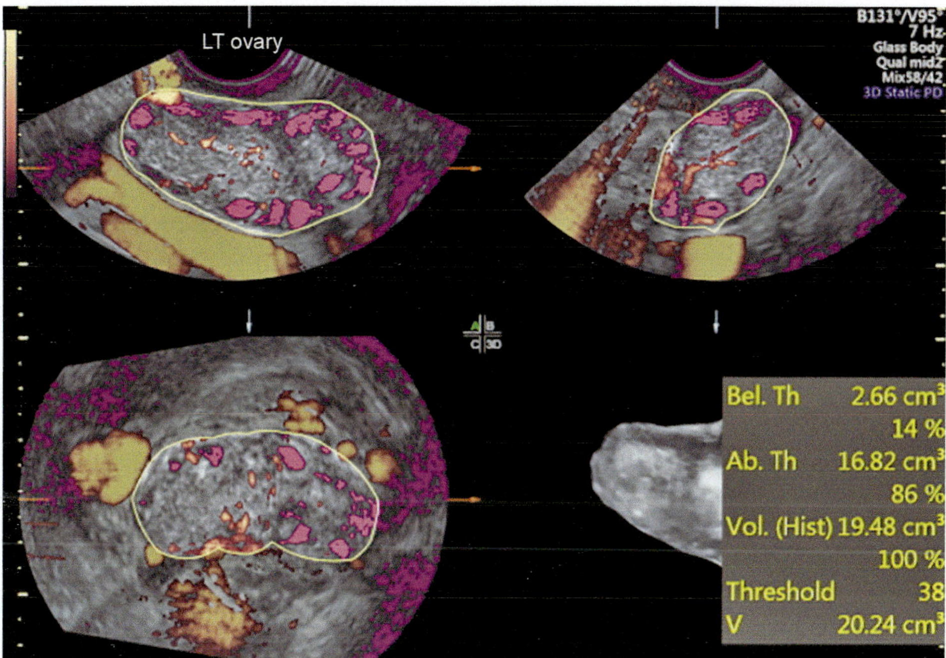

Fig. 12: Virtual organ computer-aided analysis (VOCAL)-calculated 3D power Doppler volume with threshold volume showing pink areas below the threshold and which is the total volume of the follicles, whereas the volume above the threshold is the volume of the stroma of the ovary. The values are usually in the right lower corner of the screen.

polycystic ovaries show that a longest diameter of >3.5 cm (**Fig. 13**) is diagnostic of polycystic ovary. According to Rotterdam criteria, the ovarian volume of 10 cm³ is diagnostic of polycystic ovaries.

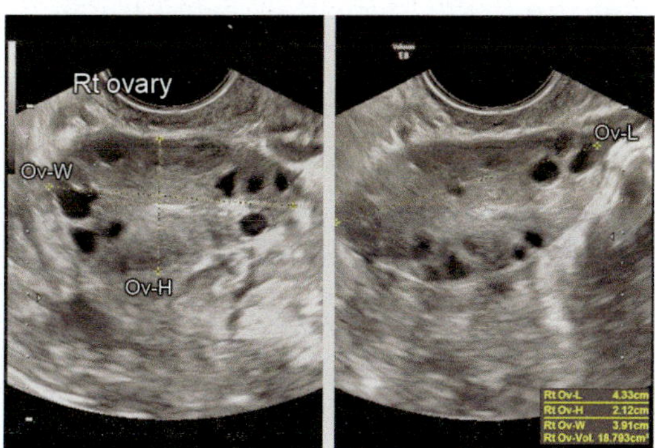

Fig. 13: B-mode ultrasound image of the ovary in dual frame showing long section of the ovary in left frame and transverse section in right frame. The longest diameter on the long section in polycystic ovary is >3.5 cm. Including three orthogonal diameters and ellipse formula for volume calculation shows volume of >10 cm³ in polycystic ovary.

Enlarged spherical ovaries >10 cm³ (**Fig. 13**) have shown good correlation between US and diagnosis of polycystic morphology and histopathological criteria for polycystic ovaries.[20] But, there are controversies regarding the ovarian enlargement in PCO. Ovarian volume 6.6 cm³ has shown 91% sensitivity and 91% specificity for polycystic ovarian syndrome[21] (**Fig. 14**).

Polycystic ovarian morphology has therefore been found to be a better discriminator than ovarian volume between women with polycystic ovarian syndrome and control women.[22]

Morphological features: These consist of number and arrangement of antral follicles, stromal echogenicity, and vascularity.

Antral Follicle Count

Antral follicle count (AFC) of 12 or more (2–9 mm) has been used as a characteristic for polycystic ovaries in Rotterdam criteria on US.

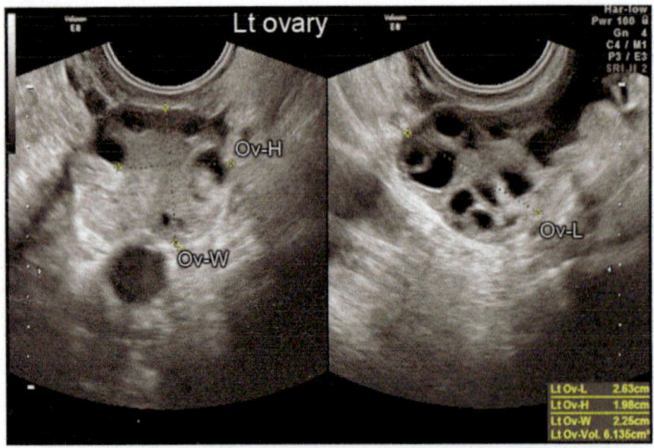

Fig. 14: B-mode ultrasound of the ovaries in dual frame showing longitudinal and transverse sections of the ovary, with multiple follicles and echogenic stroma. In spite of the typical polycystic morphology and clinical picture of polycystic ovarian syndrome in this patient, the ovarian dimensions as seen in the data in right lower corner are well within normal limits.

Setting the threshold at 12 for 2–9 mm follicle number per ovary (FNPO) offered the best compromise between specificity (99%) and sensitivity (75%)[14] (**Fig. 15**). Though polycystic histology and morphology have been found in ovaries having AFC between 5 and 15 also, as the number of follicles may decrease as age advances.

Though a study by Dewailly et al. in 2011 shows that FNPO > 19 had a sensitivity of 81% and specificity of 92% for PCO (polycystic ovaries), this study also showed that AMH (anti-Mullerian hormone) > 35 pmol/L is even more accurate with sensitivity of 92% and specificity of 97%.[23] But, this same study also quotes that this increase in number of follicles is due to changed image quality with improving technology of US scanner.

Another study shows that using ROC (receiver operating characteristics) curves, the investigators reclassified the diagnostic threshold for PCO as a mean FNPO of 20 or more [with the area under curve (AUC) of 98.7%, specificity of 100%, sensitivity of 70%, positive-predictive value (PPV) of 100%, and negative-predictive value (NPV) of 91%] and an ovarian volume of at least 13 cm^3 (with AUC of 94.8%, specificity of 100%, sensitivity of 50%, PPV of 100%, and NPV of 85%) (**Fig. 16**).[24] According to the new consensus also the number of follicles per ovary has been changed from 12 to 20.[25]

Even higher AFC threshold has been shown in a study by Lujan et al. An average value of 26 or more follicles per ovary is a reliable threshold for detecting polycystic ovaries in women with Frank manifestation of PCOS. Sensitivity and specificity for diagnosis of PCOS for FNPO of 26[26] were 85% and 94% and for OV (ovarian volume) (10 cm^3) were 81% and 84%, respectively. The higher number is because of increased resolution of new scanners to identify follicles smaller than 2 mm. But, the same study has also quoted that the lower follicle threshold may be required to detect milder variants of the syndrome.[27]

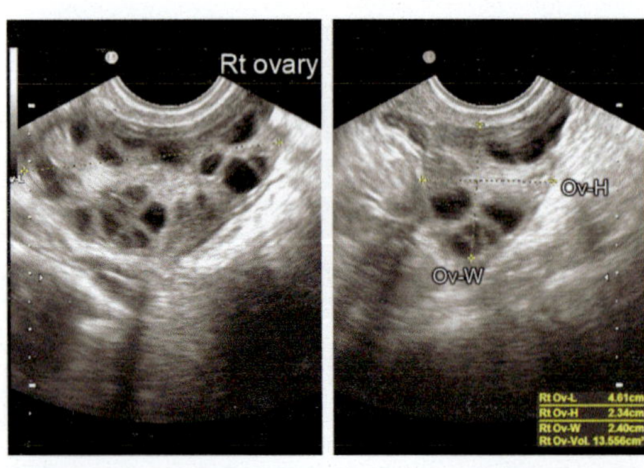

Fig. 15: B-mode ultrasound image of ovary in dual frame showing multiple small follicles suggestive of polycystic ovaries according to Rotterdam criteria of polycystic ovaries on ultrasound.

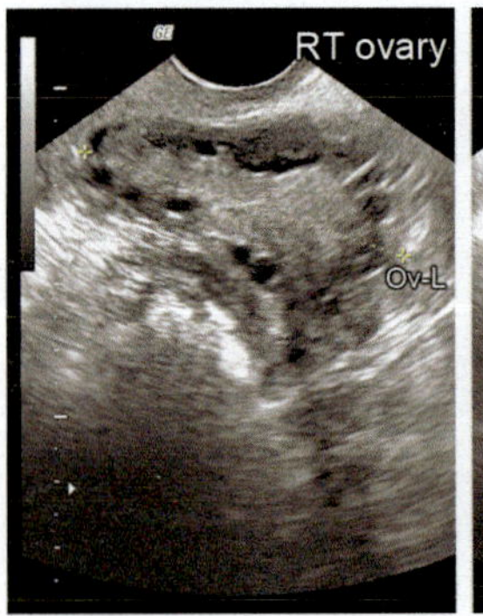

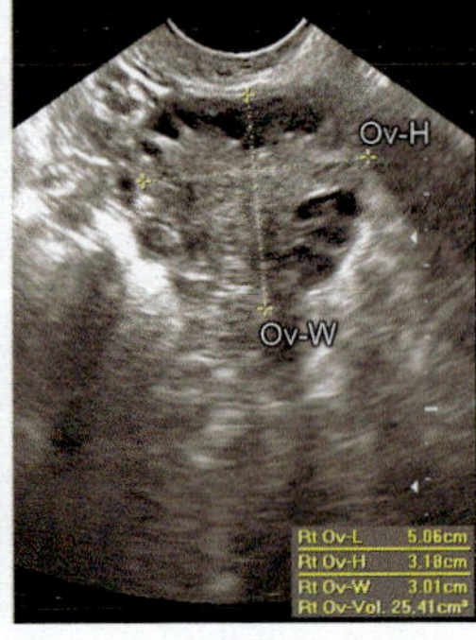

Fig. 16: B-mode ultrasound image of typical polycystic ovaries with huge volume (25 cm^3) and also multiple small uniform-sized follicles (>20).

TABLE 1: Diagnosis of polycystic ovarian syndrome (PCOS).

Age	Follicle number	Ovarian size (mL)
<24	>13	12
25–29	14	10
30–34	10	9
35–39	10	8
40–44	9	10
>44	6	7

Diagnostic potential for PCOS was highest for FNPO (0.969), followed by FNPS (follicle count in a single cross-section) (0.880), followed by ovarian volume (0.873). The US finding of polycystic ovaries in the general population is in the order of 17–22%,[26,28,29] and in women with anovulation and idiopathic hirsutism is much higher at ~90%.[30,31] The best sensitivity and specificity for diagnosis of PCOS were obtained using different threshold volume and AFC at different ages (**Table 1**).

It is important to decrease the volume and follicle number with increasing age to diagnose PCOS. This study also quoted that the polycystic ovary morphology was more accurate at predicting the PCOS diagnosis for women between 30 and 39 years of age.[32]

This means there is no universal consensus on AFC for diagnosis of PCOS. It has also been suggested that the threshold for PCOM should be revised regularly with advancing ultrasound technology and age-specific cut off values for PCOM should be defined.[32] Therefore, according to the new ESHRE 2018, guidelines for diagnosis and management of PCOS suggest that ultrasound should not be used as only one of two features to diagnose PCOS in females up to 8 years of gynecological age. That means if one wants to diagnose a young adolescent female as PCOS, she should have all the three features of PCOS according to Rotterdam criteria.

Arrangement of Follicles

The antral and atretic follicles get arranged peripherally or are dispersed in the stroma and thus may categorize polycystic ovary as peripheral and general cystic pattern. In peripheral cystic pattern, there is typical garland-like arrangement of follicles, and in generalized cystic pattern (**Figs. 17A and B**), the follicles can be seen throughout the ovary.[33] Though one school of thoughts believes that peripheral cystic pattern polycystic ovaries and generalized cystic pattern polycystic ovaries have different histopathological and endocrine bases,[34] another theory is different.

This means that ovarian size, follicle number, and arrangement of the follicles can be variable in polycystic ovaries, and a more consistent US feature should be sought

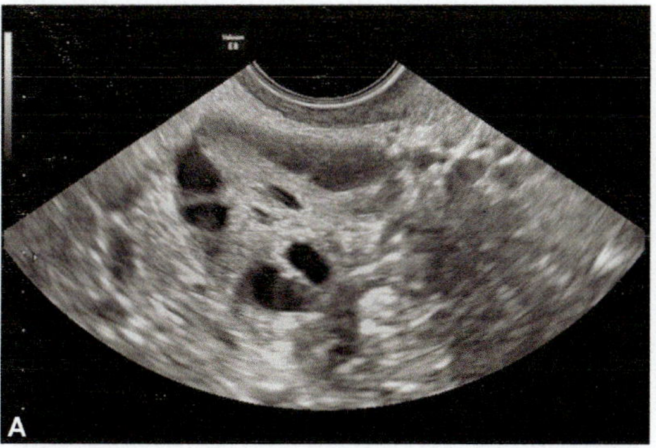

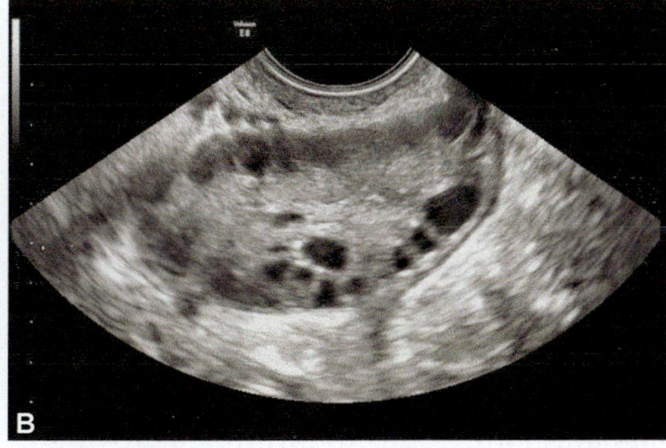

Figs. 17A and B: Longitudinal section of the ovary is seen in both parts (A) and (B). Both the ovaries show multiple follicles with echogenic stroma, but in part (A), the follicles are seen throughout the ovary, generalized cystic pattern of polycystic ovaries, whereas in part (B), these are arranged at the periphery of the ovary, peripheral cystic pattern of polycystic ovaries.

for US diagnosis of polycystic ovaries. Lam et al. have concluded in their study that the current criteria of size and follicle number will fail to identify a group of ovulatory, normoandrogenic women still at risk of complications classically associated with PCOS, such as OHSS (ovarian hyperstimulation syndrome), failed implantation, miscarriage, and hyperinsulinemia. To identify these women, further information, particularly about the ovarian stroma and the degree of vascularization, is required.[9]

At this stage, a short understanding of pathophysiology of polycystic ovarian syndrome may be of help.

PATHOPHYSIOLOGY

Polycystic ovaries are a result of chronic anovulation. Polycystic ovarian syndrome is a genetic syndrome. Its close correlation with hyperinsulinemia has been established. It is through the pathway of this that in these patients the androgen level is raised. Mildly raised basal androgen levels, in PCOS patients, lead to recruitment of several follicles from preantral to antral. Androgen leads to early follicular development (follicular growth till follicle size of 6 mm), but further progression is not normal due to hyperinsulinemia and/or other metabolic influence linked to obesity.[14] All these follicles do not become dominant. This is so because there is partial conversion of androgen to estrogen, and there is also cumulative effect of minimal estradiol production by multiple follicles leading to negative feedback for FSH (follicle stimulating hormone) and positive feedback for LH (luteinizing hormone). These factors lead to maturation arrest of these follicles and premature luteinization leading to atresia. Under the effect of LH, the granulosa cells of atretic follicles are converted into theca cells and contribute to stroma. Thus, with each anovulatory cycle, there is increase in the stromal content. As the ovary tries to accommodate this excess stroma in the same ovarian volume, there are areas in the ovary where stroma is densely packed and leads to patchy increase in echogenicity of the stroma. And, as anovulatory cycles continue and stromal abundance increases, the area of dense stroma increases till the whole stroma becomes dense, but the follicles may still be distributed throughout the ovary—generalized cystic polycystic ovary. If at this stage, the condition is left uncontrolled, gradually, the follicles in the central part of the ovary, in an effort and process of recruitment, reach the periphery or are pushed out to periphery by expanding stroma and undergo atresia ultimately leading to peripheral cystic polycystic ovary.[33,34] So, multicystic ovary to generalized cystic PCO, to peripheral cystic PCO is a process of evolution of the disease. This indicates that the patients who have more severe form of disease or a long-standing disease have a peripheral cystic pattern and evidently will have worse hormonal milieu (**Figs. 18A to D**). In patients with oligo-ovulation, instead of anovulation, though ovulation may occur, against one/two follicles matured and ruptured, there are significantly more follicles recruited, which undergo atresia as compared to normal ovaries, and so the stroma does increase.

Stromal Abundance

This explains that the stromal abundance is the most consistent and reliable feature for diagnosis of polycystic ovaries. Hyperdense stroma and stromal abundance have been described with polycystic ovaries since the first definition of the syndrome by Stein–Leventhal.

Abundance of stroma can present as increased echogenicity because stroma is densely packed, increased stromal area, or increased stromal volume in large ovary. Patients having long-standing PCOS and anovulation have more dense stroma. Since the widespread use of transvaginal US to diagnose PCOS, a cardinal feature has been shown to be the presence of a bright and

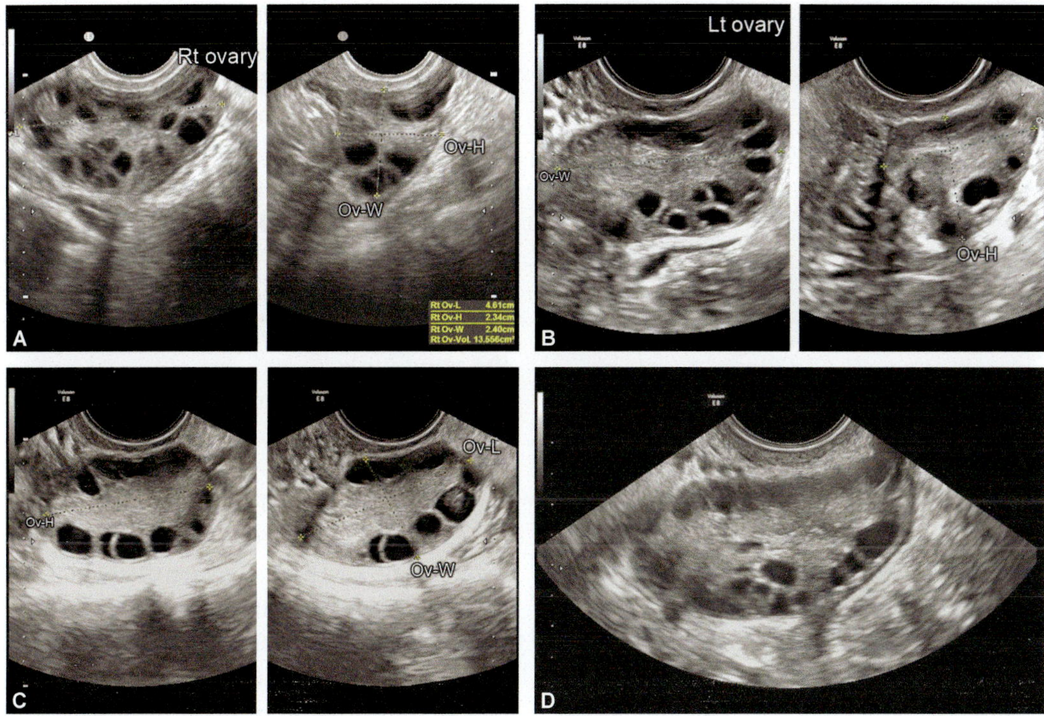

Figs. 18A to D: Polycystic ovaries have a wide range of ultrasound features on ultrasound. (A) These may be generalized cystic pattern with patchy increase in stromal echogenicity; (B) Generalized cystic pattern with generalized increase in stromal echogenicity; (C) Peripheral cystic pattern with increased stromal echogenicity with or (D) without increased ovarian volume.

highly echogenic stroma.[35] Increased stromal echogenicity and/or stromal volume are specific to PCO, but it has been shown that the measurement of ovarian volume (or area) is a good surrogate for quantification of the stroma in clinical practice.[4]

Polycystic ovaries show a hyperechoic stroma, but assessment of this hyperechogenicity is subjective not only to the operator but also to equipment settings.[36,37] The stromal echogenicity is considered to be high, if it is higher than that of normal myometrium (**Fig. 19**). This hyperechogenicity is especially useful for its differentiation from multicystic ovaries (**Fig. 20**) that are normally seen in adolescence and have multiple follicles of variable sizes and nonhyperechogenic stroma. Increased stromal echogenicity for diagnosis of PCO has a sensitivity of 94% and specificity of 90%.[38]

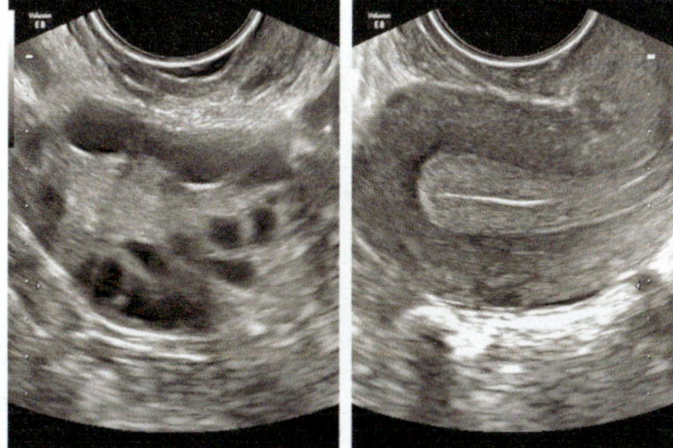

Fig. 19: B-mode ultrasound image in dual frame, showing longitudinal section of ovary in the left frame and long section of the uterus in right frame. This image is taken to compare the stromal echogenicity with echogenicity of the myometrium. Stromal echogenicity is more than the echogenicity of the myometrium in polycystic ovaries.

But, recent studies have shown that mean stromal echogenicity or total ovarian echogenicity as measured by histogram are

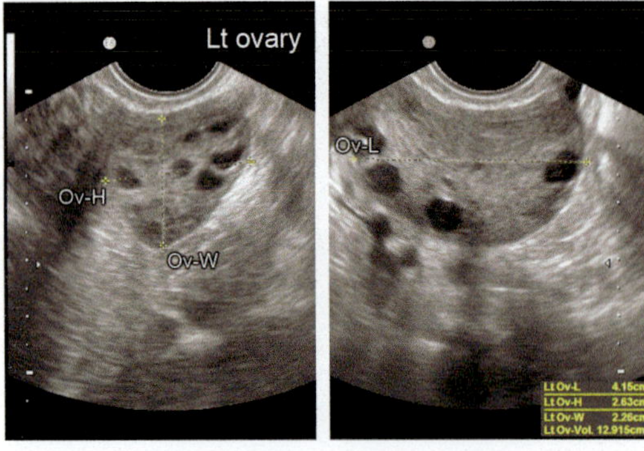

Fig. 20: B-mode image of the ovary in dual frame showing multiple follicles but the ovarian stroma is not hyperechoic. This is multicystic ovary.

not different in controls and PCOS, though stromal index (stromal echogenicity/total ovarian echogenicity) was significantly higher in PCOS than controls.[35]

Not only the echogenicity but total stromal volume is also increased in polycystic ovaries. This can be measured on US as stromal area in the most longitudinal section of ovary on 2D US. As for echogenicity, this also has been found to be effective for diagnosis of polycystic ovarian disease. Stromal area of 4.6 cm^2 has 91% sensitivity and 86% specificity for diagnosis of polycystic ovarian syndrome. The ovarian area can also be measured in this same section. Ovarian area of 5.3 cm^2 has 93% sensitivity and 91% specificity for diagnosis of polycystic ovarian syndrome[39] (**Figs. 21A and B**).

The ratio of stromal area to ovarian area has been found to be more reliable. S/A ratio also has a strongest correlation with serum androgens especially testosterone and androstenedione and insulin.[40,41]

Sensitivity for Diagnosis of PCOS (Table 2)

Mean stromal area/mean ovarian area ratio of 0.34 and above also has a specificity of 100% in the same study.[42]

The proportion revealed between the stroma and the ovary area in the median section [S/A ratio (stromal area to ovarian area ratio)] had been indicated as a reliable marker for hyperandrogenism. Hyperandrogenic subjects showed higher values of stromal area and S/A ratio, with no difference in ovarian volume and ovarian area.[43] S/A has also been found to be the best significant predictor of elevated androgen and testosterone levels. This parameter may be used in routine clinical practice for improving US diagnosis of PCOS.[42]

TABLE 2: Sensitivity for diagnosis of polycystic ovarian syndrome (PCOS).

Ovarian volume	13.21 cm^3	21%
Ovarian area	7 cm^2	4%
Stromal area	1.95 cm^2	62%
Stromal/total area	0.34	100%

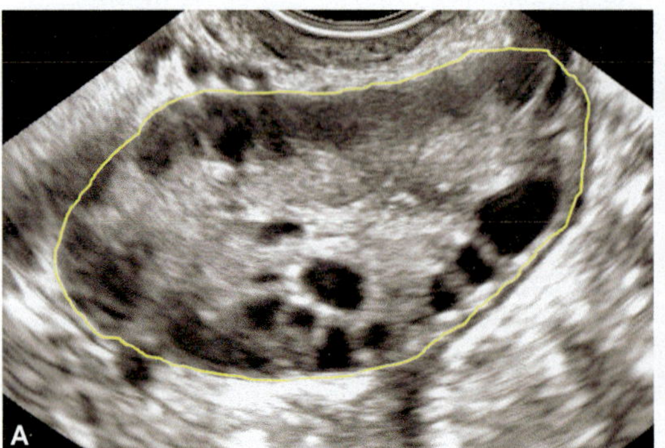

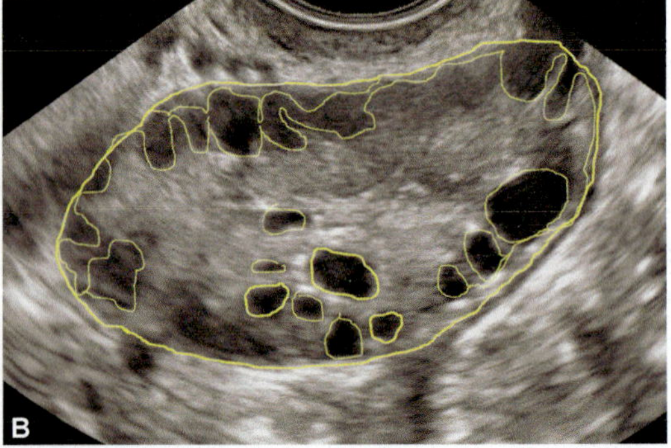

Figs. 21A and B: Both the images show B-mode image of a polycystic ovary. (A) Yellow line circumferencing the ovary to calculate the ovarian area; (B) The circumference drawn in yellow color and a yellow line also outlining the follicular area. Deducting the follicular area from the total ovarian area gives stromal area.

Stromal area to ovarian area ratio is lower in normal females.

Stromal abundance may be better assessed by stromal volume than with stromal area. Stromal volume can be assessed by using threshold volume on VOCAL-calculated ovarian volume (**Fig. 22**).

3D US provides a new method for objective quantitative assessment of follicle count, ovarian volume, stromal volume, and blood flow in the ovary.[35] 3D US is a relatively new imaging modality that has the potential to address these points and improve the sensitivity and specificity of US in the diagnosis of PCOS.[44-46] 3D US not only permits improved spatial awareness and volumetric and quantitative vascular assessment but also provides a more objective tool to examine stromal density through the assessment of the mean grayness (MG) of the ovary.[47]

TABLE 3: Ovarian volume calculation.

Ovary volume	*Right (cm^3)*	*Left (cm^3)*
Normal	5.3 ± 2.0	5.7 ± 1.6
PCOD	12.2 ± 4.7	10.5 ± 3.6[36]

(PCOD: polycystic ovarian disease)

Ovarian volume calculation by 3D US has been found to be useful over 2D evaluation of ovarian long diameter or volume by 2D US (**Table 3**).

Right ovary is larger in PCOD patients, whereas left ovary is larger in normal patients. Concerning the ovarian volume setting, the threshold at 7 cm^3 offered the best compromise between specificity (91.2%) and sensitivity (67.5%). In comparison, specificity and sensitivity were 98.2% and 45%, respectively, with threshold at 10 cm^3.[48]

Kyei-Mensah et al. showed that both total ovarian volume and stromal volume during

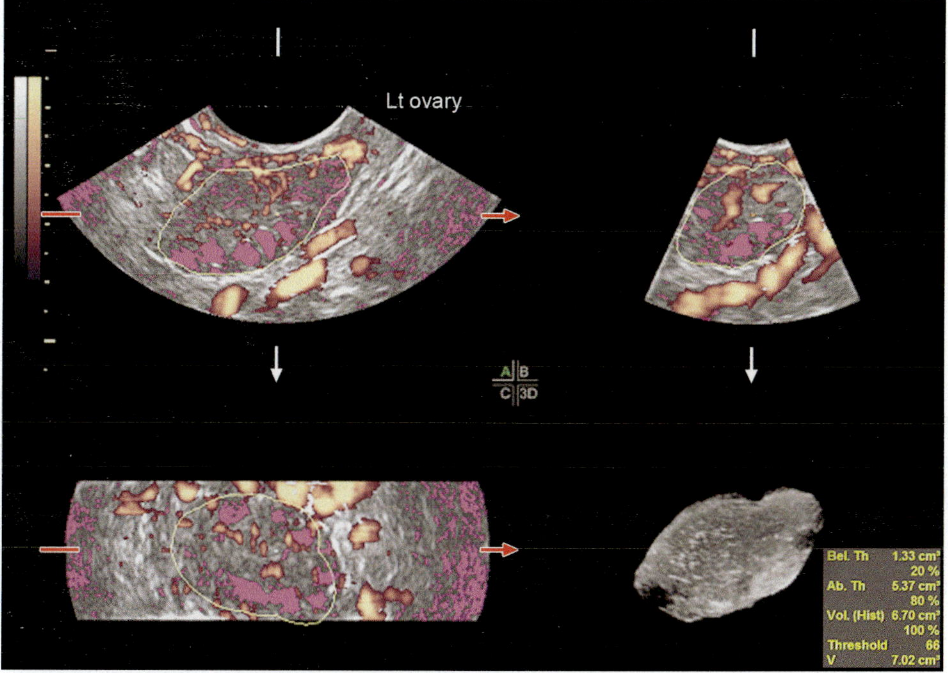

Fig. 22: 3D US-acquired image of ovary shows virtual organ computer-aided analysis (VOCAL)-calculated volume of the ovary. The pink color on the sectional planes defines the threshold level, which is set to differentiate follicles from the stroma. This software is known as threshold volume. The numbers in right lower corner show "below threshold"—the follicular volume, "above threshold"—the stromal volume and total volume of the ovary.

the early follicular phase were significantly higher in 26 women with PCOS as well as in 24 women with regular menstrual cycles but PCO on US scan, compared with 50 infertile women with regular menstrual cycles but normal ovarian morphology (16.7 ± 23.1 and 15.5 ± 20.9 mL, 15.0 ± 18.9 and 13.4 ± 18.6 mL vs 9.6 ± 20.4 and 8.6 ± 20.0 mL, respectively, all p-values < 0.05).[49]

In a study by Franks et al., it has been well derived that PCOM in normal women is not a morphological variant of normal ovaries but rather represents a functional entity—a silent form of PCOS for which serum AMH could be the best marker.[15]

Correlation of Stromal Abundance to Hyperinsulinemia

Theca cells of PCOS women hyper-respond to gonadotropins (LH) and produce excess androgens. This is due to an escape of their normal downregulation to gonadotropins. This dysregulation is linked to excess of insulin and insulin-like growth factor-1 (IGF-1). Hyperinsulinemia is a key factor to the pathogenesis of PCOS. Insulin augments LH-stimulated androgen production by stromal cells. Androgen in turn causes proliferation of stromal and theca cells. This leads to increased stroma in the PCO. Stromal volume was positively correlated with serum androstenedione concentrations in patients with polycystic ovarian syndrome.[49]

Increased androstenedione secretion as shown earlier is due to hyperinsulinemia.[50] Study by Pache et al. has shown that the degree of IR can be correlated with ovarian volume and stromal echogenicity.[51]

Some investigators showed that the correlation between ovarian stromal volume and serum androstenedione concentrations during the early follicular phase was fair though statistically significant (correlation coefficient, $r = 0.45$, $p < 0.05$). Stromal volume was not significantly correlated with the other two thecal steroid levels. Using similar methodology, Nardo et al.[52] also noted no relationship between ovarian stromal volume and serum FSH, LH, or testosterone concentrations during the early follicular phase in 23 infertile women with clomiphene-resistant PCOS, and they did not examine the serum androstenedione concentrations.[49]

Hyperinsulinemia leads to enhanced gonadotropin-stimulated steroid production in granulosa cells and theca cells, leading to increased androgen level and in turn leading to increase AMH.[53] Hyperinsulinemia in women with obesity contributes to anovulation by increased ovarian androgen secretion.[54]

A randomized study of 50 polycystic ovarian syndrome patients with 50 non-PCOS patients was done over a period 6 months with clinical examination, baseline US scan with 2D and 3D US, and fasting and postprandial insulin levels. Group A: 50 patients with normal ovulation, no hirsutism, normal menstrual cycle, and normal ovarian size; and Group B: 50 patients with PCOS, according to Rotterdam criteria. Age range of patients for both groups was between 25 and 35 with mean age for Group A was 30.4 years and mean age for Group B was 29.7 years. Mean BMI in both the groups was 28, ranges from 25 to 32 kg/m^2.

Patients with BMI < 25 kg/m^2 proved diabetes mellitus, any other endocrinological derangement (thyroid, adrenal, etc.), follicles >9 mm or residual corpus lutea on day 3 and ovarian mass lesions (cystic/solid) were excluded from the study cohort. Ovarian volume and stromal volume were calculated by applying threshold volume to the VOCAL-calculated volume. The threshold is set to differentiate follicles from stroma. Fasting and postprandial insulin levels were checked for all on the same day. Insulin estimation was done by chemiluminescence method. For postprandial insulin measurement, patient was given 75 g of glucose after fasting blood sample and then blood sample for PP insulin was taken after 2 hours. Values of ovarian and stromal volumes and AFC were all averaged for both ovaries in each patient. Two-tailed Pearson correlation was checked for ovarian volume, stromal volume, and stromal volume to ovarian volume ratio with fasting insulin and postprandial insulin level each. Ovarian and stromal volumes were compared and correlated with both fasting and postprandial insulin levels.

Positive correlation was seen between ovarian and stromal volumes and fasting and postprandial insulin levels. With Pearson correlation significance level of 0.01 (two tailed), the correlation for (**Figs. 23A and B**):

- Ovarian volume to fasting insulin was 0.651.
- Ovarian volume to PP insulin was 0.409.
- Stromal volume to fasting insulin was 0.736.
- Stromal volume to PP insulin was 0.428.

Stromal and ovarian volumes and AFC correlated significantly well with the fasting insulin levels, more than with postprandial insulin levels in obese PCOS patients. It is the stromal volume that can be best correlated with fasting insulin levels followed by ovarian volumes and AFC.

A similar study has also been done earlier. A retrospective observational study is done with 50 PCOS patients showing correlation between ovarian and stromal volumes with fasting and postprandial insulin levels. But, in this study, neither BMI nor age group was defined. This study was presented at the International Society of Ultrasound in Obstetrics and Gynecology (ISUOG) 2008, Chicago. In PCOS patients, a strong and similar correlation is seen between ovarian and stromal volumes to fasting and postprandial insulin levels. Assessing correlation between ovarian and stromal volumes and fasting and postprandial insulin levels in PCOS patients.[56]

Based on 3D US, women with PCOS have an increased stromal volume and vascularity. Even with same echogenicity, PCOS has more stromal flow. Women with PCOS had higher AFC (median 16.3 vs 5.5 per ovary), ovarian volume (12.56 vs 5.6 mL), stromal volume (10.79 vs 4.69 mL), and stromal vascularization (VI 3.85% vs 2.79%, VFI 1.27 vs 0.85),[55] though 2D power Doppler indices were not higher in PCOS than in controls (**Figs. 24A to C**).

Though a study done by Luciano et al. demonstrates that the 3D measurements of total ovarian volume, preantral follicle number, and total preantral follicular volume have better correlation with biochemical indices of PCOS, the 3D measurements of ovarian stromal volume.[52]

Kyei-Mensah et al. showed a positive correlation between stromal volume, as measured by 3D US, with serum androstenedione

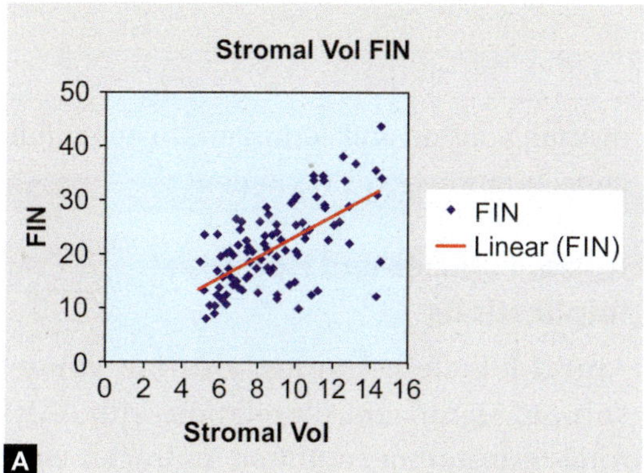

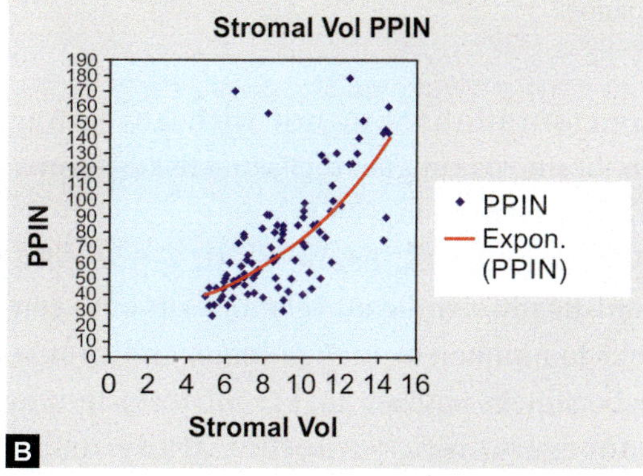

Figs. 23A and B: The graphs show correlation of the stromal volume to fasting insulin (FIN) and stromal volume to postprandial insulin (PPIN).[55]

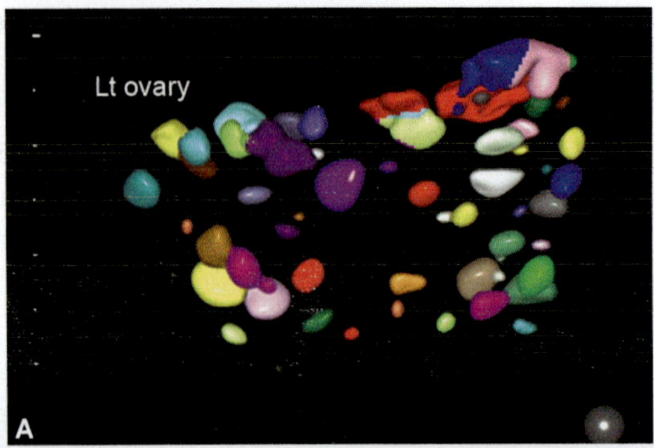

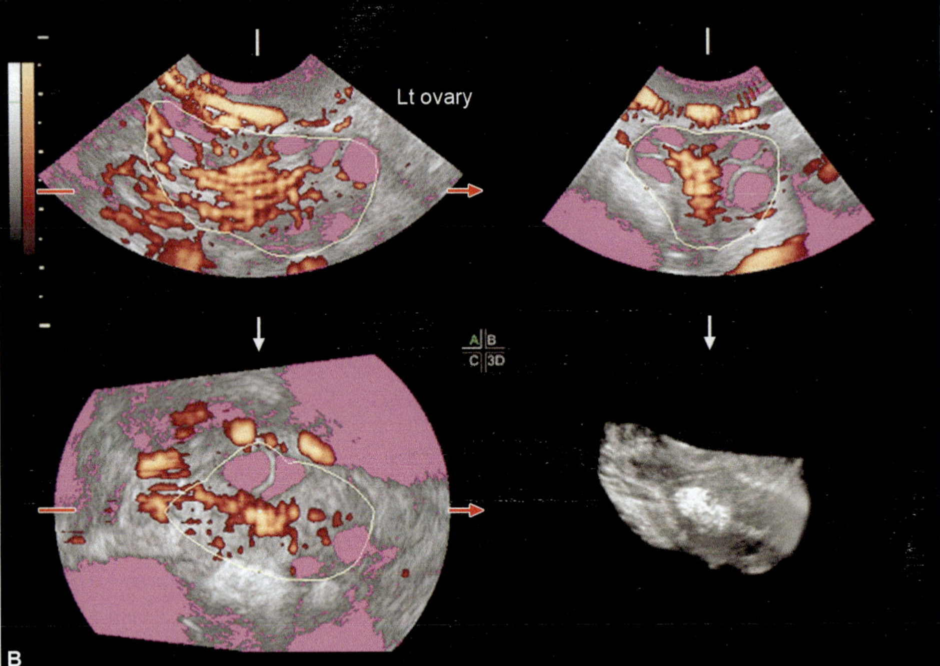

Figs. 24A and B: (A) 3D power Doppler US-acquired, virtual organ computer-aided analysis (VOCAL)-calculated, SonoAVC rendered image of polycystic ovary for calculating antral follicle count; (B) 3D US-acquired, VOCAL-calculated, and threshold volume applied image of polycystic ovary for calculating stromal volume.

concentrations, but not with any other endocrine parameter, including testosterone, in infertile women with PCOS.[49]

Using 2D US, Pache et al. reported a statistically significant relationship between follicle number, ovarian volume, and stroma echogenicity with serum LH and testosterone concentrations.[51] Another study using conventional 2D ultrasonography scanning demonstrated a significant correlation between ovarian volume and serum androstenedione concentrations in PCOS patients.[57]

Antral Follicles and Hormonal Implications

Antral follicle count and ovarian volume showed significant correlation with AMH, total testosterone, and free androgen index but not with age, BMI, or homeostasis model assessment of IR (HOMA-IR). AMH, BMI, and

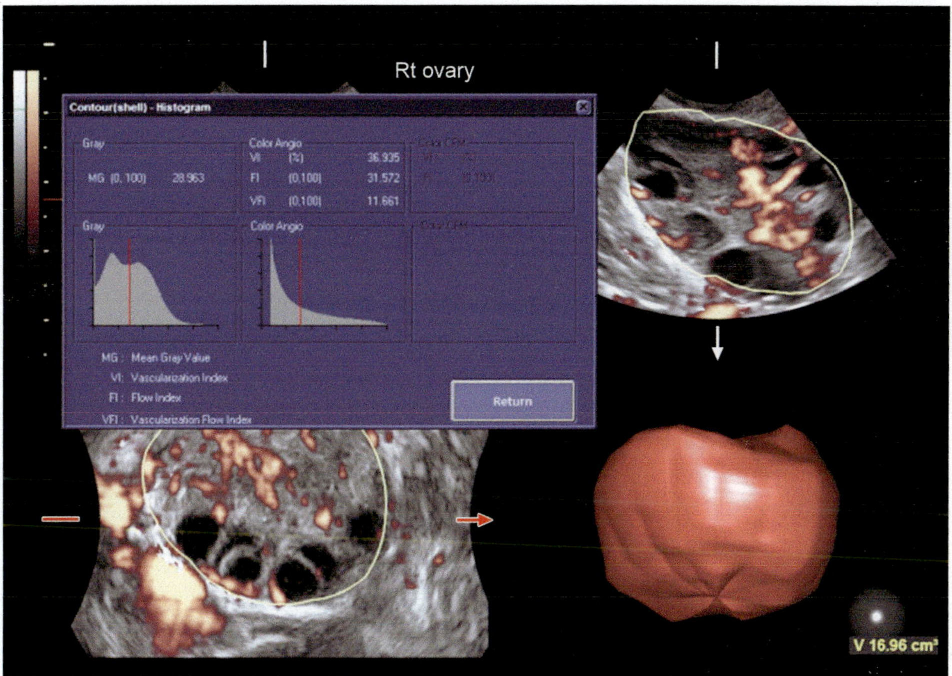

Fig. 24C: 3D US-acquired, virtual organ computer-aided analysis (VOCAL)-calculated, volume histogram applied image of polycystic ovary for assessment of global 3D power Doppler indices VI, FI, and VFI. (VI: vascularity index; FI: flow index; VFI: vascularity flow index; US: ultrasound)

total testosterone were independently related to AFC. AMH and total testosterone were main determinants for ovarian volume in stepwise regression model. AMH, obesity, IR, and high androgen levels relate to large size of antral follicle pool and ovarian volume on PCOS. Obesity and IR may enhance follicular excess by dysregulation of AMH through pathway of hyperandrogenemia.[11] Presence of PCOM is a sign of hyperandrogenism and high serum anti-Müllerian hormone levels.[58,59] When replacing PCOM with AMH, the specificity and sensitivity for identifying PCOS were 97.1% and 94.6%, respectively, according to the PCOS (Rotterdam) criteria and 97.2% and 95.5% according to the PCOS (Androgen Excess Society) criteria, respectively, at an AMH cutoff value of 20 pmol/L.[59]

This indicates that AFC and size of antral follicles can derive a lot of information about the biochemical status of the patient. The mean follicular number per ovary (FNPO) of follicles 2–5 mm in size was significantly higher in polycystic ovaries than in controls, while it was similar within 6–9 mm range. Within 2–5 mm range, significant relationship was found between FNPO and androgens but FNPO in the range of 6–9 mm was significantly and negatively related to body mass index and fasting serum insulin level.

Stromal Vascularity

Apart from an increased number of antral follicles and a larger ovarian volume, women with PCOS have also been shown to have an increased ovarian stromal volume and blood flow.[49,60] These findings were compatible with a previous study that reported a positive relationship between serum LH level and the PSV within the intraovarian stromal vessels.[61]

These are important parameters that may be relevant to our understanding of the pathogenesis and clinical presentation of PCOS and as prospective predictors of the

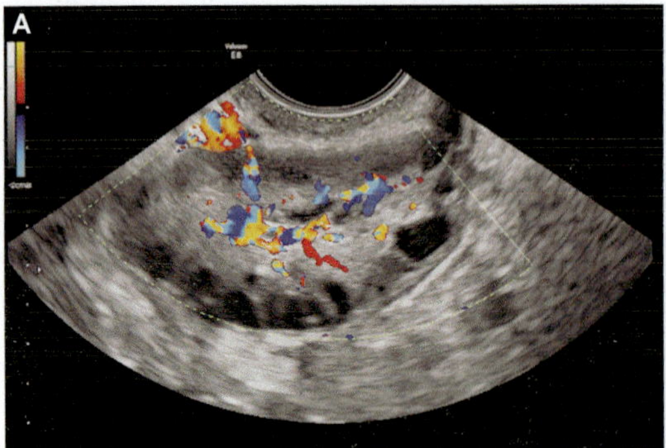

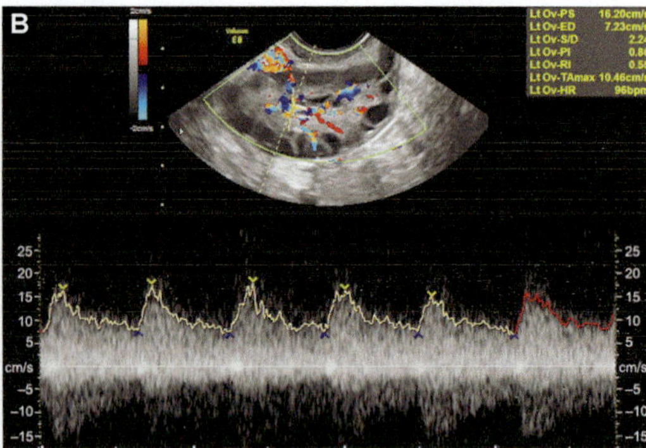

Figs. 25A and B: (A) Color Doppler ultrasound image of polycystic ovary showing ovarian stromal flow; (B) Spectral Doppler of the same ovary shows moderate-to-low resistance flow in these stromal blood vessels.

response to the various treatments used in patients with PCOS.[61,62]

Elevated LH levels may be responsible for increased stromal vascularization due to neoangiogenesis, catecholaminergic stimulation, and leukocyte and cytokine activation. In polycystic ovaries even on 3rd day of the cycle, intraovarian stromal flow is seen and has moderate-to-low resistance flow with RI of 0.50–0.58[63] (**Figs. 25A and B**). This vascularity is inversely related to LH/FSH ratio. Tonic secretion of LH in early follicular phase in PCOS is also associated with theca and stromal cell hyperplasia and consequent androgen production. This androgen hypersecretion is responsible for not only increased follicular recruitment but also for vasoconstrictive effect on the uterine arteries. This effect is thought to be due to activation of specific receptors in arterial walls and collagen and elastin deposition in smooth muscle cells. Uterine artery PI is usually >3, and sometimes, the diastolic flow is absolutely absent (**Fig. 26**). Even in later phases of the cycle, this effect continues. This leads to inadequate perfusion of the endometrium and is thought to be responsible for blastocyst implantation failure and high abortion rate in PCOS. Though stromal vascularity is high in PCOS patients, it has been shown that the ovarian vascularization per follicle, after pituitary suppression, was lower in PCO patients

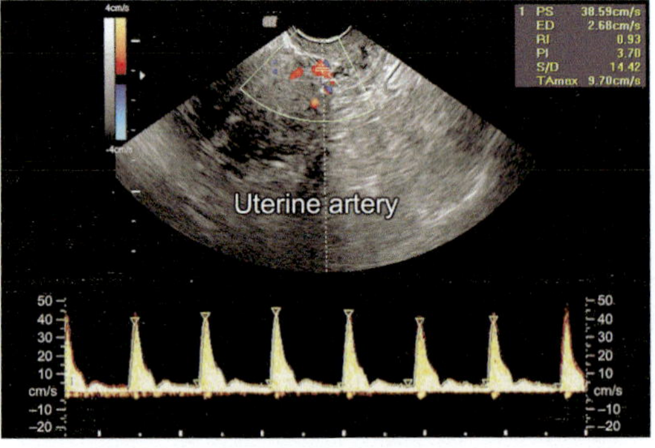

Fig. 26: Spectral Doppler of uterine artery showing high-resistance flow.

(0.02 ± 0.01 vs 0.06 ± 0.08, $p < 0.01$) and suggested that there were defects in follicular angiogenesis in PCO.[64]

Looking to the hormonal correlation with the Doppler findings, it is evident that in patients in whom the hormonal milieu is worse, the Doppler findings are more prominent. As discussed earlier, the peripheral cystic pattern of PCO is an advanced stage, then generalized cystic pattern and so the intraovarian vascularity and uterine artery resistance are more in peripheral polycystic ovaries than in generalized polycystic ovaries. In 22% of the GCP of PCO, intraovarian vessels are not recognized.[65] The vascularization indices VI, FI, and VFI are significantly higher in PCOS than in normal females, which explain excessive response to gonadotropins in PCOS females. 3D vascularization quantification has been found to be more sensitive than 2D

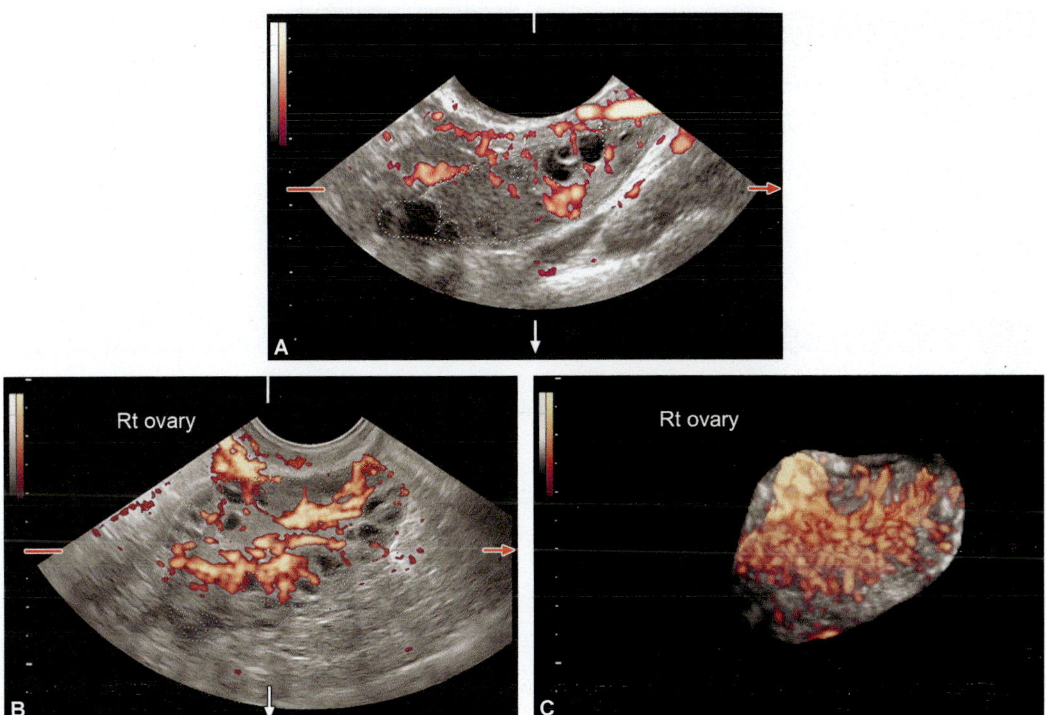

Figs. 27A to C: (A and B) Power Doppler ultrasound images of two different ovaries; (A) On the first one, the ovary shows fewer follicles and lesser color signals–lesser flow; (B) An ovary with multiple follicles and echogenic stroma—polycystic ovary and this ovary shows abundant color signals–abundant flow in the stroma; (C) This excess flow is much better appreciated on the 3D power Doppler-acquired, virtual organ computer-aided analysis (VOCAL)-calculated, and glass body-rendered image.

vascularization quantification[66] (**Figs. 27A to C**).

A study from Finland shows no difference in VI, FI, and VFI values in PCO and normal ovaries. But in normal ovaries, FI was found to be higher in left ovary.[47] In another study also, PCOS ovaries demonstrated a significantly larger ovarian volume (12.94 ± 4.27 vs 6.10 ± 3.41 mL, $p < 0.05$) and a greater ovarian blood flow as indicated by higher VI (3.99% ± 2.38% vs 1.44% ± 1.20%, $p < 0.05$), FI (50.26 ± 3.02 vs 44.44 ± 5.42, $p < 0.05$), and VFI (2.10 ± 1.32 vs 0.80 ± 0.97, $p < 0.05$) measurements in the PCOS group[60] (**Fig. 28**).

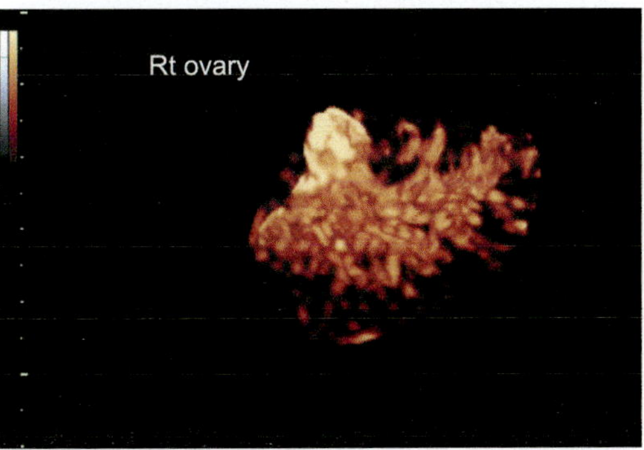

Fig. 28: The same ovary as in Figure 27C is rendered on color mode, which makes the predominance of flow even more clear.

In PCOS group, ovarian stromal artery RI values were inversely correlated with androstenedione levels ($r = -0.536$; $p < 0.05$). Also in PCOS group, uterine artery PI values were positively correlated with androstenedione levels ($r = 0.536$; $p < 0.05$).[67] This means higher androstenedione levels lead to lower RI and more flow in ovarian stromal vessels and higher resistance in uterine vessels (**Figs. 29A and B**).

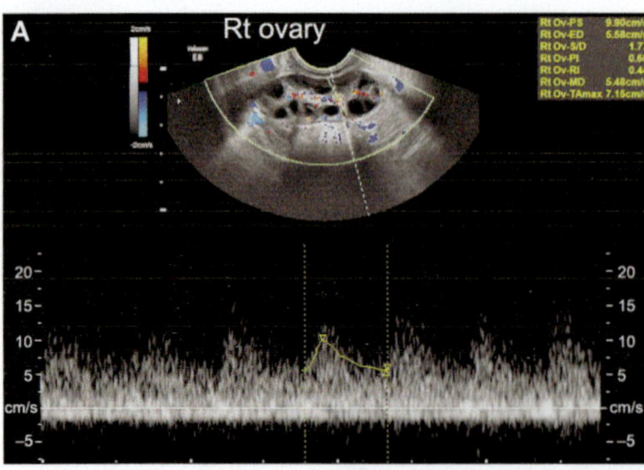

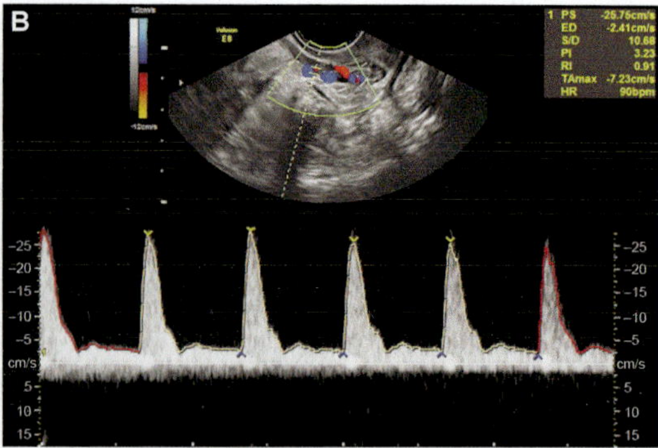

Figs. 29A and B: Spectral Doppler images of ovarian stromal vessels (A) and (B) uterine artery shows low-resistance flow in ovarian stromal vessels and higher resistance of uterine artery. Both are a response of high LH and high androgen, respectively.
(LH: luteinizing hormone)

Reduced ovarian volume (10.97 ± 0.86 vs 12.52 ± 0.61, $p < 0.01$) and a reduced stromal blood flow (VI: 0.29% ± 0.10% vs 1.01% ± 0.37%, $p < 0.05$; VFI: 0.13 ± 0.05 vs 0.49 ± 0.18, $p < 0.05$) during the early follicular phase in 40 clomiphene-resistant women with PCOS were found 3 months after laparoscopic ovarian drilling.[68] This again substantiates the fact that stromal vascularity is due to the LH excess. As drilling decreases stroma and LH, the vascularity decreases.

Stromal vascularity though may be also affected by certain other factors in PCOS patients. Stromal vascularity is significantly higher in women with PCOS who are hirsute and of normal weight rather than obese.[56] Oligoanovulatory patients with PCO but without hyperandrogenism have mild endocrine and metabolic features of PCOS.[69] Ovarian stromal FI is higher (33.94 vs 29.30) in hirsutes than in normoandrogenic PCOS women.

Ng et al. have also observed significant negative correlations between total ovarian vascular indices (VI, FI, and VFI) and BMI (correlation coefficients: –0.721, –0.698, and –0.694, respectively, all p-values <0.001). The normal weight PCOS women with BMI < 25 kg/m^2 had a significantly higher ovarian blood flow (median VI: 5.67% vs 1.82%; FI: 60.86 vs 49.50, and VFI: 1.767 vs 0.448, all p values < 0.001) than their overweight counterparts. The investigators also observed a statistically nonsignificant trend of higher serum LH level in normal weight PCOS women, although the p value was not reported.

Fertile controls and PCOS women had similar total ovarian 3D power Doppler flow indices. Normal weight PCOS women had significantly higher total ovarian 3D power Doppler flow indices than their overweight counterparts.[70] Higher age, obesity, and amenorrhea as compared to young age, normal weight, and oligomenorrhea show higher uterine artery resistance and increased ovarian stromal flow. But, in PCOS women with obesity, the vascularity was lower than in normal weight women (VI: 3.25% vs 4.51%, VFI: 1.22 vs 1.56).[55]

These are the patients who also have higher LH and higher androstenedione levels and higher ovarian volumes. Uterine artery resistance has also been found to be higher in obese than in lean patients and is also associated with hyperinsulinemia, high triglycerides, low-/high-density lipids, and higher hematocrit values. Another study that compared the blood flows in normal weight and obese PCOS also has similar findings. Comparing ovarian stromal blood flow and serum vascular endothelial growth factor (VEGF) between fertile women with normal ovaries and infertile women with PCOS, it was found that both the groups had similar total ovarian VI, FI, and VFI values after controlling for the age. Though VI, FI, and VFI were significantly higher in normal weight PCOS than in obese PCOS women.

Effect of age: Total ovarian VI and VFI were significantly lower in women aged 41 or more. AFC has the best correlation with the age, followed by serum FSH and ovarian 3D power Doppler indices. The rate of decline of total ovarian VI was 0.18% per year.[71]

Increased ovarian stromal blood flow in PCOS may be because of overexpression of VEGF, which modulates the permeability of theca cells and increases IGF-1,[72,73] which, in turn, enhances gonadotropin-stimulated steroid production in granulosa cells and theca cells resulting in increased ovarian androgen production and subsequently increased AMH production.[53]

CONTROVERSIES

- *Low flow in PCO:* Many of the PCO patients consume large doses of gonadotropins. These are the patients who on US do show multiple follicles, large ovaries, and dense stroma, and on Doppler, they do have a moderate resistance flow but have a low PSV. They may be grouped clinically as resistant PCO.
- *Moderate resistance in uterine arteries*: Not all patients with PCOS have high androgen levels, which are responsible for high uterine artery resistance, this is especially so in generalized cystic pattern of PCOS. Another cause of moderate resistance in uterine artery instead of high resistance is adenomyosis or fibroid in the fibroid commonly associated with PCOS.

Important points:

- PCOS must be diagnosed in adult women, when two of the three of Rotterdam's criteria for diagnosis of PCOS are present.
- In females up to 8 years of gynecological age, PCOS can be diagnosed only if all the three Rotterdam criteria are present.
- If one wants to use antral follicle count as ultrasound criteria for diagnosis of PCOS, this can be done only if transvaginal route of scan is used and a probe is used that has 8-MHz frequency.
- Though stromal abundance has not been included as a criterion to diagnose polycystic ovaries, this is one of the important criteria, which has a strong correlation with the pathophysiology of polycystic ovaries.

Ultrasound features of polycystic ovarian syndrome:

- *Large ovaries:* Long diameter of >3.5 cm or 10 cm3 volume correlates well with PCOS but ovaries of 6.6 cm3 also have a >90% sensitivity and specificity for PCOS.
- AFC of 20 per ovary was earlier considered as one of the diagnostic criteria for PCOS, has now moved to as high as 26 according to some studies, but it has also been shown that milder cases may have less number of follicles.
- Arrangement of antral follicles may be generalized distribution or peripheral distribution in PCOS patients.
- Stromal abundance is the most consistent feature of PCOS and is assessed by stromal echogenicity, stromal area, and stromal volume. Stromal abundance increases with severity of thedisease.
- Stromal vascularity is more in PCOS than in normal ovaries, but may be higher in PCOS with hyperandrogenemia and hyperinsulinemia, and is less in obese PCOS.
- Uterine artery resistance is high in PCOS patients more so with hyperandrogenemia.

REFERENCES

1. Aziz R, Carmina E, Dewailly D, Diamanti-Kandarakis E, Escobar-Morreale HF, Futterweit W, et al. The androgen excess and PCOS society criteria for polycystic ovary syndrome: the complete task force report. Fertil Steril. 2009;91:456-88.
2. Thatcher. Defining PCOS—a perspective. The American Infertility Association News Letter, February, 2001.

3. Irving F, Stein SR, Micheal L. The Stein–Leventhal syndrome—a curable form of sterility. N Engl J Med. 1958;259:420-3.
4. Balen AH, Laven JS, Tan SL, Dewailly D. Ultrasound assessment of the polycystic ovary: international consensus definitions. Hum Reprod Update. 2003;9:505-14.
5. Emans, SJ, Laufer MR, Goldstein DP. Chapter 9: Androgen abnormalities in the adolescent girl. Pediatric and Adolescent Gynecology, 5th edition. Philadelphia, PA: Lippincott Williams & Wilkins; 2005.
6. Norman RJ, Dewailly D, Legros RS, Hickey TE. Polycystic ovary syndrome. Lancet. 2007;370: 685-97.
7. Rotterdam ESHRE/ASRM-sponsored PCOS Consensus Workshop Group. Revised 2003 consensus on diagnostic criteria and long-term health risks related to polycystic ovary syndrome. Fertil Steril. 2004;81:19-25.
8. Balen AH, Conway G, Homburg R, Legro R. Polycystic ovary syndrome: A guide to clinical management. United Kigdom: Taylor & Francis Group; 2019.
9. Lam PM, Raine-Fenning N. The role of three-dimensional ultrasonography in polycystic ovary syndrome. Hum Reprod. 2006;21:2209-15.
10. Jayaprakasan K, Hilwah N, Kendall NR, Hopkisson JF, Campbell BK, Johnson JR, et al. Does 3D ultrasound offer any advantage in the pretreatment assessment of ovarian reserve and prediction of outcome after assisted reproduction treatment? Hum Reprod. 2007;22:1932-41.
11. Deb S, Campbell BK, Clewes JS, Rainne-Fenning NJ. Quantitative analysis of antral follicle number and size: a comparison of two dimensional and automated three dimensional ultrasound techniques. Ultrasound Obstet Gynecol. 2010;35:354-60.
12. Chen MJ, Yang WS, Chen CL, Wu MY, Yang YS, Ho HN, et al. The relationship between anti-Müllerian hormone, androgen and insulin resistance on the number of antral follicles in women with polycystic ovary syndrome. Hum Reprod. 2008;23:952-7.
13. Rainne-Fenning NJ, What is in a number? The polycystic ovary revisited. Hum Reprod. 2011;26:3118-22.
14. Jonard S, Robert Y, Cortet-Rudelli C, Pigny P, Decanter C, Dewailly D. Ultrasound examination of polycystic ovaries: is it worth counting the follicles? Hum Reprod. 2003;18:598-603.
15. Franks S, Webber LJ, Goh M, Valentine A, White DM, Conway GS, et al. Ovarian morphology is a marker of heritable biochemical traits in sisters with polycystic ovaries. J Clin Endocrinol Metab. 2008;93:3396-402.
16. Raine-Fenning N, Campbell B, Collier J, Brincat M, Johnson I. The reproducibility of endometrial volume acquisition and measurement with the VOCAL-imaging program. Ultrasound Obstet Gynecol. 2002;19:69-75.
17. Raine-Fenning NJ, Clewes JS, Kendall NR, Bunkheila AK, Campbell BK, Johnson IR. The interobserver reliability and validity of volume calculation from three-dimensional ultrasound datasets in the in vitro setting. Ultrasound Obstet Gynecol. 2003;21:283-91.
18. Riccabona M, Nelson TR, Pretorius DH. Three-dimensional ultrasound: accuracy of distance and volume measurements. Ultrasound Obstet Gynecol. 1996;7:429-34.
19. Riccabona M, Nelson TR, Pretorius DH, Davidson TE. In vivo three-dimensional sonographic measurement of organ volume: validation in the urinary bladder. J Ultrasound Med. 1996;15: 627-32.
20. Takahashi K, Eda Y, Abu Musa A, Okada S, Yoshino K, Kitao M. Transvaginal ultrasound imaging, histopathology and endocrinopathy in patients with polycystic ovarian syndrome. Hum Reprod. 1994;9:1231-6.
21. Wu MH, Tang HH, Hsu CC, Wang ST, Huang KE. The role of three-dimensional ultrasonographic images in ovarian measurement. Fertil Steril. 1998;69:1152-5.
22. Legro RS, Gnatuk CL, Kunselman AR, Dunaif A. Changes in glucose tolerance over time in women with polycystic ovary syndrome: a controlled study. J Clin Endocrinol Metab. 2005;90:3236-42.
23. Dewailly D, Gronier H, Poncelet E, Robin G, Leroy M, Pigny P, et al. Diagnosis of polycystic ovarian syndrome (PCOS): revisiting the threshold values of follicle count on ultrasound and of the serum AMH level for the definition of polycystic ovaries. Hum Reprod. 2011;26:3123-9.
24. Allemand MC, Tummon IS, Phy JL, Foong SC, Dumesic DA, Session DR. Diagnosis of polycystic ovaries by three-dimensional transvaginal ultrasound. Fertil Steril. 2006;85:214-9.
25. Monash University. (2018). International evidence based guideline for assessment and management of polycystic ovarian syndrome 2018. [online] Available from https://www.monash.edu/__data/assets/pdf_file/0004/1412644/PCOS_Evidence-Based-Guidelines_20181009.pdf. [Last accessed October, 2021].
26. Clayton RN, Ogden V, Hodgkinson J, Worswick L, Rodin DA, Dyer S, et al. How common

are polycystic ovaries in normal women and what is their significance for the fertility of the population? Clin Endocrinol (Oxf). 1992;37:127-34.

27. Lujan ME, Jarrett BY Brooks ED, Reines JK, Peppin AK, Muhn N, et al. Updated ultrasound criteria for polycystic ovary syndrome: reliable thresholds for elevated follicle population and ovarian volume. Hum Reprod. 2013;28:1361-8.
28. Polson DW, Adams J, Wadsworth J, Franks S. Polycystic ovaries—a common finding in normal women. Lancet. 1988;1:870-2.
29. Cresswell JL, Barker DJ, Osmond C, Egger P, Phillips DI, Fraser RB. Fetal growth, length of gestation, and polycystic ovaries in adult life. Lancet. 1997;350:1131-5.
30. Adams J, Franks S, Polson DW, Mason HD, Abdulwahid N, Tucker M, et al. Multifollicular ovaries: clinical and endocrine features and response to pulsatile gonadotropin releasing hormone. Lancet. 1985;2:1375-9.
31. O'Driscoll JB, Mamtora H, Higginson J, Pollock A, Kane J, Anderson DC. A prospective study of the prevalence of clear-cut endocrine disorders and polycystic ovaries in 350 patients presenting with hirsutism or androgenic alopecia. Clin Endocrinol (Oxf). 1994;41:231-6.
32. Kim HJ, Adams JM, Gudmundsson JA, Arason G, Pau CT, Welt CK. Polycystic ovary morphology: age-based ultrasound criteria. Fertil Steril. 2017;108(3):548-53.
33. Matsunaga I, Hata T, Kitao M. Ultrasonographic identification of polycystic ovary. Asia Oceania J Obstet Gynecol. 1985;11:227-32.
34. Takahashi K, Ozaki T, Okada M, Uchida A, Kitao M. Relationship between ultrasonography and histopathological changes in polycystic ovarian syndrome. Hum Reprod. 1994;9:2255-8.
35. Buckett WM, Bouzayen R, Watkin KL, Tulandi T, Tan SL. Ovarian stromal echogenicity in women with normal and polycystic ovaries. Hum Reprod. 1999;14:618-21.
36. Ardaens Y, Robert Y, Lemaitre L, Fossati P, Dewailly D. Polycystic ovarian disease: contribution of transvaginal endosonography and reassessment of ultrasonographic diagnosis. Fertil Steril. 1991;55:1062-8.
37. Robert Y, Dubrulle F, Gailandre L, Ardaens Y, Thomas-Desrousseaux P, Lemaitre L, et al. Ultrasound assessment of ovarian stroma hypertrophy in hyperandrogenism and ovulation disorders: visual analysis versus computerized quantification. Fertil Steril. 1995;64:307-12.
38. Pache TD, Wladimiroff JW, Hop WC, Fauser BCJM. How to discriminate between normal and polycystic ovaries—TVS study. Radiology. 1992;183:421-3.
39. Dewailly D, Robert Y, Helin I, Ardaens Y, Thomas-Desrousseaux P, Lemaitre L, et al. Ovarian stromal hypertrophy in hyperandrogenic women. Clin Endocrinol (Oxf). 1994;41:557-62.
40. Falghesu M, Ciampelli M, Belosi C, Apa R, Pavone V, Lanzone A. A new ultrasound criterion for the diagnosis of polycystic ovary syndrome: the ovarian stroma: total area ratio. Fertil Steril. 2001;76:326-31.
41. Belosi C, Selvaggi L, Apa R, Guido M, Romualdi D, Fulghesu AM, et al. Is PCOS diagnosis solved by ESHRE/ASRM 2003 consensus or could it include ultrasound examination of ovarian stroma? Hum Reprod. 2006;21:3108-15.
42. Fulghesu AM, Angioni S, Frau E, Belosi C, Apa R, Mioni R, et al. Ultrasound in polycystic ovary syndrome—the measuring of ovarian stroma and relationship with circulating androgens: results of multicentric study. Hum Reprod. 2007;22:2501-8.
43. Fulghesu AM, Angioni S, Spettu F, Belosi C, Apa R, Mioni R, et al. Results of multicentric study-US in PCOS—measuring of ovarian stroma and relationship with circulating androgens. Hum Report. 2007;22:2501-8.
44. Raine-Fenning NJ, Campbell BK, Clewes JS, Kendall NR, Johnson IR. The reliability of virtual organ computer-aided analysis (VOCAL) for the semiquantification of ovarian, endometrial and subendometrial perfusion. Ultrasound Obstet Gynecol. 2003;22:633-9.
45. Raine-Fenning NJ, Campbell BK, Clewes JS, Kendall NR, Johnson IR. The interobserver reliability of three-dimensional power Doppler data acquisition within the female pelvis. Ultrasound Obstet Gynecol. 2004;23:501-8.
46. Raine-Fenning NJ, Ramnarine KV, Nordin NM, Campbell BK. Quantification of blood perfusion using 3D power Doppler: an in-vitro flow phantom study. J Phys Conf Ser. 2004;1:181-6.
47. Jarvela IY, Mason HD, Sladkevicius P, Kelly S, Ojha K, Campbell S, et al. Characterization of normal and polycystic ovaries using three-dimensional power Doppler ultrasonography. J Assist Reprod Genet. 2002;19:582-90.
48. Jonard S, Robert Y, Dewailly D. Revisiting the ovarian volume as diagnostic criterion for polycystic ovaries. Hum Reprod. 2005;20:2893-8.
49. Kyei-Mensah AA, LinTan S, Zaidi J, Jacobs HS. Relationship of ovarian stromal volume to serum androgen concentrations in patients with polycystic ovary syndrome. Hum Reprod. 1998;13:1437-41.

50. Balen A, Conway G, Homburg R, Legro R. Polycystic ovary syndrome. A guide to clinical management. United Kingdom: Taylor & Francis Group CRC Press; 2006.
51. Pache TD, de Jong FH, Hop WC, Fauser BC. Association between ovarian changes assessed by TVS & clinical & endocrine signs of PCOS. Feril Steril. 1993;59:544-9.
52. Nardo LG, Buckett WM, White D, Alessandro G Digesu, Stephen Franks, Vik Khullar. Three-dimensional assessment of ultrasound features in women with clomiphene citrate-resistant polycystic ovarian syndrome (PCOS): ovarian stromal volume does not correlate with biochemical indices. Hum Reprod. 2002;17:1052-5.
53. Willis D, Mason H, Gilling-Smith C, Franks S. Modulation by insulin of follicle-stimulating hormone and luteinizing hormone actions in human granulosa cells of normal and polycystic ovaries. J Clin Endocrinol Metab. 1996;81:302-9.
54. Bohler Jr H, Mokshagundam S, Winters SJ. Adipose tissue and reproduction in women. Fertil Steril. 2010;94:795-825.
55. Lam PM, Jhonson IR, Rainne-Fenning NJ. Three dimensional ultrasound features of the polycystic ovary and the effect of different phenotypic expressions on these parameters. Hum Reprod. 2007;22:3116-23.
56. Nagori CB, Panchal SY. Correlation of Ovarian and Stromal Volumes to Fasting and Postprandial Insulin Levels in Polycystic Ovarian Syndrome Patients. Int J Infertil Fetal Med. 2014;5(1):12-14.
57. Puzigaca Z, Prelevic GM, Stretenovic Z, Balint-Peric L. Ovarian enlargement as a possible marker of androgen activity in polycystic ovary syndrome. Gynecol Endocrinol. 1991;5:167-74.
58. Dewailly D, Pigny P, Soudan B, Catteau-Jonard S, Decanter C, Poncelet E, et al. Reconciling the definitions of polycystic ovary syndrome: the ovarian follicle number and serum anti-Mullerian hormone concentrations aggregate with the markers of hyperandrogenism. J Clin Endocrinol Metab. 2010;95:4399-405.
59. Eilertsen TB, Vanky E, Carlsen SM. Anti-Mullerian hormone in the diagnosis of polycystic ovary syndrome: can morphologic description be replaced? Reprod BioMed Online. 2013;27:414-8.
60. Pan HA, Wu MH, Cheng YC, Li CH, Chang FM. Quantification of Doppler signal in polycystic ovarian syndrome using 3D power Doppler ultrasonography. Hum Reprod. 2002;17:2484.
61. Aleem FA, Predanic M. Transvaginal color Doppler determination of the ovarian and uterine blood flow characteristics in polycystic ovary disease. Fertil Steril. 1996;65:510-6.
62. Agrawal R, Conway G, Sladkevicius P, Tan SL, Engmann L, Payne N, et al. Serum vascular endothelial growth factor and Doppler blood flow velocities in in vitro fertilization: relevance to ovarian hyperstimulation syndrome and polycystic ovaries. Fertil Steril. 1998;70:651-8.
63. Battalgia C, Artini PG, D'Ambrogio G, Genazzani AD, Genazzani AR. The role of colour Doppler imaging in the diagnosis of polycystic ovarian syndrome. Am J Obstet Gynecol. 1995;172:108-13.
64. Jarvela IY, Sladkevicius P, Kelly S, Ojha K, Campbell S, Nargund G. Comparison of follicular vascularization in normal versus polycystic ovaries during in vitro fertilization as measured using 3-dimensional power Doppler ultrasonography. Fertil Steril. 2004;82:1358-63.
65. Battalgia C, Artini PG, Salvatori M, Giulini S, Petraglia F, Maxia N, et al. Ultrasonographic patterns of polycystic ovaries; colour Doppler and hormonal correlations. Ultrasound Obstet Gynecol. 1998;11:332-6.
66. Pan HA, Wu MH, Cheng YC, Li CH, Chang FM. Quantification of Doppler signal in polycystic ovary syndrome using three-dimensional power Doppler ultrasonography: a possible new marker for diagnosis. Hum Reprod. 2002;17:201-6.
67. Bostanci MS, Sagsoz N, Noyan V, Yucel A, Goren K. Comparison of ovarian stromal and uterine artery blood flow measured by colour Doppler ultrasonography in polycystic ovary syndrome patients and patients with ultrasonographic evidence of polycystic. Clin Gynaecol Obstet. 2013; 2(1):20-6.
68. Wu MH, Huang MF, Tsai SJ, Pan HA, Cheng YC, Lin YS. Effects of laparoscopic ovarian drilling on young adult women with polycystic ovarian syndrome. J Am Assoc Gynecol Laparosc. 2004;11:184-90.
69. Dewailly D, Jonard SC, Reyss AC, Leroy M, Pigny P. Oligoanovulation with polycystic ovaries but not overt hyperandrogenism. JCEM. 2006;91:3922-7.
70. Ng EHY, Chan CCW, Yeung WSB, Ho PC. Comparison of ovarian stromal blood flow between fertile women with normal ovaries and infertile women with polycystic ovary syndrome. Hum Reprod. 2005;20:1881-6.
71. Ng EH, Chan CC, Yeung WS, Ho PC. Effect of age on ovarian stromal flow measured by three-dimensional ultrasound with power Doppler in Chinese women with proven fertility. Hum Reprod. 2004;19:2132-7.

72. El Behery MM, Diab AE, Mowafy H, Ebrahiem MA, Shehata AE. Effect of laparoscopic ovarian drilling on vascular endothelial growth factor and ovarian stromal blood flow using three-dimensional power Doppler. Intern J Gynecol Obstet. 2011;112:119-21.

73. Abd El, Aal DE, Mohamed SA, Amine AF, Meki AR. Vascular endothelial growth factor and insulin like growth factor 1 in polycystic ovary syndrome and their relation to ovarian blood flow. Eur J Obstet Gynecol Reprod Biol. 2005;118:219-24.

31

CHAPTER

Baseline Scan

Sonal Panchal, Chaitanya Nagori

INTRODUCTION

Success of any assisted reproductive technology is chiefly dependent on two decisions—(1) selection of correct stimulation protocol and (2) correct timing of human chorionic gonadotropin (hCG). The stimulation protocol is to be so designed that there is no ovarian hyperstimulation and the cycle does not need to be cancelled because of poor response. This means that it should ideally be tailor-made for each patient.

Selection of correct stimulation protocol is based on prestimulation assessment of female to assess ovarian response and ovarian reserve. This is done by baseline ultrasound scan on second to third day of menstrual cycle. Ovaries must have no active follicle or corpus luteum and this confirms that estrogen and progesterone are at their low levels and, therefore, it is a baseline scan.

Route of scan has to be transvaginal always. Using transabdominal approach for ovarian assessment may miss at least 42% of the ovarian anatomical details.[1]

All the scans are done using B-mode ultrasound with color Doppler, pulse Doppler, three-dimensional (3D) ultrasound, and 3D power Doppler. Using color Doppler in this assessment is mandatory because a large number of biochemical or hormonal changes occur during the menstrual cycle, which reflect as vascular and morphological changes in the ovaries and uterus and vascular changes can be assessed by Doppler. 3D ultrasound is especially useful for volume measurements.

TECHNIQUE FOR BASELINE SCAN OF OVARIES

B-mode ultrasound assessment of the ovaries consists of assessment of ovarian diameters and volume and counting of antral follicles as quantitative assessment and qualitative assessment of stromal density.

Once ovary is located, the probe is rotated to find out the longest diameter of ovary and is stored as one frame on a dual screen. Then, probe is rotated 90° without any other probe movement to get a true transverse axis of ovary. Measure the largest longitudinal, transverse, and anteroposterior (AP) diameter of the ovary in centimeters (cm) and ovarian volume can be calculated by the formula ($x \times y \times z \times 0.523$) **(Figs. 1A and B)**.

Number of antral follicles is counted in the whole ovary by taking a two-dimensional (2D) sweep across whole ovary and eyeballing. When counting antral follicles, do not ever rotate the probe. This method is feasible and reliable when number of antral follicles is approximately 10–15. But, when number of follicles is much more as in polycystic ovaries, the calculation using B-mode scroll may be inaccurate. In these cases it is better to use 3D ultrasound with Sono AVC (automated volume calcification).

Doppler is used to see presence of vessels in ovarian stroma **(Fig. 2)**.

On color or power Doppler, box is placed on the ovary, so that whole ovary is included in color box. The vessel that is close to any of the follicles is not a stromal vessel. The

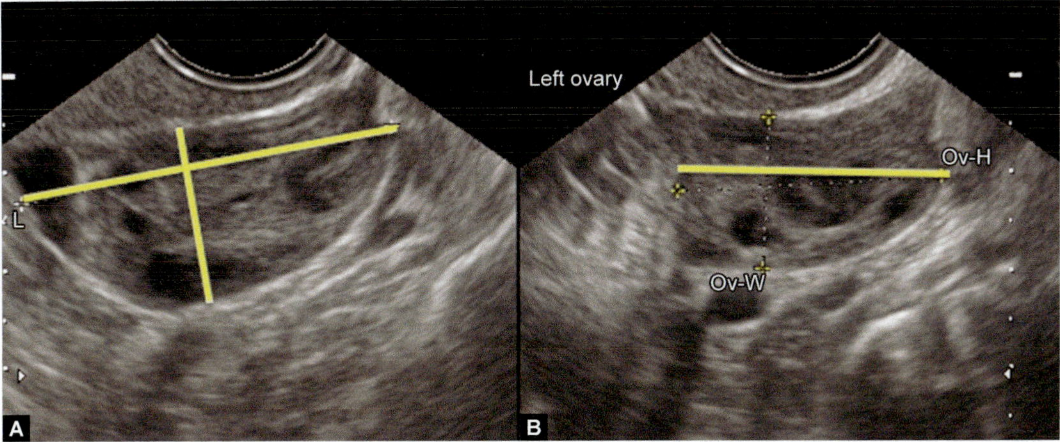

Figs. 1A and B: Measuring ovarian volume on B-mode ultrasound.

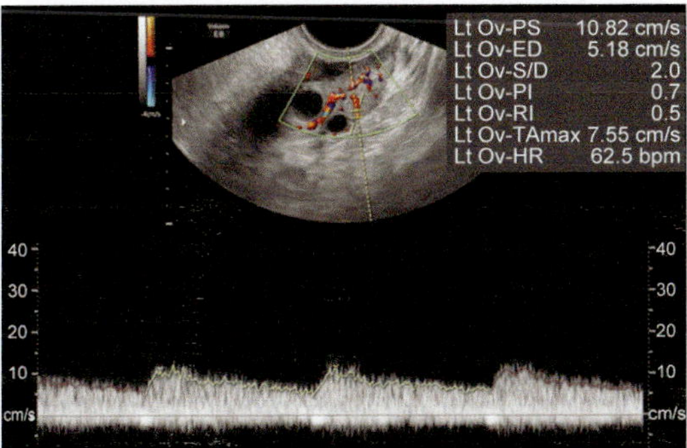

Fig. 2: Ovarian stromal flow assessment on color and spectral Doppler.

vessel selected for interrogation is a vessel that shows brightest color on color Doppler. By rotation of the probe, confirm that the vessel is not the main stem of the ovarian artery and is only its branch. Pulse Doppler is used for quantitative assessment of the flows—intraovarian resistance index (RI) and peak systolic velocity (PSV). For color Doppler, pulse repetition frequency (PRF) of 0.3, wall filters lowest with optimum gains, and balance settings are essential. For pulse Doppler, also lowest PRF and wall filters are used as stromal flow on baseline scan are low velocity flow.

Based on the above described assessment of the ovaries, these are categorized into normal, low reserve, and poorly responding or polycystic ovaries.

Normal Ovaries

Normal ovaries are the ones that have a largest diameter of 2–3 cm, ovarian volume of 3–6.6 cc, antral follicle count (AFC) per ovary of 4–19, isoechoic stroma **(Figs. 3A and B)**, stromal

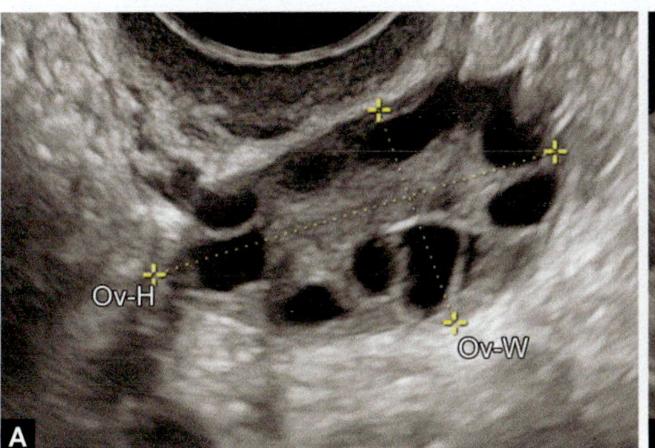

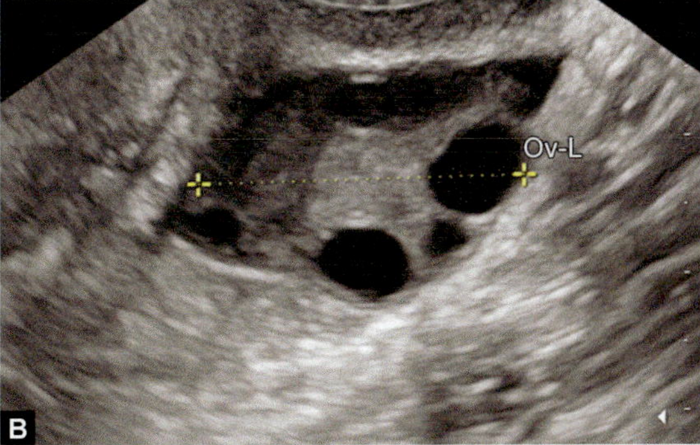

Figs. 3A and B: Normal ovary on B-mode ultrasound.

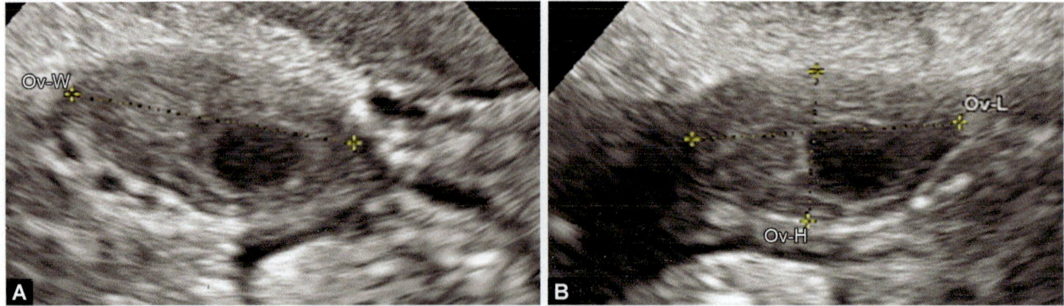

Figs. 4A and B: Low reserve ovary.

RI of 0.6–0.7, and stromal PSV of 5–10 cm/s. Ovaries with these features are categorized as normal ovaries because they respond to standard stimulation protocols and produce adequate follicles for the concerned assisted reproductive technology. These standard protocols are 75 IU of recombinant follicle-stimulating hormone (rFSH) for intrauterine insemination (IUI) cycles and 150–225 IU of rFSH for in vitro fertilization (IVF) cycles.

Low Reserve Ovaries

Low reserve ovaries are the ones that have fewer than four follicles per ovary. As these have less number of antral follicles, these are also small in size **(Figs. 4A and B)**. The largest diameter <2 cm and volume <3 cc are a low reserve ovary. These ovaries produce less number of follicles at the end of stimulation.

Although the AFC is reduced in ovaries with an endometrioma, the number of oocytes retrieved is similar suggesting that the AFC is underestimated in such ovaries. This is a consequence of an impaired ability to detect small follicles in the presence of an endometrioma.[2]

Anti-Müllerian hormone (AMH) showed a positive linear correlation to AFC in all groups.[3]

Poorly Responding Ovaries

Poorly responding ovaries are the ones that respond poorly to any stimulation. This means that these ovaries require larger doses of gonadotropins for stimulation. This poor response can be attributed to poor blood flow to these ovaries. Measurement of ovarian stromal flow in early follicular phase is related to subsequent ovarian response in IVF treatment.[4] Ovarian stromal PSV after pituitary suppression is predictive of ovarian responsiveness and outcome of IVF treatment.[5]

These ovaries show high resistance (RI > 0.7) and low velocity flow (PSV < 5 cm/s) **(Fig. 5)**.

Low reserve and poorly responding ovaries are often used as synonyms, but these are different entities. Reserve relates to AFC or ultimate yield of follicles/ova at the end of stimulation, whereas response relates to sensitivity of ovary to ovulation-stimulating agents to produce those follicles. This means that any ovary would be a permutation and combination of one of the characteristics from each of these two groups. One group

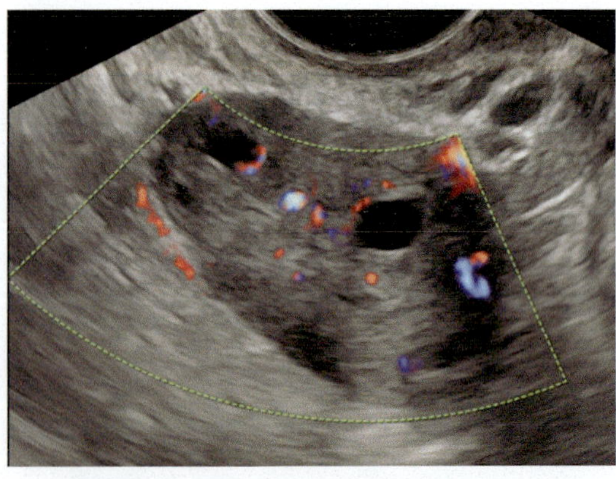

Fig. 5: Poor responding ovary with scanty ovarian stromal flow.

has normal response, poor response, and hyper response and the other group has normal reserve, low reserve, and high reserve or polycystic ovaries. It is a combination of findings such as AFC and stromal flow: RI and PSV that would ultimately decide the optimum stimulation protocol.

Deciding Stimulation Protocol

Tailor designing stimulation protocol is quite a complicated and difficult task for infertility experts and different workers have tried to simplify this by using ovarian reserve markers such as AFC, AMH, FSH, and age. But, a method that uses combination of parameters that assess reserve and response of the ovary has not been established so far. According to a study, predictors of ovarian response are:[6]

- Number of antral follicles
- Ovarian stromal flow index (FI)
- Total ovarian stromal area
- Total ovarian volume

In that order of importance.

How to decide stimulation protocol?

- *Antral follicle count and ovarian volume*: To assess ovarian reserve, AFC is the most useful marker. Doing AFC assessment alone, would be more cost-effective for predicting the ovarian response in patients undergoing controlled ovarian stimulation with gonadotropins. AFC had the highest accuracy for predicting ovarian response in patients with abnormal ovarian reserve test and was statistically significant (number of oocyte aspirated p value < 0.001) than AMH (p value = 0.06) and FSH (p value = 0.212) in predicting ovarian response. For prediction of poor ovarian reserve, a model including AFC + AMH was found to be almost similar to that of (p value = 0.001) using AFC alone.[7] Precise calculation of AFC, therefore, can help in predicting the ovarian reserve.

How to count antral follicles?

By 2D ultrasound as described earlier, scroll across the ovary and eyeball to count is the easiest method.

Three-dimensional ultrasound with inversion mode rendering and sonography-based automated volume calculation (SonoAVC) are a specialized 3D ultrasound software for calculation of antral follicle numbers and volumes. This method is more precise when follicles are multiple [>15 follicle number per ovary (FNPO)]. But, postprocessing is required for accurate calculations. Region of interest (ROI) and volume angle are selected to include the whole ovary in all three orthogonal planes on acquired ovarian volume. SonoAVC is based on inversion mode rendering. It further color codes each follicle and also shows x, y and z diameters, mean diameter, and volume of each follicle on result sheet **(Fig. 6)**.

- *Ovarian volume*: Ovarian volume correlates with oocytes retrieved.[8] Ovarian volume <3 cc was significantly predictive of higher IVF cancellation rates >50%[9] **(Fig. 2)** *and ovarian volume was also used in decision-making for stimulation protocol for ovarian induction.* A software called virtual organ computer-aided analysis (VOCAL) is used to calculate ovarian volume **(Fig. 7)**. VOCAL calculates volume of any structure by rotating it 180°. A step of rotation of 6–30° can be selected. A circumference is drawn around the structure of interest at every step of rotation and at the end of 180°, total volume is calculated.

  Ovarian volume and AFC correlate to the number of follicles matured and oocytes retrieved. AFC and ovarian volume provide direct measurements of ovarian reserve.[10]
- *Ovarian stromal flow*: To assess ovarian response—dose of gonadotropins. Measurement of ovarian stromal flow in early follicular phase is related to subsequent ovarian response in IVF

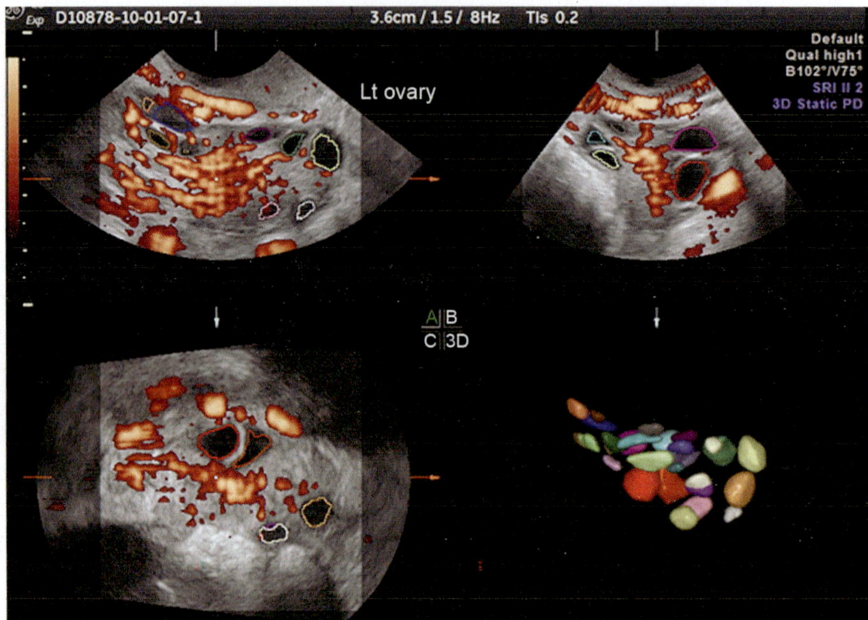

Fig. 6: 3D ultrasound image of the ovary with SonoAVC for calculating antral follicle counts.

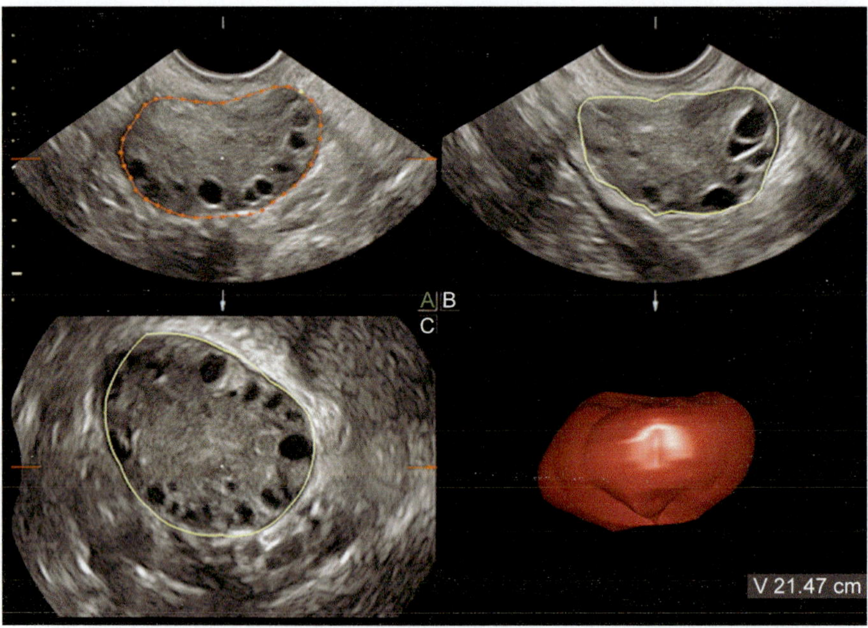

Fig. 7: 3D ultrasound calculated ovarian volume by a software called VOCAL.
(3D: three-dimensional; VOCAL: virtual organ computer-aided analysis)

treatment.[4,11] *Ovarian* stromal PSV after pituitary suppression is predictive of ovarian responsiveness and outcome of IVF treatment.[5]

The ovarian stromal blood flow was found to be negatively correlated with age. Ovarian blood flow predicts ovarian responsiveness and, hence, provides a noninvasive and cost-effective prognostic factor of IVF outcome.[5]

Kupesic has shown correlation in the ovarian stromal FI and number of mature oocytes retrieved in an IVF cycles and pregnancy rates.[6] According to this study, stromal FI [<11 low responder, 11–14 good, and >15 suggest risk of ovarian hyperstimulation syndrome (OHSS)]. On VOCAL calculated ovarian volume with power Doppler, applying volume histogram gives values of 3D power Doppler indices, vascularity index (VI), FI, and vascularity flow index (VFI) **(Fig. 8)**. VI is an index for abundance of flow in the selected volume, FI is an index for average intensity of flow in a selected volume, and VFI is a perfusion index. Applying threshold volume on the same VOCAL calculated volume will define stromal volume when threshold is set to differentiate follicles from rest of the ovarian tissue **(Fig. 9)**. This may aid in recognizing stromal abundance of polycystic ovary.

Based on all these facts and findings, we understand that ovaries that have high resistance and low velocity flow require higher doses of gonadotropins for stimulation, whereas those ovaries with low resistance and high velocity flow require lower doses of gonadotropins for stimulation.

Total number of antral follicles and ovarian stromal blood flow were the two most significant predictors of response of the ovary to ovulation induction and ovarian volume was highly significant predictor of number of follicles.[2]

Consider age and body mass index (BMI) also to calculate the stimulation dose. Freiesleben NLC et al.[12] concluded that body weight and AFC may be used to achieve appropriate ovarian response for IUI in ovulatory patients. Age is known to be one of the most important factors that reduce not only the ovarian reserve but also the oocyte quality. Ultrasound parameters with age and BMI are

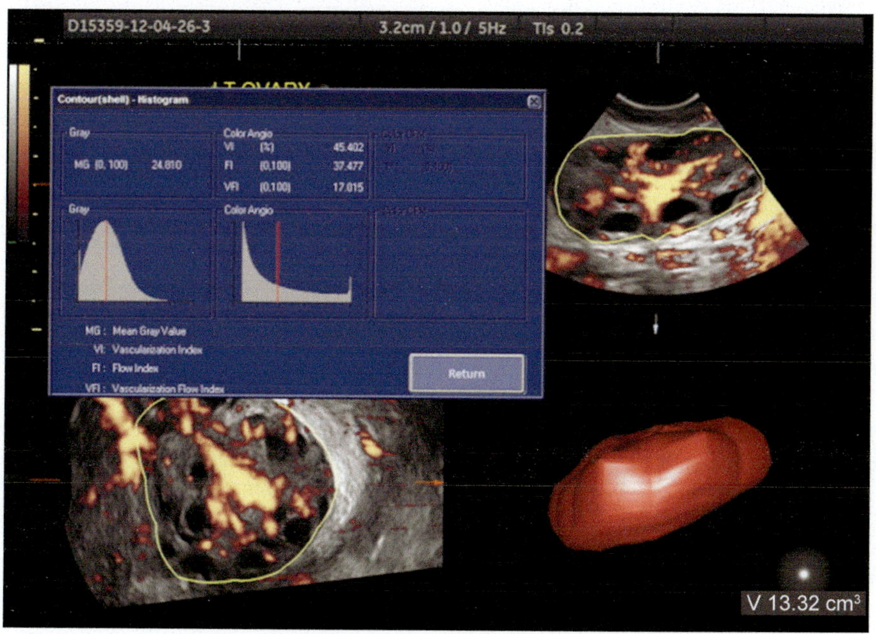

Fig. 8: 3D power Doppler ultrasound image with VOCAL calculated volume with volume histogram (blue box) showing VI, FI, and VFI parameters.
(3D: three-dimensional; FI: flow index; VI: vascularity index; VFI: vascularity flow index; VOCAL: virtual organ computer-aided analysis)

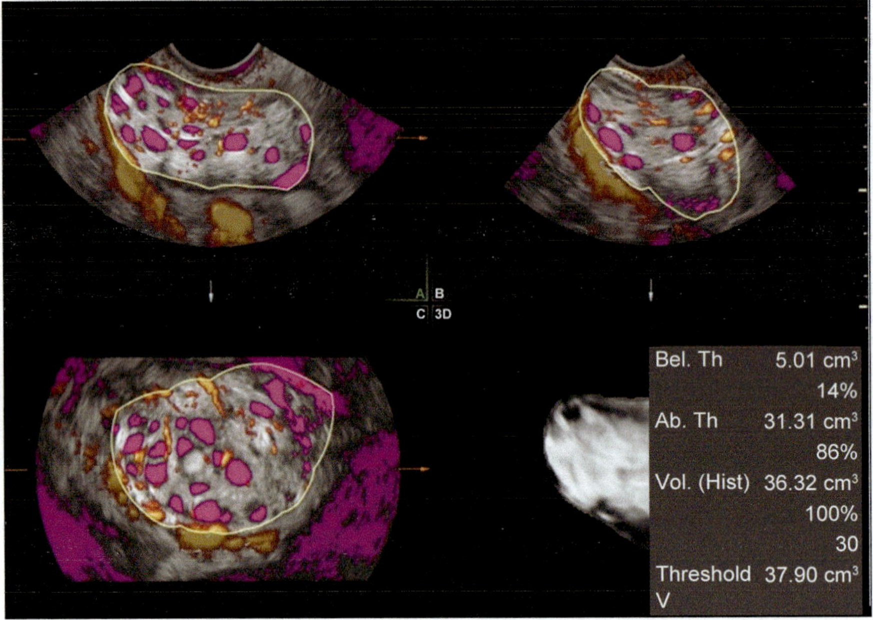

Fig. 9: 3D ultrasound acquired volume of the ovary with VOCAL calculated volume processed by threshold volume to calculate stromal volume.
(3D: three-dimensional; VOCAL: virtual organ computer-aided analysis)

reliable parameters for decision on stimulation doses.[13] AFC is predictive of number of follicles (serum estradiol level) on the day of hCG and BMI was predictive of gonadotropins dosage.[14]

As a result of several pilot studies since 2004–2012, we concluded that the final dose calculation can be based on factors given in **Table 1**.[15]

Based on the parameters that demand higher dose or lower dose in a particular patient on the baseline scan, the doses of gonadotropins for ovulation induction are modified.

Depending on the values of age, BMI, AFC, ovarian volume, ovarian stromal RI, and PSV, in a particular patient on the baseline scan, the final starting dose for IUI or IVF is calculated. Baseline scoring system is developed based on the abovementioned evidences **(Table 2)**.[16,17]

Depending on the baseline score, the doses of rFSH for ovulation induction are described in **Table 3**.

Transvaginal scan confirms that on the day when gonadotropins are started, that all the follicles are smaller than 10 mm. Follicle larger than 10 mm is dominant follicle. Follicular dominance is confirmed on day 5 of stimulation.

TABLE 1: Age, BMI, and ultrasound parameter values that may require increase or decrease in the doses of gonadotropins for ovulation induction.

	Increase the dose when..	*Decrease the dose when..*
Age	>35 years	<25 years
BMI	>28 kg/m^2	<20 kg/m^2
AFC	<3 FNPO	>12 FNPO
Stromal RI	>0.7	<0.5
Stromal PSV	<5 cm/s	>10 cm/s
Stromal FI	<11	>15
Ovarian volume	<3 cc	>10 cc

(AFC: antral follicle count; BMI: body mass index; FI: flow index; FNPO: follicle number per ovary; PSV: peak systolic velocity; RI: resistance index)

If on day 5, the follicle has not grown to dominance and the endometrium is also not growing, then it is considered as nonresponse

TABLE 2: Baseline scoring system indicating score for a particular value of different parameters used for deciding the dose of gonadotropin for ovulation induction.

Score	*1*	*2*	*3*	*4*	*5*
Age	>40	35.1–40	30.1–35	25.1–30	<25
BMI	>30	30–28.1	28–25.1	25–22.1	<22
AFC	<5	5–10	11–15	16–20	>20
Ovarian volume	<3	3.1–5	5.1–7	7.1–10	>10
Stromal RI	>0.75	0.75–0.66	0.65–0.56	0.55–0.45	<0.45
Stromal PSV	<3	3.1–5	5.1–7	7.1–10	>10

(AFC: antral follicle count; BMI: body mass index; PSV: peak systolic velocity; RI: resistance index)

TABLE 3: Doses of rFSH for IUI, IVF (fresh), and IVF-FET cycles.

Score	*IUI*	*IVF (fresh)*	*IVF-FET*
≥25	25 IU	75 IU	150 IU
21–25	37.5 IU	150 IU	225 IU
16–20	75 IU	225 IU	300 IU
11–15	112.5 IU	300 IU	375 IU
6–10	150 IU	375 IU	450 IU

(FET: frozen embryo transfer; IVF: in vitro fertilization; IUI: intrauterine insemination; rFSH: recombinant follicle-stimulating hormone)

and in these cases, dose of gonadotropin needs to be modified as mentioned below in IUI cycles depending on what was the baseline score.

Flowcharts 1 and 2 are given for dose adjustment in IUI and IVF cycles.

As per the results of our study, we believe that the scoring system devised in this study for deciding the stimulation protocol is highly reliable for safe planning of stimulation protocols in IUI cycles as the OHSS rates and

Flowchart 1: Dose adjustment algorithm for IUI cycles.

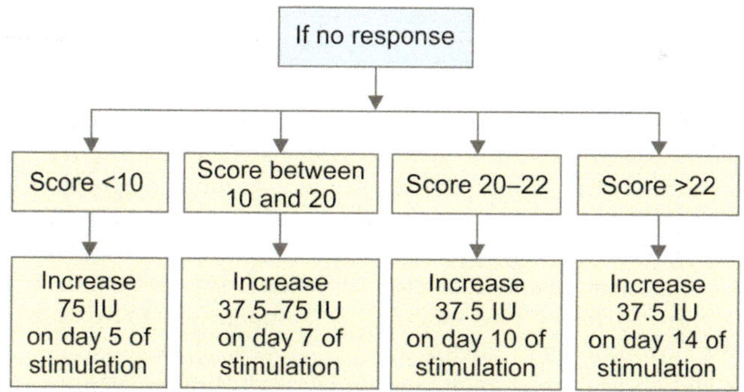

Flowchart 2: Dose adjustment algorithm for IVF cycles.

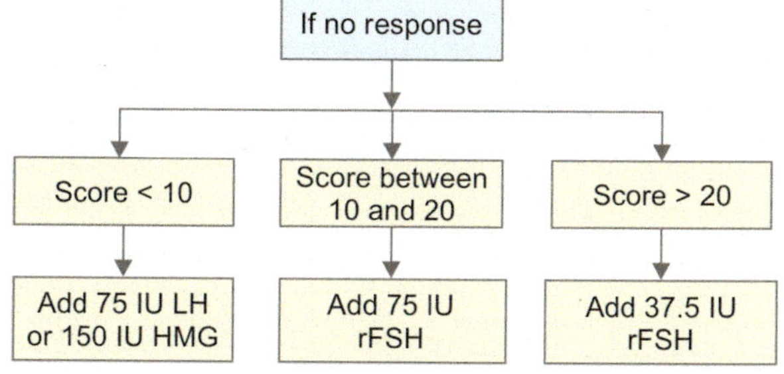

(HMG: human menopausal gonadotropin; LH: luteinizing hormone; rFSH: recombinant follicle-stimulating hormone)

cycle cancellation rates due to poor response are negligible. Multiple pregnancy rates are also acceptable. This study we believe may prove to be an important guide for safe use of gonadotropins for ovulation induction in IUI cycles.

REFERENCES

1. Hull MGR. Polycystic ovarian disease: clinical aspects and prevalence. Res Clin Forums. 1989;11:21-34.
2. Lima ML, Martins WP, Neto MAC, Nastri CO, Ferriani RA, Navarro PA. Assessment of ovarian reserve by antral follicle count in ovaries with endometrioma. Ultrasound Obstet Gynecol. 2015;46:239-42.
3. Christiansen SC, Eilertsen TB, Vanky E, Carlsen SM. Does AMH Reflect Follicle Number Similarly in Women with and without PCOS? PLoS One. 2016;11:e0146739.
4. Zaidi J, Barber J, Kyei-Mensah A, Bekir J, Campbell S, Tan EL. Relationship of ovarian stromal blood flow at baseline ultrasound to subsequent follicular response in an in vitro fertilization program. Obstet Gynecol. 1996;88:779-84.
5. Engmann L, Sladkevicius P, Agrawal R, Bekin JS, Campbell S, Tan SL. Value of ovarian stromal blood flow velocity measurement after pituitary suppression in the prediction of ovarian responsiveness and outcome of in vitro fertilization treatment. Fertil Steril. 1999;71:22-9.
6. Kupesic S, Kurjak A. Predictors of in vitro fertilization outcome by three-dimensional ultrasound. Hum Reprod. 2002;17:950-5.
7. Krishnakumar J, Agarwal A, Nambiar D, Radhakrishnan S. Comparison of antral follicle count, antimullerian hormone and day 2 follicle stimulating hormone as predictor of ovarian response and clinical pregnancy rate in patient with an abnormal ovarian reserve test. Int J Reprod Contracept Obstet Gynecol. 2016;5:2762-7.
8. Popovic-Todorovic B, Loft A, Lindhard A, Bangsbøll S, Andersson AM, Andersen AN. A prospective study of predictive factors of ovarian response in 'standard' IVF/ICSI patients treated with recombinant FSH. A suggestion for a recombinant FSH dosage normogram. Hum Reprod. 2003;18:781-7.
9. Lass A, Skull J, McVeigh E, Margara R, Winston RM. Measurement of ovarian volume by transvaginal sonography before ovulation induction with human menopausal gonadotrophin for in vitro fertilization can predict poor response. Hum Reprod. 1997;12:294-7.
10. te Velde ER, et al. Advances in fertility studies and reproductive medicine IFFS. 2007;306.
11. Arora A, Gainder S, Dhaliwal L, Suri S. Clinical significance of ovarian stromal blood flow in assessment of ovarian response in stimulated cycle for in vitro fertilization. Int J Reprod Contracept Obstet Gynecol. 2015;4:1380-3.
12. Freiesleben NLC, Lossl K, Bogstad J, Bredkjaer HE, Toft B, Loft A, et al. Predictors of ovarian response in intrauterine insemination patients and development of a dosage nomogram. Reprod Biomed Online. 2008;17:632-41.
13. Olivennes F, Howles CM, Borini A, Germond M, Trew G, Wikland M, et al. Individualizing FSH dose for assisted reproduction using a novel algorithm: the CONSORT study. Reprod Biomed Online. 2009;18:195-204.
14. Ng EHY, Tang OS, Chan CCW, Ho PC. Ovarian stromal blood flow in the prediction of ovarian response during in vitro fertilization treatment. Hum Reprod. 2005;20:3147-51.
15. Panchal S, Nagori C. Baseline scan and ultrasound diagnosis of PCOS. Donald School J Ultrasound Obstet Gynecol. 2012;6:290-9.
16. Panchal S, Nagori C. Ultrasound-based decision-making on stimulation protocol for superovulated IUI cycles. Int J Infertil Fetal Med. 2016;7:7-13.
17. Panchal S, Nagori C. Ultrasound-based decision-making on stimulation protocol in IVF. Donald School J Ultrasound Obstet Gynecol. 2016;10:330-7.

32 CHAPTER

Monitoring of Ovulation Induction by Ultrasound

Sonal Panchal, Chaitanya Nagori

INTRODUCTION

Ultrasound is the modality of choice for monitoring of the patients undergoing assisted reproductive technology (ART). It gives precise idea about the morphological changes and also about the hormonal changes occurring during the entire cycle when Doppler is also used for monitoring. The hormonal changes first reflect as vascular changes and then as morphological changes. Therefore, if vascular changes are observed with Doppler, the need of hormonal assessments for cycle monitoring can be omitted.

The purpose of follicular tracking is:

- To evaluate ovarian response to stimulation
- To decide the correct time of ovulation trigger and intrauterine insemination (IUI) or ovum pickup.

Follicles up to 2 mm in diameter grow independent of gonadotropins such as follicle-stimulating hormone (FSH).[1] These are secondary antral follicles that recruit from the primordial follicles to preantral follicles and secondary antral follicles under the effect of androgen. Further development of the follicle is only possible in the presence of appropriate levels of gonadotropins. Before day 5 of the cycle, selection of the dominant follicle occurs.

Between days 5 and 7, dominance of the follicle becomes apparent. Follicle that is 10–12 mm in size is known as a dominant follicle and it is this follicle that is most likely to grow to become a mature follicle and others become atretic **(Fig. 1)**. It is interesting to know that often first largest follicle on baseline scan is not the dominant follicle. This is possible when the follicle is a residual follicle of the previous cycle. Dominant follicle can be differentiated from the residual follicle of the previous cycle by Doppler. Blood flows close to the follicle that can be seen by Doppler when follicle becomes dominant (approximately size of 10 mm).

Scan is always done on the day when gonadotropin is started. If there is a follicle of larger than 10 mm, patient is called back when the follicle is likely to reach 18 mm. This can be estimated because a follicle that is of >10 mm in diameter is a dominant follicle and it grows at a rate of 2–3 mm/day.[2]

It has no internal echogenicity and has thin (pencil line like) walls that are not only more likely to become the leading follicle, but will also give mature healthy ovum. If all the follicles are smaller than 10 mm on the day when gonadotropin is started, the patient is called after 5 days. As the dominant follicle grows, it starts pulling vascularity toward itself.[3,4]

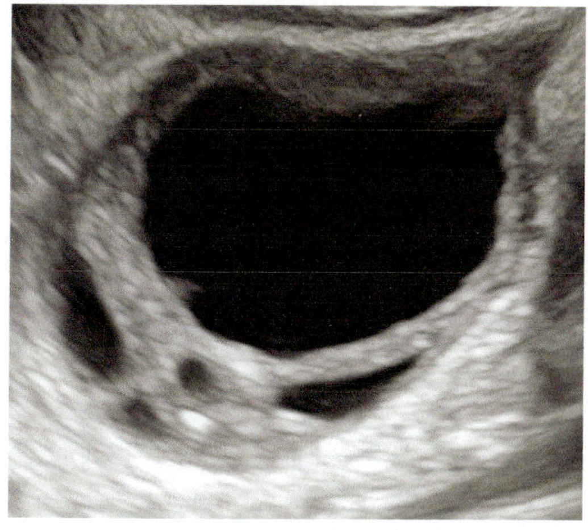

Fig. 1: 2D US image of the ovary showing one mature follicle, surrounded by small atretic follicles.

B-MODE FEATURES OF A MATURE FOLLICLE

The follicular diameter is measured as a single diameter when the follicle is seen as a round structure or three orthogonal diameters must be measured and the mean is used as follicular diameter, if it appears oval **(Figs. 2A and B)**. Anatomical maturity of the follicle may be attained from the follicular diameter of 16–18 mm **(Fig. 3)** and then onward Doppler assessment is done to assess the functional maturity of the follicle. A follicular size of 17–18 mm is considered optimum for gonadotropin-stimulated cycle, whereas for clomiphene citrate (CC)-stimulated cycles, minimum size of 18–20 mm is required.[5] It has been observed that the functional maturity in the follicle may be achieved only much later than the anatomical maturity. On B-mode ultrasound, a good quality follicle is identified by thin isoechoic walls, regular round shape, and no echogenicity in the lumen. A thin hypoechoic rim surrounding the follicle and sometimes (about 35–40%) cumulus-like shadow may be seen in the follicle approximately 24–36 hours before ovulation.

Low-level linear echoes are seen inside the follicle parallel to the wall about 6–10 hours before rupture due to separation of the inner most cell layer of the follicle, as initiation of the process of ovulation **(Fig. 4)**.[2]

DOPPLER FEATURES OF A GOOD PREOVULATORY FOLLICLE

Increase in perifollicular vascularity of dominant follicle in theca layer starts

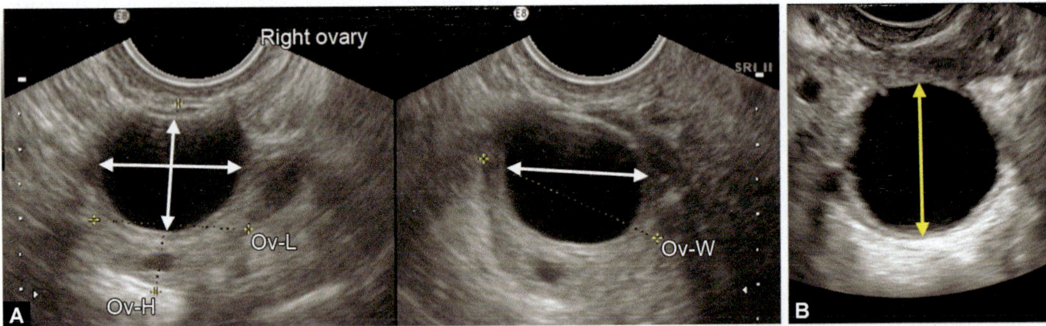

Figs. 2A and B: (A) Measurement of the mean follicle diameter; (B) Measurement of single follicle diameter in case when follicle is absolutely round.

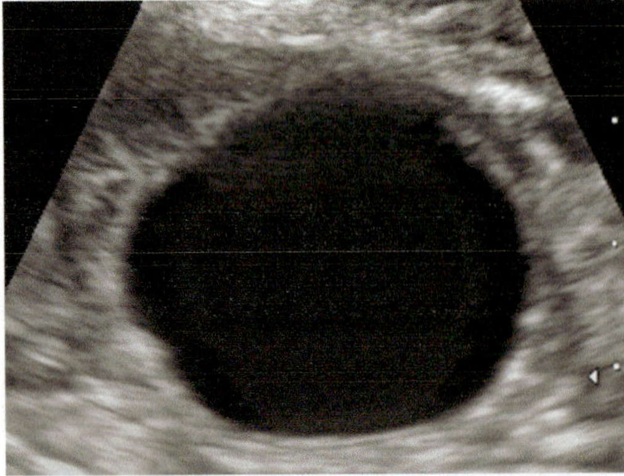

Fig. 3: B-mode ultrasound image of a mature follicle.

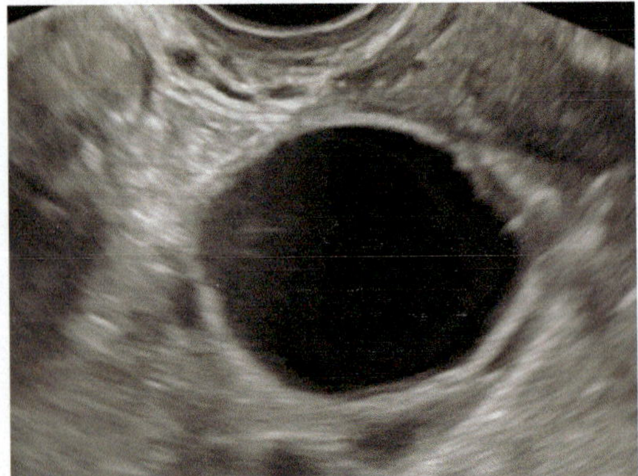

Fig. 4: B-mode ultrasound image of a follicle of which rupture is impending showing mild separation of inner wall at 2 o'clock and 6 o'clock positions.

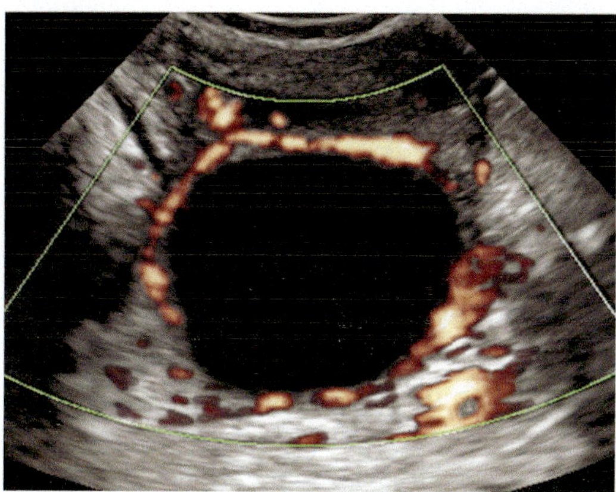

Fig. 5: Perifollicular vascularity seen on color Doppler.

developing as early as 8th day of the cycle in a normal length cycle. Fall in perifollicular resistance index (RI) starts 2 days before ovulation, reaches nadir at ovulation, remains low for 4 days, and then with gradual rise reaches 0.5 days in midluteal phase.[6]

When functionally mature on color Doppler, the follicle shows blood vessels covering at least two-thirds to three-fourths of the follicular circumference **(Fig. 5)**. Chui et al., graded the follicular flow on the day of oocyte collection as grade 1-4 when in a single cross area slice the flow covered <25%, 25–50%, 50–75%, and >75% of follicular circumference. The conception was related to grade 3-4 vascularity.[7]

On pulse Doppler, these blood vessels show RI of 0.4–0.48[7] and peak systolic velocity (PSV) of >10 cm/s **(Fig. 6)**.

The pulse repetition frequency (PRF) settings for color Doppler are set at 0.3 and wall filter at the lowest. The perifollicular vessels are only those that obliterate the follicular wall with color. If the follicular wall is seen and the vessel is seen just besides it, it is not a perifollicular vessel. Ovarian flow correlates well with oocyte recovery rates and, hence, may be useful in determining the most appropriate time to administer human chorionic gonadotropin (hCG) to optimize recovery rate. It has been quoted in a study by Nargund et al.,[7,8] that embryos produced by fertilization of the ova obtained from the follicles which had a perifollicular PSV of <10 cm/s are less likely to be grade 1 embryos and also have higher chance of chromosomal malformations. In the same study, it has been

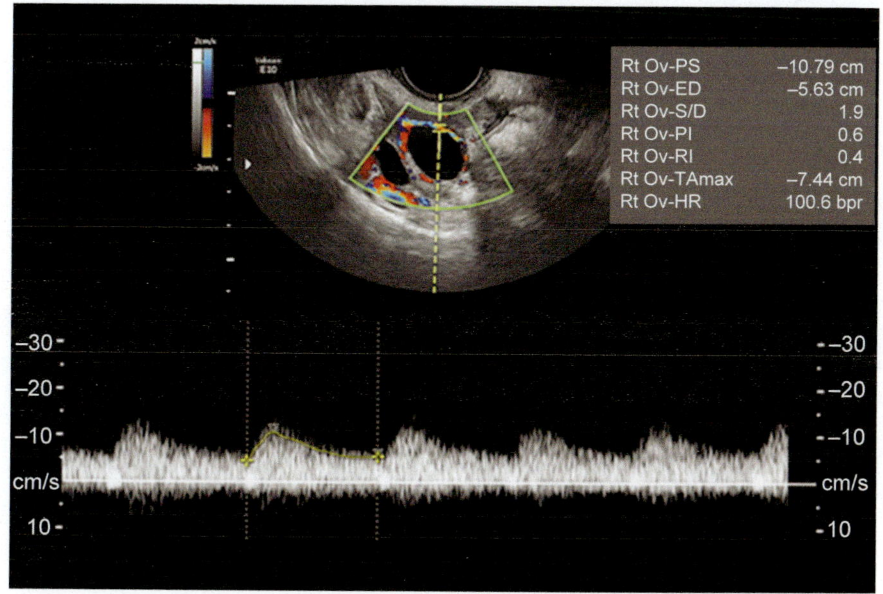

Fig. 6: Pulse Doppler image of the low resistance perifollicular flow.

shown that the probability of developing a grade 1 or grade 2 embryo is 75% if PSV was >10 cm/s, 40% if PSV was <10 cm/s, and 24% if there was no perifollicular flow. There is yet another study that supports this finding. Oocytes from severely hypoxic follicles are associated with high frequency of abnormalities of organization of chromosomes on metaphase spindle and may lead to segregation disorders and catastrophic mosaics in embryo.[9] Our data of >1,000 IUI cycles has shown that when the perifollicular RI > 0.53 and PSV < 9 cm/s 12 hours before hCG injection, the conception rates were only 8.3% and 10%, respectively, as compared to 32.8% and 28.2%, respectively, and individually when perifollicular RI < 0.50 and PSV > 11 cm/s.[10] We have, therefore, always preferred to wait with no extra medication when patient is on CC stimulation or continue with the same dose of gonadotropin till we get desired perifollicular RI and PSV, though sometimes the follicular size may reach up to 22 mm. Almost 90% of the times, the desired RI and PSV are reached by the time follicular size is 22–24 mm maximum.

In in vitro fertilization (IVF) cycles, when there are multiple follicles, trigger is planned when there are at least three follicles between 18 and 16 mm and at least three follicles in either ovary show the Doppler parameters as stated above.

On three-dimensional (3D) ultrasound, the follicular volume of 3–7.5 cc has been found to be optimum in our study.[11] This agrees with the study by Wittmaack et al.,[12] which says that in IVF-embryo transfer (ET) cycles, follicles with mean follicular diameter of 12–24 mm are associated with optimal rates of oocyte recovery, fertilization, and cleavage.[12] This corresponds to the follicular volumes of between 3 and 7 mL. The accuracy of 3D US measurement of follicular volume compared to the standard two-dimensional (2D) techniques by comparing the volume of individual follicles is estimated by both methods; 3D ultrasound with virtual organ computer-aided analysis (VOCAL) gave much more accurate measurements[13] **(Fig. 7)**.

Three-dimensional ultrasound is especially useful to assess follicular size

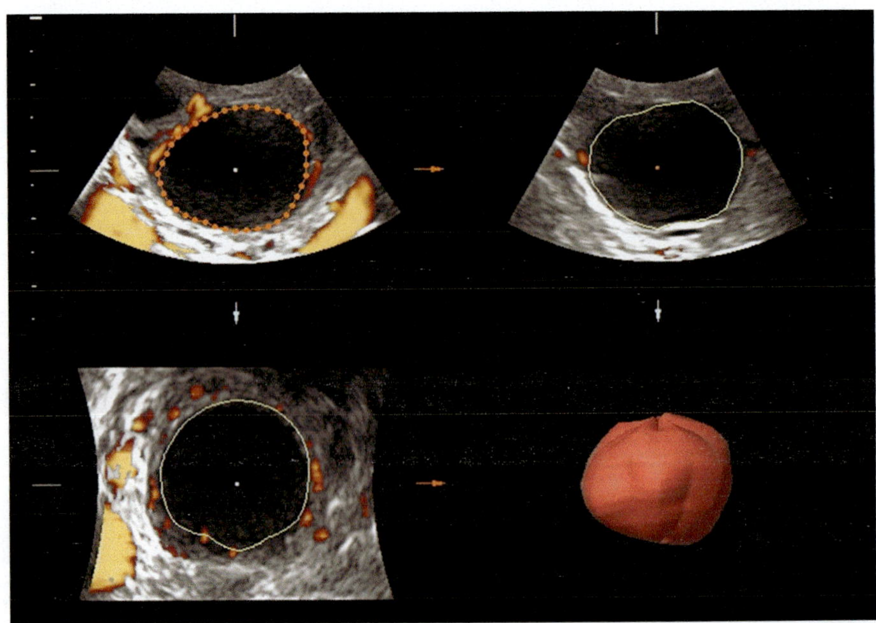

Fig. 7: 3D US acquired VOCAL calculated volume of follicle.
(3D: three-dimensional; VOCAL: virtual organ computer-aided analysis)

in IVF cycles with multiple follicles. Since there are multiple follicles and compressed by each other, these do not appear round in shape. Follicular diameter, therefore, cannot be reliable parameter for follicular size. Follicular volume can be calculated on 3D ultrasound with sonography-based automated volume calculation (SonoAVC) software. This software color codes follicles, so calculates the number of follicles correctly. Moreover, it also calculates three longest orthogonal diameters, mean diameter, and volume of individual follicle. This information is not only useful to assess the time of trigger, but is also useful to decide the type of trigger. When there are more than three follicles of between 11 and 14 mm in both the ovaries in IUI cycle stimulated with gonadotropins apart from the mature follicles and when there are more than four follicles of between 11 and 14 mm in both the ovaries apart from mature follicles of 16 mm and larger, hCG is not given as trigger.

Cumulus is a reliable sign that indicates the presence of fertilizable ovum in the follicle. Appearance of the intrafollicular cumulus-like structures by 3D US **(Figs. 8A and B)** was correlated with the recovery rate of the mature oocytes.[14]

Feichtinger et al. in their study have shown the presence of cumulus in follicles >15 mm by 3D US.[15]

It has been shown that follicular fluid concentrations of leptin, a follicular angiogenesis-related factors, are inversely related to the stromal blood flow index (FI).[16] It has also been suggested that the follicles containing oocytes capable to produce a pregnancy have a perifollicular vascular network more uniform and distinctive.[17] Quantification of power Doppler information within a 3D model of an ovarian follicle can be performed using the "histogram facility" **(Fig. 9)**. Three indices of vascularity can be generated: (1) the vascularization index (VI), which represents the ratio of power Doppler information within the total data relative to both color and gray information; (2) the FI, which is proportional to the power Doppler signal intensity; and (3) the vascularization flow index (VFI), which reflects a combination of the two.

In our study,[11] we have found perifollicular VI of between 6 and 20 and perifollicular FI > 35 as most optimum. 68.4% of patients conceived when the VI was between 6 and 18 and 50% of patients conceived when it was

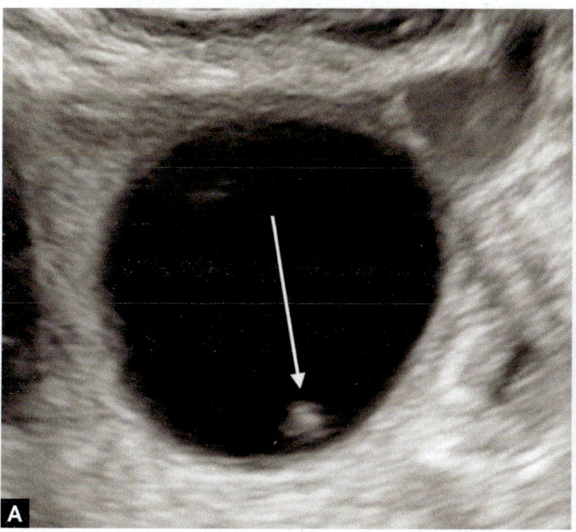

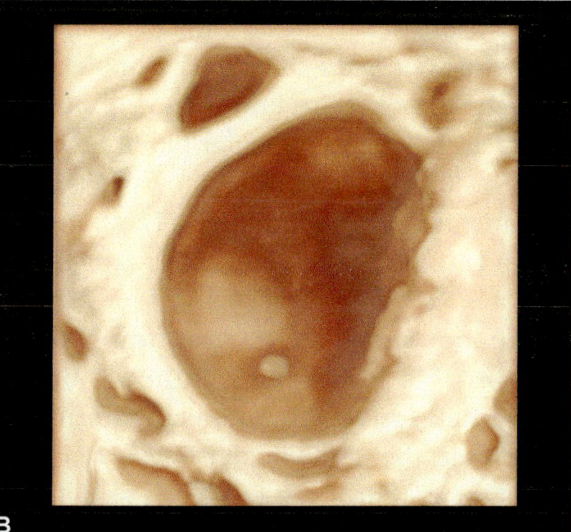

Figs. 8A and B: (A) 2D image of the follicle with cumulus like shadow; (B) 3D image of the follicle showing cumulus.

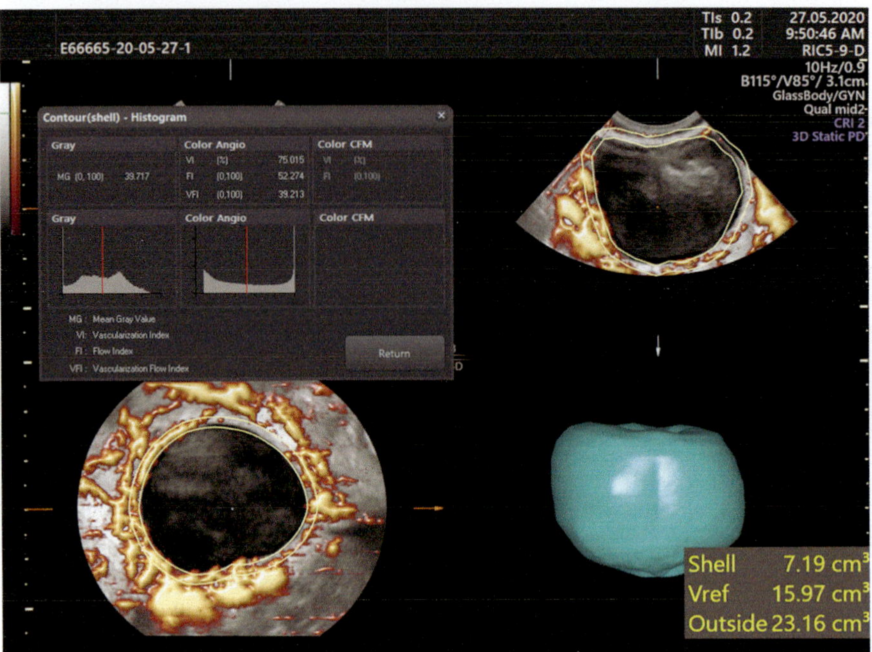

Fig. 9: 3D power Doppler of the follicle with volume histogram.

between 18 and 20. However, the pregnancy rates were <25% when VI was <6 and only 7.4% when VI was >20. It was only 7.4% of patients with FI < 27 who conceived, whereas beyond 27, the conception rates rose consistently. It was 50% with FI between 27 and 35, 70% when FI was between 35 and 43, and almost all patients had conceived when FI was >43. Although it is possible to assess the follicular flow as expressed by the PSV and perifollicular color map,[18] it is the 3D power Doppler that gives the most precise information about the vascularization and follicular blood flow.[19] A study by Kupesic and Kurjak shows that when the ratio of FV to blood FI (FV/FI) is between 0.4 and 0.6, the pregnancy rates are 39%, if >0.6, it is 52%, and when <0.4, it is only 21%.[20]

Human chorionic gonadotropin plays a major role in inducing influx of blood within follicles. At the luteinizing hormone (LH) surge, the perifollicular PSV is 10 cm/s. This means that if the follicle is said to be functionally mature when PSV is 10 cm/s, that is the time when the LH surge starts and under the effect of that LH, the perifollicular PSV keeps on rising constantly.[21] This derives that a rising PSV with steady low RI suggests that the follicle is close to rupture. Vascular changes at the time of impending ovulation include increased vascularity of the inner wall of the follicle and a coincident surge in blood velocity just prior to eruption.[21] Our unpublished study of 350 IUI cycles has shown that when the perifollicular PSV was >20 cm/s, double IUI at 12–14 hours after trigger and 36–38 hours after trigger has given much higher pregnancy rates as compared to single IUI at 36–38 hours after trigger [presented at the International Society of Ultrasound in Obstetrics and Gynecology (ISUOG), 2006].

Implantation has been the weakest link in the success of infertility treatment. Endometrium is a receptor organ for majority of the hormones involved in fertility and, therefore, study of its morphology and vascularity is thought to explain the mysteries of implantation failure. Therefore, like follicle, endometrium is also assessed by transvaginal

2D US and color Doppler before planning for hCG during any ARTs.

B-MODE FEATURES OF ENDOMETRIUM WITH GOOD RECEPTIVITY

On transvaginal sonography (TVS), endometrial thickness of minimum 6 mm is required on the day of hCG, but 8–10 mm is optimum. Endometrial thickness has more negative predictive value for implantation.[22]

In gonadotropin-stimulated cycles, the endometrial thickness is greater than in spontaneous cycles.[23] Growth rate of endometrial thickness in stimulated cycles is:

- Days 7–9 of stimulation 1.9 mm
- Days 9–11 of stimulation 0.9 mm
- Day 11 till hCG 0.6 mm
- Human chorionic gonadotropin till ET 0.5 mm.

Even when pregnancy occurs with endometrial thickness of 6–8 mm on the day of hCG, the rates of preclinical miscarriage (biochemical pregnancy) and clinical miscarriage were 21.9% and 15.6%, respectively, as compared to 0% and 12.9%, respectively, when endometrial thickness was >8 mm.[24]

It is measured from outer margin of the endometrium to outer margin of the endometrium, excluding the junctional zone and perpendicular to the long axis of endometrium and at the broadest part, which in normal endometrium is 1–2 cm inferior to the fundal end of endometrium **(Fig. 10)**.

However, in CC-stimulated cycle, the endometrial thickness may be less in the days immediately after CC is taken because of blocked estrogen receptors and its antiestrogenic effect. But, during late proliferative phase, endometrial thickness increases at a faster rate than in spontaneous cycles, as the estrogen receptors are released because of the weaning effect of CC it escapes from the antiestrogenic effect and effect of increased estrogen due to multifollicular growth.

Morphology of the endometrium is as important as thickness of the endometrium. In all the healthy endometria, the endometrial-myometrial interface is always seen as a clear hypoechoic halo surrounding the whole endometrium **(Fig. 11)**. Breach or irregularity of endometrial-myometrial junction is an indication of unhealthy endometrium and, therefore, poor receptivity.

Popularly multilayered endometrium is considered as a desired endometrial pattern. Morphologically, the endometrium is graded as the best grade A when it is a triple-line endometrium with the intervening area is as hypoechoic as the anterior myometrium. The echogenicity is attributed to the development of multiple vessels penetrating

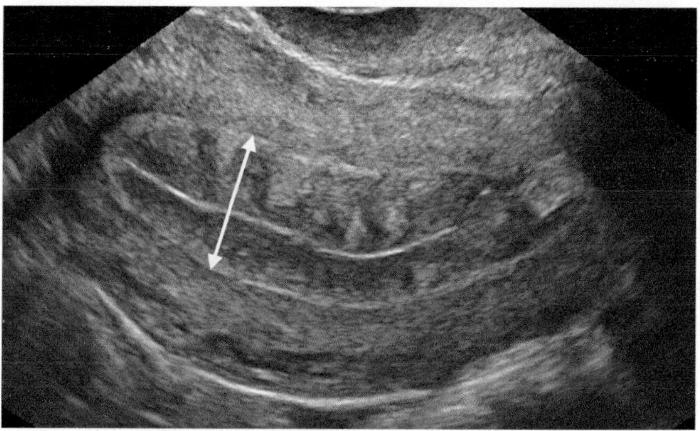

Fig. 10: Assessment of endometrial thickness.

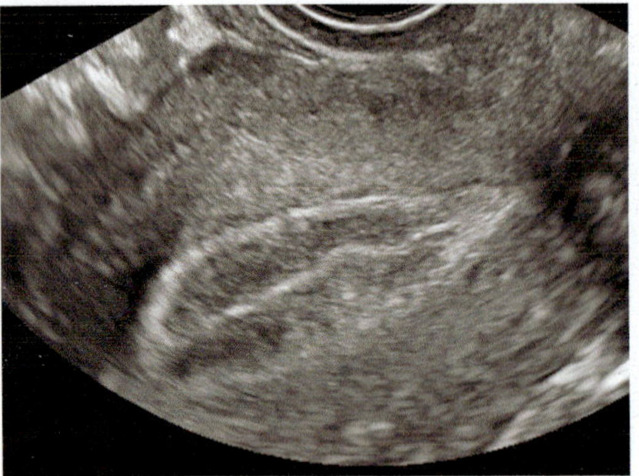

Fig. 11: B-mode ultrasound image of grade A endometrium.

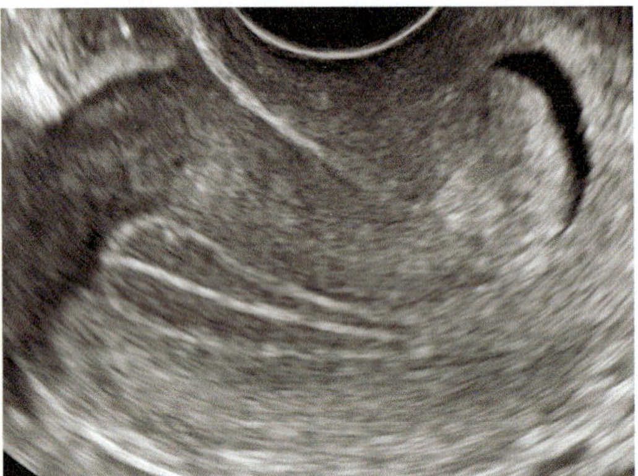

Fig. 12: B-mode ultrasound image of grade B endometrium.

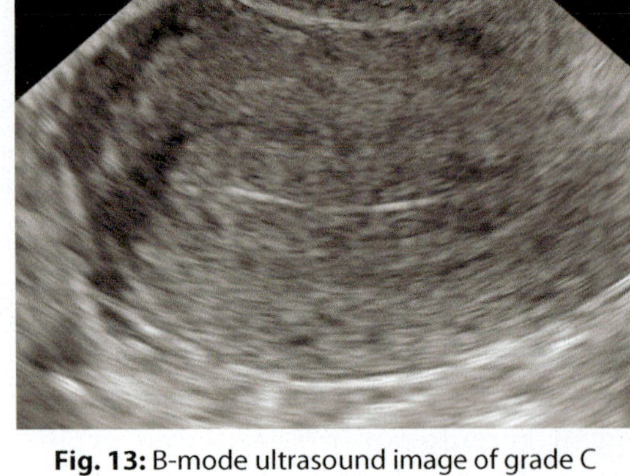

Fig. 13: B-mode ultrasound image of grade C endometrium.

in the endometrium producing multiple tissue interfaces and, therefore, causing the echogenicity and due to glycogen storage in the endometrial columnar epithelium **(Fig. 12)**. The endometrium is graded as intermediate or grade B **(Fig. 13)** when it is multilayered or triple line with hypoechoic intervening area. In grade C, the most unfavorable endometrium would be a homogeneous isoechoic endometrium,[25] though some studies have shown no significant difference in pregnancy rates among different morphological patterns. According to literature evidence and our experience, different morphological patterns of the endometrium can be related to the estradiol levels. As estradiol level increases, the endometrium becomes triple line, increases in thickness, and progresses from grade B to grade A and then to grade C with supraphysiological levels of estradiol as occurs in multifollicular development.

DOPPLER FEATURES OF ENDOMETRIUM WITH GOOD RECEPTIVITY

There are several reports by different groups[26] that agree on the fact that implantation rates can be more correlated to the vascularity of the endometrium rather than the thickness and morphology of the endometrium.

Segmental uterine artery perfusion demonstrates significant correlation with hormonal and histological markers of uterine receptivity reaching the highest sensitivity for subendometrial blood flow.[20]

On color Doppler, the endometrium, which is mature, shows vascularity in zones 3 and 4 or may be called as subendometrial and endometrial layers **(Figs. 14A to D)**.

The zones of vascularity are defined according to Applebaum[26] as: zone 1 when the vascularity on power Doppler is seen only at endometrial-myometrial junction, zone 2 when vessels penetrate through the hyperechogenic endometrial edge, zone 3 when it reaches intervening hypoechogenic zone, and zone 4 when they reach the

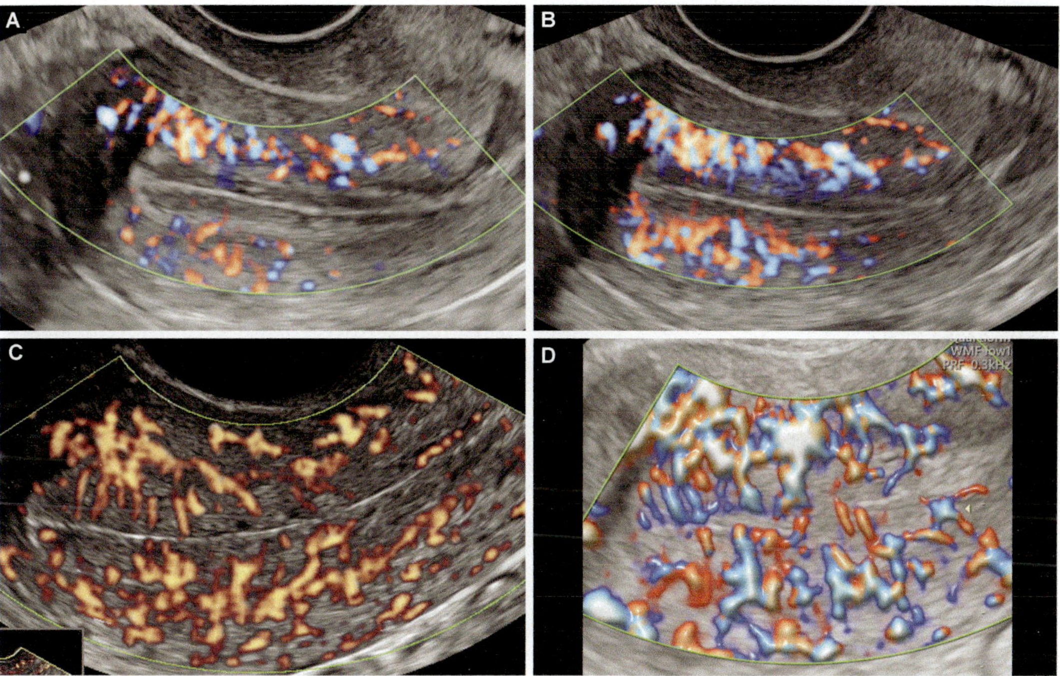

Figs. 14A to D: Power Doppler images of the zone 1–4 endometrial vascularity.

endometrial cavity. But, a particular zone can be called vascularized only when at least 5 mm^2 area of that zone is vascularized. Below this cutoff for zone 3–4, the pregnancy rates are extremely low.[27]

One more comparison of two studies has also shown similar results.[28]

- *Zone 1*: 3.5–7.5% (5.2%)
- *Zone 2*: 15.8–29.7% (28.7%)
- *Zone 3*: 24.2–47.8% (52%)
- *Zone 4*: 67.3% (74%).

ENDOMETRIAL VASCULARITY: ITS RELATION TO IMPLANTATION RATES (NAGORI AND PANCHAL)[29]

Vascularity in	*Zone 1*	*Zone 2*	*Zone 3*	*Zone 4*
Percentage of patients	6.69%	20.73%	58%	14.47%
+Beta-human chorionic gonadotropin (βhCG)	19%	21.87%	39.77%	70.14%

Vascularity in	*Zone 1*	*Zone 2*	*Zone 3*	*Zone 4*
Gestational sac	9.6%	14.58%	36.8%	68.65%
Abortions	50%	23.8%	5.6%	1.5%

Zaidi et al. found that absence of flow in the endometrial and subendometrial zones on day of trigger indicates total failure of implantation.[30]

The vessels that reach the endometrium are the spiral arteries. The pulse Doppler of these arteries should have an RI < 0.6 for the endometrium to be called mature for implantation.

While the reported correlation between vascularity in the endometrium and sub-endometrium and pregnancy rates is controversial, it has been concluded in two studies that no difference was found in patients with good prognosis for cycle outcome, but in patients with poor embryo quality, better endometrial vascularity seemed to improve the cycle outcome.[31,32]

Though yet another study has shown that when pregnancy is achieved in absence of endometrial and subendometrial flow on the day of ET, more than half of these pregnancies will finish as spontaneous miscarriage.[28]

The pulse Doppler of these arteries indicating RI between 0.49 and 0.59 and pulsatility index (PI) between 1.1 and 2.3 has also been reported to be a good prognostic factor **(Fig. 15)**.[33]

The vessels that reach the endometrium covering ≥5 mm^2 area of the endometrium are reported to be a good prognostic factor.[27]

Moreover, the pulse Doppler analysis of the uterine artery waveform is done and its PI should be <3.2 **(Fig. 16)**.

Several authors have shown that the optimum uterine receptivity was obtained when average PI of the uterine artery was between 2 and 3 on the day of transfer or on the day of trigger.[34,35]

Coulam et al., have also shown that no pregnancy was achieved after ET when uterine artery PI was above 3.3 in an IVF program also.[36]

Cacciatore et al. suggest that implantation is unlikely when PI is >3.3 and RI is >0.95 or when no velocities are seen at the end of the diastole.[37]

In such cases, therefore, in IUI cycles, hCG is withheld or postponed.

Endometrial volume by 3D US volume calculation of the endometrium may help to correlate the cycle outcome with quantitative parameter rather than endometrial thickness.[12] This is done by the software called VOCAL.

A study by Raga et al.,[38] shows that pregnancy and implantation rates were significantly lower when endometrial volume <2 mL, while no pregnancy was achieved when endometrial volume was <1 mL. Study by Kupesic et al. also shows no pregnancy when endometrial volume was <2 mL or when exceeded 8 mL.[33]

Preovulatory follicle and endometrium has been summarized in **Table 1**.

If these parameters are not reached, the cycle is not cancelled and only delayed.

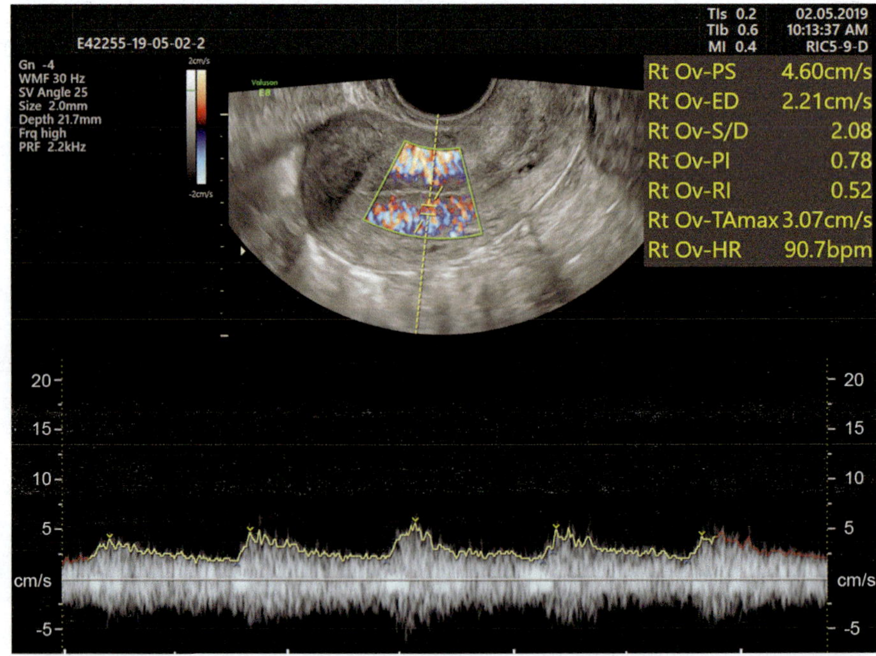

Fig. 15: Spectral Doppler image of the endometiral vascularity.

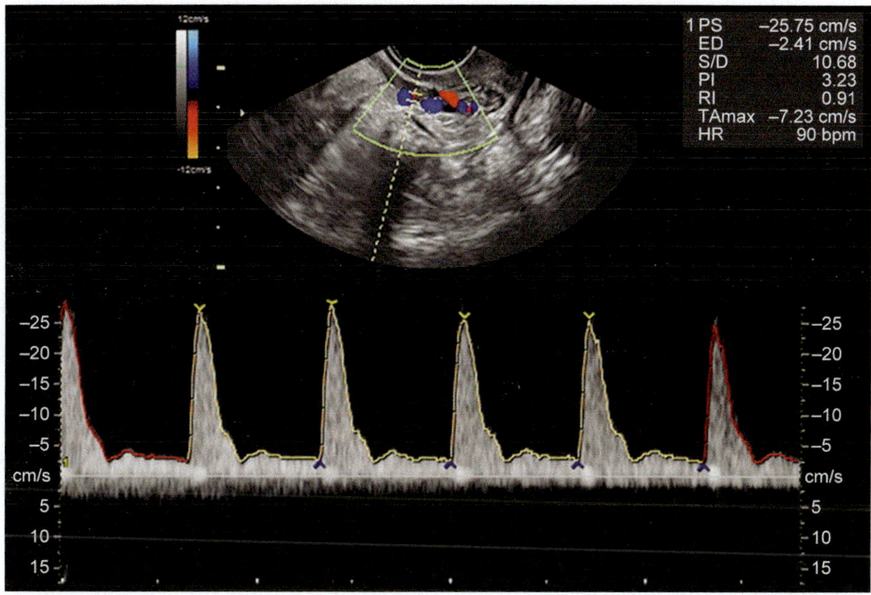

Fig. 16: Pulse Doppler image showing high resistance uterine artery flow waveform.

TABLE 1: Preovulatory follicle and endometrium.

	Follicle	*Endometrium*
Size/Thickness	16–18 mm	8–10 mm
Morphology	Thin wall, no internal echoes, and halo	Grade A/B
Vascularity	Three-fourths of circumference	Zone 3–4
RI	0.4–0.48	<0.5
PSV	>10 cm/s	–
Uterine artery PI	–	<3.2
Volume	3–7 cc	3–7 cc
3D morphology	Cumulus	Intact endometrial-myometrial junction
3D PD	More symmetrical the better	Higher the better

(3D: three-dimensional; PI: pulsatility index; PSV: peak systolic velocity; RI: resistance index)

Stimulation is continued till these parameters are achieved. In case the PSV of the follicle starts rising with low RI, it means the ovulation is impending. In such a situation, in spite of inadequate endometrial parameters, trigger is given, but the patient is also explained that the results cannot be as good as it would be if every parameter was optimal. If the follicle grows beyond 23–24 mm and still perifollicular flow is not adequate, trigger is planned and patient may be given a choice of either timed intercourse or IUI after proper explanation about the results.

SECRETORY PHASE ASSESSMENT

Rupture of the follicle leads to formation of corpus luteum. Corpus luteum is responsible for progesterone production. The functional efficacy of the corpus luteum can be assessed by Doppler by assessing the pericorpus luteal vascularity.

Segmental uterine and ovarian artery perfusion demonstrate a significant correlation with histological and hormonal markers of uterine receptivity and may aid in assessment of luteal phase defect.[39] A clear correlation between RI of corpus luteum and plasma progesterone levels has been seen in natural cycle. RI of the corpus luteum can, therefore,

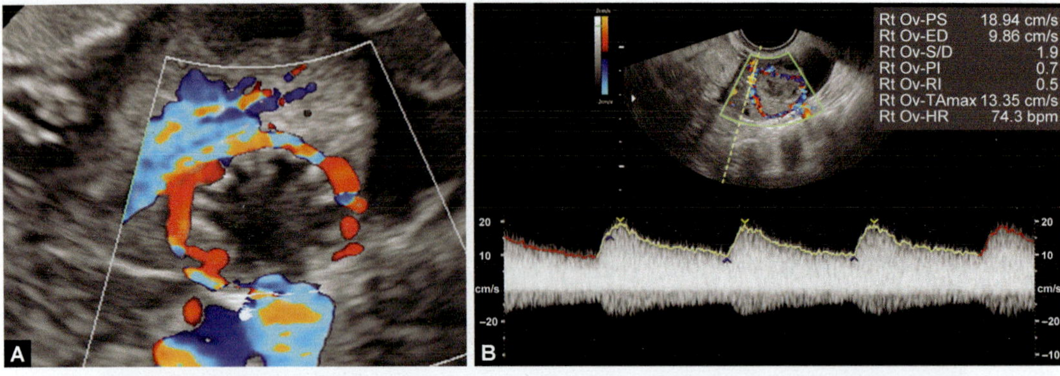

Figs. 17A and B: Normal corpus luteal flow seen on color Doppler and pulse Doppler.

be used as an adjunct to plasma progesterone assay as an index of luteal function.[40]

A corpus luteum that is functionally normal and produces adequate amount of progesterone shows corpus luteal flow: RI 0.35–0.50 and PSV 10–15 cm/s **(Figs. 17A and B)**.

The receptor organ for progesterone also (such as estrogen) is endometrium and its vascular studies can be a reliable clue to adequate progesterone production, though endometrial surface also becomes hyperechoic as a result of progesterone exposure. But, soon after rupture of the follicle, the outer margin of the endometrium starts becoming fluffy and blurred. With adequate progesterone levels that are achieved in the midluteal phase, the spiral arteries show RI of 0.48–0.52 (low resistance flow) and uterine artery shows PI of 2.0–2.5. This PI is lower than in the preovulatory phase because of smooth muscle relaxing effect of progesterone. Inadequate progesterone production and, therefore, corpus luteal inadequacy are suggested by high resistance flow in corpus luteal vessels.[40]

High spiral artery resistance would suggest inadequate response of endometrium to progesterone. This is because of inadequate progesterone receptors in the endometrium or because of local endometrial cause such as endometrial injury or chronic endometritis.

In luteal phase defect because of low progesterone levels, the resistance in the pericorpus luteal vessels is high. Because of low progesterone levels, there is inadequate relaxation of the muscularis of the uterine artery and, therefore, the uterine artery resistance is high along with higher resistance in its branches—the spiral vessels.

Corpus luteal flow and spiral artery flow in normal cycle and luteal phase defect are described in **Tables 2 and 3**.[39]

Secretory scan is especially helpful for pinpointing the cause of failure of treatment and change the protocol, if required in the next cycle, e.g., hCG for luteal support in case of corpus luteal failure, more closer monitoring of the cycle and proper time of

TABLE 2: Corpus luteal Doppler parameters throughout the cycle in normal cases and in LPD.

	Normal	*LPD*
Perifollicular	0.56 ± 0.06	0.58 ± 0.04
LH peak day	0.44 ± 0.04	0.58 ± 0.04
Midluteal phase	0.42 ± 0.06	0.58 ± 0.04
Late luteal phase	0.50 ± 0.04	0.58 ± 0.04

(LH: luteinizing hormone; LPD: luteal phase defect)

TABLE 3: Endometrial Doppler parameters throughout the cycle in normal cases and in LPD.

Phase	*Control RI*	*LPD RI*
Periovulatory	0.53 ± 0.04	0.70 ± 0.06
Midluteal	0.50 ± 0.02	0.72 ± 0.06
Late luteal	0.51 ± 0.04	0.72 ± 0.04

(RI: resistance index; LPD: luteal phase defect)

trigger for luteinized unruptured follicle and modification in the stimulation protocol for inadequate progesterone receptors in endometrium.

CORRELATION OF PROGESTERONE TO ULTRASOUND FINDINGS

Blurring of outer margin of multilayered endometrium suggests initiation of progesterone secretion **(Fig. 18)**.

Fluffiness of outer margins of multilayered endometrium.

Low resistance flow in corpus luteum with echogenic endometrium **(Figs. 19A and B)** and low resistance endometrial vascularity in midluteal phase suggest normal luteal phase.

High resistance corpus luteal flow suggests corpus luteal inadequacy.

High resistance endometrial flow in midluteal phase suggests either inadequate progesterone levels or inadequate progesterone receptors in endometrium.

CONCLUSION

Ultrasound is an excellent tool for assessment of the menstrual cycle. Hormonal changes occurring day-to-day during the menstrual cycle reflect as morphological and vascular changes in the ovary and the uterus. Assessing these changes by transvaginal ultrasound and Doppler and correctly interpreting can explain the hormonal basis of these changes. Ultrasound with Doppler can, thus, be used as the only modality for cycle assessment in patients undergoing ART and may be of help to reduce the cost of the cycle by avoiding certain hormonal assessments and still maintaining close and accurate watch on the hormonal changes occurring during treatment cycle.

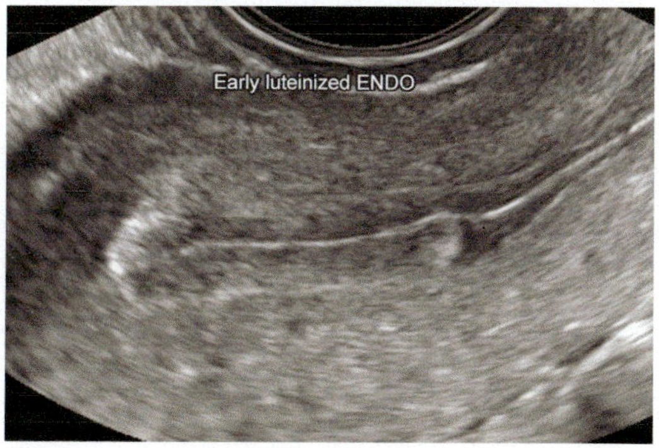

Fig. 18: Endometrium of early luteal phase seen on B-mode ultrasound.

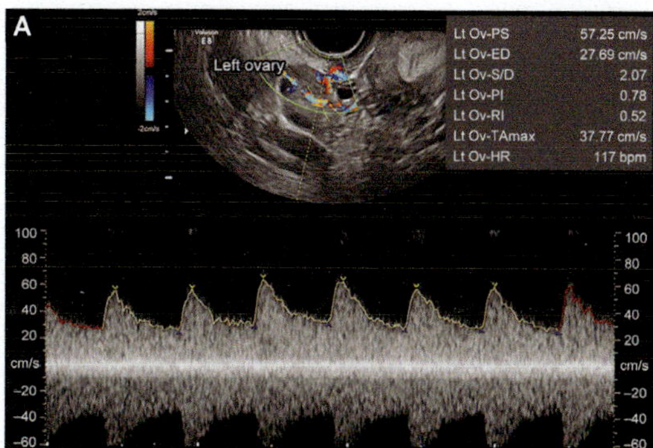

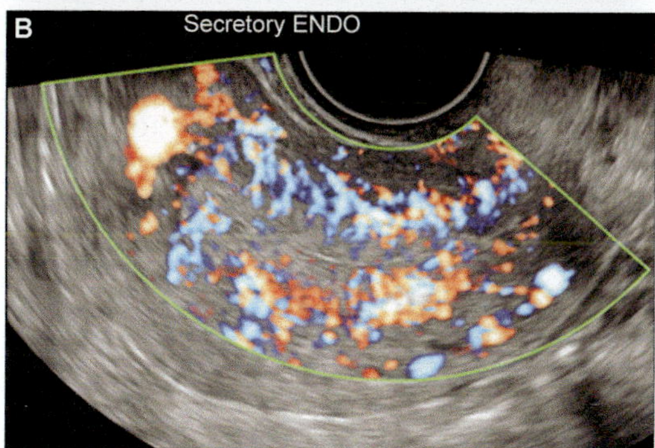

Figs. 19A and B: (A) Low resistance blood flow of the corpus luteum demonstrated on pulse Doppler; (B) High definition (HD) power Doppler showing blood flow in the secretory endometrium.

REFERENCES

1. Hackelöer BJ, Sallam HN. Ultrasound scanning of ovarian follicles. Clin Obstet Gynecol. 1983;10:603-20.
2. Hackelöer BJ, Fleming R, Robinson HP, Adam AH, Coutts JR. Correlation of ultrasonic and endocrinologic assessment of human follicular development. Am J Obstet Gynecol. 1979;135:122-8.
3. Zaidi J, Barber J, Kyei-Mensah A, Bekir J, Campbell S, Tan SL. Relationship of ovarian stromal blood flow at the baseline ultrasound

scan to subsequent follicular response in an in vitro fertilization program. Obstet Gynecol. 1996;88:779-84.

4. Engmann L, Sladkevicius P, Agrawal R, Bekir JS, Campbell S, Tan SL. Value of ovarian stromal blood flow velocity measurement after pituitary suppression in the prediction of ovarian responsiveness and outcome of in vitro fertilization treatment. Fertil Steril. 1999;71:22-9.
5. Luciano GN, Tarek AG. Ultrasonography and IVF. In: Botros RMB (Ed). Ultrasonography in Reproductive Medicine and Infertility. United Kingdom: Cambridge University Press; 2010. pp. 193-201.
6. Jokubkeine L, Sladkevicius P, Rovas L, Valentine L. Assessment of changes in volume and vascularity of ovaries during the normal menstrual cycle using three dimensional power Doppler ultrasound. Hum Reprod. 2006;21:2661-8.
7. Nargund G, Doyle PE, Bourne TH, Parsons JH, Cheng WC, Campbell S, et al. Ultrasound derived indices of follicular blood flow before HCG administration and the prediction of oocyte recovery and preimplantation embryo quality. Hum Reprod. 1996;11:2512-7.
8. Nargund G, Bourne T, Doyle P, Parsons J, Cheng W, Campbell S, et al. Associations between ultrasound indices of follicular blood flow, oocyte recovery and preimplantation embryo quality. Hum Reprod. 1996;11:109-13.
9. Van Blerkom, Antezak M, Schrader R. The developmental potential of human oocyte is related to the dissolved oxygen content of follicular fluid: association with vascular endothelial growth factor levels and perifollicular blood flow characteristics. Hum Reprod. 1997;12:1047-55.
10. Panchal SY, Nagori CB. Pre-hCG 3D and 3D power Doppler assessment of the follicle for improving pregnancy rates in intrauterine insemination cycles. J Hum Reprod Sci. 2009;2:62-7.
11. Panchal SY, Nagori CB. Can 3D power Doppler be a better tool for assessing the pre-HCG follicle and endometrium? A randomized study of 500 cases. Presented at 16th World Congress on Ultrasound in Obstetrics and Gynecology, 2006, London. J Ultrasound Obstet Gynecol. 2006;28:504.
12. Wittmaack FM, Kreger DO, Blasco L, Tureck RW, Mastroianni L, Lessey BA. Effect of follicular size on oocyte retrieval, fertilization, cleavage and embryo quality in in vitro fertilization cycles: a 6-year data collection. Fertil Steril. 1994;62:1205-10.
13. Kyei-Mensah A, Zaidi J, Pittrof R, Shaker A, Campbell S, Tan SL. Transvaginal three-dimensional ultrasound reproducibility of ovarian and endometrial volume measurements. Fertil Steril. 1996;66:718-22.
14. Poehl M, Hohlagschwandtner M, Doerner V, Dillinger B, Feichtinger W. Cumulus assessment by three-dimensional ultrasound for in vitro fertilization. Ultrasound Obstet Gynecol. 2000;16:251-3.
15. Feichtinger W. Transvaginal three-dimensional imaging for evaluation and treatment of infertility. In: Merz E (Ed). Three-dimensional Ultrasound in Obstetrics and Gynecology. Philadelphia: Lippincott Williams & Wilkins; 1998. pp. 37-43.
16. Wu MH, Tsai SJ, Pan HA, Hsiao KY, Chang FM. Three-dimensional power Doppler imaging of ovarian stromal blood flow in women with endometriosis undergoing in vitro fertilization. Ultrasound Obstet Gynecol. 2003;21:480-5.
17. Vlaisavljevic V, Reljic M, Lovrec GV, Zazula D, Sergent N. Measurement of perifollicular blood flow of the dominant preovulatory follicle using three-dimensional power Doppler. Ultrasound Obstet Gynecol. 2003;22:520-6.
18. Merce LT. Ultrasound markers of implantation. Ultrasound Rev Obstet Gynecol. 2002;2:110-23.
19. Merce LT, Barco MJ, Kupesic S, Kurjak A. 2D and 3D power Doppler ultrasound from ovulation to implantation. In: Kurjak A, Chervenak F (Eds). Textbook of Perinatal Medicine. London: Parthenon Publishing; 2005.
20. Kupesic S, Kurjak A. Prediction of IVF outcome by three-dimensional ultrasound. Hum Reprod. 2002;17:950-5.
21. Bourne TH, Jurkovic D, Waterstone J, Campbell S, Collins WP. Intrafollicular blood flow during human ovulation. Ultrasound Obstet Gynecol. 1991;1:53-9.
22. Dickey RP, Olar TT, Taylor SN, Curole DN, Harrigill K. Relationship of biochemical pregnancy to preovulatory endometrial thickness and pattern in patients undergoing ovulation induction. Hum Reprod. 1993;8;327-30.
23. Yagel S, Ben-Chetrit A, Anteby E, Zacut D, Hochner-Celnikier D, Ron M. The effect of ethinyl estradiol on endometrial thickness and uterine volume during ovulation induction by clomiphene citrate. Fertil Steril. 1992;57:33-6.
24. Boue J, Boue A, Lazar P. Retrospective and prospective epidemiological studies of 1,500 karyotyped spontaneous human abortions. Tetralogy. 1973;12:11-26.
25. Smith B, Porter R, Ahuja K, Craft I. Ultrasonic assessment of endometrial changes in stimulated cycles in an in vitro fertilization and embryo transfer program. J In Vitro Fert Embryo Transf. 1984;1:233-8.

26. Applebaum M. The 'steel' or 'teflon' endometrium—ultrasound visualization of endometrial vascularity in IVF patients and outcome. Presented at the Third World Congress of Ultrasound in Obstetrics and Gynecology. Ultrasound Obstet Gynecol. 1993;3:10.
27. Yang JH, Wu MY, Chen CD, Jiang MC, Ho HN, Yang YS. Association of endometrial blood flow as determined by a modified color Doppler technique with subsequent outcome of in vitro fertilization. Hum Reprod. 1999;14:1606-10.
28. Chein LW, Au HK, Chen PL, Xiao J, Tzeng CR. Assessment of uterine receptivity by the endometrial-subendometrial blood flow distribution pattern in women undergoing IVF-ET. Fertil Steril. 2002;78:245-51.
29. Nagori C, Panchal S. Endometrial vascularity: its relation to implantation rates. Int J Infertil Fetal Med. 2012;3:48-50.
30. Zaidi J, Campbell S, Pittrof R, Tan SL. Endometrial thickness, morphology, vascular penetration and velocimetry in predicting implantation in an in vitro fertilization program. Ultrasound Obstet Gynecol. 1995;6:191-8.
31. Merce LT, Barco MJ, Bau S, Troyano JM. Prediction of ovarian response and IVF/ICSI outcome by three-dimensional ultrasonography and power Doppler angiography. Eur J Obstet Gynecol Reprod Biol. 2007;132:93-100.
32. Merce LT, Barco MJ, Bau S, Troyano JM. Are endometrial parameters by three-dimensional ultrasound and power Doppler angiography related to in vitro fertilization/embryo transfer outcome? Fertil Steril. 2008;89:111-7.
33. Kupesic S, Bekavac I, Bjelos D, Kurjak A. Assessment of endometrial receptivity by transvaginal color Doppler and three-dimensional power Doppler ultrasonography in patients undergoing in vitro fertilization procedures. J Ultrasound Med. 2001;20:125-34.
34. Steer CV, Campbell S, Tan SL, Crayford T, Mills C, Mason BA, et al. The use of transvaginal color flow imaging after in vitro fertilization to identify optimum uterine conditions before embryo transfer. Fertil Steril. 1992;57:372-6.
35. Zaidi J, Pittrof R, Shaker A, Kyei-Mensah A, Campbell S, Tan SL. Assessment of uterine artery blood flow on the day of human chorionic gonadotropin administration by transvaginal color Doppler ultrasound in an in vitro fertilization program. Fertil Steril. 1996;65: 377-81.
36. Coulam CB, Stern JJ, Soenksen DM, Britten S, Bustillo M. Comparison of pulsatility indexes on the day of oocyte retrieval and embryo transfer. Hum Reprod. 1995;10:82-4.
37. Cacciatore B, Simberg N, Fusaro P, Tiitinen A. Transvaginal Doppler study of uterine artery blood flow in in vitro fertilization embryo transfer cycles. Fertil Steril. 1996;66:130-4.
38. Raga F, Bonilla-Musoles F, Casan EM, Klein O, Bonilla F. Assessment of endometrial volume by three-dimensional ultrasound prior to embryo transfer: clues to endometrial receptivity. Hum Reprod. 1999;14:2851-4.
39. Kupesić S, Kurjak A, Vujisić S, Petrović Z. Luteal phase defect: comparison between Doppler velocimetry, histological and hormonal markers. Ultrasound Obstet Gynecol. 1997;9:105-12.
40. Glock JL, Brumsted JR. Color flow pulsed Doppler ultrasound in diagnosing luteal phase defect. Fertil Steril. 1995;64:500-4.

33
CHAPTER

Ultrasound-guided Procedures in Assisted Reproduction

Sonal Panchal, Chaitanya Nagori

INTRODUCTION

Ultrasound has proved to be a unique noninvasive modality for diagnosis and management of subfertility and also as an aid to therapeutic procedures. Technology advancement in ultrasound has made it a modality of choice for management of subfertile patients. Moreover, ultrasound has been found to be safe for its use in peri-implantation period and early pregnancy.

The procedures in which ultrasound is being used as a guiding tool in gynecology and subfertility scenario are:

- Oocyte retrieval (OR)
- Embryo transfer (ET)
- Cyst aspiration
- Hydrosalpinx aspiration
- Aspiration of ascitic fluid in ovarian hyperstimulation syndrome (OHSS)
- Multifetal pregnancy reduction.

OOCYTE RETRIEVAL

Oocyte retrieval (OR) was done by laparotomy first and then by laparoscopy for first 10 years after the development of in vitro fertilization (IVF). Lenz and colleagues first described percutaneous transabdominal (TA)/transvesical aspiration of follicles under ultrasound guidance in 1981.[1] In 1982, transvaginal (TV) OR with TA ultrasound guidance was described.[2] TV ovum retrieval with TV ultrasound guidance with mechanical TV sector scanner was first described by Kemeter and Feichtinger in the late 1980s.[3] This was a major breakthrough in IVF treatment and was soon universally accepted. TV OR is a very simple and well-accepted method with very low complication rate.

Method

Preprocedure

Patient is asked to remain nil by mouth for ≥6–8 h. While there is no evidence that routine antibiotics reduce the risk of infection, administration of an intravenous bolus of antibiotics is generally recommended for women with history of severe pelvic inflammatory disease or if there is a risk of an endometrioma being punctured during the procedure. However, in certain units especially in the Indian subcontinent, antibiotics are routinely administered.

Premedication and Anesthesia

It is important to provide effective anesthesia and analgesia for TV OR as it is painful. No technique of anesthesia, analgesia, or sedation is free from side effects. Whatever technique is used, recognized standards of practice should be adhered to and all IVF professionals should follow the safe practice of administering sedative drugs. As little as possible should be the rule for any drugs used. Conscious sedation should be offered to all women having the procedure as it is safe and acceptable method of providing analgesia. Though there are centers that prefer only sedation for ovum pickup, in most centers, short general anesthesia is preferred **(Box 1)**. Intravenous fentanyl, propofol, and midazolam are the commonly used medications and are believed not to affect the outcome of IVF. Paracervical or preovarian blocks are also feasible options.

BOX 1: Ovum pickup.

- IV general anesthesia or local anesthesia and sedation
- Consider antibiotic cover
- Aseptic technique is a must
- Lithotomy position of the patient, clean and drape
- Cleanse TV probe and cover with sterile cover and condom with or without gel
- Set biopsy guideline on scanner and fix the biopsy guide on the probe
- Introduce the probe to image the ovary in alignment with the biopsy line
- Introduce the pickup needle through fornix
- Apply suction as the follicle is punctured
- Aspirate all follicles one after the other and repeat for the other ovary
- Remove probe and check for bleeding

For paracervical blocks, a local anesthetic agent is injected into 2–6 sites at a depth of 3–7 mm alongside the vaginal portion of the cervix in the vaginal fornices. Local anesthesia is not commonly used as it does not provide effective analgesia. Some centers have also used hypnotism for analgesia.

Technique

All sterile precautions are taken with washing hands and wearing a sterile gown. It is best to use powder-free sterile gloves. The trolley for the procedure is prepared. It should contain surgical instruments for painting and draping. Along with that, a Sims speculum, an anterior retractor, and an Alyce forceps are required in cases of unexpected bleeding or minor complications. The disposables include a sterilized probe cover and a sterilized condom without spermicidal gel. A biopsy guide is absolutely essential. Vagina is cleaned thoroughly with normal saline. No antiseptics are to be used. Some units use culture medium to cleanse the vagina. It is essential to clean the probe with the special probe cleansing solutions provided by the manufacturers before the procedure. The ultrasound transducer is enclosed in a special sterile probe cover or a plastic sleeve and then by sterile gel free condom with ultrasound gel or saline inside, prior to insertion into the vagina. The probe should be thoroughly cleaned with a damp cloth after each procedure. The biopsy guide is fixed on the probe (**Fig. 1**). Place the probe in the vagina to assess the endometrial thickness, position and accessibility of the ovaries and the number of follicles to be aspirated once the patient is anesthetized. Switch on the biopsy guide on the screen. The guide helps to identify the position of the needle and the path it will take when the needle is advanced through the vaginal fornix into the ovary. The transducer should be positioned so that the ovaries are placed closest possible to the needle tip. Oocyte pick up needle is then introduced through the needle guide to puncture the vaginal wall, through to reach the ovary. The needle and tubing are flushed with the culture media before introduction. Transducer is then manipulated to bring the follicles one after the other on the biopsy guideline with minimum possible probe movement. This is to minimize the damage to the ovarian stroma.

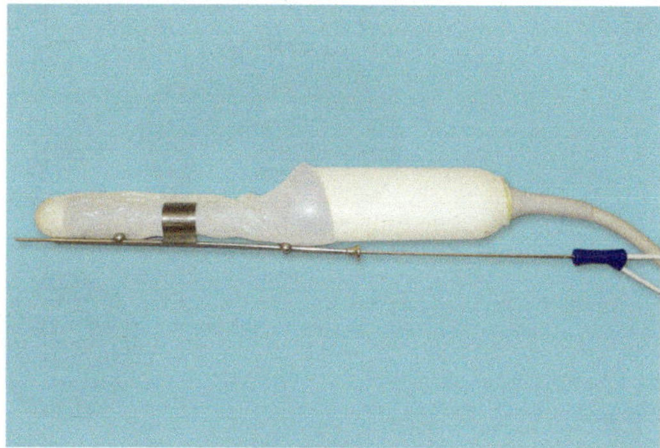

Fig. 1: Vaginal ultrasound transducer covered with sterile condom with needle guide attached. The needle tip is protruding from the proximal end of the probe.

Several designs of aspiration needles are available (**Figs. 2A and B**). They may have a single or double lumen to enable aspiration and flushing through different routes. The needle is usually 18–20 gage and must have a very sharp tip to enable easy puncture of mobile ovaries and its distal 2 cm

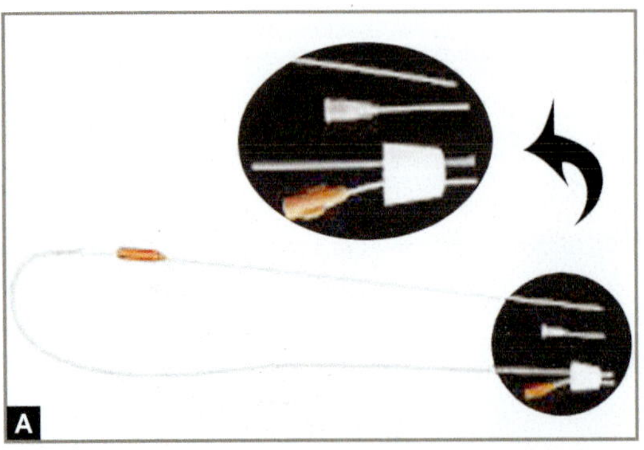

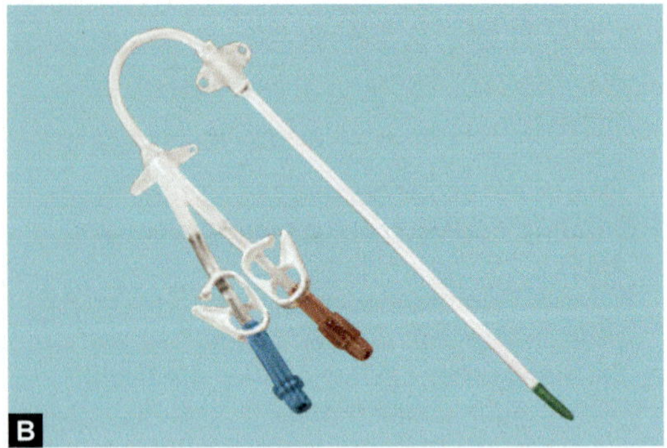

Figs. 2A and B: (A) Single-lumen ovum pickup needle with the connections in the cock to fit into the test tube and to be attached to the suction machine; (B) Double-lumen suction catheter for ovum pickup.

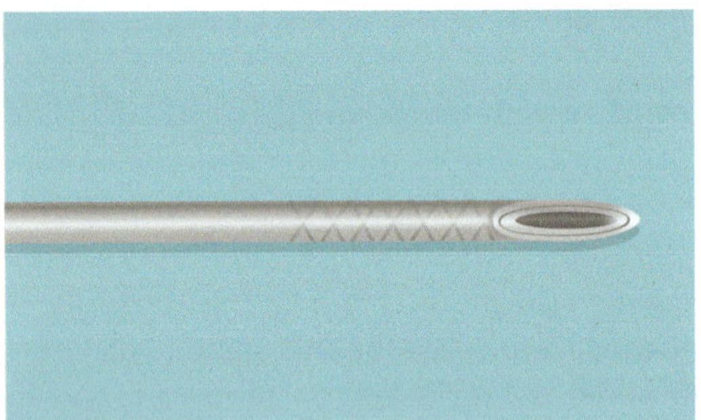

Fig. 3: Needle tip of the ovum pickup needle. The markings close to the tip make the surface rough and therefore make the needle easily visible on ultrasound.

should be roughened to enhance ultrasound visualization (**Fig. 3**). The needle is connected to a test tube, prewarmed at 37°C in hot blocks, by tubing and suction is applied either with a foot-operated pump (**Fig. 4**) or manually. Several culture media are available. One with heparin is used for this purpose. This prevents clotting of blood in the tubing that may be aspirated along with the follicular fluid. Needle is advanced from the vagina into the ovary under vision.

Needle path is usually at 2 o'clock position for puncturing the left ovary, and 10 o'clock position for left ovary in the vagina, lateral to the cervix (**Fig. 5**). But when ovaries are fixed or positioned high up in the pelvis, the path may have to be changed. If possible, the follicle should be punctured from the side of the ovary, then entering each follicle systematically with an aim to induce minimal damage to the ovary. As far as possible only single vaginal puncture with one or two ovarian punctures maximum should be done on each side. This approach reduces the risk of bleeding. Entering the ovary may be difficult in an ovary with very few follicles. In such cases, ovaries are very mobile and then pressure on the abdomen may be required to fix the ovaries. Find the nearest leading follicle and then needle must be advanced firmly and quickly into the follicle. Negative pressure is applied soon as the needle tip pierces the follicle. But the entry of the needle should be quick and with a controlled firm thrust as it has a long bevel and unless the entire bevel is not inside the follicle lumen, there is a risk of loosing the ovum. Negative pressure of 110–120 mm Hg is required. Confirm that you are puncturing the follicle and, not the vessel by manipulating the probe to view the follicle in sagittal and transverse plane if required and, if in doubt, use Doppler.

Gentle rotation of the needle helps to suck the ovum if stuck, from all the walls of the follicle. Contents are aspirated till the follicle is empty. The next follicle is entered without withdrawing the needle out of the ovary if it is in the same needle path. Keep needle in the ovary and aspirate several follicles one after another with careful gentle manipulation. The order of aspiration of different follicles should be such that the needle manipulation is the

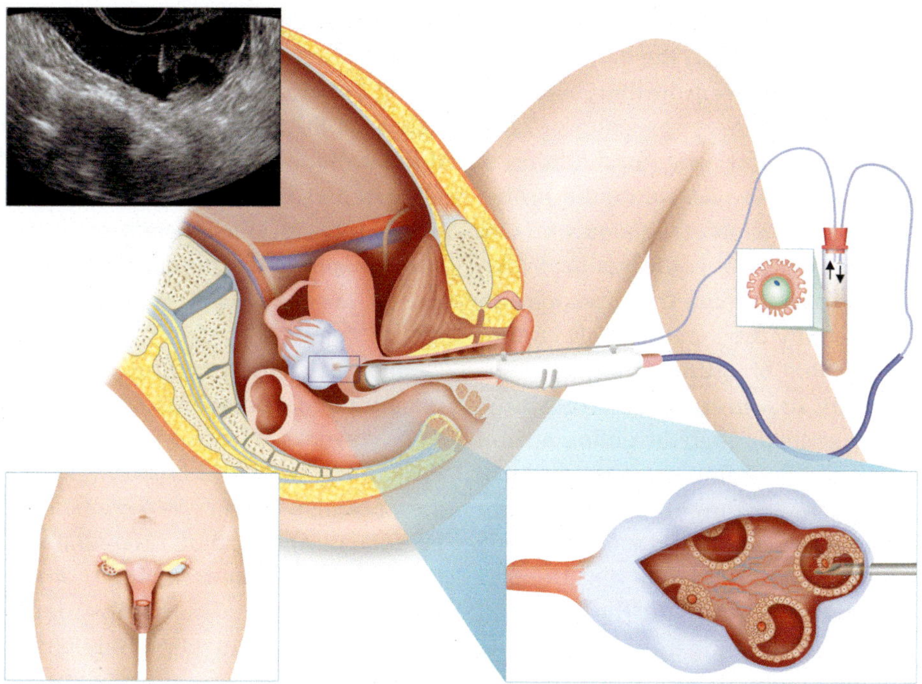

Fig. 4: Follicle aspiration equipment: An assembled follicle aspiration single-lumen needle connected to a test tube. The test tube is, in turn, connected to a suction pump. The needle is attached to the transvaginal ultrasound transducer through needle guide and bracket.

least. Follicular flushing was recommended earlier in the belief that it may improve the oocyte yield, although this may not improve the number of oocytes retrieved but increases the duration of retrieval and postoperative pain.[4,5] Flushing is recommended only if there are very few follicles and especially when the cumulus has been demonstrated in the follicle on pre-hCG scan (**Fig. 6**). All follicles till 10–12 mm size are aspirated as at times even a 10-mm sized follicle may retrieve a fertilizable follicle in aspirate. Bowels in the path of the needle can be removed by rotating and pushing movements of the probe. At times, the ovaries

Uterus
Ovary
Follicle
Egg
Vagina
Ultrasound probe
Needle passes through vaginal wall and into follicle to retrieve egg

Fig. 5: Diagram showing the needle path during ovum pickup from its site of entry from the vaginal walls to its entry into the ovary.

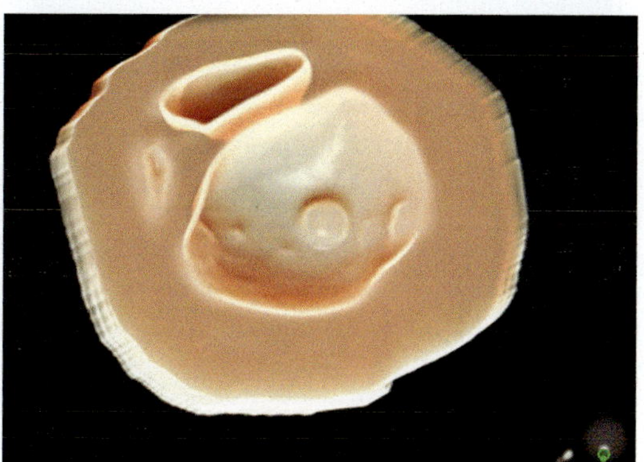

Fig. 6: 3D ultrasound picture showing a small elevation on the follicle wall, this is cumulus.

may not be accessible and rarely one may have to pass the needle through the uterus, but in such cases, one needs to ensure that vessels are avoided. Vessels on transverse section look like a follicle, and therefore when in doubt, look for pulsatility of the walls, rotate the probe, and the vessels will show elongation, and one may also use Doppler for confirmation. When the needle passes through the myometrium or cervix, piercing the small vessels cannot be avoided. This bleeding though is self-controlled by myometrial contractions. Passing the needle through the endometrium is nest avoided. After completing aspiration of all the follicles, repeat the entire procedure for the opposite ovary, confirm no active bleeding and excessive fluid in the pouch of Douglas and then remove the probe. Put the speculum and check for the bleeding from the puncture site. If required, apply pressure with a sterilized gauze for a few minutes to stop bleeding. Rarely, a vaginal pack may be required for a few minutes to control bleeding. Sometimes bleeding from the ovaries may be seen after the procedure. This usually is self-controlled.

It is best not to puncture hydrosalpinx (**Fig. 7A**) or endometriomas (**Fig. 7B**), if present, while doing OR. However, if a hydrosalpinx or an endometrioma is punctured inadvertently, prophylactic antibiotic preferably intravenous, must be administered. TA route of ultrasound guidance and puncture may be needed rarely for OR, when ovary is not approachable from vaginal route, if it is placed high up in the pelvis, as in patients with absent uterus, or if the patient has had vaginoplasty. Though none of these are absolute indications for TA oocyte retrieval as it depends on the operators' convenience and expertise for TV approach.

Complications

Generally, very few technical difficulties are encountered during vaginal egg collections. The main risks of TV oocyte recovery are pelvic infection (0.6%) and bleeding (>100 mL in 0.8% cases), which may be serious, sometimes even fatal. Appropriate preoperative vaginal preparation and minimizing the number of repeated vaginal penetrations may serve to lower the risk of infection. While there is no evidence that routine antibiotics reduce the risk of infection, the administration of an intravenous bolus of antibiotics is generally recommended to women with history of severe pelvic inflammatory disease or if an endometrioma or hydrosalpinx is punctured. Intestinal, vascular, uterine, and tubal injuries with the aspiration needle have also been reported. Bleeding and infections may be serious, sometimes, even fatal complications.

Ovaries are located close to the iliac vessels, and therefore iliac vessels are vulnerable to

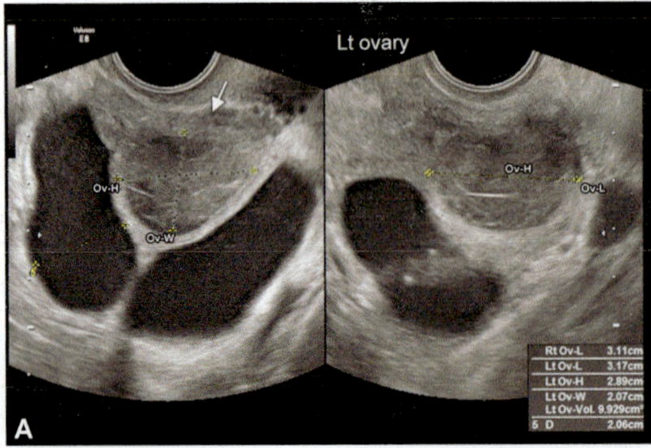

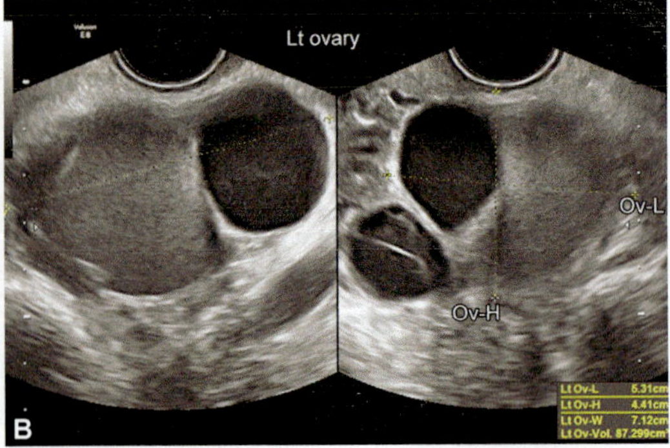

Figs. 7A and B: (A) B-mode ultrasound image of an ovary containing corpus luteum (arrow) and an anechoic sausage-shaped lesion surrounding it from below, which is a hydrosalpinx; (B) B-mode ultrasound image of ovary showing two cystic structures—one which is anechoic appears to be a follicle and the other with low-level echogenicities is most likely an endometrioma.

injury during ovum pickup by inexperienced hands. While bleeding from major vessel is a very rare occurrence in experienced hands, care must always be taken when aspirating the follicles that are close to major vessels (internal iliac vessels). It is, therefore, always safe to rotate the probe and observe for elongation of any rounded cystic structure, especially when this structure is on the deeper surface of the ovary. If elongation is seen, it is likely to be vessel and then should not be punctured. Another possible site of bleeding is from the vaginal wall. This is especially common when there is congestion of the vaginal wall. This bleeding is never severe, though may be frightening for the patient. It stops by manual pressure on the bleeding site for a few minutes or by tamponing. The third possible site from where the bleeding would occur is uterine vessels. This happens when the ovary is adherent to the uterus and placed high up in the pelvis. This can be prevented by carefully managing the needle path.

EMBRYO TRANSFER

Embryo transfer is a critical step in determining the final outcome of IVF treatment. Though evidently simple, this procedure demands a lot of perfection and precision. It is a true blend of science and art. Optimizing the technique of ET would provide the best chance of pregnancy. Ultrasound guidance in this procedure has shown advantage over clinical touch or blind ET. It has been proved that ultrasound-guided transfer significantly increases the chance of embryo implantation, ongoing pregnancy, and live birth and to improve the ease of transfer.[6,7]

Transabdominal ultrasonographic guidance is used to determine the precise depth of embryo placement within the uterus. The tip of the catheter is placed approximately 1-1.5 cm caudal to the uterine fundus, so that the embryo/s are deposited gently into the midcavity of the uterus. Apart from the depth of the uterine cavity, the curvature of uterine cavity, angle between cervix and endometrial cavity may also be visualized by ultrasound, and the angle of ET cannula may be accordingly adjusted to make the transfer easy. When the cervical canal appears curved or there is an acute angle between cervix and uterus, double-sheathed catheter or a catheter with stylet is recommended. Use of stylet under ultrasound guidance to negotiate difficult cervical passage makes ET easy and less traumatic.[8] Uterine contractions, expulsion of embryos, blood or mucus on the catheter tip, bacterial contamination of catheter, and retained embryos have all been associated with difficult ETs and also decrease the chances of conception.

Conventionally embryos were transfered on day two or three post-insemination, when the embryos are usually 2–8-cell stage of cleavage (**Figs. 8A to F**). With improvements in culture media, there is an increasing tendency for delaying ET with an aim to improve the implantation rates. While there is no improvement in live birth rates (1.07, 95% CI 0.84–1.37) with delaying ET from day 2 to day 3, transfer of embryos at blastocyst stage (day 5/6) has shown significant increase in live birth rate (OR 1.35, 95% CI 1.05–1.74) when compared with day 2–3 transfers.[9] It is a more physiological approach, allowing synchronization of the embryo with the

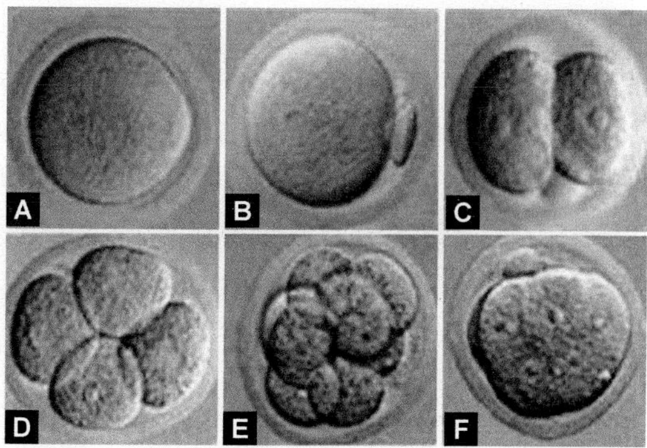

Figs. 8A to F: Development of the embryo in early stages: (A) Ovum; (B) Polar body stage; (C) Two-cell stage; (D) Four-cell stage of embryo; (E) Eight-cell embryo; (F) Blastocyst.

endometrium and the selection of viable and better embryos for transfer. These are the probable reasons for better results. However, the rates of embryos freezing are lower, and the treatment cancellation rates are higher with blastocyst transfer. The reason for this is that only the best embryos may grow to blastocyst in the laboratory. But in selected group of couples, the practice of blastocyst transfer has the potential to favor single ET without compromising the overall success rates but can significantly reduce the occurrence of multiple pregnancies. Blastocyst transfer may be a better option for the patients in whom more embryos are formed, as the cycle cancellation rate is decreased.

Technique (Figs. 9A to E)

Pretransfer ultrasound is done to check uterocervical curvature and uterocervical length. Asepsis is very essential. Patient lies in lithotomy position. Vagina is cleaned with warm normal saline. Gauze soaked in normal saline is used to wipe off all the vaginal secretions. Cusco's speculum is commonly used to visualize the cervix with minimal manipulation of cervix and uterus. Some units use Sims speculum and Ellis forceps

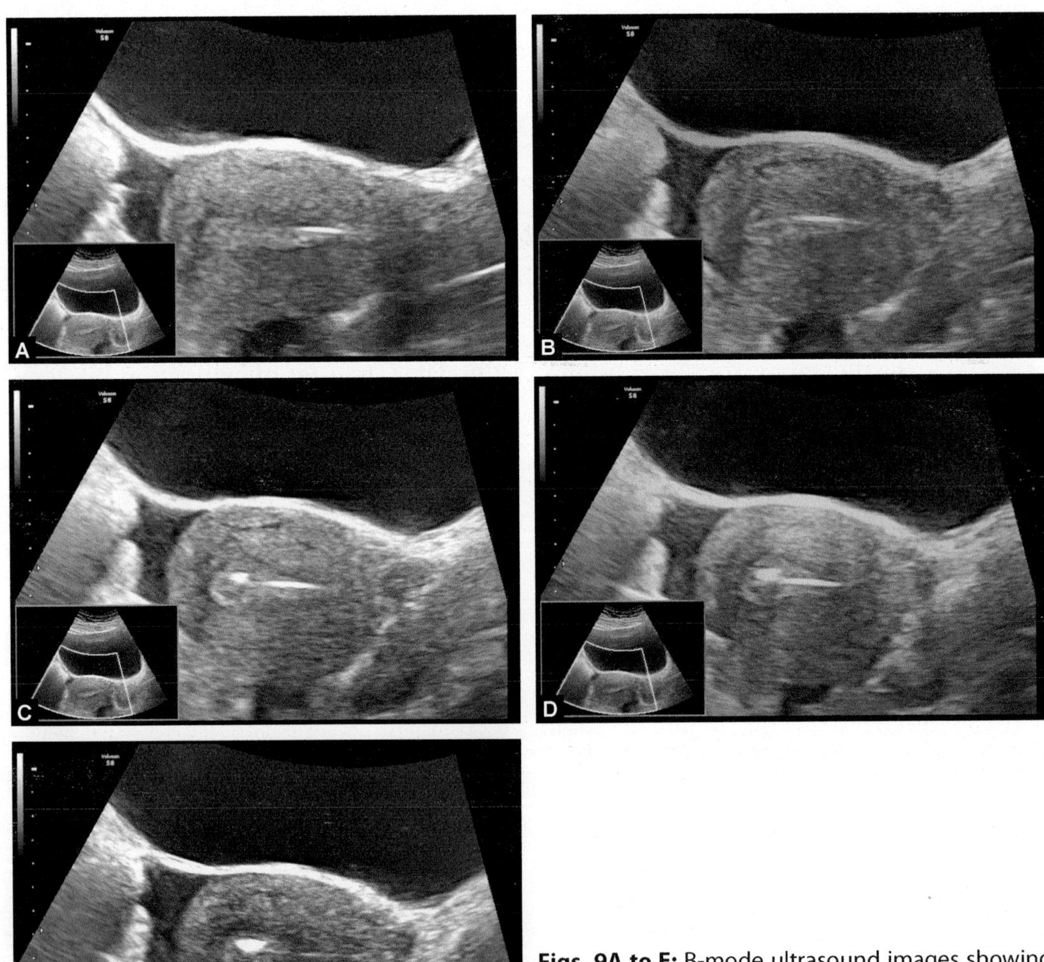

Figs. 9A to E: B-mode ultrasound images showing progression of the embryo transfer catheter and release of embryo with air bubble in the uterus demonstrated as progress of the procedure from A to E.

or tenaculum to visualize and stabilize the cervix. With this approach, the uterocervical angle is straightened to make the ET easier. Though Cusco's speculum is commonly recommended, the passage of catheter is much easier when Sims speculum is used. However, it has been reported that this may lead to uterine contractions and may expel out the embryos and compromise the treatment outcome. But it is important to remember, on the other hand, that if the transfer is difficult, chance of implantation may be compromised. Sims speculum does help in a smooth passage of the ET catheter and may not compromise the conception rates.

Soft catheters are preferred over rigid ones as these are less likely to traumatize the cervix and endometrium and to invoke any uterine contractions. The commonly used soft catheters (Wallace) have a softer inner cannula and a stiffer outer sheath (**Fig. 10**). Occasionally, resistance to pass the soft inner cannula into the uterus usually at the level of internal os is encountered, and in these cases, the stiffer outer sheath is advanced in the cervical canal to negotiate the resistance at the internal os, and the inner cannula can then be advanced into the uterine cavity. A firmer malleable catheter with a stylet and an outer sheath is another option in difficult cases (**Fig. 11**), where the catheter is advanced up to the level of the internal os. The inner stylet is then removed, and the softer cannula with embryos loaded is fed through the outer

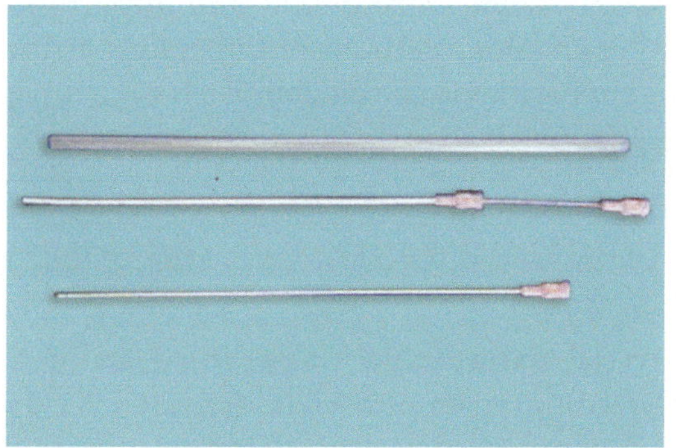

Fig. 10: Single-sheathed (lower most) and double-sheathed (the middle one) embryo transfer catheters.

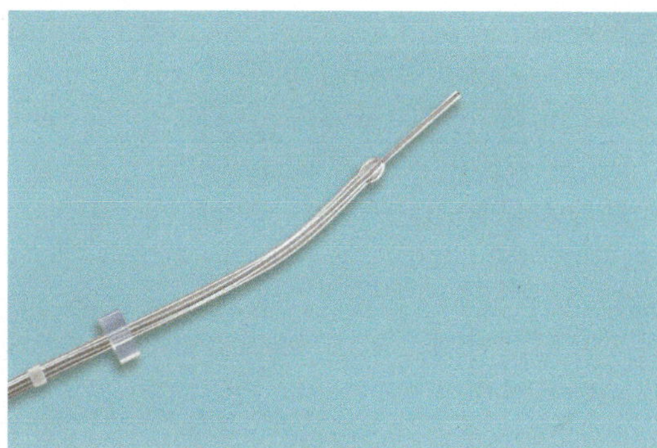

Fig. 11: Embryo transfer catheter with outer stiff, but malleable sheath and inner very thin and non-traumatic catheter.

sheath to be advanced into the uterine cavity for transfer. The outer sheath or the malleable catheter should never be advanced beyond the internal os.

Embryo-loaded catheter is brought to the transfer room only when everything is set. Keep the theater lights dimmed when loaded ET catheter is brought to the ET theater. Introduce the transfer catheter into the cervix, under TA ultrasound guidance. If uterocervical canal on pretransfer ultrasound is not straight, one may electively use a stiff outer sheath or a cervical cannula for introduction of the transfer catheter through it as discussed earlier. In any case, the embryo is not retained in the catheter for >2 min. If it takes longer, the embryos are replaced back into the culture dish and reloaded later. Double-sheathed embryo-transfer catheter is to be used in such cases. After introducing the outer sheath, which is firm in consistency, its position is confirmed beyond the internal os. The inner cannula is introduced through this sheath later on. Cannula tip is kept 1–1.5 cm away from the tip of the endometrial cavity (**Fig. 12**). Embryos in the catheter are loaded in 15–25 μL of medium. Volumes of 50 μL or larger lead to lower pregnancy rates, as this fluid may either flow out of the uterus or may fill up the tubes. Once the cannula is introduced to the desired level in the uterus, the piston of the syringe is pushed to introduce the desired amount of fluid containing embryos into the uterus.

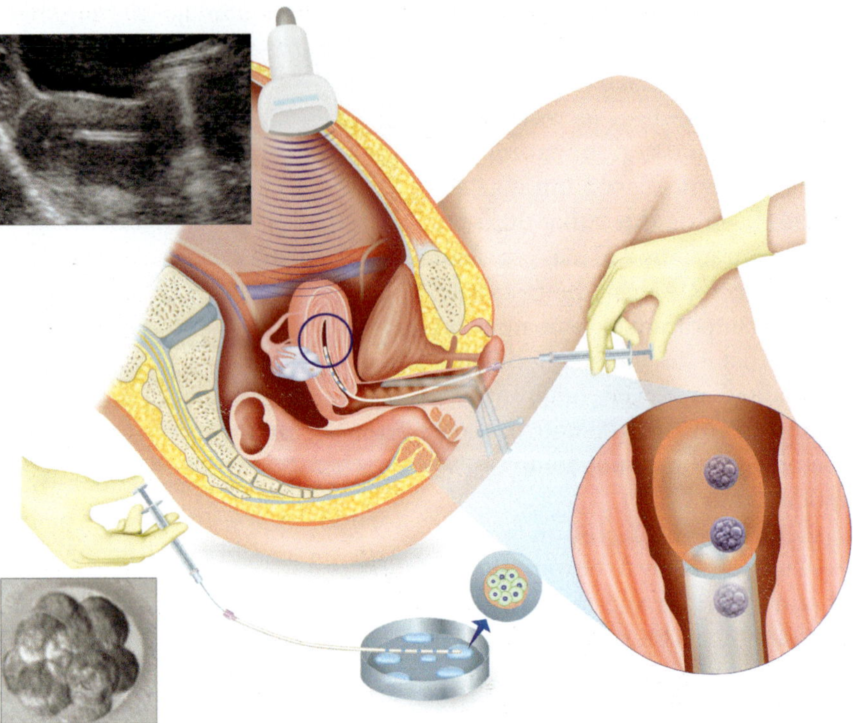

Fig. 12: Diagrammatic presentation of ultrasound-guided embryo transfer.

The ET cannula is seen as an echogenic line and can be traced from the internal os into the endometrial cavity, and when the tip is placed ≥1 cm proximal to the fundal end of the endometrium, the passage of embryos with the air bubble is seen as a release of echogenic spot into the endometrial cavity and is also known as "bullet sign" (**Fig. 8E**). Then the cannula is steadily held in position for a few seconds. After that it is gently pulled out with the piston pressed not to cause a suction action. Fluid remaining in the cannula is checked under the microscope to confirm that embryos are not stuck and held up in the cannula. Patient may be gently shifted into the bed and allowed to rest for 15–30 minutes. Success rates are similar regardless of the time for which the patient is kept motionless.

Bleeding at the time of the transfer may adversely affect the embryos. In difficult transcervical transfers, either transfer under anesthesia, or a surgical transfer transfundally under laparoscopic guidance may be done.

Variables affecting implantation rates and success of ET are:

- Ease of transfer
- Presence of blood or mucus on transfer catheter
- Type of catheter used
- Catheter loading
- Technique of transfer
- Uterine depth and precise depth of ET in uterine cavity
- Avoiding uterine contractions
- Physician's experience and physician's perception of transfer difficulty was the most important variable.[10]

Variations in Embryo Transfer Technique (Box 2)

Ultrasound-guided Instead of Clinical Touch Method

In an exhaustive Cochrane Database Systematic Review that included 13/15 randomized controlled trials only, Brown et al.,[6] reported significantly higher live birth/

BOX 2: Steps to optimize embryo transfer.

- Pretransfer assessment of uterine cavity and cervical canal
- Gentle removal of cervical mucus if abundant
- Avoid touching the endometrium to:
  - Avoid cervical bleeding
  - Avoid endometrial damage
  - Avoid initiation of uterine contractions
- Confirm proper delivery of embryos inside the uterine cavity, this can be done by:
  - Confirming the location of catheter tip
  - Visualize the easy passage of drop of media containing embryos followed by air bubble in the endometrial cavity

ongoing pregnancies per woman randomized associated with USG-ET (ultrasound-guided ET) (452/1,376 compared with 353/1,338 for clinical touch; odds ratio 1.40; 95% confidence interval (CI) 1.18–1.66; ($p < 0.001$) in six studies. This suggested that a population of women with 25% chance of pregnancy using clinical touch would be increased to 32% (28–46%) using USG-ET. Ultrasound guidance for ET is therefore recommended.

Ultrasound-guided ET enables the visualization of:[11]

- Guiding cannula and transfer catheter placement in relation to the endometrial surface and uterine fundus during ET
- The position and movement of a air bubble transfered with the embryo
- The impact of subendometrial myometrial contractions leading to endometrial movement.

Studies have shown that no significant changes in results have been observed whether TA or TV ultrasound is used for guidance.[11] However, TA ultrasound is preferred as it does not interfere with the TV/transcervical procedure of ET.

Advantages of ultrasound-guided ET:

- Helps placement of soft catheters
- Confirms the position of catheter tip
- Allows to guide the direction of the catheter along the contour of the endometrial cavity especially in uteri with acute curves
- Prevents damage to endometrium and plugging of catheter
- Full bladder that is required for TA ultrasound, straightens the uterocervical angle and helps catheter passage
- Helps to negotiate the catheter through difficult cervical canal.

Catheter Types

Catheters with echogenic tips are better appreciated on ultrasound guidance and therefore reduce the time taken from loading the catheter to depositing the embryos in endometrial cavity. Coaxial catheter system has been preferred by some and has been claimed to be of help in difficult transfers. But in a prospective randomized study of 251 patients, no significant change was found in implantation rate, clinical pregnancy rate, or ongoing pregnancy rate between the two catheters.[12] Another group compared soft catheters and catheters with echogenic tip and concluded that catheters with echogenic tip simplify the ET and also improve implantation rates.[13]

Transfer at the Point of Maximal Implantation Potential

A large observational retrospective study by Gergely et al., has shown that if point of maximum implantation potential (MIP) is individually found in each patient by the help of 3D ultrasound and embryos are deposited at this point, it can improve the implantation rates.[14] Point of MIP can be calculated by 3D ultrasound. On coronal section of the uterus, two lines are drawn, one on each side parallel to the cornu. The point at which these lines intersect is the point of maxi mal implantation potential (**Figs. 13A and B**).

CYST ASPIRATIONS

Cysts in the ovary before starting stimulation are not desired and may delay or cancel stimulation. Follicular or simple cysts (**Fig. 14**)

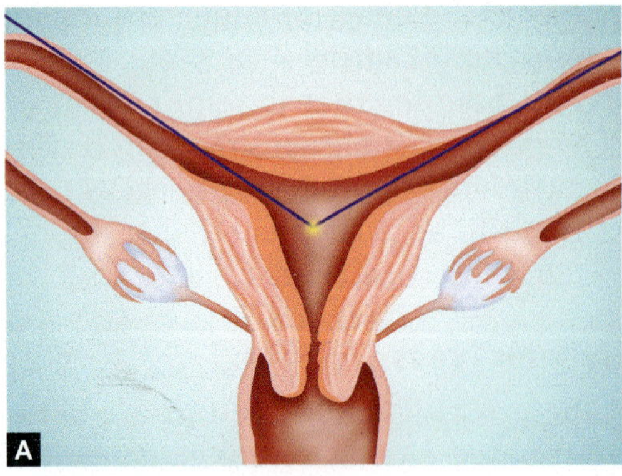

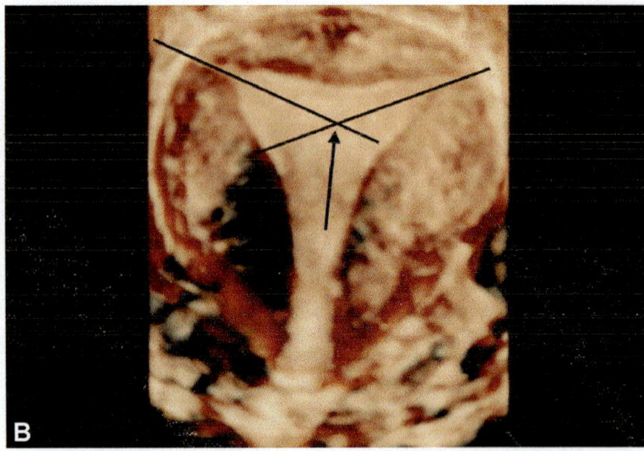

Figs. 13A and B: (A) Diagrammatic presentation of how to calculate the point of maximum implantation potential; (B) 3D ultrasound image of coronal section of uterus with lines showing calculation of point of maximum implantation potential where the two lines passing through the cornu and cutting across perpendicularly cross each other.

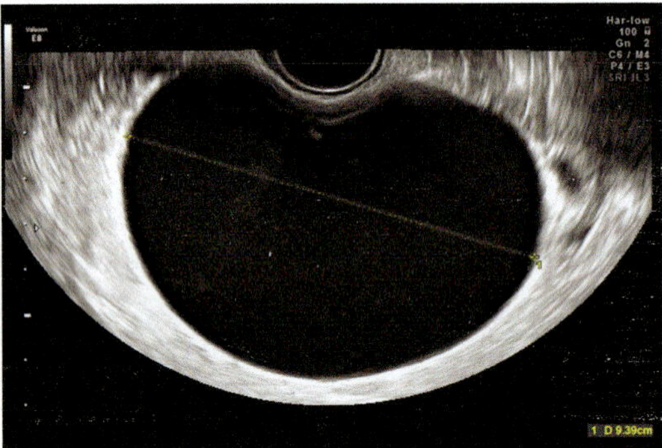

Fig. 14: B-mode ultrasound image of thin-walled anechoic ovarian cyst.

BOX 3: Cyst-aspiration technique.

- Lithotomy position for patient with empty bladder
- Cleanse and drape parts including vagina with antiseptic solution
- TV probe is cleansed and covered with a sterile probe cover
- Biopsy guide is attached and long 17–20 gage needle is attached with teflon tubing to suction pump, is introduced into the cyst
- Aspiration is done till the cyst is empty
- Remove needle and check for bleeding

of the ovaries can be aspirated transvaginally under ultrasound guidance. Cysts with internal echogenicities should not be aspirated under ultrasound guidance. These are treated by laparoscopic procedures as these are usually not simple cysts.

Procedure

A thorough ultrasound evaluation and diagnosis must be done before planning the procedure. It is done in the operation theater. Proper asepsis is to be maintained. Patient is positioned in lithotomy-like position or the same position in which TV scans are done. Short general anesthesia with propofol or local paracervical block with sedation may be used depending on operator's comfort and patient's cooperation (**Box 3**).

We usually prefer a 5–9 MHz TV probe with the biopsy attachment. The probe is thoroughly cleaned and disinfected. The disinfectants used depend on the manufacturer's recommendations. Probe is then covered with a sterile probe cover. Jelly is put on the probe, and the probe is covered with a sterile condom. The biopsy guide is attached to the probe 17–20 gauge long needle with Teflon tubing is used. The tubing is attached to the aspiration (suction pump). When all the fluid is aspirated and the cyst is empty, the needle is removed. Scan is done to rule out any bleed or fluid collection in pelvis. Perioperative antibiotics are given generally. Usually, postoperative pain is very little but, if required, analgesics may be given. Sclerosant agents may be injected in the cyst immediately after aspiration. But this is usually preferred in patients with recurrence of the cyst after aspiration.

ASPIRATION OF HYDROSALPINX

It has been proved beyond doubts in several studies that hydrosalpinx (**Fig. 15**) has a negative impact on IVF outcome.[15] This is due to the toxic effect of infected tubal fluid on the implanting embryo. This is why hydrosalpinx needs to be managed before ET. Salpingectomy or tubal ligation/clipping has been used as surgical therapy for hydrosalpinx in patients with subfertility. Ultrasound-guided TV aspiration has also been recommended as a treatment option to remove hydrosalpingeal fluid. Fluid would reaccumulate if the procedure is done before starting stimulation. Because of fast refilling tendency, hydrosalpinx aspiration is not a therapy of choice, generally. However, many times, hydrosalpinx may be diagnosed on ultrasound scan, while undergoing ovarian stimulation, and in these cases, hydrosalpinx aspiration can be offered and performed immediately after OR. Clinical pregnancy rates for aspiration versus control groups were 31.3% and 17.6%, respectively, in a small study.[16] The procedure is same as that for cyst aspiration.

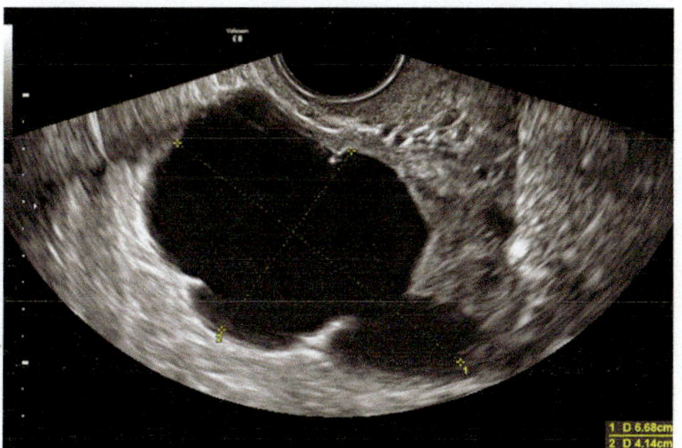

Fig. 15: B-mode ultrasound image of anechoic adnexal cystic lesion with incomplete septae, typical of hydrosalpinx.

Alternatively, hydrosalpinx may also be removed or clipped on laparoscopy.

ASPIRATION OF ASCITIC FLUID IN OVARIAN HYPERSTIMULATION SYNDROME

Ovarian hyperstimulation syndrome (OHSS) is one of the most dreaded complications of subfertility treatment. Various protocols have been devised to prevent it, but it still occurs, and the incidence is higher in IVF cycles than in patients on ovulation induction for IUI (intrauterine insemination). Fluid collection in the third space; peritoneal, pleural, and pericardiac spaces, is one of the consequences. Pleural and pericardial fluid aspirations must be done by subspecialists, but the aspiration of peritoneal fluid is generally done by experienced radiologists and gynecologists. This procedure reduces the patient's weight, leg edema, abdominal circumference and improves the derangements of renal function.[17] Aspiration may be done repeatedly at intervals, or an indwelling catheter may be placed. Whatever the technique is, ultrasound guidance for the placement of the needle and the catheter is absolutely essential. Al-Ramahi et al. have described placing an indwelling catheter (closed-system Dawson-Mueller catheter with "simp-loc" locking design) for continuous drainage.[18] Abuzeid et al., used a pigtail catheter for the same purpose.[19] A watch on serum protein balance and albumin supplementation are required as there is significant protein loss. Koike et al. developed a continuous autotransfusion system of ascites (CATSA). This eliminated the need of protein supplementation because the ascites fluid itself was again transfused. It was done for 5 h every day at a rate of 100–200 mL/h.[20] TV approach was thought to be better than TA approach. This approach is very convenient for those who are conversant

TABLE 1: Risks of prematurity associated with multiple pregnancy.[23]

Type of multiple pregnancy	*Average gestational age at delivery*	*Perinatal mortality (%)*	*Respiratory distress syndrome (%)*	*Intracranial hemorrhage (%)*	*Retinopathy (%)*
Triplet	31 + 5	14	23	14	10
Quadruplet	29 + 5	36	65	15	9
Quintuplet	28 + 4	40	75	10	25

with TV ultrasound.[21] Ultrasound guidance helps to prevent ovarian injury as ovaries are otherwise also large in OHSS.

FETAL REDUCTION

The twin pregnancy rates and higher order pregnancy rates have significantly increased due to infertility treatments.[22] Prematurity and associated neurological sequelae can occur as a complication of multiple pregnancies, and these complications become worse with rising order of pregnancy **(Table 1).** The risk of cerebral palsy is high in these patients. Its incidence in survivors is 2.3 in singletons, 12.6 in twins, and 44.8 in triplets per 1000. More than 20% of babies with birth weight <750 g develop cerebral palsy, and it is 4.6% higher in twin pregnancies. Apart from risks of mortality and morbidity to the fetus, maternal risk of hypertension, other cardiovascular and pulmonary complications, gestational diabetes, and postpartum hemorrhage are also significantly increased in multiple pregnancies. While the best approach to reduce the prevalence of multiple pregnancies is to limit the number of embryos transferred to one or two, and fetal reduction may be required in rare situations, single ET is now implemented in most countries and in most centers. This is probably a solution to control the multiple pregnancy rates. Generally, twin pregnancies are managed conservatively in most cases, but for triplets and higher order pregnancies, fetal reduction is recommended and offered to the couple.

The procedure of fetal reduction may be done:

- To reduce the number of fetuses (multifetal pregnancy reduction—MFPR) to reduce prematurity and its complications. Whatever be the cause before planning as to which fetus to reduce, it is essential to confirm that the fetus that is not to be reduced is normal. MFPR may also be done in some cases for the maternal cause. Mother's health, if is thought not able to support multiple fetuses, is also one of the indications to opt for fetal reduction.

Karyotype by chorion villous biopsy should be offered to all before performing MFPR. If not possible, at least nuchal translucency (NT) screening is performed before reduction. This is to assure that after MFPR, the prognosis for the remaining fetus/es is good.

- To eliminate the fetus with abnormality (selective reduction).

  As stated earlier, selective reduction is opted when one of the fetuses of multifetal pregnancy is abnormal. When any chromosomal abnormality is detected by ultrasound, it must be confirmed by karyotyping before the procedure. Legally, confirmation after termination is also required for assurance that the abnormal fetus was terminated.

The procedure and technique of embryo reduction may change depending on the age of gestation, ease and expertise of the operator, and the location of the fetus to be reduced in the uterus.

Preprocedure

Appropriate counseling must be done for every patient/couple before the procedure. That should include the risks of multiple pregnancies in terms of incidence of prematurity and associated complications of prematurity including miscarriage and neurological sequelae on the other hand, and also about procedure-related risks such as infection and miscarriage. It must be emphasized that miscarriage may occur even after 4–8 weeks of a successful procedure and risk of pregnancy loss before 24 weeks is about 9%–15%. The short- and long-term sequelae of prematurity must also be discussed with the couple. They should be explained about immediate consequences of prematurity like respiratory distress syndrome, intracranial hemorrhage, necrotizing enterocolitis, and retinopathy and also about late consequences like neurological deficits, cerebral palsy, recurrent hospitalization in infancy, neonatal and infant mortality. Benefits of MFPR should be weighed against potential risks of procedure, including fetal loss and maternal stress.

After the couple has consented for the procedure, a detailed ultrasound scanning of all the fetuses is done to assess the fetal anatomy and growth in detail including NT if possible. Proper mapping of the sac positions by ultrasound is a must, if possible, using 3D ultrasound (**Figs. 16 and 17**). Laboratory investigations (blood and urine) for minor surgeries are also done.

There are lots of views as to what is the best time and best method for the procedure. Some people may reduce as early as 8 weeks and claim that it causes less maternal psychological trauma, and some may prefer waiting till 14 weeks arguing that MFPR can be done after ruling out anomalies in detail. We prefer to do it around 11–12 weeks as it is possible that before 9 weeks, a spontaneous miscarriage or missed miscarriage may occur even otherwise. There is also a scope to rule out major structural or chromosomal anomalies in the fetus before reduction, when done at 11–12 weeks of gestation.

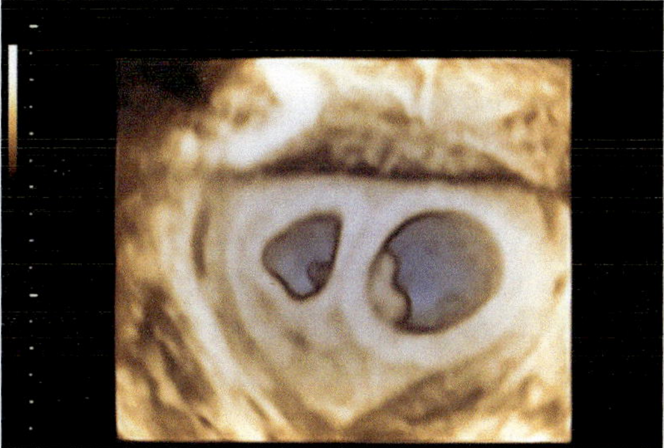

Fig. 16: 3D ultrasound image of coronal section of uterus showing twin pregnancy with two sacs located side by side.

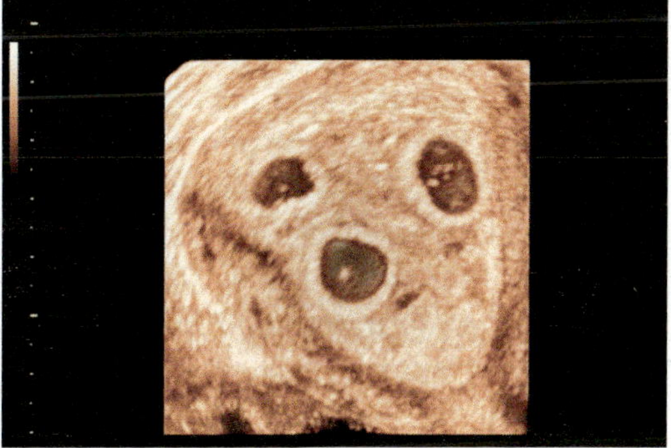

Fig. 17: 3D ultrasound image of coronal section of uterus showing triplet pregnancy with two sacs located side by side and the third sac above the two.

Various methods and routes have been tried by different workers for the procedure. Choice depends on the gestational age, chorionicity, and the operator's expertise. The most widely used method for dichorionic twins is intracardiac/intrathoracic potassium chloride injection. Some workers also prefer methotrexate. Methods like transcervical aspiration and mechanical trauma are used to reduce one of the fetuses as early as 7–8 weeks of pregnancy and are too crude and not widely accepted.

KCl (potassium chloride) injection

This can be done by TA/TV approach under ultrasound guidance. Preferred time to do this procedure is 11–12 weeks of gestation.

Procedure done later than 12 weeks has higher risk of coagulation disorders in mother. When reduction is done, after 15 weeks,[24] risk of preterm delivery at <33 weeks is three times higher. Asepsis is of prime importance. When reduction is done to decrease the order of pregnancy, fetus close to the probe is selected for reduction. Transcervical or TV reduction may be safer very early in gestation and TA safer later in first trimester.[25]

Transvaginal approach

The procedure is preferably done under short general anesthesia, though some may prefer a local anesthesia with sedation. Patient is placed in lithotomy position. Parts are cleaned and painted with povidone-iodine solution or savlon, and the patient is draped with sterilized towels. TV ultrasound probe is cleaned and prepared for the procedure. It is covered by a sterile cover/jelly-free condom. The biopsy guide is attached to the probe, and the probe is placed in vagina. Scanning is done to map the positions of the sacs and to find out the most easily approachable embryo or an abnormal embryo, that is to be reduced. The biopsy guideline is switched on, on the scanner. The embryo desired to be reduced is brought in alignment with this line. A 20–21 gauge long needle is introduced through the needle guide.

Attach needle to 2 cm^3 syringe, filled with 1.3–2 mEq/L or 2–7 mmol of KCl to the needle and prefill the needle also before it enters the gestational sac. Once the needle enters the sac, it is placed close to the embryo. Insert needle with a controlled thrust and with slight depression, check that the needle is in the embryo. Gentle in and out movement of the probe will move the embryo also along with it, if the needle is in the embryo. The needle must enter the embryo in its thorax. Intracardiac location of the needle tip is the best, but intrathoracic location would also serve the purpose (**Fig. 18**). In case of doubt, 4D biopsy guide may be more useful. Once the position of the needle tip is confirmed to be in the heart or close to the heart of the embryo, slowly inject 1–2 mL of KCl. A forceful injection may push away the embryo. Injection jet can be seen on B-mode and confirmed by color Doppler. Sometimes, injected KCl may also be seen as lucency in the fetal thorax. Wait patiently for a few minutes, without changing the position of the needle. Heart stops beating in a few seconds. Monitor for asystole for 60 s, remove needle. Fetus sinks in the amniotic cavity. Recheck after a few hours and on the next day. Close observation of the maternal heart must be done when KCl is injected.

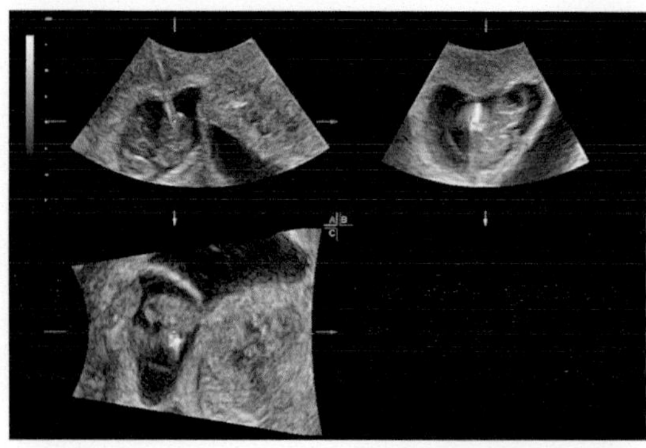

Fig. 18: 3D ultrasound sectional plane image confirming the needle position in the fetal thorax in all three sections (orthogonal planes).

Postoperative spotting is not known except for the transcervical approach. Observe for leakage of liquor amnii.

Antibiotic cover is given for 7 days, tocolytics for 72 hours, and rest for 48 hours though some studies have shown that prophylactic antibiotics, tocolytics, or cervical suturing have no role.

Risks of the Procedure

- Premature rupture of membranes.
- Intra-amniotic infection—chorioamnionitis.
- Clinical/laboratory evidence of disseminated intravascular coagulation, of which some cases may also require monitoring for decreasing fibrinogen levels and

prolonged PTT (partial thromboplastin time) and heparin therapy.

- Rarely after initial asystole immediately after injection, the heart may again start beating, and in such cases repeat KCl injection may be needed. Repeat procedure after 1 week may be required if the termination has not occurred. But this is a controversial issue.

Transabdominal approach: When TA approach is used, either free-hand technique or needle guide may be used, depending on operator's convenience. The procedure otherwise remains the same. Whatever route and whatever technique are used, extensive perinatal follow-up is essential to prevent premature delivery. MFPR reduces but does not eliminate the risk of prematurity associated with higher-order pregnancies. Postprocedure prognosis is worse depending on the degree of higher-order pregnancies,[26] and the number of pregnancies that are reduced.[24-26]

Reduction of triplets to twins significantly reduces the risk of prematurity in terms of gestational age at delivery, birth weight, overall pregnancy loss which makes it a medically justifiable procedure.[27] In spite of all care taken, MFPR has been quoted as "a therapy to achieve most good for least harm." In spite of all available methods to reduce multifetal pregnancies, there is still a significant risk to the fetus and the mother. It is, therefore, insisted that single ET is the safest and the most desirable practice. The fact remains for all ultrasound-guided procedures. It has a steep learning curve and success of the procedure increases with experience.

KEY POINTS

- Ultrasound has proved to be reliable as a guiding tool for several procedures for managing the patients with subfertility.
- Ultrasound-guided procedures are less invasive and have significantly reduced the postoperative hospital care.
- Though minimally invasive, these procedures must be done in operation theaters, and all emergency fighting drugs and gadgets must be readily available.
- Adequate asepsis, adequate anesthesia, and antibiotic cover are a must.
- It is essential to master the scanning technique before trying these procedures.
- Ultrasound-guided procedures have a steep learning curve.
- No ultrasound-guided procedure must be attempted if the ultrasound image quality is inadequate.
- TV ultrasound-guided procedures must not be attempted in presence of any vaginal infection.

ACKNOWLEDGMENT

We are obliged to Dr Jayaprakasan K for his support in refinement of this chapter.

REFERENCES

1. Lenz S, Lauritsen JG, Kjellow M. Collection of human oocytes for in vitro fertilization by sonographically guided follicular puncture. Lancet. 1981;23:1163.
2. Lenz S, Lauristen JG. Ultrasonically guided percutaneous aspiration of human follicles under local anesthesia: a new method of collecting oocytes for in vitro fertilization. Fertil Steril. 1982;38:673-7.
3. Feichtinger W, Kemeter P. Transvaginal sector can sonography for needle guided transvaginal follicle aspiration and other applications in gynecologic routine and research. Fertil Steril. 1986;45: 722-5.
4. Bagtharia S, Haloob AR. Is there a benefit from routine follicular flushing for oocyte retrieval? J Obstet Gynecol. 2005;25:374-6.
5. Kingsland CR, Taylor CT, Aziz N, Bickeston N. Is follicular flushing necessary for oocyte retrieval? A randomized trial. Hum Reprod. 1991;6:382-3.
6. Brown J, Buckingham K, Abou-Setta AM, Buckett W. Ultrasound versus 'clinical touch' for catheter guidance during embryo transfer in women. Cochrane Database Syst Rev. 2010;(1):CD006107.
7. Porter MB. Ultrasound in assisted reproductive technology. Semin Reprod Med. 2008;26:266-76.
8. Allahbadia GN, Kadam KS, Gandhi GN, Arora S, Mhatre YP, Virk S. The stilette for a Sure-view. Fertil Steril. 2006;86(Suppl 3):S252.

9. Blake DA, Farquhar CM, Johnson N, Proctor M. Cleavage stage versus blastocyst stage embryo transfer in assisted conception. Cochrane Database Syst Rev. 2007;17:CD002118.
10. Lass A, Abusheikha N, Brinsden P, Kovacs GT. The effect of a difficult embryo transfer on the out- come of IVF. Hum Reprod. 1999;14:2417.
11. Woolcott R, Stanger J. Potentially important variables identified by transvaginal ultrasound-guided embryo transfer. Hum Reprod. 1997;12:963-6.
12. Karande V, Hazlett D, Vietzke M, Gleicher N. A prospective randomized comparison of the Wallace catheter and the Cook Echo-Tip catheter for ultrasound-guided embryo transfer. Fertil Steril. 2002;77:826-30.
13. Coroleu B, Barri PN, Carreras O, Belil I. Buxaderas R, Veiga A, et al. Effect of using an echogenic catheter for ultrasound-guided embryo transfer in an IVF programme a prospective, randomized, controlled study. Hum Reprod. 2006;21:1809-15.
14. Gergely RZ, DeUgrate CM, Danzer H, Surrey M, Hill D, Decherney AH. Three dimensional/four dimensional ultrasound- guided embryo transfer using the maximal implantation potential point. Fertil Steril. 2005;84:500-3.
15. Camus E, Poncelet C, Goffinet F, Wainer B, Merlet F, Nisand I, et al. Pregnancy rates after in-vitro fertilization in cases of tubal infertility with and without hydrosalpinx a meta-analysis of published comparative studies. Hum Reprod. 1999;14:1243-9.
16. Hammadieh N, Coomarasamy A, Ola B, Papaioannou S, Afnan M, Sharif K. Ultrasound-guided hydrosalpinx aspiration during oocyte collection improves pregnancy outcome in IVF a randomized controlled trial. Hum Reprod. 2008;23:1113-7.
17. Thaler I, Yoffe N, Kaftory J, Brandes JM. Treatment of ovarian hyperstimulation syndrome the physiologic basis for modified approach. Fertil Steril. 1981;36:110-3.
18. Al-Ramahi M, Leader A, Claman P, Spence J. A novel approach to the treatment of ascites associated with ovarian hyperstimulation syndrome. Hum Reprod. 1997;12:2614-6.
19. Abuzeid MI, Nassar Z, Massaad Z, Weiss M, Ashraf M, Fakih M. Pigtail catheter for the treatment of ascites associated with ovarian hyperstimulation syndrome. Hum Reprod. 2003;18:370-3.
20. Koike T, Araki S, Minakami H, Ogawa S, Sayama M, Shibahara H, et al. Clinical efficacy of peritoneovenous shunting for the treatment of severe ovarian hyperstimulation syndrome. Hum Reprod. 2000;15:113-7.
21. Aboulgar MA, Mansour RT, Serour GI, Amin Y. Ultrasonically guided vaginal aspiration of ascites in the treatment of ovarian hyper-stimulation syndrome. Fertil Steril. 1990;53:933-5.
22. Chauhan SP, Scardo JA, Hayes E, Abuahmed AZ, Berghella V. Twins prevalence, problems and preterm births. Am J Obstet Gynecol. 2010;203(4):305-15.
23. Strauss A, Paek BW, Genzel-Boroviczeny O, Schulze A, Janssen U, Hepp H. Multifetal gestation-maternal and perinatal outcome of 112 pregnancies. Fetal Diagn Ther. 2002;17:209-17.
24. Antsaklis A, Souka AP, Daskalakis G, Papantoniou N, Koutra P, Kavalakis Y, et al. Pregnancy outcome after multifetal pregnancy reduction. J Matern Fetal Neonatal Med. 2004;16:27-31.
25. Evans MI, Dommergues M, Timor-Tritsch I, Zador IE, Wapner RJ, Lynch L, et al. Transabdominal versus transcervical and transvaginal multifetal pregnancy reduction: international collaborative experience of more than one thousand cases. Am J Obstet Gynecol. 1994;170:902-9.
26. Evans MI, Littman L, Richter R, Richter K, Hume RF Jr. Selective reduction for multifetal pregnancy. Early opinions revisited. J Reprod Med. 1997;42:771-7.
27. Yaron Y, Bryant-Greenwood PK, Dave N, Moldenhauer JS, Kramer RL, Johnson MP, et al. Multifetal pregnancy reduction (MFPR) of triplets to twins comparison of nonreduced triplets and twins. Am J Obstet Gynecol. 1999;180: 1268-71.

34
CHAPTER

Transvaginal Assessment of the Cervix

Sonal Panchal, Chaitanya Nagori

INTRODUCTION

Cervix is an organ easily assessable by direct visualization and examination by per speculum and per vaginal examination, but as is well known these chiefly assess only the external os and the distal part of the cervix **(Figs. 1A and B)**. Especially, the supravaginal part of the cervix and the internal os cannot be assessed by per vaginal or per speculum examination. Moreover, lesions in the cervical canal can also not be diagnosed by this method.

Cervical assessment is important for gynecological and obstetric indications. Assessment of cervix is indicated for gynecological indications such as cervical polyp, cervical fibroids, cervical malignancies, and cervical ectopic pregnancy. In obstetric cases, of course, the major concern is the cervical competence and the length to assess the risk of premature labor. Of course, the cervical assessment is also important to assess the progress of the labor. But, in this chapter, we shall limit our discussion to the gynecological and prelabor indications of cervical assessment. Cervix has homogeneous echogenicity and has same echotexture like that of myometrium. Endocervical glands appear as a hypoechoic band on both the sides of the cervical angle tapering at the level of internal os. The echogenicity of the endocervical glands changes especially in the preovulatory phase and becomes hyperechoic **(Figs. 2A and B)**. On transverse section at the level of internal os, both the uterine arteries are seen entering the uterus **(Fig. 2A)**. External os is identified on sagittal plane as a dip between the anterior and the posterior lip of the cervix. But, it can be well identified on transverse section also **(Fig. 2C)** and even better on three-dimensional (3D) ultrasound rendering **(Fig. 2D)**.

Visualization of the cervix can be improved by withdrawing the probe a little once it touches the cervix. One may also move in the anterior or the posterior fornix depending on the position of the cervix. It is preferable

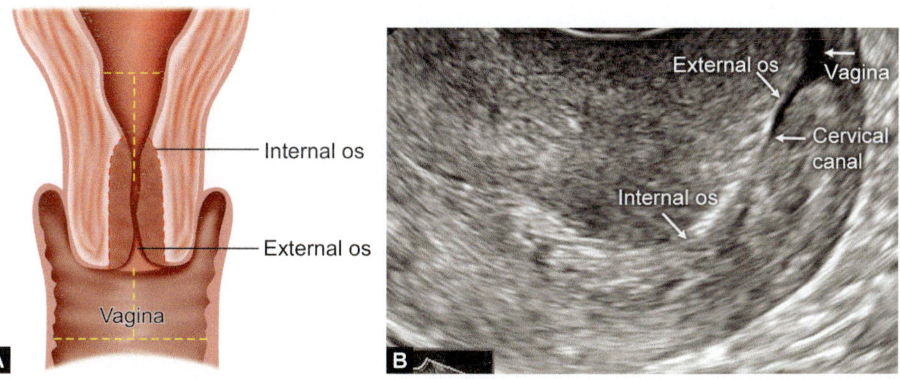

Figs. 1A and B: (A) Diagrammatic representation; (B) B-mode ultrasound image showing anatomy of cervix.

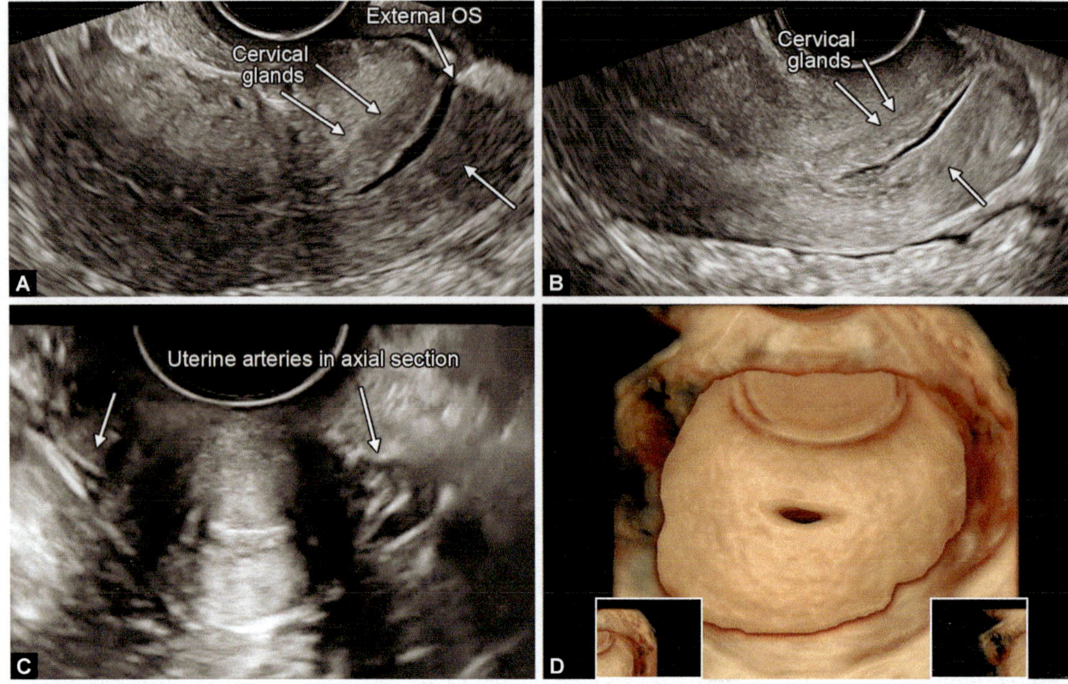

Figs. 2A to D: B mode images of sagittal section of cervix with cervical mucus and paired arrows show the cervical glands that appear as hypoechoic layer on both sides of the cervical canal (A) and hyperechoic (B) (periovulatory phase of cycle). (C) Transverse section of cervix. (D) 3D rendered image of cervix.

to manipulate the probe, so that the cervical canal becomes perpendicular to the sound beam.

Gel sonovaginography is a useful outpatient department (OPD)-based investigation for better evaluation of cervical lesions. 20 mL of ultrasound gel is instilled preferably into the posterior fornix before introduction of the probe. This facilitates the visualization of the cervix and the vaginal wall.

CERVICAL POLYPS

The polyps appear as solid echogenic lesions in the cervical canal and are usually associated with fluid in the cervical canal and so are easy to identify **(Figs. 3A to E)**. When there is no fluid in cervical canal, these are difficult to identify but are suspected when the cervical canal shows irregularity. Polyps appear as teardrop solid lesions and may be sessile or pedunculated. On color or power Doppler, these polyps typically show single-feeding vessel pattern such as endometrial polyps **(Figs. 4A and B)**. Cervical polyps, when small, are not of much clinical significance; but, when large, it may lead to obstruction for the passage of intrauterine insemination cannula or embryo transfer cannula. Cervical polyps may also present as intermenstrual bleeding, postcoital bleeding in premenopausal age, and in bleeding per vaginum in postmenopausal women. In these cases, especially pulsed wave Doppler plays an important role to assess the possibility of malignancy. If resistance index (RI) of these vessels is <0.45, the chances of atypia and malignancy are significantly increased. On B-mode ultrasound, it is not possible to differentiate between benign and malignant lesion, though the later may show heterogeneous echogenicity and at times also show cauliflower-like margins.

CERVICAL FIBROIDS

Cervical fibroids are not very common. When the entire fibroid or >50% of the fibroid is below the level of the internal os,

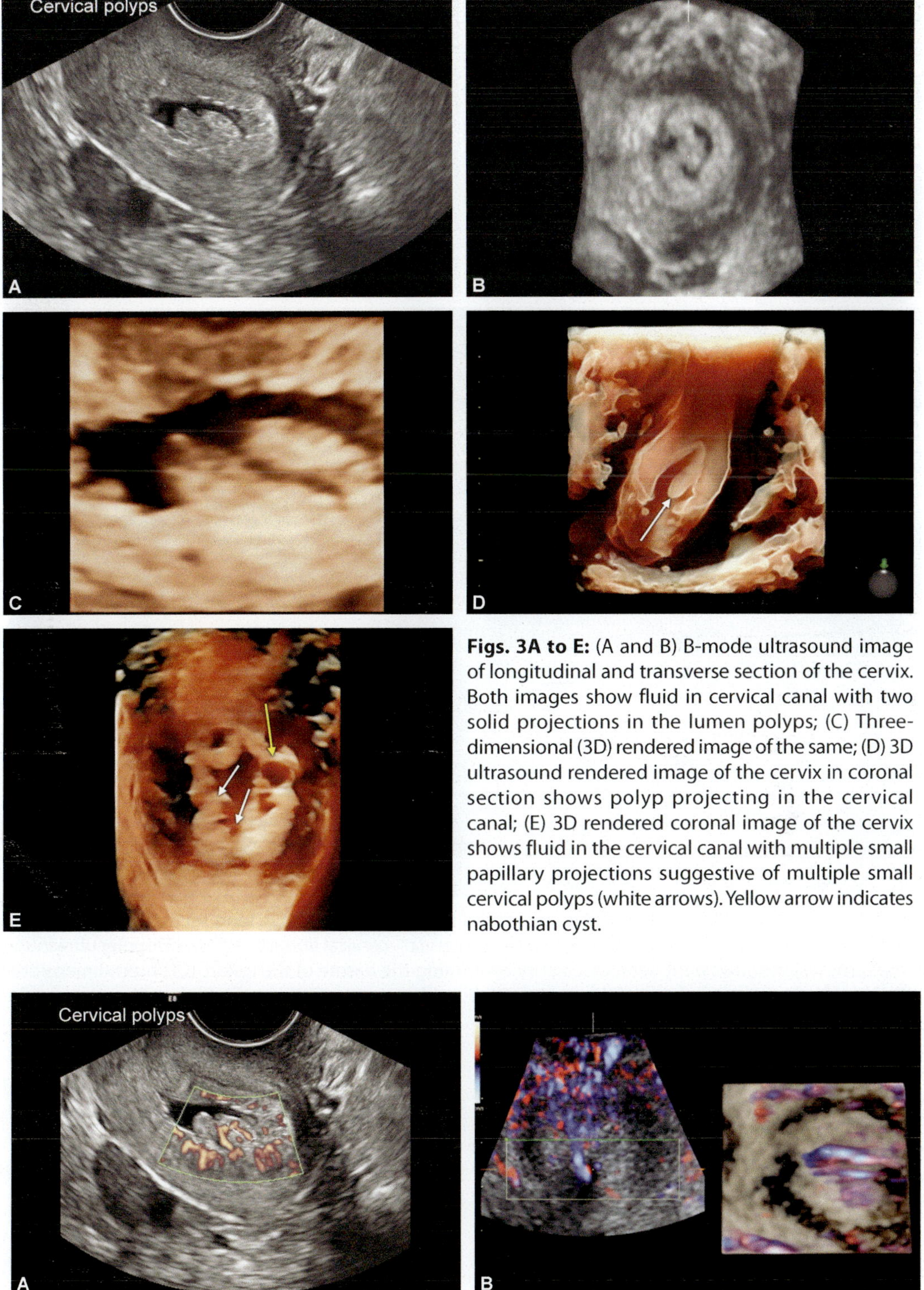

Figs. 3A to E: (A and B) B-mode ultrasound image of longitudinal and transverse section of the cervix. Both images show fluid in cervical canal with two solid projections in the lumen polyps; (C) Three-dimensional (3D) rendered image of the same; (D) 3D ultrasound rendered image of the cervix in coronal section shows polyp projecting in the cervical canal; (E) 3D rendered coronal image of the cervix shows fluid in the cervical canal with multiple small papillary projections suggestive of multiple small cervical polyps (white arrows). Yellow arrow indicates nabothian cyst.

Figs. 4A and B: (A) Power Doppler ultrasound image of cervix showing fluid in lumen with two polyps on B-mode. Power Doppler shows single vessel feeding each polyp: (B) Three-dimensional (3D) power Doppler and glass body rendered image of the same case as in (A) showing polyps with single-feeding vessel.

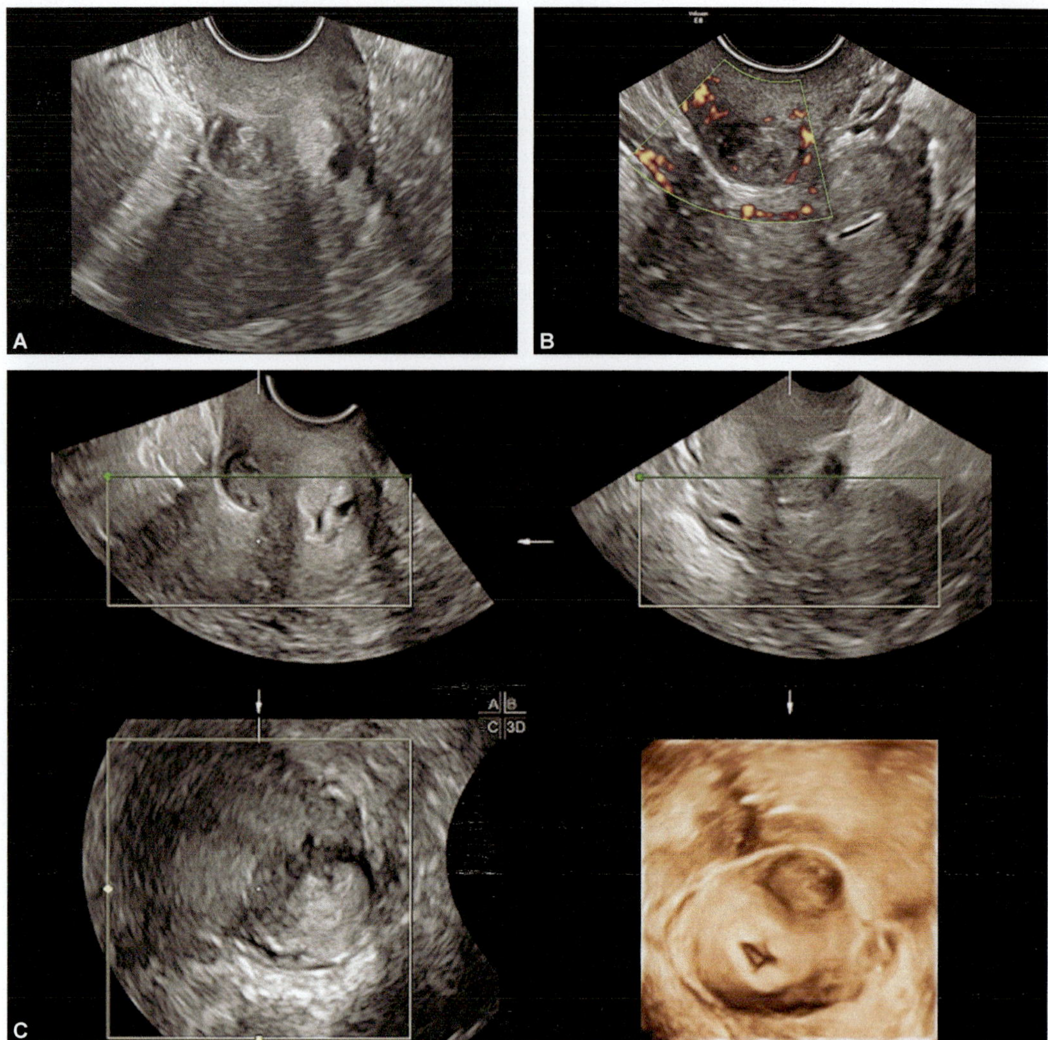

Figs. 5A to C: Cervical fibroid. (A) B-mode ultrasound image of the uterus in long section showing a well-defined hypoechoic round lesion in anterior wall of the cervix—cervical fibroid; (B) Power Doppler ultrasound of the same lesion shows peripheral vascularity confirming the nature of the lesion; (C) Three-dimensional (3D) ultrasound-acquired volume of the cervix with fibroid, also part (C) shows multiplanar images and the rendered image.

it is named as cervical fibroid. Fibroids are also hypoechoic, round, or oval well-defined lesions such as uterine fibroids and also show peripheral rim-like vascularity **(Figs. 5A to C)**. Like the fibroids in the uterus, these fibroids also show fan shadows and edge shadows. These fibroids when large may lead to difficulty in visualization of the uterine body. If these fibroids are degenerated, intralesional vascularity is also seen and in these cases, it is difficult to differentiate from cervical malignancy.

NABOTHIAN CYSTS

The cysts are very common in cervix **(Figs. 6A to F)**. These are well-defined roundish or oval cystic lesions. These are dilatation of cervical glands due to collection of secretions of cervical glands usually as a result of inflammation of the cervical glands.

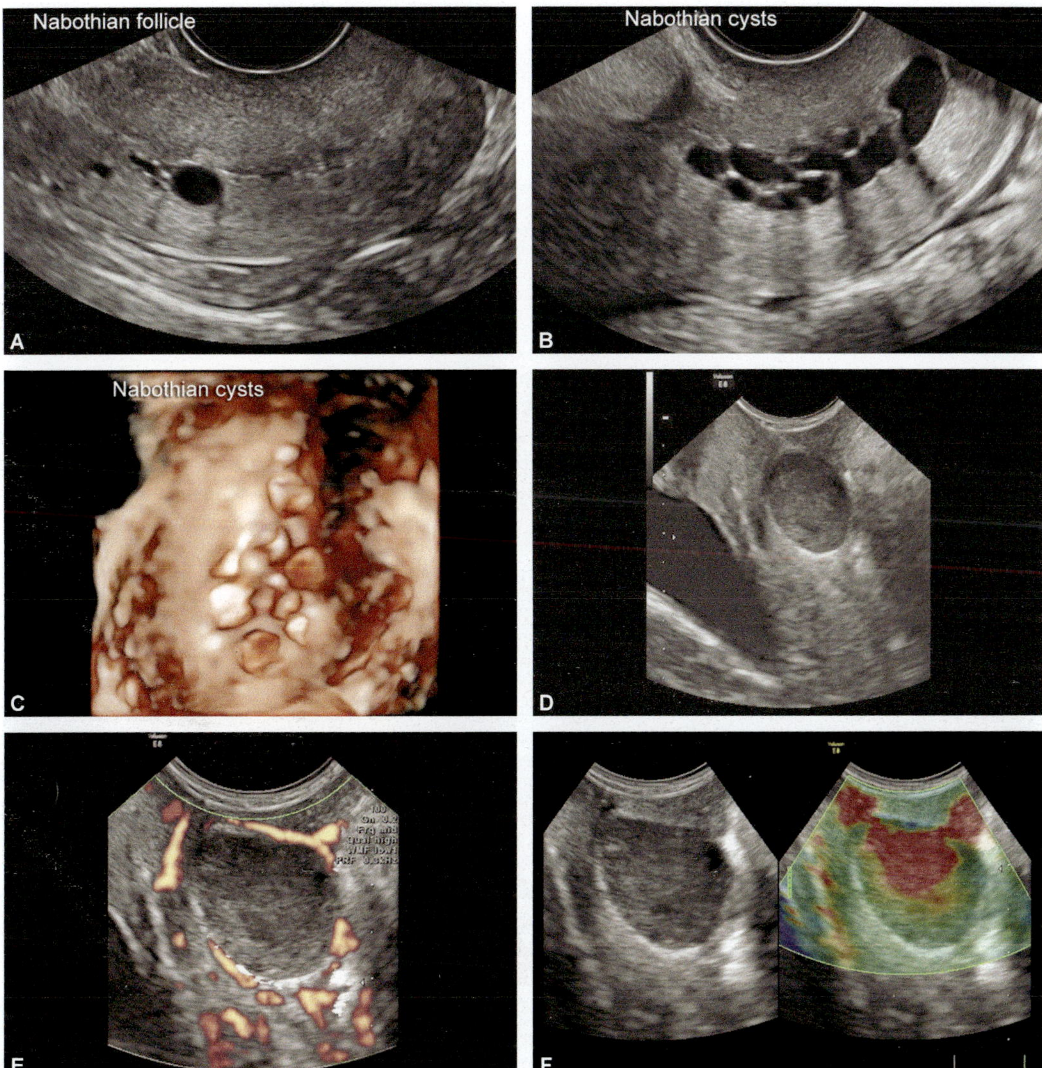

Figs. 6A to F: Nabothian cysts. (A) B-mode ultrasound image of long axis of uterus showing an anechoic round lesion in posterior wall of the cervix, just caudal to internal os, with posterior acoustic enhancement suggestive of nabothian cyst; (B) B-mode ultrasound image of long axis of uterus showing multiple anechoic areas in posterior wall of the cervix with posterior acoustic enhancement. These are multiple nabothian cysts; (C) 3D ultrasound HD live rendered image of multiple nabothian cysts seen in (B); (D) B-mode ultrasound image of cervix with a round cystic lesion with low-level echogenicities in the lumen. Posterior acoustic enhancement suggests cystic nature of the lesion and internal echogenicities suggest thick fluid-like pus inside—infected nabothian cyst; (E) Power Doppler shows peripheral vascularity due to inflammation; (F) Infected nabothian cyst seen in the previous figure when assessed by elastography, fills with red color, confirming the fluid content.
(3D: three-dimensional; HD: high-definition)

CERVICAL ECTOPIC PREGNANCIES

These pregnancies are extremely rare **(Figs. 7A and B)**. Anechoic gestational sac with dense echogenic rim of decidual reaction is seen in one of the cervical lips and so gestational sac is seen eccentrically in the cervix. This leads to thickening of the cervical lip leading to bulky cervix and, therefore, hourglass shape

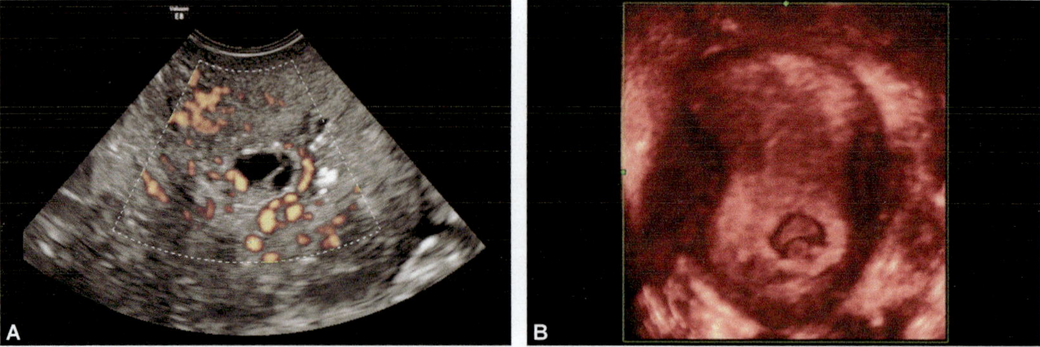

Figs. 7A and B: (A) B-mode ultrasound image of longitudinal section of the uterus showing a round anechoic structure with hyperechoic margins in cervical wall. On power Doppler, the structure shows peripheral vascularity. Findings suggest ectopic pregnancy in cervix; (B) This is a three-dimensional (3D) rendered image of the same pathology leading to typical hourglass uterus because of bulky cervix.

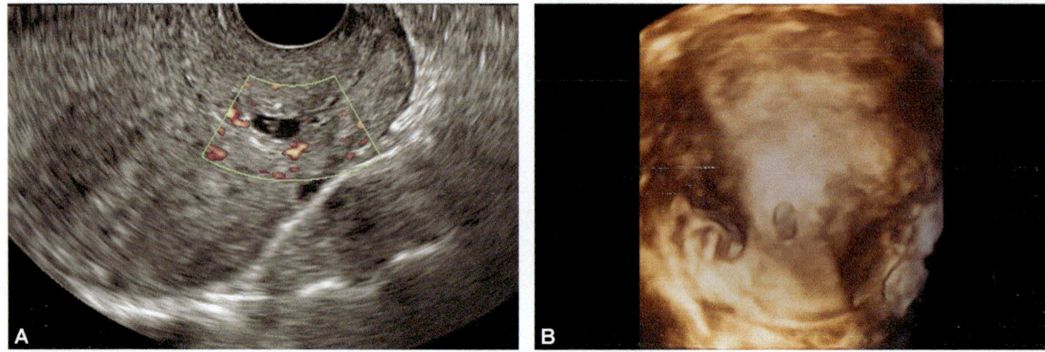

Figs. 8A and B: (A) Similar lesion as seen in **Figures 6A and B**, but the lesion does not show significant peripheral vascularity and the lesion is central in the cervix; (B) Figure shows the same lesion on three-dimensional (3D) ultrasound rendered image, cystic lesion, placed central in cervical canal. Findings suggest gestational sac in the process of expulsion (abortion in process).

of the uterus. The gestational sac shows a rim of low-resistance vascularity. This has to be differentiated from a gestational sac, which is in process of abortion **(Figs. 8A and B)**. The latter shows the sac in the cervical canal (located central in the cervix) and shows no or only scanty peripheral vascularity of cervical pregnancy. Cervical pregnancies are difficult to treat and if the diagnosis is late, it may demand hysterectomy due to bleeding. Early diagnosis and treatment with local methotrexate is almost always a preferred scenario.

CERVICAL MALIGNANCY

Cervical malignancies take one of the highest tolls on women. It is more commonly seen in the women of reproductive age group and is believed to be primarily due to human papillomavirus (HPV). Screening for cervical carcinoma has been widely propagated throughout the world and that has helped to decrease the mortality because of cervical cancer. Screening is chiefly done by Pap smear and this is of help for early detection of squamous cell carcinoma. Carcinomas are more common among the malignant lesions of the cervix and histopathologically these may be squamous cell carcinoma or adenocarcinoma. Unfortunately, these lesions are diagnosed late. The symptoms usually appear late. Common presentation mimics that of a cervical polyp, intermenstrual, postcoital, or postmenopausal

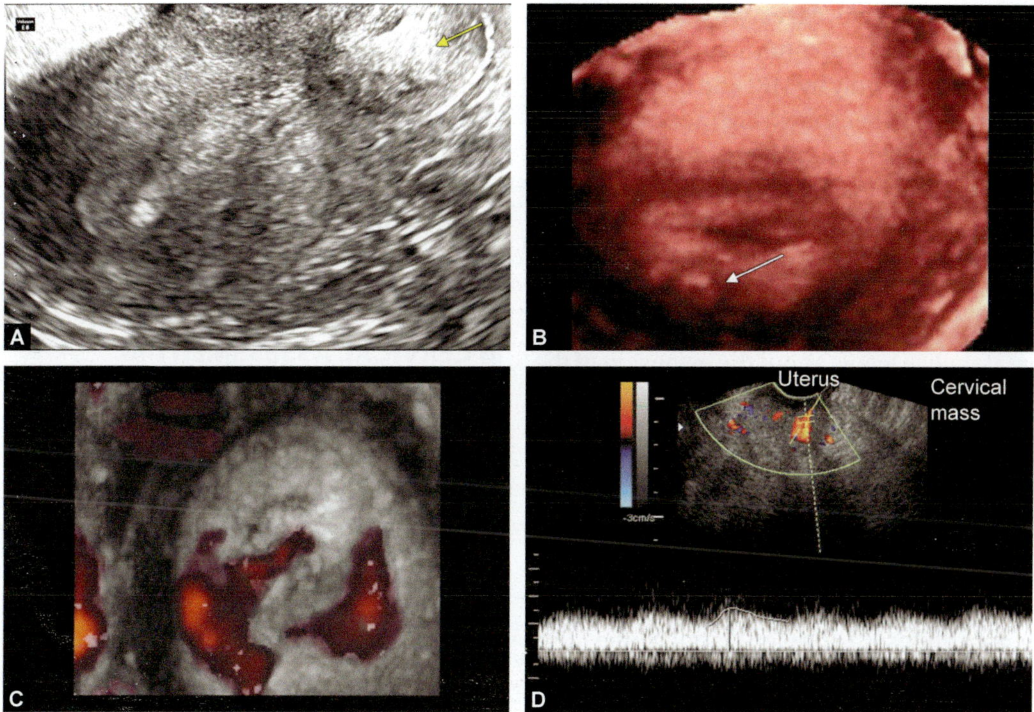

Figs. 9A to D: (A) B-mode ultrasound image of long section of uterus and cervix showing thickened posterior lip of cervix with heterogeneous hyperechoic mass in it (arrow); (B) Three-dimensional (3D) rendered image of the same cervix shows irregularity on the posterior lip of the cervix (arrow); (C) The same lesion on 3D power Doppler, glass body rendered image shows locally increased vascularity as color blobs; (D) On spectral Doppler, these vessels show low-resistance vascularity typical of malignant neoangiogenesis.

bleed. Pain is not common except in advanced cases. In advanced cases when the disease extends beyond cervix in the parametrium and into bowel or bladder, i.e., patient will complain of pain and bowel and bladder symptoms. Asymmetrical thickening of the cervical lips is the earliest sign of the cervical neoplasm **(Figs. 9A to D)**. Like malignancies anywhere, the cervical malignant mass also shows heterogeneous echogenicity, irregular margins, and increased vascular density, but squamous cell carcinoma more often appear hypoechoic whereas adenocarcinomas are isoechoic. Lesions may be exophytic or endophytic and its exact site of origin is important to document. This can be done by in and out movement of the probe. Three information can be achieved by this: (1) site of origin and its base and distance from internal os, (2) firmness of the lesion (higher indicates possibility of malignancy, and (3) surrounding penetration and adhesions. On reporting, it is essential to mention the distance of the upper margin of the lesion to internal os and its extension into the myometrium or body of the uterus, its extension into the cervical stroma, and tumor-free cervical strip or parametrial, bladder, or bowel infiltration. Loss of normal tissue interfaces between cervix and vagina, bladder, and bowel and extension of the isoechoic, hypoechoic but more commonly heterogeneous lesion indicate extracervical extension of the tumor. Endometrial blood collection (hematometra) is a common finding with cervical malignancy. Extension of the cervical lesion into the surrounding tissues is best appreciated on tomographic ultrasound imaging (TUI).

Though in all cases with suspicion of cervical carcinoma, confirmation of diagnosis is always done only by MRI and biopsy. Lately, 3D ultrasound has shown high accuracy for the diagnosis of cervical malignancy. Ultrasound also has an advantage of seeing the relationship of the mass with surrounding tissues, integrity, or invasion of tissue planes. 3D ultrasound is, therefore, used to assess the extension of cervical malignancies into bladder, rectum, or laterally. Details about the extension of the lesion are more clear and confirmed on MRI. Ureteric involvement is quite common with advanced cervical carcinoma and, therefore, when assessing the patient with ultrasound or MRI, assessment of the kidneys for back pressure changes is essential. Similarly, it is also essential to search for enlarged pelvic lymph nodes. 3D power Doppler may also show the typical vascular pattern with caliber variations, microaneurysms, arteriovenous fistulae, and heterogeneously distributed vascularity **(Figs. 10A to C)**. In all cases with cervical enlargement or a mass lesion or a history of intermenstrual or postmenopausal bleeding, it is essential to evaluate the anterior, posterior tissue interfaces and fornices to exclude the possibility of extension of the lesion. In and out movement of the probe to assess the mobility or otherwise gives an important clue to the nature and extension of the lesion **(Figs. 11A and B)**.

CERVICAL ASSESSMENT IN PREGNANCY

Assessment of the cervix for obstetric indications is one of the assessment of cervical insufficiency and risk of preterm delivery. Ultrasound is used as a basis for deciding for therapeutic cerclage, observation of patients after cerclage, differentiating true and false labor, and predicting success full labor induction in patients with cervical insufficiency.

Cervical insufficiency is defined on transvaginal sonography (TVS) as cervical

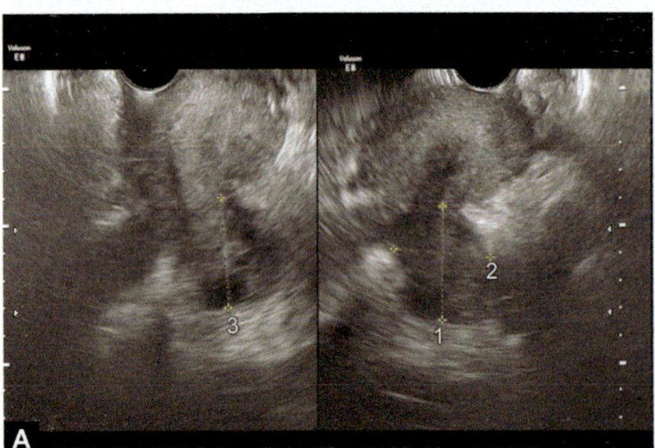

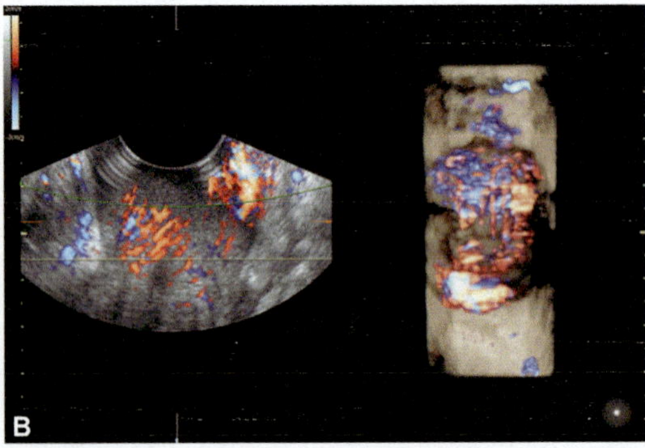

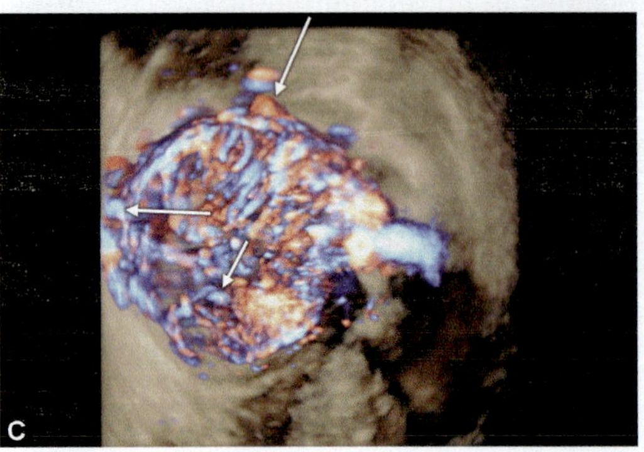

Figs. 10A to C: (A) B-mode ultrasound image of the cervix on transvaginal scan shows a heterogeneously hypoechoic solid exophytic mass lesion arising chiefly from posterior surface of the cervix. It has defined but irregular margins. Findings strongly suggest a cervical malignant mass lesion; (B) Three-dimensional (3D) power Doppler—acquired volume of the same lesion shows marked increased and heterogeneously distributed vascular density; (C) Color mode—angio mode rendered image of the same volume shows a large fireball of color. The vessels cannot be identified individually but show irregular caliber as marked by arrows.

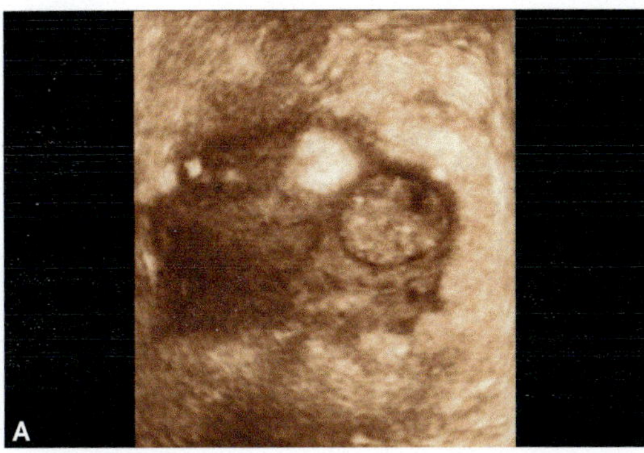

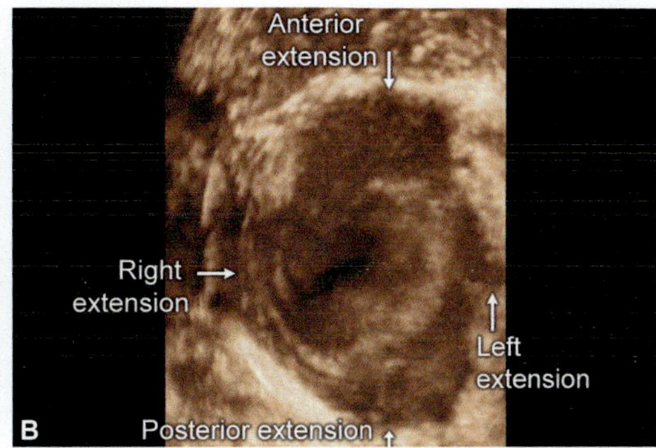

Figs. 11A and B: Three-dimensional (3D) ultrasound surface rendered image of a cervical malignancy. (A) The lesion has heterogeneous echogenicity and irregular margins. At a more caudal level, no cervical margins are identified. This is because of extension of the lesion into surrounding structures; (B) A more cephalic section shows faint cervical margins and extension of hypoechoic lesion on all sides. 3D ultrasound can be a valuable tool to assess the extent of malignant lesion.

length <25 mm and/or advanced cervical changes on physical examination before 24 weeks of gestation in women with either one or more prior pregnancy losses or preterm births at 14–36 weeks **(Figs. 12A and B)**.

High-risk population for preterm delivery includes women with:

- History of preterm delivery
- Rupture of membranes
- Repeated midtrimester pregnancy losses
- Cervical surgery
- Congenital uterine abnormalities
- Diethylstilbestrol exposure.

Ultrasound examination of the cervix provides an objective and noninvasive method for assessment of the cervix. It gives information about cervical length and also about cervical dilatation. This can be done by transabdominal, transperineal, translabial, or transvaginal route. Translabial or transperineal ultrasound is not always able to provide adequate information of the cervix because of maternal obesity or because of acoustic shadowing from rectum or symphysis pubis. This acoustic shadowing, even when does not obliterate the visualization completely, may obscure the cervical canal partially and

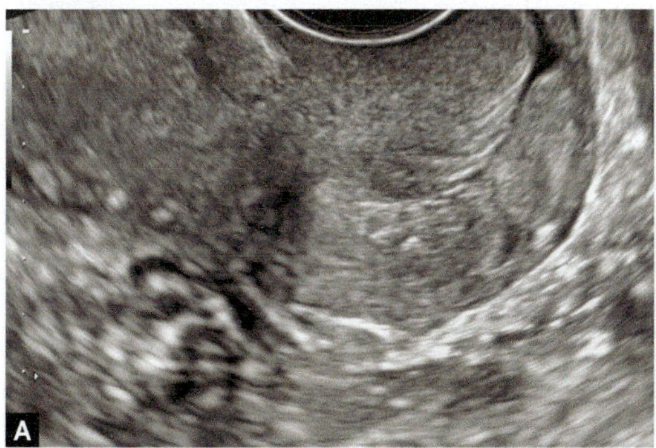

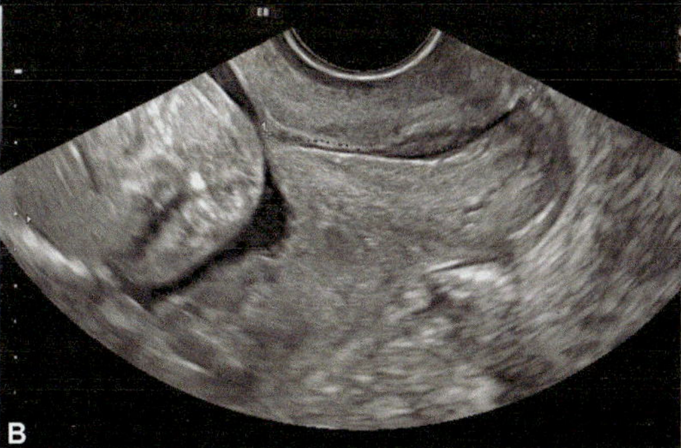

Figs. 12A and B: B-mode ultrasound image of long section of cervix on transvaginal scan. (A) Figure shows its normal curved long axis in nonpregnant or pregnant state; (B) This is longer than the cervix that is seen in figure, which is a straight cervix in a gravid uterus. Straightening itself may be an indication of its shorter length.

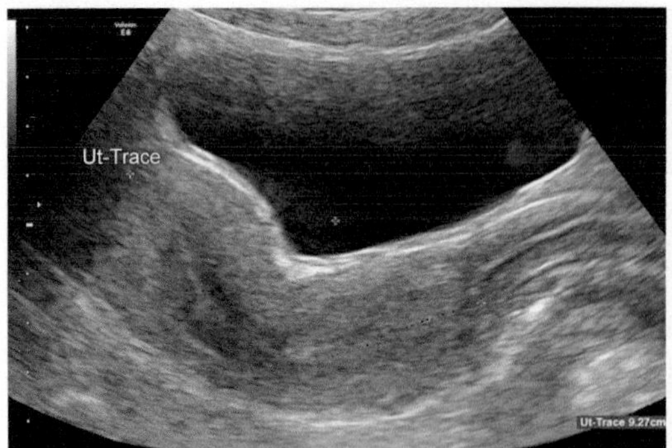

Fig. 13: B-mode ultrasound image of long axis of uterus and cervix. Anechoic full bladder is seen anterior to the uterus. Uterus and cervix follow the curve of the full bladder leading to stretching and false lengthening of the cervix. Anatomical details of cervical anatomy are also markedly masked because of inherent less resolution of transabdominal scan as compared to transvaginal scan for pelvic organs.

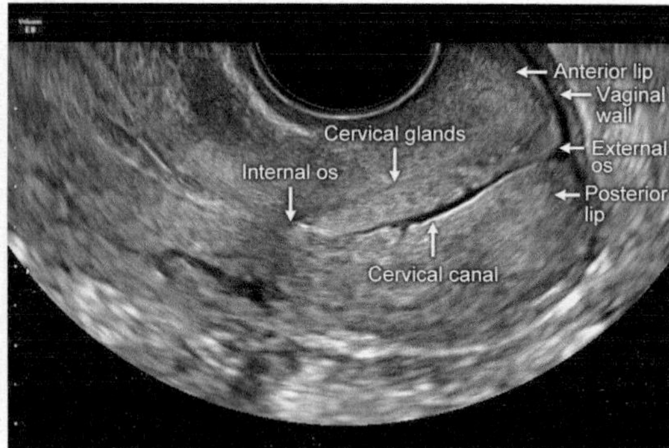

Fig. 14: B-mode ultrasound image of cervix on transvaginal scan showing all anatomical details.

result in false shortening of cervical length.[1] For transabdominal assessment of the cervix, the bladder needs to be full; this stretches the cervix resulting in apparent lengthening of the cervix[2] **(Fig. 13)**.

Transvaginal ultrasound is the modality of choice for assessment of the cervix.

The advantage is that with the complete length of the cervix, internal and external os and the canal can be studied by transvaginal ultrasound without interference from fat, bowel gas, or fetal parts[3] **(Fig. 14)**. When using transvaginal route for assessment of cervical length, it must be kept in mind that if any pressure is exerted while scanning, pressure on the cervix can distort it and this will result into false measurement of cervical length.

So, once the cervix is seen, pull the probe a bit out and then measure the straight distance from external os to internal os. Moreover, transvaginal ultrasonography can help to identify the presence of other ultrasound risk markers for preterm delivery such as the presence of intraamniotic debris (a possible sign of intrauterine microbial colonization) and choriodecidual separation[4] **(Figs. 15A and B)**.

A dynamic assessment of the cervical length with and without fundal pressure is a more reliable method for assessment of

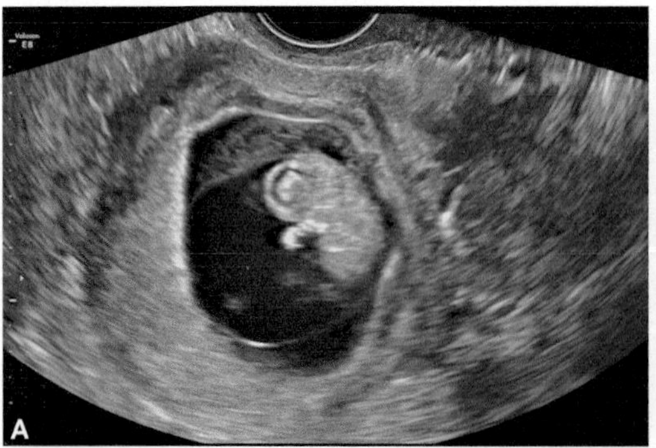

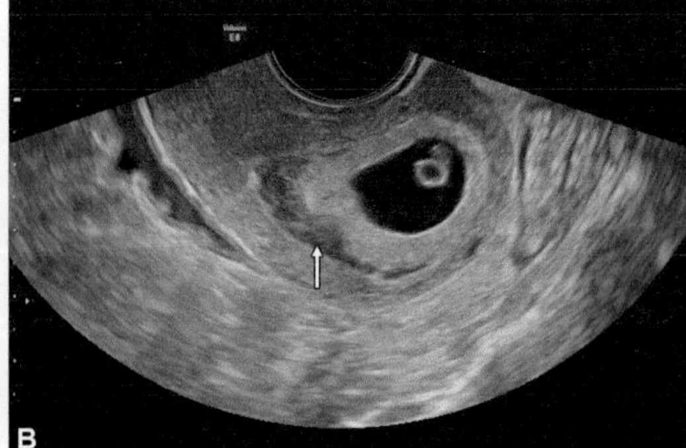

Figs. 15A and B: (A) First trimester scan on transvaginal B-mode ultrasound shows low-level echogenicities in gestational sac but outside amniotic sac. Possible cause may be infection or hemorrhage; (B) Hypoechoic area (arrow) is seen around the chorionic plate on first trimester transvaginal B-mode scan—choriodecidual separation and hemorrhage.

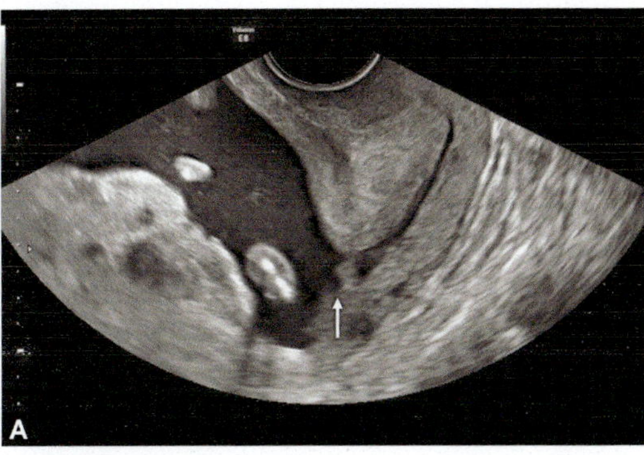

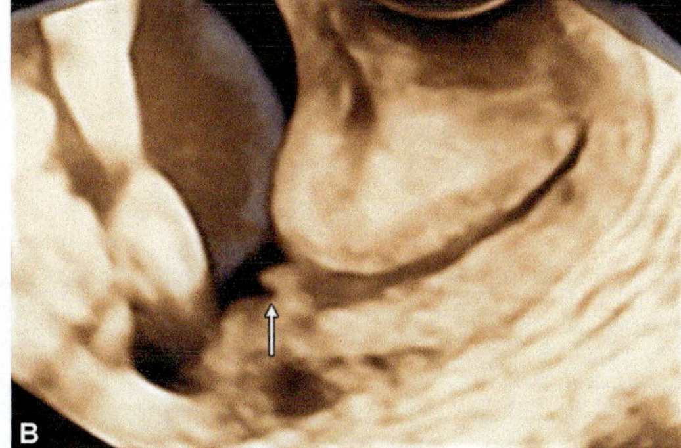

Figs. 16A and B: Open internal os and cervical canal seen on fundal pressure on the gravid uterus indicates: (A) Incompetence on B-mode; (B) Surface rendered three-dimensional (3D) image by arrow.

cervical incompetence in women at high risk at 15–24 weeks.[5] MacDonald et al. reported that opening of the internal os at rest or in response to transfundal pressure was the earliest ultrasound feature of cervical incompetence[6] **(Figs. 16A and B)**.

TECHNIQUE OF TRANSVAGINAL ULTRASOUND METHOD FOR CERVICAL ASSESSMENT

- Bladder should be empty
- Patient is in supine position with hip and knee flexed
- Probe in anterior fornix
- Do not exert undue pressure
- Picture should be magnified to ≥75% of the screen
- Correct image should show endocervical mucosa along the cervical canal.

Calipers are placed at internal os and external os. The caliper for internal os is placed at the apex of V-shaped notch and for external os is placed at the apex of triangular echodensity of external os **(Fig. 17)**.

- Each examination is done for 3–5 minutes to observe any dynamic cervical changes
- Shortest of three diameters is taken as cervical length[7]
- Funneling must be documented. Funneling is described as Y or U shape of cervix **(Figs. 18 and 19)**
- Cervical index can be measured as: (Funnel length + 1)/Cervical length

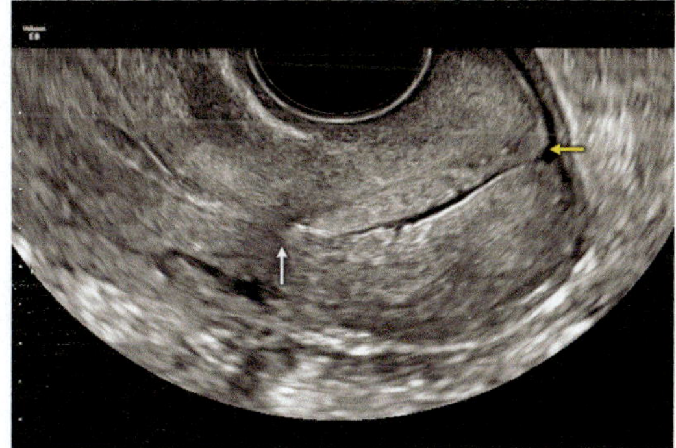

Fig. 17: B-mode transvaginal scan of cervix showing exact location of internal os (white arrow) and external os (yellow arrow).

- Funnel length, funnel width, and percentage of funneling [Funnel length/ (Funnel length + Cervical length) × 100] is also evaluated by different workers
- When this technique for cervical length assessment is followed, the interobserver error is 5–10%.

The criteria that are mandatory for cervical length assessment are as follows:

- Internal os should be clearly visible as flat dimple or as hypoechoic triangle
- Whole length of cervical canal should be clearly visible
- External os appears symmetrical
- External surface of the cervix should be clearly identified
- Distance between posterior lip of cervical canal should be identical to distance from anterior lip.

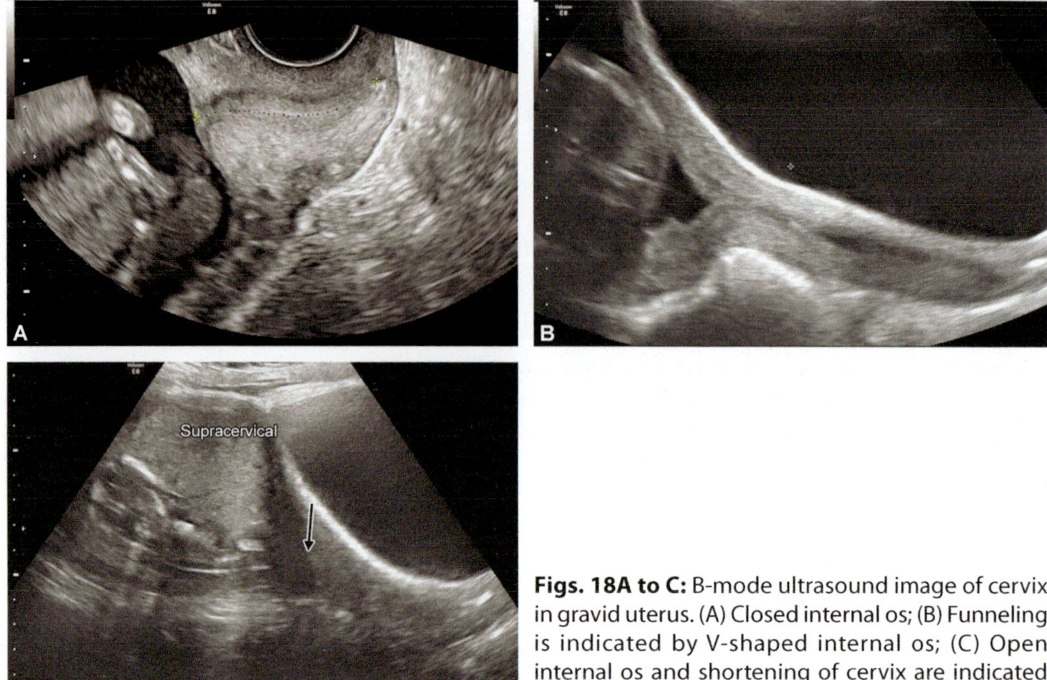

Figs. 18A to C: B-mode ultrasound image of cervix in gravid uterus. (A) Closed internal os; (B) Funneling is indicated by V-shaped internal os; (C) Open internal os and shortening of cervix are indicated by deep "V".

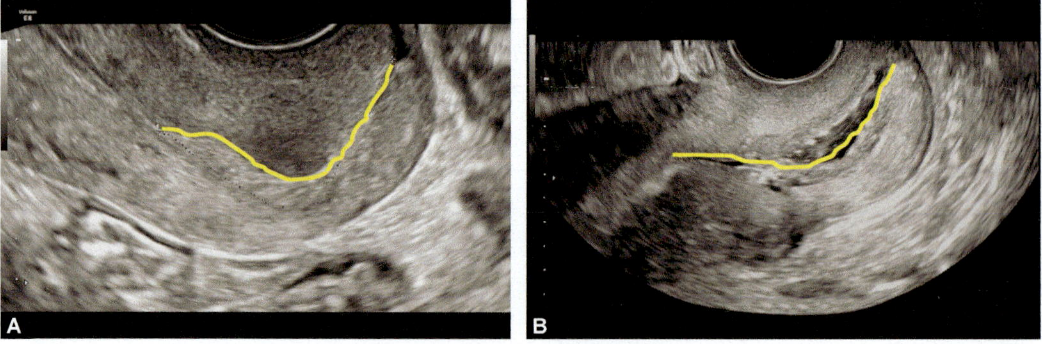

Figs. 19A and B: B-mode ultrasound image of curved cervices. Yellow lines demonstrate tracing of cervical canal to assess correct length of cervix from internal os to external os.

The anatomical difficulties for cervical assessment are identification of internal os due to undeveloped lower uterine segment, focal myometrial contraction, rapid and spontaneous cervical change, and endocervical polyps. The technical problems are incorrect interpretation for dilatation of internal os due to vaginal probe orientation and artificial lengthening of cervical canal due to distortion of cervix by the transducer.[8]

If the cervix is to be measured in first trimester, the suggested method is to measure the linear distance between the two ends of glandular area of cervix and then measure the shortest distance between the glandular area and the gestational sac (isthmic length).[9] Serial measurements of cervix in first and second trimester and rate of decrease in cervical length may be useful to assess the risk of preterm delivery.

Cervical assessment has been tried with 3D ultrasound by several workers, but with no advantage over 2D ultrasound.

Transvaginal cervical assessment for prediction of preterm birth was first documented by Anderson et al. This study had shown that a cervical length of <39 mm before 30 weeks of pregnancy was a significant risk factor for early delivery.[10] There have been several studies since the noncervical length and funneling of internal os and the risk of preterm delivery. The incidence of premature deliveries is increasing especially because of iatrogenically increased incidence of multiple gestations due to assisted reproductive techniques.

In women with symptoms of preterm labor, it is not possible by frequency or intensity of contractions to differentiate between true and false preterm labor.[11] Transvaginal ultrasound can assess the cervix and differentiate between the two and can also predict preterm delivery. In patients with threatened preterm labor, cervical length of <30 mm had a high risk of preterm delivery and those with <20 mm of cervical length delivered preterm,[12] whereas another study showed a sensitivity of 56%, PPV of 90%, specificity of 96%, and NPV of 79% for preterm delivery with cervical length of ≤20 mm. Barghella et al. reported that funneling was a good predictor of preterm delivery in second trimester, but may be normally seen after 32 weeks.[13] Short cervix and/or funneling can be used as a guide to decide for tocolytic therapy. In one of the largest studies of 3,694 singleton pregnancies, cervical assessment was done between 18 and 22 weeks. When cervical length was <29 mm, the relative risk for delivery before 35 weeks was 8 as compared to 28 when internal os was dilated to 5 mm,[14] although To et al. concluded that funneling did not provide significant additional contribution to cervical length in prediction of delivery before 33 weeks.[15]

In women with a history of spontaneous preterm birth, a systematic review of controlled studies showed that measurement of cervical length in the second trimester, especially before 24 weeks, predicted the risk of recurrent preterm birth.[16]

On TVS, cervical length <25 mm at <24 weeks to predict preterm birth at <35 weeks yield sensitivity of 65.4%, specificity of 75.5%, PPV of 33.0%, and NPV of 92.0%. The shorter the cervical length, the higher the positive likelihood ratio for spontaneous preterm birth <35 weeks.[17]

This means that though the cervix is measured as normal length, this is not an assurance that pregnancy problems of abortions or preterm labor will not occur. However, if the cervix is short, it definitely depicts early abortion or labor.

Presence of cervical funneling of >75% or a cervical shortening of <10 mm was predictive of preterm premature rupture of membranes (PPROM).[18] In patients with PPROM, cervical length of <20 mm and/or funneling was associated with short time interval from admission to delivery.[19]

In women with prior preterm birth at 28–36 weeks, it is recommended to initiate screening at 16 weeks. Ultrasound examination is generally repeated every 2 weeks until 24 weeks as long as the cervical length is ≥30 mm and increased to weekly if cervical length is 25–29 mm with the expectation that preterm cervical changes will precede overt preterm labor or membrane rupture symptoms by 3–6 weeks.[17] Cervical ultrasonography appears to be more efficient as a short term than as a long-term predictor, so serial examinations in a time interval of 10–14 days for women with short cervical length should be recommended.[20]

Multiple regression analysis has confirmed that cervical length was a significant predictor of preterm birth before 35 weeks and that multiparous had a 43% greater risk compared with nulliparous.[21] Transvaginal scan for cervical measurement is at 22–24 weeks has shown TVS to be superior to Bishop score and fetal fibronectin in cervicovaginal secretion. But, at 31–32 weeks, no one method is better than the other for predicting preterm delivery.[22]

Before 16 weeks, internal os is difficult to identify and lower segment of the uterus is also not formed, so cervical measurement before 16 weeks is not a reliable screening method for assessing the risk of preterm delivery.[23] In multiple pregnancies, cervical measurement is more important than singleton pregnancy. For singleton pregnancy, the cutoff for exponential rise in risk of preterm delivery is 15 mm, whereas for multiple pregnancies, it is 25 mm.[24] Ultrasonographic cervical length measurements may predict the latency period between admission and delivery without increasing the risk of neonatal sepsis or chorioamnionitis.[25] Elective cervical cerclage has a significant effect in preventing spontaneous preterm birth before 34 weeks of gestation.[26] Placement of cervical cerclage before 27 weeks of gestation in women who have a cervix shorter than 25 mm may reduce the incidence of preterm delivery before 34 weeks of gestation among high-risk patients.[27] Although when the cervix is shorter than 15 mm at the time of cerclage at 22–24 weeks, the risk of delivery before 33 weeks cannot be substantially reduced.[28]

In a nonhigh-risk population, a single TVS cervical length measurement should be done at 18–24 weeks in women with risk factors for cervical insufficiency and no prior delivery and treat those with a short cervix (≤20 mm) with vaginal progesterone supplementation.

Because of poor PPVs and sensitivities and lack of proven effective interventions, routine transvaginal cervical length assessment is not recommended in women at low risk. However, depending on the setup and the type of practice, one TVS at 18 weeks seems no harm rather it may pick up a woman who has short cervix.

To summarize for assessment of the cervix in pregnant women for the risk of preterm labor, it includes cervical length, funneling of internal os, and shortening of the cervix on dynamic examination.

REFERENCES

1. Carr DB, Smith K, Parsons L. Ultrasonography for cervical length measurement: agreement between transvaginal and translabial techniques. Obstet Gynecol. 2000;96:554-8.
2. To MS, Skemtou C, Cicero S. Cervical assessment at the routine 23 weeks scan: problems with transabdominal sonography. Ultrasound Obstet Gynecol. 2000;15:292-6.
3. Doyle NM, Monga M. Role of ultrasound in screening patients at risk for preterm delivery. Obstet Gynecol Clin North Am. 2004;31:125-39.
4. Kusanovic JP, Espinoza J, Romero R. Clinical significance of the presence of amniotic fluid "sludge" in asymptomatic patients at high risk for spontaneous preterm delivery. Ultrasound Obstet Gynecol. 2007;30:706-14.
5. Guzman ER, Pisatowski DM, Vintzileos AM, et al. A comparison of ultrasonographically detected cervical changes in response to transfundal pressure, coughing and standing in predicting cervical incompetence. Am J Obstet Gynecol. 1997;177:660-5.
6. MacDonald R, Smith P, Vyas S. Cervical incompetence: the use of transvaginal sonography to provide an objective diagnosis. Ultrasound Obstet Gynecol. 2001;18:211-6.
7. Owen J, Iams JD, National Institute of Child Health and Human Development Maternal-Fetal Medicine Units Network. What we have learned about cervical ultrasound. Semin Perinatol. 2003;27:194-203.
8. Yost NP, Bloom SL, Twickler DM. Pitfalls in ultrasonographic cervical canal length measurement for predicting preterm birth. Obstet Gynecol. 1999;93:510-6.
9. Greco E, Lange A, Ushakov F, Rodriguez J, Nicolaides KH. Prediction of spontaneous preterm delivery from endocervical length at 11–13 weeks. Prenat Diagn. 2011;31:84-9.
10. Anderson HF, Nugent CE, Wanty SD. Prediction of risk of preterm delivery by ultrasonographic measurement of cervical length. Am J Obstet Gynecol. 1990;166:859-67.
11. Iams JD, Casal D, McGregor JA, Goodwin TM, Kreaden US, Lowensohn R, et al. Fetal fibronection improves the accuracy of diagnosis of preterm labor. Am J Obstet Gynecol. 1995;173:141-5.
12. Murakawa H, Utumi T, Hasegawa I. Evaluation of threatened preterm delivery by transvaginal

ultrasonographic measurement of cervical length. Obstet Gynecol. 1993;82:829-32.
13. Barghella V, Kuhlman K, Weiner S, Texeira L, Wapner RJ. Cervical funneling: sonographic criteria predictive of preterm delivery. Ultrasound Obstet Gynecol. 1997;10:161-6.
14. Taipale P, Hiilesmaa V. Sonographic measurement of uterine cervix at 18–22 weeks' gestation and the risk of preterm delivery. Obstet Gynecol. 1998;92:902-7.
15. To MS, Skentuo C, Liao AW. Cervical length at 23 weeks of gestation in the prediction of spontaneous early preterm delivery. Ultrasound Obstet Gynecol. 2001;18:200-3.
16. Crane JM, Hutchens D. Transvaginal sonographic measurement of cervical length to predict preterm birth in a symptomatic women at increased risk: a systematic review. Ultrasound Obstet Gynecol. 2008;31:579.
17. Iams JD, Cebrik D, Lynch C, Behendt N, Das A. The rate of cervical change and the phenotype of spontaneous preterm birth. Am J Obstet Gynecol. 2011;205:130.e1-6.
18. Obido AO, Berghella V, Reddy U. Does transvaginal ultrasound of the cervix predict preterm premature rupture of membranes in a high-risk population? Ultrasound Obstet Gynecol. 2001;18:223-7.
19. Carlan SJ, Richmond LB, O'Brien WF. Randomised trial of endovaginal ultrasound in preterm premature rupture of membranes. Obstet Gynecol. 1997;89:458-61.
20. Heath VC, Southall TR, Souka AP. Cervical length at 23 weeks of gestation: prediction of spontaneous preterm delivery. Ultrasound Obstet Gynecol. 1998;12:312-7.
21. Fujita MM, Brizot de L, Liao AW. Reference range for cervical length in twin pregnancies. Acta Obstet Gynecol Scan. 2002;81:856-9.
22. Hoesli I, Tercanli S, Holzgreve W. Cervical length assessment by ultrasound as a predictor of preterm labor—is there a role for routine screening? BJOG. 2003;110:61-5.
23. Conoscenti G, Meir YJ, D'Ottavio G. Does cervical length at 13–15 weeks gestation predict preterm delivery in the unselected population. Ultrasound Obstet Gynecol. 2003;21:128-34.
24. Berghella V, Talucci M, Desai A. Does transvaginal sonographic measurement of cervical length before 14 weeks predict preterm delivery in high-risk pregnancies? Ultrasound Obstet Gynecol. 2003;21:140-4.
25. To MS, Skentou C, Cicero S. Cervical length at 23 weeks in triplets: prediction of spontaneous preterm delivery. Ultrasound Obstet Gynecol. 2000;16:515-8.
26. Palma-Dias RS, Fonesca MM, Stein NR. Relation of cervical length at 22–24 weeks of gestation to demographic characteristics and obstetric history. Braz J Med Biol Res. 2004;37:737-44.
27. Heath VC, Southall TR, Souka AP, Novakov A, Nicolaides KH. Cervical length at 23 weeks of gestation: relation to demographic characteristics and previous obstetric history. Ultrasound Obstet Gynecol. 1998;12:304-11.
28. Crane J, Scott H, Stewart A. Transvaginal ultrasonography to predict preterm birth in women with bicornuate or didelphys uterus. J Matern Fetal Neonatal Med. 2012;25:1960-4.

35

CHAPTER

Ultrasound in Urogynecology

Sonal Panchal, Chaitanya Nagori

INTRODUCTION

Urogynecology deals with urinary dysfunction, bowel dysfunction, and prolapse of anterior compartment, posterior compartment, or vault. The most common cause for urogynecological abnormalities is pelvic floor trauma during labor. 10–30% of all women having delivered normally have some avulsion of puborectalis. Over 40% of women undergoing normal labor suffer from either frank tears or irreversible overdistension of hiatus.[1]

Common complaints are recurrent urinary tract infection, persistent dysuria, urgency, frequency, urinary incontinence (UI), genitourinary prolapse, flatus, and fecal incontinence. These commonly affect postmenopausal females resulting into a lot of restriction to activities, decreased self-esteem, lack of confidence, depression, and also deterioration of lifestyle.

Complaints and clinical history often help to direct to the correct diagnosis, especially in cases of stress urinary incontinence (SUI). Important points in history are duration and the severity of incontinence. It is also important to listen to the patient's perception of symptoms carefully with differentiation between incontinence, urgency, and difficulty in voiding. Symptoms must be evaluated in light of obstetric history, history of previous surgeries, present or previous medications, fluid intake and schedule of food, etc., and details of how many times does she have to void and the quantity of urine. Complaint of fecal incontinence is evaluated with food habits, changes in food habits, history of medications, stool frequency, and consistency.

PHYSICAL EXAMINATION

This chiefly includes assessing for vulvovaginitis, atrophic changes, prolapse of bladder, bowel or vault, and presence of pelvic masses. Neurological disease may often be the basis for the complaints and detailed history and examination are essential to rule out the same. Patients with incontinence and prolapse must be assessed also with coughing or Valsalva. Inspection for narrowing of vaginal introitus and lifting up of posterior wall of vagina and anus is helpful to establish the diagnosis.

General condition of the patient should also be assessed that may be the cause of all the symptoms and this also includes tone and strength of the muscles including those of the pelvic floor. Tone of the pelvic floor muscles is assessed with digital palpation, but one may also use electromyography or perineometry.

INVESTIGATIONS

- Urine analysis
- Transabdominal ultrasound for kidneys, ureters, and bladder
- Transvaginal ultrasound for uterus, adnexa, and ovaries
- *Transperineal ultrasound for assessment of the pelvic floor*: B-mode ultrasound allows us to evaluate the internal pelvic anatomy, but not the pelvic floor muscles, as these are perpendicular to the probe surface
- *Three-dimensional-four-dimensional (3D-4D) transperineal ultrasound*: 3D pelvic

floor ultrasound enables us to evaluate the levator ani with much less cost to the health care provider and minimal discomfort to the patient.[2,3]

Method:

- With empty bladder
- With transvaginal probe with probe placed in the introital area in midsagittal plane
- Acquisition angle of 80° or more to include the entire pelvis
- One volume at rest and one on Valsalva
- One may also use 4–7 MHz convex probe with a volume angle of 70°.

Tomographic ultrasound imaging (TUI) or omniview with volume contrast imaging (VCI) on 3D ultrasound can also be used to assess the pelvic floor muscles.[4] At least three central slices are taken. Plane of minimum hiatal dimensions and two slices 2.5 mm and 5 mm are cranial to it. Lowermost slice is just below the insertion of puborectalis muscle[5] **(Fig. 1)**. Tomographic ultrasound imaging may also be a valuable and time-saving option.

- *MRI*: Major advantage of ultrasound is that it is a dynamic study and so effect of stress, coughing, and Valsalva can be better demonstrated. It has been documented that 3D ultrasound to be superior especially for prolapse assessment mentioning that ultrafast acquisition MRI may be required for this purpose.[6,7]

Patients in whom surgical management is required:

- Uroflowmetry
- Urethral pressure profilometry
- Videocystourethrography.

ANATOMY

Endopelvic fascia is made of smooth muscle and fibrous connective tissue. It inserts into fascial coverings of obturator internus and levator ani. Increased intra-abdominal pressure compresses urethra against this. Pubocervical fascia supports bladder and is between vagina and bladder. Weakness of any of these support systems leads to prolapse and incontinence. Separation of pubocervical fascia (unilateral or bilateral) from arcus tendineus fascia covering obturator internus and levator ani muscles (pelvic diaphragm) leads to stress incontinence and cystourethrocele.[8-10] Levator ani consists of pubococcygeus, puborectalis, and iliococcygeus muscles. These muscles span between obturator internus laterally and pubic symphysis anteriorly. The second layer is superficial to this and is urogenital diaphragm made of ischiocavernosus, bulbospongiosus, and transversus perinei superficialis.[11] Levator hiatus is space between these various muscles and through that are urethra, vagina, and anus.[12] Puborectalis extends from pubic symphysis till behind the anus.[13] The latter is the most important muscle to maintain continence and control.

Structures of the lower genitourinary tract and pelvic floor can be visualized from different approaches: transperineal, introital, transvaginal, abdominal, or endoanal.

Method

Patient is placed in semireclining position. Bladder is partially filled. Filling the bladder

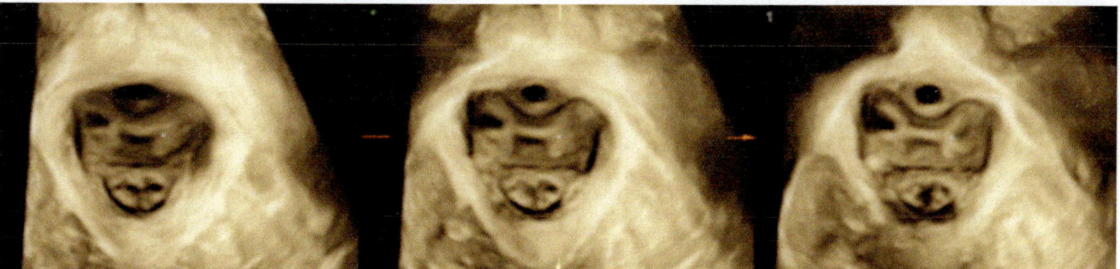

Fig. 1: 3D ultrasound TUI image of the pelvic floor showing plane of minimum hiatal dimensions and two slices 2.5 mm and 5 mm are cranial to it.

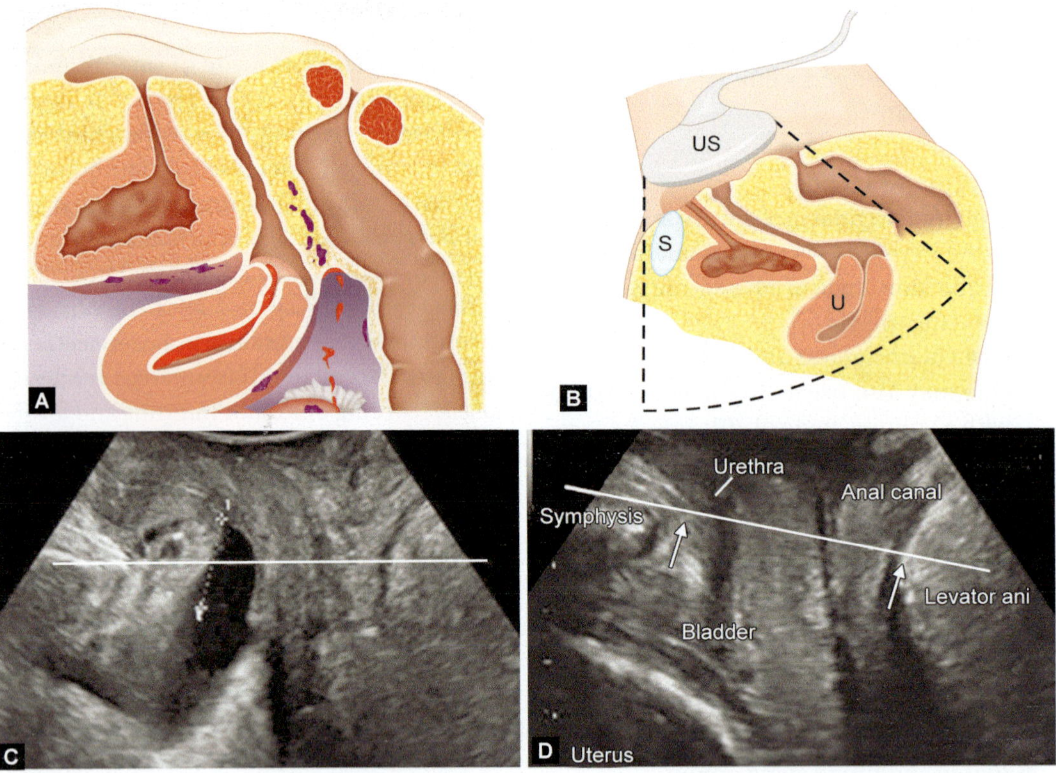

Figs. 2A to C: (A) Diagrammatic representation of the anatomy of the pelvis as seen from the introitus; (B) Diagrammatic representation of the 2D ultrasound image of the pelvis as seen on introital scan; (C and D) 2D ultrasound image of the pelvis as seen on introital scan showing plane of minimal diameter at rest (C) and on Valsalva.

may lead to incontinence and may show funneling that is more pronounced.[14] Prolapse also becomes more evident when pressure is applied with full bladder.[15] This position is convenient for the patient when pressure is to be exerted during assessment of the pelvic floor.[16]

Transperineal Ultrasound

Transperineal ultrasound (TUS) is carried out with a 3.5–6 MHz curved array transducer placed on the perineum in the midsagittal line. Transducer is covered with nonpowdered glove. Examination is usually performed in the dorsal lithotomy position with the hips flexed and abducted. For perineal ultrasound, probe is placed over the labia. Parting of labia may be required for better image quality. Transducer is placed firmly on symphysis pubis (SP) and perineum. This shows entire SP.

The resulting image shows the SP, urethra, bladder, vagina, rectum, and anal canal **(Figs. 2A to C)**. Other findings include the uterus, the cul-de-sac with bowels and fluid as well as synthetic implants or pelvic pathologies. The SP is used as a stable landmark serving as a reference for evaluation of the bladder neck position and mobility. Full rectum, gas in rectum, pelvic organ prolapse (POP), vaginal scar tissue, or synthetic implants may impair visibility.[17-20]

Dietz et al., using 3D/4D introital scan identified specific labor-related damage to the puborectalis muscle termed as avulsion. It is the result of the detachment of the muscle from its insertion on the inferior pubic ramus and the pelvic side as a consequence

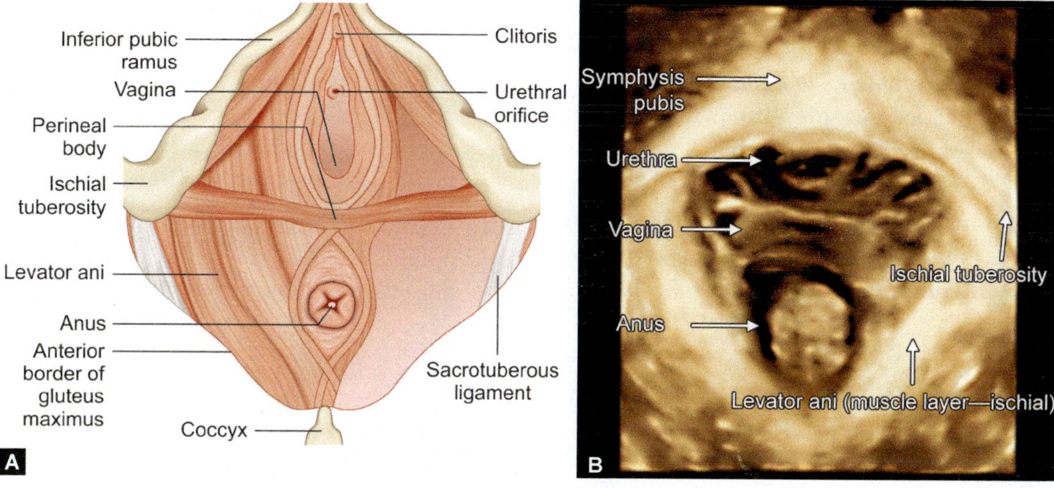

Figs. 3A and B: Coronal plane anatomy of the pelvic floor: (A) Diagrammatic presentation; (B) As seen on 3D ultrasound.

of overstretching of the levator during the second stage of labor and may be detected in up to 36% of women following their first vaginal delivery. Damage to the levator muscle leads to enlargement of the levator hiatus, which on 4D introital ultrasound is observed as "hiatus ballooning." Both levator avulsion and ballooning are associated with prolapse of the pelvic organs.[17,19,21] Since the technique enables one to obtain tomographic or multislice scans, the whole puborectalis muscle and its attachments to the pubic rami can be visualized **(Figs. 3A and B)**.

Introital Ultrasound (Figs. 4A and B)

This technique involves the use of front-firing endovaginal probes (5–7.5 MHz) placed on the vaginal introitus. It provides higher resolution of images but reduced penetration into the tissues. The effect of the Valsalva maneuver on proximal urethral mobility may be evaluated analogously to transperineal ultrasound (TPUS) using the inferior margin of the SP as a reference.[19,20] For introital scan, the probe is placed over external urethral orifice, with long axis of the probe, along the long axis of the body. This scan shows only

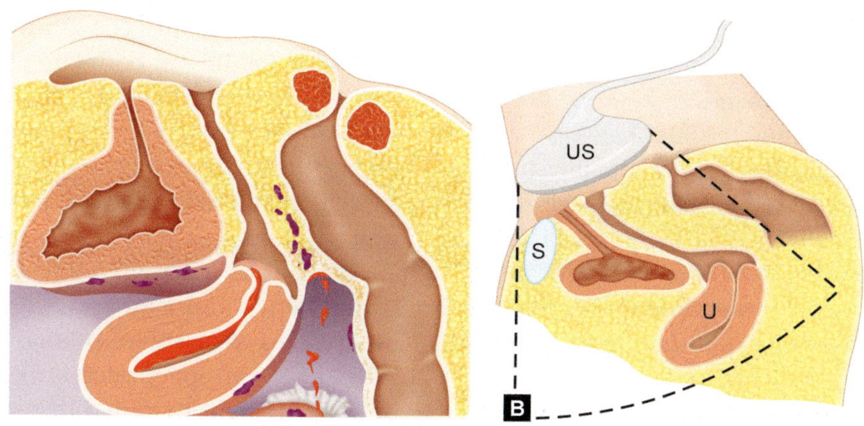

Figs. 4A and B: (A) Diagrammatic presentation of female pelvic anatomy; (B) Diagrammatic presentation of female pelvic anatomy on translabial scan.

lower end of SP. Primarily assessment of the urethra, urinary bladder, periurethral tissues, endopelvic fascia, vagina, and rectum is assessed. Excessive pressure is never exerted on the probe. This may displace the bladder neck. Dynamic assessment is essential when assessing pelvic floor. The assessment is done at rest, on coughing, on Valsalva maneuver, and with pressure.

Measurements

- *Height*: Vertical distance between lower end of SP to the bladder neck (20.6 mm at rest and 14 mm on pressing).[22-24]
- *Angle* β: It is a posterior urethrovesical angle between long axis of urethra and bladder neck. Assessment is done at rest, during contraction, coughing, and pressing[25] (normal at rest 96.8° and on pressure 108.1°).[22-24]
- *Bladder wall thickness*: It is best measured after micturition in lithotomy position with transvaginal image.[26] Measurement is done at the thickest part of the trigone dome and anterior wall of urinary bladder.
- *Bladder neck funneling*: It is not seen at rest. Morphological layers of urethra are not seen in midsagittal plane due to artifact. But, if incontinence is present, funneling must be seen, unless examination is done in lying down position, with empty bladder or with inadequate Valsalva pressure.[16] Funneling and increased bladder neck mobility are commonly seen in patients with incontinence.[27-29]

Bladder neck mobility may be:

- Check for bladder neck mobility. It may be influenced by pregnancy and delivery apart from body habitus. Mobility can decrease with pelvic floor awareness education[30,31]
- Rotational posteroinferior descent—with inferior margin of symphysis acting as a pivot
- Vertical descent along urethral axis[32]
- *Bladder neck and pubic point movement*:[33]
  - *Strain and bladder neck*: 16.9 mm ± 6.1
  - *Pubic point*: 4.8 mm ± 3.9
  - *Cough bladder neck*: 10.2 mm ± 5.4
  - *Pubic point*: 2.9 mm ± 3.4.

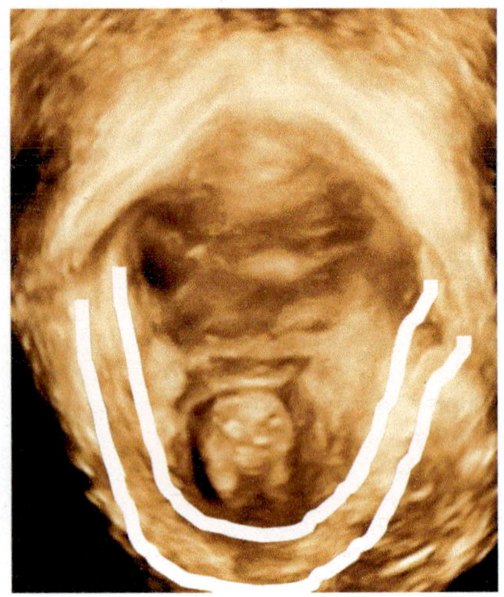

Fig. 5: Measurement of the maximum muscle levator ani thickness.

Some workers also assess the levator ani thickness. In the axial view, maximum diameters of the pubovisceral muscle in two locations bilaterally and muscle area by tracing its outline at the level of maximal muscle thickness can also be assessed **(Fig. 5)**. Maximum levator thickness is determined by slowly moving the plane of minimal hiatal dimensions cranially until the plane of maximal thickness of the pubovisceral muscle is reached. This is usually located about 1–1.5 cm above the actual levator hiatus. Though measures of muscle mass did not correlate with levator function as determined by displacement of the bladder neck on levator contraction, a finding that agrees with clinical impressions: a bulky levator may not necessarily contract well.[34]

Endoanal route is used for anal incontinence and anal tumors. It can also be used for assessment of anal sphincter. Ultrasound is an optional test in the evaluation of patients with complex or recurrent UI and/or POP (level of evidence 3, grade of recommendation C).

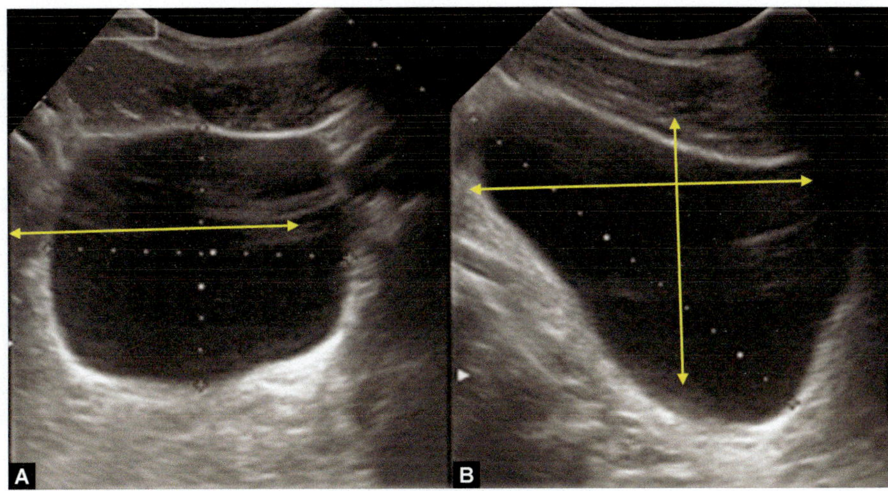

Figs. 6A and B: Transverse and longitudinal sections of the bladder on transabdominal scan with measurement of maximum orthogonal diameters, to assess the bladder volume.

B-mode ultrasound is done to look for:

- Bladder volume
- Bladder wall thickness
- Bladder tumors
- Urethral diverticula (UD)
- Hematomas
- Bladder neck mobility
- Cystocele/cystourethrocele
- Enterocele/rectocele
- Rectal intussusception (RI).

BLADDER VOLUME MEASUREMENT

This is especially done in cases of:

- Overactive bladder syndrome
- Neurogenic bladder
- Pelvic prolapse
- Voiding symptoms
- After incontinence surgeries.

It is always done on transabdominal scan.

The recent International Federation of Gynecology and Obstetrics (FIGO) group guidelines, in concert with other recommendations, advise that volumes greater than 150 mL should be regarded as abnormal.[35]

Higher incidence of elevated postvoid residual (PVR) is observed among patients with stress urinary incontinence (SUI), previous incontinence surgery, overactive bladder, multiple sclerosis, and POP stage 2 or greater.[36]

According to Tseng et al., almost 16% of women with SUI have PVR > 100 mL.[37]

Therefore, measurement of PVR is recommended as a standard workup in patients with urinary incontinence (UI) or POP before and after the treatment. Due to high prevalence of urine retention and frequent need for clean intermittent catheterization, evaluation of PVR is of pivotal. Ultrasound estimations may be performed using either three diameters (length, height, and width) or the surface area in the transverse image and the length obtained in the longitudinal image **(Figs. 6A and B)**. Although >20 different formulae for PVR calculation have been proposed over the years, the inaccuracy of ultrasound measurements may be as high as 20–25%. However, this level of accuracy is sufficient for clinical purposes.

BLADDER WALL THICKNESS AS A MARKER OF DETRUSOR OVERACTIVITY

Numerous studies using abdominal, transperineal, introital, or endovaginal ultrasound have shown increased bladder wall thickness (BWT) or detrusor wall thickness (DWT) in patients with detrusor overactivity (DO). This phenomenon is

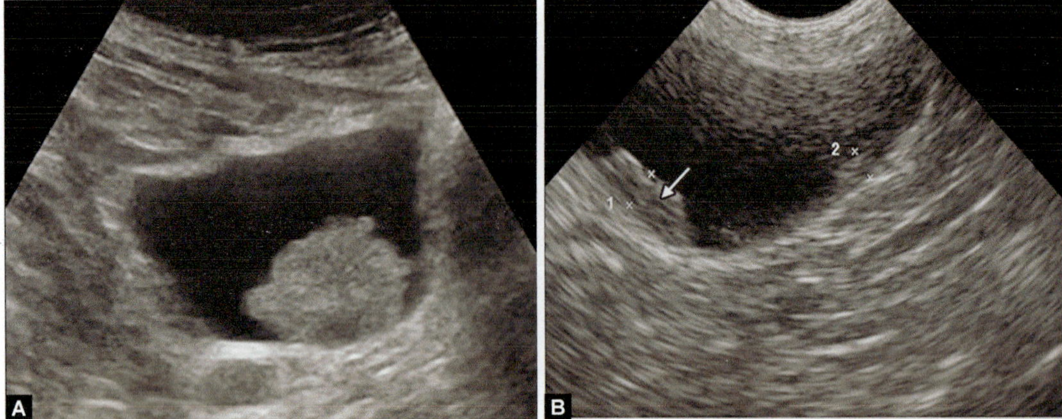

Figs. 7A and B: (A) Solid projection like bladder tumor with irregular margins; (B) Plaque like bladder neoplasm.

believed to reflect bladder wall hypertrophy secondary to frequent detrusor contractions during the storage phase. A systematic review performed by Latthe et al.,[38] after assessment of the methodological quality of 190 studies included only five studies for further analysis. Using a 5 mm cutoff for BWT for identifying DO, the sensitivity and specificity of this marker were 85% and 89% in one study,[39] but 40% and 79% in another study.[40] BWT is measured at three places—anterior wall, trigone, and the dome and take a mean value of this, though there are insufficient data to reliably estimate accuracy of BWT in DO. Bladder wall thickening is also seen with infection after radiation or surgery, in neurological bladder, detrusor instability, outflow tract obstruction, and neoplasm.

BLADDER TUMORS

These are polypoid/sessile solid projections or plaque like with regular or irregular surface and with or without calcifications **(Figs. 7A and B)**. Bladder wall invasion is checked by sliding organ sign.[41] It may also be used in cervical malignancies to detect bladder invasion. Bladder endometriotic nodule may also look very similar to plaque-like tumor growth.

URETHRAL DIVERTICULA

Urethral diverticula (UD) affect 6–20 in 1,000,000 of the general population, but may be observed in up to 1.4% of those with UI.[42-44] Most probably, UD develops from the periurethral glands obstructed and dilated as a consequence of chronic inflammation.[45,46] The majority of diverticula are in the form of a simple pouch, but some can have complex morphology such as saddlebag or circumferential **(Fig. 8)**. The classic presentation of UD includes the “three Ds”: dysuria, dyspareunia, and postvoid dribbling. However, many nonspecific complains such as frequency, urgency, UI, pain, or discharge

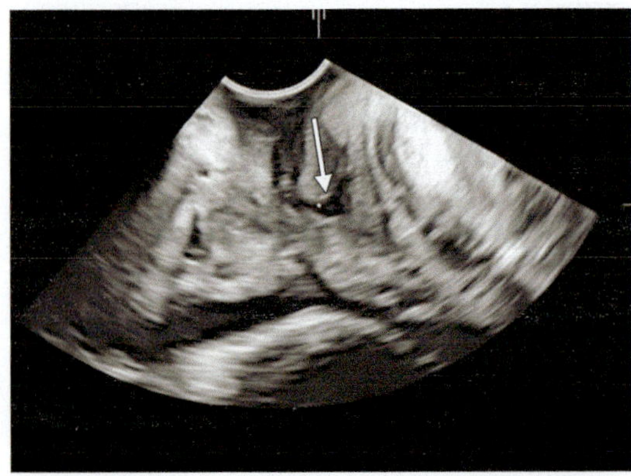

Fig. 8: 3D ultrasound multiplanar image of pelvic floor with VCI showing urethral diverticulum (arrow).

may be reported. On physical examination, a periurethral mass, sometimes mimicking cystocele, can be palpated.[45,46] On transvaginal ultrasound, these are seen as cystic lesions (single/multiple) around the urethra.[47]

RETROPUBIC HEMATOMA

It is seen following retropubic urethropexy or suburethral sling procedure and also in cases with successful surgery and satisfactory healing.[48] On transvaginal scan, it appears as hypoechoic or mixed echogenic area between SP, urethra, and bladder.

Bladder Neck Funneling

Opening of the bladder neck on Valsalva or coughing is a typical finding in women with SUI, but can be seen in asymptomatic women as well.[28,49,50]

It is also observed in urge UI and, thus, cannot be regarded as diagnostic for any of these conditions.[50]

There is insufficient evidence for clinical benefit of standard evaluation of bladder neck funneling in patients with UI **(Fig. 9)**. Descent of pelvic organs in cases of mild or moderate prolapse can be easily visualized by ultrasound during the Valsalva maneuver or coughing. Ultrasound imaging enables one to discriminate between cystourethrocele and isolated cystocele in the anterior compartment and between rectocele and enterocele in the posterior compartment.[16]

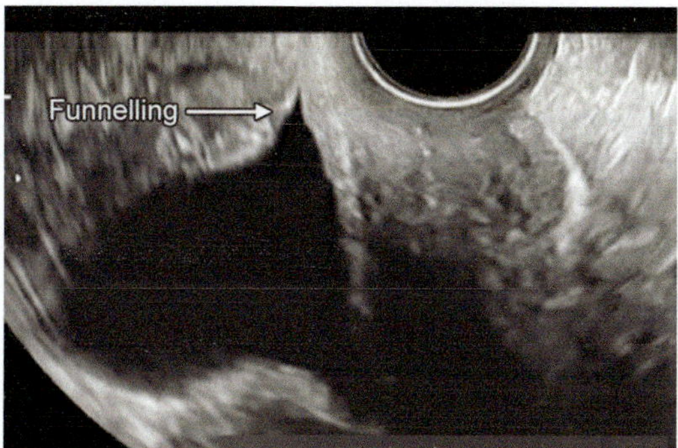

Fig. 9: B mode ultrasound image of the pelvic floor, on introital scan done with endocavitary probe, showing funelling of the vesicourethral junction on Valsalva.

Transperineal ultrasound can be used to quantify the degree of prolapse. A fairly good correlation between ultrasound and clinical prolapse assessment has been demonstrated.

URETHRAL MOBILITY (BLADDER NECK MOBILITY)

On transperineal or introital ultrasound, the position of the bladder neck at rest and on maximal Valsalva may be determined relative to the central line of the SP or its inferoposterior margin. Since the entire SP is rarely visualized, drawing of the central line (axis) may be difficult.[20] Hennemann et al.,[51] managed to draw the central line in only 12% of transperineal images. Therefore, using the inferoposterior margin of the SP, a reference is recommended, but care must be taken not to change the ultrasound position during the maneuver.[20] On Valsalva, the bladder neck and proximal urethra rotate in the posteroinferior direction. The distal urethra remains stable due to the fact that together with the anterior vaginal wall, it is tethered to the SP and pelvic sidewalls. This results in either urinary retention or an urge to pass urine immediately after voiding once. Valsalva maneuver is forced expiration against closed glottis and contracted diaphragm and abdominal wall and must be continued for at least 5 seconds. It is important that the maneuver is properly explained to the patient and rehearsed because most of the times when patient is asked to exert pressure in downward direction, such as in Valsalva, she actually uplifts the pelvic floor and holds it tight. This may mask both the hypermobility of bladder neck as well as the prolapse. This is called levator coactivation. Levator coactivation can be differentiated from the Valsalva on imaging by assessing the anteroposterior diameter of the pelvic orifice or distance from the

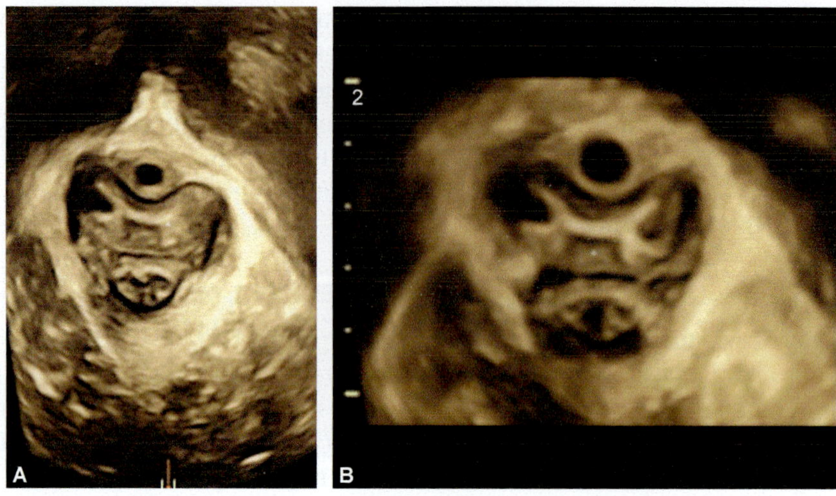

Figs. 10A and B: 3D ultrasound rendered image of pelvic floor at rest (A) and on levator coactivation showing reduced anteroposterior diameter of levator hiatus (B).

posterior most margin of symphysis pubis and anterior margin of anorectal flexure. Reduced anteroposterior diameter of levator hiatus with elevation of anorectum and change in the angle between levator plate and SP suggests levator coactivation **(Figs. 10A and B)** and increase in anteroposterior diameter of the levator hiatus with downward movement of anorectum suggests Valsalva. Anterior vaginal wall prolapse and SUI are at least partly due to disruption of paravaginal and/or paraurethral support structures, i.e., the endopelvic fascia and pubourethral ligaments at the time of vaginal delivery.[52]

Measurements are taken at rest and on maximal straining **(Figs. 11A to C)**. The hypermobility of the urethra is not well defined and different cutoffs of 20, 25, or 30 mm have been proposed.[18,19] The angle ≥30° defines urethral hypermobility.[35] In one study among nulliparous continent women of approximately 20 years of age, the bladder neck descent varied between 1 and 40 mm.[53] Interestingly, a study on a twin model suggested that bladder neck mobility may be due to some extent determined genetically.[54]

Urethral hypermobility is considered to be related to SUI. This is mainly due to the fact that urethral mobility is a prerequisite for suburethral sling action.

Endopelvic fascia and anterior vaginal wall form a supportive layer on which urethra course.[55,56] Reactivity of the pelvic floor can be assessed by measuring the distance from lower margin of pubic symphysis to bladder neck (H). Increased distance reflects good levator ani reactivity **(Figs. 11A to C)**.[57]

CYSTOCELE

With hypermobility of the urethra, there may also be hypermobility of the bladder. This allows a pouch of the bladder descending below the level of the bladder neck and this result into urinary retention. This urine-filled pocket of bladder protrudes on the anterior vaginal wall as cystocele. Vertical descent of the urethra may also be associated with descent of bladder and cystocele.

VAGINAL WALL OR VAULT PROLAPSE

It is defined as descent of anterior urethrovesical junction or any point on the anterior vaginal wall <3 cm from the hymenal ring.[58] Low uterus may compress posteriorly and obscure rectocele. Retroverted uterus with uterine descent may lead to voiding dysfunction.

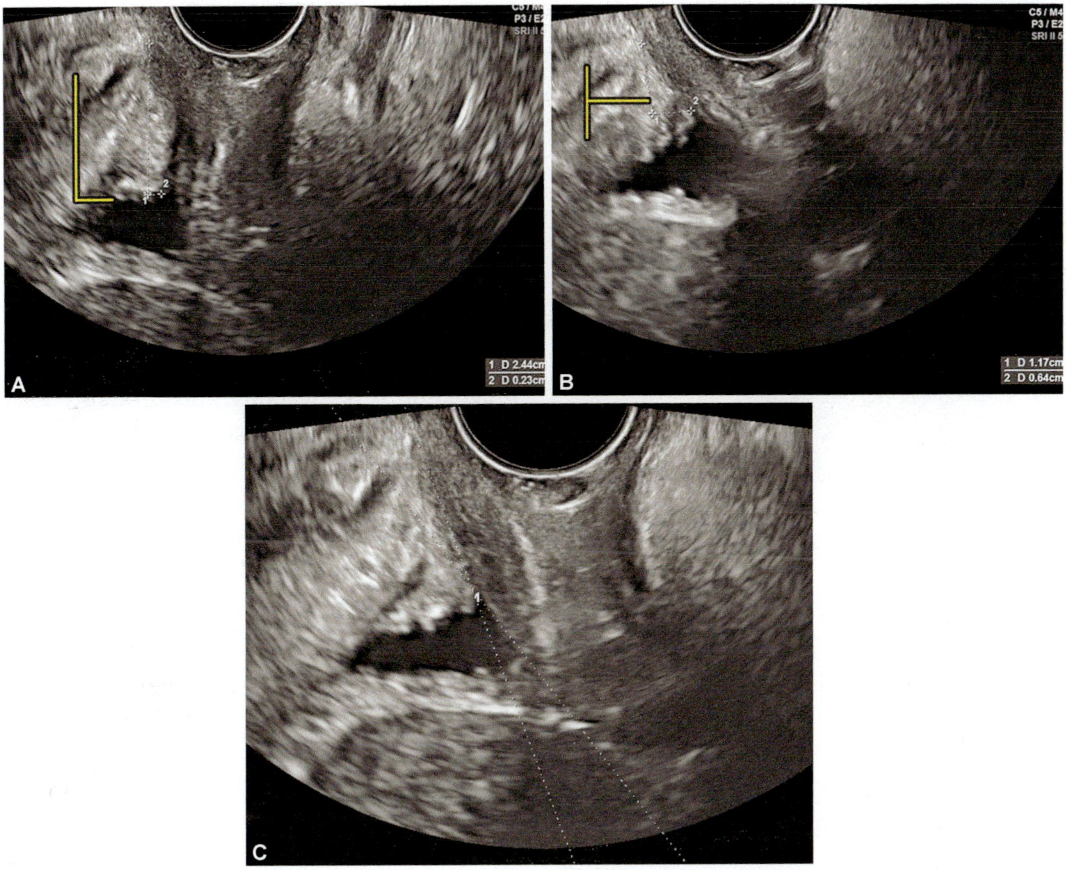

Figs. 11A to C: B mode ultrasound images of the pelvic floor (A). At rest, (B) on Valsalva, showing the downward and posterior displacement of the bladder neck. (C) Measurement of the posterior vesicourethral angle on this image.

For the prolapse or descent, it has been shown that the levator hiatal size at rest closely correlates with the possibility of descent even in absence of trauma.[59] The hiatal size is measured as shown in **Figure 12**. Significant correlations exist between hiatal area and pelvic organ descent. Levator ani anatomy plays an independent role in determining pelvic organ support. Hiatal overdistension may be present due to microtrauma even in absence of avulsion. It is diagnosed by increase in >20% hiatal area even 4 months after delivery (hiatus >25 cm^2). 25 cm^2 is the upper limit of normal ballooning. Larger hiatal area than this indicates hiatal overdistension and risk of prolapse.

- Mild (25–29.9 cm^2)

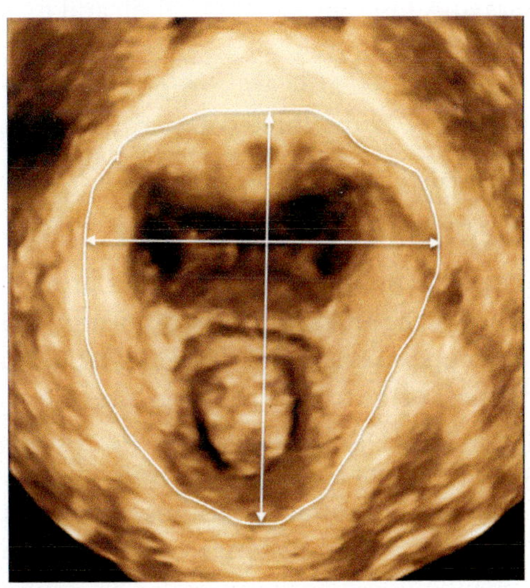

Fig. 12: 3D rendered image of the pelvic floor showing measurements of the hiatus.

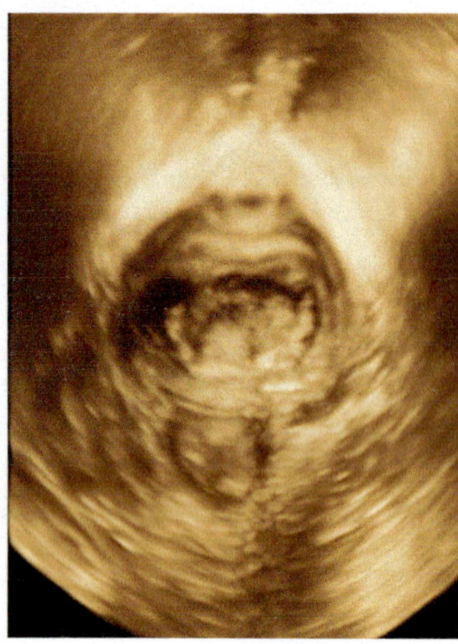

Fig. 13: 3D rendered image of the pelvic floor showing bilaterally atrophied levator ani muscle.

- Moderate (30–34.9 cm^2)
- Marked (35–39.9 cm^2)
- Severe (40 cm^2)

Posterior compartment assessment:

- Rectoenterocele
- Enterocele
- Rectal prolapse
- Rectal intussusception.

Rectoceles are associated with intact but abnormally distensible rectovaginal septum. These commonly present as incomplete bowel emptying, futile straining for stool, and rectal prolapse.

Bilateral levator ani atrophy results in prolapse of all the three compartments **(Fig. 13)**.

RECTAL INTUSSUSCEPTION

It refers to the invagination of the proximal portion of the intestine into its distal portion in a telescope-like fashion.[60] In case of RI, the full thickness of the rectal wall invaginates into the anal canal[61] **(Fig. 5)**. This may produce a bulge of the posterior vaginal wall easily mistaken for rectocele or enterocele. Ultrasound studies showed the RI prevalence of 3.9% among urogynecologic patients and 4.3% among patients with obstructed defecation.[61,62]

It is more common in patients with a clinical diagnosis of rectocele. It is more common in patients with a clinical diagnosis of rectocele or enterocele.[62]

For enterocele,[62] defecation proctography is a standard method for detection of RI. However, this condition may be detected by two-dimensional or 3D transperineal ultrasound with satisfactory levels of sensitivity and specificity.[63] Since transperineal ultrasonography is better tolerated than defecation proctography, this modality may well replace defecography as the initial examination of choice.[64]

TAPE POSITION AND OUTCOME OF SUBURETHRAL SLING

Synthetic implants are easily seen on TPUS, IUS, or TVUS. In case of suburethral slings, ultrasound imaging enables precise localization of the tape position in relation to the urethra and other structures. Position of the tape relative to the urethra is one of the most important factors determining sling outcome. The most common indications for sling incision are overactive bladder, voiding dysfunction, and recurrent urinary tract infections.[65] A key role of the tape inserted under the urethra is to reinforce weakened pubourethral ligaments. The tape positioned under the urethra creates a fulcrum on which the urethra angulates (kinks) on straining.[66]

Urethral "kinking" is observed in approximately 90% of cured patient after retropubic slings, but only in 24–50% of cured patients after transobturator tapes.[67-70]

Other modes of action have been proposed: compression of the urethra and surrounding tissue against the SP or protrusion of the tape into the posterior wall of the urethra with transient narrowing of its lumen ("urethral encroachment").[70]

It is not surprising that in case of location of a tape close to the bladder neck or immobile urethra, functioning of these mechanisms may be invalid. An optimal distance between 3 and 5 mm from the implant to the urethral lumen, as measured on IUS, has been proposed. A distance shorter than 3 mm is associated with a greater risk of complications.[71] It is obvious that too much tension applied to the tape may cause voiding difficulties. In patients subjected to a repeat sling for recurrent or persistent SUI, limited mobility of the urethra detected by the Q-tip test or by ultrasound increases the risk of an unfavorable outcome more than four times.[72] Patients treated with tension-free vaginal tape (TVT) with postoperative bladder neck mobility ≤10 mm had a 2.6-fold higher risk of failure, whereas postoperative bladder neck mobility >15 mm significantly reduced the risk of failure [relative risk (RR) = 0.4]. On balance, recognition of urethral hypomobility (or lack of hypermobility) puts patient at higher risk of sling failure and prompts consideration of other treatment options.

Clear relationships between ultrasound findings and patients' complaints have not been established and data available in the literature are rarely directly applicable to individual cases. Attempts have been undertaken to improve the efficacy of sling procedures by preoperative measurement of the urethral length and revising the site for the beginning of the suburethral incision of the vaginal wall. The one-third rule for retropubic and two-third rule for transobturator procedures have been proposed.[73,74]

ULTRASOUND FOR EVALUATION OF PATIENTS TREATED WITH VAGINAL MESH

Ultrasound is the best imaging modality for visualization of mesh implants. A significant reduction in mesh dimensions (termed as retraction, shrinkage, or contraction), up to 60% of its original length, has been reported on ultrasound examination months or even days after surgery. The severity of retraction was associated with increased risk of prolapse recurrence, postoperative vaginal pain, and de novo urgency.[75-79]

Although these findings reasonably explain the pathogenesis of some unfavorable surgical outcomes, their value in everyday practice has not been demonstrated. Up to 7.8% of mesh procedures are complicated by voiding dysfunction and urinary retention.[80]

Occasionally, these complaints may be secondary to a retroperitoneal hematoma, which can be easily diagnosed by ultrasound. Thus, ultrasound imaging may be recommended as an examination supplementary to physical assessment when formation of a hematoma is suspected such as in cases of postoperative voiding dysfunction, defecatory dysfunction, excessive pain, vaginal bleeding, or decreasing hemoglobin level.[81] Injury to the urethra, bladder, or ureter usually is recognized and managed during surgery. On rare occasions, patients with unrecognized injuries may present with fistulas, voiding disturbances, or pelvic pain.

CORRELATION WITH SYMPTOMS AND GUIDE TO TREATMENT[82]

- *Recurrent lower urinary tract infections*: Atrophied endopelvic fascia and increased residual urine—cystocele/overcorrection of urethra. It may also be associated with bladder or UD, intravesical calculi, foreign body, or abnormally located intrauterine device
- *Urgency and frequency of urine*: Periurethral or intravesical masses, bladder and UD, anterior uterine fibroids, and funneling of proximal urethra
- *Dysuria and dyspareunia*: UD, periurethral masses, and migrating mild intrauterine contraceptive device
- *Urge*: Thick bladder wall
- *Stress urinary incontinence*: Hypermobile urethra, reduced or absent pelvic floor activity, cystocele, and funneling.

SUMMARY

Availability of pelvic floor ultrasound has revolutionized the understanding of morphological anomalies of levator ani. The cause of these abnormalities is now understood to be due to injury to the muscles of pelvic floor—traumatic avulsion of the muscles. This is most commonly due to birth trauma and is associated with anterior and central compartment prolapse. 3D ultrasound helps to evaluate pelvic floor anatomy better.

Levator ani trauma leads to anterior and middle compartment prolapse.[83] Abnormal puborectalis may lead to fecal incontinence.[84] If avulsion is bilateral, it may lead to effect on sexual function.

Ultrasound may be proposed as the initial examination of choice. Ultrasound may be used for assessment of bladder neck mobility before anti-incontinence procedures. On rare occasions, it is helpful in recognition of pathologies mimicking vaginal prolapse such as vaginal cyst, UD, or RI. In patients subjected to suburethral slings, causes of surgery failure or postsurgical voiding dysfunctions can be revealed by imaging. Many reports link the location of a tape close to the bladder neck to unfavorable outcomes of sling surgery. Some postoperative complications such as urinary retention, mesh malposition, hematoma, or urinary tract injury can be diagnosed by ultrasound.

REFERENCES

1. Shek K, Deitz H. Intrapartum risk factors of levator trauma. Br J Obstet Gynecol. 2006;26:710-6.
2. Dietz HP, Steensma AB, Hastings R. Three-dimensional ultrasound imaging of pelvic floor: the effect of parturition on paravaginal support structures. Ultrasound Obstet Gynecol. 2003;21:589-95.
3. Dietz HP. Ultrasound imaging of the pelvic floor: Part II: three-dimensional or volume imaging. Ultrasound Obstet Gynecol. 2004;23:615-25.
4. Youssef A, Montaguti E, Sanlorenzo O, Cariello L, Salsi G, Morganelli G, et al. Reliability of new three-dimensional ultrasound technique for pelvic hiatal area measurement. Ultrasound Obstet Gynecol. 2016;47:629-35.
5. Deitz H, Shek KL. Tomographic ultrasound imaging of the pelvic floor: which level matters most? Obstet Gynecol. 2009;33:698-703.
6. Dohke M, Mitchell DG, Vasavada SP. Fast magnetic resonance imaging of pelvic organ prolapse. Tech Urol. 2001;7:133-8.
7. Lienemann A, Sprenger D, Anthuber C, Baron A, Reiser M. Functional cine magnetic resonance imaging in women after abdominal sacrocolpopexy. Obstet Gynecol. 2001;97:81-5.
8. Gosling JA. The structure of the bladder neck, urethra, and pelvic floor in relation to female urinary continence. Int Urogynecol J. 1996;7:177-8.
9. Monga A. Fascia—defects and repair. Curr Opin Obstet Gynecol. 1996;8:366-71.
10. Martan A, Masata M, Halaska M, Voigt R. Ultrasound imaging of the urethral sphincter. Ceska Gynekol. 1997;62:330-2.
11. Unger CA, Weinstein MM, Pretorius DH. Pelvic floor imaging. Ultrasound Clin. 2010;5:313-30.
12. Kruger JA, Heap SW, Murphy BA, Dietz HP. Pelvic floor function in nulliparous women using three-dimensional ultrasound and magnetic resonance imaging. Obstet Gynecol. 2008;111:631-8.
13. Weinstein MM, Jung SA, Pretorius DH, Nager CW, den Boer DJ, Mittal RK. The reliability of puborectalis muscle measurement with 3-dimensional ultrasound imaging. Am J Obstet Gynecol. 2007;197:68.e1-6.
14. Schaer GN, Koechli OR, Schuessier B, Haller U. Perineal ultrasound: determination of reliable examination procedures. Ultrasound Obstet Gynecol. 1996;7:347-52.
15. Deitz HP, Wilson PD. The influence of bladder volume on the position and mobility of the urethrovesical junction. Int Urogynecol J Pelvic Floor Dysfunct. 1999;10:3-6.
16. Tunn R, Petri E. Introital and transvaginal ultrasound as the main tool in the assessment of urogenital and pelvic floor dysfunction: an imaging panel and practical approach. Ultrasound Obstet Gynecol. 2003;22:205-13.
17. Santoro GA, Wieczorek AP, Dietz HP, Mellgren A, Sultan AH, Shobeiri SA, et al. State of the art: an integrated approach to pelvic floor ultrasonography. Ultrasound Obstet Gynecol. 2011;37:381-96.
18. Dietz HP. Ultrasound imaging of the pelvic floor. Part I: Two-dimensional aspects. Ultrasound Obstet Gynecol. 2004;23:80-92.
19. Dietz HP. Pelvic floor ultrasound: a review. Am J Obstet Gynecol. 2010;202:321-34.

20. Tunn R, Schaer G, Peschers U, Bader W, Gauruder A, Hanzal E, et al. Updated recommendations on ultrasonography in urogynecology. Int Urogynecol J Pelvic Floor Dysfunct. 2005;16:236-41.
21. Dietz HP. Ultrasound imaging of the pelvic floor. Part II: three-dimensional or volume imaging. Ultrasound Obstet Gynecol. 2004;23:615-25.
22. Weber AM, Abrams P, Brubaker L, Cundiff G, Davis G, Dmochowski RR, et al. The standardization of terminology for researchers in female pelvic floor disorders. Int Urogynecol J Pelvic floor Dysfunct. 2001;12:178-86.
23. Khullar V, Cardozo LD, Salvatore S, Hill S. Ultrasound: a noninvasive screening test for detrusor instability. Br J Obstet Gynaecol. 1996;103:904-8.
24. Schaer GN, Koechli OR, Schuessler B, Haller U. Perineal ultrasound for evaluating the bladder neck in urinary stress incontinence. Obstet Gynecol. 1995;85:220-4.
25. Schaer G, Koelbl H, Voigt R, Merz E, Anthuber C, Niemeyer R, et al. Recommendations of the German Association of Urogynecology on functional sonography of the lower female urinary tract. Int Urogynecol J Pelvic floor Dysfunct. 1996;7:105-8.
26. Khullar V, Salvatore S, Cardozo LD, Bourne TH, Abbott D, Kekkeher C. A novel technique for measuring bladder wall thickness in women using transvaginal ultrasound. Ultrasound Obstet Gynecol. 1994;4:220-3.
27. Tunn R, Perucchini D. Morphological assessment for diagnosing urogynecological disorders. Zentraili Gynakol. 2001;123:672-9.
28. Schaer GN, Perucchini D, Munz E, Peschers U, Koechli OR, Delancey JO. Sonographic evaluation of the bladder neck in continence and stress incontinence women. Obstet Gynecol. 1999;93:412-6.
29. Schaer GN, Koechli OR, Schuessler B, Haller U. Improvement of perineal sonographic bladder neck imaging with ultrasound contrast medium. Obstet Gynecol. 1995;86:950-4.
30. Peschers UM, Vodusek DB, Fanger G, Schaer GN, De Lancey JO, Schuessler B. Pelvic muscle activity in nulliparous volunteers. Neurourol Urodyn. 2001;20:269-75.
31. Miller JM, Perucchini D, Carchidi LT, DeLancey JO, Miller JA. Pelvic floor muscle contraction during a cough and decreased vesical neck mobility. Obstet Gynecol. 2001;97:255-60.
32. Yang JM, Yang SH, Huang WC. Dynamic morphological changes in the anterior vaginal wall before and after laparoscopic Burch colposuspension in primary urodynamic stress incontinence. Ultrasound Obstet Gynecol. 2005;25:289-95.
33. Martan A, Masata M, Halaska M, Otcenásek M, Svabik K. Ultrasound imaging of paravaginal defects in women with stress incontinence before and after paravaginal defect repair. Ultrasound Obstet Gynecol. 2002;19:496-500.
34. Tunn R, Paris S, Fischer W, Hamm B, Kuchinke J. Static magnetic resonance imaging of the pelvic floor muscle morphology in women with stress urinary incontinence and pelvic prolapse. Neurourol Urodyn. 1998;17:579-89.
35. Medina CA, Costantini E, Petri E, Mourad S, Singla A, Colorado SR, et al. Evaluation and surgery for stress urinary incontinence: A FIGO working group report. Neurourol Urodyn. 2017;36:518-28.
36. Fitzgerald MP, Jaffar J, Brubaker L. Risk factors for an elevated postvoid residual urine volume in women with symptoms of urinary urgency, frequency and urge incontinence. Int Urogynecol J Pelvic Floor Dysfunct. 2001;12:237-9.
37. Tseng LH, Liang CC, Chang YL, Lee SJ, Lloyd LK, Chen CK, et al. Postvoid residual urine in women with stress incontinence. Neurourol Urodyn. 2008;27:48-51.
38. Latthe PM, Champaneria R, Khan KS. Systematic review of the accuracy of ultrasound as the method of measuring bladder wall thickness in the diagnosis of detrusor overactivity. Int Urogynecol J. 2010;21:1019-24.
39. Khullar V, Cardozo LD, Salvatore S, Hill S. Ultrasound: a noninvasive screening test for detrusor instability. Br J Obstet Gynecol. 1996;103:904-8.
40. Lekskulchai O, Dietz HP. Detrusor wall thickness as a test for detrusor overactivity in women. Ultrasound Obstet Gynecol. 2008;32:535-9.
41. Huang WC, Yang JM, Yang YC, Yang SH. Ultrasonographic characteristics and cystoscopic correlates of bladder wall invasion by endophytic cervical cancer. Ultrasound Obstet Gynecol 2006;27:680-6.
42. El-Nashar SA, Bacon MM, Fine SK, Weaver AL, Gebhart JB, Klingele CJ. Incidence of female urethral diverticulum: a population-based analysis and literature review. Int Urogynecol J. 2014;25:73-9.
43. Burrows LJ, Howden NL, Meyn L, Weber AM. Surgical procedures for urethral diverticula in women in the United States, 1979–1997. Int Urogynecol J Pelvic Floor Dysfunct. 2005;16:158-61.
44. Aldridge CW, Beaton JH, Nanzig RP. A review of office urethroscopy and cystometry. Am J Obstet Gynecol. 1978;131:432-7.

45. Crescenze IM, Goldman HB. Female urethral diverticulum: current diagnosis and management. Curr Urol Rep. 2015;16:71.
46. Rovner ES. Urethral diverticula: a review and an update. Neurourol Urodyn. 2007;26:972-7.
47. Gerrard ER, Lloyd LK, Kubricht WS, Kolettis PN. Transvaginal ultrasound for the diagnosis of urethral diverticulum. J Urol. 2003;169:1395-7.
48. Tseng LH. Wang AC, Lin YH, Li SJ, Ko YJ. Randomized comparison of the suprapubic arc sling procedure vs. tension-free vaginal taping for stress incontinent women. Int Urogynecol J Pelvic Floor Dysfunct. 2005;16:230-5.
49. Huang WC, Yang JM. Bladder neck funneling on ultrasound cystourethrography in primary stress urinary incontinence: a sign associated with urethral hypermobility and intrinsic sphincter deficiency. Urology. 2003;61:936-41.
50. Digesu GA, Khullar V, Cardozo L, Salvatore S. The open bladder neck: a significant finding? Int Urogynecol J Pelvic Floor Dysfunct. 2004;15:336-9.
51. Hennemann J, Kennes LN, Maass N, Najjari L. Evaluation of established and new reference lines for the standardization of transperineal ultrasound. Ultrasound Obstet Gynecol. 2014;44:610-6.
52. DeLancey JO. The anatomy of pelvic floor. Curr Opin Obstet Gynecol. 1994;6:313-6.
53. Dietz HP, Steensma AB, Vancaillie TG. Levator function in nulliparous women. Int Urogynecol J Pelvic Floor Dysfunct. 2003;14:24-6.
54. Dietz HP, Hansell NK, Grace ME, Eldridge AM, Clarke B, Martin NG. Bladder neck mobility is a heritable trait. BJOG. 2005;112:334-9.
55. DeLancy JOL. Structural support of the urethra as it relates to stress urinary incontinence: the hammock hypothesis. Am J Obstet Gynecol. 1994;170:1713-20.
56. DeLancy JOL. Stress urinary incontinence. Where are we now, where should we go? Am J Obstet Gynecol. 1996;175:311-9.
57. Dietz HP, Wilson PD, Clarke B. The use of perineal ultrasound to quantify levator activity and teach pelvic floor muscle exercises. Int Urogynecol J Pelvic floor Dysfunct. 2001;12:166-8.
58. Abrams P, Cardozo L, Fall M, Griffiths D, Rosier P, Ulmsten U, et al. The standardisation of terminology in lower urinary tract function: report from the standardisation sub-committee of the International Continence Society. Am J Obstet Gynecol. 2002;187:116-26.
59. Delancey JO. Anatomy. In: Cardozo L, Staskin D (Eds). Textbook of Female Urology and Urogynecology. London: Isis Medical Media; 2001. pp. 112-24.
60. Barbete P. Ouevres Chirurgiques et Anatomiques. Geneva: Francois Miege; 1674. p. 5221.
61. Rodrigo N, Shek KL, Dietz HP. Rectal intussusception is associated with abnormal levator ani muscle structure and morphometry. Tech Coloproctol. 2011;15:39-43.
62. Rojas RG, Atan IK, Shek KL, Dietz HP. The prevalence of abnormal posterior compartment anatomy and its association with obstructed defecation symptoms in urogynecological patients. Int Urogynecol J. 2016;27:939-44.
63. Beer-Gabel M, Carter D. Comparison of dynamic transperineal ultrasound and defecography for the evaluation of pelvic floor disorders. Int J Colorectal Dis. 2015;30:835-41.
64. Dietz HP. Translabial ultrasound in the assessment of pelvic floor and anorectal function in women with defecatory disorders. Tech Coloproctol. 2014;18:481-94.
65. Viereck V, Rautenberg O, Kociszewski J, Grothey S, Welter J, Eberhard J. Midurethral sling incision: indications and outcomes. Int Urogynecol J. 2013;24:645-53.
66. Kuronen M, Schaer GN, Long C, et al. Clinical and ultrasonographic comparison of tension-free vaginal tape and transobturator tape procedure for the treatment of stress urinary incontinence. J Minim Invasive Gynecol. 2008;15:425-30.
67. Long CY, Hsu CS, Lo TS, Liu CM, Chen YH, Tsai EM. Ultrasonographic assessment of tape location following tension-free vaginal tape and transobturator tape procedure. Acta Obstet Gynecol Scand. 2008;87:116-21.
68. Foulot H, Uzan I, Chopin N, Borghese B, Chapron C. Monarc transobturator sling system for the treatment of female urinary stress incontinence: results of a post-operative transvaginal ultrasonography. Int Urogynecol J Pelvic Floor Dysfunct. 2007;18:857-61.
69. Yang S, Huang W. Dynamic interaction involved in the tension-free vaginal tape obturator procedure. J Urol. 2008;180:2081-7.
70. Lo TS, Wang AC, Horng SG, Liang CC, Soong YK. Ultrasonographic and urodynamic evaluation after tension free vagina tape procedure (TVT). Acta Obstet Gynecol Scand. 2001;80:65-70.
71. Kociszewski J, Rautenberg O, Perucchini D, Eberhand J, Geissbühler V, Hilgers R, et al. Tape functionality: sonographic tape characteristics and outcome after TVT incontinence surgery. Neurourol Urodyn. 2008;27:485-90.
72. Lo TS, Pue LB, Tan YL, Wu PY. Risk factors for failure of repeat midurethral sling surgery for recurrent or persistent stress urinary incontinence. Int Urogynecol J. 2016;27:923-31.
73. Kociszewski J, Rautenberg O, Kuszka A, Eberhand J, Hilgers R, Viereck V. Can we place tension-free vaginal tape where it should be? The one-third rule. Ultrasound Obstet Gynecol. 2012;39:210-4.

74. Viereck V, Kuszka A, Rautenberg O, Wlaźlak E, Surkont G, Hilgers R, et al. Do different vaginal tapes need different suburethral incisions? The one-half rule. Neurourol Urodyn. 2015;34:741-6.
75. Rogowski A, Bienkowski P, Tosiak A, Jerzak M, Mierzejewski P, Baranowski W. Mesh retraction correlates with vaginal pain and overactive bladder symptoms after anterior vaginal mesh repair. Int Urogynecol J. 2013;24:2087-92.
76. Svabík K, Martan A, Masata J, El-Haddad R, Hubka P, Pavlikova M. Ultrasound appearances after mesh implantation—evidence of mesh contraction or folding? Int Urogynecol J. 2011;22:529-33.
77. Velemir L, Amblard J, Fatton B, Savary D, Jacquetin B. Transvaginal mesh repair of anterior and posterior vaginal wall prolapse: a clinical and ultrasonographic study. Ultrasound Obstet Gynecol. 2010;35:474-80.
78. Tunn R, Picot A, Marschke J, Gauruder-Burmester A. Sonomorphological evaluation of polypropylene mesh implants after vaginal mesh repair in women with cystocele or rectocele. Ultrasound Obstet Gynecol. 2007;29:449-52.
79. Feiner B, O'Rourke P, Maher C. A prospective comparison of two commercial mesh kits in the management of anterior vaginal prolapse. Int Urogynecol J. 2012;23:279-83.
80. Kannan K, Rane A. Pelvic hematoma after Perigee™ procedure for cystocele. J Obstet Gynecol. 2010;30:524-5.
81. Huang WC, Yang JM. Voiding dysfunction related to a vaginal hematoma after a Perigee™ procedure. Ultrasound Obstet Gynecol. 2013;41:230-1.
82. Khurana A. Ultrasound in urogynecology. In: Kurjak A, Chervenak F (Eds). Donald School Textbook of Ultrasound in Obstetrics and Gynecology, 4th edition. New Delhi: Jaypee Brothers Medical Publishers (P) Ltd; 2017.
83. Deitz H, Simpson JM. Levator trauma is associated with pelvic organ prolapse. Br J Obstet Gynecol. 2008;115:979-84.
84. Chantarasorn V, Shek KL, Dietz HP. Sonographic detection of puborectalis muscle avulsion is not associated with anal incontinence. Aust N Z J Obstet Gynecol. 2011;51:130-5.

Index

Page numbers followed by *b* refer to box, *f* refer to figure, *fc* refer to flowchart, and *t* refer to table.

A

B

C

F

G

H

I

J

K

L

M

S

U

V

W

Y

Z